פק

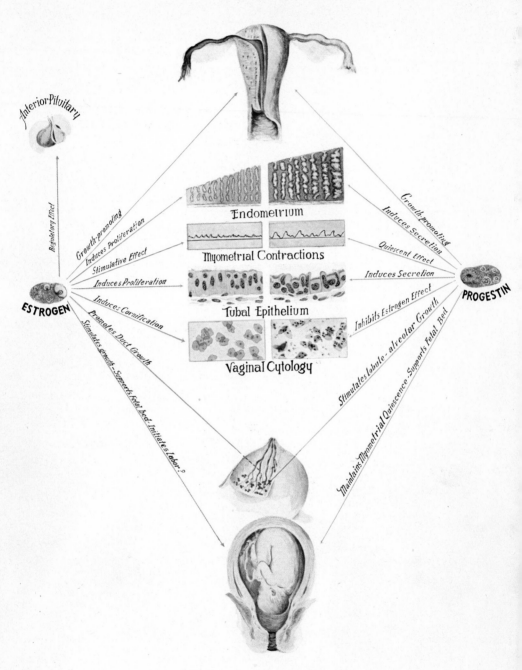

Anterior Pituitary

ESTROGEN

PROGESTIN

Regulatory Effect

Growth-promoting

Induces Proliferation

Stimulative Effect

Induces Proliferation

Induces Cornification

Promotes Duct Growth

Stimulates growth - Supports fetal bed - Initiates labor?

Endometrium

Myometrial Contractions

Tubal Epithelium

Vaginal Cytology

Growth promoting

Induces Secretion

Quiescent Effect

Induces Secretion

Inhibits Estrogen Effect

Stimulates Lobule-alveolar Growth

Maintains Myometrial Quiescence - Supports Fetal Bed

Biology of estrogen and progestin.

FEMALE ENDOCRINOLOGY

INCLUDING SECTIONS ON THE MALE

By

JACOB HOFFMAN, A.B., M.D.

Demonstrator in Gynecology, Jefferson Medical College; Pathologist in Gynecology,
Jefferson Hospital; Formerly Research Fellow in Endocrinology
and Director of the Endocrine Clinic, Gynecological
Department, Jefferson Hospital,
Philadelphia

FULLY ILLUSTRATED
INCLUDING SOME IN COLORS

W. B. SAUNDERS COMPANY
PHILADELPHIA AND LONDON
1944

DEDICATED TO MY WIFE
WHOSE ENCOURAGEMENT AND ACTIVE ASSISTANCE
MADE THIS BOOK POSSIBLE

FOREWORD

Even a casual observer will be struck with the frequency of endocrine disorders. Possibly a third of the gynecologist's patients suffer from functional ailments and some of them demand the utmost in diagnostic study and therapeutic management.

For these women, the manifestations of the generative function are associated with distressing symptoms of one sort or another. They become painfully aware of a disturbance in their functional powers which makes menstruation a monthly ordeal or hinders their powers of reproduction. Maladjustment of the ductless glands accordingly produces so much suffering, physical and mental, that it ranks, so far as the happiness of the individual is concerned, with some of the more important organic lesions of the generative organs, and unfortunately is often more difficult to relieve or cure.

It is therefore not surprising that endocrine disorders have become the target of many investigators. Their studies bearing on physiology, pathology, symptoms, diagnosis, and therapy have produced many conclusions that are contradictory or are soon supplanted by others whereas comparatively few endure as unquestioned facts. The words of the Psalmist "I am fearfully and wonderfully made" are exemplified by the apparently mysterious jumbling of the associated endocrine activities in the individual.

We may well ask why two women with the same aberrations of endocrine function, so far as we can determine, should differ so much in the manifestations of the disorder: one will have too little, the other too much, uterine bleeding; one will have painful and the other painless periods; one will be fertile, the other infertile. While an explanation in individual instances may be forthcoming upon other grounds, the difficulty of satisfactorily reconciling the endocrinologic studies with the clinical picture often seems insurmountable.

Busy practitioners of medicine are apt to forego the time-consuming study necessary to a real understanding of a given endocrinologic problem. Being more concerned with the remedy, they eagerly grasp at the promise afforded by the use of hormones, which has increased to tremendous proportions. These are selected in many instances on the strength of statements that they are "good" for certain symptoms. Consequently they may be given unwisely and, sad to relate, sometimes with distinctly harmful results. A glaring example of the latter is hormonal therapy to stop menopausal bleeding when an unlooked-for and undiscovered malignant growth is actually the cause.

The importance of the subject with which Dr. Hoffman's book is concerned cannot therefore be gainsaid. His qualifications for undertaking such a work began with his pupilage under Robert Meyer in the normal and pathologic histology of the generative organs, and his directly pertinent studies with Aschheim and Zondek soon after they helped to launch what may be spoken of as modern female endocrinology.

Dr. Hoffman has been associated in pathology with the Gynecological Department of the Jefferson Medical College and Hospital for the greater part of my professorship. He brought to us at the start the benefit of his understanding of the newer concepts of the physiology and histopathology of the generative organs.

In 1931, he organized an endocrine clinic in connection with our out-patient department. Since then, in this clinic as well as in private practice, he has been an indefatigable worker and at all times has maintained a conservative and critical attitude in the management of endocrine disorders. His wide acquaintance with the work of others in the field has given him an advantageous point of view from which he has sought to distinguish between the good and the bad. His reluctance to accept the conclusions sometimes reached is not surprising in view of the frequency with which the results of one observer have been negatived by another of equal ability.

The reader will find an exhaustive and critical review of the literature from which he may derive information that will be conducive to a well-grounded appreciation of any endocrinologic problem that concerns him.

Full discussion is made of the treatment of endocrinologic disorders, not only with hormones, but also with gynecologic and general medical measures. The prevailing and authoritative practice in all three are fully set forth with an appraisal of their value based upon the clinical experience and observation of the author.

Laboratory methods are clearly described with practical detail. The subject matter is well arranged and covers the entire field of endocrinology as it affects the generative organs. A complete analytical index will enable the reader to find readily the subject matter he desires.

The composition of the text is excellent. There is necessarily in such a work passages that have required meticulous care in construction and that must be thoughtfully digested by the reader. In this book, however, the burden of the reader's thorough understanding will be lightened by a happy phrasing and choice of words.

BROOKE M. ANSPACH

PREFACE

The literature on sex endocrinology has grown so rapidly during the past two decades that the average physician finds it almost impossible to keep pace with even the more fundamental advances. The problem of digesting this large mass of data has been rendered especially difficult by the many controversial issues that have arisen in both the laboratory and the clinic.

While this volume is primarily concerned with the clinical aspects of gonadal and reproductive endocrinology, a proper appreciation of the etiology and management of endocrine disorders requires a working knowledge of the fundamentals of glandular physiology. For this reason, a separate section covering the more important contributions to the subject has been included. Well aware of the complex and often conflicting nature of the subject-matter, the author has tried to give the reader a concise, simple, and clear exposition, avoiding purely speculative and ill-founded concepts, and emphasizing what appear to be the sounder views. Full cognizance has been taken of data derived from animal experimentation, but, in view of the wide gap existing between the laboratory animal and man, analogies and inferences have been drawn with caution and only when the findings appeared to be in harmony with impressions gained through clinical observation and parallel studies in man.

In presenting the clinical material, emphasis is placed on disturbances of functional origin, because these make up by far the larger part of all endocrine disorders. Though the average practitioner is only rarely confronted with the classical endocrinopathies, these are included because of their profound effect on the sexual sphere.

The flood of endocrine literature and availability of hormonal preparations has made the clinician so "endocrine conscious" as to distort his perspective and lead him often to overlook other potent factors of a non-endocrine nature residing in the organism. To counteract this bias, it was deemed necessary to stress nervous and constitutional factors in the etiology and to give general physical and mental hygiene its deserved place in the therapeutic armamentarium. This should not be interpreted as the negative viewpoint of the therapeutic nihilist. Actually this approach is a positive one, for it stresses the existence of endogenous forces which may, if given full expression, permit the ultimate attainment of normal function. By eradicating depressive states and fortifying the resources of the organism, it is often possible to insure maximum expression of the individual's inherent incretory potentialities.

It is not our purpose to discourage those whose hopes have been raised by the promise of a more direct and specific approach. The author, for one, would be very grateful if that approach were possible. At the present time, however, there are very few conditions where the available gonadotropes or gonadal hormones can with certainty be said to be of benefit. Moreover, their promiscuous use may disturb the delicate and complex endocrine mechanism in the young and encourage dangerous delay in the recognition and control of organic lesions in the old.

Diagnostic aids adapted for use in endocrine disorders are described. Mention is made of the more important tests designed for the determination of the gonadal and gonadotropic hormones in the blood and urine. The results obtained with them in health and disease are given, and their limitations as practical aids are considered. Their value is fairly well established in conditions, such as pregnancy or syndromes due to hormone-secreting tumors, where marked deviations from normal hormone levels are demonstrable. In functional disorders, where only minor deviations occur, these tests are of little consequence and may often be misleading unless viewed in the light of other findings.

The hormonal preparations now available for the treatment of gonadal and reproductive disorders are described and tabulated. Their indications and contraindications are fully considered in the discussion of the individual clinical entities.

The author is deeply indebted and sincerely grateful for the many helpful suggestions and valuable criticisms offered him by Dr. Brooke M. Anspach, Dr. Abraham Cantarow, Dr. James B. Collip, Dr. George W. Corner, Dr. Robert L. Dickinson, Dr. Robert T. Frank, Dr. Max A. Goldzieher, Dr. Frederick L. Hisaw, Dr. David Marine, Dr. Thaddeus L. Montgomery, Dr. Emil Novak, Dr. Hugo R. Rony, Dr. Isadore C. Rubin, Dr. Lewis C. Scheffey, Dr. Howard C. Taylor, Jr., Dr. Charles W. Turner, Dr. Phillip F. Williams, and Dr. Emil Witschi.

The author wishes to thank the members of the staff of the W. B. Saunders Company for their patient and helpful cooperation, and for the many courtesies extended to him. For the art work, he is indebted to Katharine McGarrity, Karl Sherman, and Maxim Gottlieb. Thanks are also due the staff of the Library of the College of Physicians of Philadelphia for their many favors.

JACOB HOFFMAN

CONTENTS

PART I. PHYSIOLOGY

CHAPTER I

PAGE

DEVELOPMENT OF THE FEMALE REPRODUCTIVE ORGANS 1
Embryonic Period 1
Period from Birth to Puberty 4
Puberal Period 5
Maturity 7
Cyclic Changes in the Uterine Mucosa 16
Cyclic Changes in the Tubal Mucosa 25
Cyclic Changes in the Cervical Mucosa 25
Cyclic Changes in the Vaginal Mucosa 27

CHAPTER II

ENDOCRINE ROLE OF THE OVARY: THE FOLLICLE 32
Introduction 32
Endocrine Role of the Follicle 34
Biology of Estrogen 34
Effects of Chronic Estrogen Stimulation 37
Effect of Estrogen on the Ovary 41
Effect of Estrogen in the Male 42
Cells of the Ovary Secreting Estrogen 43
Secretion of Androgen by the Ovary 47

CHAPTER III

ENDOCRINE ROLE OF THE OVARY: THE CORPUS LUTEUM 50
Introduction 50
Biology of Progesterone 50

CHAPTER IV

THE TIME OF OVULATION AND THE "SAFE PERIOD" 64
Introduction 64
Methods of Ascertaining Ovulation Time 64
Evaluation of the Knaus-Ogino Theory 68

CHAPTER V

ENDOCRINE FACTORS IN MENSTRUATION 76
Introduction 76
Causation of Menstrual Bleeding 77
Hormonal Factors in Menstruation 78
Sequence of Events Shortly Before and During Menstruation 85
Uterine Factors Controlling Amount and Duration of the Menstrual Flow 92
Comparison of Changes During Menstruation and Pseudomenstruation 94
The Central Nervous System and Menstruation 96
Summary 97

CHAPTER VI

PAGE

ENDOCRINE CONTROL OF UTERINE MOTILITY 101
  Methods of Study 101
  Role of the Ovarian and Hypophyseal Hormones 102
  Motility of the Gravid Uterus 108
  Role of the Hypophysis, Adrenals and Thymus 111

CHAPTER VII

ENDOCRINE ROLE OF THE UTERUS 115
  Hysterectomy Experiments 115
  Uterine Implants and Extracts 116

CHAPTER VIII

ENDOCRINE ROLE OF THE PLACENTA 119
  Estrogen in the Placenta 119
  Progesterone in the Placenta 120
  Gonadotropic Hormones 121

CHAPTER IX

PARTURITION 123
  Factors Initiating and Maintaining Labor 123

CHAPTER X

THE PHYSIOLOGY OF THE BREAST 129
  Anatomy of the Mammary Glands 129
    Formative Phase 129
    Functional Phase 131
    Involutional Phase 132
  Hormonal Factors in Mammary Development and Function 132
    Proliferative Phase 132
    Secretory Phase: Endocrine Control of the Mammary Gland During Late Pregnancy and Lactation 135
    Factors Controlling the Initiation of Milk Secretion 140
    Factors Controlling the Maintenance of Lactation 145
  Effect of Lactation on the Reproductive Organs 149

CHAPTER XI

THE PHYSIOLOGY OF THE TESTIS 155
  Spermatogenic Function 155
  Endocrine Function of the Testis 155
    Effects of Androgens in the Male 157
    Effects of Androgens in the Female 160
  The Testis and Anterior Hypophysis 162

CHAPTER XII

THE PHYSIOLOGY OF THE ANTERIOR HYPOPHYSIS 167
  Cytology 167
  The Anterior Hypophysis and the Gonads 169
  Sex Hormones of the Anterior Hypophysis 172
  Gonadotropes of Extra-Hypophyseal Origin 179
  Response of the Human Ovary to the Gonadotropes 187
  Response of the Human Testis to the Gonadotropes 190
    The Age Factor in the Gonadal Response to the Gonadotropes .. 191
  Effect of the Gonads on the Anterior Hypophysis 194

CHAPTER XIII

PAGE

THE ANTERIOR HYPOPHYSIS IN GROWTH AND METABOLISM 204
    The Anterior Hypophysis and the Other Endocrine Glands 205
    Role of Anterior Hypophysis in Metabolism 211

CHAPTER XIV

THE PHYSIOLOGY OF THE POSTERIOR HYPOPHYSIS 220
    Incretory Function of the Posterior Hypophysis 220
    Pharmacologic Effects of Posterior Lobe Extracts 222
    Clinical Aspects of Posterior Pituitary Disease 224

CHAPTER XV

THE HYPOTHALAMICO-HYPOPHYSEAL SYSTEM 226
    Introduction 226
    Anatomy 227
    Functions of the Hypothalamus 229

CHAPTER XVI

THE PHYSIOLOGY OF THE THYROID GLAND 234
    Experimental Studies of Thyroid Function 234
    Present Concept of Thyroid Function 235
        Relation of the Thyroid to the Anterior Hypophysis 238
        Relation of the Thyroid to the Gonads 239

CHAPTER XVII

THE PHYSIOLOGY OF THE SUPRARENAL GLANDS 244
    Physiology of the Adrenal Medulla 244
    Pharmacology of Epinephrine 246
    Physiology of the Adrenal Cortex 248
    Adrenal-Anterior Hypophysis Relationship 252
    Adrenal-Thyroid Relationship 253
    Relation of the Adrenal Cortex to the Sexual Sphere 254

CHAPTER XVIII

THE PHYSIOLOGY OF THE PARATHYROIDS 262
    Experimental Studies of Parathyroid Functions 262
    Parathyroid-Gonadal Relationship 264

CHAPTER XIX

THE PANCREAS AND THE GONADS 268
    Effect of the Pancreas on Gonadal and Reproductive Function 268
    Effect of the Gonads on the Pancreas 270

CHAPTER XX

THE PHYSIOLOGY OF THE THYMUS GLAND 272
    The Thymus and Growth 272
    Thymus-Gonadal Relation 274
    The Relation of the Thymus to Other Glands 276

CHAPTER XXI

PAGE

THE PHYSIOLOGY OF THE PINEAL BODY 282
   Experimental Studies of Pineal Function 282
   Pineal Tumors 284

CHAPTER XXII

THE ANTI-HORMONES 286
   The Nature of the Anti-Hormones 286

PART II. CLINIC

CHAPTER XXIII

ADOLESCENCE 291
   Sexual Alterations 291
   Somatic Alterations 294
   Troublesome Puberal Manifestations 295

CHAPTER XXIV

AMENORRHEA, OLIGOMENORRHEA, AND HYPOMENORRHEA 297
   Introduction 297
   Etiology of Pathologic Amenorrhea 298
      Uterine Causes 299
      Ovarian Causes 300
      Role of the Anterior Hypophysis 305
      Role of Other Endocrine Glands 306
      Nonendocrine Causes of Amenorrhea 306
   Symptomatology and Diagnosis 310
   Prognosis 317
   Treatment 317

CHAPTER XXV

FUNCTIONAL UTERINE BLEEDING 326
   Introduction 326
   Anovulatory Bleeding 328
      Anatomical and Histological Characteristics 328
      Clinical Characteristics 334
      Etiology 335
      Diagnosis and Differential Diagnosis 345
      Treatment 346
   Abnormal Bleeding from an Atrophic Endometrium 353
   Ovulatory Bleeding 354
   Intermenstrual Bleeding 358

CHAPTER XXVI

DYSMENORRHEA 362
   Introduction 362
   Etiology 362
      Etiology of Functional Dysmenorrhea 364
   Diagnosis and Differential Diagnosis 378
   Treatment 380
      Treatment of the Immediate Attack 380
      Treatment of the Underlying Cause 381

CHAPTER XXVII

STERILITY 387
  Etiology 387
  Diagnosis 394
    Investigation of the Male Partner 394
    Investigation of the Female Partner 397
  Treatment 405
    Treatment of the Male Partner 405
    Treatment of the Female Partner 405

CHAPTER XXVIII

SPONTANEOUS AND HABITUAL ABORTION 412
  Etiology 412
    Fetal Faults 412
    Maternal Faults 413
  Treatment 419
    Preconceptional Treatment 419
    Postconceptional Treatment 420
    Treatment of Impending Abortion 422

CHAPTER XXIX

THE CLIMACTERIC 425
  Symptomatology 425
    Sexual Symptomatology 425
    Nonsexual Symptomatology 427
  Etiology 429
  Diagnosis 436
  Treatment 436
    Medical Treatment 436
    Organotherapy 438

CHAPTER XXX

TROUBLESOME MANIFESTATIONS ASSOCIATED WITH THE MENSTRUAL
  CYCLE 443
  Intermenstrual Pain 443
  Premenstrual Tension 446
  Migraine 449
  Periodic Extragenital Hemorrhage ("Vicarious Menstruation") 451

CHAPTER XXXI

ABNORMAL MANIFESTATIONS ARISING DURING GESTATION 456
  Hyperemesis Gravidarum 456
  Late Toxemias of Pregnancy 457
    Etiology 457
    Treatment 461
  Endocrine Aspects of Dystocia 461
    Etiology 461
    Diagnosis 464
    Treatment 464
  Maternal Tetany 466
    Etiology 466
    Clinical Manifestations 467
    Diagnosis 468
    Course and Prognosis 470
    Treatment 470

CHAPTER XXXII

PAGE

ABNORMALITIES OF THE BREAST 475
Pre-adolescent Abnormalities of the Breast 475
Abnormalities in Mammary Growth 475
    Mammary Hypoplasia 476
    Mammary Hypertrophy 479
    Mammary Hyperplasia (Chronic Mastitis) 480
Abnormalities in Mammary Function 489
    Deficient Milk Secretion (Hypogalactia) 489
    Galactorrhea 491
    Postpartum Breast Engorgement and Undesired Lactation 492

CHAPTER XXXIII

OBESITY 496
Etiology 496
    Control of Energy Intake 498
    Control of Energy Expenditure 499
Heredity and Constitution 505
    The Endocrine Glands in Obesity 506
Complications and Sequelae 518
Prognosis 519
Diagnosis 519
Treatment 521

CHAPTER XXXIV

CONSTITUTIONAL TYPES 528
Description of Types 528
Significance of Constitution in Gynecology 534
Treatment of Constitutional Inferiority 535

CHAPTER XXXV

ENDOCRINOPATHIES 537
Hypophyseal Infantilism 537
Hypophyseal Giantism 544
Acromegaly 548
    Etiology and Pathology 552
    Diagnosis and Differential Diagnosis 554
    Course and Prognosis 555
    Treatment 555
Dystrophia Adiposogenitalis (Fröhlich's Syndrome) 556
    Clinical Characteristics 556
    Etiology and Pathology 560
    Diagnosis 562
    Course and Prognosis 563
    Treatment 563
Simmonds' Disease (Hypophyseal Cachexia) 564
    Clinical Characteristics 565
    Etiology and Pathology 567
    Diagnosis and Differential Diagnosis 568
    Course and Prognosis 571
    Treatment 571
Cushing's Syndrome (Pituitary Basophilism) 573
    Symptomatology 574
    Pathology 576
    Etiology 576
    Diagnosis and Differential Diagnosis 580

                                                                              PAGE
      Course and Prognosis 581
      Treatment 581
    The Adrenogenital Syndrome 581
      Clinical Characteristics 582
      Etiology and Pathology 584
      Diagnosis and Differential Diagnosis 586
      Prognosis 587
      Treatment 587
    Chronic Adrenal Insufficiency (Addison's Disease) 588
      Clinical Characteristics 588
      Etiology and Pathology 589
      Diagnosis 590
      Course and Prognosis 591
      Treatment 592
    Hormone Secreting Tumors of the Ovary 595
      Granulosa Cell Tumor 595
      Theca Cell Tumor (Thecoma) 598
      Arrhenoblastoma 600
      Gynandroblastoma 602
      Luteal Cell Tumor (Luteoma) 603
    Precocious Puberty (Macrogenitosomia Praecox) 605
      Etiology 605
      Diagnosis 609
      Prognosis and Treatment 610
    Lipodystrophia Progressiva 610
    Dercum's Disease (Adiposis Dolorosa) 612

                              CHAPTER XXXVI

CRYPTORCHIDISM AND MALE HYPOGONADISM 620
    Cryptorchidism 620
    Male Hypogonadism 623

                              CHAPTER XXXVII

SEX DETERMINATION AND DIFFERENTIATION OF SEX CHARACTERS 631
    Introduction 631
    Prevailing Theories on the Control of Sex 632

                              CHAPTER XXXVIII

HERMAPHRODISM 641
    Causes of Hermaphrodism 641
    Clinical Management of Intersexuality 647

                    PART III. LABORATORY

                              CHAPTER XXXIX

DIAGNOSTIC AIDS 649
    Endometrial Biopsy and Curettage 649
    The Vaginal Smear 650
    Sex Hormone Tests 654
      Quantitation of Estrogens in the Blood and Urine 655
      Quantitation of Pregnanediol in the Urine 662
      Quantitation of Androgens in the Urine 664
      Quantitation of Gonadotropic Hormones in the Blood and Urine 670

CHAPTER XL

PAGE

SEX HORMONE FINDINGS IN THE BLOOD AND URINE 681
    Estrogen Findings in Normal and Abnormal Conditions 681
    Pregnanediol Findings in Normal and Abnormal Conditions 686
    Androgen Findings in Normal and Abnormal Conditions 689
    Gonadotropic Hormone Findings in Normal and Abnormal Conditions 692

CHAPTER XLI

HORMONAL PREPARATIONS 705
    Estrogenic Substances 705
    Progestational Substances 711
    Androgenic Substances 713
    Gonadotropic Substances 714
    Lactogenic Substances 717
    Adrenal Cortical Substances 718
    Tables 719

BIBLIOGRAPHICAL INDEX 734

SUBJECT INDEX 764

PART I

PHYSIOLOGY

CHAPTER I

DEVELOPMENT OF THE FEMALE REPRODUCTIVE ORGANS

EMBRYONIC PERIOD

The Ovary.—Development of the ovary during the embryonic period falls into two stages:[1, 2, 3] an indifferent phase, when the gland presents no features by which its future sex can be established; and the phase of differentiation, when the ovary becomes recognizable as such.

The *undifferentiated gonad* is first discernible in embryos 5 mm. long as a thickening of the celomic epithelium on the ventromedian surface of the urogenital fold. A solid mass of epithelial cells is laid down, which soon separates into a superficial epithelial layer, the *germinal epithelium,* and an inner mass or epithelial core, containing large genital cells and smaller indifferent cells. The germinal epithelium, separated from the inner mass by a distinct basement membrane, is composed of cuboidal or columnar cells and an occasional primordial germ cell. Steadily deepening grooves on each side of the mass gradually separate it from the neighboring structures in the urogenital fold, with which it remains connected only at the hilum. As the phase of differentiation approaches, the epithelial core assumes a looser texture which distinguishes it from the denser superficial layer.

Differentiation begins in the latter part of the second fetal month, when most of the cells in the inner loose epithelial mass are transformed into young ova. Simultaneously, blood vessels and connective tissue strands grow in from the hilum, the connective tissue strands subdividing into innumerable septa which radiate toward the surface and form a fine network throughout the extent of the gland. Those which reach the surface eventually form the dense layer known as the *tunica albuginea.* Invading the medullary and cortical zones, these delicate septa separate the epithelial cells into numerous small islands, each containing a young ovum surrounded by a single layer of follicle cells. At the same time the size of the gland is greatly increased by formation of new cells in the periphery. As the latter make their appearance, the old cells in the medulla degenerate and are replaced by a dense connective tissue stroma. This makes for a more or less equal division between primordial follicles and connective tissue stroma.

While the sequence of events described above is recognized by most authorities, there is uncertainty as to the *identity of the parent cells* from which the definitive germ cells are derived, and the age at which production of new germ cells ceases. According to one view, the sex cells that are

1

to become functional stem from large genital cells discernible during the latter stages of cell cleavage and distinguishable from the somatic cells by their pale granular cytoplasm and the large size of their bodies and nuclei. These "sex" cells are believed to migrate by way of the entodermal gut and dorsal mesentery to the genital ridge. Another view holds that all ova destined to mature originate in the germinal epithelium. This theory is based on the finding of Pflüger's plugs, proliferations from the germinal epithelium which contain epithelial and germinal cells surrounded by a basement membrane. These plugs or cords dip into the stroma and eventually break up into islands, each harboring an oocyte enveloped by a single layer of epithelial cells, recognizable as the granulosa cells. Protagonists of this theory are not agreed as to when the germinal epithelium ceases to deliver potential germ cells to the ovarian stroma. Some believe that oogenesis ceases at birth or earlier, and that germ cells which develop during reproductive life are derived from potential gonocytes delivered to the ovarian stroma before birth. Others, notably Allen[4] and Evans and Swezy,[5] deny that any of the ova formed before birth become functional, and maintain that the germinal epithelium supplies new germ cells cyclically as they are needed throughout reproductive life. Though the latter view finds support in recent studies in the mouse[6] and guinea pig,[7] its applicability to the human being is not yet established.

The Tubular Tract.—During the indifferent period, which extends to approximately the middle of the second fetal month, the *wolffian* and *müllerian ducts* are laid down. The wolffian ducts appear somewhat earlier (3 mm. embryo), and are formed by fusion of the collecting tubules of the pronephros. Growing caudally, they extend to the cloaca where they establish independent openings into the urogenital sinus. The müllerian ducts are first seen in embryos 7 to 8 mm. long. Each appears as a shallow depression in the celomic epithelium on the lateral aspect of the wolffian body, lateral to the cranial extremity of the wolffian duct. As the groove deepens, its edges separate from the neighboring celomic epithelium, fold towards each other and, except for the cranial end, become fused. The duct thus formed is trumpet-shaped, tapering down from its wide, gaping cranial extremity to its closed caudal tip, which is composed of a solid aggregation of cells. Each duct extends caudally, the tip boring its way through the mesenchyme of the urogenital fold.

The *position* of the müllerian ducts with relation to each other and to the wolffian ducts, varies at different levels. In their cranial portion, they are separated and lie lateral to the wolffian ducts, closely following the latter's course. As both pairs of ducts approach the lateral wall of the contracted part of the celomic cavity (the future pelvis), their course is deflected towards the mid-line. At this point, the müllerian ducts cross the path of the wolffian ducts and continue medial to them within the so-called genital cord. Thenceforth, they again run vertically in close proximity to each other and continue their course toward the urogenital sinus. In embryos 30 mm. long, the solid tips of the ducts finally reach the epithelial wall of the sinus. Pushing it forward, they cause it to bulge into the sinus, forming the eminence known as the müllerian tubercle.

In the meantime, the caudal portions of the müllerian ducts, which have been brought into contact with each other, begin to fuse in a caudal direction. When fusion is complete, *three divisions* are distinguishable: (1) a paired, cranial, vertical portion; (2) a paired, intermediate, transverse portion, and (3) a single fused, caudal, vertical portion, the uterovaginal primordium.[3]

By the middle of the second month, the wolffian ducts gradually begin to regress, and eventually leave only vestigial remnants throughout the length of the tubular tract (*epoophoron, paroophoron,* and *Gärtner's* ducts). The müllerian ducts develop rapidly, and the various constituents of the genital tract gradually begin to be distinguishable. They derive their epithelial lining from the müllerian ducts, and their muscular and connective tissue from the surrounding tissue of the genital cord. The upper unjoined portions of the müllerian ducts become the fallopian tubes, the open cranial end forming the ostium abdominale, with tubal fimbria already discernible in embryos 30 mm. long. The subsequent development of the müllerian ducts consists mainly of a lengthening and increased tortuosity, with differentiation of the tubal epithelium and muscularis.

The unfused transverse portions of the ducts combine with the upper part of the fused, caudal, vertical portion to form the *fundus* and *corpus* of the uterus. As differentiation proceeds, the wall of the uterus thickens and division into a serous, muscular, and mucosal layer gradually takes place. By the seventh month, the *uterine glands* appear.

The remainder of the uterovaginal primordium is transformed into the *cervix* and, according to the recent studies of Koff,[3] into all but the distal end of the vagina. Vilas[8] and Meyer[2] believe that the entire vaginal mucosa is derived from entodermal epithelium of the urogenital sinus, which invades the genital cord and replaces the müllerian epithelium. After the fourth fetal month, in contrast to the rest of the tubular tract, the *vagina* begins to be lined by stratified squamous epithelium. At first there forms a solid plug, the caudal end of which widens and lengthens, invaginating the posterior wall of the urogenital sinus into which it opens. By the fifth month, the epithelial cells degenerate and desquamate in a cranial direction, thus creating the vaginal lumen. At the same time, the urogenital sinus becomes relatively shorter, gradually lessening the distance between its outer opening and the vaginal orifice. From the seventh month to birth, the müllerian apparatus shows evidence of stimulation and marked activity. This expresses itself in an increased length of the uterus, which grows from 8.2 mm. in the sixth month to 18.4 mm. in the eighth month, and finally to 30 mm. at birth. The increase in length is largely due to elongation of the cervix, which at birth is approximately twice as long as the corpus. At this time, the uterus appears as a pear-shaped organ high up in the pelvis. Folding of the cervical mucosa and increased prominence of the cervical glands occur during this late fetal period.

The Hymen.—The hymen appears as a transverse, perforated membrane which incompletely covers the external opening of the vagina. Theories concerning its origin vary, depending on which view is accepted as to the derivation of the vagina's distal end. According to Koff[3] and

Meyer,[2] both the unpaired posterior segment and anterior paired lips are derived from the mesenchyme of the genital cord and covered with sinus epithelium.

The External Genitalia.—Primordia of the external genital organs are the genital tubercle, the margins of the urethral groove, and the labio-scrotal or genital swellings. Up to the seventh fetal week, these structures appear alike in both sexes. In embryos 8 mm. long, the *genital tubercle* becomes distinguishable in the ventral body wall midway between the umbilical cord and the tail and cranial to the urethral groove. It appears as a cylindrical protuberance, formed by a proliferation of the connective tissue of the abdominal wall and covered by ectodermal epithelium. The shallow *urethral groove* lies on its caudal incline and is separated from the anal pit by a transverse ridge, the primordium of the perineum. The margins of the urethral groove are slightly elevated to form the so-called urethral folds, the primordia of the labia minora. Towards the end of the second month, the genital tubercle enlarges and thickens to form the phallus. This is crowned by the glans, a knob-like tip clearly set off from the stalk of the phallus by a constriction. On each side of the phallus, but separated from it by a furrow, lie lateral elevations known as the *labio-scrotal swellings*, the primordia of the scrotum in the male, and of the labia majora in the female.

After the middle of the third month, these undifferentiated structures undergo marked changes and by the end of the fourth month, are distinguishable as male or female organs. The female phallus, in contrast to that of the male, is retarded in its development, becoming the clitoris with its glans clitoridis and prepuce. The female urethral groove does not extend to the tip of the glans, as in the male, but remains patent in its original position, constituting the future vaginal vestibule. The lips of the urethral groove are transformed into labia minora, while the labioscrotal swellings develop into the labia majora, fusing in front of the anal pit to form the posterior commissure. Shortly before birth the labia majora partly cover the labia minora and clitoris, evidence that the acme of fetal sexual differentiation has been achieved.

PERIOD FROM BIRTH TO PUBERTY

The Ovary.—At birth, the ovaries lie high up against the posterior abdominal wall. They are composed of a central core containing blood vessels and nerves, and a dense stroma which harbors the primary follicles. Estimates of the number of ova present in the ovaries at birth vary from 70,000 to 400,000. According to Simkins,[9] two types of follicles are distinguishable: *primordial follicles,* which he describes as large "genitaloid" cells surrounded by an incomplete layer of ellipsoidal cells, and found only in the cortex of the ovary of fetuses and young infants; and *primary follicles,* which are always surrounded by at least a single row of large, round, and regular nuclei. "Primary follicles" are present only in the peripheral margin of the medullary zone, and are larger, less numerous, and take a deeper stain than the "primordial" cells.

As the ovary matures, the number of "primordial follicles" decreases steadily, while the total number of "primary follicles" remains fairly constant (about 30,000). The latter eventually develop into definitive structures, but only a small proportion (at most 500) reach full maturity. The rest develop to a certain extent, but ultimately undergo regressive changes at some point before rupture. In some cases, a few follicles reach the graafian stage, but under normal conditions they rarely rupture before the advent of puberty. Graafian follicles essentially similar to those seen in the adult ovary may be observed occasionally in infants, and rarely in fetuses.

The process by which an enormous number of follicles develop only to degenerate, has provoked much speculation. Some interpret it as a struggle for mastery wherein the best eggs survive. Others believe the purpose of wholesale follicular destruction is to provide space and formative stuff for the growth of follicles destined to attain full maturation and ovulation. A third possibility is that this is simply another example of the generosity of nature, which creates an overabundance of germ cells in order to insure ultimate maturity of a sufficient number for reproductive purposes.

As regression of the "primordial follicles" and development of the "primary follicles" proceeds, the peripheral part of the medulla becomes increasingly prominent, encroaching on the cortical portion until, with the onset of puberty, the latter is markedly attenuated and appears as a thin zone of connective tissue surrounded by a layer of epithelium. In the meantime, the amount of connective tissue stroma increases and by the third year of life it constitutes the major part of the gland. Thereafter its absolute amount increases steadily.

Internal and External Genitalia.—During childhood, the reproductive organs gradually descend into the pelvis, but their growth is very slow as compared with that of the rest of the body. Except for a slight increase in size of the endometrial glands, some straightening of the convoluted uterine tubes, and some enlargement of the external genitalia, there is very little change. It is noteworthy that ovarian and uterine growth during this period do not run parallel, the ovary developing slowly and steadily, while the uterus grows in spurts.

PUBERAL PERIOD

This epoch, which occupies a period of years (see Chap. XXIII), is marked by rapid development of the entire reproductive apparatus.

The Ovary.—The ovary is transformed from a thin, elongated structure with a smooth surface, to a larger, oval-shaped organ, composed of a deep or medullary, and a superficial or *cortical layer*. The latter is composed of a surface epithelium, tunica albuginea, and a parenchymatous zone. The surface or germinal epithelium appears as a single layer of low cuboidal cells, with small nuclei and a granular protoplasm. This epithelial zone is a continuation of the peritoneal epithelium and, except at the hilum, entirely envelops the ovary in horse-shoe fashion. Immediately beneath the germinal epithelium is the tunica albuginea, a dull white band of condensed fibrous stroma, free of follicles. The parenchymatous zone, which varies from 1 to 3 mm. in thickness, is composed largely of a cellular connective tissue stroma in which spindle cells predominate. It harbors the ovarian vesicles as well as the primary and growing follicles. The *medullary layer* is a loose connective tissue, which harbors the arteries, veins, lymphatics, and nerves, as well as the tubules of the rete ovarii, the female homologue of the testis.

Internal and External Genitalia.—Although the absolute size of the internal and external genital organs increases during the puberal period, the *uterus* shows the most striking changes. This organ, which begins to grow after the eighth year, does not attain full maturity for several years after the onset of the puberal epoch. Growth of the corpus is more rapid than that of the cervix, so that by the end of the puberal epoch, it is approximately twice as long as the cervix. Histologically, the mature uterus is composed of a well differentiated covering of serosa (perimetrium), a muscular coat (myometrium), and a lining mucous membrane (endometrium).

The *serosa* or perimetrium, which is well defined where it covers the dorsal and ventral surfaces of the uterus, merges into the broad ligaments on each side of the organ, forming the parametrium. Here are found the main trunks of the uterine vessels as well as the utero-vaginal plexus. The latter, together with the third and fourth sacral nerves, innervate the uterus.

Beneath the perimetrium is the *myometrium*, composed of interwoven bundles of muscle and fibrous tissue. It may be divided roughly into a subserous layer, where the direction of the muscle fibers follows that of the long axis of the uterus; a middle or vascular layer, where the muscle fibers are so arranged as to encircle each vein and artery as it passes through the myometrium to the mucosa; and an innermost stratum, whose muscle fibers follow a circular path around the uterine cavity.

The *endometrium* begins abruptly at the internal os and lines the entire uterine cavity. Its importance lies in the fact that it is the source of periodic menstrual bleeding and forms the fetal bed in the event of conception. It is about 1 mm. thick and is composed of a surface epithelium and cellular connective tissue which harbors the tubular uterine glands, each enclosed by a delicate basement membrane and surrounded by a spiral arteriole derived from the stratum vasculare.

During the puberal period, the *tubes* grow straighter and wider, while the mucosal plicae become more clearly differentiated and lined by a low cylindrical epithelium composed of ciliated and non-ciliated cells. At the same time growth of the circular and long muscles occurs. The vagina lengthens and widens, its mucosa becomes more vascular and velvety, and the posterior fornices grow deeper. At maturity, it appears as a fibromuscular tube lined by stratified squamous epithelium, devoid of glands.

The *external genitalia* likewise increase in size. The mons veneris becomes more prominent, owing to a deposit of fatty tissue. The labia majora become larger and take on fat, thus obscuring the labia minora.

MATURITY

Beginning at some time during the puberal epoch and continuing throughout reproductive life, barring pregnancy and lactation, the ovary, uterus and possibly other parts of the müllerian tract undergo significant modifications at cyclic intervals.

The Ovarian Cycle.—In the mature ovary, at approximately 28 day intervals, a number of follicles begin to grow, but as a rule only one is destined to achieve complete development. The series of complex changes through which it passes may be divided into a follicular and a corpus luteum phase, separated by the event of ovulation.

Follicular Phase.—A primary *follicle* lying just beneath the tunica albuginea begins to enlarge. Changes occur simultaneously in its three components: the ovum, the granulosa, which is a single layer of flat epithelial cells surrounding the ovum, and the theca interna, a specialized zone

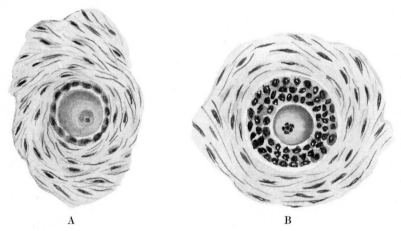

A   B

Fig. 1.—Early development of follicle. (A) Ovum surrounded by single layer of granulosa cells. (B) Proliferation of granulosa cells.

of ovarian stroma, which envelops the follicle. As the follicle matures, the *granulosa cells* multiply by mitosis, become stratified, and assume cuboidal and columnar shapes. Vacuolation and liquefaction of some of the granulosa cells create a crescent-shaped cavity on one side of the follicle. This hollow is soon filled with a clear serous fluid, the liquor folliculi. As the liquor accumulates, the cavity enlarges and assumes a spherical shape. On the side opposite to that at which the cavity first appears, the granulosa cells are piled up in a mound, which is attached to the wall of the follicle and harbors the ovum. This is called the cumulus oophorus or discus proligerus.

At this point in the follicle's development the *egg* becomes surrounded by several radiating layers of granulosa cells, the corona radiata, from which it is separated by an innermost perivitelline space containing fluid, and by a strong homogeneous capsule, the zona pellucida.

Coincident with these changes within the follicle, it becomes enveloped

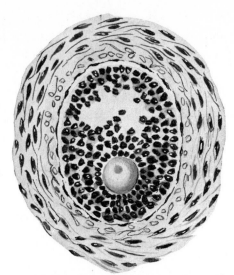

Fig. 2.—Early development of follicle. Further proliferation of granulosa cells with beginning antrum formation.

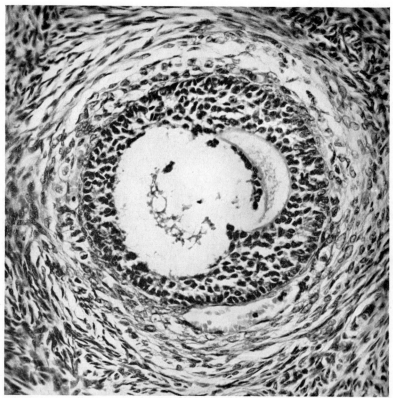

Fig. 3.—Microphotograph of developing follicle showing proliferation of granulosa cells and antrum formation.

by a zone of connective tissue, the so-called *theca layer*. This is composed of two concentric strata: the *theca interna* and *theca externa*. The former, immediately adjacent to the granulosa layer, is cellular in texture and contains round and polygonal cells rich in protoplasm, which later assume an epithelioid character. Unlike the granulosa, this layer is endowed with a capillary network, which is constantly enriched as the follicle matures. The outer zone, or theca externa, is almost indistinguishable from the surrounding ovarian stroma, and is composed of a less cellular fibrous connective tissue containing small spindle cells. This layer harbors blood vessels, lymph channels and nerves. As the follicle matures and the time of rupture approaches, the capillary net work of the theca layer becomes more prominent and the large spindle cells begin to take on fat and yellow pigment, preparatory to their post-ovulatory conversion into prominent theca lutein cells.

The *position* of the follicle, with relation to the surface of the ovary, changes in the course of its development. At first it moves towards the medulla, but when about 0.5 cm. in diameter begins to grow outward towards the periphery. According to Strassmann,[10] the migration of the follicle towards the surface is facilitated by the theca interna and externa. The former grows eccentrically, its one-sided proliferation being always directed towards the surface. This results in a wedge-shaped cone which infiltrates and penetrates the surrounding tissues, thus opening a path for the enlarging follicle. The follicle proper follows the line of least resistance, its progress being further facilitated by edema of the surrounding tissues. At the same time that the theca interna cone is forming, the theca externa, rich in connective tissue fibers, prevents expansion of the follicle in any direction except towards the periphery by remaining thick on the side towards the medulla and thinning out on the side towards the ovarian surface. When the follicle reaches the surface, it measures 1 to 1.5 cm. in diameter and is known as the ripe or *graafian follicle*.

Ovulation.—After reaching the periphery, the follicle begins to protrude. The theca interna flattens out, forming a straight line, and proliferation ceases. As a result of cellular degeneration, the membrane between the interior of the follicle and the peritoneal cavity becomes progressively attenuated.

In the meantime, the ovum gradually becomes detached from the wall of the follicle. Some believe this is accomplished by fatty degeneration of the cells in the cumulus oophorus; others attribute it to secretion of secondary liquor folliculi in the intercellular spaces of this aggregation of cells.

Direct observation of ovulation has thus far been accomplished in the rabbit[11, 12] and ewe.[13] In the rabbit, the ovulatory act has been described[12] as follows: Shortly before rupture, the follicle is projected well above the surface of the ovary and appears markedly distended. A fine network of capillaries is seen working in from the edge towards the center of the protruding part of the follicle. These gradually become more numerous, thicker, and branched. There now appears near the apex of the follicle a pale avascular spot, the so-called stigma, which soon develops into a papilla. At the tip of this nipple-shaped protuberance, a minute, oval-

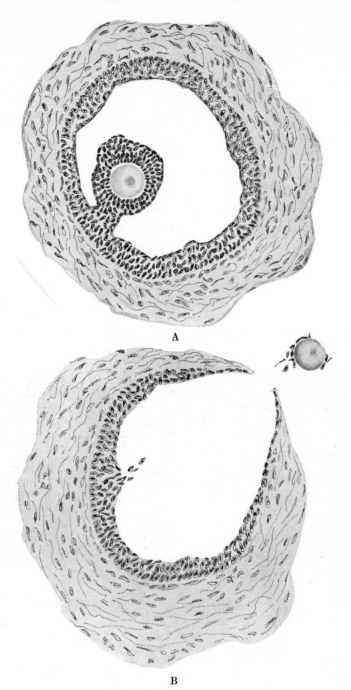

A

B

Fig. 4.—Later development of follicle. A, Mature graafian follicle; egg is surrounded by discus proligerus and projects into follicular cavity. B, Act of ovulation; ovum is catapulted from follicular cavity.

shaped opening with smooth unbroken edges becomes discernible. A fine trickle of blood is seen, followed by a minute current of thick, viscid, blood-tinged fluid. The act of rupture occupies a period of 5 to 7 seconds. Discharge of the liquor folliculi, and the ovum with its surrounding corona radiata occurs within 30 to 60 seconds. The viscosity of the follicular

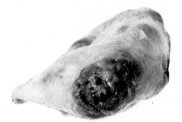

Fig. 5.—Human ovary showing recently ruptured follicle.

fluid checks the ovum's exit, thus preventing it from being catapulted into the abdominal cavity beyond the reach of the tubal fimbriae.

In the human, as in the rabbit, the protruding surface of the follicle, because of cellular degeneration, becomes attenuated and there appears the pale, translucent spot which is to provide the exit for the ovum.

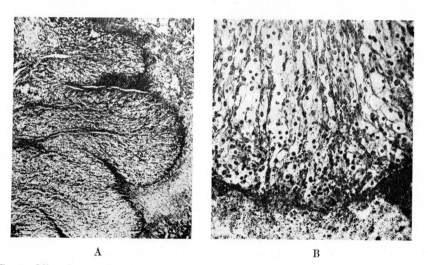

A   B

Fig. 6.—Microphotograph of human corpus luteum in the early stage of organization. Tissue removed on eighteenth day postmenstruum. A, Low power. B, High power.

Whether the events which follow the appearance of the stigma are identical with those observed in the rabbit is not certain. It has been suggested that follicular rupture in the human is probably more precipitous, since the liquor folliculi is less viscid and apparently under greater pressure than in the rabbit.

Corpus Luteum Phase.—Formation of the corpus luteum begins immediately following ovulation. The ruptured follicle, after discharge of its contents, constitutes the inconspicuous foundation upon which the yellow body is built. The size of the collapsed follicle varies considerably and depends upon that attained by the mature graafian follicle before rupture. Gray at first, it soon assumes its characteristic yellow color. According to Robert Meyer,[14] the development and decline of the corpus luteum may be divided into four stages as follows:

Proliferation.—Immediately following rupture and extrusion of the ovum, the follicle appears as a flaccid, collapsed, folded structure lined by granulosa cells of a loose texture and surrounded by the theca interna. The point of rupture soon becomes filled with a soft fibrinous plug, and, in the course of several days, becomes sealed by connective tissue derived

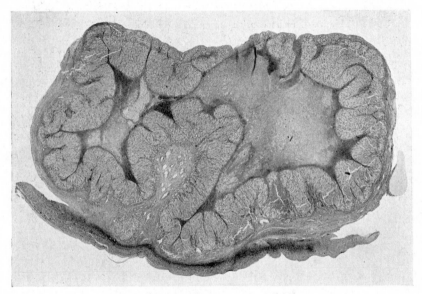

Fig. 7.—Fresh corpus luteum in full bloom.

from the theca interna. Contrary to an earlier belief, hemorrhage does not occur immediately after rupture, and very little or no blood is found in the collapsed follicle at this time. The theca layer, with its rich blood supply, proliferates rapidly and plays an important role in the development of the yellow body, for it is from this layer that the granulosa derives the blood supply so essential for its subsequent function as an endocrine gland. In the early stages of corpus luteum development, the theca cells are much more prominent than the granulosa cells. Large and polyhedral in shape, they contain large amounts of lipoid substance and are described as *theca lutein* cells to distinguish them from the granulosa lutein cells which they closely resemble but which appear later.

The granulosa cells multiply rapidly, but because of a limited blood supply, contain relatively little lipoid material. Though no definite capillary formations are seen in the granulosa layer during this phase, pools of blood become apparent by the third day after rupture.

Vascularization.—During the latter half of the first, and the first half of the second week after rupture, numerous capillaries spring from the theca interna and begin to invade the granulosa. As this process continues, blood is poured into the central cavity and mixes with the residual liquor folliculi to form a pale, red, jelly-like coagulum. So great is this capillary proliferation that in a very short time each granulosa cell is endowed with its own capillary.

Some of the blood vessels, after penetrating the granulosa layer, run along its inner margin and soon invade the central core as well. As they invade the granulosa layer, they are trailed by delicate connective tissue

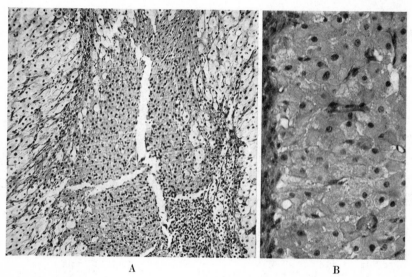

A   B

Fig. 8.—Microphotograph of mature corpus luteum. A, Magnified 125 ✕; B, magnified 400 ✕.

septa, which also spread along the inner margin of the granulosa, some entering the inner core, others extending outward into the granulosa layer.

With the marked increase in the blood supply, the granulosa cells take on large amounts of fat and pigment, become large and polyhedral in shape. As they grow more prominent, the theca cells become correspondingly less conspicuous.

Maturity.—At the height of development, the granulosa cells, now rich in lipoid and yellow pigment (carotin), give the corpus luteum its characteristic yellow color. The mature granulosa lutein cell is large, well defined, polyhedral in shape, and contains a palely staining, centrally situated, round or oval-shaped nucleus, and a fairly prominent nucleolus. Because of the marked increase in number and size of the cells, the granulosa layer becomes crenated and assumes a ruff-like, serrated pattern. By this time, the connective tissue along the inner margin of the granulosa has sent into the granulosa layer numerous fibrillar septa. These combine with the septa which stem directly from the theca interna, to form an interdigitating connective tissue structure that supports the luteal cells. The theca interna cells are now relatively inconspicuous, appearing mainly in the septa, and are distinguishable from the granulosa lutein cells by their smaller size and darker color.

The subsequent course of the corpus luteum depends upon the fate of the ovum. Should it die, regressive changes set in rapidly, but in the event

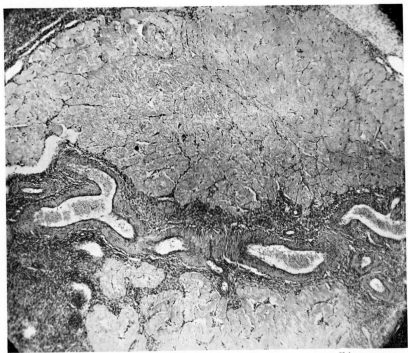

Fig. 9.—Microphotograph of human ovary showing a corpus albicans.

of conception, the yellow body persists and continues to function as the corpus luteum of pregnancy.

Retrogression.— (Corpus luteum of menstruation). Regressive changes first appear at approximately the eighth to the tenth day after rupture.[46] The granulosa lutein cells become vacuolated and disappear. The nuclei, suspended by strands of cytoplasm, are eventually destroyed by pyknosis and chromatolysis, the disintegrated fragments being then carried away by macrophages and leucocytes. The theca persist longer than the granulosa cells and, as the latter degenerate, become more prominent by contrast. Later they, too, undergo fatty and hyaline degeneration. As a result, the structure as a whole becomes smaller and is replaced by fibrous tissue, appearing by the end of six to ten weeks as a homogeneous hyalinized mass. Still later, it is invaded by fibroblasts, and progressive organization ensues, culminating in scar tissue formation. The resulting structure, the so-called corpus fibrosum or albicans, assumes various shapes and eventually becomes fused with the ovarian stroma.

Corpus Luteum of Pregnancy.—In the event of conception and implantation, the ripe corpus luteum increases in size to about 3 cm. in diameter, and continues to function at least until the fourth month of gestation. Regression sets in after this point, but proceeds very slowly, the structure often remaining intact until the end of pregnancy. Histologically, the degenerating corpus luteum of pregnancy differs from that of menstruation in that it contains colloid and calcific deposits.

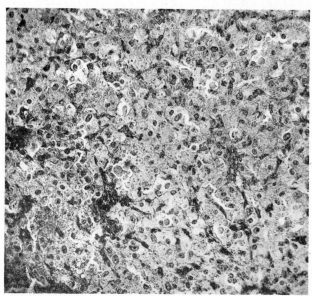

Fig. 10.—Corpus luteum of pregnancy. Microphotograph of tissue obtained at the twenty-third week of gestation.

Follicular Atresia.—Throughout reproductive life, numerous follicles undergo some degree of development, but as a rule only one matures during each menstrual cycle, while the others undergo atresia. The type of atresia varies according to the degree of follicular development achieved at the time regression begins. In general, it is possible to distinguish between the *obliterative form,* which occurs in the early stages of development, and the *cystic form,* seen in larger follicles whose growth has progressed further towards the point of rupture. The latter sometimes eventuate in retention cysts which may have a pathologic significance (see Uterine Bleeding, Chap. XXV).

The process of follicular atresia involves destruction of the ovum by pyknosis and chromatolysis, absorption of the liquor, and fatty degeneration of the granulosa cells. The follicle collapses coincident with a marked proliferation of theca lutein cells which grow centrifugally, invading the

2

granulosa and cavity, and eventually obliterating it. The resulting structure has been described as the connective tissue counterpart of the corpus luteum. At a later stage, the theca lutein cells atrophy, and eventually merge imperceptibly with the ovarian stroma to form the corpus fibrosum or atreticum.

Follicular atresia is particularly marked in pregnancy, when the theca interna cells hypertrophy, take on much fat and pigment, and become even more prominent than the theca lutein cells of the corpus luteum at the outset of its development.

CYCLIC CHANGES IN THE UTERINE MUCOSA

We owe our present concept of the endometrial cycle and its correlation with the cyclic alterations in the ovary to the epoch-making work of Hitschmann and Adler,[15] and the subsequent studies of Robert Meyer,[16] Schröder,[17] Shaw[18] and others.[19] These observers found that coincident with follicular maturation and corpus luteum formation in the ovary, characteristic cyclic changes take place in the endometrium of the fundus uteri, and to a lesser extent in that of the isthmus.

The endometrial cycle consists of an anabolic and a catabolic phase. The former involves a progressive growth and preparation of the uterine mucosa for nidatory purposes, in the event that conception occurs. The latter phase, clinically manifested in menstrual bleeding, consists of a breakdown or dismantling of the highly prepared and sensitized mucosa, and betokens failure of fertilization.

The changes of the uterine mucosa during the menstrual cycle are continuous and overlap so that there is no clear-cut point at which one phase ends and the other begins. Nevertheless, it is customary for descriptive purposes to divide the endometrial cycle into various phases, as follows:

Anabolic Phase	Proliferative Phase	Early—2nd to 5th day / Late—6th to 14th day
	Secretory Phase	Early—15th to 21st day / Late—22nd to 28th day

Catabolic Phase (Menstruation)   1st and 2nd day

Early Proliferative Phase.*—At the beginning of the cycle, and following menstrual disintegration which terminates the preceding one, the endometrium appears as a thin, denuded membrane measuring only about 1 mm. in thickness. It is composed of a dense, cellular, poorly vascularized, spindle-celled stroma, which harbors the basal parts of the endometrial glands. The latter consist of tubular stumps with narrow lumina and show only slight branching. They are widely separated from one another and at first run either perpendicularly, obliquely or parallel to the surface. Few or no mitotic figures are observed during this early phase. The glands are lined by epithelial cells which contain elongated, oval-shaped, darkly-staining, basally situated nuclei. The protoplasmic zone of the glandular

---

* This is sometimes termed the postmenstrual phase or the period of regeneration or repair.

epithelium is sharply demarcated, and the lumina of the glands are empty. Veins and arterioles project freely into the uterine cavity and, like the stumps of the glands, are enveloped by a dense sheath of reticulum.

According to Schröder,[20] re-epithelization of the denuded surface normally begins by the third day and is complete by the end of the first week. It is apparently accomplished by radial migration of the epithelial cells which line the wide-mouthed glandular stumps. Simultaneously, a new growth of capillaries appears, and the arterioles and veins become elongated, running parallel to the uterine glands and perpendicular to the surface epithelium.

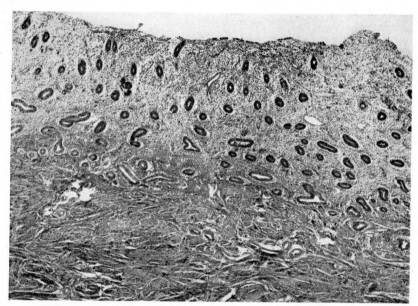

Fig. 11.—Early postmenstrual endometrium. Microphotograph of tissue obtained four days postmenstruum. Note that the surface is already partially epithelized.

These changes coincide with development of a primordial follicle in the ovary and continued regression of the corpus luteum of the preceding menstrual cycle.

Late Proliferative Phase.*—This part of the cycle extends from about the 6th to the 14th day and is marked by proliferative changes in both the glands and stroma. Mitotic activity is marked, and the mucosa steadily increases in thickness until it measures about 3 mm. by the end of the second week. As the glands become longer and wider, they assume a course perpendicular to the surface. Towards the end of the second week they assume mild serpentine formations. The cells lining the glands are higher, and their long oval nuclei are basally or centrally situated. The stroma gradually becomes looser in texture and more and more vascu-

---

* This, together with the early secretory phase, is sometimes described as the "interval phase."

larized as the blood vessels grow steadily longer. Considerable branching
of blood vessels occurs in the superficial zone, forming a subepithelial
capillary network. The individual capillaries run a straight course parallel
to the surface. In the deeper zone of the endometrium they closely sur-
round the uterine glands, with the long axis of the capillary mesh paralleling the glands. The basalis is supplied by capillaries derived from
vessels of the submucosal layer of the myometrium. These capillaries
apparently undergo no cyclic changes, and are independent of the vascular
apparatus which nourishes the functional layers.

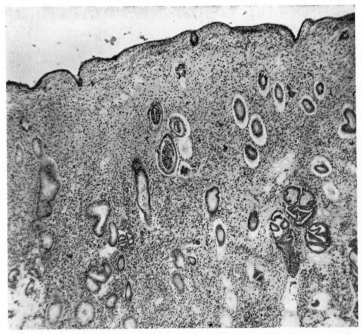

Fig. 12.—Proliferative type of endometrium. Microphotograph of tissue obtained ten days
postmenstruum.

The height of the late proliferative phase coincides with full maturation
of the graafian follicle. At the end of this period, ovulation occurs. This
marks the beginning of the corpus luteum phase and the initiation of
secretory activity in the endometrium.

Early Secretory Phase.—During the third week, the mucosa becomes
thicker, the glands more tortuous, and the stroma better vascularized and
edematous. Mitotic activity gradually ceases. Within 48 hours after ovulation, the glandular nuclei are displaced toward the lumen side of the cell,
so that a clear space is left at the basal portion. This constitutes the earliest
sign of secretory function. Globules of glycogen now appear in the cells.

At this time, the corpus luteum is developing, but has not yet attained
full maturity.

Late Secretory Phase.*—During the fourth week, the mucosa thickens to approximately 5 mm. For the first time, the functional layer of the

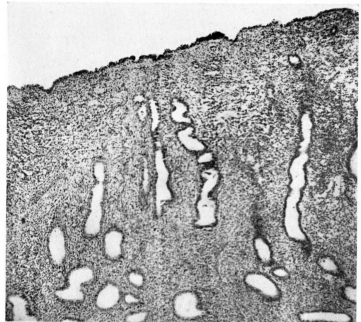

Fig. 13.—Proliferative type of endometrium. Microphotograph of tissue obtained twelve days postmenstruum.

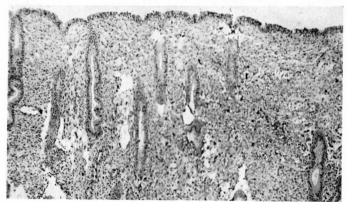

Fig. 14.—Early pregravid endometrium. Microphotograph of endometrial tissue obtained fifteen days postmenstruum.

mucosa is clearly demarcated from the basal or foundation layer, whence it is derived. Histologically, *three strata* are distinguishable: (1) An outer zone or *compacta* lies immediately beneath the surface epithelium and is

*Otherwise known as premenstrual, pregravid or progravid phase.

composed largely of an edematous stroma, which harbors the relatively narrow terminal parts of the uterine glands. (2) A middle zone or *spongiosa*, which is approximately twice as thick as the compacta, contains the most dilated portions of the glands and comparatively little stroma. These two layers make up four-fifths of the endometrium. (3) The remaining fifth is made up of the innermost zone, the *basalis*. This is sometimes termed the non-functioning layer since it takes no part in the cyclic changes. It lies adjacent to the myometrium and is made up of a dense cellular stroma containing the narrow basal ends or fundi of the uterine glands.

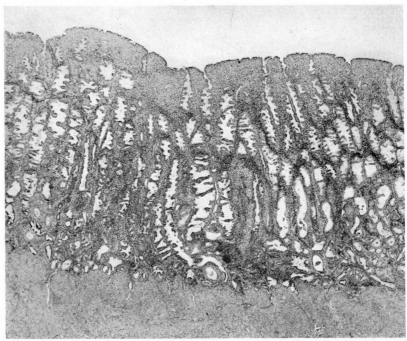

Fig. 15.—Pregravid endometrium. Microphotograph of tissue obtained twenty-seven days postmenstruum.

The glands, stroma, and blood vessels present striking morphologic and functional alterations, as follows:

Glandular Changes.—The glands, particularly those in the spongiosa, become sacculated and assume cork-screw or serrate formations. The columnar cells which line them take on more glycogen and become distended with protoplasm. The nuclei are oval-shaped, stain palely, and are more basally situated. As the secretions pour into the lumen, the free surface of the protoplasmic zone becomes increasingly irregular and eventually assumes a wavy, frayed, tuft-like appearance. The lumina of the glands become distended with fresh protoplasm containing glycogen and, according to some, fat droplets. The terminal parts of the glands situated in the compacta layer are now more tortuous and actively secreting.

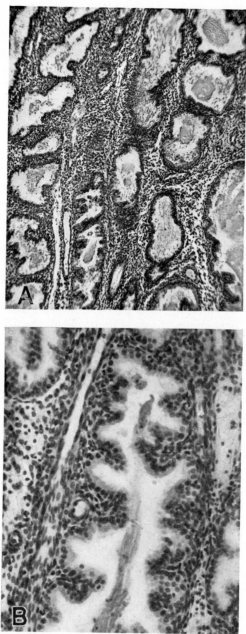

Fig. 16.—Pregravid endometrium. Spongiosa layer. A, Microphotograph of tissue obtained on the twenty-seventh day postmenstruum (× 125). B, Section of gland from same layer. Gland is lined by a single layer of secreting cells with basally situated nuclei. Note wavy protoplasmic zone.

As active secretion proceeds and the time of the flow draws near, signs of cellular degeneration appear. Many of the cells, emptied of their secretions, undergo chromatolysis and nuclear degeneration. These involutionary changes may precede the appearance of blood in the vagina by one or more days. Observing such changes during the fourth week of the cycle, Sturgis and Meigs[21] have criticized the custom of designating the endometrial changes just before the flow as the "active secretory" phase. They contend that the immediately premenstrual endometrial alterations are actually involutional in nature, contrasting with the actively secreting mucosa during pregnancy. Shortly before the flow, the glands are distended, the papillary infoldings of the lining are flattened out, the epithelial cells are frayed at the edges and reduced in height, and many of the nuclei shrunken and pyknotic. During pregnancy, on the other hand, active secretion is evidenced by the crowded, tremendously convoluted glands, and by the swollen, round epithelial cells, bulging with glycogen globules. They conclude, with apparent justification, that involutionary changes foreshadowing the menstrual phase appear before extravasation of blood begins.

Stromal Changes.—The stroma of the functional layers, and especially that of the compacta, becomes progressively looser in texture. The cells take on much plasma, swell, and become polygonal in shape. Their nuclei are rounder and stain poorly. Towards the end of the cycle, the stroma becomes markedly edematous, and its cells often resemble decidual cells. The stroma of the spongiosa shows only a mild degree of edema which is most pronounced around the blood vessels. The connective tissue of the basalis remains closely packed and takes no part in this process.

Blood Vessel Changes.—During the late secretory phase,[22] the arterioles continue to grow for a longer time than the other constituents of the mucosa, become increasingly tortuous and assume spiral patterns. That portion of the arteriole which transverses the spongiosa is of a larger calibre, more winding and has thicker walls, while that which passes through the compacta is less serpentine and more of a capillary nature. As the end of the cycle nears, the blood vessels become very much dilated and engorged. Varicose swellings of the veins appear in the border zone between the compacta and spongiosa, and shortly before the flow, those in the spongiosa become abruptly dilated.

During the late secretory phase, a mature corpus luteum is present in the ovary.

Menstrual Phase.—It is generally conceded [16, 17, 23] that menstrual disintegration of the superficial layer is characterized by (1) cessation of secretory activity, (2) discharge of the glandular contents, (3) absorption of the stromal fluid, (4) destruction and sequestration of part or all of the functional layers and (5) bleeding into the endometrial stroma and uterine cavity. The basalis is not involved in this regressive process and remains unaltered. Even before hemorrhage occurs, the glands begin to discharge their secretions and collapse. The surface epithelium and the cells lining the glands become detached, undergo degeneration, and are gradually cast off. This is followed by a progressive diapedesis and rhexis of the markedly dilated and engorged capillaries. Numerous polymorphonuclear leucocytes and lymphocytes, probably derived from the blood, invade the functional layers. Small localized hemorrhages appear in the spongiosa, and soon the entire functionalis is infiltrated with blood. The pools of blood which form between the compacta and spongiosa tend to separate the two layers, forming an irregular or ragged line of cleavage.

Within a few hours, or in some instances, a few days, fragmentation of the upper layers of the mucosa ensues. This is localized at first, but soon becomes general until the entire functionalis disintegrates. The mucosa

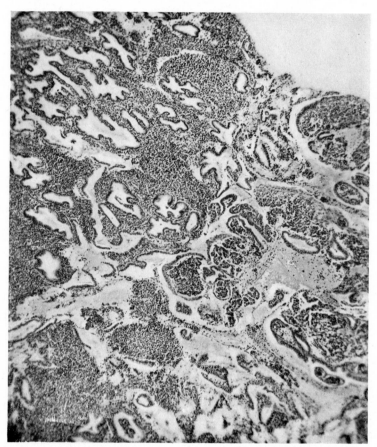

Fig. 17.—Menstruating endometrium. Microphotograph of tissue obtained on first day of the flow.

during this phase presents a bizarre appearance. Well preserved intact glands appear side by side with collapsed or fragmented acini. Here and there, clumps of desquamated epithelial cells surrounded by blood and leucocytes are seen in the same field. In some instances, fragmentation, necrosis, and hemorrhage are confined to the zone between the compacta and spongiosa layers, the compacta being cast off in relatively large, well preserved pieces.

The amount of blood and tissue loss, as well as the time required for completion of the dismantling process show wide individual variations. In some cases only small fragments of tissue are lost, while in others the

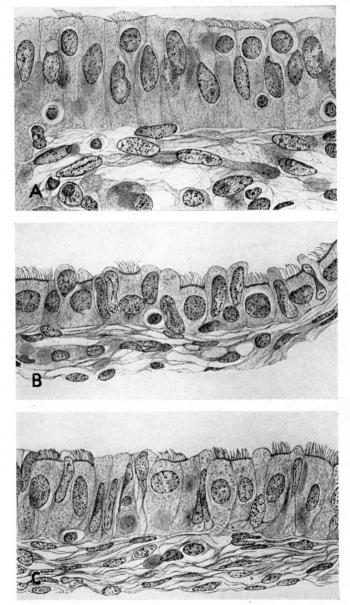

Fig. 18.—Cyclical changes in the human tubal epithelium. A, Mid-interval. B, Premenstrual. C, Late interval. (F. F. Snyder, Johns Hopkins Hosp. Bull., Vol. 35.)

entire compacta and spongiosa is destroyed. Where the tissue loss is relatively small, involution of the mucosa is apparently accomplished largely by absorption of the stromal edema fluid, and by collapse of the glands after discharge of their secretions.[23]

CYCLIC CHANGES IN THE TUBAL MUCOSA

The tubal plicae in the mature organ are lined by a single layer of epithelium, composed of approximately equal numbers of ciliated (non-secretory) and non-ciliated (secretory) cells, supported by a connective tissue stroma. Recent studies suggest that the tubal epithelium undergoes demonstrable modifications which can be correlated with events in the ovary.

Postmenstrual Phase.—Cyclic changes in the human tubal mucosa were first described by Snyder[24] in 1924. His findings have since been corroborated and extended by Novak and Everett[25] and others.[26, 27] The ciliated cells, except for variations in height, undergo no conspicuous alterations. During the postmenstrual phase, the tubal epithelium is low and somewhat uneven, but by the third or fourth day the cells are taller, more uniform in height, narrow, and closely situated. In the course of the second and third week, the epithelium reaches its maximum height. At this time, the ciliated and non-ciliated cells are of equal height, and the surface of the mucosa is consequently even. The ciliated cells are broad, and contain rounded nuclei which are situated close to the outer margin of the cell. The non-ciliated cells, which take a darker stain, are narrow and possess elongated nuclei which lie nearer the base of the cell. Because of the difference in the position of their nuclei, the epithelium appears to be two layered.

Premenstrual Phase.—During the premenstrual phase, the epithelium becomes progressively lower and cytoplasmic processes jut out from the non-ciliated cells as far as the tips of the cilia or even beyond. The nuclei often project into these processes, which may be pedunculated. Because of these protruding cells, the surface of the mucosa is uneven and contrasts with the even surface seen during the second and third week. According to Scaglione,[28] the cells now are actively secreting and contain lipoid granules. Novak and Everett[25] speak of a great loss of cells, but Snyder[24] makes no mention of this.

Menstrual Phase.—During the menstrual phase, the ciliated cells remain broad and low, while the non-ciliated cells, now emptied of their secretions, are lower than in the premenstruum. So-called "peg cells," interpreted by Novak and Everett[25] as emptied secretory cells, are present in fairly large numbers.

CYCLIC CHANGES IN THE CERVICAL MUCOSA

That the cervical mucosa undergoes rhythmic modifications related to the ovarian and uterine cycle, has recently been suggested by Wollner.[29] On the basis of biopsy studies in twenty normally menstruating women, this observer describes the changes in the cervical mucosa as follows:

Postmenstrual Phase.—The cervical epithelium, during the postmenstrual phase, consists of a continuous layer of low, columnar, sharply de-

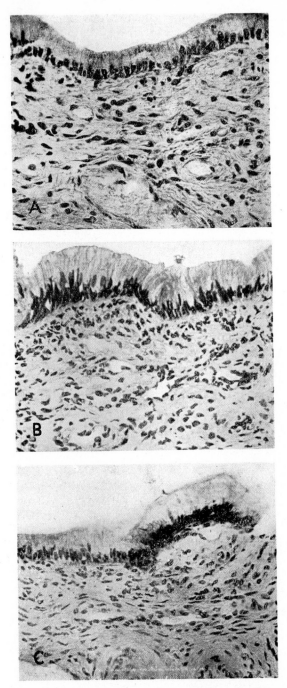

Fig. 19.—Microphotographs of human cervical epithelium. A, Seven days after onset of menstruation. B, Twenty-three days after onset of flow. C, Second day of menstruation. (Wollner in Surg., Gyn. and Obst., Vol. 64.)

fined cells with small, oval-shaped, deeply staining, basally situated nuclei. By the sixth day after the onset of the flow, these cells completely cover the surface of the mucosa. The stroma is composed of dense, fibrous, connective tissue with widely spaced cells containing small nuclei and very little cytoplasm. The few tubular glands present are lined by cells similar to those which compose the surface epithelium. Their lumina are narrow and contain no mucus.

Interval Phase.—In the interval phase of the cycle, the cells gradually become higher and broader, the nuclei larger and elongated, and the cytoplasm more abundant. The nuclei are spindle-shaped, deeply staining, and basally situated. Toward the end of this phase, there appear signs of secretion. At the same time the blood vessels become engorged. The stroma now is more cellular, loose, edematous and its cells larger and contain more cytoplasm. The glands are irregular, show profuse branching, and project into the surrounding stroma.

Premenstrual Phase.—During the premenstrual phase, the surface epithelium becomes more prominent, while the cells lining the glands increase in height, become irregular, and bulge into the lumen. Evidence of active secretory activity is now apparent.

Menstrual Phase.—After the onset of the flow, the surface epithelium becomes denuded. Re-epithelization soon begins, starting at the broken ends of the glands. At the same time, the glandular epithelium shows extensive destruction and exfoliation, some of the glands becoming entirely denuded. When exfoliation is complete, the glands collapse and return to their original outline, whereupon rapid regeneration of their lining epithelium occurs. In a more recent communication, Wollner[30] states that the cervix apparently contributes to the menstrual flow. Free blood is found in the lumina of exfoliating glands and some of the tremendously dilated blood vessels near the surface are seen opened up after the exfoliation of the surface epithelium.

A cervical cycle has also been observed by Sjövall,[31] whose description differs in certain details from that of Wollner. While these findings are interesting, further confirmation is desirable.

CYCLIC CHANGES IN THE VAGINAL MUCOSA

The studies by which Stockard and Papanicolaou[32] demonstrated cyclic changes in the vagina of the guinea pig have stimulated similar investigations in the human. Though some observers are convinced that the human vaginal mucosa undergoes cyclic morphologic and functional changes during the menstrual cycle, others question this, particularly in view of recent evidence[2] casting doubt on its müllerian origin.

In 1927, Dierks[33] described cyclic vaginal alterations which could be correlated with the ovarian cycle. He distinguished *three vaginal zones:* (1) a basalis, (2) a middle or cornified layer, and (3) a superficial zone or functionalis. According to his description, the two upper zones are cast off during menstruation, leaving only a thin basal layer. After the flow, the basalis grows progressively thicker and by the seventh day a new cornified zone and functionalis form. The new functionalis continues to proliferate and becomes increasingly hyperemic. Just before the flow, the cornified zone is composed of flattened cells with shrunken pyknotic nuclei. The cells of the functionalis, fairly large with round nuclei, undergo

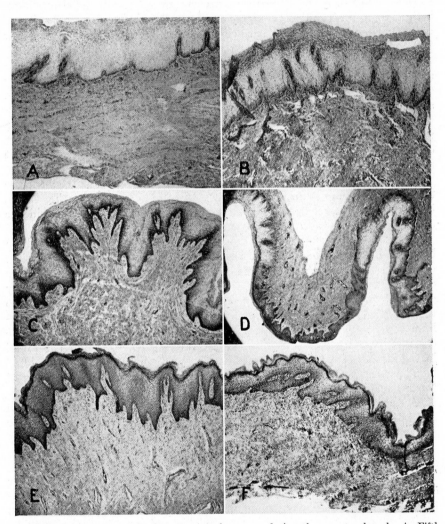

Fig. 20.—Changes in the human vaginal mucosa during the menstrual cycle. A, Fifth day after onset of menstruation. B, Second week postmenstrual. C, Beginning of third week postmenstrual. D, Third week postmenstrual. E, End of third week postmenstrual. F, Beginning of fourth week postmenstrual. (Geist in Surg., Gyn. and Obst., Vol. 51.)

extensive karyopyknosis and chromatolysis, which extends towards the cornified zone.

The results of similar studies since carried out have been conflicting. Some workers have been unable to demonstrate cyclic modifications of any kind. In a recent study, Zondek and Friedmann[34] found it impossible to ascertain the day or the phase of the menstrual cycle from the histologic appearance of the vaginal mucosa. On the other hand, several observers[35, 36] have described variations in the thickness of the mucosa, and the occurrence of vacuolization in the basalis, particularly during the postmenstrual and premenstrual phases. In 1933, Papanicolaou[37] demonstrated cyclic variations in the cellular contents of the human vaginal lumen which could be correlated with events in the ovary. He was forced to admit, however, that considerable variability exists between different individuals and different areas of the same mucosa.

More recently, Traut, Block, and Kuder,[38] using the biopsy method, were unable to confirm Dierks' observation that the loose zone of the functionalis shows cyclic variations in height. Nor could they find anything resembling a regular evolution of a cornification zone which might be

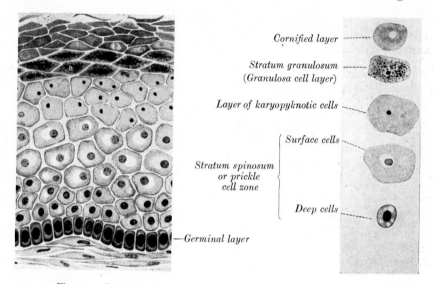

Cornified layer

Stratum granulosum
(Granulosa cell layer)

Layer of karyopyknotic cells

Surface cells

Stratum spinosum
or prickle
cell zone

Deep cells

—Germinal layer

Fig. 21.—Cytology of human vaginal epithelium. (E. G. Murray.)

correlated with the ovarian cycle. According to these observers, the only constant cyclic changes occur in the basalis. The cells in this zone are relatively quiescent except for a brief period of six or seven days during the week preceding or following the flow. At this time they show increased proliferative activity associated with dilatation of the capillaries and an increase in the number of leucocytes.

During the past few years, through the work of Papanicolaou, Shorr,[39, 40, 41] Rubenstein,[42, 43] and others, some progress has been made in improving the histological methods available for the study of the vaginal mucosa and the cellular contents of the vagina. Their use has yielded evidence tending to confirm the earlier impression that the vaginal mucosa undergoes cyclic changes which keep pace in a general way with events in the ovary and uterus.[44] It is still difficult, however, to accord each picture its place in the cycle. Unlike the endometrium, in which modifications characteristic of the luteal phase are clearly distinguishable from those which characterize the follicular phase, the vaginal mucosa, with the methods thus far devised, presents no change associated exclusively with luteal activity. The changes which occur during the luteal phase, namely increased desquamation and decreased cornification, may occur in the absence of a functioning corpus luteum. According to some observers,[45] either change alone is not significant, but if both coincide, they constitute reliable evidence of ovulation and corpus luteum formation. On the whole, it would appear that the cyclic changes in the vaginal mucosa are such that their correct interpretation is possible only in the hands of a thoroughly experienced investigator, and only if they are followed continuously throughout the cycle. (For description and evaluation of vaginal smear techniques as a diagnostic aid and therapeutic guide, see Chap. XXXIX.)

BIBLIOGRAPHY

1. Gray, H.: Anatomy. 24th ed., ed. by W. H. Lewis, Philadelphia, Lea & Febiger, 1942.
2. Meyer, R.: Arch. f. Gynäk. 158:639, 1934; ibid. 163:205, 1936; ibid. 164:207, 1937; ibid. 165:504, 1938; Zentralbl. f. Gynäk. 61:2846, 1937.
3. Koff, A. K.: Contrib. to Embryol. 24:59, 1933. In: Obstetrics and Gynecology, ed. by A. H. Curtis. Philadelphia and London, W. B. Saunders Co., 1933, vol. 1, chap. 17.
4. Allen, E.: Am. J. Anat. 31:439, 1923.
5. Evans, H. M., and Swezy, O.: Mem. Univ. Calif. 9:119, 1931.
6. Allen, E., and Creadick, R. N.: Anat. Rec. 69:191, 1937.
7. Schmidt, I. G., and Hoffman, F. G.: Am. J. Anat. 68:263, 1941.
8. Vilas, E.: Ztschr. f. Anat. u. Entwicklungsgesch. 98:263, 1932.
9. Simkins, C. S.: Am. J. Anat. 51:465, 1932.
10. Strassmann, E. O.: Arch. f. Gynäk. 119:168, 1923; Surg., Gynec. & Obst. 67:299, 1938; Am. J. Obst. & Gynec. 41:363, 1941.
11. Walton, A., and Hammond, J.: Brit. J. Exp. Biol. 6:190, 1928.
12. Smith, J. T.: Am. J. Obst. & Gynec. 27:728, 1934.
13. McKenzie, F. F., and Berlinger, V.: Mo. Agr. Sta. Res. Bull. No. 264, 1937.
14. Meyer, R.: Arch. f. Gynäk. 100:1, 1913.
15. Hitschmann, F., and Adler, L.: Monat. f. Geburtsh. u. Gynäk. 27:1, 1908.
16. Meyer, R.: Henke and Lubarsh Handb. d. spez. Path., Anat. u. Hist. Uterus und Tuben, 1930, vol. 7, part 1.
17. Schröder, R.: Monat. f. Geburtsh. u. Gynäk. 39:3, 1914; Arch. f. Gynäk. 104:27, 1915.
18. Shaw, W.: J. Obst. & Gynec. B.E. 32:679, 1923.
19. Novak, E., and TeLinde, R. W.: J.A.M.A. 83:900, 1924.
20. Schröder, R.: Veit-Stoeckel Handb. d. Gynäk. vol. 1, pt. 2, Munchen, Bergmann, 1928.
21. Sturgis, S. H., and Meigs, J. V.: Am. J. Surg. 33:369, 1936.
22. Saito, O.: Okayama Igakki Zasshi, 1926, pp. 470–471.
23. Bartelmez, G. W.: Carnegie Inst. Wash. Pub. Anat. 1933, No. 443, p. 183.
24. Snyder, F. F.: Bull. J. Hopkins Hosp. 35:141, 1924.
25. Novak, E., and Everett, H. S.: Am. J. Obst. & Gynec. 16:499, 1928.
26. Joël, C. A.: Monatschr. f. Geburtsh. u. Gynäk. 110:252, 1940.
27. Winge, M., and Winkel Smith, C. C.: Nord. Med. (Hospitalstid.) 5:434, 1940.
28. Scaglione, S.: Riv. ital. Ginec. 7:107, 1928.
29. Wollner, A.: Surg., Gynec. & Obst. 64:758, 1937.
30. Wollner, A.: Am. J. Surg. 57:331, 1942
31. Sjövall, A.: Acta obst. & gynec. Scandinav. 18:4, 1938.
32. Stockard, C. R., and Papanicolaou, G. N.: Am. J. Anat. 22:225, 1917.
33. Dierks, K.: Arch. f. Gynäk. 130:46, 1927; ibid. 138:111, 1929.
34. Zondek, B., and Friedmann, M.: J.A.M.A. 106:1051, 1936.
35. Stieve, H.: Zentralbl. f. Gynäk. 55:194, 1931.

36. Smith, B. G., and Brunner, E. K.: Am. J. Anat. *54*:27, 1934.
37. Papanicolaou, G. N.: Am. J. Anat. *52* (Suppl.) : 519, 1933
38. Traut, H. F., Block, P. W., and Kuder, A.: Surg., Gynec. & Obst. *63*:7, 1936
39. Papanicolaou, G. N., and Shorr, E.: Am. J. Obst. & Gynec. *31*:806, 1936.
40. Shorr, E., and Papanicolaou, G. N.: Proc. Soc. Exper. Biol. & Med. *41*:629, 1939.
41. Shorr, E.: Proc. Soc. Exper. Biol. & Med. *43*:501, 1940; ibid. *46*:330, 1941; Science *94:* 545, 1941.
42. Rubenstein, B. B.: Endocrinol. *27*:843, 1940.
43. Rubenstein, B. B., and Duncan, D. R. L.: Endocrinol. *28*:911, 1941.
44. Geist, S. H.: Surg., Gynec. & Obst. *51*:848, 1930.
45. Krohn, L., Harris, J., and Hechter, O.: Am. J. Obst. & Gynec. *44*:213, 1942.
46. Brewer, J. I.: Am. J. Obst. & Gynec. *44*:1048, 1942.

3

CHAPTER II

ENDOCRINE ROLE OF THE OVARY: THE FOLLICLE

INTRODUCTION

Excretory and Incretory Functions.—The ovary performs both an excretory and incretory function. Nature's ingenuity and economy are well exemplified in the mechanism by which these two functions are carried out. The vehicle, the follicle, which bears the excretory product, the ovum, also provides the material necessary to prepare for its future nourishment and growth in the event of conception. These functions are so coordinated that nourishment comes neither too soon nor too late. Ovulation is the starting point for two processes: transport of the ovum into the abdominal cavity, where it may pursue its course and be fertilized or not, as the case may be, and formation of the corpus luteum, which helps prepare the uterus to receive the ovum, should fertilization take place.

In most species, though less conspicuously in man, provision is also made for the sperm to be somewhere along the path of the ovum, so that its extrusion from the follicle will not be in vain. To accomplish this, the follicle, which bears the ovum, also secretes a hormone capable of inducing a willingness or desire to copulate. In some animals optimal conditions for fertilization are assured by the fact that ovulation occurs only following coitus and rarely, if ever, at any other time.

Following *ovulation*, the ovary stands at the fork of two roads. If the ovum dies, there is no longer need for a nidatory bed and the corpus luteum becomes superfluous and regresses. On the other hand, if conception occurs, the corpus luteum becomes essential, and therefore enlarges and continues to function. In animals which normally ovulate only in response to coitus, all waste is avoided, for a corpus luteum forms only when the deposition of sperm in the female genitalia is assured. In species which ovulate spontaneously regardless of coitus, the corpus luteum of the infertile cycle is dispensed with more or less rapidly. In the rodent, for example, its life span is very short and its function almost negligible. In man, its existence is brief compared with the duration of pregnancy, but its development is nevertheless considerable.

The corpus luteum of pregnancy, in the various species, differs also in the length of time it is needed. In smaller mammals, such as the rat, mouse and rabbit, it remains indispensable up to term. On the other hand, in larger mammals, such as the horse, and man, auxiliary forces are provided by the growing placenta, so that the corpus luteum may safely relinquish its task early in pregnancy.

With this general outline of the ovary's task and how it accomplishes it, we may now present a more detailed description of the endocrine role of the ovary, or more specifically of its chief constituents, the *graafian follicle* and *corpus luteum.* The *time of ovulation,* long a subject of speculation and a point of great practical and academic interest, will likewise receive attention.

The ovary produces hormones essential for the development and function of the accessory genitalia and secondary sex characters. The endocrine role of the ovary has been greatly clarified through ablation experiments and studies with ovarian transplants and extracts.

Effects of Ovariectomy.—The effects of ovariectomy in the mature woman are well known. In the juvenile subject, on the other hand, the sequelae of this operation have been inferred largely from degenerative experiments in the immature laboratory animal. The status of the "eunuchoid" female is suggestive of what may be expected in the ovariectomized prepuberal girl. Unfortunately, such evidence is not altogether satisfactory because of the possibility that the gonadal and somatic retardation are independent manifestations of some inherited or acquired abnormality.

The effect of ovarian ablation in the lower animal varies according to the *age,* and *degree of genital development* attained at the time of operation. If performed before puberty, the accessory genitalia and secondary sex characters do not develop. In the sexually mature rodent, ovariectomy is followed by cessation of the estrus cycles, progressive involution of the accessory genitalia and mammae, diminished sex drive, and a slowing up of voluntary activity. In the mature rhesus monkey, this operation causes retrogressive modifications of the accessory genitalia and fading of the sexual skin. Except for the premature onset of uterine bleeding, where ovariectomy is performed at the height of the follicular phase or later in the cycle (see Chap. V), there is no subsequent menstruation. In the mature woman, as in the monkey, involutionary changes in the accessory genitalia and cessation of menstrual function are inevitable.

Ovarian Transplants.—Ovarian transplants in the human have proved unsuccessful, and the available information regarding their efficacy as replacement therapy is based largely on studies in the ovariectomized laboratory animal. The observation that, in such species as the rabbit, guinea pig, and rodent, ovarian transplants postpone or prevent post-castration changes in the accessory genitalia and secondary sex characters, made it clear that the gonads act through hormonal and not through nervous pathways. The positive results obtained with transplants encouraged attempts to isolate the active principle of the ovary and determine its efficacy for the control of the symptoms of ovarian deficiency.

Ovarian Extracts.—The effects reported with the older ovarian extracts were varied and unconvincing. The impurity of the extracts, failure to use controls, and lack of reliable criteria of physiologic effect combined to confuse earlier observers. The discovery, in 1923, that the accessory genitalia and particularly the vagina of the guinea pig,[1] rat,[2] and mouse,[3] undergo cyclic alterations which can be correlated with events in the ovary, was the starting point for intensive studies which have greatly clarified the physiology of the ovary. It is now established that the graafian follicle produces the hormone responsible for estrus, while the corpus luteum supplies the active principle which elicits the characteristic modifications of the accessory genitalia during pseudopregnancy and pregnancy. In 1929, [4, 5] crystalline estrogen was prepared for the first time (see Chap. XLI). Shortly after this, investigators[6] succeeded in preparing a corpus luteum extract capable of eliciting in the accessory genitalia modifications like those seen during the luteal phase of the infertile and fertile cycle.

ENDOCRINE ROLE OF THE FOLLICLE

Follicular Functions.—The specific functions of the follicle have been ascertained by observing the alterations of the accessory genitalia which appear coincident with follicular maturation, or following the administration of follicular extracts in the castrate.

Through the histologic study of human ovaries, uteri and uterine curettings simultaneously removed at operation, Hitschmann and Adler,[7] Schröder,[8] Meyer[9] and others demonstrated that proliferative changes of the uterine mucosa coincide with follicular maturation, while secretory activity of the endometrium is invariably associated with a functioning corpus luteum. Studies in the rat, mouse, rabbit and guinea pig revealed that estrus and ovulation are synchronous, and that the ovarian and estrus cycles begin and end simultaneously in animals with a limited breeding season. A relationship between the follicle and estrus was further suggested by the observation that in the rabbit, failing copulation, maturation of follicles and estrus persist throughout the breeding season. Also significant was the fact that the slow but progressive growth of the accessory genitalia in the juvenile animal coincides with maturation of follicles only, corpora lutea appearing for the first time when puberal development is fairly well advanced.

Though these findings made it clear that the proliferative changes of the accessory genitalia coincide with follicular development, and the two phenomena are causally related, experimental proof of this relationship, and identification of the hormone concerned was not achieved until potent follicular extracts, containing what is now generally referred to as the estrogenic hormone, were prepared and their specific effects determined.

BIOLOGY OF ESTROGEN

It is now well established that the estrogenic hormone is essential for development of the accessory genitalia and secondary sex characters at puberty, and their maintenance and function during maturity.

Effects on Uterus.—Under its influence, the uterus of the infantile or spayed rodent rapidly enlarges, becomes markedly hyperemic and distended with a serous fluid. The glandular and stromal elements of the endometrium become well differentiated and the myometrium hypertrophies, so that the uterus morphologically and histologically resembles that of the mature intact animal during estrus. In the intact immature, or spayed adult monkey, estrogen causes hypertrophy of the uterine musculature, and marked proliferation of the endometrium equivalent to the modifications seen during the follicular or pre-ovulatory phase of the menstrual cycle. Cessation of the estrogen treatment, as a rule, is soon followed by bleeding from the estrogen-prepared mucosa (see Chap. V), after which the uterus reverts to its infantile proportions. Similar effects have been obtained in the mature human castrate. Marked development and growth of hypoplastic uteri has been produced in man with relatively large doses of estrogenic substance over a protracted period. Dodds[10] and Clauberg[11] found 500,000 to 1,000,000 rat units necessary for this effect. The latter observed that proliferation of the mucosa occurred only after an appreciable increase in the size of the uterus had been achieved. The effect was transient and cessation of injections was soon followed by regressive changes and reversion of the uterus to its previous immature proportions.

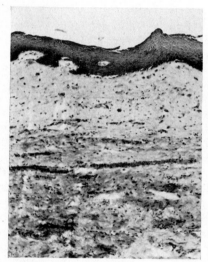 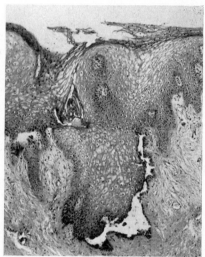

Fig. 22.—Human vaginal epithelium before and after estrogen stimulation. A, Microphotograph of tissue obtained by biopsy from thirty-two-year-old woman with amenorrhea for four years. Note atrophic changes. B, Vaginal epithelium of same patient following subcutaneous injection of 2000 r.u. estradiol benzoate twice weekly for six weeks. Note marked proliferation and cornification.

Effects on Vagina.—In the mature spayed rodent, estrogen repairs the vaginal atrophy and causes the typical changes of estrus to reappear within seventy-two hours. Whether it is also responsible for the vaginal mucification seen in the rodent during pregnancy and pseudopregnancy, is still controversial. In the intact immature or spayed adult monkey, it causes progressive proliferation of the vaginal epithelium.

Effects on Fallopian Tubes.—Estrogen stimulates growth of the tubes in the immature intact animal. In the mature castrate it prevents their involution or, if regression has already set in, restores them to their precastration state. In the spayed adult rodent and monkey,[12] mitosis, cell division and secretory activity of the tubal epithelium have been observed following estrogen treatment. This hormone apparently also influences the activity of the tubal musculature. In the intact animal, the tubal contractions reach their height at estrus.[13] Their dependence on estrogen is indicated by the fact that they disappear following ovariectomy and can be restored by administering estrogenic substance.[14, 15] In the mouse,[16] moderate doses may lead to "tube-locking" which interferes with the transport of ova. On the other hand, large doses relax the tubes and hasten the passage of the eggs into the uterus.[17] Tubal motility in the human being is also dependent on the estrogenic hormone. In cyclically menstruating women, the tubes show regular, rhythmic contractions which increase at the time of ovulation. After the menopause, these become weaker and less frequent, finally ceasing entirely. Estrogen injections restore them within a short period of time.[18, 19]

Effects on Secondary Sex Characters.—The estrogenic hormone is essential for development of the secondary sex characters. In certain species of birds, plumage changes have been noted following its administration. Its role in mammary development and function is discussed in detail elsewhere (see Chap. X). In certain subhuman primates, this hormone is apparently responsible for the swelling and reddening of the sexual skin seen during the follicular phase of the menstrual cycle. These modifications are absent in the ovariectomized animal, but can be made to reappear by administering estrogen.[20]

Effects on the Mating Instinct.—There is evidence that the mating instinct, also referred to as sexual drive, heat or libido, depends on hormonal as well as nervous factors. That estrogen plays an important role is indicated by the fact that most of the lower mammals experience heat at the height of estrus, and show little or no desire to copulate following ovariectomy.[21] Estrogen's ability to stimulate sexual behavior has been demonstrated in the rodent, cat, dog, sheep and monkey. While the desire to copulate in the lower mammal and subhuman primate is evinced during a limited period which coincides with the peak of the follicular phase of the cycle, there is no clearcut evidence that the periods of sexual desire in man are likewise circumscribed. The human female is apparently receptive to the male at almost any time. Whether this diffuse libido is an expression of hormonal impulse present throughout the cycle, or is purely dependent upon nervous factors, is not clear. Systematic investigations of the sexual urge in man are beset with difficulties, for the investigator must depend entirely on information volunteered by his patient. Unfortunately, such testimony is often distorted by conscious or unconscious misstatements, faulty memory, or undue prominence of certain experiences in the individual's consciousness. Her concept of sexual desire, and ability to distinguish true libido from related impulses, such as affection, will materially influence the value of such information. The intervention of exogenous aphrodisiacs may further confuse the picture.

Granting that sex desire is designed to insure union of the gametes, we should expect that in man, as in the lower mammal, libido would be at its height during the optimal time for conception, namely the period shortly before and after ovulation. From the results of studies carried out thus far, sex desire would appear to be increased several days before the calculated optimal time for ovulation (see Chap. IV), and also shortly before the flow. Davis,[22] who interviewed 2200 women by the questionnaire method, found that less than 20 per cent were conscious of regular periods of sex desire. The majority of these experienced a rise in libido shortly before, after and, in some cases, during the flow. In a group of women observed by Dickinson,[23] the peak of sex desire tended to precede the flow by six or seven days. These and other studies[24, 25] suggest that the sex urge in man shows wide individual variations with a tendency to rise during the premenstruum and following the flow.

The heightened sex desire experienced by some women during the premenstruum may be due to the large quantities of estrogen then present in the body fluids (see Chap. XL). On the other hand, it is conceivable that in man, as in the guinea pig,[26] this instinct depends on the luteal hormone, which reaches its highest concentration at this phase of the cycle. Tinkelpaugh[24] believes that the emotion experienced by some women during the premenstruum is not sex desire but a craving for affection created by the general depression and physical and nervous instability which characterizes this phase of the cycle. Moreover, it is possible that the prominent position which the menstrual flow holds in the individual's consciousness may lead her to fix evidence near or following this event.

It is evident, then, that proof of a periodic rise in sex desire in man and its dependence on estrogen in the body fluids is still lacking. Reports that estrogen therapy is effective in elevating or depressing the libido are not convincing because of the subjective nature of this manifestation and the prominence of nervous and psychic factors in its causation. The author has noted a striking increase in libido in both sexes following the injection of sterile saline solution, employed as a psychotherapeutic measure.

EFFECTS OF CHRONIC ESTROGEN STIMULATION

Protracted treatment with large doses of estrogen may induce abnormal changes in the accessory genitalia. The nature of these modifications apparently depends on the dosage, length of treatment and inherited predisposition of the test animal.

Hyperplasia of the Internal Genitalia.—The term "hyperplasia" describes an abnormal multiplication or increase in the number of normal cells, in normal arrangement, in a tissue. Varying degrees of benign hyperplasia of the accessory genitalia of castrate and intact mammals and man have been observed following estrogen treatment. The proliferation of the epithelial and connective tissue elements thus induced is particularly striking in the *uterine mucosa*. Typical cystic hyperplasia of the endometrium has been noted in the estrogen-treated mouse,[27] guinea pig,[28] rabbit,[29] monkey[30] and man.[31]

Hyperplasia of the myometrium and *cervix* have also been induced with estrogen. According to Wollner,[32] excessive estrogen stimulation may be an etiologic factor in endocervicitis and cervical erosion. Confirmatory evidence is still lacking. The *vaginal response* to nonphysiologic doses of this hormone varies considerably, depending on the length of treatment, and species of the test animal. In the rodent,[27] estrogen first elicits pronounced proliferation and cornification of the vaginal epithelium, so that the lumen becomes filled with desquamated cornified cells. If treatment is unduly prolonged, the vagina ceases to respond, gradually becomes thinner, and mitotic activity ceases. The cells of the basalis show extensive leucocytic infiltration and become vacuolated. Localized areas of degeneration appear and this sometimes eventuates in myxomatous changes of the vaginal connective tissue. In the monkey and human being,[33] protracted estrogen treatment causes proliferation and stratification of the vaginal epithelium.

There is a growing body of evidence that under certain conditions, estrogen may be a factor in the etiology of benign and malignant neoplasms of the accessory genitalia.

Fibromyomata.—Witherspoon[34] maintains that protracted estrogen stimulation plays a part in the etiology of uterine fibroids. As proof he offers the observation that such tumors rarely develop before puberty or after the menopause, undergo marked enlargement during gestation, when the organism is flooded with estrogen, tend to regress following extinction of ovarian function, and are frequently associated with endometrial hyperplasia. Experimental proof is provided by the observation[35, 36] that multiple tumors, resembling fibromyomata, can be produced in the guinea pig by administering large doses of estrogen over a protracted period of time. Since such tumors seldom form spontaneously in this species, their experimental production is especially significant.

Endometriomata.—There is evidence that endometriomata, which undergo the same cyclic modifications as the endometrium proper, regress after ovarian ablation. This would imply that their proliferative and secretory activity depends on the ovarian sex hormones. Whether these hormones also contribute to the formation of these growths, is not agreed. That chronic hyperestrinism may be an etiologic factor is suggested by the observation[37, 38, 39] that endometriomata are frequently associated with follicular cysts and endometrial hyperplasia, and themselves often present hyperplastic changes. Experimental support for this view is provided by the observation[29] that mice subjected to prolonged estrogen treatment may develop growths resembling endometriomata at one stage of the treatment. On the other hand, Payne's[40] observation that additional pelvic pathology was present in four-fifths of a group of cases with endometriosis, suggests that the latter condition, and the cystic follicles and endometrial hyperplasia which often accompany it, are independent manifestations of a common cause.

Granting that chronic hyperestrinism contributes to the formation of fibromyomata and endometriomata, it must be emphasized that the tissues' inherent susceptibility to tumor formation is of considerable importance. It is noteworthy that the response of the accessory genitalia to a given dose of estrogen varies widely not only as between one strain and another of the same species, but also between different members of the same strain, and different areas of the same organ.

Estrogen and Cancer.—*Experimental Evidence.*—In some mammals, persistent estrogen treatment produces atypical or so-called "precancerous" lesions of the accessory genitalia. Genital lesions, histologically suggesting malignancy, have only occasionally been demonstrated in the estrogen treated animal. McEuen[41] observed a carcinoma surrounding a perirenal abscess in a female rat, following the vaginal application of estrone for 698 days. A cervical lesion, diagnosed as carcinoma, was noted by Overholser and Allen[42] in a castrate rhesus monkey given 2000 I. U. of estrogen over a period of 51 days. Especially significant is the report of Gardner and coworkers[43] that cervical neoplasms, histologically diagnosed as carcinoma, appeared in 20 mice following prolonged stimulation with huge doses of estrogen. In one instance a total of 1050 gamma of estradiol benzoate was given over a period of 319 days. When pieces of the tumor tissue were transplanted to male or female mice, they continued to grow despite the fact that the hosts received no estrogen, thus substantiating the histological diagnosis of carcinoma. Since no case of spontaneous cervical carcinoma has thus far been encountered in this species, a causal relationship between the protracted estrogen treatment and the malignant neoplasms can hardly be doubted. In contrast to these positive findings, several workers have reported a complete absence of malignant changes in the accessory genitalia of their test animals despite the use of larger doses and more prolonged treatment. Smith and Engle[44] observed metaplasia without evidence of cancer in 7 monkeys, following treatment with a total of 33,000 to 95,000 I. U. of estrogen over a period of 60 to 170 days. Zuckerman's[45] monkeys showed no evidence of genital carcinoma even after a total of 265,000 I. U. of estrone in the course of 565 days.

Clinical Evidence.—The available evidence relating to the role of estrogen in the etiology of human cancer is limited and inconclusive. In three women given as high as 6,000,000 I. U. of estradiol benzoate over periods up to one year, Zondek[31] found cervical erosions but no evidence of malignant change. Geist and his associates[33] could detect no evidence of pathologic change in the genitalia of a group of women receiving doses up to 53,400,000 I. U. over periods ranging from 6 months to five and one-half years. On the other hand, Dockerty[46] noted endometrial carcinoma in three out of thirty-two women harboring granulosa cell tumors, which are known to be associated with a high estrogen concentration of the body fluids. Gemmell and Jeffcoate[47] found cervical carcinoma in three out of forty-three women given estrogen for the relief of kraurosis vulva or senile vaginitis. Allaben and Owen[48] have reported a case in which breast cancer developed following estrogen therapy. Auchincloss and Haagensen[49] have described a case, with a family history of cancer, particularly of the breast, in which mammary cancer developed after the administration of 79.067 mg. of estradiol benzoate over a period of two years and three months. Of interest is the observation[50] that the incidence of mammary cancer is higher in women with a late menopause, and conversely[51] that bilateral oophorectomy apparently exerts a protective influence against mammary carcinoma.

Though the available evidence indicates that genital cancer may sometimes result from protracted stimulation by nonphysiologic quantities of estrogen, the fact that such treatment has no apparent carcinogenic action in some subjects, suggests that the reactivity of the tissues plays an important part in determining whether or not malignant lesions will result

Recognition of this interplay between the estrogens and certain unidentified endogenous factors which predispose to malignancy is of the utmost clinical importance. This should be borne in mind when contemplating the use of estrogen for the treatment of menstrual disturbances or the symptomatic menopause. It has been argued that estrogen, in the doses and for the length of time it is generally used clinically, is unlikely to do harm, particularly in view of evidence that much of the hormone is inactivated or excreted shortly after entering the body. Since the response to treatment in a given case is unpredictable, because of wide individual variations in cancer susceptibility, such therapy should be instituted with full consciousness of the danger that it may encourage a latent, unrecognized genital or mammary neoplasm. This is especially important when the patient is at the cancer age, has a family history of genital or mammary cancer, or harbors cervical erosions, polyps or other genital lesions which might conceivably provide a fertile soil for cancer.

Relation of Naturally Occurring Estrogens to the Carcinogenic Hydrocarbons.—Considerable interest has been aroused by recent studies suggesting a close chemical and biological relationship between the naturally occurring estrogens and certain organic compounds, the so-called "carcinogens." The latter produce cancerous lesions when repeatedly applied to the skin or injected subcutaneously, and in addition possess varying degrees of estrogenic activity. The molecular structure of the naturally occurring estrogens, and such carcinogenic hydrocarbons as $1:2:5:6$, dibenzanthracene, $1:2$ benzpyrene and $5:6$ cyclopenteno–$1:2$ benzanthracene show only minor differences in the character of their polar groups, sidechains and degree of aromatization. All are saturated hydrocarbons possessing the phenanthrene nucleus. It is significant that synthetic estrogenic compounds have been obtained from the carcinogens, and both estrogens and carcinogens have been prepared from the sterols. Also noteworthy is the finding of appreciable quantities of sterols and estrogens in tumor tissue. It has been suggested that the carcinogens may be formed within the organism as a result of disturbances in the metabolism of the sex hormones or bile salts.

Though it might be supposed from the foregoing observations that there is a direct connection between the carcinogenic activity of the natural estrogens and carcinogenic hydrocarbons, there is reason to believe that the relationship is actually indirect. Though alike in certain respects, there are several important differences between them which make it unlikely that the same chemical group is responsible for their carcinogenic activity. The *similarities and dissimilarities* may be summarized as follows:

1. Both the natural estrogens and carcinogenic hydrocarbons operate as stimulants to growth, and the cancerous change which they induce depends on proliferative processes persisting over a considerable fraction of the test animal's life span. With both, hyperplasia and cellular proliferation precede the appearance of cancer.

2. The carcinogenic hydrocarbons can produce cancer in any epithelial tissue to which they are directly applied, and also in remote organs and tissues. The estrogens, on the other hand, do not produce cancer of the

skin when locally applied. They can induce cancerous changes only in the accessory genitalia and breasts, which normally possess a specific physiological sensitiveness to them. This is due to the fact that the estrogens are strictly stimulants of sexual tissues.

3. The carcinogens regularly produce malignant lesions, provided that the dose is adequate and the treatment sufficiently prolonged. The ability of the estrogens to induce cancer depends not only on the dosage and length of treatment, but even more on the tissue's inherent predisposition to malignancy.

4. Though the estrogens and carcinogenic hydrocarbons are chemically closely related, the chemical groups responsible for these types of activity are not the same. As Loeb[52] states, there are substances with estrogenic but no carcinogenic properties, others with carcinogenic but no estrogenic activity, and some possessing both types of activity. The fact that either type of activity may exist independently of the other and that, even where both are present, the strength of the two activities shows no parallelism, suggests that a different chemical group is responsible for each.

It would thus appear, to use the words of Loeb, "that estrin causes cancer formation in certain tissues because it acts as a specific and very potent growth stimulus on these tissues, and that its chemical relationship to some carcinogenic hydrocarbons is not the essential factor in this respect. It is probable that specific growth stimuli, acting over a long period of time, ultimately change the cell equilibrium in such a way that certain substances inducing cell proliferation are propagated in an autocatalytic manner. The essential factor in the cancerous formation is the action of growth stimuli in cooperation with hereditary and constitutional factors."[53]

Effect of Estrogen on the Ovary

Though estrogenic substances, given continuously over a protracted period of time, tend to suppress gonadal function indirectly through their effect on the anterior pituitary gland (see Chap. XII), recent studies indicate that under certain circumstances appropriate doses exert a direct stimulating effect on the ovary. That estrogen plays a part in the formation and function of the *corpus luteum* was first suggested by Westman's[54] observation that destruction of the follicles by cauterization interferes with corpus luteum formation in the rabbit. More recent studies in this species have shown that estrogen prolongs the life span of the corpus luteum of pregnancy and pseudopregnancy[55, 56] and prevents the rapid involution which would otherwise follow ablation of the adenohypophysis[57] or extirpation of the pregnant uterus with its contents.[58] In hypophysectomized mice, estrogen failed to sustain the function of the corpora lutea, according to Allen.[59] Williams[60] found the ovarian weight appreciably greater in hypophysectomized rats bearing implants of crystalline estrogen than in hypophysectomized controls. There is some evidence[61, 62] that this substance augments existing luteal function in the human subject.

A synergism between estrogen and the *gonadotropes* is evident in the observation of Pencharz[63] that a combination of stilbestrol (see Chap. XLI) and chorionic gonadotropin (see Chap. XII) caused a marked augmentation of ovarian weight and the formation of large follicles and corpora lutea, in the hypophysectomized rodent. Simpson and associates[64] found that stilbestrol alone, in the hypophysectomized animal, caused growth of many follicles, which did not develop antra though they were increased in size. When chorionic gonadotropin, which alone caused only a slight increase in ovarian weight due to interstitial cell hypertrophy, was supplemented by stilbestrol, the gonads were much larger than could be expected on the basis of a mere additive effect. This increase was due to the development of large follicles, thecal luteinized follicles, corpora lutea, and hypertrophy of interstitial tissue.

These observations suggest that a local effect of estrogen is an essential link in the chain of effects through which the anterior pituitary gland brings about normal cyclic ovarian activity. Attempts to stimulate the hypofunctioning human ovary by combined estrogen and gonadotropin therapy have thus far yielded inconstant results.[65] It would seem wise to refrain from the indiscriminate use of such combined therapy until more is known of the quantitative and temporal relationships involved, since estrogen, under certain circumstances, may adversely affect ovarian function.

EFFECT OF ESTROGEN IN THE MALE

The sex specificity of the natural estrogens has been questioned on the ground that they also occur in the male organism. The significance of their presence here is not certain. Whether they are essential for normal sexual development and function, or are merely by-products or intermediate compounds produced by the testicle and adrenal cortex, is not established.

Effect on the Testis.—The effect of the estrogens on the male gonad is inhibitory. In the immature rat, adequate doses prevent testicular growth and descent into the scrotum. The effect is temporary, recovery being complete within a short time after injections are stopped.[66, 67] In the mature rodent, similar treatment causes atrophy of the seminiferous tubules, interferes with spermatogenesis, and if sufficiently intensive and prolonged leads to atrophy of the interstitial cells. Degenerative changes have also been observed in the human testis following estrogen therapy.[68] Whether these substances directly inhibit testicular function, or act by suppressing the anterior pituitary, is uncertain. The latter possibility was first suggested by Moore and Price[69] on the basis of their observation that the testicular atrophy which follows prolonged estrogen treatment can be prevented by simultaneously administering a potent gonadotropic extract. On the other hand, Korenchevsky and his associates[70] question this interpretation on the ground that the pituitaries of male rats, in which testicular atrophy has been induced with estrogen, present gross modifications indicative of activation rather than suppression.

Effects on Accessory Genitalia.—The response of the male accessory genitalia to estrogen varies according to the tissues involved. Intensive and prolonged estrogen administration in the rodent causes pronounced hyperplasia of the fibromuscular tissue of the seminal vesicles and prostate, a response sometimes referred to as the "paradoxical phenomenon."[71] In some species, particularly the mouse,[72] dog, ground squirrel and monkey, protracted estrogen treatment causes metaplasia of the epithelium of the prostatic utricle, colliculus seminalis, and of the bulbous and cavernous portion of the urethra. Other modifications described in the estrogen treated male animal, include a myxomatous change in the connective tissue of the ampullary portion of the vas deferens, metaplasia of the bulbo-urethral and stromal elements of the hydatids of Morgagni, scrotal hernia, and retention of urine with dilatation of the bladder. A feminizing and hermaphrodizing effect has been recorded in the rat and rabbit.[73] Following persistent estrogen stimulation in the male rabbit, the penis becomes softened and eventually disappears, so that the whole genital area resembles the female pudenda with its clitoris and common urogenital vestibulum. It would thus appear that estrogen affects the persistent müllerian contributions to the male genital tract, and derivatives of the urogenital sinus. As David[74] points out, it apparently promotes growth of smooth muscle tissue and interstitium, and of the submucosal and undifferentiated cylindrical epithelium in non-tubular organs.

Estrogen and the male sex hormone are apparently both synergistic and antagonistic in their effect on the male accessory genital organs. When given simultaneously in moderate doses, they act synergistically on both the smooth muscle and epithelium of the seminal vesicles. Freud[71] believes that estrogen increases the activity of the male sex hormone, causing harmonious development of the substratum and wolffian duct epithelium. He suggests that estrogen's role in the male organism is to prepare the musculature and connective tissue of the wolffian duct for the activity of the male sex hormone.

Large doses and more protracted estrogen administration suppresses the secretory activity of the seminal vesicle epithelium, which is normally dependent on the testicular hormone. The latter in turn is capable of checking the effect of excessive estrogen on the fibromuscular tissue and epithelium of the seminal vesicle and prostate. This is implied in the observation[75] that estrogen produces hyperplasia of the connective tissue and smooth muscle, and metaplasia of the epithelium of these structures more readily in the castrate than in the intact animal. If testicular hormone is administered together with estrogen, it partly or completely prevents these changes.

CELLS OF THE OVARY SECRETING ESTROGEN

Granulosa versus Theca Cells.—Though it is generally agreed that the maturing follicle secretes estrogen, the fact that this structure is composed of both granulosa and theca cells has made for much controversy as to which of the two is the site of estrogen production. According to some observers,[54] the granulosa cells, which stem from epithelial structures, secrete the estrogenic hormone, while the theca cells, which are of connective tissue origin and are derived from the cells of the stroma, constitute at best only a storage depot for this hormone. Others[76] maintain that estrogen secretion is a function of the theca and a few go so far as to state that the theca cells secrete estrogen not only when they form part of the maturing follicle, but also when they occur independently in the form of disorganized masses, the so-called "interstitial tissue."

Experimental Evidence.—To determine what part the granulosa and theca cells play in the production of estrogen, attempts have been made to destroy by cauterization certain constituents of the ovary, while leaving others intact. The evidence thus obtained is not very reliable, because of the technical difficulties involved. Some have tried to solve this problem by comparing the estrogen content of the granulosa and theca cells, as determined by bioassay, but this method of study is likewise unsatisfactory because of the possibility that the hormones may seep through from the cells which secrete them to adjacent cells which merely store them. For this reason, the presence of estrogen in a tissue is not conclusive proof that it is produced there. On the other hand, valuable information has been obtained by observing the cytology of the granulosa and theca cells of the developing follicle. Studies of the ovarian response to gonadotropic extracts, or to sub-castration doses of x-ray, and observations in patients bearing granulosa and theca cell tumors have also yielded significant clues.

Allen and coworkers[77] were unable to demonstrate estrogen in cortical stroma free of visible follicles, though they obtained as much as 5 rat units per gram from the walls of large follicles composed mainly of granulosa cells. They concluded that the latter are the probable site of estrogen production. On the other hand, Zondek and Aschheim[78] could detect no estrogen in granulosa cells scraped from the wall of large follicles, but obtained a positive Allen-Doisy response with the theca cells.

Participation of the granulosa cells in estrogen production has been questioned by Mossman,[79] on the basis of his observations in the pocket gopher. He points out that the granulosa cell layer is essentially a serous epithelium and is not cytologically like that of a gland of internal secretion. Moreover, it lacks the rich vascular supply and histological arrangement of a true endocrine gland. Mossman considers it unlikely that the granulosa cells produce estrogen up to the time of rupture, and then secrete a second hormone, progesterone, when, as part of the corpus luteum, they assume the characteristics of an endocrine gland. He points out that in contrast to the "obviously non-glandular epithelium," the theca layer of the maturing follicle possesses the cytologic characters, as well as the rich blood supply of a true incretory gland. Significantly, the height of theca cell activity exactly coincides with the height of estrus in the pocket gopher. He concludes that the theca cells are the source of estrogen.

There is some evidence to support the contention that the *theca cells* are capable of secreting estrogen even when they occur in disorganized masses, in which no ovum or granulosa is distinguishable. Such collections of theca cells were first noted in the lower mammal by Bouin and Ancel,[80] and Limon.[81] They are indistinguishable from the hypertrophied, epithelioid, lipoid-laden theca-lutein cells of the graafian follicle and have, therefore, been termed "theca-lutein," "stroma-lutein," or "lutein" cells. When present in large collections, they are spoken of as "interstitial cell masses" or *interstitial tissue*. Some observers apply the term "interstitial gland" to all epithelioid and sudanophile cells of the theca interna and stroma. Others apply this term only to that tissue which is derived by hypertrophy from the theca interna cells. Mossman[79] maintains that "interstitial tissue" stems from the theca interna of atretic and ruptured follicles. According to Seiferle,[82] the female "interstitial gland" embodies no fixed cells, but is rather a variegated group consisting as a rule of more or less lipoid-rich connective tissue cells of epithelioid, fibrocytic or histocytic character. These cells, he believes, represent various reaction-forms and work-forms of the stroma spindle cells. In their classic epithelioid form, they appear only in the theca interna of the large graafian follicle and developing corpus luteum. They may form the parenchyma of corpora atretica, but are only rarely present in the cortical stroma.

Interstitial cells occur in varying amounts in different species. In the horse, for example, they appear only during fetal life, in the rodent only during adult life, and in the cat during fetal and postnatal life. In man, their number shows wide individual variations. According to Wallart,[83] they are well developed at birth, gradually increase up to puberty, and may persist in some instances as late as the third decade of life. Freimann,[84] on the other hand, found that such cells appear only during childhood and even then are not a constant finding. Seitz[85] has called attention to the presence of large numbers of "interstitial" cells during pregnancy, while Meyer[86] and others have found them in abundance in hydatid mole and chorionepithelioma. Aschner[87] could demonstrate such tissue in multiparae but not nulliparae.

Though a secretory function has long been ascribed to these cells, some support for this assumption has only recently been provided. Zondek[88] found appreciable amounts of estrogen in the cortex of the ovary during pregnancy, when it is rich in theca-lutein cells, but not in the nonpregnant state, when such cells are scant or absent. He could also demonstrate estrogen in the fluid and wall of ovarian cysts composed entirely of theca lutein cells, but not in ordinary ovarian cysts.

Significant in this connection is the observation that rodent ovaries, which are completely or almost completely devoid of granulosa cells but contain hypertrophied, lipoid-rich theca cells, secrete estrogen. Such modifications have been experimentally produced by exposing the ovaries to subminimal doses of x-ray,[102] or by administering chorionic gonadotropin before the eighteenth day of life, when it evokes luteinization of the theca but does not cause maturation of the granulosa cells (see Chap. XII). The use of x-rays in the mouse has been reported by Parkes and coworkers,[89] who found that follicles become atretic and are destroyed without undergoing complete degeneration. The large mature follicles survive and may eventually ovulate, while the smaller ones become entirely disorganized and fragmented so that the ovaries ultimately consist of a more or less uniform tissue apparently derived from the interfollicular cells. The ovaries of both immature and mature animals so treated apparently retained their endocrine function, as shown by the appearance of cornification in the vaginal epithelium. Parkes concluded that the graafian follicle is not indispensable for the secretion of the estrus inducing hormone. In a subsequent study in the guinea pig, Genther[90] found that animals subjected to castration doses of x-ray showed follicular development without ovulation or corpus luteum formation. The ovaries degenerated to form "interstitial gland" tissue, which apparently remained in a healthy condition. Vaginal smears showed a state of continuous estrus, and assays of the urine revealed the presence of 1 rat unit of estrogen in a three day specimen. Noting that the number of developing follicles present was not sufficient to account for the amount of estrogen present, Genther concluded that it is at least partly derived from the "glandular" tissue.

Commenting on Parkes' findings and conclusions, Moricard,[91] on the basis of a cytologic study of the developing follicle, maintains that the follicular fluid is produced apart from the estrogen it contains, which is elaborated in part at least by the theca interna. The estrogen present in the circulating blood before the occurrence of follicular rupture is derived from the theca interna, which, unlike the granulosa, is in intimate contact with the capillaries. X-ray irradiation, he believes, suppresses secretion of follicular fluid but not the elaboration of estrogen. This, Moricard believes, accounts for the continuance of cyclic changes of the accessory genitalia despite failure of follicular maturation.

Selye and his coworkers[92] first demonstrated that the ovaries of rats under eighteen days of age respond to pregnancy urine gonadotropin with thecal luteinization. The granulosa is apparently unresponsive to the chorionic hormone at this time, and with continued treatment the ovaries become filled with masses of theca lutein cells in which no ova or functioning granulosa cells are distinguishable. That such ovaries secrete estrogen is indicated by the appearance of persistent estrus changes in the vaginal epithelium.

Recent studies with fractionated anterior pituitary extracts have provided additional evidence suggesting that the theca cells play an important and perhaps the primary role in estrogen production. Greep and his associates[93] found that in immature, hypophysectomized rats receiving follicle-stimulating extract ("thelykentrin"), the interstitial cells underwent complete atrophy. Though the ovaries contained maturing follicles, many with large antra, healthy looking granulosa cells, and normal ova, no estrogen was secreted, as shown by the state of the uterus and vagina. When the follicle stimulating extract was supplemented by the interstitial cell stimulating fraction (luteinizer, "metakentrin"), the interstitial cells were repaired and hypertrophied, and large amounts of estrogen were secreted, as shown by the associated changes in the accessory genitalia.

On the basis of the evidence at hand, it would appear that epithelioid cells of connective tissue origin, whether they exist independently, or are part of the organized follicle, are capable of secreting an estrogenic substance. Those who favor the granulosa cells as the primary site of estrogen production under normal conditions, argue that their view is not necessarily invalidated by proof that other ovarian tissues are also able to assume this function under certain circumstances.[94] Thus far, the most convincing evidence pointing to the granulosa cells as the primary source of estrogen has been provided by the recent study of Traut and Marchetti.[95] Among a group of fifty-four patients with granulosa and theca cell tumors, they found four "pure" theca cell tumors and one "pure" granulosa cell neoplasm. Clinical evidence pointing to estrogen production appeared in none of the cases with a pure theca cell tumor, but was encountered in the single instance with a pure granulosa cell tumor. In the remaining cases with tumors containing both granulosa and theca cells, they observed that the higher the proportion of theca cells, the less the likelihood of encountering clinical manifestations of estrogenic activity.

SECRETION OF ANDROGEN BY THE OVARY

It is now well established that the female excretes androgenic substances in amounts approaching those found in the male (see Chap. XL). That these are largely if not solely of adrenal cortical origin is suggested by their absence in women with Addison's disease,[96] and their continued appearance despite bilateral ovariectomy.[97] These observations suggest that under normal conditions, the ovary produces little or no androgenic hormone. That it may acquire this function under certain circumstances is indicated by clinical and experimental evidence. Masculinization is a characteristic manifestation of arrhenoblastomata, and may occasionally accompany granulosa or theca cell tumors (see Chap. XXXV). In the very young, or the mature suckling rodent, equine or chorionic gonadotropin causes thecal luteinization associated with evidence of masculinization.[98, 99, 100] In Genther's[90] mature female guinea pigs, following subcastration doses of x-ray to the ovaries, the formation of "interstitial gland tissue" was associated in some cases with psychic and physical evidence of masculinization. Hill[101] observed that ovarian implants in the ears of castrate male mice secreted androgenic substances, as shown by the condition of the accessory genitalia of the hosts.

In view of the close chemical relationship existing between the ovarian and testicular hormones, it is not surprising that perversion of ovarian function, as seen in certain ovarian neoplasms or as is the case with ear transplants, may result in the production of substances possessing androgenic activity. While it would appear that the ovary may produce androgens under certain conditions, the available evidence does not warrant the conclusion that androgen production is a normal function of the female gonad.

BIBLIOGRAPHY

1. Stockard, C. R., and Papanicolaou, G. N.: Am. J. Anat. 22:225, 1917.
2. Long, J. A., and Evans, H. M.: Mem. Univ. California 6:1, 1922.
3. Allen, E.: Am. J. Anat. 30:297, 1922.
4. Doisy, E. A., Veler, E. D., and Thayer, S.: Am. J. Physiol. 90:329, 1929.
5. Butenandt, A.: Deut. med. Wchnschr. 55:2177, 1929.
6. Corner, G. W., and Allen, W. M.: Am. J. Physiol. 88:326, 1929.
7. Hitschmann, F., and Adler, L.: Monatschr. f. Geb. u. Gynäk. 27:1, 1908.
8. Schröder, R.: Monatsch. f. Geburtsh. u. Gynäk. 39:3, 1914.
9. Meyer, R.: Arch. f. Gynäk. 93:354, 1911.
10. Dodds, E. C.: Lancet 1:931, 987, 1048, 1934.
11. Clauberg, C.: Zentralbl. f. Gynäk. 57:1991, 1933.
12. Allen, E., Smith, G. M., and Gardner, W. U.: Am. J. Anat. 61:321, 1937.
13. Seckinger, D. L., and Snyder, F. F.: Bull. Johns Hopkins Hosp. 39:371, 1926.
14. Manzi, L.: Arch. di ostet. e ginec. 17:253, 1930.
15. Wimpfheimer, S., and Feresten, M.: Endocrinol. 25:91, 1939.
16. Whitney, R., and Burdick, H. O.: Endocrinol. 20:643, 1936.

4

17. Burdick, H. O., and Whitney, R.: Endocrinol. *21*:637, 1937.
18. Geist, S. H., Salmon, U. J., and Mintz, M.: Am. J. Obst. & Gynec. *36*:67, 1938.
19. Bernstein, P., and Feresten, M.: Endocrinol. *26*:946, 1940.
20. Bachman, C., Collip, J. B., and Selye, H.: Proc. Roy. Soc., London s.B. *117*:16, 1935.
21. Hemmingsen, A. M.: Scandinav. Arch. f. Physiol. *65*:97, 1933.
22. Davis, K. B.: Factors in the Sexual Life of 2200 Women, New York, Harper & Brothers, 1929.
23. Dickinson, R. L.: Am. J. Obst. & Gynec. *14*:718, 1927.
24. Tinklepaugh, O. L.: Am. J. Obst. & Gynec. *26*:335, 1933.
25. Billings, E. G.: Bull. Johns Hopkins Hosp., *54*:440, 1934.
26. Young, W. C., Dempsey, E. W., Myers, H. I., and Hagquist, C. W.: Am J. Anat. *63*: 457, 1938.
27. Gardner, W. U., Allen, E., and Strong, L. C.: Anat. Rec. *64* (Supp.):17, 1936.
28. Nelson, W. O.: Anat. Rec. *68*:99, 1937.
29. Lacassagne, A.: Compt. rend. Soc. de biol. *120*:1156, 1935.
30. Zuckerman, S.: J. Obst. & Gynec. Brit. Emp. *44*:494, 1937.
31. Zondek, B.: J.A.M.A. *114*:1850, 1940.
32. Wollner, A.: Am. J. Obst. & Gynec. *37*:947, 1939.
33. Geist, S. H., and Salmon, U. J.: Am. J. Obst. & Gynec. *41*:29, 1941; ibid. *42*:242, 1941.
34. Witherspoon, J. T.: Am. J. Cancer *24*:402, 1935.
35. Marx, R., Glass, S. J., and Shulman, A.: Am. J. Obst. & Gynec. *44*:259, 1942.
36. Lipschutz, A.: J.A.M.A. *120*:171, 1942.
37. Jeffcoate, T. N. A., and Potter, A. L.: J. Obst. & Gynec. Brit. Emp. *41*:684, 1935.
38. Witherspoon, J. T.: Arch. Path. *20*:22, 1935.
39. Frank, I. L., and Geist, S. H.: Am. J. Obst. & Gynec. *44*:652, 1942.
40. Payne, F. L.: Am. J. Obst. & Gynec. *39*:373, 1940.
41. McEuen, C. S., Selye, H., and Collip, J. B.: Lancet *1*:775, 1936.
42. Overholser, M. D., and Allen, E.: Surg., Gynec. & Obst. *60*:129, 1935.
43. Gardner, W. U., Allen, E., Smith, G. M., and Strong, L. C.: J.A.M.A. *110*:1182, 1938.
44. Engle, E. T., and Smith, P. E.: Anat. Rec. *61*:471, 1935.
45. Zuckerman, S.: Lancet *1*:435, 1937.
46. Dockerty, M. B.: Am. J. Obst. & Gynec. *37*:425, 1939.
47. Gemmell, A. A., and Jeffcoate, T. N. A.: J. Obst. & Gynec. Brit. Emp. *46*:985, 1939.
48. Allaben, G. R., and Owens, E.: J.A.M.A. *114*:1517, 1940.
49. Auchincloss, H., and Haagenson, C. D.: J.A.M.A. *114*:1517, 1940.
50. Heiberg, B., and Heiberg, P.: Acta Chir. Scandinav. *83*:479, 1940.
51. Herrell, W. E.: Am. J. Cancer *29*:659, 1937.
52. Loeb, L.: Estrogenic Hormones and Carcinogenesis, in, Glandular Physiology and Therapy, Chicago, American Medical Association, 1935, Chap. 13, pp. 177–192.
53. Loeb, L., Burns, E. L., Suntseff, V., and Moskop, M.: Am. J. Cancer *30*:47, 1937.
54. Westman, A.: Arch. f. Gynäk. *158*:476, 1934.
55. Westman, A., and Jacobsohn, D.: Acta Obst. & Gynec. Scandinav. *17*:1, 13, 235, 1937.
56. Heckel, G. P., and Allen, W. M.: Endocrinol. *24*:137, 1939.
57. Robson, J. M.: J. Physiol. *90*:435, 1940.
58. Greep, R. O.: Anat. Rec. *76* (Supp.):25, 1940.
59. Allen, E.: Anat. Rec. *79* (Supp.):2, 1941.
60. Williams, P. C.: Nature, London *145*:388, 1940.
61. Browne, J. S. L., and Venning, E. H.: Am. J. Physiol. *123*:26, 1938.
62. Hamblen, E. C.: Endocrine Gynecology, Springfield, Ill., Chas. C. Thomas, 1939.
63. Pencharz, R. I.: Science *91*:554, 1940.
64. Simpson, M. E., Evans, H. M., Fraenkel-Conrat, H. L., and Li, C. H.: Endocrinol. *28*:37, 1941.
65. Geist, S. H., Gaines, J. A., and Salmon, U. J.: Am. J. Obst. & Gynec. *42*:619, 1941.
66. Golding, G. T., and Ramirez, F. T.: Endocrinol. *12*:804, 1928.
67. Lipschutz, A.: Quart. J. Exper. Physiol. *25*:109, 1935.
68. Heckel, N. J.: Tr. Am. A. Genito-Urin. Surgeons *34*:237, 1941.
69. Moore, C. R., and Price, D.: Am. J. Anat. *50*:13, 1932.

70. Korenchevsky, V., and Dennison, M.: Biochem. J. *28*:1474, 1486, 1934.
71. Freud, J., deJongh, S. E., and Laqueur, E.: Nederl. tydschr. u. geneesk. *77*:1109, 1933.
72. Lisco, H., and Biskind, G. R.: Endocrinol. *29*:772, 1941.
73. Kun, H.: Endokrinol. *13*:311, 1934.
74. David, K., Freud, J., and deJongh, S. E.: Biochem. J., *28*:1360, 1934.
75. Waterman, L.: Acta brev. Neerland. *6*:56, 1936.
76. Geller, F. C.: Arch. f. Gynäk. *139*:530, 1930.
77. Allen, E., Doisy, E. A., Francis, B. F., Gibson, H. V.: Robertson, L. L., Colgate, C. E., Kountz, W. B., and Johnston, C. G.: Am. J. Anat. *34*:133, 1924.
78. Zondek, B., and Aschheim, S.: Klin. Wchnschr. *6*:248, 1927.
79. Mossman, H. W.: Am. J. Anat. *61*:289, 1937.
80. Bouin, P., and Ancel, P.: Compt. rend. Soc. de biol. *67*:466, 1909.
81. Limon: Arch. Anat. Microsc., 1902.
82. Seiferle, E.: Ztschr. f. Zellforsch. u. mikr. Anat. *25*:421, 1936.
83. Wallart, J.: Arch. f. Gynäk. *81*:271, 1907; Ztschr. f. Geburtsh. u. Gynäk. *63*:520, 1908.
84. Freimann, S. C.: Monatschr. f. Geburtsh. u. Gynäk. *104*:224, 1937.
85. Seitz, L.: Arch. f. Gynäk. *77*:203, 1905.
86. Meyer, R.: Verhandl. d. deut. path. Gesellsch. *16*:398, 1913.
87. Aschner, B.: Ztschr. f. Geburtsh. u. Gynäk. *76*:304, 1914.
88. Zondek, B.: Die Hormone des Ovariums und des Hypophysenvorderlappens, Berlin, J. Springer, 1931.
89. Brambell, F. W. R., and Parkes, A. S.: Proc. Roy. Soc. London s.B. *101*:316, 1927.
90. Genther, I.: Am. J. Anat. *55*:1, 1934.
91. Moricard, R.: Progrès méd. *40*:1538, 1934.
92. Selye, H., Collip, J. B., and Thomson, D. L.: Proc. Soc. Exper. Biol. & Med. *30*:780, 1933.
93. Greep, R. O., Van Dyke, H. B., and Chow, B. F.: Endocrinol. *30*:627, 1942.
94. Allen, E.: J.A.M.A. *116*:405, 1941.
95. Traut, H. F., and Marchetti, A. A.: Surg., Gynec. & Obst. *70*:494, 1933.
96. Fraser, R. W., and Smith, P. H.: Quart. J. Med. *10*:297, 1941.
97. Hamblen, E. C., Cuyler, W. K., Wilson, J. A., and Pullen, R. L.: J. Clin. Endocrinol. *1*:777, 1941.
98. Rutishener, E.: Deut. Arch. f. Klin. Med. *175*:640, 1933.
99. Selye, H., and Collip, J. B.: Proc. Soc. Exper. Biol. & Med. *30*:647, 1933.
100. Pfeiffer, C. A.: Anat. Rec. *77* (Supp.):59, 1941.
101. Hill, R. T.: Endocrinol. *21*:495, 1937.
102. Geist, S. H., Gaines, J. A., and Escher, G. C.: Endocrinol. *29*:59, 194`

CHAPTER III

ENDOCRINE ROLE OF THE OVARY: THE CORPUS LUTEUM

INTRODUCTION

While the existence of the corpus luteum in both the pregnant and nonpregnant woman has long been recognized, its functions have only recently been established. At the close of the last century, Beard[1] suggested that this structure may be concerned with nidation. He interpreted menstruation as an "abortion" precipitated by degeneration of the yellow body, just as parturition is caused by retrogression of the corpus luteum of pregnancy. In the following year, Prenant[2] and Born,[3] working independently, pointed out that the yellow body possesses the histologic characteristics of an endocrine gland. Fraenkel,[4] in 1903, demonstrated that ablation of the corpus luteum of pregnancy in the rabbit invariably leads to resorption or abortion of the fetuses, depending on whether operation is performed early or late in gestation. This observation, together with the important studies subsequently carried out by Loeb,[5] Bouin and Ancel,[3] Fellner,[7] and Herrmann,[8] made it increasingly evident that the corpus luteum is an endocrine organ vitally concerned with the reproductive processes.

For a time, it was thought that the yellow body performs the major functions of the ovary. After 1923, when estrogen, the active principle of the follicle, was isolated, some suggested that this hormone may be responsible for all the sexual phenomena attributed to the ovary. Their assumption that the follicle and corpus luteum produce their effects through the same hormone was further strengthened when estrogenic activity was demonstrated in luteal extracts. This confusion was dispelled in 1929, when progestin, the specific hormone of the corpus luteum was isolated in relatively pure form. The preparation of progesterone, crystalline form of the luteal hormone, in 1934, enabled investigators to study its effects unobscured by estrogen, which contaminated the earlier luteal extracts.

BIOLOGY OF PROGESTERONE

Inhibition of Ovulation.—Beard[1] and Prenant[2] first suggested that the corpus luteum may inhibit ovulation. Tandler,[9] in 1910, called attention to the fact that persistence of the yellow body in cattle retards ovulation and renders them temporarily sterile. Experimental proof was provided by Loeb,[10] who demonstrated that corpus luteum ablation in the nonpregnant guinea pig accelerates the appearance of the succeeding estrus phase. Hammond[11] noted a similar effect in the nonpregnant cow after squeezing out the corpus luteum. Loeb,[12] working with the guinea pig, and Drummond-Robinson and Asdell,[13] who studied the goat, found that corpus luteum ablation during pregnancy is soon followed by ovulation, regardless of whether the fetuses are expelled immediately or retained temporarily.

The corpus luteum apparently inhibits ovulation in man, for its removal during the menstrual cycle causes the premature appearance of the flow.[14] Since the next menstrual period after the induced flow occurs at the normal interval, as calculated from the date of the induced bleeding, it may be assumed that a new ovarian cycle is initiated on removal of the yellow body.

There is ample evidence that the premature occurrence of ovulation following corpus luteum ablation is due to withdrawal of its active principle, progestin. Papanicolaou,[15] in 1926, inhibited ovulation in the guinea pig with an extract of corpus luteum tissue. A similar effect has since been obtained in the rat[16] and mouse.[17] Mahnert[18] and later Fels[19] found their luteal extracts effective in preventing the follicular rupture which would otherwise follow coitus in the rabbit. Studies[20, 21, 22] with progesterone have confirmed the earlier experiments. Selye,[20] and Phillips[21] inhibited estrus and produced ovarian atrophy in the mature rat by administering 4 mg. of progesterone daily.

Action on Hypophysis.—The available evidence indicates that progestin inhibits ovulation indirectly by suppressing the hypophyseal sex principles, and not through any direct effect on the follicle. Makepeace and associates[22] found that the pseudopregnant rabbit responds with follicular rupture to a dose of gonadotropic hormone equivalent to that present in the hypophysis at the tenth and fifteenth day of pseudopregnancy. They concluded that ovulation does not follow coitus during pseudopregnancy because the yellow body prevents discharge of luteinizer by the hypophysis. Their observation[22] that progestin does not interfere with the ovulatory response to exogenously supplied gonadotropin tends to bear out this assumption. Of interest also is Selye's[23] observation that 1 milligram of progesterone daily for 5 days caused ovarian atrophy in the nonpregnant adult mouse, but even larger doses failed to produce this effect in the pregnant animal. Since hypophysectomy also leads to ovarian atrophy in the nonpregnant but not the pregnant animal, Selye suggests that the luteal hormone probably acts by preventing release of luteinizer by the hypophysis. Its failure to cause ovarian atrophy in the pregnant animal, he believes, is due to its inability to inhibit secretion or release of gonadotropin by the placenta.

Action on Follicular Growth.—Though progestin inhibits ovulation, it apparently has no effect on the development of the follicle up to the point where it begins to undergo changes preparatory to rupture. Dempsey[24] found that the corpus luteum hormone does not retard the rate of follicular growth but does prevent preovulatory swelling and rupture. Conversely, corpus luteum ablation does not speed up the rate of follicular growth, but permits ovulation at an earlier stage. Tietze and his associates[25] noted that in the pregnant woman, the follicles grow to the 5 mm. stage, and then invariably undergo atresia. On the basis of this observation, Tietze divides follicular development into a "vegetative" and a "generative" phase. The first covers development of the follicle up to the 5 mm. stage, and is apparently a continuous process. The "generative" phase includes development of the follicle from the 5 mm. stage to rupture, and is a periodic process requiring an additional hormonal impulse. It is the latter phase which is inhibited by the corpus luteum.

Progestational Modifications of the Uterine Mucosa.—In a series of experiments between 1906 and 1911, Bouin and Ancel[6] found that when ovulation and corpus luteum formation were induced in mature rabbits through sterile coitus, the endometrium presented modifications histologically similar to those seen in early pregnancy. Noting that removal of the corpora lutea thus induced prevented the appearance of the mucosal changes, they concluded that they were caused by some stimulus emanating from the yellow body. In 1911, R. Meyer[26] described the various stages

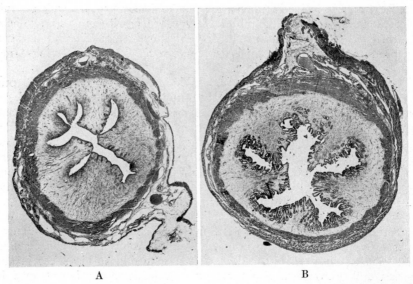

A   B

Fig. 23.—Uterine horn of mature castrate rabbit: A, Following stimulation with estrogen. B, After stimulation with estrogen followed by progesterone.

of corpus luteum formation in the human and correlated them with the changes in the uterine mucosa. He stressed the fact that pregravid, secretory modifications of the endometrium appear premenstrually only when a functioning corpus luteum is present. More recently Hisaw,[27] and Corner and Allen[28] demonstrated that the rat and rabbit castrated during estrus respond to extracts of sow corpora lutea with mucosal alterations like those associated with early gestation or pseudopregnancy. Corner and Allen applied the term "progestational" to the mucosal modifications because of their resemblance to those seen at the time of implantation. These observers also coined the name "progestin" for the specific luteal principle responsible for this effect. Pregravid, secretory changes like those seen premenstrually in the presence of a functioning corpus luteum (see Chap. I) were first induced in the human castrate by Kaufmann,[29] in

1932. He accomplished this by inducing growth of the endometrium with large doses of estrogen, and then administering a series of injections of a potent corpus luteum extract. Kaufmann's observation, soon confirmed by Clauberg,[30] Loeser[31] and many others, established beyond doubt the universality and specificity of progestin.

Estrogen and Progesterone.—In the earlier experiments, it was repeatedly stressed that the endometrium must first be primed by estrogen before it can respond to the luteal hormone with progestational modifications. This has been questioned by Hisaw,[27, 32] who was able to induce a full progestational reaction in the atrophic endometrium of the castrated monkey, rabbit and rat, by administering relatively large amounts of the corpus luteum hormone in crude or crystalline form. To explain the apparent non-essentiality of estrogen in this effect, he suggested that progesterone's close chemical relationship to the follicular hormone enables it, when given in sufficiently large doses, to induce the preparatory changes which are necessary for a progestational reaction and are ordinarily dependent on estrogen. It should be pointed out that Hisaw's experiment was carried out in animals whose uteri had at some previous time been subjected to the influence of estrogen. Whether a similar effect can be produced with progesterone alone in uteri never before stimulated by estrogenic substance was not established by his study. This is also true of similar experiments since carried out by other investigators in the rabbit,[33] rat,[34] and monkey.[35] Even if it is granted that progestational modifications can be experimentally induced with progesterone alone, it does not necessarily follow that estrogen plays no essential role. Its participation in this effect under normal conditions is implied in the observation that the progestational reaction obtained with a given dose of progesterone is distinctly enhanced if moderate doses of estrogen precede it or are given simultaneously.[36] The recent studies of Black and his associates,[37] and of Gilbert,[38] indicate that an optimal luteal effect requires that estrogen precede and accompany progesterone.

While moderate doses of estrogen augment the endometrial response to the luteal hormone, massive doses may partially or completely suppress its progestational effect. This has been demonstrated in the rabbit[39, 40] and rat.[41] Attempts to demonstrate the ability of large doses of estrogen to inhibit the effect of progesterone in the primate have thus far yielded negative results.[35, 36, 41, 42] Whether primates differ in this respect from the lower mammals, or failure to obtain inhibition was due to inadequate dosage, we cannot say. The ability of estrogen to interfere with the response to progesterone is not due to an antagonism in the sense of an ability to neutralize, but arises out of the fact that one stimulates growth while the other promotes secretory activity. If the growth stimulus is excessive, transition of the cells to the secretory phase of their life cycle is hindered or prevented. As emphasized by Gilbert,[38] to insure an optimal luteal effect a delicate balance between the two hormones must be preserved.

Deciduomata Formation.—Loeb,[43] in 1908, found that in rabbits rendered pseudopregnant by sterile coitus, traumatization of the uterus resulted in the formation at the site of injury of peculiar tumefactions

which persisted about two weeks. He named these transient tumors decid-
uomas because of their histologic semblance to the true decidua of pregnancy. Since none appeared when the corpora lutea of pseudopregnancy
were removed, he concluded that functioning luteal tissue is essential for
their formation.[44] That a hormonal stimulus is responsible for this effect
became clear when he succeeded in producing it in uterine autotransplants.
His investigations also revealed that the uterus of the pseudopregnant
animal is able to respond to irritation with deciduoma formation for a

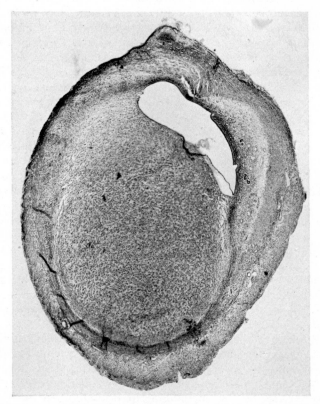

Fig. 24.—Deciduoma produced in the uterine horn of a castrate rat by administering estrogen, then traumatizing the uterus and following with corpus luteum extract.

limited period, approximately corresponding to the time when a fertilized
ovum would normally enter the uterus.

Experimental proof that the decidua, the maternal part of the placenta,
is dependent on hormonal stimuli arising in the corpus luteum, was
provided by Weichert[45] in 1928. This observer produced deciduomata in
ovariectomized guinea pigs and rats by inducing estrus with estrogen,
traumatizing the uterus, and then administering an extract of sow's corpora lutea. This experiment has since been repeated in the rat[46] and
rhesus monkey.[47] Here, as with the progestational modifications of the
uterine mucosa, the preliminary action of estrogen is important but not

indispensable. Rothschild and Meyer[46] observed that the rat's uterus responds to trauma with deciduomata formation if primed by estrogen and progestin. If estrogen is omitted and 0.6 rabbit units of progestin administered daily, no deciduomata form, but if 2 rabbit units are given daily, tumors appear. An excess of estrogen may nullify the effect of progestin, as shown by the observation that this hormone causes regression of experimentally induced deciduomata.

Limitations of the Endometrial Response to Progestin.—Hisaw and Leonard[48] first pointed out that the mucosal response to progestin cannot be maintained indefinitely. They found that the progestational modifications induced with progestin in the estrogen-primed uterus of the castrate rabbit, regress after the tenth day despite continued administration of the luteal hormone. Several investigators have confirmed this observation and in addition have demonstrated that the mucosal modifications in the pseudopregnant rabbit, which normally regress after the seventeenth day following sterile coitus, cannot be maintained beyond this time by administering progestin.[49] In an attempt to postpone regression of the mucosa in the pseudopregnant animal, some observers have employed gonadotropic extracts with the aim of producing a fresh crop of corpora lutea and thus insuring a continued supply of progestin. Courrier and Kehl[50] found that the mucosa regressed at the usual time despite daily injections of gonadotropic substance. McPhail,[51] on the other hand, postponed regression until the end of five weeks after sterile mating by injecting a gonadotropic preparation at ten day intervals. Klein[52] observed degeneration of the mucosa after the seventeenth day despite gonadotropic hormone administration, but progestational modifications reappeared on the twenty-second day with continued treatment. He concluded that the rabbit decidua cannot persist longer than seventeen days in the absence of some extra-ovarian factor, presumably the fetus or placenta. Further stimulation with progestin is apparently of no avail, and only after the mucosa has regressed is it once again capable of responding to this hormone. Selye and his co-workers[53] found that experimentally induced deciduomata in rats regressed despite continued administration of progesterone. In this connection, Lyon and Allen[54] observed in the rat that deciduomata experimentally induced in the sterile horn of a unilateral pregnancy undergo degenerative changes after the twelfth day. Since the hormones secreted by the corpora lutea of pregnancy act on both horns equally, the fact that the decidua in the pregnant horn persists beyond the twelfth day must be attributed to the presence of the products of conception. The latter may conceivably exert some direct effect on the mucosa, prolonging its responsiveness to the luteal hormone, or the fetal placenta may produce progestin which, combined with that from the corpus luteum, is sufficient to maintain the decidua of the pregnant horn. Courrier[55] has suggested that progestin's inability to maintain progestational modifications indefinitely is due to the fact that it requires the support of small amounts of estrogen. That this is at least partly explanatory is suggested by his observation that the addition of small quantities of estrogen definitely retarded regression of a progestational mucosa.

Maintenance of Pregnancy.—*Corpus Luteum Ablation and Abortion.*
—A protective influence of the yellow body on pregnancy was first suggested by Born.[3] Fraenkel[4] in 1903, observed that castration or destruction of all the corpora lutea in the pregnant rabbit before the eighteenth day of gestation was invariably followed by resorption or abortion of the embryos. When operation was delayed until after the twentieth day, most of the animals aborted. Subsequent studies showed that the rat, mouse, goat, ground squirrel and opossum also apparently require the yellow body throughout gestation, since its ablation at any stage invariably leads to abortion.

In the human, on the other hand, pregnancy may continue to a normal conclusion despite corpus luteum ablation performed after the first few weeks of gestation. Pratt[56] has recorded two cases in which the yellow body was removed as early as the twentieth day after the last flow without ill effects. Asdell,[57] in a review of the literature to 1928, found only four abortions among a group of 34 cases subjected to bilateral oophorectomy some time between the first and seventh month of gestation. DeWit and Oppers[58] collected 131 cases of which only 23.7 per cent aborted following removal of the corpus luteum during the first four months of gestation. As summed up by Sturgis,[59] the available reports suggest that the corpus luteum may often be removed after the second month without interrupting pregnancy, while before the second month abortion may ensue in 10 to 33 per cent of the cases.

Why some individuals abort and others remain unaffected by corpus luteum ablation is not clear. Conceivably, operative trauma may account for some of the abortions, particularly in women with an unstable nervous system. Individual differences in the placenta's ability to take over the burden of progestin production may also explain the varied responses to loss of the yellow body. In this connection, Selye and associates[60] observed that ovarian ablation in the pregnant rat was followed by partial involution of the uterus, but the progestational modifications persisted for several days wherever the placentae remained intact. They concluded that the fate of the products of conception, following ovariectomy, depends on how well the fetus resists the increased pressure exerted by the partially involuted uterus, and also to what extent progestin production is assumed by the placenta.

That a *deficiency of progestin* is responsible for the *abortion* which follows ovarian or corpus luteum ablation was experimentally demonstrated by Allen and Corner[61] in 1929. By administering an extract of sow's corpora lutea, these workers were able to maintain pregnancy to term in rabbits ovariectomized shortly after mating. Luteal extracts have been shown to be equally effective for this purpose in the rat,[62] mouse,[63] and ground squirrel.[64] Robson[65] observed that the abortion which follows hypophysectomy in the pregnant rabbit and is apparently due to corpus luteum regression, can be prevented by administering progesterone. The luteal hormone does not invariably constitute complete replacement therapy in the castrate pregnant animal. Klein[52] could not maintain pregnancy with a luteal extract in the rabbit. According to Allen and Heckel,[66] progesterone must be supplemented by small quantities of estrogen to prevent abortion following ovariectomy performed on the first few days of pregnancy. If operation is postponed until the eleventh day, progesterone alone suffices to insure the continuance of gestation.[67] Why estrogen is essential before the eleventh day and not after that point is not clear, unless it is assumed that the placenta is sufficiently well developed after the eleventh day to fully compensate for the ovarian supply of this hormone.

It would seem then that the successful maintenance of pregnancy depends on an adequate supply of progestin and probably also estrogen. Some mammals depend for their supply of progestin largely, if not entirely, on the corpus luteum of pregnancy, while others, including man, are supplied after the earliest stages by some extra-ovarian source, probably the placenta (see Chap. XIII).

There is evidence that the luteal hormone contributes to the maintenance of pregnancy through its *protective action on the fetal bed*, rather than through any direct effect on the developing embryo. This was first demonstrated by Corner,[68] who found that if the corpora lutea of the pregnant rabbit are excised 14 to 18 hours after mating, the fertilized ova develop to the blastocyst stage and are then transported to the uterine cavity where they soon die. More recently, Pincus and Werthessen[69] found that if ovariectomy is performed shortly after mating in the rabbit, ovum growth ceases at the blastocyst stage, but if luteal hormone is administered postoperatively, it promotes ovum growth in proportion to the amount of hormone given. The degree of endometrial proliferation was found to be correlated with the growth of the ovum. Since they could also promote growth of such ova by keeping them in a proper culture medium, they concluded that arrest of ovum growth following oophorectomy is due to the absence of special uterine conditions. It would thus appear that the luteal hormone maintains pregnancy by creating in the uterine mucosa favorable conditions, probably nutritive, which are essential for nidation and retention of the developing ovum.

Inhibition of Uterine Motility.—There is evidence that in some of the lower mammals, and possibly man, the progestational principle inhibits the spontaneous rhythmic activity of the uterine muscle and its reactivity to pituitrin (for details see Chap. VI). These effects were at first thought to be produced by a specific luteal principle distinct from that responsible for the progestational reaction of the endometrium, but studies with crystalline progesterone have demonstrated that the endometrial and myometrial effects are due to a single hormone. The luteal hormone's inhibitory effect on the uterine musculature is apparently designed to keep the pregnant uterus in a quiescent state, thus favoring the continuance of gestation. Its withdrawal is believed by some to be one factor in the initiation of parturition (see Chap. IX).

Effect on the Uterine Blood Vessels.—Champy and Keller,[70] in 1928, prepared a corpus luteum extract which produced vasodilatation and hyperemia of the uterus. Later, Fels and associates[71] claimed to have isolated from corpus luteum tissue two chemically distinct principles, *luteosterone C*, which caused vasodilatation and hyperemia of the uterus, and *luteosterone D*, which elicited progestational modifications of the endometrium. Their contention that these two effects are produced by distinct luteal hormones has not been corroborated.

The active principle of the corpus luteum is apparently also responsible for the growth of the endometrial arteries normally seen in the monkey uterus during the luteal phase of the cycle.[72]

In a recent study, Hechter and his coworkers[73] observed that progesterone, in common with estrogen and certain other steroids, increases the permeability of the uterine capillaries.

Effect on the Uterine Tubes.—The progestational principle exerts a specific effect on the tubal epithelium and musculature. Histologic studies indicate that the tubal mucosa undergoes cyclic changes in the course of the estrual and menstrual cycle (see Chap. I). During the luteal phase of the infertile cycle and also during gestation, it presents changes which have been interpreted as evidence of secretory activity. This interpretation is borne out by Joël's[74, 75] observation that the glycogen and ascorbic acid content of the human tubal mucosa reaches its height during the luteal phase, and that its lipoid content is highest at the beginning of this phase. That the progestational hormone is responsible for the tubal modifications seen during the luteal phase has been demonstrated in the rabbit by Westman[76] and Caffier.[77]

Cyclic variations in the activity of the tubal musculature have also been described. There occur rhythmic contractions whose amplitude is greatest at the height of the follicular phase and least during the luteal phase of the cycle. Studies in the rabbit[78, 79] and man[80] indicate that the relative quiescence of the tubal musculature during the period of corpus luteum function is due to its progestational principle.

Recent studies[81] suggest that the relative quiescence of the tubal musculature induced by the luteal hormone plays an important part in insuring transport of the fertilized ova to the uterine cavity. Whether the secretory activity of the tubal mucosa, which occurs under the influence of this hormone, is essential for their proper development during their stay in the tubes, is not certain.[82]

Effect on the Uterine Cervix.—Evidence relating to the activity of the cervical mucosa and its dependence on the ovarian sex hormones is still fragmentary and conflicting. According to some investigators,[83, 84] the human cervical mucosa undergoes cyclic changes which parallel those in the endometrium. Secretory activity becomes apparent at the midcycle and reaches its height during the premenstruum, when there is an increase in cervical discharge. This description is in line with Westman's[85] observation that the monkey cervix secretes abundant mucus during the luteal phase of the cycle. The implication that mucus secretion is due to the action of progestin is borne out by Cesa's[86] report that estrogen plus crude luteal extract possessing progestational activity, increased the number and secretory activity of the cervical glands in the guinea pig. It also finds support in the observation[87] that a progressive increase in mucus secretion occurs during pregnancy when large amounts of estrogen and progestin are known to be present.

Apparently contradicting these observations are the reports of Seguy[88, 89] and Lamar[90] that secretion of cervical mucus is highest at the midcycle and lowest during the premenstruum. These observers also noted that at the midcycle the mucus reaches its peak as regards alkalinity, fluidity, freedom from leucocytes, and permeability to spermatozoa. At other times, particularly during the premenstruum, the secretions are scanty, viscid, full of leucocytes, and impermeable to spermatozoa. The conditions prevailing at the midcycle are apparently due to the estrogenic hormone, for they could be duplicated in castrate and menopausal women by administering stilbestrol.[91] This effect of estrogenic substances has also been demonstrated by Watson.[92]

In a recent study, Birnberg[93] found that *pregneninolone,* an orally active compound with progestational activity, increased the alkalinity and permeability of the cervical mucus in 5 out of 6 sterile women. No mention was made of the quantity of mucus secreted before and after treatment.

In contrast to the confusion which surrounds its effect on mucus secretion, progestin's ability to check the effect of an excess of estrogen on the cervical mucosa is well established. The epithelial metaplasia which follows protracted estrogen stimulation[94, 95] can be prevented by the simultaneous administration of progesterone.[96] In this connection, Wollner[97] has suggested that so-called cervical "erosions" may be due in many instances to chronic stimulation by estrogen unopposed by progestin.

Effect on the Vagina.—Progesterone alone, without previous estrogen stimulation, has no effect on the vaginal mucosa unless very large doses are used.[98, 99] In the monkey, Hartman and Speert[100] could elicit epithelial growth and cornification by administering 10 to 20 mg. of progesterone daily for 19 to 32 days. In the rodent,[101] the vaginal cornification elicited with estrogenic substance can be prevented by administering adequate doses of progesterone at the same time. Under the combined treatment, the vagina shows the mucification which characterizes the diestrous phase. Observers differ as to whether this effect is due to the combined action of the two hormones acting synergistically, or is to be interpreted as a subthreshold estrogen effect, attributable to an antagonism between estrogen and progestin with consequent partial nullification of estrogen. The latter view is based on the observation that mucification can be induced with estrogen alone in doses below those required for cornification. This evidence has been criticized on the ground that the mucification produced with subthreshold doses of estrogen is not comparable to that obtained with a combination of estrogen and progesterone, nor equivalent to that seen during gestation.[102] In a recent study, Jones and Astwood[103] observed that rats receiving progesterone, followed by a combination of estrogen and progesterone, first showed vaginal cornification which was subsequently replaced by diestrous changes. When the dose of progesterone was kept at the level necessary to induce mucification, the effect could be intensified by increasing the dose of estrogen. They concluded that mucification is not the result of progesterone neutralizing estrogen, but represents the combined effect of the two hormones acting synergistically.

Effect on the Pelvic Ligaments.—During the terminal phase of gestation *in the guinea pig*, the pubic joints relax, widening the pelvic outlet. This enlargement, which is apparently designed to facilitate birth, is accomplished by separation of the iliosacral union and symphysis pubis, permitting free and independent movement of the two ossa. That these alterations are under luteal control was demonstrated by Hisaw,[104] who prepared a relatively pure pelvis-relaxing extract of sow's corpora lutea, which he named *"relaxin."* This hormone is distinct from the progestational principle. Their separate existence first became apparent when Corner and Allen's luteal extract, which could elicit definite modifications in the rabbit endometrium, was found to be without effect on the pelvic ligaments of the guinea pig.[105] Confirmatory evidence was subsequently provided by Brouha,[106] who prepared a luteal extract which caused pelvic relaxation but had no effect on the rabbit endometrium.

The observation[107] that loosening of the pelvic ligaments can be induced with estrogen alone has led some workers to suggest that the pelvic modifications produced with luteal extracts are due to their estrogen content and not to some specific luteal hormone. Though estrogen alone can undoubtedly cause some degree of pelvic relaxation, the observation[102] that its effect is greatly augmented by a single dose of relaxin suggests that the latter hormone plays an important part in this phenomenon.

Pelvic modifications identical with those in the pregnant guinea pig have not been observed *in the gravid woman.* There is evidence that there occurs in the latter a thickening, softening and increased vascularization of the tissues in and about the pelvic joint.[108] Whether these changes are produced by the same hormonal factors that operate in the guinea pig is not certain. The demonstration of a relaxin-like substance in the blood serum of pregnant women[109] suggests this hormone helps prepare the birth canal for parturition in the human as it does in the guinea pig.

Effect on the Sexual Skin of the Monkey.—The progressive reddening and swelling of the sexual skin of the monkey during the follicular phase of the menstrual cycle which can be produced with estrogen (see Chap. II), gradually subsides after ovulation. That its regression during the luteal phase is at least partly due to progestin was first demonstrated by Engle and Smith[110] in 1932. Their findings have since been confirmed by Hisaw and associates,[111] who inhibited the sex skin response to 300 rat units of estrogen by administering 1 rabbit unit of progestin.

Effect on the Mating Instinct.—Until recently, it was generally believed that the mating instinct depends on estrogen. Studies in the rat and guinea pig suggest that, at least in these species, the copulatory reflex requires the synergistic action of estrogen and progestin. Sexual behavior has been induced in the ovariectomized guinea pig by administering estrogen followed by progesterone.[112, 113, 114] Dempsey and his associates[112] suggest that estrogen, acting before ovulation, sensitizes the animal for sexual receptivity, but the determining factor is progesterone, which they believe is secreted by the unruptured follicle during the period of preovulatory enlargement. Though there is some indirect evidence suggesting that progesterone or a substance closely related to it is secreted before ovulation,[115, 116] conclusive proof is still lacking. Boling and Blandau[117] found a small dose of estrogen followed by progesterone more effective than a large dose of estrogen alone in inducing the mating response in the spayed female rat. The heat induced by the combined treatment more closely resembled spontaneously occurring heat in length and intensity.

Effect on Estrogen Metabolism.—Smith and Smith,[118] in 1931, observed that when estrogen and progestin were administered simultaneously some of the injected estrogen could be recovered from the urine. On the other hand, when estrogen was given alone in the same amounts, none was demonstrable. They concluded that progestin promotes the excretion of estrogen. In 1937, Pincus and Zahl[116] described similar findings and, in explanation, suggested that progestin gives estrogen partial protection against destruction. In addition, they presented evidence indicating that progestin also facilitates the conversion of estrone to estriol. Smith and Smith's[119] recent study of the estrone and estriol level during the menstrual cycle in the human being suggests that the luteal hormone performs a similar function in the primate.

The role of the progestational hormone in menstruation, and the development and function of the breast is discussed elsewhere (see Chap. V, X).

BIBLIOGRAPHY

1. Beard, J.: The Span of Gestation and the Cause of Birth, Jena, G. Fischer, 1897.
2. Prenant, A.: Rev. gen. d. Sc. *9*:646, 1898.
3. Born, G.: cited by L. Fraenkel (*infra* 4).
4. Fraenkel, L.: Arch. f. Gynäk. *68*:438, 1903.
5. Loeb, L.: Zentralbl. f. allg. Path. u. path. Anat. *18*:563, 1907.
6. Bouin, P., and Ancel, P.: Compt. rend. Soc. de biol. *61*:417, 1906; ibid. *66*:505, 689, 1909; J. de physiol. et de path. gén. *13*:31, 1911.
7. Fellner, O. O.: Arch. f. Gynäk. *100*:641, 1913.
8. Herrmann, E.: Monatschr. f. Geburtsh. u. Gynäk. *41*:1, 1915.
9. Tandler, J.: Wien. Klin. Wchnschr. *23*:459, 1910.
10. Loeb, L.: Deut. med. Wchnschr. *37*:17, 1911.
11. Hammond, J.: The Physiology of Reproduction in the Cow, New York, The Macmillan Co., 1927.
12. Loeb, L.: Am. J. Anat. *32*:305, 1923.
13. Drummond-Robinson, G., and Asdell, S. A.: J. Physiol. *61*:608, 1926.
14. Seitz, L., and Wintz, H.: Monatschr. f. Geburtsh. u. Gynäk. *49*:1, 1919.
15. Papanicolaou, G. N.: J.A.M.A. *86*:1422, 1926.
16. Gley, P.: J. de physiol. et de path. gén. *27*:528, 1929.
17. Parkes, A. S., and Bellerby, C. W.: J. Physiol. *64*:233, 1927.
18. Mahnert, A.: Zentralbl. f. Gynäk. *54*:2283, 1930.
19. Fels, E.: Arch. f. Gynäk. *158*:364, 1934.
20. Selye, H., Browne, J. S. L., and Collip, J. B.: Proc. Soc. Exper. Biol. & Med. *34*:472, 1936.
21. Phillips, W. A.: Am. J. Physiol. *119*:623, 1937.
22. Makepeace, A. W., Weinstein, G. L., and Friedman, M. H.: Am. J. Physiol. *119*:512, 1937.
23. Selye, H.: Anat. Rec. *75*:59, 1939.
24. Dempsey, E. W.: Am. J. Physiol. *120*:126, 1937.
25. Tietze, K., and Wegener, R.: Zentralbl. f. Gynäk. *59*:1097, 1935.
26. Meyer, R.: Arch. f. Gynäk. *93*:354, 1911.
27. Hisaw, F. L.: Anat. Rec. *64* (Suppl.):54, 1935; Am. J. Anat. *61*:483, 1937.
28. Corner, G. W., and Allen, W. M.: Am. J. Physiol. *88*:326, 1929.
29. Kaufmann, C.: Zentralbl. f. Gynäk. *56*:2058, 1932.

30. Clauberg, C.: Zentralbl. f. Gynäk. *57*:1461, 1933.
31. Loeser, A.: Zentralbl. f. Gynäk. *57*:1704, 1933.
32. Hisaw, F. L., Greep, R. O., and Fevold, H. L.: Proc. Soc. Exp. Biol. & Med. *36*:840, 1937.
33. Allen, W. M.: Cold Spring Harbor Symposia on Quant. Biol. *5*:66, 1937.
34. Selye, H.: Anat. Rec. *78*:253, 1940.
35. Hartman, C. G., and Speert, H.: Endocrinol. *29*:639, 1941.
36. Engle, E. T., and Smith, P. E.: Am. J. Anat. *63*:349, 1938.
37. Black, J., Heynes, O. H., and Gillman, J.: J. Clin. Endocrinol. *1*:547, 1941.
38. Gilbert, C.: Endocrinol. *30*:773, 1942.
39. Robson, J. M.: J. Physiol. *92*:371, 1938.
40. Gillman, J., and Stein, H. B.: Endocrinol. *31*:167, 1942.
41. Courrier, R., and Gros, G.: Compt. rend. Soc. de biol. *125*:746, 1937.
42. Gillman, J., and Stein, H. B.: Endocrinol. *28*:274, 1941.
43. Loeb, L.: Zentralbl. f. Physiol. *17*:498, 1908.
44. Loeb, L.: Zentralbl. f. Physiol. *18*:73, 1909.
45. Weichert, C. K.: Proc. Soc. Exper. Biol. & Med. *25*:490, 1928.
46. Rothschild, I., and Meyer, R. K.: Proc. Soc. Exper. Biol. & Med. *44*:402, 1940.
47. Rossman, I.: Anat. Rec. *70* (Suppl.): 67, 1938.
48. Hisaw, F. L., and Leonard, S. L.: Am. J. Physiol. *92*:574, 1930.
49. Fremery, P. de, Luchs, A., and Tausk, M.: Arch. f. d. ges. Physiol. *231*:341, 1932.
50. Courrier, R., and Kehl, R.: L'Algérie Médicale, Jan., 1930.
51. McPhail, M. K.: J. Physiol. *79*:118, 1933.
52. Klein, M.: Arch. d'anat., d'hist., et d'embryol. *18*:1, 1934.
53. Selye, H., Borduas, A., and Masson, G.: Endocrinol. *30*:71, 1942.
54. Lyon, R. A., and Allen, W. M.: Anat. Rec. *65*:351, 1936.
55. Courrier, R.: Compt. rend. Soc. de biol. *127*:140, 1938.
56. Pratt, J. P.: Endocrinol. *11*:195, 1927.
57. Asdell, S. A.: Physiol. Rev. *8*:313, 1928.
58. Duyvene de Wit, J. J., and Oppers, V. M.: Nederl. tijdschr. v. geneesk. *83*:4001, 1939.
59. Sturgis, S. H.: Am. J. Obst. & Gynec. *35*:752, 1938.
60. Selye, H., Collip, J. B., and Thomson, D. L.: Endocrinol. *19*:151, 1938.
61. Allen, W. M., and Corner, G. W.: Am. J. Physiol. *88*:340, 1929.
62. Harris, R. G., and Pfiffner, J. J.: Anat. Rec. *44*:205, 1929.
63. Robson, J. M.: J. Physiol. *92*:371, 1938.
64. Johnson, G. E., and Challans, J. S.: Anat. Rec. *47*:300, 1930.
65. Robson, J. M.: J. Physiol. *86*:415, 1936.
66. Allen, W. M., and Heckel, G. P.: Science *86*:409, 1937.
67. Allen, W. M., and Heckel, G. P.: Am. J. Physiol. *125*:31, 1939.
68. Corner, G. W.: Am. J. Physiol. *86*:74, 1928.
69. Pincus, G., and Werthessen, N. T.: Anat. Rec. *67* (Suppl.): 34, 1936.
70. Champy, C., and Keller, T.: Arch. de morphol. gén. et expér. vol. 27, 1928.
71. Fels, E., Slotta, K. H., and Ruschig, H.: Klin. Wchnschr. *13*:1207, 1934.
72. Daron, G. H.: Am. J. Anat. *58*:349, 1936.
73. Hechter, O., Krohn, L., and Harris, J. M.: Endocrinol. *30*:598, 1942.
74. Joël, C. A.: J. Obst. & Gynec. Brit. Emp. *46*:721, 731, 1939.
75. Joël, C. A.: Schweiz. med. Wchnschr. *71*:1286, 1941.
76. Westman, A., Jorpes, E., and Widstrom, G.: Acta obst. & gynec. Scandinav. *11*:279, 1931.
77. Caffier, P.: Zentralbl. f. Gynäk. *62*:1024, 1938.
78. Binder, A.: Arch. f. Gynäk. *168*:744, 1939.
79. Anderes, E.: Schweiz. med. Wchnschr. *71*:364, 1941.
80. Geist, S. H., Salmon, U. J., and Mintz, M. E.: Proc. Soc. Exper. Biol. & Med. *38*:783, 1938.
81. Burdick, H. O., Whitney, R., and Emerson, B.: Endocrinol. *31*:100, 1942.
82. Alden, R. H.: J. Exper. Zool. *90*:159, 171, 1942.
83. Wollner, A.: Surg., Gynec. & Obst. *64*:758, 1937.

84. Sjövall, A.: Acta obst. & gynec. Scandinav. *18*:4, 1938.
85. Westman, A.: Acta obst. & gynec. Scandinav. *12*:282, 1932.
86. Cesa, I.: Compt. rend. Soc. de biol. *122*:1237, 1936.
87. Stieve, H.: Zentralbl. f. Gynäk. *52*:218, 1928.
88. Séguy, J., and Vimeux, J.: Gynéc. et Obst. *27*:346, 1933.
89. Séguy, J., and Simonnet, H.: Gynéc. et Obst. *28*:657, 1933.
90. Lamar, J. K., Shettles, L. B., and Delfs, E.: Am. J. Physiol. *129*:234, 1940.
91. Guttmacher, A. F., and Shettles, L. B.: Human Fertility *5*:4, 1940.
92. Watson, M. C.: Can. M. A. J. *40*:542, 1939.
93. Birnberg, C. H., Kurzrok, L., and Weber, H.: Am. J. Surg. *57*:180, 1942.
94. Wollner, A.: J. Clin. Endocrinol. *1*:3, 1941.
95. Zuckerman, S.: Lancet *1*:435, 1937.
96. Hisaw, F. L., and Lendrum, F. C.: Endocrinol. *20*:228, 1938.
97. Wollner, A.: Am. J. Surg. *57*:180, 1942.
98. Allen, W. M., and Meyer, R. K.: Anat. Rec. *61*:427, 1935.
99. Hisaw, F. L., Greep, R. O., and Fevold, H. L.: Proc. Soc. Exper. Biol. & Med. *36*: 840, 1937.
100. Hartman, C. G., and Speert, H.: Endocrinol. *29*:639, 1941.
101. Courrier, R., and Cohen-Solal, G.: Compt. rend. Soc. de biol. *124*:961, 1937.
102. Brouha, L., and Desclin, L.: Arch. internat. de pharmacodyn. et de thérap. *48*:147, 1934.
103. Jones, G. E. S., and Astwood, E. B.: Endocrinol. *30*:295, 1942.
104. Hisaw, F. L.: Physiol. Zool. *2*:59, 1929.
105. Corner, G. W., and Allen, W. M.: Am. J. Physiol. *88*:326, 1929.
106. Brouha, L.: Compt. rend. Soc. de biol. *109*:548, 1932.
107. Tapfer, S., and Haslhofer, L.: Arch. f. Gynäk. *159*:313, 1935.
108. Abramson, D., Roberts, S. M., and Wilson, P. D.: Surg., Gynec. & Obst. *58*:595, 1934.
109. Abramson, D., Hurwitt, E., and Lesnick, G.: Surg., Gynec. & Obst. *65*:335, 1937.
110. Engle, E. T., and Smith, P. E.: Proc. Soc. Exper. Biol. & Med. *29*:1225, 1937.
111. Hisaw, F. L., Greep, R. O., and Fevold, H. L.: Am. J. Anat. *61*:483, 1937.
112. Dempsey, E. W., Hertz, R., and Young, W. C.: Am. J. Physiol. *116*:201, 1936.
113. Hertz, R., Meyer, R. K., and Spielman, M.: Endocrinol. *21*:533, 1937.
114. Collins, V. J., Boling, J. L., and Young, W. C.: Anat. Rec. *70* (Suppl.) :17, 1938.
115. Astwood, E. B.: Am. J. Physiol. *126*:162, 1939.
116. Pincus, G., and Zahl, P. A.: J. Gen. Physiol. *20*:879, 1937.
117. Boling, J. L., and Blandau, R. J.: Endocrinol. *25*:359, 1939.
118. Smith, G. V. S., and Smith, O. W.: Am. J. Physiol. *98*:578, 1931.
119. Smith, G. V. S., Smith, O. W., and Pincus, G.: Am. J. Physiol. *121*:98, 1938.

5

CHAPTER IV

THE TIME OF OVULATION AND THE "SAFE PERIOD"

INTRODUCTION

A reliable method of determining the time of ovulation would be of distinct value in defining the limits of the "safe period" for women who do not desire pregnancy, and insuring optimal conditions for conception in those who wish to conceive. In addition, it could serve as a valuable adjunct in the investigation of female sterility. Lack of such a method is responsible for the confusion that has long existed regarding the chronological relationship between follicular rupture and menstruation. The earlier impression that the two phenomena are synchronous was shown to be erroneous by Hitschmann and Adler,[1] R. Meyer,[2] Schröder,[3] and others, who correlated events in the ovary and endometrium, and demonstrated that ovulation normally precedes the onset of the flow. Their findings initiated a long series of studies which have formed the basis of two opposing views. One, the so-called "Knaus-Ogino theory," holds that the time of ovulation bears a fairly constant chronological relationship to the menstrual flow and fluctuates within narrow limits; the other maintains that ovulation may occur at any time during the menstrual cycle, though it is most likely to take place midway between the flows. Considerable clinical data has been presented in support of both views. It must be emphasized that the relative merits of each should not be judged merely by the number of reported cases which apparently substantiate it, but also by the reliability of the methods employed to ascertain the time of ovulation.

METHODS OF ASCERTAINING OVULATION TIME

The following are some of the more important methods employed to determine the time of ovulation:

1. Macroscopic and microscopic examination of ovaries.
2. Microscopic examination of the endometrium.
3. Recovery of tubal ova.
4. Analysis of cases where conception followed a single coitus.
5. Bimanual palpation of the ovaries and uterus.
6. Uterine reactivity to pituitrin (Knaus test).
7. Estrogen and gonadotropin in the blood and urine.
8. Pregnanediol excretion studies.
9. Detection of changes in electrical potential.
10. Vaginal smear studies.

Macroscopic and Microscopic Examination of the Ovary.—The presence of a mature follicle on the verge of rupture, a recently ruptured follicle, or a fresh corpus luteum is used by some workers[4, 5, 6, 7] as a basis for estimating the time of ovulation. The difficulty of judging the precise moment of rupture from such evidence alone is generally conceded by competent histologists. In many of the cases so studied, reliable information as to the date of the preceding menstrual period was not available. This method has the disadvantage that where the ovaries are removed for examination, the flow which follows is usually premature and the relation of rupture to the cycle as a whole must therefore remain uncertain. Even where the ovaries are inspected in situ, there is no assurance that the shock incident to abdominal section has not prematurely precipitated or delayed the succeeding menses, thus obscuring the position of ovulation in the cycle. Since the opportunity to inspect the ovaries in most instances arises because of some pelvic pathology, the findings may not be truly representative of what occurs under normal conditions.

Microscopic Examination of the Endometrium.—The uterine mucosa, except in occasional instances where some inherent defect makes it refractory to the ovarian sex hormones, accurately reflects events in the ovary. For this reason, it has been employed by some investigators[8, 9, 10] as a means of determining ovulation time. It is generally believed that early pregravid or secretory changes in the endometrium normally follow follicular rupture and coincide with beginning corpus luteum formation. Accordingly, the approximate position of the ovulatory act in the menstrual cycle may be ascertained by determining when early secretory modifications first appear and obtaining the dates of the preceding and succeeding flow.

The accuracy of this method is assailable on the ground that there is no definite information as to the length of the interval between follicular rupture and the appearance of early secretory changes in the endometrium. Since the mucosal response depends on the amount of progestin present and the reactivity of the mucosa to this hormone, it may be expected that this interval will vary in different individuals and at different times in the same individual. It therefore follows that, while the presence of secretory changes is usually reliable evidence that ovulation has occurred, the exact time of ovulation cannot be ascertained from this finding alone.

Recovery of Tubal Ova.—The recovery of live ova from the fallopian tubes was first accomplished in the monkey[11] and man[12] by Allen and associates. In view of the difficulties inherent in this procedure, it is not surprising that only a limited number of human ova have thus far been recovered from the tubes.[13] While the presence of live ova in the tubes is incontrovertible evidence that follicular rupture has recently taken place, the precise moment of its occurrence cannot be deduced without definite knowledge of the life span of the unfertilized human ovum (see below).

Conception Following a Single Coitus.—During the first World War, when coitus was presumably limited to the duration of the soldier's furlough, a number of investigators[14, 15] sought to ascertain the time of ovulation in women conceiving following a single coitus. Each patient provided the date of her last menstrual period, while the government records fixed the dates of the furloughs. In calculating the probable ovulation time, it was assumed that the ovum and sperm remain viable for no longer than thirty-six hours, and that coitus, ovulation and conception, therefore, take place within an interval of several hours. The earlier studies were open to the criticism that the possibility of extra-marital relations was not definitely excluded, and that the date of the last flow and information relating to the length and regularity of previous cycles was furnished largely from the patient's memory. Efforts to eliminate these sources of error have been made in more recent investigations,[16, 17, 18] which have tended to confirm the results of the earlier studies.

It must be emphasized that the data obtained by this method can only indicate what days of the cycle are fertile. Whether the fertile period bears a constant relationship to the time of ovulation depends to a large extent on the validity of the premise that the life span of the male and female germ cells is short and varies within narrow limits (see below).

Bimanual Palpation of the Ovaries and Uterus.—Several workers have attempted to ascertain ovulation time in the monkey[19] and human[20, 21] on the basis of alterations in the size and consistency of the ovaries and uterus, as ascertained by bimanual palpation. As Dickinson[20] points out, the accuracy of this method depends on the proper choice of subjects and the examiner's ability to detect minor modifications in these organs through his sense of touch.

Uterine Reactivity to Pituitrin (Knaus Test).—The Knaus[22] ovulation test is based on the assumption that uterine reactivity to pituitrin, as determined by the intrauterine bag method (see Chap. VI), is lost within forty-eight hours after follicular rupture. Aside from the technical difficulties of the test, it is open to the objection that loss of myometrial reactivity to pituitrin does not invariably accompany corpus luteum formation. Even where this occurs, repeated tests must be performed to determine the exact moment when refractoriness to pituitrin sets in. Granting that this may be determined with accuracy, there is no convincing proof that the interval between ovulation and loss of reactivity to pituitrin is, as Knaus assumes, invariably forty-eight hours.

Estrogen and Gonadotropin in the Blood and Urine.—A clue to the time of ovulation has been sought in the estrogen and gonadotropin content of the blood and urine during the course of the menstrual cycle. The results of such studies have been too variable to permit definite conclusions. Smith and Smith[23] found that the maximal excretion of estrogen occurs on the twelfth to the thirteenth day before the flow, regardless of the length of the cycle. The gonadotropic hormone, according to their experience, is consistently demonstrable in the urine only immediately before the onset of the flow. Kurzrok[24] observed a rise in gonadotropin excretion midway between the flows in 9 out of 10 cases. On the basis of subsequent events, he calculated that the rise had preceded the occurrence of ovulation by 24 hours. Frank[25] also noted a peak in gonadotropin excretion during the second week of the cycle, but hesitated to accept this as a reliable criterion of ovulation, because of the possibility that rupture depends on other factors besides a hormonal impulse from the adenohypophysis. According to the recent studies of D'Amour and his associates,[26, 27, 28] a rise in gonadotropic hormone excretion occurs between the twelfth and sixteenth day before the flow. In some, though not all cycles, this is followed by a second rise shortly before the onset of bleeding. They also detected two peaks of estrogen excretion, which usually preceded the gonadotropin peaks. They suggest that the rise in estrogen stimulates the anterior pituitary to release its gonadotropic hormones which in turn cause ovulation, but concede that proof of this is still lacking. Until such proof is available, and more is known of the length of the interval between the midcycle estrogen and gonadotropin peak and the occurrence of ovulation, data derived from such studies can be of only limited value.

Pregnanediol Excretion Studies.—Browne and Venning[29] first demonstrated that pregnanediol, an excretion product of progestin, rises to a plateau after ovulation and falls abruptly shortly before the onset of the flow. Granting that its appearance in the urine is fairly reliable evidence that ovulation has occurred, the exact time of follicular rupture cannot be calculated from this finding alone. Information as to the length of the interval between ovulation and the appearance of pregnanediol in the urine, and proof that it is constant, are not yet available.

Changes in Electrical Potential.—The observation[30] that ovulation in the rabbit is an explosive act suggested the possibility that changes in electrical potential may prove an accurate criterion of follicular rupture in man. With this in mind, Burr and his associates[31] employed a vacuum tube microvoltmeter equipped with a photoelectric recorder, connected through silver, silver chloride electrodes and salt bridges to the symphysis pubis and vagina. In the rabbit, this apparatus registered a distinct rise in electrical potential at the moment of follicular rupture. In a rabbit with ovaries exposed to view, Reboul and his coworkers[32] noted a rise in electrical potential at the moment of, or within a few seconds after, follicular rupture.

Use of this method in the human being has thus far been attempted in only a small number of cases. In one patient observed by Burr and his associates,[33] the apparatus was attached as the expected time of ovulation drew near. During the ensuing fifty-seven hours, the following changes were recorded: At first the vagina was negative to the symphysis, the apparatus registering only about 10 millivolts. It then gradually became positive, reaching 30 millivolts within seven hours. During the next five minutes, it fluctuated between 70 and 80 millivolts. Laparotomy performed on the following day revealed a freshly ruptured follicle. Rock[34] employed this method in a group of patients about to undergo laparotomy, and found that a rise in electrical potential may precede rupture by several hours. Of nine patients who showed a rise before operation, evidence of rupture was found in only six. In the remaining three cases, there was evidence of follicular maturation, but ovulation had not occurred.

According to Burr and Musselman,[35] changes in electrical potential, apparently related to events in the ovary, may be detected by attaching the apparatus to the index fingers of both hands. In one case, between the fourteenth and seventeenth day before the onset of the flow, the right index finger showed an increase in positive polarity amounting to several thousand microvolts. Repeated tests over a period of nine months revealed that the electrical cycle repeated itself with surprising regularity. In a pregnant woman, the monthly cyclic phenomena were entirely absent. In a further study[36] of fourteen women, these observers found the peaks to be much less regular, occurring most often in the middle of the cycle or immediately after menstruation, but in no case before the flow. More recently, Langman and Burr[37] reported that when a microvoltmeter with photoelectric recorder is attached to the cervix and ankle, the cervix is usually positive to the ankle but becomes negative on one day during each cycle. They suggest that this negative shift may be associated with ovulation but offer no proof to substantiate this.

Vaginal Smear Studies.—Recent interest in the vaginal smear as a diagnostic aid has led some observers to employ it as a means of ascertaining ovulation time. Its value for this purpose is not established (see Chap. XXXIX).

EVALUATION OF THE KNAUS-OGINO THEORY

The contention of Knaus[38] and Ogino[39] that ovulation occurs within a circumscribed period which bears a constant relationship to the flow, has

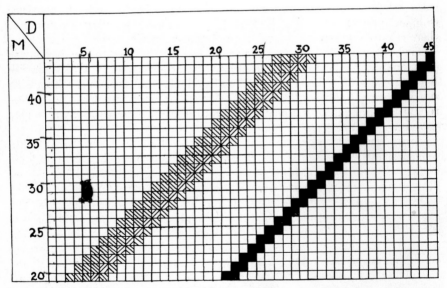

D = Number of days after onset of last flow
M = Length of the menstrual cycle
≈≈≈ = Fertile period
////, = Time of ovulation
■■■ = Menses

Fig. 25.—Fertile period of the menstrual cycle (Knaus).

renewed the hope that natural control of conception may be achieved by limiting coitus to periods of the cycle when no ovum is available for fertilization. Since this theory relates ovulation to the expected rather than the preceding flow, its practical application necessarily depends on an accurate knowledge of the individual's menstrual habit. To acquire this information, and ascertain to what extent the length of the cycle deviates from the twenty-eight day norm, a careful record of the menstrual dates during the preceding eight to twelve months is indispensable. In calculating the limits of the fertile period of the cycle, Knaus assumes that ovulation always occurs fourteen days before the onset of the flow, and that the maximum life span of the ovum and sperm is twenty-four and forty-eight hours respectively. The *method of calculation* can best be understood by taking a hypothetical case. In a woman whose cycles vary in length from twenty-six to thirty-two days, the fertile period may be calculated as follows: 14 (constant in 28 day cycle) plus (26 — 28) equals 12, the earliest day on which ovulation could occur: 14 plus (32 — 28) equals 18, the latest day on which it may take place. Counting back two days to allow for the life span of the sperm, and one day forward to allow for that of the ovum, the fertile period is found to extend from the tenth to the nineteenth day of the cycle.

Positive proof of the validity of this theory would be its successful use as a contraceptive measure in a large series of cases. The available reports permit no conclusions. Some observers[18] claim almost 100 per cent success, while others[40, 41] report conception in an appreciable number of cases where coitus was limited to the supposed sterile phase of the cycle.

The weakness of the Knaus-Ogino theory lies in the fact that it rests on assumptions for which there is as yet no conclusive proof. It assumes that (1) the length of the postovulatory phase of the menstrual cycle is constant; (2) the ovum is fertilizable only 24 hours after its extrusion from the follicle; (3) the spermatozoa lose their fertilizing capacity within 48 hours after their deposition in the female genitalia; (4) if the cycle has tended to be a certain length for a period of one year, it will continue so thereafter; and (4) ovulation occurs only once during each cycle and is unaffected by coitus or other extraneous stimuli. The available evidence relating to each of these assumptions will be considered briefly.

Length of the Postovulatory Phase of the Menstrual Cycle.—Earlier estimates of the length of the postovulatory or luteal phase of the cycle varied from nine to over twenty days. Ogino[39] believes that it is fairly constant, varying from twelve to sixteen days. Knaus[38] maintains that it has a constant length of fourteen days, on the basis of his studies of uterine reactivity to pituitrin in the human being, and by analogy to the rabbit. in which pseudopregnancy is always the same length. Hartman,[19] who ascertained the time of ovulation in the monkey by bimanual rectal palpation, found that variations in the length of the cycle were due to changes in the length of the luteal rather than the follicular phase, which remained fairly constant. Knaus[38] encountered a few instances among his human material in which the follicular phase was constant while the luteal phase varied, but dismissed them as exceptional, blaming an inadequate blood supply. Rock and Bartlett,[10] who used the endometrial picture as an index of events in the ovary, found that the length of the preovulatory phase varied within extremely wide limits in all their cases, while the luteal phase was fairly constant in all but 25 per cent. Vollmann[42] has reached a similar conclusion on the basis of calendar records made in the course of 200 cycles in four women with intermenstrual pain. Taking this symptom as evidence of the occurrence of ovulation, he found that the preovulatory phase varied from thirteen to fifteen days in 81.5 per cent of the cycles. Variations in the length of the cycle were apparently due to changes in the length of the follicular phase.

Life Span of the Unfertilized Ovum.—According to a view sponsored earlier by R. Meyer,[43] the unfertilized human ovum remains viable until shortly before the flow, a period of approximately two weeks after its expulsion from the follicle. This concept has been questioned by a number of competent workers, whose studies in the human being[44, 45] and lower mammal indicate that the life span of the ovum is relatively short. In the ferret,[46] for example, the unfertilized ovum remains viable for less than thirty hours, in the guinea pig,[47] up to twenty-six hours, in the opossum[48] and sow,[49] less than twenty-four hours, while in the rabbit[50] it survives only five to six hours. Though precise information regarding the human ovum is lacking, the observation that degenerative changes are discernible in human ova removed from the fallopian tubes, tends to bear out the assumption that their life span is short.

Life Span of the Deposited Spermatozoa.—Spermatozoa apparently remain motile for a relatively long time if kept in an environment similar to that prevailing in the scrotum. Brault[51] found that sperms kept in the fluid of an extirpated spermatic cyst at 37° C. remained motile for almost two weeks. Whether they also retained their fertilizing capacity was not ascertained. According to Stokes,[52] active spermatozoa may be found in the male ejaculate two to three weeks after vasectomy. After isolation of the tail of epididymus, the sperms retain their fertilizing power up to forty days in the rabbit,[53] and thirty days in the guinea pig.[54] Motility persists under these conditions up to sixty days in the rabbit,[53] and fifty-nine days in the guinea pig.[54]

Sperm survival is considerably curtailed after deposition *in the female genitalia*. According to Moench,[55] the sperms are all killed off by the heat and environment of the female genital tract in less than forty-eight hours. Besides the unfavorable effect of body heat, the female genitalia offer obstacles of a chemical, mechanical, and bacterial nature. Sperms have been reported to retain their motility in the female genitalia for ten hours in the mouse, twelve to sixteen hours in the rat, forty-one hours in the guinea pig and sow, and forty-eight hours in the rabbit and horse. Studies of the life span of human sperms, after deposition in the female genitalia, have yielded varying results. The general impression is that they survive for only a relatively short time. Cary[56] could find no viable sperm *in the vagina* later than two hours after coitus. *In the cervix*, on the other hand, motility persisted for a longer period, though here again there is considerable individual variation. In five women artificially impregnated from one donor, Seymour[57] found that the sperms retained their motility from forty-five to one hundred and ten hours. That the cervical secretions contribute in a positive way to the sperms' survival is suggested by Cary's[56] observation that locomotion persists in normal cervical mucus many hours longer than in the direct specimen kept at room or body temperature. Moench[55] ascribes this to the fact that they are in a strongly alkaline medium where little oxygen is available. This slows up their activity and preserves their power of locomotion. When placed under the microscope, the greater oxygen supply then available permits renewed activity and shortens their life span.

Runge[58] was unable to recover motile sperms from the *uterus* after the second day post-coitum. Haussmann,[59] on the other hand, observed actively motile sperm on the third and a slight degree of locomotion as late as the seventh day. Ohlin[60] investigated the *effect of the tubal secretions* on the male germ cell by mixing sperms with tubal scrapings obtained at operation. Observing no significant alterations in the sperms, he concluded that the tubal secretions are indifferent to them, offering no conserving or nourishing medium to counteract the adverse effects of heat and phagocytosis.

Though significant, the fragmentary evidence at hand provides no definite information as to how long the sperms retain their fertilizing power after reaching the female genitalia. As emphasized elsewhere (see Chap. XXVII), motility per se does not necessarily imply ability to fertilize.

Variability in the Length of the Menstrual Cycle.—The assumption that most normal women menstruate at twenty-eight day intervals has been disproved by ample evidence. Most authorities now agree that, though the average length of the menstrual cycle approximates this figure, wide variations may be encountered between different individuals and at different times in the same individual (see Table 1).

Coitus-Induced Ovulation.—Proponents of the view that the fertile phase of the cycle is limited to a brief period midway between the flows, explain instances of fertile coitus early or late in the cycle by assuming that ovulation in the human can be induced by coitus or other extraneous stimuli.[61] Data supporting this assumption are necessarily limited. *In the lower mammal,* two types of ovulation have been described. In most species the ovulatory act is controlled by endogenous factors and is independent of external stimuli. In others, notably the rabbit, this phenomenon depends on the stimulus of coitus, and may also be experimentally induced by mechanical or electrical stimuli applied to the cervix, provided the animal is in heat. That the coital act does not stimulate ovulatory function in species which normally ovulate spontaneously, has been demonstrated in the ewe[62] and guinea pig.[63]

Whether ovulation *in primates* can be induced by coitus is not certain. In one monkey observed by Hartman[64] for three successive cycles, ovulation occurred at approximately the same time in each cycle, that is, on the fourteenth or fifteenth day, despite the fact that the animal copulated frequently during the first and third, and not at all during the second cycle. Knaus[38] made a similar observation in a woman who carefully recorded the dates of coitus and menstruation. In this instance, the menstrual rhythm remained unaltered regardless of whether or not coitus was practiced. An additional argument against coitus-induced ovulation *in man*

TABLE 1

VARIABILITY IN LENGTH OF MENSTRUAL CYCLE

Author	No. of cases	Nationality	Occupation	Age at start of study	Total number of cycles	Length of cycles
Foster (1889)........	56	American	Selected patients		380	Shortest—16, longest—46 days. 45 cycles 28 days long; 110 cycles 29–46 days long; 225 cycles 16–27 days long.
Issmer (1889)........	12	German	Housewives	19–39	120	Shortest—20, longest—40 days. None absolutely regular; deviations from individual means vary from 2 to 12 days.
King (1926, 1933)....	54	American	College women and industrial workers	17–35	877	Shortest—16; longest—53 days. None absolutely regular; deviations from individual means vary from 1 to 26 days.
Pratt et al. (1929)....	50	American	Nurses and office workers	12–36	301	Shortest—17, longest—36 days. None absolutely regular.
Geist (1930).........	200	American	Selected patients			Variable. Flow appears from 5 days before to 10 days after expected time.
Allen (1933).........	131	American	Student nurses		1522	Shortest—13, longest—84 days.
Engle and Shelesnyak (1934)............	100	American–Jewish	Orphanage girls	11–16	3140	Shortest—7, longest—256 days. None absolutely regular. Deviations from individual means vary from 6 to 211 days.
Fluhmann (1934).....	76	American	Student nurses	18–27	747	Shortest—11, longest—144 days. None absolutely regular. Deviations from individual means vary from 2 to 69 days.
Weinstock (1934).....	416	German	Selected patients	16–40		Shortest—14, longest—56 days. Majority 26–30 days.
Scipiades (1935)......	51	Hungarian	University students	18–34	386	Shortest—20, longest—91 days. None absolutely regular; average 30 days.
Latz and Reiner (1935, 1937)............	202	American Canadian	Housewives	20–49	2449	Shortest—15, longest—101 days. Deviations from individual means vary from 1 to 53 days.
Gunn et al. (1937) ..	479	British	Professional and other women	13–51	6000	Majority (90%) 25 to 36 days. None absolutely regular. Most vary 8 to 9 days.

is provided by the observation that in most instances virgins show no significant change in the menstrual rhythm after marriage.

The view that coitus or other extraneous stimuli may induce follicular rupture *in man* finds some support in the observation that conception may follow dilatation and curettage in some cases of functional sterility. It is tempting to explain such cures by assuming that mechanical stimulation of the cervix induced ovulation in the same way that a similar procedure produces this effect in the rabbit. This is purely speculative, for the cures may as reasonably be attributed to correction of some local defect, or spontaneous adjustment of the underlying cause. Of interest in this connection is Birnberg's[65] report that twenty-three out of thirty women showed a rise in gonadotropin excretion within thirty hours after cervical dilatation, and three of the women who were sterile conceived shortly afterward. If it is granted that a rise in the gonadotropin content of the urine heralds ovulation, as some believe, then Birnberg's findings imply that cervical dilatation may induce ovulation. Unfortunately, this observer gave no information as to the date of the next period in his cases. Nor did he attempt to ascertain whether early secretory modifications of the endometrium followed the rise in the gonadotropin level. His failure to use controls to determine whether a similar rise would occur on the same days of the cycle in untreated cases also detracts from the value of his study. Carefully controlled studies along these lines may eventually furnish valuable information, but for the present the question of coitus-induced ovulation in man must remain open.

Summary.—In summation, it may be stated that the Knaus-Ogino theory cannot be accepted unreservedly because of the many unproved assumptions on which it rests. Only this is certain, that ovulation tends to occur at approximately the midphase of the cycle, so that this time is most fertile, while other days in the cycle are relatively less so. Whether a period of absolute sterility (safe period) exists is still uncertain. In view of the conflicting evidence on this point, it is unwise to rely solely on the Knaus-Ogino method where contraception is desired. Its application in a given case should be undertaken with full cognizance of its limitations. Where it is desirable to insure optimal conditions for conception, coitus should be practiced during the midphase of the cycle, for all agree that ovulation is most likely to occur at this time. On the other hand, where natural contraception is the objective, the physician may only assure his patient that she is comparatively safe if coitus is limited to those days of the cycle which are sterile according to Knaus' method of calculation. She should be warned, however, that conception at such times, though improbable, is not impossible. The variability in the length of the menstrual cycle is perhaps the greatest stumbling block in predicting the limits of the fertile period, for unexpected irregularities may occur at any time and in any cycle. When calculating the limits of the "safe" period in a specific instance, cognizance should be taken of such factors as illness, undue excitement, nervous shock, use of certain drugs, strenuous exercise and change of environment and climate, for these may alter the normal menstrual rhythm and the time of ovulation. Under such conditions, caution should be exercised until sufficient time has elapsed to show what trend the subsequent cycles will take.

BIBLIOGRAPHY

1. Hitschmann, F., and Adler, L.: Monatschr. f. Geburtsh. u. Gynäk. *27*:1, 1908.
2. Meyer, R.: Zentralbl. f. Gynäk. *37*:50, 1913.
3. Schröder, R.: Monatschr. f. Geburtsh. u. Gynäk. *39*:3, 1914.
4. Halban, J., and Koehler, R.: Arch. f. Gynäk. *103*:575, 1914.
5. Schröder, R.: Arch. f. Gynäk. *101*:1, 1914.
6. Schickele, G.: Gynec. et Obst. *3*:170, 1921.

7. Ogino, K.: Japanese Med. World *8*:147, 1928.
8. Novak, E., and TeLinde, R. W.: J.A.M.A. *83*:900, 1914.
9. Schröder, R.: Veit's Handb. d. Gynäk. *6*:84, 1928.
10. Rock, J., and Bartlett, M. K.: J.A.M.A. *108*:1022, 1937.
11. Allen, E.: Anat. Rec. *37*:351, 1923.
12. Pratt, J. P., Allen, E., Newell, Q. U., and Bland, L. J.: J.A.M.A. *93*:834, 1929.
13. Lewis, W. K.: Bull. Johns Hopkins Hosp. *48*:368, 1931.
14. Siegel, P. W. Zentralbl. f. Gynäk. *45*:984, 1921.
15. Zangemeister, W.: Arch. f. Gynäk. *107*:405, 1917.
16. Weinstock, F.: Zentralbl. f. Gynäk. *58*:2947, 1934.
17. Miller, A. G.: Surg., Gynec. & Obst. *66*:723, 1938.
18. Latz, L. J., and Reiner, E.: Am. J. Obst. & Gynec. *43*:74, 1942.
19. Hartman, C. G.: Am. J. Obst. & Gynec. *26*:600, 1933.
20. Dickinson, R. L.: Am. J. Obst. & Gynec. *33*:1027, 1937.
21. Stapfer: cited by H. Vignes and M. Robey, in Périodes de fécondité et de stérilité chez la femme, Paris, Masson, 1936
22. Knaus, H.: Zentralbl. f. Gynäk. *59*:2642, 1935.
23. Smith, G. V. S., and Smith, O. W.: New England J. Med. *215*:908, 1936.
24. Kurzrok, R.: Am. J. Obst. & Gynec. *28*:319, 1934.
25. Frank, R. T.: J.A.M.A. *103*:393, 1934.
26. Gustavson, R. G., Mason, L. W., Hays, E. E., Wood, T. R., and D'Amour, F. E.: Am. J. Obst. & Gynec. *35*:114, 1938.
27. D'Amour, F. E.: Am. J. Obst. & Gynec. *40*:958, 1940.
28. D'Amour, F. E., and Woods, L.: J. Clin. Endocrinol. *1*:433, 1941.
29. Venning, E. H., and Browne, J. S. L.: Endocrinol. *21*:711, 1937.
30. Hill, R. T., Allen, E., and Kramer, T. C.: Anat. Rec. *63*:239, 1935.
31. Burr, H. S., Hill, R. T., and Allen, E.: Proc. Soc. Exper. Biol. & Med. *33*:109, 1935.
32. Reboul, J., Davis, H., and Friedgood, H. B.: Am. J. Physiol. *120*:724, 1937.
33. Burr, H. S., Musselman, L. K., Barton, D. S., and Kelly, N. B.: Science *86*:312, 1937.
34. Rock, J., Reboul, J., and Wiggers, H. C.: New England J. Med. *217*:654, 1937.
35. Burr, H. S., and Musselman, L. K.: Yale J. Biol. & Med. *9*:155, 1936.
36. Burr, H. S., and Musselman, L. K.: Am. J. Obst. & Gynec. *44*:223, 1942.
37. Langman, L., and Burr, H. S.: Am. J. Obst. & Gynec. *44*:223, 1942.
38. Knaus, H.: Periodic Fertility and Sterility in Women, Vienna, W. Maudrich, 1934.
39. Ogino, K.: Conception Period in Women, English trans. by Mujigawa, Harrisburg, Pa., Medical Arts Publication Co., 1934.
40. Boas, C. van E.: Nederl. tijdschr. v. geneesk. *78*:1938, 1934.
41. Schumacher, P. H.: Monat. f. Geburtsh. u. Gynäk. *110*:193, 1939.
42. Vollmann, R.: Monat. f. Geburtsh. u. Gynäk. *110*:193, 1939.
43. Meyer, R.: Arch. f. Gynäk. *100*:1, 1913.
44. Bryce, T. H., and Teacher, J. H.: Contributions to the Study of the Early Development and Embedding of the Human Ovum, Glasgow, J. Maclehose & Sons, 1908.
45. Triepel, H.: Anat. Anz. *46*:385, 1914; ibid. *48*:133, 1915.
46. Hammond, J., and Walton, A.: J. Exper. Biol. *11*:307, 1934.
47. Young, W. C.: Anat. Rec. *67*:305, 1937.
48. Hartman, C. G.: Am. J. Obst. & Gynec. 7:40, 1924.
49. Lewis, L. L.: Okla. Agr. Exper. Sta. Bull. *96*:3, 1911.
50. Hammond, J.: J. Exper. Biol. *11*:140, 1934.
51. Brault, P.: Bull. Soc. d'obst. et de gynec. *23*:35, 1934.
52. Stokes, W. R.: Biological and Medical Aspects of Contraception, Washington, D. C., Nat'l Comm. of Fed. Legis. for Birth Control, 1934, p. 56.
53. Hammond, J., and Asdell, S. A.: Brit. J. Exper. Biol. *4*:155, 1926.
54. Young, W. C.: J. Morphol. & Physiol. *48*:475, 1929.
55. Moench, G. L.: Am. J. Obst. & Gynec. *38*:153, 1939.
56. Cary, W. H.: J.A.M.A. *106*:2221, 1936.
57. Seymour, F. I.: J.A.M.A. *106*:1728, 1936.
58. Runge, E.: Arch. f. Gynäk. *87*:572, 1909.

59. Haussmann, D.: Uber das Verhalten der Samenfaden in den Geschlechtsorganen des Weibes, Berlin, A. Hirschwald, 1879.
60. Ohlin, C. A.: Acta obst. & gynec. Scandinav. *15*:50, 1935.
61. Grosser, O.: Med. Klin. *56*:706, 1932.
62. McKenzie, F. F., and Terrill, C. E.: Mo. Agr. Sta. Res. Bull. No. 264, 1937.
63. Young, W. C., Dempsey, E. W., and Myers, H. I.: J. Compt. Psychol. *19*:313, 1935.
64. Hartman, C. G.: Sex and Internal Secretions, ed. by E. Allen, Baltimore, Williams, Wilkins Co., 1932, chap. 14.
65. Birnberg, C. H.: Endocrinol. *21*:294, 1937.

References for Table 1

Foster, F. P.: New York Med. J. *49*:610, 1889.
Issmer, E.: Arch. f. Gynäk. *35*:310, 1889.
King, J. L.: Carnegie Contrib. Embryol. *18*:79, 1926; Am. J. Obst. & Gynec. *25*:583, 1933.
Geist, S. H.: Am. J. Obst. & Gynec. *20*:320, 1930.
Allen, E.: Am. J. Obst. & Gynec. *25*:705, 1933.
Engle, E. T., and Shelesnyak, M. C.: Human Biol. *6*:431, 1934.
Fluhmann, C. F.: Am. J. Obst. & Gynec. *27*:73, 1934.
Weinstock, F.: Zentralbl. f. Gynäk. *58*:2947, 1934.
Scipiades, E.: Arch. f. Gynäk. *159*:360, 1935.
Latz, L. J., and Reiner, E.: J.A.M.A. *105*:1241, 1935; Illinois M. J. *71*:210, 1937.
Gunn, D. L., Jenkin, P. M., and Gunn, A. L.: J. Obst. & Gynec. Brit. Emp. *44*:839, 1937.
Pratt, J. P., Allen, E., Newell, Q. U., and Bland, L. J.: J.A.M.A. *93*:834, 1929.

CHAPTER V

ENDOCRINE FACTORS IN MENSTRUATION

INTRODUCTION

Definition.—The application of the term "menstruation" has been the subject of much controversy. Such authorities as R. Meyer,[1] Schröder[2] and Shaw[3] use it to describe periodic uterine bleeding which accompanies disintegration of a pregravid mucosa. These observers maintain that ovulation and corpus luteum formation are necessary precursors of the menstrual process, and that bleeding not preceded by these events in the ovary is not true menstruation. During the past two decades American investigators, particularly Novak,[4] Corner,[5] and Allen,[6] have taken the stand that menstruation should be more broadly defined to include cyclic bleeding, which clinically resembles hemorrhagic disintegration of a pregravid mucosa, but occurs from a proliferative type of endometrium and is preceded by follicular maturation without ovulation or corpus luteum formation. *Menstruation* will be employed here in the narrower sense and *pseudomenstruation* will be applied to menstruation-like bleeding from a proliferative type of mucosa. As will be shown later, though the two forms of bleeding may clinically resemble one another, the features which distinguish them are sufficiently important to warrant their being considered distinct entities.

Significance of the Menstrual Process.—Since ancient times, observers have pondered the purpose of the menstrual flow in the body economy. Perhaps the oldest recorded theory considered it a means whereby the organism rids itself of harmful impurities. Another early belief held that the periodic hemorrhage serves to relieve the body of an excess of blood. An association between this phenomenon and reproductive function was first considered early in the nineteenth century. The observation that periodic uterine bleeding ceases after ovariectomy and during pregnancy, prompted a few investigators to assume that it is dependent upon the presence of the ovaries, and occurs because of failure to conceive. That the ovaries act through hormonal rather than nervous pathways became clear when menstrual bleeding was shown to occur in ovariectomized monkeys bearing ovarian implants or transplants. The meaning of the menstrual phenomenon remained vague, however, largely because its temporal relationship to events in the ovary was not known. Some observers erroneously assumed that menstruation coincides with ovulation and corresponds to estrus in the lower animal. Heape believed it to be the analogue of proestrus bleeding in the dog and cow.

The error of these views was established by Hitschmann and Adler,[7] R. Meyer,[8] and Schröder,[9] who correlated the histologic changes in the ovaries, uteri and uterine curettings during the menstrual cycle. Their findings led them to conclude that menstruation follows ovulation and corpus luteum formation, and ensues only in the absence of conception and following corpus luteum regression. These observations are the basis for the *present conception of menstruation as representing frustration of a physiologic effort to achieve fertility*. It is now generally agreed that it is a degenerative process which marks the end of the anabolic phase of the ovarian and endometrial cycle, and is not analogous to estrus, which represents the acme of growth in the sex cycle.

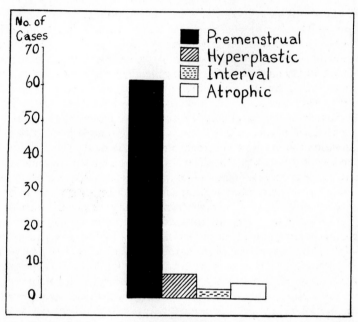

Fig. 26.—Graph showing endometrial findings in seventy-five women with what appeared clinically to be normal periods. It is noteworthy that while 81 per cent showed premenstrual (pregravid) changes before the expected flow, hyperplastic, interval (proliferative), or atrophic changes were encountered in 19 per cent. The terms "pseudomenstruation" or "anovulatory menstruation" have been adopted to describe such cases.

Hartman[10] and Bartelmez[11] believe menstrual bleeding has a physiologic significance, and is analogous to bleeding into the brood-chamber, which occurs in certain species at the time of implantation. This analogy is unconvincing in view of the fact that implantational bleeding occurs in the presence of a fertilized ovum and is presumably intended to nourish it, while menstruation occurs when fertilization has failed, and accompanies destruction of the fetal bed.

CAUSATION OF MENSTRUAL BLEEDING

A discussion of the factors controlling menstruation entails a consideration of the hormonal stimuli which induce the uterine changes that precede and accompany menstruation. In addition it is necessary to consider the role of the uterus per se, whose response to these stimuli determines the onset, amount and duration of the bleeding.

HORMONAL FACTORS IN MENSTRUATION

Some observers maintain that menstruation is a negative phenomenon precipitated by withdrawal of some hormonal stimulus operating during the anabolic phase of the cycle. Others interpret it as a positive phenomenon elicited by some specific substance that acts directly upon the site of the bleeding.

Menstruation as a Negative Phenomenon: Role of the Ovarian Hormones.—The knowledge that the onset of the flow coincides with regression of the corpus luteum was largely responsible for the assumption that menstruation is precipitated by loss of some substance secreted by the yellow body. This belief was strengthened by the observation that, in the monkey and man, excision of a functioning corpus luteum is soon followed by uterine bleeding. The identity of the hormone whose withdrawal leads to menstruation has been the subject of much controversy, for the human corpus luteum contains both estrogen and progestin, and the bleeding which follows its spontaneous regression or destruction may therefore conceivably be due to withdrawal of either or both hormones.

Estrin-Deprivation Theory.—The theory that estrogen withdrawal is the cause of menstruation was first suggested by the observation[12] that bleeding clinically resembling menstruation may follow within a few days after bilateral oophorectomy performed at a time when neither ovary contains a functioning corpus luteum. In support of this view, it has also been pointed out that cyclic bleeding clinically identical with menstruation but not preceded by ovulation or corpus luteum formation occurs during the summer months in certain primates, and occasionally may be encountered in man.[5] Since such bleeding ensues from a mucosa subjected to the action of the follicular hormone alone, it was proposed that periodic uterine hemorrhage, whether from a proliferative or pregravid endometrium, may be accounted for solely on the basis of a withdrawal of estrogen, active principle of the follicle.

Experimental evidence tending to support this so-called "estrin-deprivation" theory of menstruation accumulated rapidly. It has been shown that the bleeding which follows ovariectomy performed during the follicular phase of the cycle can be prevented by administering *estrogen*; or if already started, its amount and duration can be materially reduced.[13] It has been repeatedly demonstrated that menstruation-like bleeding from a proliferative type of mucosa can be induced in the castrate monkey and woman by administering a series of *estrogen injections* and then abruptly stopping treatment. The bleeding thus induced follows the last injection after a latent period, which may vary from five to twenty days or longer. On the basis of the experimental evidence presented thus far,[14] it would appear that the length of the latent period, and the amount and duration of the induced flow, depend to a certain extent on the *dosage and duration of the treatment.* To insure the occurrence of bleeding, the subject must have achieved a certain degree of sexual maturity, and minimum requirements as to daily dosage and length of treatment must be fulfilled. This would imply that the endometrium must attain a certain minimal degree of growth before withdrawal of hormonal support can lead to bleeding. Withdrawal of the hormone must be relatively abrupt; if the daily dose of estrogen is reduced very gradually, the endometrium regresses without bleeding.[15] Complete withdrawal is not essential, mere reduction of the daily dose being sufficient. The extent to which the dose must be reduced apparently does not depend upon the quantity of hormone administered to build up the mucosa. This is evident in Zuckerman's observation[16] that castrate monkeys, receiving doses ranging from 850 to 3000 I.U. daily, did not bleed when the dose was reduced to 200 I.U., but a reduction to 150 I.U. was followed by bleeding within a few days. The fact that the same dose permitted bleeding in animals which had received 850 I.U. and those previously given 3000 I.U. daily may perhaps be explained by assuming that, where large doses are used to build up the mucosa, only part of the hormone is utilized. The amount utilized by the mucosa in Zuckerman's animals probably did not greatly exceed 200 I.U., since this proved sufficient to maintain the integrity of the mucosa and prevent bleeding. On the other hand, 150 I.U. was apparently sufficiently below the minimum requirements for preserving the integrity of the endometrium to permit bleeding. It would appear then that the extent to which the estrogen level must drop to permit bleeding is related to the maximum amount which the endometrium is capable of utilizing and not to the amount of hormone made available for its use.

The validity of the estrin-priva hypothesis has been questioned on the ground that uterine bleeding may occur without estrin deprivation, as indicated by the presence of large amounts of this hormone in the body fluids,[17] or by the absence of any morphologic change in the ovary which might be taken to signify a drop in estrogen production.[18] In experiments involving protracted estrogen stimulation, in the monkey[19] and man,[20] it has been observed that uterine bleeding occurred one or more times during the course of injections, although the supply of the hormone was maintained at a constant level.

Several explanations have been offered in an attempt to reconcile these observations with the estrin-priva theory. The existence of some excretory mechanism which periodically increases estrogen destruction or elimination, has been considered but it still remains unidentified. Zuckerman[21] has suggested that cyclic variations in the activity of the adrenal cortex may, because of its effect on water metabolism, lead to a cyclic rise and fall in the threshold for estrogen stimulation. Corner[18] has stated that it is conceivable that "fluctuations of estrin level can occur without morphologic variation in the ovary, and perhaps . . . the give and take of the pituitary-ovarian (or of the pituitary-ovarian-adrenal) relationship does produce in cyclic fashion an actual estrin deprivation." That the pituitary is not implicated is indicated by Zuckerman's observation[19] that hypophysectomy does not prevent the periodic uterine bleeding which occurs in spayed monkeys receiving daily injections of a "threshold" dose of estrone. This investigator also found[22] that adrenalectomy makes it difficult but not impossible to induce periodic estrus in spayed rats by keeping them at a critical and constant threshold level of estrogenic stimulation. This would seem to exclude the adrenal cortex as the cause of cyclic estrin deprivation, or a cyclic rise and fall in the threshold for estrin stimulation.

The cause of the *bleeding during chronic estrogen administration* may perhaps be found in the endometrium. Of interest is the observation of Allen and associates[23] that the mucosa thickens under the repeated stimulus of the hormone and eventually reaches a point where the original dose becomes inadequate to preserve mucosal integrity and postpone disintegration and hemorrhage. Another explanation is implied in Hisaw's observation[13] that the endometrium of animals receiving chronic estrogen treatment proliferates and thickens very rapidly at first, but soon reaches a point beyond which it ceases to grow. This would suggest that during estrogen treatment, the uterine mucosa cannot proliferate indefinitely, but sooner or later becomes exhausted and disintegrates despite continued adequate hormonal support.

It is also possible that the bleeding noted during chronic estrogen treatment is due to *mechanical rupture of the blood vessels*. The persistent action of the hormone may result in excessive enlargement and disorganization of the vascular apparatus of the endometrium, making for the eruptive type of bleeding. This may account for at least some of the episodes of bleeding which occur in the presence of large amounts of estrogen. It is significant in this connection that abnormal changes of the endometrial blood vessels are a characteristic finding in irregular uterine bleeding from a hyperplastic endometrium,[24] a condition generally attributed to excessive or protracted estrogen stimulation (see Chap. XXV).

In the light of the foregoing discussion, we would not be justified in accepting the occurrence of bleeding in the presence of a constant supply of estrogen as damaging evidence against the estrin-priva theory.

This theory has also been attacked on the ground that *some women may fail to bleed despite a fall in the estrogen level*, as judged by the estrogen content of the body fluids. Fluhmann[25] performed several hundred blood estrogen tests in a group of mature women and found that some experienced no flow despite a recurring rise and fall in the estrogen level of the blood. His findings do not necessarily disprove the estrin-priva theory, for failure to bleed under such circumstances may conceivably be due to a refractory state of the endometrium, which prevents a growth response sufficient to insure the occurrence of bleeding in the event that the estrogen supply is reduced. It is also possible that some of his patients failed to bleed because the drop in the estrogen level was not sufficiently marked to permit endometrial disintegration.

Some observers believe that the long latent period which intervenes between estrogen administration and the onset of bleeding argues against estrin deprivation as the immediate cause of menstrual bleeding. As shown by Engle and Crafts,[26] bleeding may begin as late as thirty to seventy days after a single injection of estrogen in castrate monkeys. It must be emphasized, however, that estrogen deprivation does not necessarily coincide with cessation of injections. It is necessary to take into consideration the time required for complete absorption of the hormone and its utilization by the endometrium. It is also conceivable that actual deprivation of hormonal support may be further delayed by the presence in the castrate organism of substances, possibly of adrenal cortical origin (see Chap. XVI), which are closely related chemically to the estrogens, so that the estrogen-stimulated mucosa can convert them to its use. This possibility is suggested by recent reports that an endometrium which has been developed to the proliferative phase with estrogen, can be maintained in this condition and prevented from disintegrating by adequate doses of *testosterone*.[27] The small amounts available for this purpose in the castrate organism may be sufficient to postpone bleeding for a time, particularly where the endometrial structure built up by exogenous estrogen is small.

On the whole, though many questions still remain unanswered, and others are likely to arise as experimental investigations proceed, estrogen withdrawal appears to offer a reasonable explanation for bleeding from an estrogen-stimulated mucosa. It does not necessarily follow that it can also account for bleeding from a pregravid mucosa, on which both estrogen and progestin have acted. That another factor, namely progestin deprivation, plays an important part in such bleeding has become increasingly apparent during the past decade.

Progestin-Deprivation Theory.—Zuckerman[28] was among the first to take a firm stand against the suggestion that true menstruation may be explained on the basis of estrin deprivation. Earlier attempts to prove that progestin withdrawal is an important factor in the causation of bleeding from a pregravid endometrium were unconvincing. Many investigators[13, 29] succeeded in inducing bleeding from a pregravid mucosa by administering a series of estrogen injections followed by a course of progestin injections. These results failed to establish the precise role of the progestational hormone, because the effect of the estrogen required to prepare the endometrium for progestin could not be excluded. Despite this difficulty, Zuckerman, Hisaw, Engle and others have succeeded, through painstaking studies with various combinations of estrogen and progestin, in throwing considerable light on the relative importance of each in the menstrual process.

Zuckerman[30] has demonstrated that *the normal menstrual rhythm can be mimicked by controlling the level of estrogen and progestin* in the body. This observer induced cyclic bleeding at twenty-eight day intervals in castrate monkeys by administering increasing doses of estrogen up to 3000 I.U. daily for fourteen days, and then giving about 100 I.U. daily during the following two weeks. This monthly rhythm was not significantly altered when progestin was administered daily during the first ten to twelve days of the period when the animals were receiving 100 I.U. of estrogen daily.[31] Zuckerman concluded that a wave of estrogenic stimulation must be regarded as the basic mechanism of the menstrual cycle. His observation that a phase of luteal activity may be superimposed upon a threshold level of estrogen without affecting the periodicity of the bleeding, may account for the observation that, in some women, ovulatory cycles may alternate with anovulatory cycles without any noticeable change in the periodicity of the bleeding.

At first sight, Zuckerman's findings suggest that estrogen withdrawal is the essential factor in inducing periodic bleeding from a pregravid mucosa, while progestin withdrawal plays at best only a minor role. Were this true, it might be expected that estrogen would be more effective than progestin in preventing or postponing bleeding from a pregravid mucosa. Actually, however, the situation is reversed. It has been repeatedly shown that *adequate amounts of progestin can delay mucosal disintegration and bleeding* for long periods of time.[32] Such postponement can be achieved whether the mucosa has previously been stimulated by estrogen alone, or by estrogen and progestin. On the other hand, while estrogen can postpone bleeding from an estrogen-stimulated mucosa, its ability to do so is markedly diminished, if not completely lost, when the mucosa is converted to the pregravid phase.[33] Thus, there is evidence that *normal menstruation may occur in the presence of large quantities of estrogen* in the body fluids, uterine mucosa, and the menstrual blood.[34] A number of investigators have reported failure to delay menstrual bleeding in women with large amounts of estrogen given during the luteal phase of the menstrual cycle. In monkeys and women[35] receiving a series of estrogen injections followed by enough progestin to induce full pregravid changes, estrogen administered thereafter cannot further postpone bleeding, though the amount used would have delayed the bleeding for a long time had progestin been omitted. Recent studies[36] have shown that a short series of progestin injections, given mid-way between the flows in normally menstruating women, may induce intracyclic bleeding. In monkeys under chronic estrogen treatment, a short series[18] or even a single injection of progestin[37] is followed within a few days by bleeding despite continued administration of estrogen. These observations have done much to convince protagonists of the estrin-deprivation theory that its application is limited to pseudomenstruation, and that bleeding from a pregravid endometrium is due in part at least to progestin withdrawal.

The work of Hisaw and Greep[33] in castrated monkeys indicates that, though difficult, it is not impossible to *postpone bleeding from a progestin-stimulated mucosa with estrogen.* According to these investigators, such bleeding can be postponed by administering several times the daily dose needed to bring the endometrium to the proliferative phase. For example, when 100 rat units of estrogen were given daily for twenty-one days, followed by 25 or 50 rat units of estrogen plus 0.5 rabbit unit of progestin daily for eighteen to twenty-one days, and then 500 rat units of estrogen daily for ten to eighteen days, no bleeding occurred at any time during the treatment, although the mucosa had presumably passed successively through a proliferative, a secretory, and again through a proliferative phase. This may explain why some women fail to menstruate for long periods of time, despite normal cyclic events in the ovary and endometrium, as revealed by repeated endometrial biopsies (see Chap. XXIV). The transition of the mucosa from secretory to proliferative activity, without interruption by bleeding, may conceivably be due to the presence of unusually large amounts of estrogen at the time of corpus luteum regression.

There has been much speculation as to why *estrogen partially or completely loses its ability to postpone bleeding when the endometrium is subjected to the action of progestin.* Hisaw suggests that estrogen and progestin compete physiologically for mastery of the cells of the endometrium. Corner[35] considers direct chemical antagonism unlikely because of the close chemical similarity between the two hormones. He reasons that the blockade set up in the receptor tissues by the action of progestin may be either on a physiochemical level, depending on molecular states in the tissue, or at a morphological level, the histological effects of progestin being so different from those of estrogen that the latter cannot avert their retrogression. It seems likely that the competition between estrin and progestin is physiological and arises out of the fact that the former stimulates growth, the latter, secretory activity in the endometrium. As pointed out by Loeb,[38] there is an antagonism between mitotic cell proliferation (growth) and function (secretory activity) which is "due mainly to a differentiation which takes place in the cell in the course of time and which is prevented or delayed by the effect of growth stimuli. The antagonism is reciprocal. Growth inhibits those alterations in the cell which tend to initiate certain functional activities like secretion, and progressive differentiation is unfavorable to the development of those changes on which mitotic division depends. . . . We find the same phenomena in growth of glandular structures in general. Growth stimuli of embryonal or regenerative character induce cells which are yet less differentiated to proliferate. This growth is accompanied by differentiation which itself limits growth and prepares the cells for secretory activity."

If it is granted that this principle is applicable to the uterine mucosa, it becomes clear why estrin and progestin are at once synergistic and antagonistic in their effect on the endometrium. As shown elsewhere (see Chap. II), if the *dose of estrogen* is kept within certain limits, it enhances the action of progestin on the mucosa, but if these limits are exceeded, it may interfere with the secretory response.[31] Conversely, as Hisaw[33] and Zuckerman[28] have shown, where secretory activity of the mucosa has been induced by *progestin*, it becomes progessively more difficult for estrogen to exert its specific growth-promoting effect. As a result, it gradually loses its ability to maintain the mucosa and a daily dose equivalent to that used to develop the endometrium is no longer effective in postponing the flow.

It is not yet certain whether *the action of progestin on the glandular elements, stroma, blood vessels* or all three is the decisive factor in determining whether or not withdrawal of this hormone will cause bleeding despite the presence of estrogen. According to Hisaw,[33] the increased resistance to the hemorrhage-inhibiting action of estrogen, created by progestin stimulation, is not closely correlated with the histological status of the glands. He found that a daily dose of 500 rat units of estrogen postponed bleeding from endometria in which a typical pregravid reaction had presumably been elicited by daily injections of 25 or 50 rat units of estrogen plus 0.5 rabbit unit of progestin. On the other hand, the same amount of estrogen failed to postpone bleeding from endometria in which presumably only early secretory activity had been induced by administering 100 rat units of estrogen plus 1 rabbit unit of progestin daily for ten days. Hisaw concluded that the particular effect of progestin which makes the mucosa resistant to the hemorrhage-inhibiting action of estrogen occurs independently of, and much earlier than, the glandular changes, and probably involves the stroma and vascular apparatus of the endometrium.

Noteworthy in this connection is Watson and McHenry's observation[39] that the administration of estrogen followed by progestin in the castrate monkey is followed by bleeding associated with necrosis limited to the epithelium of those glands which have been fully activated by progestin, and to the stroma surrounding them. These observers suggest that "during the functional stage, the internal economy of the epithelial cells in the endometrium is so altered by the accumulation within the cell of the secretion to be elaborated, that a return to their former state after the stimulus to the formation of secretion has been withdrawn is impossible."

In the light of the available evidence, it seems reasonable to conclude that *bleeding from a pregravid mucosa is due to withdrawal of progestin and,* to a lesser extent, *of estrin.* The relative importance of each probably varies according to the completeness of the pregravid transformation. This in turn apparently depends on the extent of the endometrial structure built up under the influence of estrogen, the amount of progestin available, the length of time during which it is permitted to act, and the reactivity of the mucosa to the two hormones. Estrogen probably loses its ability to prevent endometrial bleeding when the area modified by progestin and no longer responsive to the influence of estrogen is so extensive that its dissolution, upon progestin withdrawal, brings in its wake a destruction of the supporting stroma and blood vessels sufficiently far-reaching to result in outwardly visible bleeding.

If this is conceded to be the mechanism involved, it would explain why estrogen injections fail to postpone the expected flow if treatment is begun during the luteal phase, but may do so if begun during the follicular phase of the cycle, in the monkey[40] and man.[41] By administering adequate amounts of estrogen before progestin has gained a foothold, it is possible to check conversion of the endometrium to the secretory phase. As a result, the mucosa remains responsive to estrogen despite the intervening luteal phase in the ovary. The observation that, in the normal ovulatory cycle, menstrual bleeding follows corpus luteum regression despite the presence of large amounts of estrogen also becomes understandable. Estrogen, in the quantity available, is apparently incapable of causing the fully converted progestational mucosa to retrace its steps to the proliferative phase, and at best can enact merely a supplementary role in maintaining the integrity of the endometrium. Upon withdrawal of the main support, progestin, the structure falls, and only after it is removed by desquamation and the way cleared for a new growth, can estrogen reassert its supremacy and induce proliferative changes once more.

Menstruation as a Positive Phenomenon.—Hartman and his associates[42] first suggested that menstrual bleeding may be due to the direct action of a *bleeding factor* elaborated by the adenohypophysis. This was based on their observation that the bleeding which follows estrin depriva-tion in the castrate monkey can be prevented by hypophysectomy. On the other hand, the ovariectomized, hypophysectomized monkey responds with microscopic bleeding to gonadotropic extracts of anterior lobe tissue or human pregnancy urine. This theory was subsequently questioned by Saiki[43] on the ground that he could not induce bleeding in hypophysec-tomized monkeys with anterior pituitary or pregnancy urine extracts unless the ovaries were intact. He concluded that the bleeding which follows administration of anterior lobe extract depends on the presence of func-tioning ovaries and therefore may not be considered the effect of a pitui-tary "bleeding hormone," acting directly on the uterus. Engle[44] pointed out that Hartman succeeded in inducing bleeding in the absence of ovarian tissue only when he administered crude pregnancy urine gonadotropic extract, which is known to produce local congestion in the primate uterus. This, coupled with the fact that the monkey uterus can readily be made to bleed by non-specific substances, led him to conclude that the bleeding noted by Hartman in hypophysectomized, ovariectomized monkeys was a non-specific effect. His interpretation was subsequently conceded by Hartman.[45]

Prompted by Markee's observation[46] that vasoconstriction is a constant precursor of menstrual bleeding (see below), Hartman and Firor[47] at-tempted to demonstrate that the *vasoconstrictor principle* of the posterior hypophysis is the "bleeding factor." Their findings in estrogen-treated monkeys, from which the whole hypophysis, or all except the posterior lobe and pars intermedia had been removed, seemed to support this possi-bility. To test it further, Hartman and Geiling[48] administered pituitrin continuously to cyclically bleeding monkeys, but though a vasoconstrictor effect was produced, the onset of the flow was not hastened. In a similar experiment, Markee[49] observed blanching but no bleeding in ocular endo-metrial transplants of pituitrin-injected monkeys. These negative findings, together with the observation of Smith and his associates[50] that estrin-priva bleeding can be induced in completely hypophysectomized monkeys, finally convinced Hartman that the "bleeding factor," if it exists at all, does not originate in the hypophysis. As an alternative possibility, he has suggested that a vasoconstrictor substance produced within the uterus may be the immediate cause of menstrual bleeding.[51]

That the positive and negative theories of menstruation are reconcil-able is suggested by recent evidence relating to the sequence of events in the uterus leading to menstrual bleeding.

Sequence of Events Shortly Before and During Menstruation

The available information concerning events in the menstruating human uterus is derived mainly from studies of uteri and uterine curet-tings. The first important contributions to this subject were made by Hitschmann and Adler,[7] Schröder,[9] and others whose findings have since been amply confirmed. While these observers were fully cognizant of the essential changes which characterize the menstrual process, they could only surmise, from their histologic material, the normal sequence of these

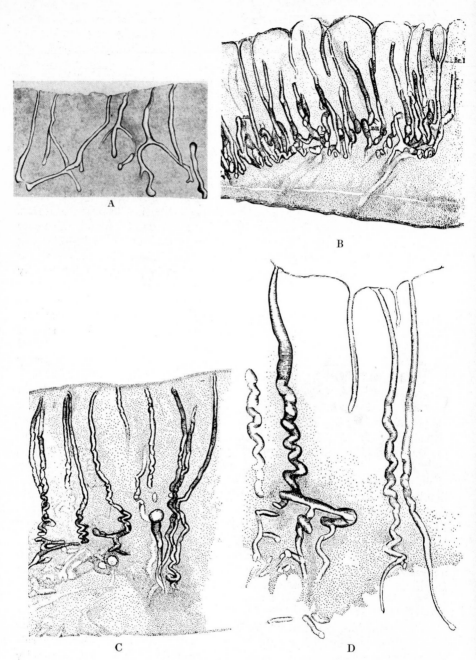

Fig. 27.—Reconstruction of human uterine glands (O'Leary). A, Transition between phase of repair and that of proliferation (tissue obtained nine days postmenstruum); B, early proliferative phase (tissue obtained thirteen days postmenstruum); C, early proliferative phase (tissue obtained eleven days postmenstruum); D, transition between proliferative and pregravid phase (tissue obtained ten days postmenstruum).

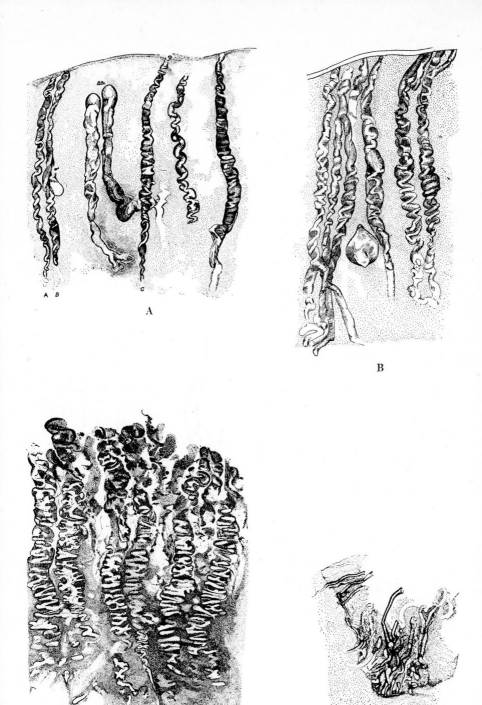

Fig. 28.—Reconstruction of human uterine glands (O'Leary). A, Early pregravid phase (tissue obtained twenty days postmenstruum); B, height of pregravid phase; endometrium is approaching menstruation (tissue obtained thirty days postmenstruum); C, menstruation (first day); D, menstruation (second day).

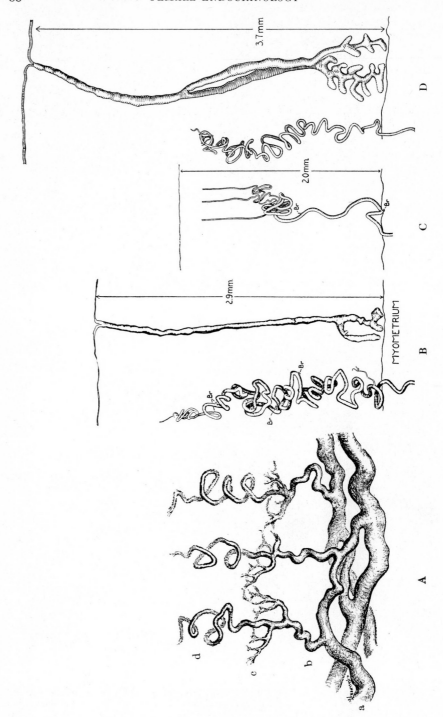

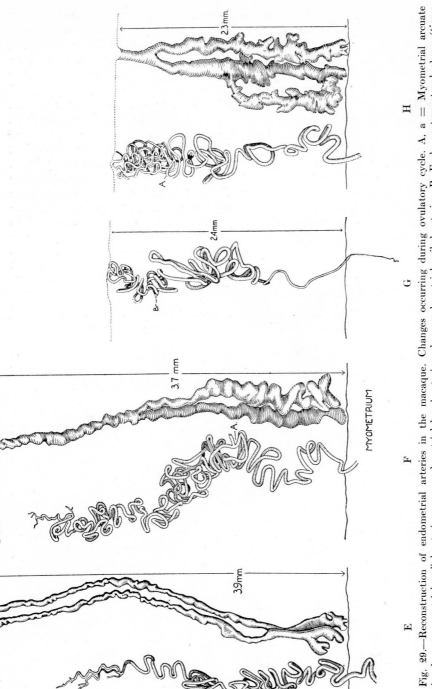

Fig. 29.—Reconstruction of endometrial arteries in the macaque. Changes occurring during ovulatory cycle. A, a = Myometrial arcuate arteries; b = myometrial radial arteries; c = endometrial basal arteries; d = endometrial coiled arteries. B, Early postmenstrual phase (tissue obtained four days postmenstruum). C, Early proliferative phase (tissue obtained eight days postmenstruum). D, Proliferative phase of ovulatory cycle (tissue obtained eleven days postmenstruum). E, Early progravid phase (tissue obtained sixteen days postmenstruum). F, Late progravid phase (tissue obtained thirteen days postmenstruum). G, Menstrual phase of ovulatory cycle (early first day). H. Menstrual phase of ovulatory cycle (third day). (A. after Okkels and Engel; B–H, after Daron.)

changes and their relation to each other. Such information is obviously best obtained by directly observing the menstrual process in vivo. Markee[46] recently accomplished this in the macaque by microscopically examining ocular endometrial transplants. Although such transplants cannot exactly duplicate conditions existing in the uterus in situ, they have nevertheless yielded significant information. Markee's observations in vivo,[52] coupled with Bartelmez'[11] histologic studies of the menstruating human uterus, and Daron's[53] description of the endometrial blood vessels in the monkey, have contributed greatly to our present understanding of the sequence of events in the primate uterus shortly before and during menstruation. Daron[53] distinguished two types of arteries in the uterine mucosa: large, tortuous, coiled arteries, and small arteries which extend only into the basal zone of the mucous membrane. The coils of the first type are closely wound, forming a radial column through the mucosa. They have very few branches along their course but divide peripherally, rather abruptly, into numerous pre-capillary arterioles. In ovulatory cycles, the coiled arteries exhibit a progressive increase in extent toward the uterine lumen and also an increase in tortuosity, so that in the late pregravid phase, they are immediately under the surface epithelium. The second type of arteries, which extend only into the basal zone of the mucous membrane, are not involved in the cyclic changes (see Fig. 29). Daron[59] has also described small veins coursing parallel to each other in a centrifugal fashion from the uterine lumen, without uniting to form larger trunks basalward. Anastomoses at acute angles between parallel veins are very numerous, while in the middle third of the endometrium there appear larger "venous lakes," that is, greatly dilated veins at the site of certain anastomoses.

Changes Preceding Bleeding.—On the basis of the available data, events in the primate uterus at the end of the anabolic phase are thought to proceed as follows: With the onset of the catabolic phase, endometrial activity gradually ceases and extensive and rapid regression occurs. The result is a disproportion between the length of the coiled arteries and the thickness of the endometrium. By reason of this disproportion, additional coils form, retarding the blood flow through the arteries and their branches. This results in stasis, which precedes the onset of bleeding by one to three days. From four to twenty-four hours before the onset of the flow, that portion of the coiled arteries located in the deepest part of the endometrium or adjacent uterine muscle, becomes constricted. Daron[53] observed such constriction only in pregravid endometria, but Markee[52] noted it also during estrin-priva bleeding. This produces an *ischemic necrosis* of the superficial part of the endometrium. Degenerative changes follow with crumbling of tissue which, localized at first, eventually becomes generalized. The glands and supporting stroma, as well as the terminal branches of the arterioles and parts of the coiled arteries proper are involved in this destructive process. The degenerative process is checked at the point where the glands and coiled arterioles enter the basalis, probably because this area possesses an independent blood supply, provided by the small arteries which extend into this region alone.

Bleeding.—Bleeding does not begin at the same time in all parts of the mucous membrane, and normally occurs only once in a given region during any menstrual period. Because of the constriction of the radial myometrial arteries, and the marked coiling of the arterioles as they pass through the endometrium, no blood circulates through them except in individual arteries which may relax for a time and then contract once more. Blood escapes from the capillaries and arterioles by diapedesis, or through breaks or defects in their degenerating walls. It may pass directly through the stroma and surface epithelium into the uterine cavity, or may collect in subepithelial lakes that bulge and finally rupture.

In addition to the blood derived from the capillaries and arterioles, the menstrual discharge may be amplified by "direct" or *"reflux" hemorrhages* from the veins, which apparently remain patent during menstruation. As Daron[53] has emphasized, bleeding from the ends of the coiled arteries is rare, but bleeding veins are a frequent finding in the menstruating uterus.

Cessation of Bleeding.—Menstrual bleeding is normally terminated when an adequate circulation is established by dilation of the straight arteries, growth of some of them, and development of a new capillary bed from the portion of the coiled arteries just proximal to their necrotic tips. After menstruation ceases in a given region, the denuded stroma once again becomes covered by epithelium that grows from the tips of the remaining portions of the glands.

Factors Precipitating Menstruation.—From the foregoing description, it is apparent that the initial step in the menstrual process is *regression and shrinkage of the mucosa*. Since this is clearly traceable to the loss of hormonal support which occurs at this time, *hormone withdrawal* may reasonably be regarded as the precipitating cause of menstruation. The fact that vasoconstriction is a constant precursor of actual bleeding lends support to Hartman's suggestion[51] that some *vasoconstrictor substance* produced by the uterus participates in the menstrual process. However, this hypothetical substance probably plays at best only a secondary role, for, as demonstrated in pituitrin-treated monkeys,[48, 49] vasoconstriction per se does not cause menstrual bleeding. Since vasoconstriction occurs only after stasis has produced an injurious anoxemia, it may be as Markee has suggested, that the uterus produces a vasoconstrictor during the period of stasis. There is reason to believe that *chemical changes* actually occur during this period, for blood which remains long in the degenerating mucosa loses its coagulability, while that which passes through it quickly, retains this property. Moreover, blood present in the endometrium first begins to take on the color and composition of menstrual blood while it remains stagnant in the endometrial blood vessels, the extent to which it is modified depending on how long it is permitted to stagnate.[54] Thus, it would seem that formation of a vasoconstrictor substance within the uterus, if it occurs at all, is merely a secondary effect of hormone withdrawal and constitutes simply one step in the chain of events leading to desquamation and bleeding.

The identity of this hypothetical vasoconstrictor substance is not yet known and proof that it originates within the endometrium is still lacking. Brewer's observation[55] that spasm of the skin capillaries occurs premenstrually at approximately the same time that vasoconstriction takes place in the endometrium, suggests that a vasoconstrictor substance is present in the circulating blood at this time. Whether the same substance is responsible for both effects, and whether the uterus produces it or derives it from the circulating blood cannot be decided from the evidence at hand.

UTERINE FACTORS CONTROLLING AMOUNT AND DURATION OF THE MENSTRUAL FLOW

There is reason to believe that the amount and duration of the flow are controlled to a large extent by the activity of the endometrial blood vessels and uterine musculature.

Blood Vessels.—The *spiral shape* of the endometrial arterioles has frequently been emphasized as an important factor in minimizing the blood loss during menstruation. It also seems fairly certain that the *vasoconstriction* characteristic of the menstrual phase not only favors tissue necrosis, but also prevents excessive blood loss. It is not certain whether this constriction is due solely to the independent activity of the blood vessel walls, or is at least partly attributable to changes in the activity of the *muscle fibers* that envelope these vessels as they pass through the myometrium on their way to the mucosa. Bucura[56] and, more recently, Joachimowitz,[57] and Bartelmez[11] have described longitudinal bundles of muscle fibers which are situated immediately beneath the tunica intima of the arteries, usually on one side of the vessel, and may conceivably influence the flow of blood. In the middle zone of the myometrium, at the point where the arteries branch into arterioles, Keiffer[58] has observed groups of arterioles surrounded by bundles of muscles so arranged that they can either promote or impede the blood flow.

There is evidence indicating that the activity of the *uterine veins* may also influence the amount and duration of the menstrual flow. Daron[59] observed that bleeding veins are a frequent finding in the menstruating mucosa and concluded that, after the initial rupture of subepithelial hematomata and general denudation, much blood is lost by regurgitation from a source deep in the endometrium. He suggests that, while the initiation of menstruation depends primarily upon the arterioles, the total amount of blood lost is controlled by the veins. Keiffer[54] has described what he calls *venous hearts*, valvular and contractile modifications of the venous walls which show rhythmic dilatation and contraction related to the contractions of the uterus as a whole. To them he ascribes the dominant role in producing the characteristic vascular changes incident to menstruation.

Myometrium.—A number of observers have attempted to relate the activity of the endometrial blood vessels to that of the myometrium. Lahm[60] attributed premenstrual venous congestion to an atonia of the uterine muscle. Marlow[61] has likewise stressed the importance of myometrial activity, pointing out that "in the premenstrual phase, while the high pressure arterial system distributes blood to the endometrium, the low pressure valveless venous outflow system becomes more and more embarrassed because of myometrial grasp." Westman[64] maintains that the influence of changes in the contractility of the uterine muscle on the blood flow is a factor in the mechanism of menstruation which is too often overlooked.

Bartelmez[11] has suggested that venous drainage may depend on rhythmic uterine contractions which, if retarded or inhibited before menstruation, may conceivably cause venous congestion.

In a study of menstruating human endometria, Bartelmez could find no evidence of constriction of the arterioles in the mucosa, and concluded that we must look to the myometrium for the cause of menstrual ischemia. Noteworthy in this connection is Daron's observation[53] that the arteries in the menstruating macaque's uterus are constricted as they pass through the myometrium, but enlarge abruptly as they enter the mucous membrane. Also significant is Markee's[52] statement that the vasoconstriction seen during menstruation is confined to that part of the artery which is located in the deepest portion of the endometrium or in the adjacent uterine muscle.

Interrelation of Vascular and Myometrial Activity.—Recent studies indicate that vascular and myometrial activity, if not causally related, are at least closely correlated, not only during menstruation but throughout the menstrual cycle. Fagin and Reynolds[62] observed that no congestion occurs during the follicular phase of the cycle because of the small but steady contractions which occur at this time. They found that estrogen causes dilatation of the endometrial blood vessels and increases their permeability, with the result that the endometrium becomes edematous. As estrogen treatment is continued, it initiates intermittent contractility of the uterus which serves to increase the volume of blood flow through the dilated endometrial vessels, thus preventing undue congestion. There is evidence (see Chap. VI) that, during the luteal phase, the tonus of the uterine muscle is lowered and the contractions are slower but more ample, a fact which probably accounts for the edema and congestion of the endometrium at this time. Shortly before and during menstruation there occur increasingly powerful myometrial contractions which, according to Moir,[63] may become so powerful as to obliterate completely the pulsations of the arteries.

Compression of the radial myometrial arteries may be at least partly attributable to the fact that the muscle fibers, which grow longer and looser during the luteal phase, under the influence of *progestin*, shrink when this hormone is withdrawn. This possibility is suggested by Westman[64] on the basis of the observation that, in the pseudopregnant rabbit, within a short time after corpus luteum ablation, the previously relaxed uterus becomes markedly contracted and pale.

In the light of the foregoing discussion, it seems likely that all constitutents of the uterus participate in the menstrual process, though the relative importance of each is still uncertain. On the whole, the available evidence indicates that the response of the glandular elements to *changes in the level of the two ovarian hormones* determines whether growth or secretory activity shall continue, or cease and be followed by regression, shrinkage, and eventually by tissue dissolution and bleeding. The endometrial blood vessels, built up during the anabolic phase by estrogen and progestin, are a source of menstrual blood but, because of their coiled form, also aid in checking the further flow of blood into the uterine cavity.

The resulting ischemia favors tissue necrosis and speeds up the process of desquamation which clears the endometrium for a new growth. The response of the myometrium to variations in the level of estrogen and progestin (see Chap. VI) probably also influences the amount and duration of the flow.

COMPARISON OF CHANGES DURING MENSTRUATION AND PSEUDOMENSTRUATION

Tissue Loss.—Systematic attempts to compare the events in the uterus during menstruation and pseudomenstruation have thus far been limited. According to Markee,[52] essentially the same vascular alterations precede bleeding from a proliferative and from a pregravid mucosa. He could observe striking differences only between ovulatory cycles with maximum growth and anovulatory cycles with minimum growth. He lists the following ten differences: "In ovulatory cycles (1) the period of vasodilatation is more marked; (2) greater regression occurs in the transplant; (3) the coiled arteries are more highly developed; (4) additional coils appear earlier during regression; (5) the ends of the coiled arteries approach nearer the surface of the endometrium before the onset of bleeding, and during it more of them project above the denuded surface; (6) there is greater loss of blood; (7) a larger proportion of the hemorrhages are from the arterioles and capillaries; (8) a smaller proportion are from the veins; (9) more of the endometrium is desquamated; and (10) the fragments are larger." The reports of Bartelmez[11] and Daron[53] also reveal certain differences between the two types of bleeding. Bartelmez[11] noted varying degrees of tissue loss during bleeding from a pregravid mucosa, in contrast to little or no loss during bleeding from a proliferative type of endometrium. This is consistent with the observation that there is comparatively little tissue loss in *hyperplastic bleeding*, which likewise occurs from a mucosa stimulated by estrogen alone (see Chap. XXV). As R. Meyer[65] has pointed out, it is very unusual for a hyperplastic endometrium to be desquamated to the same extent as a menstruating mucosa. Frankl[24] has also called attention to the fact that only partial desquamation occurs in bleeding from a hyperplastic endometrium. A possible explanation is suggested by Watson and McHenry's observation[39] that tissue loss during true menstruation is limited to that tissue which has completed its life cycle, so to speak, by undergoing complete transformation to the pregravid, secretory phase. Since no such transformation occurs in the mucosa stimulated by estrogen alone, it is not surprising that the tissue is not desquamated in the same manner or to the same extent as in true menstruation.

Blood Vessel Destruction.—Daron[53] observed that the blood vessels are much more extensively involved in the destructive process in ovulatory than in anovulatory bleeding. A possible explanation is suggested by his observation that, in the monkey uterus, the arterioles lie immediately beneath the surface in the pregravid mucosa, but extend only part way through the endometrium in the proliferative mucosa, whose superficial portion is supplied only by capillaries and veins. This difference in the extent of tissue loss and blood vessel destruction during bleeding from a proliferative and secretory type of mucosa may possibly account for the observation[66] that bleeding begins much sooner after progestin than after estrogen withdrawal.

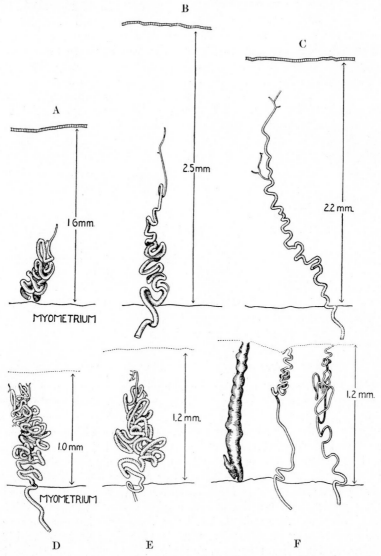

Fig. 30.—Reconstruction of endometrial arteries in the macaque. Changes occurring during anovulatory cycle (Daron). A, Nineteenth day postmenstruum; B, twenty-first day postmenstruum; C, twenty-sixth day postmenstruum; D, first day of menstrual phase; E, second day of menstrual phase; F, second day of menstrual phase.

Although destruction of the blood vessels would seem to be more extensive in true menstrual bleeding, Hartman's observations[67] in the monkey indicate that the amount of blood lost is not appreciably greater. In explanation, Daron[53] has suggested that the vasoconstriction and the resulting menstrual blanch are more prolonged in true menstrual bleeding. His observation that evidence of constriction was present in most of his menstrual (ovulatory) and in only a few of his pseudomenstrual (anovulatory) specimens apparently supports this possibility. It is also significant that Bartelmez[11] found no sign of a capillary circulation in his menstrual (ovulatory) specimens, but did find evidence of blood in the superficial capillaries of a few of the pseudomenstrual (anovulatory) endometria. Markee,[52] on the other hand, could observe no appreciable difference between the degree of vasoconstriction in the two types of bleeding.

Myometrial Activity.—Comparative studies of myometrial activity during menstruation and pseudomenstruation are limited. Wilson and Kurzrok[68] found that during anovulatory cycles the uterus shows the high tonus and small, rapid contractions which characterize the follicular phase of the normal menstrual cycle. In the ovulatory cycle, on the other hand, this type of activity is replaced during the luteal phase by slow contractions of considerable amplitude and an associated fall in tonus. The amplitude of the contractions increases steadily as the time of the flow approaches, and reaches a maximum height on the first or second day of menstruation. These observers failed to state whether, in the anovulatory cycle, any appreciable change occurs in the rapidity of the contractions or in the tonus of the musculature as the bleeding phase approaches. Theoretically, if it is true that the bleeding in such cycles is due to a drop in the estrogen level, a coincident diminution in myometrial activity might be expected. Findings similar to those of Wilson and Kurzrok have been more recently described by Henry and Browne.[72]

THE CENTRAL NERVOUS SYSTEM AND MENSTRUATION

It is well known that emotional shock, such as great joy or fright, may delay or precipitate the menstrual flow. The mechanism involved has not yet been defined. Bleeding from the uterus has been observed following transection of the nervous connections of the ovary, either peripherally or in the spinal cord. Van Wagenen,[69] who transected the spinal cord at different levels between the eighth and twelfth thoracic segment in monkeys, found that uterine bleeding occurred after a latent period which was progressively shortened as the level of transection was lowered. The effect apparently depended on the presence of the ovaries, since no bleeding occurred when castrate animals were used. The ovarian change produced by the operation was apparently transient, for the postoperative bleeding was followed by normal menstrual periods. Markee and his associates[70] found that in most cases transection induced bleeding in the uterus in situ, but not in ocular endometrial transplants, which had bled cyclically before the operation. In the few instances where the transplant bled following transection, hemorrhage began after bleeding from the uterus in situ had ceased, whereas before operation menstrual bleeding had occurred simultaneously in both. The latent period between operation and the onset of bleeding was shorter after transection than following ovariectomy. They concluded that local congestion of the vascular bed, rather than a drop in the estrogen level, was responsible for the induced bleeding.

Granting that nervous stimuli may either precipitate or postpone the menstrual flow, it does not follow that the nervous system participates in the control of the menstrual process. Reports of menstruation in endometrial transplants in the monkey's eye[52] and the human vagina[71] provide convincing evidence that menstruation is not dependent on nervous factors.

SUMMARY

Although our understanding of menstruation is still far from complete, we now possess sufficient information upon which to base a working hypothesis as to the causation of menstrual bleeding and deviations from the normal. It is evident that numerous factors are implicated. An important link in the chain of effect, and one which has been too often overlooked in the enthusiasm of seeking out some hormonal cause, is the uterus itself, with its complex neuromuscular and vascular system. There is no doubt that the ovarian sex hormones and, indirectly, the anterior pituitary sex principles play a leading role in the menstrual process, but it is equally clear that the response of the uterus is likewise important. In seeking to explain the mechanism of menstrual bleeding and disorders of menstruation, two groups of factors must be considered: the hormonal stimuli emanating from the ovary, which are in turn directly dependent upon anterior lobe function; and the endometrial, neuromuscular and vascular constituents of the uterus.

It would appear that the withdrawal of estrogen in the anovulatory cycle, and of estrogen and progestin in the ovulatory cycle precipitates bleeding from the uterus. Withdrawal of hormonal support is followed by regression of the endometrial structure built up by the ovarian hormones. The blood vessels developed during the cycle for the nourishment of the mucosa are directly affected by loss of hormonal support, and indirectly by the glandular and stromal degeneration which is simultaneously initiated. These one-way circuits, once opened, have no recourse except to empty their contents into the uterine cavity. Contraction or recoil of the uterine musculature and vaso-constriction of the endometrial arterioles interfere with the further entrance of blood into the mucosal blood vessels until a new cycle is initiated. Growth of new blood vessels associated with endometrial growth then closes the blood circuit so that bleeding does not occur again until a degenerative phase is reached once more.

On the basis of our present knowledge, the prerequisites for normal menstruation may be listed as follows:

1. A normally functioning anterior pituitary gland which produces the follicle-stimulating and luteinizing fractions in the proper amount and at the appropriate time of the cycle (see Chap. XII).

2. A responsive ovary which is capable of follicular maturation, ovulation, and corpus luteum formation under the influence of the anterior pituitary gonadotropic hormones.

3. A responsive uterus with:

   (a) A normal mucosa capable of proliferation and secretory activity under the influence of estrogen and progestin respectively.

   (b) A normal vascular system which, under the influence of the ovarian sex hormones, estrin and progestin, develops and brings an adequate supply of blood to the uterine mucosa; and, on withdrawal of these hormones, responds with constriction of the arterioles to some substance, possibly of uterine origin.

   (c) A normally developed myometrium with a neuromuscular system capable of helping to check the flow of blood to the endometrial blood vessels during the catabolic phase.

The ovarian and endometrial events leading to bleeding from a pregravid mucosa apparently differ in certain respects from those culminating in bleeding from an estrogenic type of endometrium. Because of these differences, and despite recent evidence indicating that the vascular alterations immediately preceding the onset of bleeding are the same in both, the use of the terms "menstruation" and "pseudomenstruation" to distinguish between them, would appear to be justified.

BIBLIOGRAPHY

1. Meyer, R.: Ber. u. d. ges. Gynäk. u. Geburtsh. 26:268, 1934.
2. Schröder, R.: Am. J. Obst. & Gynec. 16:155, 1928.
3. Shaw, W.: Brit. Med. J. 1:7, 1934.
4. Novak, E.: Am. J. Obst. & Gynec. 16:155, 1939.
5. Corner, G. W.: J.A.M.A. 89:1838, 1927.
6. Allen, E.: Carnegie Inst. Wash. Pub. No. 380, Contrib. Embryol. No. 98, 19:1, 1927.
7. Hitschmann, F., and Adler, L.: Monatschr. f. Geburtsh. u. Gynäk. 27:1, 1908.
8. Meyer, R.: Arch. f. Gynäk. 100:1, 1913.
9. Schröder, R.: Zentralbl. f. Gynäk. 38:1321, 1914.
10. Hartman, C. G.: J.A.M.A. 92:1992, 1929.
11. Bartelmez, G.: Carnegie Inst. Wash. Pub. No. 443, Contrib. Embryol. No. 142, 24:141, 1933; J.A.M.A. 116:702, 1941.
12. Allen, E.: Carnegie Inst. Wash. Pub. No. 380, Contrib. Embryol. No. 98, 29:1, 1927.
13. Hisaw, F. L.: Am. J. Obst. & Gynec. 29:638, 1935.
14. Engle, E. T.: Am. J. Obst. & Gynec. 38:600, 1939.
15. Markee, J. E.: Unpubd. communication, cited by Hartman, C. G., and Firor, W. M.: Quart. Rev. Biol. 12:85, 1937.
    Hisaw, F. L., and Greep, R. O.: Endocrinol. 23:1, 1938.
16. Zuckerman, S.: J. Physiol. 87:51P, 1936.
17. Siebke, H.: Zentralbl. f. Gynäk. 54:1601, 1930.
18. Corner, G. W.: Am. J. Obst. & Gynec. 38:862, 1939.
19. Engle, E. T., and Smith, P. E.: Anat. Rec. 61:471, 1935.
    Zuckerman, S.: J. Endocrinol. 2:263, 1941.
20. Reynolds, S. R. M., Kaminester, S., and Schloss, S.: Proc. Soc. Exper. Biol. & Med. 45: 749, 1940.
    di Paola, G., and del Castillo, E. B.: J. Clin. Endocrinol. 2:215, 1942.
21. Zuckerman, S.: Proc. Roy. Soc., London, s.B. 123:457, 1937; J. Physiol. 89:49P, 1937.
    Long, C. N. H., and Zuckerman, S.: Nature, London, 139:1106, 1937.
22. Zuckerman, S., and Bourne, G.: J. Endocrinol. 2:268, 1941.
23. Allen, E., Hisaw, F. L., and Gardner, W. U.: Sex and Internal Secretions, Baltimore, Williams & Wilkins Co., 1939, chap. 8, p. 452.

24. Frankl, O.: Wien. med. Wchnschr. *84*:570, 1934.
25. Fluhmann, C. F.: Endocrinol. *30*:318, 1936.
26. Engle, E. T., and Crafts, R. C.: Proc. Soc. Exper. Biol. & Med. *39*:564, 1938.
27. Engle, E. T., and Smith, P. E.: Endocrinol. *25*:1, 1939.
     Duncan, P. A., Allen, E., and Hamilton, J. B.: Endocrinol. *28*:107, 1941.
28. Zuckerman, S.: Proc. Zool. Soc., London, p. 691, 1930; Brit. Med. J. *2*:1093, 1932.
29. Kaufmann, C.: Zentralbl. f. Gynäk. *56*:2058, 1932; ibid. *57*:42, 1933.
30. Zuckerman, S.: Proc. Roy. Soc., London, s.B. *123*:441, 1937.
31. Zuckerman, S.: Proc. Roy. Soc., London, s.B. *124*:150, 1937.
32. Wiesbader, H., Engle, E. T., and Smith, P. E.: Am. J. Obst. & Gynec. *32*:1039, 1936.
33. Hisaw, F. L., and Greep, R. O.: Endocrinol. *23*:1, 1938.
     Kaufmann, C.: Zentralbl. f. Gynäk. *59*:1508, 1935.
     Gillman, J.: S. African J. Med. Sci. *3*:66, 1938.
34. Frank, R. T.: The Female Sex Hormone, Springfield, Ill., Chas. C. Thomas, 1929.
     Yerby, L. D.: Proc. Soc. Exper. Biol. & Med. *36*:496, 1937.
35. Corner, G. W.: Am. J. Physiol. *124*:1, 1938.
36. Zondek, B., and Rozin, S.: J. Obst. & Gynec. Brit. Emp. *45*:918, 1938.
     Gillman, J.: J. Clin. Endocrinol. *1*:331, 1941; Endocrinol. *30*:54, 1942.
37. Hisaw, F. L.: Ann. Rev. Physiol. *4*:503, 1942.
38. Loeb, L.: Special Cytology, ed. by E. V. Cowdry, New York, Paul Hoeber, Inc., 1932, vol. 3, sect. 41.
39. Watson, M. C., and McHenry, E. W.: Am. J. Obst. & Gynec. *35*:316, 1937.
40. Hartman, C. G.: Am. J. Obst. & Gynec. *27*:564, 1934.
     Zuckerman, S.: Proc. Roy. Soc., London, s.B. *118*:13, 1935.
     Corner, G. W.: Am. J. Physiol. *113*:238, 1935.
41. Tietze, K.: Zentralbl. f. Gynäk. *60*:88, 1936; Arch. f. Gynäk. *161*:284, 1936.
42. Hartman, C. G., Firor, W. M., and Geiling, E. M. K.: Am. J. Physiol. *95*:662, 1930.
43. Saiki, S.: Am. J. Physiol. *100*:8, 1932.
44. Engle, E. T.: Proc. Soc. Exper. Biol. & Med. *29*:447, 1932.
     Engle, E. T., Smith, P. E., and Shelesnyak, M. C.: Am. J. Obst. & Gynec. *29*:787, 1935.
45. Hartman, C. G.: Am. J. Obst. & Gynec. *27*:564, 1934.
46. Markee, J. E.: Anat. Rec. (Suppl.) *55*:66, 1933.
47. Hartman, C. G., and Firor, W. M.: Anat. Rec. *61*:55, 1935.
48. Hartman, C. G., and Geiling, E. M. K.: Proc. Soc. Exper. Biol. & Med. *35*:383, 1936.
49. Markee, J. E.: Unpubd. communication, cited by Hartman, C. G., and Firor, W. M.: Quart. Rev. Biol. *12*:85, 1937.
50. Smith, P. E., Tyndale, H. H., and Engle, E. T.: Proc. Soc. Exper. Biol. & Med. *34*: 245, 1936.
51. Hartman, C. G., and Firor, W. M.: Quart. Rev. Biol. *12*:85, 1937.
52. Markee, J. E.: Anat. Rec. *70* (Suppl.) : 54, Abst. No. 85, 1938; Carnegie Inst. Wash. Pub. No. 518, Contrib. Embryol. No. 177, *28*:219, 1940.
53. Daron, G. H.: Am. J. Anat. *58*:349, 1936.
54. Keiffer, H.: Bruxelles-méd. *16*:1028, 1936; Bull. Acad. roy. de méd. de Belgique *13*:253, 1933; Bull. Acad. de méd., Paris *110*:217, 1933.
55. Brewer, J. I.: Am. J. Obst. & Gynec. *36*:597, 1938.
56. Bucura, C. J.: Zentralbl. f. Gynäk. *34*:561, 1910.
57. Joachimowits, R.: Biol. Gen. *4*:447, 1928.
58. Keiffer, H.: Bull. Acad. roy. de méd. de Belgique *2*:355, 1937.
59. Daron, G. H.: Anat. Rec. *67* (Suppl.) : 13, Abst. No. 28, 1937.
60. Lahm, W.: Zentralbl. f. Gynäk. *50*:2699, 1926.
61. Marlow, F. W.: Canad. J. Med. & Surg. *77*:134, 1935.
62. Fagin, J., and Reynolds, S. R. M.: Am. J. Physiol. *117*:86, 1936.
63. Moir, C.: Tr. Edinburgh Obst. Soc. 1933–34, p. 93.
64. Westman, A.: Acta Obst. et Gynec. Scand. *12*:282, 1932.
65. Meyer, R.: Arch. f. Gynäk. *113*:259, 1920.
66. Smith, P. E., and Engle, E. T.: Anat. Rec. *70* (Suppl.) : 73, Abt. 75, 1938.

67. Hartman, C. G.: Carnegie Inst. Wash. Pub. No. 433, Contrib. Embryol. No. 134, *23*:1, 1932.
68. Wilson, L., and Kurzrok, R.: Endocrinol. *23*:79, 1938.
69. Van Wagenen, G.: Anat. Rec. *52*:40 (Abst.), 1932; Am. J. Physiol. *105*:473, 1933.
    Van Wagenen, G., and Zuckerman, S.: Am. J. Physiol. *106*:416, 1933.
70. Markee, J. E., Davis, J. H., and Hinsey, J. C.: Anat. Rec. *64*:231, 1935.
71. Roberg, O. T., Jr.: West. J. Obst. & Gynec. *45*:1, 1937.
72. Henry, J. S., and Browne, J. S. L.: Am. J. Obst. & Gynec. *45*:927, 1943.

CHAPTER VI

ENDOCRINE CONTROL OF UTERINE MOTILITY

The factors responsible for the changing behavior of the uterine musculature, under various physiologic conditions, are of interest because they may throw some light on the etiology of dysmenorrhea, the mechanism of normal labor, and the cause of disturbances in parturition. The dependence of myometrial activity on hormonal stimuli is now well established, but precise definition of their effects has been hampered by species differences and difficulties inherent in the methods of study employed in the laboratory animal and human being.

METHODS OF STUDY

The spontaneous activity of the myometrium and its reactivity to various hormones and drugs have been studied both in vitro and in vivo. Investigation in vitro is accomplished by the Magnus-Kehrer method.[1, 2] The uterine muscle strip is immersed in physiological salt solution, and its movements are recorded by a special apparatus to which it is attached. This is unsatisfactory because it cannot recreate conditions prevailing in the living organism. Moreover, the response of the muscle strip may be materially affected by variations in the ionic concentration of the solution, which may thus obscure the result. The in vivo methods of study are generally conceded to be more satisfactory, for the uterine muscle may be observed under normal conditions, at body temperature, with its own blood supply, and its innervation intact. Moreover, controlled experiments may be carried out with the same organ from day to day, for extended periods of time. Of the numerous methods devised for use in the experimental animal, the more important ones are the uterine fistula technique of Reynolds and Friedman,[3] direct inspection of the uterus through an abdominal window or by means of a laparoscope, and electrical methods based on the "action current" of the contracting muscle.[4, 5]

For the study of the human uterus, both external and internal hysterography has been employed, the former being particularly suited for the study of the gravid uterus.[6, 7] In the earlier studies of the non-gravid uterus, it was filled with water or lipiodol and connected with a recording manometer by means of a tube.[8] This method was open to the objection that some of the fluid might be forced through the fallopian tubes, leaving the uterus incompletely filled. To eliminate this source of error, observers adopted the use of a rubber bag which is inserted into the uterine cavity and then inflated with air or water.[9, 10] While this method has many advantages, it is not infallible, as indicated by the varied and conflicting findings reported from different laboratories. Tension or distention resulting from the presence of a foreign body, nervousness or impatience of the subject during the course of the investigation, and other as yet undefined variables may account for the divergent results.

ROLE OF THE OVARIAN AND HYPOPHYSEAL HORMONES

In seeking to identify the forces governing myometrial activity, particular attention has been directed to the ovarian and hypophyseal hormones.

The Estrogenic Hormone.—There is a considerable body of evidence indicating that the estrogenic hormone produces changes in the myometrium, which heighten its motility, as judged by its spontaneous activity and reactivity to posterior lobe extract. A correlation between the estrogen level in the body and the degree of myometrial activity has been established by recording the movements of the uterus in the immature and mature nonpregnant subject, and in the castrate animal before and after the administration of estrogenic substances.

Observations in Lower Mammals.—Studies in the immature animal are limited, but are of interest because of the complete lack of information relating to the prepubertal human subject. The excised uterus of the immature guinea pig and rabbit shows no spontaneous activity, but that of the immature rat is active as early as the third day after birth. During the first few weeks of life in the latter species, there occur longitudinal rhythmic contractions which are slight at first but gradually increase in amplitude. Harne and Painter[11] believe this type of myometrial activity expresses an inherent characteristic of uterine muscle which is independent of hormonal stimuli. This they base on their observation that during active sexual life, when the uterus is presumably under hormonal control, its activity changes to a wavelike or nodal type, while at the termination of the reproductive period, it once again reverts to the type of activity seen in the immature animal. Whether the immature human uterus is quiescent, like that of the immature rabbit or guinea pig, or contracts like that of the prepubertal rat, has not been ascertained.

In the mature intact rat, mouse, rabbit and guinea pig, estrus is associated with both qualitative and quantitative alterations in myometrial activity. As Pompen[12] has pointed out, otherwise uncoordinated movements over the entire surface of the uterus are coordinated at this time, producing rhythmical waves of contraction, which pass from the tubal to the cervical end of the organ. In the estrus rat, the continuous wavelike motion of the rapidly contracting uterus contrasts with the ample, but slow and scattered movements seen in the various segments of this organ during the diestrus phase. In the rabbit, Reynolds[13] recorded intense, coordinated activity during estrus, in contrast to feeble, uncoordinated contractions or none at all during the diestrus phase. Morgan[14] observed a waxing and waning of uterine activity in rabbits in a state of continuous estrus. This is probably due to the fact that the persistent estrus is not due to a single persistent follicle, but to successive crops of maturing follicles which develop up to a certain point and then regress. This might be expected to result in a rise and fall in the estrogen level with consequent waxing and waning of uterine motility.

In the monkey, an increase in myometrial activity, rhythmic in nature, has been recorded at the height of the follicular phase. A progressive increase in motility apparently also occurs in the human being during the follicular phase of the menstrual cycle. Dickinson,[15] who followed the movements of the uterus by bimanual palpation, found it quiescent from the fifth to the ninth day, after which it showed increasingly marked contractions that persisted to the sixteenth day. Falk and Nahon[4] also reported a definite increase in myometrial activity from the ninth to the eighteenth day. The results of studies by the intra-uterine bag method vary somewhat in detail but in general indicate that the movements of the uterus during the period of follicular activity are rhythmic, frequent, of small amplitude and high tonus.[16, 17, 18, 19]

Sokoloff[20] first pointed out that the motile uterus of the mature animal becomes quiescent after bilateral ovariectomy. His observation has been fully corroborated. In the rabbit, some workers[13, 21] have described increasingly uncoordinated, irregular and smaller movements, culminating in complete quiescence within less than a month after operation. Others[14] have recorded infrequent, prolonged and regular contractions of fairly constant amplitude as late as four weeks after castration. In the rat, a nodal type of activity resembling that seen shortly before maturity, has been observed within two days after operation.[11] In the guinea pig, castration is followed by uterine movements similar to, but smaller and more sluggish than those seen in the intact, virgin animal, and a state of complete quiescence is reached within three months after ovarian ablation.[22] These variations in the interval between operation and complete loss of uterine motility are probably due to individual and species differences in the rate at which postcastration atrophy of the uterus proceeds. The infrequent but regular contractions seen a month after castration in some species, may be an expression of the inherent contractility of the uterus, or represent a stage in the transition from full activity to complete quiescence.

Observations in the Human.—The human uterus also shows a gradual loss of motility following ovarian ablation. Wittenbeck[23] detected only slight spontaneous myometrial activity six months after the natural or artificial menopause, and found the uterus completely quiescent by the end of the first year. Kraul and Simon[24] noted a diminution or loss of uterine motility following the menopause, while Miller and associates[25] found the tone unstable and the rhythmic contractions feeble or lacking. Recent studies have confirmed these reports.[19, 26]

The effect of estrogen on the quiescent uterine muscle of the castrate has been investigated in vivo and in vitro. In the earlier in vitro studies with crude estrogen, some reported stimulation, others depression or no effect whatsoever. When crystalline estrogen became available, it was found to have no effect in vitro, suggesting that the stimulative effects previously reported were due to impurities in the crude extracts. In vivo studies have yielded more uniform results. It has been shown that in the castrate rabbit, rat, mouse and guinea pig,[22, 27, 28] as well as in the human castrate,[19, 29] estrogen treatment causes the quiescent uterus to revert to the type of activity seen in the presence of a functioning follicle.

The Progestational Hormone.—The effect of the progestational principle of the corpus luteum on myometrial activity has been the subject
of considerable controversy. Ancel and Bouin[30] first pointed out that
spontaneous myometrial activity in the rabbit ceases with the formation
of the corpus luteum of pseudopregnancy and remains in abeyance until
the end of the luteal phase, when the myometrium again shows the type
of activity characteristic of the follicular phase. Their observation was
later confirmed by Knaus,[31] who described the rabbit uterus during the
luteal phase as flaccid and completely quiescent, showing no spontaneous
activity or reactivity to pituitrin.

The apparent motility inhibiting effect of the corpus luteum began to
arouse wide interest when Knaus[16] presented evidence suggesting that it
performs a similar function in man. According to his description, the
uterus, after the sixteenth day of the normal menstrual cycle, shows a
decreased capacity for spontaneous contractions, is flaccid and sluggish,
and does not respond to posterior lobe extract. He proposed that loss of
reactivity to this substance may serve as a test for ovulation.

Attempts to confirm his findings and extend them to other species,
have yielded varied results. Reynolds[13] confirmed his observations in the
rabbit, and studies with progesterone have established the responsibility
of the progestational principle for the quiescence of the luteal phase.[32]
That the quiescence is not complete has been suggested by Bell,[33] who followed the movements of the rabbit uterus by serial x-ray photographs of
silver wire stitches, placed in the mesometrium along the uterine border.
He observed periods of quiescence lasting 10 to 15 minutes, with intervening large contractions.

In the rat, mouse, guinea pig,[34] sow,[35] and monkey,[36] it has been shown
that the contractions slow down but do not cease in the presence of progestin, and reactivity to pituitrin persists. Some observers conclude from
this that the role of progestin in the regulation of myometrial activity is
not the same in all species. Reynolds[37] questions this conclusion and suggests that "failure to demonstrate inhibition by means of the tests thus
far used, particularly that of pituitrin inhibition, betokens a lack of sensitivity to the test rather than a physiological difference in the several
species studied."

Studies in the human being have also yielded results at variance with
those of Knaus. Schultze[38] and Tachezy[39] found the reactivity to pituitary
extract greater during the latter part of the menstrual cycle than in its
earlier phases. Their conclusion that loss of pituitrin reactivity is not a
reliable test for ovulation is now generally conceded. Moir[17, 40] challenged
Knaus' findings as regards both spontaneous activity and reactivity to
pituitrin. He was able to demonstrate spontaneous contractions throughout the cycle. After about the sixteenth day, the small, regular and frequent contractions which characterize the early part of the cycle, were
replaced by less regular but stronger movements, that gradually increased
in force with the approach of menstruation. Just before the onset of bleeding, they occurred at three minute intervals and reached a force as great
as 100 mm. of mercury. During menstruation, they occurred at two minute

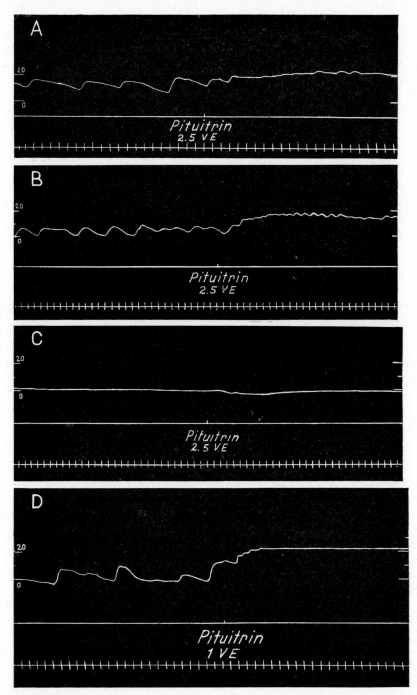

Fig. 31.—Reactivity of human uterus to pituitrin during the course of the menstrual cycle. A, On second day; B, on eighth day; C, on fourteenth day; D, on sixteenth day; E, on twenty-ninth day of the cycle. (Knaus, H.: Periodic Fertility and Sterility in Woman, Wilhelm Maudrich.)

intervals and created an intra-uterine pressure up to 120 mm. of mercury. Posterior lobe extract, he found, elicited a contraction at all times during the cycle. Tests with the oxytocic and vasopressor fractions showed that the former could elicit no response at any time, while an equivalent dose of vasopressin produced a delayed positive reaction, regardless of when it was given.

Kurzrok,[41, 42] Bickers,[19, 43] and Henry and Browne[80] have confirmed Moir's description of spontaneous activity and reactivity to whole posterior lobe extract during the normal menstrual cycle. Kurzrok observed small, regular and frequent contractions beginning about the seventh day after the onset of the last flow and persisting until about the seventeenth or twentieth day. After this point, he noted slower, less frequent contractions, of greater amplitude and lower tonus. These steadily increased in amplitude to a peak on the first or second day of the flow and then gradually became less ample. They were not replaced by small, regular, rapid contractions until almost a week after the onset of bleeding. He described the small movements as "follicular type" contractions, to distinguish them from the large, slow "luteal type" contractions, on the assumption that they are caused by estrogen and progestin, respectively. To account for the fact that the transition from the follicular to the luteal phase occurs a week sooner than the change from "follicular" to "luteal type" contractions, and that the latter persist for a week after progestin secretion has ceased, he assumes that there is a lag in the response of the myometrium to the ovarian sex hormones. He could elicit a response with whole pituitary extract at any time in the cycle and found it especially marked during the latter half. The injection of progesterone seemed to increase the amplitude and tonus of the contractions and the reactivity to pituitrin. When this hormone was administered during the follicular phase, there followed within a short time severe cramping unassociated with any significant change in the contractions.

Moir's study of the uterine response to oxytocin and vasopressin has been repeated and extended by McLellan.[44] This observer obtained a response to vasopressin at all times during the menstrual cycle. Equivalent doses of oxytocin were without effect at any time except during the flow. Much larger quantities elicited a reaction during the intermenstrual phase, but this McLellan attributes to the effect of small amounts of vasopressin present in the extract.

In an extensive study of myometrial reactivity to oxytocin, Kneer[45] observed that the myometrium became responsive to this substance a few days before the onset of the flow, and remained so for about a week after its onset. At all other times, the response was negative, regardless of whether the endometrium showed proliferative or pregravid changes. On correlating the response to oxytocin with the estrogen level, he was led to conclude that loss of reactivity coincides with a rise in this hormone, while renewal of reactivity is associated with estrogen withdrawal. Where this hormone remains absent for a protracted period, reactivity is lost once more, due to regression which culminates in a state analogous to that of the castrate.

Knaus' conclusions have not altogether lacked supporters. Kraul and Simon[24] noted a loss of myometrial reactivity to pituitrin in ten out of fourteen women during the premenstruum. Lackner and his coworkers[46, 47, 48] found that, though there is a wide range in the motility of the uterus of normal women at various parts of the cycle, the percentage of positive reactions to whole pituitary extract, and its oxytocic and vasopressor fractions, is much less during the second half of the cycle than during the first half and the last two days. In their experience, the administration of progesterone shortly before the flow seemed to decrease the size of the contractions, and lessen the reactivity to pituitrin. In dysmenorrheic women, this hormone relieved the pain, in some cases coincident with lessening of the contractions, in others without any significant change in motility. Daels[49] found that 10 mg. of progesterone was followed by a decrease in spontaneous activity after a latent period of twenty-four hours, but no significant loss of reactivity to pituitrin could be demonstrated.

The explanation of these divergent findings is not clear. Variations in technique, individual differences in spontaneous activity and reactivity to posterior lobe extract, and variations in the proportion of oxytocin and vasopressin present in the extracts used, may be partly responsible. Observers are apparently in accord on only one point, namely that spontaneous activity, and reactivity to pituitrin or its oxytocic and vasopressor principles, are greatest just before and during the menstrual flow. Though the evidence is still too confused to permit any conclusion, taken as a whole, it suggests the following hypothesis. In the lower mammal, where menstruation and the changes incident to this process do not enter to complicate the picture, the presence of progestin is clearly associated with large, slow contractions and varying degrees of myometrial sluggishness. In the human being, the presence of this hormone is likewise associated with large, slow movements, and a loss of tonus which suggests some degree of flaccidity. A significant deviation from conditions observed in the lower mammal occurs with the approach of menstruation. This is heralded by an increase in the power and amplitude of the contractions, and increasing reactivity to oxytocin. If this is due to the luteal hormone, as some assume, it is difficult to understand why it reaches its climax during the flow and persists for several days after its onset. The assumption of a myometrial lag is convenient but lacks proof. While there is good reason to believe that the change from small, rapid contractions to large, slow ones is due to progestin, the increasing power of the contractions with the approach of the flow, when the corpus luteum is regressing, must be explained on some other basis. As shown elsewhere (see Chap. V), it would appear that true menstruation, and the endometrial and vascular changes which precede it, are due primarily to progestin deprivation and secondarily to withdrawal of estrogen. There is also evidence suggesting that the vasoconstriction, which is an invariable precursor of menstrual bleeding, is due to some substance formed, possibly within the uterus, as regression of the endometrium proceeds. It is conceivable that this hypothetical substance, or a second one formed with it in the course of this process, is responsible for the change in myometrial activity which occurs at this time. For the present, this must remain purely speculative.

MOTILITY OF THE GRAVID UTERUS

Characteristics in Lower Mammals.—Studies in the rat, rabbit, guinea pig and dog, indicate that early gestation is marked by comparative myometrial quiescence, and late pregnancy by increasing uterine contractions. In the rabbit, Knaus[50] noted only slight movements during the first half of gestation, but with the approach of term, the contractility, tonus, and spontaneous activity of the uterus showed a steady rise. He observed a partial or complete loss of reactivity to pituitrin during the first 18 days, followed by increasing reactivity which reached its climax at term. In the rat, mouse and guinea pig, spontaneous myometrial activity is slight or absent in early pregnancy and increases with term's approach, but *reactivity to pituitrin* is demonstrable throughout gestation. A detailed description of the activity of the pregnant rabbit uterus has been given by Reynolds,[51] on the basis of an extensive study. During early pregnancy, he observed slow, leisurely, uncoordinated contraction waves, which passed up and down part or all of the uterus. Later, as the organ enlarged with the growing fetus, these movements gradually faded away, reaching their lowest ebb on the twentieth day. During late pregnancy, he noted spontaneous movements, which increased in frequency and amplitude, but remained local and uncoordinated. As term approached, these movements remained local in character but became increasingly vigorous. During labor, the contractions were coordinated like those of estrus, but differed in that they were independent of the tubal contractions and stronger at the cervical end. The characteristic contractions of labor did not begin in a cataclysmic manner, but were rather a gradually increasing manifestation of the segmental activity which began before the last week of gestation.

Characteristics in Monkey and the Human.—Studies of myometrial activity during pregnancy in the monkey and human are limited. During labor in the monkey, Hartman[52] and his associates observed coordinated wavelike movements, which passed from the fundus to the vaginal end of the uterus, and were comparable to the peristaltic action involved in the propulsion of a foreign body through a hollow viscus. In the human being, Robson[53] could observe no significant difference between the spontaneous activity of uterine strips removed during the eighth week of gestation and those obtained at term. According to Kreis,[54] the movements of the human uterus after the eighth month of gestation are very much like those seen in the rabbit at term. Bourne and Bell,[55] and Moir[56] recorded rhythmical movements punctuated by periods of complete relaxation at the thirty-sixth week of gestation. The contractions were equivalent in force to those noted during the first stage of labor, but were not accompanied by pain or cervical relaxation.

The pregnant human uterus is relatively refractory to whole posterior pituitary extract during early gestation, but becomes increasingly responsive with the approach of term. Reactivity is highest during labor and quickly diminishes following delivery. The oxytocic principle can elicit no response during the early months, but as pregnancy advances, the reaction to this principle becomes increasingly marked, reaching its peak during parturition. Vasopressin, surprisingly, evokes a response at all stages of gestation.

The activity of the human uterus, as determined by external hysterography, has recently been followed throughout gestation by Wilson[57] and Murphy.[7] Wilson noted the same irregular type of motility that is seen during the luteal phase of the menstrual cycle. Two types of contraction wave could be distinguished: large, arrhythmic waves, lasting one to five minutes, which apparently represented a mass contraction in which all uterine fibers participate, and small waves, lasting one minute or less, which seemed to represent regional myometrial activity. He could detect no periodic variations in contractility corresponding to the time when the menses would occur if the patient were not pregnant. Nor could be observe any evidence of increasing activity with advancing gestation. Murphy found that spontaneous contractions first appeared on the one hundred and sixty-sixth day, and increased progressively thereafter, the increase being especially marked in the thirty-second week. The approach of term was marked by increasing tension, and the contractions showed a tendency to become stabilized during the last month. In the thirty-seventh and thirty-eighth week, contractions were absent or were of unusually small magnitude, but in the thirty-ninth and fortieth week, long, strong movements appeared. *Reactivity to pituitrin* showed individual variations, in some cases being absent. Though a positive reaction could be obtained in some cases in early pregnancy, the number of positive responses increased steadily as pregnancy advanced. In early pregnancy, pituitrin induced intermittent contractions, while later it produced this effect plus increased tension. The contractions were like those which occur spontaneously during gestation, but differed from those of labor, which have a slower contractile phase.

The large general and small localized contractions described by Wilson have also been noted by Fenning,[58] whose observations led him to conclude that labor motility is inaugurated in advance of the development of pains.

Role of Estrogen in Myometrial Activity.—The progressive increase in the motility of the human uterus during the latter half of gestation coincides with a steady rise in the estrogen level of the blood and urine. This would suggest that estrogen stimulates myometrial activity during pregnancy just as it does in the infertile cycle. Attempts to demonstrate its ability to increase the motility of the pregnant uterus, with a view of proving that it plays a positive role in initiating labor, have yielded equivocal results. According to some investigators, estrogen has an abortifacient effect in the mouse and rat only if given early in gestation.[59, 60] Others report that it induces abortion in the rabbit and mouse at any point in gestation, but the dosage required for this effect decreases with the approach of term.[61, 62] In the guinea pig, on the other hand, abortion has been induced with estrogen at any phase of gestation, but the required dose increased as the animals approached term.[63, 64]

These divergent reports may possibly be accounted for by the fact that estrogen not only stimulates the activity of the uterine muscle but also plays an important part in producing the endometrial modifications essential for implantation and retention of the embryo. An excess of this hormone may conceivably induce abortion by increasing the irritability of the uterine musculature, or impairing the nidatory bed and thus causing fetal death. The abortion or resorption of the products of conception noted following estrogen injections early in gestation may be due largely, if not wholly, to impairment of the fetal bed. In this connection, D'Amour[65] observed fibrotic changes in the uterine mucosa, and a thinning out of the uterine secretions essential for implantation and retention of the fetus, in animals aborting after estrogen treatment. Abortion which follows estrogen injections late in pregnancy may be traceable to increased myometrial irritability as well as impairment of the fetal bed.

Heckel and Allen[66] observed postponement of parturition in experimental animals following estrogen injections begun shortly before term. They attribute this effect to this hormone's ability to prolong the life span of the corpus luteum of pregnancy. To reconcile their observation with reports of abortion following estrogen treatment, they suggest that the abortion thus induced is due to placental or fetal damage rather than increased myometrial motility. Proceeding on the assumption that the fetus, placenta, or both, normally produce a substance which maintains the corpus luteum, they reason that limited treatment with estrogen damages the placenta but cannot prolong the life of the corpus luteum. Premature expulsion of a dead fetus therefore follows. On the other hand, prolonged estrogen administration injures the placenta and fetus but at the same time prolongs the life of the yellow body. Under such conditions, retention of a dead fetus results. According to this theory, therefore, the dosage and length of treatment determines whether estrogen will precipitate or postpone parturition.

The role of estrogen in the regulation of uterine motility in the pregnant woman cannot be decided from the limited evidence at hand. Some observers claim that this hormone is effective in initiating or accelerating labor, while others could see no effect even with massive doses. The positive reports are inconclusive because the possibility that the increase in uterine activity was spontaneous cannot be ruled out.

Role of Progesterone in Myometrial Activity.—Since the uterus tends to be quiescent during early gestation, when the activity of the corpus luteum of pregnancy is at its height, and becomes increasingly active with the approach of term, when the yellow body regresses, it would seem reasonable to suppose that the luteal hormone inhibits myometrial activity during gestation as it does in the infertile cycle. The effects noted after corpus luteum ablation or progestin administration in the pregnant animal are suggestive but not conclusive, since this hormone is not concerned solely with myometrial motility but also plays an important part in maintaining the fetal bed.

Corpus Luteum Ablation During Pregnancy.—Wide species differences have been noted in the response to corpus luteum ablation during pregnancy. In some species, gestation proceeds normally no matter when operation is performed. In others, abortion occurs only if the yellow body is removed during the early stages of gestation. A third group invariably abort whether the operation is performed early or late in gestation. In the human being, removal of the corpus luteum alone, or with all remaining ovarian tissue, during the early months of gestation, is followed by abortion in less than one-fourth of the cases.[67] At first sight, these variations would seem to imply that the need for the luteal hormone varies considerably between one species and another. In view of recent evidence that the placenta produces progestin (see Chap. VIII), it seems more likely that these variations are due to differences in the placenta's ability to replace the yellow body as a source of this hormone.

Prevention of Abortion.—That progestin can prevent the abortion which would otherwise follow ovariectomy in the pregnant animal was first demonstrated in the rabbit by Corner and Allen.[68] A number of clinical reports[69, 70] have testified to the efficacy of progesterone for the prevention of spontaneous or habitual abortion (see Chap. XXVIII). Whether the good effects noted are coincidental or due to its ability to inhibit myometrial motility or preserve the fetal bed, we cannot say. Several observers have reported postponement of parturition in experimental animals following the administration of luteal extract. Of interest also is Hammond's[71] observation that a prolonged pregnancy results if the number of functional corpora lutea is made to exceed the number of fetuses by permitting only part of the released ova to be fertilized. Presumably, parturition is delayed because more luteal hormone is thus made available to each fetus.

Though the evidence is still incomplete, it would appear that both estrogen and progestin influence myometrial activity in the nongravid and gravid subject. The effect of estrogen on the nonpregnant uterus is fairly well established; that of progestin still requires clarification. How each affects the activity of the gravid uterus, and what part it plays in determining how the pregnancy shall terminate, is difficult to decide, because of the multiplicity of their effects in the pregnant organism, and the complexity of the mechanism involved in the maintenance of gestation and initiation of labor.

ROLE OF THE HYPOPHYSIS, ADRENALS AND THYMUS

The Anterior Hypophysis and Uterine Motility.—It is obvious that the adenohypophysis, whose gonadotropic principles stimulate the secretion of estrogen and progestin by the ovary, indirectly controls uterine motility. The possibility that this gland may also directly affect myometrial activity was first suggested by Reynolds and Friedman.[3] Observing that the rabbit's uterus becomes quiescent shortly after coitus and before corpus luteum formation, and that initiation of the quiescent state coincides with the coitus-induced release of the anterior hypophyseal luteinizing principle, these observers concluded that this hormone is probably responsible for the quiescent effect. As proof that it acts independently of the ovary, they offered their observation that a luteinizing extract of human pregnancy urine induced uterine quiescence in the castrate rabbit. Similar findings have been reported by Sager and Leonard,[72] but Gustavson and Van Dyke,[73] Morgan,[74] and Robson,[75] on the basis of studies in

8

the cat, rabbit and guinea pig, deny that the adenohypophysis has any direct effect on myometrial activity. They found pregnancy urine gonado-tropic extract without any effect whatsoever on the uterine musculature in the absence of the ovary. Uterine quiescence could only be induced in the intact animal, and then only if the extract elicited corpus luteum formation.

The Anterior Hypophysis and Progesterone.—Reynolds[37] has also sug-gested that the anterior lobe acts synergistically with progestin in inhibit-ing uterine motility. This he bases on the observation that more progestin is required to induce uterine quiescence in the hypophysectomized than in the intact animal. Since the amount of estrogen required to induce endo-metrial proliferation is not affected by removal of the hypophysis, he con-cludes that the lessened reactivity to progestin is not due to the general systemic depression, but to loss of a pituitary principle which directly influences the uterine cells and increases their receptivity to progestin. This theory still awaits corroboration.

The Posterior Pituitary and Uterine Motility.—As already shown, posterior pituitary extracts are capable of stimulating myometrial contrac-tions which vary in intensity according to the initial spontaneous activity of the organ. This in turn depends at least partly on the concentration of estrogen and progestin in the body. Though the oxytocic activity of its extracts is well established, there is no convincing proof that this gland is normally concerned with myometrial activity in the nonpregnant animal, or that it contributes to the spurt of activity which occurs in the pregnant animal at term and culminates in labor (see Chap. IX).

The Adrenal Medulla and Uterine Motility.—Adrenalin, the active principle of the adrenal medulla, may either stimulate or inhibit the activ-ity of the uterine muscle. In the rabbit, squirrel, hedgehog, monkey, and man, it has a stimulative effect on both the gravid and nongravid uterus. In the guinea pig, rat, mouse, and sow, its effect on the gravid and non-gravid uterus is inhibitory. The nonpregnant cat and dog respond to it with relaxation, but during pregnancy, it has a motor effect. Adrenalin appar-ently acts by way of the nervous system, for its effect is similar to that obtained by stimulating the hypogastric nerves, which carry both motor and inhibitory fibers to the uterus. The response to adrenalin is apparently determined by the relative strength of these fibers. That this in turn is influenced by the ovarian hormones is suggested by the observation that progesterone administration in the nonpregnant cat causes the uterus to respond to adrenalin with contraction instead of relaxation.[76]

Though the adrenal medulla yields a substance capable of influencing the activity of the uterine musculature, there is nothing to indicate that this gland participates in the regulation of myometrial activity.

The Thymus and Uterine Motility.—Müller,[77] in 1917, reported that an extract prepared from thymus tissue increased myometrial contractions and could also prevent fatigue if the muscle was not already exhausted. Later Temesvary,[78] in his search for a means of shortening labor, noted that large doses of thymus extract slightly increased the contractions of the excised uterus. The myometrial movements, though less powerful than those induced with posterior lobe extract, were more rhythmical and continued for a longer time. On combining thymus extract with an equal amount of pituitrin, he found they had a complementary effect, producing contractions which were more rhythmical and prolonged, and at the same time stronger, though not too powerful. Subsequent experiments with this combined extract, known as "thymophysin," have yielded conflicting results. Competent investigators now agree that the addition of a thymus extract in no way alters the oxytocic and vasopressor properties of posterior lobe extract. Most observers accept Nelson's[79] conclusions, based on a careful pharmacologic study, that the effect of thymophysin on the uterus is due to its pituitrin content, its action being merely that of a dilute posterior pituitary preparation.

BIBLIOGRAPHY

1. Magnus, R.: Pflüger's Arch. f. d. ges. Physiol. *102*:123, 1904.
2. Kehrer, E.: Arch. f. Gynäk. *81*:160, 1907.
3. Reynolds, S. R. M., and Friedman, M. H.: Am. J. Physiol. *94*:693, 705, 1930.
4. Falk, H. C., and Nahon, R.: Am. J. Obst. & Gynec. *30*:403, 1935.
5. Jacobson, E., Lackner, J. E., and Sinykin, M. B.: Am. J. Psychol. *53*:407, 1940.
6. Lorand, S.: Monatschr. f. Geburtsh. u. Gynäk. *103*:137, 1936.
7. Murphy, D. L.: Surg., Gynec. & Obst. *73*:175, 498, 1941; Am. J. Obst. & Gynec. *42*. 281, 1941.
8. Knaus, H.: Zentralbl. f. Gynäk. *35*:2193, 1929.
9. Knaus, H.: Zentralbl. f. Gynäk. *57*:2658, 1933.
10. Moir, C.: Brit. Med. J. *1*:1022, 1932.
11. Harne, O. G., and Painter, E. E.: Am. J. Physiol. *105*:566, 1933.
12. Pompen, A. W. M.: Acta brev. Neerland. *2*:13, 1932.
13. Reynolds, S. R. M.: Am. J. Physiol. *97*:706, 1931.
14. Morgan, T. N.: J. Obst. & Gynec. Brit. Emp. *40*:1196, 1933.
15. Dickinson, R. L.: Am. J. Obst. & Gynec. *33*:1027, 1937.
16. Knaus, H.: Periodic Fertility and Sterility in Women, Vienna, W. Maudrich, 1934.
17. Moir, C.: Trans. Edinburgh Obst. Soc. *41*:93, 1934.
18. Wilson, L., and Kurzrok, R.: Endocrinol. *23*:79, 1938.
19. Bickers, W., and Main, R. J.: J. Clin. Endocrinol. *1*:992, 1941.
20. Sokoloff, A.: Arch. f. Gynäk. *51*:286, 1896.
21. Hartmann, H., and Störring, F.: Arch. f. Gynäk. *145*:757, 1931.
22. Newton, W. H.: J. Physiol. *79*:301, 1933.
23. Wittenbeck, F.: Arch. f. Gynäk. *142*:446, 1930.
24. Kraul, L., and Simon, S.: Wien. klin. Wchnschr. *47*:1505, 1934.
25. Miller, E. G., Jr., Cockrill, J. R., and Kurzrok, R.: Am. J. Obst. & Gynec. *28*:319, 1934.
26. Lackner, J. E., and Tulsky, A. S.: J. Clin. Endocrinol. *1*:415, 1941.
27. Marrian, G. F., and Newton, W. H.: J. Physiol. *78*:19P, 1933.
28. Robson, J. M.: J. Physiol. *79*:139, 1933.
29. Krohn, L., Lackner, J. E., and Soskin, S.: Am. J. Obst. & Gynec. *34*:379, 1937.
30. Ancel, P., and Bouin, P.: Compt. rend. Acad. d. sci. *154*:1633, 1912.
31. Knaus, H.: Arch. f. Gynäk. *138*:201, 1929.
32. Tsutsulopulos, G.: Arch. f. Gynäk. *171*:81, 1941.
33. Bell, G. H.: J. Physiol. *99*:352, 1941.
34. Bell, G. H., and Robson, J. M.: J. Physiol. *88*:312, 1936.
35. Adams, E.: Endocrinol. *26*:891, 1940.
36. Bell, G. H.: J. Endocrinol. *3*:87, 1942.
37. Reynolds, S. R. M.: Physiology of the Uterus with Clinical Correlations, New York, Paul B. Hoeber, Inc., 1939.
38. Schultze, G. K. F.: Zentralbl. f. Gynäk. *55*:3042, 1931.

39. Tachezy, R.: Zentralbl. f. Gynäk. *58*:266, 1934.
40. Moir, C.: Proc. Roy. Soc. Med. *29*:950, 1936.
41. Kurzrok, R., Wiesbader, H., Mulinos, M. G., and Watson, B. P.: Endocrinol. *21*:335, 1937.
42. Wilson, L., and Kurzrok, R.: Endocrinol. *23*:79, 1938; ibid. *26*:587, 1940; ibid. *27*:23, 1940.
43. Bickers, W.: Am. J. Obst. & Gynec. *43*:663, 1942.
44. McLellan, A.: Lancet *1*:919, 1940.
45. Kneer, M.: Arch. f. Gynäk. *170*:483, 1940.
46. Falls, F. H., Lackner, J. E., and Krohn, L.: J.A.M.A., *106*:271, 1936.
47. Krohn, L., Lackner, J. E., and Soskin, S.: Am. J. Obst. & Gynec. *34*:379, 1937.
48. Lackner, J. E., Wachtel, H., and Soskin, S.: Am. J. Obst. & Gynec. *36*:612, 1938.
49. Daels, J.: Schweiz. med. Wchnschr. *71*:1249, 1941.
50. Knaus, H.: Arch. f. exper. Path. u. Pharmacol. *124*:152, 1927.
51. Reynolds, S. R. M.: Anat. Rec. *70*(Suppl.):65, 1935.
52. Ivy, A. C., Hartman, C. G., and Koff, A.: Am. J. Obst. & Gynec. *22*:388, 1931.
53. Robson, J. M.: J. Physiol. *79*:83, 1933.
54. Kreis, J.: Bull. Soc. d'obst. & de gynéc. *22*:231, 1933.
55. Bourne, A. W., and Bell, A. C.: J. Obst. & Gynec. Brit. Emp. *40*:423, 1933.
56. Moir, C.: Lancet *1*:414, 1936.
57. Wilson, L.: Am. J. Obst. & Gynec. *43*:955, 1942.
58. Fenning, C.: Am. J. Obst. & Gynec. *43*:791, 1942.
59. Parkes, A. S.: J. Physiol. *69*:463, 1930.
60. Katzman, P. A., and Doisy, E. A.: Endocrinol. *15*:207, 1931.
61. Kehl, R.: Compt. rend. Soc. de biol. *112*:675, 1933.
62. Tschaikowsky, W. K.: Zentralbl. f. Gynäk. *56*:395, 1932.
63. Parkes, A. S., and Bellerby, C. W.: J. Physiol. *62*:562, 1926.
64. Kelly, G. L.: Surg., Gynec. & Obst. *52*:713, 1931.
65. D'Amour, F. E., and Gustavson, R. G.: J. Pharmacol. & Exper. Therap. *51*:353, 1934.
66. Heckel, G. P., and Allen, W. M.: Am. J. Physiol. *123*:353, 1934.
67. Duyvene de Wit, J. J., and Oppers, V. M.: Nederl. tijdschr. f. geneesk. *83*:4001, 1939.
68. Allen, W. M., and Corner, G. W.: Am. J. Physiol. *88*:340, 1929.
69. McGregor, T. N., and Stewart, C. P.: J. Obst. & Gynec. Brit. Emp. *46*:857, 1939.
70. Campbell, R. E., and Sevringhaus, E. L.: Am. J. Obst. & Gynec. *39*:573, 1940.
71. Hammond, J.: J. Exper. Biol. *11*:140, 1934.
72. Sager, V., and Leonard, S. L.: Proc. Soc. Exper. Biol. & Med. *35*:242, 1936.
73. Gustavson, R. G., and Van Dyke, H. B.: J. Pharmacol. & Exper. Therap. *41*:139, 1931.
74. Morgan, T. N.: J. Obst. & Gynec. Brit. Emp. *42*:79, 1935.
75. Robson, J. M.: J. Physiol. *84*:296, 1935.
76. Kennard, J. H.: Am. J. Physiol. *118*:196, 1937.
77. Müller, H.: Ztschr. f. Biol. *67*:489, 1917.
78. Temesvary, N.: Zentralbl. f. Gynäk. *40*:322, 1926; ibid. *56*:1333, 1932.
79. Nelson, E. E.: J.A.M.A., *96*:352, 1931
80. Henry, J. S., and Browne, J. S. L.: Am. J. Obst. & Gynec. *45*:927, 1943.

CHAPTER VII

ENDOCRINE ROLE OF THE UTERUS

Removal of the uterus, with retention of one or both adnexa, may sometimes be followed within a short time by degenerative changes in the ovaries, and typical climacteric symptoms. From this some workers infer that the uterus produces an internal secretion essential for the maintenance of ovarian function. This assumption, if true, would imply that, where hysterectomy is indicated, little is to be gained by retaining part or all of the ovarian parenchyma. On the other hand, if unfounded, it would follow that the practice of making uterine implants in the hysterectomized individual, with the object of preventing a premature menopause, must be considered worthless.

To test the validity of this hypothesis, experiments have been carried out to determine what modifications in ovarian function follow hysterectomy, and what effect uterine implants or extracts have in preventing these changes. In addition, investigators have compared the incidence and severity of climacteric symptoms in untreated hysterectomized women and those in whom part of the uterus had been retained, a uterine implant has been made, or uterine extract administered.

HYSTERECTOMY EXPERIMENTS

Effects in Animals.—The effect of hysterectomy in the rat, mouse, rabbit, guinea pig, ferret and dog has been ascertained by microscopic examination of ovaries removed at varying intervals after operation, or by repeated vaginal smears which more or less accurately reflect the status of ovarian function. The results of such studies have been varied and conflicting, some reporting persistent estrus, others complete cessation of the estrus cycles in hysterectomized animals. The ovaries have been described by some as normal, while others observed cystic follicles, thecal cell hypertrophy with formation of true or false corpora lutea, or interstitial cell invasion. Luteinization of the theca cells has been the most common finding. In the pseudopregnant guinea pig[1] and rabbit,[2] hysterectomy prolongs the life of the corpus luteum. In the pregnant guinea pig, removal of the products of conception is followed by regression of the corpus luteum of pregnancy; but if the uterus is removed together with its contents, the corpus luteum persists and continues to function.[3, 4] These observations suggest that the presence of the uterus favors corpus luteum regression. A possible explanation has been offered by Heckel[5] on the basis of his observation that estrogen prolongs the life of the corpus luteum. This observer suggests that hysterectomy produces the same effect by removing tissue which would utilize much of the endogenous estrogen. The unused hormone can then act on the yellow body, prolonging its life span.

In the immature and mature monkey, Burford and Diddle[6] could see no significant ovarian alterations as late as four to seven months after hysterectomy. More recently, Van Wagenen and Catchpole[7] found that the reestablishment of ovarian function in postpartum monkeys was not significantly affected by hysterectomy immediately after delivery.

Effects in the Human.—In humans, the reported effects of hysterectomy have been as varied as in the lower mammals. Some find that the ovary becomes slightly smaller but retains all its functions. Others have described an increase in the number of follicles, cystic degeneration, follicular enlargement, or atresia. Thecal luteinization comparable to that seen in the laboratory animal has not been observed. It should be emphasized that hysterectomy in the human is usually performed because of pelvic pathology. Under such conditions, it is difficult to ascertain whether the ovarian alterations are attributable to loss of the uterus or the associated pathology.

Studies of the estrogen and gonadotropin content of the body fluids in hysterectomized women indicate that cyclic ovarian function may persist in the absence of the uterus. Krane[8] could detect no increase in the follicle stimulating hormone, which might indicate ovarian failure. The excretion of estrogen was within normal limits and showed a cyclic rise and fall as late as six years after hysterectomy. In one case observed by Frank,[9] similar findings were obtained.

UTERINE IMPLANTS AND EXTRACTS

Effects in Animals.—Takakusu[10] and Fellner,[11] working with the rat and guinea pig respectively, found uterine implants effective in preventing the formation of corpora lutea, which would otherwise appear after hysterectomy in these species. Winter,[12] on the other hand, has reported negative results with uterine implants and extracts in the hysterectomized rat. Loeb[13] found that the presence of uterine transplants did not prevent persistence of the corpus luteum after hysterectomy in the pseudopregnant guinea pig. Hirtz[14] observed that corpora lutea did not form in the rabbit following ablation of the uterus, unless uterine extract was administered. Mishell and Motyloff,[15] working with the same species, found that extract of cow endometrium seemed to check the degenerative changes initiated by hysterectomy, and tended to prolong the life of any corpora lutea that chanced to form after operation. This subject has been further complicated by reports that luteinization, like that produced with hypophyseal or chorionic gonadotropin, can be elicited in the guinea pig and dog with uterine implants or extracts. Fellner[11] suggests that there may be two distinct uterine hormones, one favoring, the other inhibiting luteinization. He believes that they act by way of the adenohypophysis, since hysterectomy in immature animals is followed by the premature appearance of estrus associated with cellular changes in the adenohypophysis similar to those seen in the mature gland. A somewhat similar view has been expressed by Herlant,[16] on the basis of his observation that hysterectomy is followed by corpus luteum formation, and hyperplasia of the acidophilic cells resembling that seen in the adenohypophysis during gestation. He suggests that the uterus produces a hormone which inhibits the production and release of the anterior pituitary luteinizing hormone.

Effects in the Human.—According to some,[17, 18, 19, 20] hysterectomy with retention of the ovaries or implantation of ovarian tissue is less likely to be followed by vasomotor symptoms in women with endometriosis or those receiving uterine implants, than in cases where no functioning endometrial tissue is present. Several workers[21, 22, 23] claim that troublesome symptoms can often be alleviated or prevented by retaining part of the fundus, or implanting uterine tissue into the vaginal wall or cervical stump, so as to permit periodic menstrual bleeding.

On the whole, the evidence thus far presented as proof of the existence of a uterine hormone leaves much to be desired. On the other hand, there is good reason to believe that posthysterectomy sequelae may as reasonably be accounted for on the basis of a disturbance of the vascular and possibly also the nervous connections of the ovary. Keitler[24] has shown that in the rabbit, where the ovarian blood supply is practically independent of that of the uterus, ovarian atrophy does not occur following hysterectomy. Kross[25] observed that removal of one uterine horn in the rat was followed by degenerative changes in the ovary corresponding to the extirpated horn, while the opposite ovary remained normal. Wang and Guttmacher[26] investigated the ovarian response to traumatization without actual removal of the uterus. They interrupted the blood supply of the ovary by ligating the uterine artery or excising the uterine mesentery at the junction of the oviduct and uterine horn. On subsequent examination, some of the ovaries appeared normal, while others contained cystic follicles. Neugebauer[27] found that ovarian degeneration invariably ensued when the ovarian arteries were ligated. Some ovaries contained cystic follicles or luteinized cysts, while others were transformed into a mass of interstitial tissue. The severity of the degenerative changes varied according to the extent to which the ovaries developed a collateral circulation.

Studies in the monkey[6] and the human[28] also suggest that injury to the ovarian vascular connections rather than loss of a hypothetical uterine hormone is responsible for posthysterectomy sequelae. Of interest is Dippel's[29] observation that hysterectomy before the age of forty was followed by annoying symptoms in only 16.6 per cent of the cases where no pelvic pathology was present, and the condition of the ovarian and infundibulopelvic ligaments was such as to minimize the likelihood of injuring the ovarian blood supply. On the other hand, where the uterus was removed because of fibromyoma or pelvic inflammatory disease, which increases the technical difficulties of operation and the likelihood of injuring the ovarian blood supply, symptoms appeared in 57.8 per cent.

It has been suggested that mutilation of important nervous pathways may contribute to the ovarian degeneration which follows extirpation of the uterus. Such damage may conceivably affect the function of the ovary directly, or may act indirectly by severing nervous pathways which regulate the interplay between the adenohypophysis and ovary. The latter possibility has been suggested by Siegmund,[30] on the basis of his observation that after hysterectomy, ovarian activity is depressed but its reactivity to exogenous gonadotropin remains unaltered. This evidence is contradicted by the report of Palmer and Fulton[31] that the ovaries of their hysterectomized mice showed loss of reactivity to chorionic gonadotropin, though they presented no evidence of surgical trauma or degeneration. While destruction of the ovary's nervous connections may be a contributory factor, the fact that ovarian transplants may function normally so long as they possess an adequate blood supply, would seem to justify the conclusion that injury to the vascular tree is the chief cause of ovarian regression following hysterectomy.

In the light of the available evidence, it is apparent that no endocrine role may as yet be ascribed to the uterus.

BIBLIOGRAPHY

1. Loeb, L.: Proc. Soc. Exper. Biol. & Med. *20*:441, 1923.
2. Asdell, S. A., and Hammond, J.: Am. J. Physiol. *103*:600, 1933.
3. Desclin, L.: Compt. rend. Soc. de biol. *109*:972, 1932.
4. Klein, M.: Compt. rend. Soc. de biol. *130*:1393, 1939.
5. Heckel, G. P.: Surg., Gynec. & Obst. *75*:379, 1942.
6. Burford, T., and Diddle, A. W.: Surg., Gynec. & Obst. *62*:701, 1936.
7. Van Wagenen, G., and Catchpole, H. R.: Proc. Soc. Exper. Biol. & Med. *26*:580, 1941.
8. Krane, W.: Zentralbl. f. Gynäk. *63*:457, 1939.
9. Frank, R. T., Goldberger, M. A., and Spielman, F.: J.A.M.A. *103*:393, 1934.
10. Takakusu, S.: Arch. f. mikro. Anat. u. Entwcklngm. *102*:1, 1924.
11. Fellner, O. O.: Pflüger's Arch. f. d. ges. Physiol. *231*:410, 1932.
12. Winter, E. W.: J. Obst. & Gynec. Brit. Emp. *43*:113, 1936.
13. Loeb, L.: Am. J. Physiol. *83*:202, 1927.
14. Hirtz, G.: Rev. franç. de gynéc. et d'obst. *33*:860, 1938.
15. Mishell, D. R., and Motyloff, L.: Endocrinol. *28*:436, 1941.
16. Herlant, M.: Compt. rend. Soc. de biol. *114*:273, 1933.
17. Mayer, L.: Bruxelles méd. *14*:1170, 1934.
18. Cheval, M.: Proc. Roy. Soc. Med. *27*:1395, 1934.
19. Shaw, H. N.: West. J. Surg. *44*:165, 1936.
20. Tonkes, E.: Zentralbl. f. Gynäk. *60*:35, 1936.
21. Fuchs, H.: Zentralbl. f. Gynäk. *59*:914, 1935.
22. Marx, R., Catchpole, H. R., and McKennon, B. J.: Surg., Gynec. & Obst. *63*:170, 1936.
23. Roberg, O. T., Jr.: West. J. Surg. *45*:1, 1937.
24. Keitler, H.: Monat. f. Geburtsh. u. Gynäk. *20*:686, 1904.
25. Kross, I.: Am. J. Obst. & Gynec. *4*:408, 1922.
26. Wang, G. H., and Guttmacher, A. F.: Am. J. Physiol. *82*:335, 1927.
27. Neugebauer, K.: Compt. rend. Soc. de biol. *123*:260, 1937.
28. Fredet, P.: Mem. Acad. de Chir. *62*:666, 1936.
29. Dippel, A. L.: Am. J. Obst. & Gynec. *37*:111, 1939.
30. Siegmund, H.: Arch. f. Gynäk. *160*:472, 1936; ibid. *165*:155, 1937.
31. Palmer, A., and Fulton, L.: Nature, London *148*:596, 1941.

CHAPTER VIII

ENDOCRINE ROLE OF THE PLACENTA

Halban,[1] in 1905, first suggested that the placenta may be a gland of internal secretion. Studies since carried out have demonstrated that it harbors hormonal substances biologically similar to the anterior hypophyseal luteinizing hormone, and the active principles of the follicle and corpus luteum. Whether it secretes or merely stores them has been the subject of much discussion. The suggestion that the placenta produces these substances has been resisted on the ground that it lacks secretory elements and other characteristics of an incretory gland. As Blair-Bell[2] has pointed out, true endocrine glands have ancient ontogenetic and phylogenetic histories, while the placenta is of comparatively recent origin. Moreover, all hormonopoietic organs elaborate their own specific secretions, whereas the hormones found in the placenta are like those of the ovarian follicle, corpus luteum and anterior hypophysis. Even if it is conceded that the placenta plays an endocrine role, it is difficult to accept the proposition that it at once duplicates the functions of two such dissimilar glands as the ovary and hypophysis. Though due weight must be given to these objections, the available evidence nevertheless suggests that this structure may serve as a temporary organ of internal secretion.

ESTROGEN IN THE PLACENTA

Estrogen was first demonstrated in the human placenta by Fellner.[3] As proof that it is secreted there, it has been pointed out that the placenta contains more estrogen than the graafian follicle; the increase in its estrogen content with advancing gestation roughly parallels the rise in the estrogen level of the blood and urine and its expulsion at term is followed by rapid disappearance of this hormone from the body fluids. That the greater part of the estrogen present in the pregnant woman is produced outside the ovary is indicated by the observation that bilateral ovariectomy is followed by only a slight drop in the estrogen level of the body fluids.[4, 5, 6]

In this connection, it is significant that in the pregnant mare, as in man, estrogen is demonstrable in the placenta, and bilateral oophorectomy does not interrupt pregnancy or cause the disappearance of estrogen from the body fluids.[7] On the other hand, in the mouse, rat and rabbit, where no estrogen is demonstrable in the placenta, castration is invariably followed by resorption or abortion of the fetuses. From this it would appear that, in the larger mammals and man, at an early stage of gestation, some extra-ovarian source assumes the ovary's task of secreting estrogen and thus helps maintain pregnancy. Though it seems likely that this extra-ovarian source is the placenta, a decision is not justified in view of recent evidence pointing to the adrenal cortex as a source of estrogen (see Chap. XVI). The fact that a rise in the estrogen level is not a constant finding in chorionepithelioma,[8, 9, 10] where a considerable amount of actively proliferating chorionic tissue is present, also raises a doubt as to the placenta's role in estrogen production. Noteworthy is the recent report[28] that placental cells maintained in continuous culture produce gonadotropic but not estrogenic hormone.

PROGESTERONE IN THE PLACENTA

Attempts to demonstrate progestin in the human placenta were unsuccessful at first because of the presence of relatively large amounts of estrogen in the extracts prepared from such tissue. This difficulty was overcome when Meyer and Allen[11] evolved a method of separating the two hormones. Utilizing this technique, several observers[12, 13, 14, 15] have succeeded in detecting small quantities of progestin in human placental tissue.

That the placenta secretes the progestin found therein is indicated by clinical and experimental evidence. The demonstration that progestin is essential for the maintenance of pregnancy (see Chap III), coupled with the observation that pregnancy may often proceed normally despite ablation of the corpus luteum in man, would imply that this hormone is supplied by some structure other than the ovary. The existence of an extra-ovarian source is also suggested by Selye's observation[16] that the endometrium and mammae of the pregnant rat continue to show evidence of progestin effect following bilateral oophorectomy. Similarly, Courrier and Gros[17] found that following ovarian ablation in the pregnant cat, the fetuses were reabsorbed but the placentae remained viable. The endometrium, as late as three weeks after operation, presented histologic modifications typical of pregnancy and known to be dependent on progestin. Of interest in this connection is Haterius' observation[18] that the pregnant rat may carry to term despite bilateral oophorectomy, if most of the fetuses are removed and the placentae retained, thus assuring a high placenta-fetal ratio. The explanation apparently is that the progestin content per placenta in this species is not adequate to carry the fetuses to term, without assistance from the corpora lutea of pregnancy. If, on the other hand, several placentae are available for the support of a single fetus, an adequate supply of progestin is assured despite removal of the ovaries. Jones and Weil[19] ascertained the daily excretion of pregnanediol, a degradation product of progesterone, in a patient from whom the corpus luteum of pregnancy was removed on the fifty-eighth day after the last menstrual flow without interrupting gestation. They found no pregnanediol for twelve days after the operation, after which it reappeared in the urine in increasing amounts. From this they concluded that progestin is produced during early gestation by the corpus luteum of pregnancy, but beginning about the end of the second month, an additional supply of the hormone is provided by the placenta.

Though the foregoing evidence strongly indicates that progestin, or a substance biologically identical with it, is produced outside the ovary during gestation, positive proof that the placenta is the extra-ovarian source is still lacking. In view of the evidence that substances possessing progestational properties can be obtained from the adrenal cortex under certain conditions (see Chap. XVI), and that pregnanediol is excreted in adrenal cortical hyperplasia and certain cortical neoplasms, there remains the possibility that the adrenal cortex, either alone or with the placenta, supplements the ovarian supply of progestin during pregnancy.

GONADOTROPIC HORMONES

The Anterior Hypophysis in Pregnancy.—Whether the gonadotropic substances present in the body fluids during pregnancy are derived from the anterior hypophysis, placenta, or both, is still controversial. It is generally agreed that little or no gonad-stimulating hormone is demonstrable in the human adenohypophysis during pregnancy. Some observers interpret this as evidence that the gonadotropic activity of the gland is greatly diminished at this time. Another view, based on morphologic and cytologic evidence, holds that the hypophysis is hyperactive during gestation, its low hormone content being due to rapid discharge of its incretory products. This interpretation seems plausible in view of the analogous situation existing in hyperthyroidism, where the thyroid contains little or no stored thyroxin. Though incontrovertible evidence is lacking, it seems likely that the anterior pituitary gland supplies at least a part of the gonadotropes which flood the organism during gestation.

Placental Source of Pregnancy Gonadotropes.—That the larger part of the pregnancy gonadotropes are derived from an extrahypophyseal source, probably the placenta, is suggested by the observation that the gonadotropes of glandular origin are not biologically identical with those found in the human placenta (see Chap. VIII). It should be emphasized, however, that differences in their biologic activity do not necessarily imply different sites of origin. The chorionic gonadotropes may conceivably represent derivatives of the hypophyseal hormones, which have become modified in the pregnant organism. Perhaps the most cogent argument thus far presented in favor of their placental origin is the observation[20, 21, 28] that gonadotropic hormone is produced in vitro, in placental culture tissues. Kido's[22] observation that gonadotropic hormone appeared in the urine of rabbits bearing placental tissue implants is not conclusive, since intervention of the hypophysis was not excluded. Newton and his associates[23, 24] recently showed that the activity and histological structure of the corpus luteum of pregnancy in the mouse is maintained after hypophysectomy and removal of the fetuses with retention of the placentae. Regression follows removal of the placentae, whether or not the hypophysis is present. Though this suggests that the placenta produces a substance capable of maintaining corpus luteum function, it does not necessarily follow that this is a gonadotropin, for estrogen may have a similar effect.[25]

There is some evidence that the placenta contains small quantities of *androgen*[26] and a substance which is capable of inducing full mammary development and secretion of milk,[27] but there is no proof that these substances are secreted and not merely stored there.

BIBLIOGRAPHY

1. Halban, J.: Arch. f. Gynäk. 75:353, 1905.
2. Blair-Bell, W.: J. Obst. & Gynec. Brit. Emp. 40:1579, 1933.
3. Fellner, O. O.: Biochem. Ztschr. 147:185, 1924.
4. Waldstein, E.: Zentralbl. f. Gynäk. 53:1305, 1929.
5. Brindeau, A., Hinglais, H., and Hinglais, M.: Compt. rend. Soc. de biol. 115:1509, 1934.
6. Probstner, A.: Endokrinol. 8:161, 1931.
7. Hart, G. H., and Cole, H. H.: Am. J. Physiol. 109:320, 1934.
8. Smith, G. Van S., and Smith, O. W.: Proc. Soc. Exper. Biol. & Med. 32:847, 1935.
9. Siegmund, H.: Arch. f. Gynäk. 149:498, 1932.
10. de Snoo, K.: Zentralbl. f. Gynäk. 52:2703, 1928.
11. Meyer, R. K., and Allen, W. M.: Anat. Rec. 56:321, 1933.
12. Ehrhardt, C., and Fischer-Wasels, H.: Zentralbl. f. Gynäk. 60:787, 1936.
13. Haffner, J.: Acta obst. & gynec. Scandinav. 18:125, 1938.
14. Smith, G. Van S., and Kennard, J. H.: Proc. Soc. Exper. Biol. & Med. 36:508, 1937.
15. McGinty, D. A., McCullough, N. B., and Wolter, J. G.: Proc. Soc. Exper. Biol. & Med. 34:176, 1936.
16. Selye, H., Collip, J. B., and Thomson, D. L.: Endocrinol. 19:151, 1935.
17. Courrier, R., and Gros, G.: Compt. rend. Soc. de biol. 121:1517, 1936.
18. Haterius, H. O.: Am. J. Physiol. 114:399, 1936.
19. Jones, H. W., and Weil, P. G.: J.A.M.A. 111:519, 1938.
20. Nogayama, A.: Nagasaki Igakkwai Zassi 15:2707, 2727, 1937.
21. Gey, G. O., Seegar, G. E., and Hellman, L. M.: Science 88:306, 1938.
22. Kido, I.: Zentralbl. f. Gynäk. 61:1551, 1937.
23. Newton, W. H., and Beck, N.: J. Endocrinol. 1:65, 1939.
24. Deanesly, R., and Newton, W. H.: J. Endocrinol. 1:65, 1939.
25. Heckel, G. P., and Allen, W. M.: Am. J. Physiol. 123:353, 1934.
26. Cunningham, B., and Kuhn, H. H.: Proc. Soc. Exper. Biol. & Med. 48:314, 1941.
27. Newton, W. H., and Richardson, K. C.: J. Endocrinol. 2:322, 1941.
28. Seegar Jones, G. E., Gey, G. O., and Gey, M. K.: Bull. Johns Hopkins Hosp., 72:26, 1943.

CHAPTER IX

PARTURITION

Many theories have been proposed at one time and another to explain the phenomenon by which, with dramatic suddenness, the mature products of conception are expelled from the uterus. Recent studies of the hormonal control of reproductive function and uterine motility (see Chap. VI) have thrown some light on this intriguing problem.

There is evidence that, in the course of gestation, under the influence of estrogen, progestin, and possibly also relaxin, the generative tract undergoes progressive structural modifications designed to facilitate expulsion of the fetus at term. With advancing pregnancy, the uterine musculature hypertrophies and the pelvic ligaments become loosened. The cervix enlarges and becomes progressively vascularized. The increasing number of blood vessels separate the muscle fibers so that at the end of gestation the cervix is spongy, readily compressible, and therefore easily obliterated by the descending passenger. The cervical dilatation incident to labor would thus appear to be at least partly dependent on hormonal forces operating throughout gestation.

FACTORS INITIATING AND MAINTAINING LABOR

In seeking to identify the factors immediately concerned with the initiation and maintenance of labor, observers have directed their attention to the uterus, its contents, and extra-uterine factors which may directly or indirectly help precipitate expulsive uterine contractions.

Role of the Fetus—Though labor is often spoken of as a response to the fetus' call for a change of environment, there is as yet no satisfactory explanation of how the fetus enforces its demand. Whether it acts through mechanical or chemical stimuli, or a combination of both, is not known. It has been suggested that the birth mechanism is set in motion by fetal metabolic products acting on the medulla, or by a hypothetical fetal antigen which circulates in the maternal blood. Some observers believe that the fetus, at term, ceases to produce some inhibitory substance, or secretes increased amounts of a stimulating substance which elicits expulsive uterine contractions. Pressure of the presenting part on the lower uterine segment has also been considered as a possible precipitating cause. This is thought to induce uterine contractions through a local reflex, or by nervous impulses which pass from the cervical ganglia to the posterior hypophysis, stimulating it to discharge its oxytocic principle.

Doubt is cast on the importance of the fetus as a factor in the initiation of labor by the observation[1, 2] that removal of the fetuses of pregnant rats does not precipitate expulsion of the placentae. Instead, complete emptying of the uterus takes place spontaneously at the time when parturition would normally occur. This phenomenon, termed "pseudoparturition,"[2] suggests that the placenta rather than the fetus controls the birth mechanism.

Role of the Placenta.—Though the available evidence strongly suggests that the placenta plays an essential role in the chain of events leading to labor, the mechanism involved is not clear. Infarcts and senility of the placenta, and increased venosity or gaseous alterations in the placental blood have been mentioned as possible causes of parturition. A more recent theory proposes that the placenta sets the birth mechanism in motion by secreting effective amounts of an oxytocic substance. Attempts to demonstrate a significant difference between the oxytocic properties of blood from parturient and nonparturient women have thus far yielded inconstant results.

Role of the Uterus.—The suggestion that loosening, thinning, and thrombosis of the decidua may precipitate labor has been discarded because these modifications are too inconstant to be significant. It has long been recognized that the uterine muscle becomes increasingly irritable with the approach of term. Whether labor is the natural outcome of this growing irritability, or some additional force must be brought to bear, is not known. *Heightened myometrial irritability* is thought to be at least partly due to increasing uterine distention. According to Reynolds,[3] uterine growth ceases with the approach of term and coincident with the period of most rapid fetal growth; the resulting distention evokes powerful uterine contractions which culminate in labor. In view of the fact that distention occasioned by an oversized fetus is more likely to delay than precipitate parturition, uterine distention would appear to play at best only a minor role in the initiation of labor.

The *shape* of the uterus is also thought to play a part. Laferty[4] points out that the powerful intermittent contractions which precede labor can exert no expulsive force on the fetus so long as it is surrounded by amniotic fluid. Only when the increasing size of the fetus, near term, causes the presenting part to come in contact with the converging walls of the uterus, is sufficient force exerted on the fetus to enable it to enter the pelvic outlet, and initiate true labor.

The importance of local factors in the initiation of labor is emphasized by Kross'[5] observation that when two pregnant animals were joined by parabiosis, labor in one did not initiate expulsive contractions in the other. Significant also is Markee and Hinsey's[6] observation that a cat, in which superfetation had occurred, first gave birth to the older fetuses. Following their expulsion, the emptied horn regressed but the full horn continued to show the characteristic changes of pregnancy until two weeks later, when it expelled its contents.

Nervous Factors.—There is reason to believe that the activity of the human uterus during labor is largely independent of its extrinsic nerve supply. Normal labor has been recorded in women with transverse myelitis, acute myelitis and paraplegia. Moreover, there is experimental evidence that parturition proceeds normally despite severance of the cerebrospinal and sympathetic nervous connections of the uterus. Particularly striking is Kurdinowski's[7] description of normal labor in the extirpated uterus of the rabbit. These observations imply that the central nervous system is not essential for labor. That the pregnant human uterus is not wholly insensitive to powerful nervous stimuli, is indicated by the observation that labor may be prematurely precipitated by powerful emotional states. In the words of Bourne and Bell,[8] "labor is largely a matter of local myogenic contractions and reflex activity of the uterus, while external stimuli such as emotion are able, by the nervous supply, to modify the contractile activity of the uterus."

To what extent the intrinsic nervous connections of the uterus participate in the expulsion of the ripe products of conception is not clear. In the rabbit, Reynolds and his associates[9] could induce rhythmic contractions with estrogen in transplants of uterine tissue of which virtually all the intrinsic nerves were destroyed. Whether this holds only for the rabbit, whose uterus has relatively few intrinsic nerves, or also applies to man and other species, where the intrinsic nerve supply of this organ is richer, is not known.[10]

Hormonal Factors.—On the basis of recent studies of the uterine response to various hormonal substances (see Chap. VI), observers have sought to explain labor on the basis of an altered hormonal environment.

Estrogen.—Particular emphasis has been placed on the role of estrogen. It is generally agreed that this hormone, through its growth promoting and vascularizing effect, acts throughout pregnancy to prepare the uterus for parturition. According to Reynolds,[3] it also contributes indirectly by inhibiting the growth-promoting effect of distention. As a result, growth of the uterus at term ceases to keep pace with that of the fetus, causing increasing distention which in turn gives rise to expulsive contractions. That estrogen contributes directly to the initiation and maintenance of labor, is suggested by the observation that it is the only known substance capable of inducing coordinated rhythmic myometrial contractions. Moreover, its concentration in the body fluids increases steadily as gestation advances and reaches its peak at term.[11] An appreciable rise in the estrogen level has been observed not only shortly before the onset of normal labor but also preceding threatened abortion.[12] Reports that estrogen may induce abortion in the experimental animal,[13] and is sometimes effective for the induction or acceleration of labor in the human[14, 15] have been offered as further proof that it plays a positive role in the initiation of labor.

On the other hand, opponents of this view argue that the pattern of estrogen-induced uterine contractions differs from that incident to labor; that its abortifacient action is attributable to the toxic effect of the large doses used, and that reports that estrogen induces or shortens labor in the human are unconvincing because they were not well controlled. The fact that labor does not occur before term, despite the presence of large quantities of this hormone in the body fluids, would also seem to argue against this theory. According to Cohen and associates,[16] however, most of the estrogen excreted during the first eight months of gestation is in a "combined" or inactive form. About one week before parturition, the amount of "combined" estrogen decreases, while the "free," or active, form increases, and the total amount of estrogen excreted drops. These observers postulate the existence of some mechanism which controls the quantity of active estrogen present during gestation and increases it at the time of labor. They propose that the production of large amounts of free estrogen of a high physiological potency is a factor in parturition. This, they believe, is due to hydrolysis of the "combined" estrogen, or to some interference with the normal mechanism of inactivation after it is produced. They attribute the drop in total estrogen excreted to utilization of the

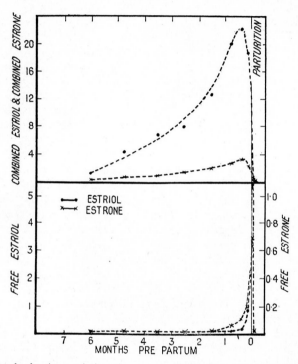

Fig. 32.—Graph showing variations in amount of "free" and "combined" estrogen excreted preceding and during parturition (average curves). The figures relate to milligrams excreted per twenty-four hours. (Cohen, S. L., Marrian, G. F., and Watson, M. E.: Lancet, Vol. 228.)

"free" form, the increase in the amount of active estrogen representing the unutilized excess. Though their findings have been confirmed,[17, 18] their conclusions require further substantiation. As Robson[19] has pointed out, the peak of estrogen excretion in the mare is reached some time before term, but no increase in the "free" form occurs before or at term. This may signify that the rise demonstrated in man has no significance so far as the initiation of labor is concerned, or that estrogen plays a more important part in some species than in others. A theory diametrically opposed to that of Cohen and his associates has been advanced by Kneer[20] on the basis of an extensive study of the reactivity of the human uterus to oxytocin. Correlation of the reactivity to this substance with the level of estrogen in the body led him to conclude that loss of reactivity coincides with a rise in the estrogen level, while increasing reactivity occurs when this hormone is withdrawn. He suggests that labor is due to withdrawal of estrogen. Smith and his associates[21] have recently reached a somewhat similar conclusion on the basis of their studies of estrone and estriol excretion. Observing that the changes in the ratio of these substances before labor are similar to those which precede menstruation, they suggest that labor, like menstruation, is due to withdrawal of estrogen and progesterone.

Protagonists of the view that estrogen contributes directly to the initiation and maintenance of labor are not agreed as to its mode of action. It has been suggested that it stimulates the posterior hypophysis to secrete its oxytocic principle, but convincing proof of this is still lacking. The available evidence suggests that it may produce expulsive contractions either through a direct pharmacodynamic action on the uterine musculature or by sensitizing it to some other substance, possibly pituitrin.

Progesterone.—The view that progestin withdrawal is at least partly responsible for the onset of labor is based on evidence (see Chap. VI) that this hormone exerts an inhibitory effect on the uterine musculature. Support for this theory is provided by the observation that a drop in the pregnanediol level of the urine is demonstrable in some cases of threatened abortion and preceding labor. Clinical reports that progesterone therapy is sometimes apparently effective for the control of threatened abortion (see Chap. XXVIII) have also been offered as proof of this assumption. According to Rosenkranz,[22] parturition is not due so much to a drop in progestin as to a change in the estrogen-progestin balance in favor of the former. Study of the estrogen and progestin content of placentae of thirty cases of prolonged labor revealed the presence of a normal amount of progestin and about half the normal amount of estrogen.

Oxytocins.—Increased production of an oxytocic, possibly by the posterior pituitary gland, is thought by some workers[23] to contribute in a positive way to the initiation of labor. It is significant that the pregnant human uterus, which is refractory to pituitrin during early gestation, becomes highly sensitive to it at term, and then loses this reactivity within a few days postpartum. There is, however, no satisfactory evidence that the oxytocin content of the posterior lobe increases during parturition. Nor has a significant rise in its concentration been demonstrated in the body fluids of the parturient woman. On the other hand, Fisher and his associates[24] have described disturbances of parturition in a large proportion of pregnant guinea pigs with hypothalamic lesions so placed as to interrupt at least some of the fibers of the supraoptico-hypophyseal tract. In view of their previous experiment[25] demonstrating that complete interruption of this tract in the cat is followed by posterior lobe atrophy and almost complete loss of its antidiuretic, vasopressor, and oxytocic hormone content, they suggest that a deficiency of oxytocin may be responsible for the difficult and prolonged, or delayed parturition in their guinea pigs. They attribute the normal labor observed by some investigators in

9

hypophysectomized animals to failure to destroy all neural tissue capable of secreting the oxytocic principle. Their studies, though not conclusive, have reopened the question of the posterior pituitary's participation in labor. Further investigation is necessary before any conclusion may be reached.

That the oxytocic substance which precipitates labor may be of placental origin has been suggested by Fontes[26] on the basis of his observation that an oxytocic effect could be produced with the blood and urine of women in labor, but not with the cord blood. Significant in this connection is Fomina's[27] observation that the amniotic fluid contains a substance with oxytocic activity which increases in amount with advancing gestation.

It is apparent that the evidence is still too limited to permit any conclusion as to the identity of the factors controlling parturition. It strongly suggests, however, that a number of factors of intra- and extra-uterine origin are concerned in this physiologic process.

BIBLIOGRAPHY

1. Kirsch, R.: Am. J. Physiol. *122*:86, 1938.
2. Selye, H., Collip, J. B., and Thomson, D. L.: Endocrinol. *19*:151, 1935.
3. Reynolds, S. R. M.: Physiology of the Uterus with Clinical Correlations, New York. Paul B. Hoeber, Inc., 1939.
4. Laferty, J. M.: Am. J. Obst. & Gynec. *28*:582, 1934.
5. Kross, P. L.: Am. J. Obst. & Gynec. *10*:64, 1926.
6. Markee, J. E., and Hinsey, J. C.: Anat. Rec. *61*:241, 1935.
7. Kurdinowski, E. M.: Arch. f. Gynäk. *73*:425, 1904; Arch. f. Physiol. Suppl. *28*:23, 1904.
8. Bourne, A. W., and Bell, A. C.: J. Obst. & Gynec. Brit. Emp. *40*:423, 1933.
9. Reynolds, S. R. M., and Kaminester, S.: Am. J. Physiol *112*:640, 1935.
10. Danforth, D. N., and Ivy, A. C.: Surg., Gynec. & Obst. *69*:351, 1939.
11. Goldberger, M. A., and Frank, R. T.: Am. J. Obst. & Gynec. *43*:865, 1942.
12. Jeffcoate, T. N. A.: J. Obst. & Gynec. Brit. Emp. *39*:67, 1932.
13. Parkes, A. S., and Bellerby, C. W.: J. Physiol. *62*:562, 1926.
14. Jeffcoate, T. N. A.: Lancet *1*:1045, 1940.
15. Friedrich, H.: Zentralbl. f. Gynäk. *65*:613, 1941.
16. Cohen, S. L., Marrian, G. F., and Watson, M. C.: Lancet *1*:674, 1935.
17. Smith, G. V., and Smith, O. W.: Am. J. Physiol. *121*:98, 1938.
18. Palmer, A.: Am. J. Obst. & Gynec. *36*:1005, 1938.
19. Robson, J. M.: Recent Advances in Sex and Reproductive Physiology, Philadelphia. Blakiston, 1934.
20. Kneer, M.: Arch. f. Gynäk. *170*:483, 1940.
21. Smith, O. W., Smith, G. V., and Schiller, S.: J. Clin. Endocrinol. *1*:461, 1941.
22. Rosenkranz, K. D.: Arch. f. Gynäk. *168*:51, 1939.
23. Bell, G. H., and Robson, J. M.: J. Physiol. *88*:312, 1936.
24. Fisher, C., Magoun, H. W., and Ransom, S. W.: Am. J. Obst. & Gynec. *42*:459, 1941.
25. Dey, F. L., Fisher, C., and Ranson, S. W.: Am. J. Obst. & Gynec. *36*:1, 1938.
26. Fontes, J. M.: Compt. rend. Soc. de biol. *114*:855, 1933.
27. Fomina, P. I.: Arch. f. Gynäk. *160*:333, 1936.

CHAPTER X

THE PHYSIOLOGY OF THE BREAST

Lactation, the final contribution of the maternal organism to the new-born, constitutes an important step in the reproductive process. Recent research has shown that the mammary glands are not only functionally allied with reproductive activity, but are also intimately associated, through hormonal and nervous pathways, with the gonads and gonad-governing glands. It has been recognized for some time that characteristic changes occur synchronously in the breast and generative organs during the various phases of sex life. The nature of the mammary alterations and the hormonal stimuli responsible for them are our main concern here.

ANATOMY OF THE MAMMARY GLANDS

In the course of a lifetime, the mammae pass through the following phases: [1, 2, 3, 4]

    I. Formative phase
        a. Embryonic period
        b. Postnatal development (birth to puberty)
        c. Maturity (menstrual life)
    II. Functional phase
        a. Pregnancy
        b. Lactation
   III. Involutionary phase
        a. Postpartum and post-lactational involution
        b. Menopausal and senile involution

FORMATIVE PHASE

Embryonic Period.—The anlage of the mammary gland appears at the sixth week of fetal life, and consists then of an ectodermal thickening which extends vertically as a narrow ridge along both sides of the body wall. As this ridge becomes more prominent, it is readily distinguishable as the so-called "milk-line." In man, all but the cranial third eventually disappears. In human embryos 26 to 60 mm. long, the "milk-line" breaks up into a series of swellings composed of ectodermal cells. These constitute the "mammary buds," primordia of the future mammary gland. The number of glands which eventually develop from these swellings varies according to the litter number characteristic of the particular species. In man, normally only one pair develops.

The primitive gland appears during the fourth fetal month as a thickening and down-growth from the milk line in the region of the future breast. Lens shaped at first, it gradually becomes globular, then bulbous, and finally lobed. By the first fetal month, long, solid epithelial cords begin to extend down from the ectoderm in the mammary area which is later to become the areola. The central cords undergo further differentiation, grow broader and longer, and ultimately form milk ducts, the future mammary parenchyma. The peripheral cords, which are shorter and narrower, in time develop into the glands of Montgomery. In the center of the milk bud, there appears a slight depression surrounded by unstriped muscle tissue which, on contracting, creates a small elevation forming the nipple.

Postnatal Development (Birth to Puberty).—In man, at birth the breast appears as a somewhat elevated, small, rounded node, situated in the center of the pectoral region. Histologically, it is seen to consist of slender cylinders, composed of close-lying epithelial cells. These cylinders

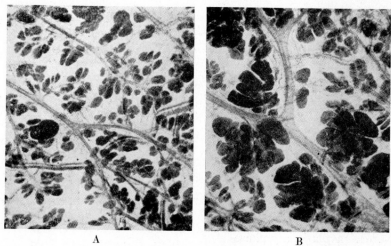

A   B

Fig. 33.—*A*, Biopsy specimen of monkey mammary gland at day twenty-two of cycle, eleven days after the occurrence of ovulation. *B*, Mammary biopsy specimen, same animal five days later, showing lobular enlargement during premenstruum of ovulatory cycle. (Speert, H.: Surg., Gynec. & Obst. Vol. 73.)

thread their way through the fibrillar tissue, blood vessels, lymphatics and muscular tissue comprising the nipple, and branch out and dilate at the ends to form acini.

A few days after birth, the breast in both sexes may become swollen and tender, and secrete a milky fluid (witches' milk). Except for this transient activation, now generally attributed to hormones derived from the maternal circulation before birth, the breast remains relatively quiescent during childhood, the only change being an increase in the number and complexity of the tubules. Although duct development occurs in some species during this period, any increase in the size of the breast in the larger mammals and man, barring precocious puberty, is due to an increase in fat and connective tissue.

Maturity (Menstrual Life).—With the onset of puberty and recurring menstrual cycles, there is a gradual and progressive enlargement of the mammary gland. This is due to the formation of new ducts and lobules, hyperplasia of the connective tissue, and deposition of fat. Now, for the first time, the female breast becomes distinguishable from that of the male. The transition is gradual and the age at which it occurs depends upon the same constitutional, endocrine and environmental factors that determine the initiation of menstrual function (see Chap. XXIII). When full sexual maturity is attained, the breast appears as a compound tubulo-alveolar gland, composed of lactiferous or lobar ducts, which radiate from the nipple and subdivide in an arborescent fashion into numerous intra-lobar and interlobular ducts. From the latter stem the intralobular ducts along which develop alveoli, the true secretory elements. A group of alve-oli constitutes a lobule, and a number of lobules form a lobe.[5]

Cyclic Changes.—That the breast of the mature woman undergoes cyclic alterations paralleling events in the ovary was first suggested by Rosenburg.[6] According to this observer, the breast at the intermenstrual period consists of ducts but no acini. Following ovulation, and as the corpus luteum forms, the epithelium multiplies rapidly and there appear out-growths from the ducts with large numbers of small lobules. As the corpus luteum regresses, these lobules also regress and vanish during the postmenstrual period, so that the gland is in a state of rest at the time of the next ovulation. Unlike Rosenburg, Dieckmann,[7] Dawson,[8] and Taylor[9] hold that lobule development is a gradual but progressive process and that acini, once formed, persist and, with recurring cycles, ultimately achieve adult form. Cyclic changes have also been described in the human mam-mary gland with respect to the size of the epithelial cells, the lipoid gran-ules within the cells, and the degree of edema and cellular infiltration within the stroma. Speert[145] has recently shown that distinct enlargement of the lobules occurs cyclically during the premenstruum in the monkey breast (see Fig. 33).

FUNCTIONAL PHASE

Pregnancy.—During pregnancy, the breast enlarges and acquires a firmer consistency. At the same time, the nipple increases in size and is more sensitive and erectile; the pigmentation of the areola becomes darker and more extensive, and the glands of Montgomery more prominent.

The histologic alterations in the mammae during gestation may be divided into a proliferative and secretory phase. During the initial or *proliferative phase*, which extends through the first half to two-thirds of pregnancy, there occurs progressive proliferation of ducts and especially alveoli, and the individual glandular elements attain full maturity. The proliferation of the glandular elements is so marked that the connective tissue appears diminished, although actually its total amount may be in-creased because of the greater size of the breast as a whole. The adipose tissue is decreased in amount and, in some instances, may almost dis-appear. The *secretory phase* is characterized by enlargement of the epithe-lial cells lining the alveoli, and the initiation of secretory activity. This activity shows a steady crescendo as the individual approaches term. Colostrum formation becomes progressively more marked and its accumu-lation in the alveoli distends the entire glandular system. As emphasized by Turner,[10] these changes are in the nature of hypertrophy rather than hyperplasia, the increased size of the breast being due to the presence of secretory products rather than an increase in the amount of secretory tissue.

Lactation.—Following delivery, colostrum secretion continues for a few days regardless of whether suckling is instituted. The breasts become engorged, giving rise to a sense of distention. The mammary swelling reaches its height on the third to the seventh postpartum day, and then recedes. The breast undergoes progressive involution, unless suckling is instituted, in which case it acquires the doughy consistency characteristic of the lactating gland. This alteration marks the transition from colostrum formation to milk secretion.

Except for an increase in the size of the acini and their lining epithelium, the lactating breast differs from that of late pregnancy only in that epithelial activity is more uniform throughout the gland. According to Jaschke,[11] the lactating breast presents all stages of secretory activity. Side by side within the same lobe may be seen alveoli showing evidence of beginning or active secretion, and others in a state of rest preparatory to regeneration and renewed activity.

INVOLUTIONAL PHASE

Postpartum and Post-lactational Involution.—On weaning, or following the termination of pregnancy without lactation, the mammae gradually return to a state of comparative quiescence. The breast becomes smaller and flabbier because of diminished vascularity and shrinkage of the parenchyma. Secretory activity ceases gradually, the acini and their epithelial lining undergo progressive shrinkage until they disappear and are replaced by adipose tissue.

Menopausal and Senile Involution.—The involutionary mammary alterations seen at the end of reproductive life, parallel the regressive changes in the gonads incident to this period. The parenchyma undergoes atrophic changes and is eventually replaced by fibrillar connective tissue. With advancing age this tissue is replaced by fat. The dilated alveoli and lactiferous ducts, which may be present in large numbers after the menopause, gradually disappear with advancing age.

HORMONAL FACTORS IN MAMMARY DEVELOPMENT AND FUNCTION

Reports that severance of the nervous connections of the breast has no apparent deleterious effect upon its subsequent growth or function, led earlier investigators to postulate a hormonal rather than a nervous control of this gland. The identity of the hormones involved, and their role in mammary growth and function have inspired extensive investigations. Considerable progress has been made but much has yet to be learned concerning this complex subject.

PROLIFERATIVE PHASE

Endocrine Control of Mammary Growth Outside of Pregnancy.— A causal relationship between ovarian function and mammary growth was

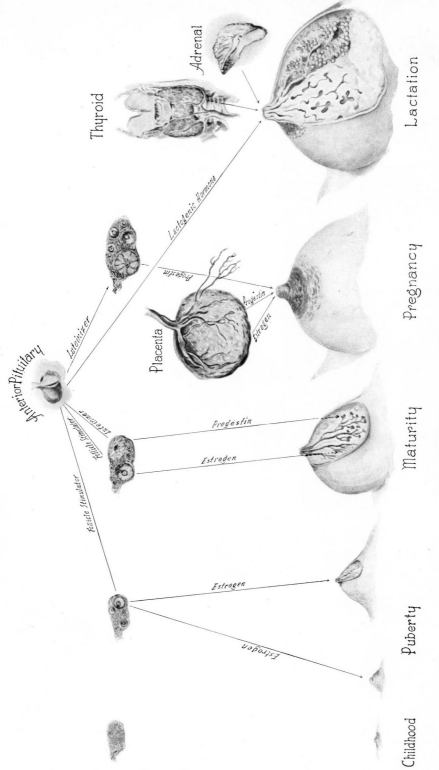

Fig. 34.—Endocrine control of the breast.

early inferred from the observation[12, 13] that breast atrophy follows bilateral oophorectomy, and that such glands can be restored to normal by ovarian implants. Lacking potent extracts of the follicle and corpus luteum, earlier workers could only deduce their role in mammary activity from studies correlating the changes occurring simultaneously in the ovary and mammae of various species during the sex cycle. Duct growth was observed in all species with recurring follicular cycles. On the other hand, lobule-alveolar formation was noted only in the presence of a functioning corpus luteum, the degree of such proliferation being proportional to the length of the luteal phase. These observations furnished presumptive evidence that the duct system is dependent upon the follicle, and the lobule-alveolar system upon the yellow body. Proof of this assumption and identification of the active hormonal principles involved first became possible with the isolation of estrogen and progestin, specific hormones of the follicle and corpus luteum respectively.

Role of Estrogen.—There is ample evidence that estrogenic substances, both natural and synthetic,[14] are capable of inducing normal *duct growth* in the male and spayed female animal. Their role in lobule-alveolar growth, on the other hand, is not clear. In such species as the cat and dog, true lobule development has not been elicited with any of the available estrogens. In the mouse, rat, rabbit, goat and monkey, the reported effects of various estrogens range from marked lobule-alveolar proliferation to no alveolar response whatsoever. Of the species studied, the guinea pig alone invariably responds to the estrogens with marked alveolar growth. These varied effects may perhaps be attributed, as Nelson[5] suggests, to species differences, the use of different estrogenic compounds, or to variations in dosage, length of treatment and the route of administration.

Whatever the explanation may be, the available evidence obviously permits no conclusion as to estrogen's role in lobule-alveolar growth. Though varying degrees of lobule-alveolar proliferation can be induced in some species with certain estrogens, this is not conclusive proof that lobule development normally depends upon this hormone alone. Nor does it necessarily follow that progestin plays no part. There is evidence (see below) that most species require progestin in addition to estrogen to insure full lobule-alveolar development. This, together with the observation that estrogen and progestin are closely related chemically, and that some estrogenic compounds evoke a more marked alveolar response than others, suggests that in all species, including even the guinea pig, lobule-alveolar development is normally at least partly dependent on progestin. The fact that marked growth of alveoli can be induced in the guinea pig with estrogen alone may merely indicate that in this species the mammae are peculiarly adapted to utilize, for purposes of lobule-alveolar development, not only the specific lobule-stimulating hormone, progestin, but also certain estrogens which are chemically closely related to the luteal hormone.

Role of Progesterone.—The results of experiments with crude and crystalline progestin indicate that the luteal hormone stimulates *proliferation of the lobule-alveolar system* in the breast previously developed by estrogen. In species which respond to estrogen with some lobule-alveolar growth, the addition of progestin greatly augments the effect. The luteal hormone is apparently most effective when it is preceded by estrogen and accompanied by small doses of this hormone. When acting alone on a breast not previously stimulated by estrogen, it is without effect unless massive doses are used.[15, 16]

The available evidence relating to the effect of progestin on the human breast is unsatisfactory, since no attempt was made to ascertain the histologic status of the lobule-alveolar system before and after treatment.[17, 18] In the absence of proof to the contrary, however, it seems likely that in the primate, as in most of the lower mammals, the luteal hormone is essential for lobule-alveolar growth.

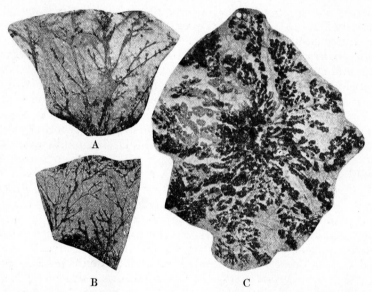

Fig. 34a.—Mammary gland of castrate rabbit. *A*, After estrogenic hormone followed by progestin for twenty days. No lobule proliferation. *B*, Second check gland removed after progestin injections for thirty days. Note further involution of duct system. *C*, After daily injection of progestin plus estrogen for eighteen days. Note lobule proliferation. (Turner: in Allen: Sex and Internal Secretions, Williams and Wilkins Co.)

Endocrine Control of the Mammary Gland in Early Pregnancy.— Breast development in man during the first half of gestation differs only quantitatively from that of the luteal phase of the normal menstrual cycle. The evidence at hand indicates that identical hormonal stimuli, which differ only in their intensity, are concerned in both conditions. As early as 1911, Ancel and Bouin[19] demonstrated that in the rabbit, the characteristic mammary alterations of early pregnancy can be duplicated by inducing pseudopregnancy through sterile coitus. Since a fertilized ovum and placenta are absent in this condition, their experiment eliminated these structures as the cause of the mammary changes of early pregnancy. At the same time it suggested that the corpus luteum may be the source of the growth stimulus, since the mammary modifications appeared coincident with its formation and disappeared with its regression.

Experiments with the specific hormones of the follicle and corpus luteum have fully substantiated the implications of Ancel and Bouin's studies. It is now fairly well established that *progestin*, acting with small quantities of estrogen on the estrogen-primed breast of male or spayed female rabbits, induces lobule-alveolar proliferation without secretion, an effect comparable to that seen at the end of pseudopregnancy or the middle of true pregnancy.

SECRETORY PHASE: ENDOCRINE CONTROL OF THE MAMMARY GLAND DURING LATE PREGNANCY AND LACTATION

The mechanism which controls colostrum formation during the latter half of gestation, and milk secretion following parturition is not yet completely understood. Identification of the factors responsible for mammary secretion constitutes a fascinating chapter in reproductive physiology.

Role of the Corpus Luteum.—A view, widely accepted until recently, attributed the mammary alterations of late pregnancy to the action of the corpus luteum. At first it was believed that breast development in the pseudopregnant animal falls short of that of true pregnancy because the life span of the corpus luteum is shorter. Apparently supporting this assumption was the observation that species in which pseudopregnancy and pregnancy are of equal length, achieve the same degree of mammary development under both conditions.

To determine the role of the corpus luteum in mammary development of late pregnancy, observers have noted the effect of removing the corpus luteum of pregnancy, or extending the luteal phase in pseudopregnant animals by hysterectomy, or by administering progestin or gonadotropic hormone. Ablation of the corpus luteum in pregnant animals failed to yield unequivocal results. In many of the species studied, the occurrence of abortion shortly after operation made it uncertain whether the ensuing interruption of mammary development was caused by loss of the yellow body or expulsion of the products of conception. In such species as the guinea pig, horse and man, pregnancy and mammary development continued normally despite removal of the yellow body. This would seem to permit the inference that, in some species at least, the corpus luteum is not essential for the mammary changes of late pregnancy, but it does not exclude the possibility that a progestin-like substance, possibly of placental origin (see Chap. VIII), is essential for mammary development throughout pregnancy.

Hysterectomy in pseudopregnant animals, in some as yet undetermined way, causes persistence of the corpus luteum. In guinea pigs subjected to this operation, Loeb[20] observed that the life span of the yellow body exceeded that of true pregnancy, and the mammae presented alterations comparable to those of late pregnancy. In pseudopregnant rabbits,[21] on the other hand, hysterectomy does not greatly prolong corpus luteum function, and the mammary development does not exceed the pseudopregnant level. These experiments suggest that the yellow body can produce mammary changes equivalent to those of late pregnancy, provided that its functional span is sufficiently long. This is also implied in Turner and Gardner's[22] observation that considerable secretory activity occurs in the mammae of rabbits receiving corpus luteum extract combined with relatively large doses of estrogen. It should be emphasized, however, that since intact animals were used in these investigations, they failed to exclude the possibility that the corpus luteum acts through or with the assistance of some other agent. That the *anterior pituitary gland* is an essential contributing factor was established by chance when investigators attempted to prolong luteal activity in pseudopregnant animals by administering gonad-stimulating extracts.

Role of the Anterior Hypophysis.—Evans[23] and Parkes,[24] in 1929, reported that the pseudopregnant rat and rabbit respond to anterior pituitary extracts with formation of fresh crops of corpora lutea and mammary alterations equivalent to those of late pregnancy. On the other hand, Jares[25] found that a gonadotropic extract of pregnancy urine induced formation of fresh corpora lutea, but did not carry mammary development beyond that of pseudopregnancy. Since the conditions of Parkes' and Jares' experiments were substantially the same, their results could be reconciled only by assuming that the characteristic secretory activity of the breast in late pregnancy requires not only the prolonged activity of the corpus luteum, but also some factor which is present in the anterior pituitary gland but not in pregnancy urine. Proof of this was provided by Stricker and Grueter,[26] whose experiments demonstrated that the anterior hypophysis elaborates a hormone which is not only essential for the secretory activity of late pregnancy, but for milk secretion as well.

Investigations since carried out have greatly clarified the hormonal mechanism governing the mammary changes of late pregnancy and the initiation and maintenance of lactation, but there are still many controversial problems whose solution is necessary to fill the gaps in our knowledge of this important subject.

Hypophyseal Lactogenic and Mammotropic Factors.—(a) *The Lactogenic Hormone.* The existence of a specific *anterior pituitary lactation-promoting principle* has been confirmed by many competent observers. Variously designated "lactation-promoting hormone," "lactogenic hormone," "prolactin," "galactin," and "lactogen," it has been shown to be distinct from the growth, gonadotropic and corticotropic factors of the anterior lobe.

(b) *Mammogen I and II.*—That the adenohypophysis also produces a *substance which directly stimulates duct and lobule growth* was first suggested by Corner,[27] in 1930. As proof he offered his observation that rabbits, castrated during estrus, responded to anterior pituitary extract with mammary changes which he interpreted as evidence of alveolar proliferation and secretory activity. His suggestion was subsequently questioned by Turner[10] and Gardner,[28] who could observe neither duct nor lobule development in castrate animals receiving anterior lobe extract. They suggested that the mammary changes, interpreted by Corner as evidence of an increase in the number of alveoli, were actually due to heightened secretory activity of previously formed alveoli which were so distended by the accumulated secretions as to give the erroneous impression of increased numbers of secreting units. More recently, however, Turner and his associates have carried out an extensive series of experiments which they believe demonstrate the existence of what they term *mammogen I and mammogen II*. The former stimulates duct growth, the latter lobule-alveolar proliferation. *Estrogen* stimulates production and release of mammogen I, while *progestin* stimulates secretion of mammogen II by the anterior pituitary. According to this theory, the ovarian hormones exert no direct effect on mammary growth but act by way of the hypophysis.[29, 30, 31]

Opinion is still divided regarding the validity of this hypothesis. Turner's report that estrogen increases the duct growth-promoting activity of the anterior pituitary could not be confirmed by Nelson[32] or by Reece and Leonard.[33] Studies of the efficacy of the ovarian hormones in the hypophysectomized animal have yielded conflicting results. Some investigators[34, 35, 36] have observed a complete absence of mammary response to estrogen in the absence of the adenohypophysis, while others[37, 38, 39] report that its effect is diminished but not completely abolished under such conditions. All appear to agree that mammary involution is less marked in the hypophysectomized castrate animal receiving anterior lobe implants or extracts than where such treatment is withheld.[32, 33] They differ, however, as to whether this is due to the favorable systemic effect of the anterior pituitary hormones, or to a direct stimulative effect on the mammae. Comparative studies of the duct growth response of the hypophysectomized animal to estrogen, anterior pituitary extract, and a combination of both, have failed to provide a definite answer to this problem. Turner's group[29] found that the addition of the thyrotropic, lactogenic or adrenocorticotropic principles of the anterior hypophysis, failed to increase the mammary response to estrogen. On the other hand, Uyldert[39] found that the addition of an anterior pituitary extract, with gonadotropic but no growth-promoting activity, appreciably increased the effect of estrogen on mammary duct growth. More recently, Reece and Leonard[40] reported that though estrogen had no effect in the hypophysectomized animal, estrogen plus a growth-promoting extract of anterior lobe tissue caused duct growth equivalent to that produced with estrogen alone in the intact animal.

The observation of Astwood and his associates[41] that inanition results in the same lack of response to estrogen as hypophysectomy, has been offered as proof that general systemic depression and not lack of some specific mammotropic hormone is responsible. This has been challenged by Samuels and his associates,[42] who found that the response of the hypophysectomized animal to estrogen could not be improved by forced feeding and the administration of thyroxin, salt and cortical hormone. Trentin and Turner[43] showed that estrogen will stimulate duct growth in underfed animals provided that sufficiently large doses are given.

As a further argument against Turner's hypothesis, it has been pointed out that the local application of estrogen causes duct growth in the treated breast, while distant glands show little or no evidence of stimulation.[44, 45]

In answer to this, Leonard and Reece[46] have reported that estrogen produces no growth effect when applied locally in the hypophysectomized animal, although it is effective in the normal and partially hypophysectomized animal. This does not constitute a complete answer, but merely demonstrates that the pituitary deficiency which prevents a response to injected estrogen is equally effective whether the hormone is administered by injection or local application. Turner's group[47] suggests that the localized response to topical application may be due to estrogen's ability to produce hyperemia and increase metabolism, thus aiding the anterior pituitary mammogen in producing localized mammary hyperplasia.

A specific mammotropic hormone has not yet been isolated. The claim of Turner's group[47] that this principle is present in lipid extracts of anterior pituitary gland tissue has been questioned by Greep and Stavely,[48] who could not duplicate their results.

As the evidence now stands, it would appear that the ovarian sex hormones require the presence of the adenohypophysis for a complete effect on duct growth and lobule-alveolar development. For a decision as to the manner and extent of this gland's contribution, further investigation is necessary.

Prerequisites for Mammary Response to the Lactogenic Hormone.—The conditions which must prevail to insure a mammary response to the lactogenic hormone have been the subject of extensive investigation. Particular attention has been directed to the importance of estrogen and progestin in preparing the breast for lactation, and to the question whether the lactogenic hormone requires the presence of the ovary or hypophysis in order to induce milk secretion.

Estrogen and Progestin in Preparing the Breast for Lactation.— Stricker and Grueter[26] emphasized the need for priming the breast with both estrogen and progestin before it can respond to the lactogenic hormone. They based this on their observation that anterior lobe extract induced milk secretion in rabbit breasts primed by estrogen and progestin, but not in those stimulated by estrogen alone. Corner,[27] on the other hand, suggested that milk secretion can be induced in mammae primed by estrogen alone, and that the preliminary action of progestin is not essential. As proof, he offered his observation that anterior pituitary extract induced milk secretion in mature, virginal rabbits castrated during estrus. Since ovulation and corpus luteum formation normally occur in this species only after coitus, he assumed that the mammae of his virginal animals had at no previous time been subjected to the influence of progestin. More recently Gardner and his coworkers[49] observed limited secretion of milk or a milk-like substance following the administration of anterior pituitary lactogenic hormone in rabbits whose mammae had been primed by estrogen alone, and contained ducts but no alveolar formation. To explain the occurrence of secretory activity in such glands, these observers point out that the epithelium of the smaller ducts is identical with that lining the alveoli, and they are apparently capable of serving as producers as well as conductors of milk. It must be emphasized, however, that the amount of secretion noted in Gardner's test animals was limited and hardly comparable to that seen in the postpartum lactating animal, or that induced with lactogenic hormone in mammae previously primed by estrogen and progestin.

It would seem, therefore, that though Stricker and Grueter erred in assuming that no milk secretion can occur in glands prepared by estrogen alone, they were correct in stating that full secretory activity is possible only if the breast has been stimulated by both ovarian hormones. Their completely negative results in estrogen prepared mammae may be attributable to inadequate dosage or the relative impotency of their lactogenic extract. On the other hand, though Corner was correct in assuming lactation can occur in the rabbit breast primed only by estrogen, he was not justified in concluding that progestin plays a negligible role in preparing the gland for milk secretion.

The available evidence, though limited, suggests that in other species, as in the rabbit, the estrogen-primed breast is capable of limited secretory activity, but maximum milk production requires preliminary growth of alveoli under the influence of progestin. An apparent exception is the guinea pig, whose breast responds with full secretory activity to the lactogenic hormone, though previously primed only by estrogen. The reason for this probably lies in the fact that in this species the breast responds to estrogen with full lobule-alveolar proliferation and is thus amply provided with the secretory structures essential for lactation. The extent of the breast's response to the lactogenic hormone is apparently proportional to the amount of secretory epithelium present. This in turn depends on estrogen and, to a varying extent, on progestin. Insofar as the latter hormone is required for lobule-alveolar development, to that extent is it important in preparing the breast for milk secretion comparable to that which follows pregnancy.

Efficacy of the Lactogenic Hormone.—(*a*) *In the Absence of the Ovary.*—Stricker and Grueter's[26] studies demonstrated that the hypophyseal lactogenic hormone can induce milk secretion in castrate rabbits whose mammae have previously been subjected to the influence of estrogen and progestin. Secretory activity was elicited as late as three months after ovarian ablation, suggesting that, once properly primed, the rabbit breast remains responsive to the lactogenic principle for a considerable period. In the castrate guinea pig and rat, on the other hand, the breast fails to respond with milk secretion even when the lactogenic extract is administered immediately after castration. From this, some workers inferred that the lactogenic principle can act only in the presence of the ovary. This was subsequently disproved by the observation that the ovariectomized rat responds with milk secretion if the lactogenic extract is immediately preceded by injection of the ovarian sex hormones. In the light of this observation, it seems likely that diminished reactivity to the lactogenic hormone was responsible for the negative results obtained in recently castrated rats not given estrogen and progestin. It appears then that the lactogenic hormone can induce milk secretion in the properly prepared breast, despite absence of the ovary. In species whose mammae regress rapidly on withdrawal of the ovarian sex hormones, a continuous exogenous supply up to the moment when the lactogenic principle is brought to bear, is apparently essential to keep the breast in a receptive state and make milk secretion possible.

(b) *In the Absence of the Hypophysis.*—Riddle and his associates[50] found that the ability of the lactogenic hormone to stimulate the crop-gland of the pigeon and ring-dove is unimpaired in the absence of the hypophysis. On the other hand, Gomez and Turner[51] could obtain no response with purified lactogenic extract in the hypophysectomized pigeon, cat, rat or guinea pig, even when the lactogenic hormone was administered immediately after operation. These divergent findings are apparently attributable to differences in the purity of the lactogenic extracts used, for while the purified lactogenic preparations are as a rule without effect in the hypophysectomized animal, crude anterior pituitary extracts have been reported to induce milk secretion in many instances. As Gomez and Turner[51] have pointed out, hypophysectomy not only removes the lactogenic principle, but also other important hypophyseal hormones which control vital metabolic processes. The loss of these hormones and the accompanying general depression probably decreases the concentration of the available precursors of milk in the blood. The greater effectiveness of crude lactogenic preparations, they believe, is due to the presence of metabolic principles needed to restore the supply of milk precursors to normal. As proof they offer their observation that lactation could be induced in hypophysectomized animals by administering a relatively pure lactogenic preparation, combined with adrenal cortical extract and glucose,[52] or with anterior pituitary adrenocorticotropic extract.[53]

The participation of the adrenocorticotropic and possibly other metabolic principles of the adenohypophysis in inducing lactation is now generally conceded.[54, 55] Some observers[56] maintain that since pure lactogenic hormone is ineffective in the hypophysectomized subject and requires the assistance of other pituitary principles to induce milk secretion, all the factors required for this effect should be termed lactogenic. Meites and Turner[57] oppose this suggestion and insist that the lactogenic factor is the hormone specifically concerned with the initiation of lactation. In support of their view, they offer the observation[58] that, though less lactogen is required to induce milk secretion in pseudopregnant rabbits if other anterior pituitary principles are added, large amounts of the latter without lactogen cannot initiate lactation.

FACTORS CONTROLLING THE INITIATION OF MILK SECRETION

Observers have long sought an answer to the question why milk secretion is absent during pregnancy and what causes its appearance following parturition. In the light of recent evidence, it would appear that milk production requires a properly prepared breast and an adequate supply of lactogenic hormone. Since the breast during late pregnancy is adequately prepared, its failure to secrete milk must be assumed to be due either to lack of an adequate supply of lactogenic hormone, or to the presence of some inhibitory substance or substances which prevent a response to an adequate supply of this hormone.

The lactogenic hormone is apparently present during gestation, for substances possessing lactogenic activity have been found during late pregnancy in the hypophysis,[59, 60] placenta,[61, 62] blood[63, 64] and urine.[65] That these substances may be at least partly derived from the pregnant uterus has been suggested by Collip and his associates,[66, 67] on the basis of their observation that rats hypophysectomized shortly before term secrete milk for a few hours following parturition. Whether the substance responsible for this brief period of lactation is secreted by the pregnant uterus or its contents, or merely stored there, cannot be decided from the available evidence.

The Supply of Lactogenic Hormone.—According to Turner and Meites,[68] absence of milk secretion during pregnancy is due to lack of an adequate supply of lactogenic hormone, while its initiation postpartum is due to a marked increase in the supply of this hormone. They base their view on the observation that in the rat,[69] guinea pig,[60] and rabbit,[68] the lactogen content of the pituitary remains as low during pregnancy as in the nonpregnant state, while immediately postpartum, a 200 to 400 per cent increase is demonstrable. As proof that pregnancy does not inhibit the lactogenic hormone of the pituitary, they offer their observation that the high lactogen content of the pituitary of lactating rabbits persists despite the simultaneous occurrence of pregnancy. They conclude that the primary reason lactation does not occur during pregnancy is because the lactogenic hormone in the pituitary is too low to support lactation. No suggestion is offered as to the cause of the increased elaboration of lactogenic hormone following parturition.

Lactation-Inhibiting Factors.—These findings do not necessarily exclude the possibility that some inhibitory factor or factors present during gestation are responsible for the absence of milk secretion. The sudden increase in lactogen content of the pituitary noted postpartum is subject to two possible interpretations. It may represent increased storage of the hormone, due to removal of some factor which stimulates its discharge from the gland. On the other hand, it may be the result of an increased rate of production, due to removal of some inhibiting factor, or the intervention of some positive force which stimulates lactogen production. Except for suckling, there is no evidence that such a positive force comes into play at this time. On the other hand, there is evidence that the postpartum increase in pituitary lactogen is independent of suckling in the rat[59] and guinea pig,[70] though this would not appear to be true in the rabbit.[70] It seems likely, therefore, that there is some inhibitory influence operating during pregnancy, which can prevent the establishment of full lactogenic activity, though it is not adequate to suppress it after it is once established, as is true where pregnancy occurs in a lactating animal.

The Placenta in Lactation Inhibition.—The existence of some lactation-inhibiting factor or factors during pregnancy has been suspected for some time, but attempts to identify them have only recently borne fruit. The first clue to their identity was provided in 1905, when Halban[71] called attention to the inhibition of lactation in parturient women with retained *placental* remnants. Frankl[72] later reported that placental grafts made near term prevented postpartum lactation as long as they remained viable. In the rabbit, Smith and Smith[73] noted that the retention of viable placental tissue prevented milk secretion, while Nelson[74] demonstrated that removal of the ovaries and embryos without disturbing the placentae inhibited lactation during but not beyond the period of placental retention.

Studies in nonpregnant and pseudopregnant animals suggest that the lactation-inhibiting effect of functioning placental tissue is due to its estrogen content. Whether progestin also plays a part is not certain.

Progesterone as the Lactation-Inhibiting Factor.—The possibility that the inhibition of milk secretion during pregnancy is due to a substance present in the corpus luteum was earlier suggested by Hammond.[75] Observing milk secretion in rabbits following caesarian section performed after the twelfth day of gestation, he concluded that the initiation of lactation is due to regression of the yellow body following the interruption of pregnancy. His view finds support in the observation[76] that milk secretion can be initiated in the pregnant goat by removing the corpus luteum after full lobule-alveolar development is achieved. This evidence is not conclusive, for degeneration and detachment of the products of conception was not excluded and it is therefore possible that the yellow body was not the only factor withdrawn. Collip[66] has more recently adopted Hammond's view on the basis of his observation that, though pregnancy urine gonadotropin elicited marked duct and alveolar development in intact animals, lactation did not occur until the intensely luteinized ovaries of the test animals were removed. Anselmino and his associates[77, 78] have presented evidence suggesting that the corpus luteum produces a lactation-inhibiting substance distinct from progestin. According to Folley and Kon,[79, 146] crystalline progesterone neither increased nor diminished milk secretion in the lactating rat, while Selye[80] found that massive doses of this hormone failed to prevent the initiation of lactation in the mouse. Negative results have also been reported in man.[81]

Estrogen as the Lactation-Inhibiting Factor.—The observation that large quantities of estrogen are present in the body fluids during pregnancy, and that the onset of milk secretion coincides with an abrupt drop in the estrogen level, suggest that this hormone may be the factor which holds milk secretion in abeyance until parturition. Of interest is Bruhl's[82] report that "witches' milk" is secreted in the newborn only after the estrogens derived from the maternal circulation disappear from the body fluids. Recent investigations in the rabbit, rat, guinea pig, cow and man have uniformly shown that estrogen is an effective agent in preventing the initiation of milk secretion, and may be at least partially effective in suppressing established lactation.

Mechanism of Estrogen's Lactation-Inhibiting Effect.—Some hold that estrogen acts indirectly by restraining production or release of the lactogenic hormone. Others believe it hinders milk secretion directly by interfering with the action of the lactogenic hormone on the breast.

Growth Stimulus Incompatible with Secretory Activity.—According to Nelson[74] it acts both directly and indirectly. He points out that estrogen induces growth while the lactogenic hormone evokes a secretory response, and suggests that the mammae are physiologically incapable of responding to a secretory stimulus while under the influence of growth-promoting stimuli. In the struggle for physiologic supremacy, the occurrence of milk secretion depends on which of the two is in the ascendancy. Nelson's suggestion is in line with an interpretation offered earlier by Loeb: [83]

Recognizing an antagonism between mitotic cell proliferation and function, this observer states that it "is mainly due to a differentiation which takes place in the cell in the course of time and which is prevented or delayed by the effect of growth stimuli. The antagonism is reciprocal. Growth inhibits those alterations in the cell which tend to initiate certain functional activities like secretion, and progressive differentiation is unfavorable to the development of those changes in the cell on which mitotic division depends. However, this antagonism is not absolute. We may still find mitosis in cells in which the presence of fat droplets indicates some secretion, and especially soon after labor, we may find in the mammary gland mitotic proliferation due perhaps to the influence of the follicular hormone; but as the secretion becomes more and more fully established, mitoses are rarer or are lacking altogether . . . it is possible that the deficient secretion during the later periods of pregnancy notwithstanding far advanced development of the alveoli, is due to a certain inhibiting effect in the gland cells of the growth stimuli emanating from the corpus luteum. In the same sense we may interpret the fact that in lactating cows castration may prolong the milk secretion for a long period of time. This effect is presumably made possible by the elimination of the growth stimuli emanating from the ovary, which tend to counteract the secretory function. . . . In general, the mammary gland begins to produce a characteristic secretion, milk or a material more or less closely resembling milk, as soon as the growth substances have produced a certain amount of tissue and a sudden cessation of the proliferative activity has taken place. This cessation of growth processes is again conditioned by two factors: (1) by a discontinuance of the production of the specific hormone, and (2) by processes of cell differentiation which accompany proliferative activity in the mammary gland, and which lead to limitation of further growth activities with the setting up in their places of certain functional phenomena, as for instance, secretion. We find the same phenomena in growth of glandular structures in general. Growth stimuli of embryonal or regenerative character, induce cells which are as yet less differentiated to proliferate. This growth is accompanied by differentiation which itself limits growth and prepares the cells for secretory activity. While thus in the mammary gland certain secretory processes may be observed even while the corpus luteum is continuing to give off the specific growth substance—still the active secretion takes place only after a large mass of tissue has been built up which has undergone this differentiating growth and then suddenly experiences a lack in the supply of the growth substance."

The assumption that estrogen prevents milk secretion during pregnancy by promoting growth processes which are incompatible with secretory activity, is borne out by the observation that this hormone is much more effective in preventing the initiation of lactation than in suppressing established lactation. Frankl[72] was able to prevent lactation by making placental implants before term, but Selye[84] found such implants without effect in lactating animals. Smith and Smith[73] could prevent the onset of milk secretion in postpartum rabbits by administering 2,000 rat units of estrogen daily, but after lactation was well established, as much as 4,000 rat units daily were without effect. The explanation may lie in the fact that cells which have achieved full secretory activity are no longer capable of responding to a growth stimulus. This may at least partly explain why established lactation may continue undiminished in animals which become pregnant while lactating.

10

Action on Lactogenic Hormone.—That estrogen prevents lactation through a direct effect on the breast is also implied in the observation that the response to the lactogenic effect of whole anterior lobe extract in the hypophysectomized guinea pig can be prevented by simultaneously administering estrogenic substance.[73] It is also noteworthy that milk secretion cannot be induced during pregnancy despite an adequate exogenous supply of lactogenic hormone.[74]

The theory that estrogen prevents milk secretion during gestation by inhibiting lactogen production by the adenohypophysis, is not borne out by the available evidence. On the contrary, recent studies point to a possible stimulative effect of this hormone on pituitary lactogenic activity. Turner and his associates observed that the lactogen content of the pituitary dropped after ovariectomy and increased following the administration of various estrogens.[85, 86] This apparently denotes increased production, for it is associated with a rise in the lactogen content of the blood.[87] It is of interest in this connection that the so-called "pregnancy cells," which normally appear in the hypophysis during gestation, are also present in lactating animals, where they persist until weaning.[88] Since they are present during the period of active milk secretion and disappear with its termination, it is possible, as Kraus[89] has suggested, that they are the source of the lactogenic principle, and that their presence in the pregnant, as well as the lactating animal signifies accelerated production of this hormone. That their appearance during pregnancy is due to the action of estrogen is suggested by the observation that they can be induced with this hormone in the nonpregnant animal,[88] and that such animals may lactate following a course of estrogen injections.[90] The fact that secretory activity, as evidenced by colostrum formation, is greatest during late pregnancy, when the estrogen level is at its height, would also seem to point to a stimulative rather than an inhibitory effect of this hormone on lactogen production. The observation that pregnant lactating animals may show an increase in milk production near term may possibly be explained by the formation of additional secretory structures in the breast, under the influence of estrogen and progestin, and increased lactogen production, due to the rising tide of estrogen. A similar explanation may account for the observation that estrogen administration during lactation may increase the milk yield.[91, 92] This is not necessarily inconsistent with the assumption that growth activity is incompatible with secretory function, but may be explained by assuming that estrogen stimulates growth of new structures, while preexisting structures, which have already achieved secretory activity, continue to produce milk. Thus, while growth and secretion cannot occur simultaneously within the same cell, they apparently can occur at the same time in different areas of the same breast.

Conclusion.—If it is granted that estrogen has a two-fold action, at once stimulating lactogen production and preventing this hormone from exerting its full effect on the breast, the mammary changes during pregnancy may possibly be explained as follows: During early gestation, when the estrogen level is just beginning to rise, the quantity of lactogen produced by the pituitary is limited and the growth stimulus, estrogen, is dominant. As pregnancy advances and the estrogen level rises, lactogen production increases until it is present in sufficient concentration to super-impose its secretory effect on the continued growth effect of estrogen, and colostrum forms. After this point, estrogen and lactogen apparently strike a balance calculated to permit the secretion of colostrum, without allowing this secretory process to culminate in the production of true milk. Only after delivery, when expulsion of the uterine contents results in an abrupt withdrawal of estrogen, does full secretory activity, as manifested in milk production, become possible. How expulsion of the products of concep-tion leads to the marked increase in the lactogen content of the pituitary noted by Turner,[68] is still unknown. If it is true that estrogen stimulates lactogen production, this increase can hardly be attributed to removal of the placental estrogens. Meites and Turner[93] have suggested that the low lactogen content of the pituitary during gestation may be due to the presence of progestin, which prevents estrogen from exerting its full stimu-lative effect on lactogen production. They base this on their observation that the simultaneous administration of progesterone partially or com-pletely prevents the increase in the lactogen content of the pituitary which would otherwise follow the administration of estrogen. Withdrawal of progesterone at term could hardly account for the rise in pituitary lactogen noted postpartum, for estrogen, whose positive influence it is presumably inhibiting, is withdrawn at the same time.

That the inhibitory influence, from which the pituitary is released, may be nervous rather than hormonal in nature, is suggested by the observation of Selye[84] that milk secretion failed to occur in rats when the young were removed by Caesarian section and the uterus was immediately distended with paraffin.

FACTORS CONTROLLING THE MAINTENANCE OF LACTATION

There would seem to be no doubt that lactation depends on the presence of a properly prepared breast and an adequate supply of lac-togen.[68] Both requisites are apparently fulfilled in the postpartum subject. Substances possessing lactogenic activity have been found in the body fluids of the lower mammals during lactation.[63] In postpartum women, an increased lactogen content of the urine has been demonstrated.[64] These substances are apparently derived solely from the hypophysis, for its removal during lactation is invariably followed by abrupt cessation of milk secretion.[94] In order that lactation may continue, it is necessary to insure a continued adequate supply of lactogen and to keep the breasts in a receptive condition. This in turn apparently depends on suckling and conditions inherent in the breast.

Role of Suckling.—While the lactogenic hormone is conceded to be a sine qua non of milk production, the mere presence of an intact pituitary and fully primed breasts in the postpartum individual are not of them-selves sufficient for the maintenance of lactation. It is well known that regression of the mammary gland sets in following parturition, unless suckling is instituted. Although it has long been recognized that suckling plays an important part in lactation, its mode of action has not yet been fully clarified. Some believe its effect is simply to remove the products of secretion. By preventing their accumulation in the alveoli, pressure atrophy of the secretory epithelium is avoided and further secretory activity is assured. This interpretation finds support in the observation that, in the guinea pig[95] and rabbit,[96] cutting the nipple to prevent withdrawal of milk led to mammary regression despite continued suckling of other uncut glands, which remained normal and continued to secrete milk. On the other hand, Selye and his associates[84, 97, 98] maintain that the maintenance of milk secretion through suckling is not due to the fact that it insures milk withdrawal. These observers found that when the *galactophores* of lactating rats or mice were cut to prevent the escape of milk, lactation could nevertheless be maintained for three weeks by suckling or gentle manipulation of the nipple. When the galactophores were cut on only one side and suckling confined to this side, secretory activity continued on both sides. They concluded that nursing promotes milk secretion by reflexly stimulating the hypophysis to secrete its lactogenic hormone, rather than by withdrawing the accumulated secretions or initiating a local reflex in the suckled breasts. This finds some support in the observation of Reece and Turner,[99] that the lactogen content of the pituitary rises when suckling is withheld and falls once more when it is resumed. This occurs regardless of whether or not milk is removed.

The identity of the nervous pathways which carry the stimulus initiated by suckling to the pituitary, is not known. Doubt is cast on the existence of such pathways by reports that lactation proceeds normally after severing all the nerves of the breast,[100] or cutting the entire spinal cord.[101] On the other hand, Ingelbrecht[102] has shown that milk secretion ceases when suckling is confined to nipples paralyzed by severing the spinal cord between the last dorsal and first lumbar vertebrae; but if it is applied to normal nipples, secretion occurs in both the normal and paralyzed glands.

Local Factors Controlling the Amount and Duration of Milk Secretion.—As previously stated, the quantity of milk secreted depends partly on the amount of mammary parenchyma and the degree to which it has been developed. The quantity of mammary parenchyma is apparently genetically controlled and varies according to the inherited constitution of the individual. The extent of its development, on the other hand, is determined by the supply of estrogen and progestin. A fully developed breast, an intact hypophysis and an adequate suckling stimulus, though sufficient to initiate and maintain lactation for a varying period of time, cannot prolong it indefinitely. This has been demonstrated in the rat by Parkes[103] and Selye,[98] who attempted to prolong lactation beyond its normal duration by supplying fresh litters. Though the lactation period was extended somewhat, milk secretion ceased after a time, despite continued suckling.

Exhaustion of the supply of lactogenic hormone is apparently only partly responsible for the cessation of milk production, for efforts to prolong lactation indefinitely by administering potent lactogenic preparations have proved unsuccessful. Turner[104] found that lactating goats "go dry" despite persistent suckling and continued administration of a lactogenic extract. Further secretory activity could be induced only if a new growth of secreting structures was brought about by administering estrogen and progestin. Grant[105] found that as much as 800 Riddle units of lactogenic substance daily only reinstated a limited milk secretion in the regressing mammae of female guinea pigs. Like Turner, he found the acinar tissue of such regressing glands must be reconditioned by estrogen and progestin before it can enter upon another cycle of secretion. These observations are of distinct importance from the clinical standpoint, for they indicate that the limiting factor may reside in the milk secreting structures and that consequently the efficacy of lactogenic preparations is necessarily limited by the condition of the receptor organ.

Role of the Adrenal Cortex in Lactation.—Participation of the adrenal cortex in lactation is indicated by the observation that in many, though not all, species, adrenalectomy prevents milk secretion or suppresses it after it is established.[106] It is also implied in the observation that the addition of adrenocorticotropic or adrenal cortical extract is necessary to insure a response to the lactogenic hormone in the hypophysectomized animal (supra). It is likewise significant that lactation can be induced in the adrenalectomized animal with adrenal cortical extract plus lactogenic hormone, but not with lactogenic hormone alone.[107]

The identity and mode of action of the *adrenal cortical factor* which helps maintain lactation is not certain. The use of the life-sustaining principle, *cortin*, to induce lactation in the adrenalectomized animal, yielded inconstant results. Secretion of milk was noted in some of the cases so treated, but in others it was without effect, although sufficient cortical extract was administered to keep the test animals in a state of good health. Hartman and his associates[108, 109] have postulated the existence of a specific lactogenic factor, which they have named *cortilactin*. They maintain that it is one-tenth as potent as purified prolactin when measured by the crop-gland response, and plays no role in gluconeogenesis. This has been questioned by Gaunt,[110] who showed that cortin can maintain lactation in the adrenalectomized animal if given in sufficiently large doses. He suggested that the negative results obtained by Hartman's group with this hormone were due to inadequate dosage, and not to lack of a specific mammotropic hormone in the extract. According to Gaunt, the adrenal cortex helps maintain lactation indirectly through its regulatory effect on salt and water metabolism. Its removal, he believes, prevents lactation by causing depletion of the fluid and salt content of the blood, thus preventing the large fluid shifts essential for milk production. His view receives support from Leventein's[111] observation that adrenalectomy in lactating animals causes only slight structural changes in the mammae, which differ from those of intact animals only in that the alveoli are less distended and contain a more dense secretion. Levenstein found that salt therapy restored such glands to normal, and the changes which appear in the mammae after adrenalectomy could be duplicated by simply restricting the fluid intake.

Recent studies with the various active compounds derived from the adrenal cortex indicate that the adrenal cortical factor which maintains lactation in the adrenalectomized animal is not desoxycorticosterone, but some compound related to *17–hydroxy–11–dehydrocorticosterone* and *dehy-drocorticosterone*.[112, 113] In view of the evidence (see Chap. XVII) that the adrenal cortex is concerned with carbohydrate metabolism, it seems likely that the disturbance of sugar metabolism, which follows its removal, also contributes to the suppression of lactation seen in the adrenalectomized animal. The inconstant results obtained with cortin may be attributable to the fact that it exerts only a slight effect on sugar metabolism.

Role of the Thyroid in Lactation.—It has often been observed that women with hyperthyroidism lactate poorly. On the assumption that excessive secretion of thyroid hormone lowers milk production, some clinicians have resorted to thyroid feeding to check excessive or undesired milk secretion. Conversely, antithyroidal treatment has been employed with the hope of improving deficient milk secretion. The reported results of such therapy are conflicting and permit no conclusions.

Experimental studies of the role of the thyroid in lactation have yielded varied results. Thyroidectomy in the lactating cow[114] and goat[115] has been found to reduce without completely suppressing milk secretion. In the dog and rat, some workers could demonstrate no unfavorable effect on established lactation, while others report a drop in milk production. Houssay[116] found that thyroid ablation in dogs did not interfere with the response of the breast to the lactogenic principle. In the rat and guinea pig, Nelson and Tobin[117] observed that thyroidectomy during pregnancy or before conception did not interfere with postpartum lactation. Nor did it prevent the secretion of milk which occurs when a series of estrogen injections are given and then abruptly stopped. The lowered activity of the thyroid which follows hypophysectomy, is apparently not responsible for the inefficiency of lactogenic hormone in the hypophysectomized animal, for the addition of thyroxin fails to improve the response.[117]

The effect of thyroid feeding has been investigated in the rat, guinea pig, goat and cow. Where thyroid substance has been used, the results have varied considerably, due possibly to variations in the potency of the materials. In general, such investigations have failed to demonstrate a stimulative effect on milk production. On the other hand, studies with thyroxin, a chemically pure synthetic product, suggest that moderate doses of this substance may increase the rate of milk and fat production in the cow and goat.[118, 119] If given in large doses, this substance has a depressive effect on milk production. Siegert[120] suggests that this may be due to the fact that it prevents access of a sufficient amount of water and salt to the breast. To account for the stimulative effect of moderate doses, it has been suggested that it may act either by stimulating general metabolism and incidentally that of the mammary gland, by increasing lactogenic hormone production, improving the flow of blood through the breast, or maintaining the level of milk precursors in the blood.

Role of the Posterior Hypophysis in Lactation.—In 1910, Ott and Scott[121] called attention to an increased flow of milk following the administration of posterior pituitary extract. This has been corroborated by numerous observers. Most authorities believe that the increased flow of milk thus induced is not due to increased milk secretion but to accelerated expulsion of secretions already formed. This is apparently the result of the oxytocic action of the extract on the smooth muscles of the breast, whose function is to facilitate the expression of milk. Whether the oxytocic factor of the posterior lobe normally plays an essential role in the removal of milk during nursing is not certain. Gomez[122] found that while anterior lobe extract maintained lactation in hypophysectomized rats, the young could not obtain the milk present in the gland unless injections of pituitrin were also given. Turner and Cooper[123] have postulated the existence of a posterior pituitary factor, distinct from pitocin and pitressin, which causes contraction of smooth muscle elements around the alveoli during the milking process. The validity of their suggestion cannot be decided from the evidence at hand. Though there are reports that lactation may proceed normally despite removal of the posterior hypophysis,[124] these are inconclusive because there is no proof that all tissue, now known to form part of the posterior lobe, was destroyed (see Chap. XIV).

Role of the Parathyroids and Pancreas in Lactation.—Evidence relating to the role of the parathyroids, pancreas, and other glands in lactation is limited. Chaikoff and Lyons[125] found that removal of the pancreas interfered with the response to the lactogenic hormone in only one out of six dogs. On the basis of a survey of the literature and his own findings, Nelson[126] concluded that this gland is not essential for lactation. In the absence of evidence to the contrary, it seems reasonable to suppose that the pancreas and parathyroids influence the process of milk secretion to the extent that the elements, whose metabolism they control, enter into the composition of true milk.

EFFECT OF LACTATION ON THE REPRODUCTIVE ORGANS

Lactation and Gonadal Function.—In the absence of suckling, the estrual or menstrual cycle is normally reestablished soon after parturition. If lactation intervenes, recurrence of the sex cycle may be delayed to a varying extent. In man, lactation is associated with *amenorrhea* which may persist from six weeks to a year or longer. In some women, menstruation is delayed until weaning, while in others it may recur despite continued suckling, particularly if the amount of milk secreted is deficient. Ovulation is usually, but not invariably, inhibited during the period of amenorrhea and may sometimes remain absent for several months after the appearance of cyclic uterine bleeding.[127]

To account for *lactation anestrus* in the lower mammals, it has been suggested that the genital tissues are refractory to stimulation at this time. Selye[128] was unable to induce estrus in lactating animals with estrogenic hormone. Parkes[129] and Votquenne[130] were more successful, but found the amount of estrogen required for this effect proportional to the number of young suckled. On removing the corpus luteum, Parkes was able to induce estrus in lactating animals with practically the same amount of estrogen required for this effect in the nonlactating animal. He therefore suggested that the absence of estrus during lactation may be due to the inhibitory influence of the yellow body. This is borne out by the observation of Selye[131] that nonpregnant rats, when suckled, go into diestrus which is associated with formation of corpora lutea like those of pregnancy, and progestational modifications of the uterine mucosa. The mammae of such animals present pseudopregnant changes and, if they have recently been weaned, secretion occurs. Since they could not elicit this phenomenon ("suckling pseudopregnancy") in hypophysectomized animals, it would appear that suckling in some way stimulates the pituitary gland to release its luteinizing principle, which in turn induces corpus luteum formation and prevents further estrus cycles.

Desclin and Gregoire[132] believe that suckling not only stimulates production of the luteinizing hormone, but also simultaneously suppresses production of the follicle-stimulating factor. In this connection, Nathanson and Fevold[133] observed that the urine of lactating amenorrheic women induced diestrus in rats and mice, while commercial lactogenic preparations were only slightly effective. They concluded that the estrus-inhibiting activity of the urine was due to its luteinizing hormone content rather than to the presence of a lactogenic substance. Studies since carried out with various lactogenic preparations[134, 135] indicate that the lactogenic principle, or a closely related fraction in the pituitary lactogenic preparations, causes maintenance of the corpus luteum and progestin secretion in the rat. Follicular development is apparently held in abeyance during such treatment.

The theory that lactation prevents the appearance of estrus by stimulating luteinizing hormone production cannot account for the absence of estrus in certain species where the corpus luteum regresses sometime before weaning and the recurrence of estrus. Nor can it account for the observation that corpus luteum ablation in lactating rats is not followed by estrus as long as suckling continues.[136]

It has been suggested that the absence of estrus or menstruation during lactation may be due to an *inhibitory effect of the lactogenic hormone* on the ovaries or on the production and release of gonadotropin by the anterior pituitary.[137] Lactogenic extracts have been found to cause gonadal atrophy in male[138] and female[139] birds and fowl, have no effect in male rats,[140] and only a transient inhibitory effect in female rats or mice.[141] That no actual antagonism exists between the lactogenic principle and the ovary is suggested by Allen's[142] observation that the menses appeared at the normal time in a monkey which was made to secrete milk by means of a lactogenic extract.

The absence of estrus or menstruation during lactation is attributed by some to the *drain upon the nutritional resources* of the organism. Selye and McKeown[98] question this view on the basis of their observation that their test animals remained anestrus despite the fact that the galactophores were cut to prevent the escape of milk, thus minimizing the burden on the metabolism. It has also been criticized by McKeown and Zuckerman,[136] who point out that, when foster-mothering is employed to extend the period of lactation, estrus recurs before weaning.

It is possible that suppression of the sex cycle during lactation is due to the fact that *nursing strains the hormonal resources of the anterior pituitary gland*, which supports both milk secretion and gonadal function.

It is conceivable that the hypophysis, which is called upon to produce its lactogenic hormone and other essential metabolic principles required for milk secretion, is incapable of simultaneously supporting gonadal function. When weaning occurs, or milk secretion diminishes despite continued suckling and the breast "goes dry," the hypophysis is relieved of its burden of maintaining lactation and can then again divert its energies in the direction of the gonadal sphere.

Lactation and Uterine Involution.—It is well recognized that lactation promotes involution of the uterus. Of interest is Moir's[143] observation that increased uterine contractions can be recorded coincident with suckling, in the human being. The mechanism involved in this effect is not clear. Loeb[144] observed that the guinea pig uterus atrophies during lactation, although follicular maturation and ovulation continue. He suggested that suckling sets up a nervous impulse which directly stimulates uterine contractions, thus promoting involutionary changes. Others maintain that though the uterine contractions induced by stimulating the breast are probably of simple reflex origin, some hormonal factor is responsible for the uterine atrophy which may follow prolonged lactation.

BIBLIOGRAPHY

1. Arey, L. B.: Developmental Anatomy, 3rd ed., Philadelphia, W. B. Saunders Co., 1934.
2. Fitzwilliams, D. C. L.: On the Breast, London, Wm. Heinemann, 1924.
3. Deaver, J.: The Breast, Philadelphia, P. Blakiston's Son & Co., 1917.
4. Cheatle, G. L., and Cutler, M.: Tumours of the Breast, London, Edw. Arnold & Co., 1931.
5. Nelson, W. O.: Physiol. Rev. *16*:488, 1936.
6. Rosenburg, A.: Frankfurt. Ztschr. f. Path. *27*:466, 1922.
7. Dieckmann, H.: Arch. f. path. Anat. u. Physiol. *256*:321, 1925.
8. Dawson, E. K.: Edin. Med. J. *41*:653, 1934.
9. Taylor, H. C., Jr.: Surg., Gynec. & Obst. *62*:129, 1936.
10. Turner, C. W.: Sex and Internal Secretions, ed. by E. Allen, Baltimore, Williams & Wilkins Co., 1932, chap. 12, p. 544.
11. von Jaschke, R. T.: Die Weibliche Brust, in Halban and Seitz, Biologie u. Pathologie des Weibes, 1926, vol. 5, pt. 2, p. 1338.
12. Knauer, E.: Arch. f. Gynäk. *60*:322, 1900.
13. Halban, J.: Monatschr. f. Geburtsh. u. Gynäk. *12*:496, 1900.
14. Lewis, A. A., and Turner, C. W.: J. Dairy Sci. *24*:845, 1941.
15. Selye, H.: Proc. Soc. Exper. Biol. & Med. *43*:343, 1940.
16. Hartman, C. G., and Speert, H.: Endocrinol. *29*:639, 1941.
17. Werner, A. A.: Endocrinol. *19*:2, 1935; ibid. *24*:119, 1939.
18. Guldberg, E.: Zentralbl. f. Gynäk. *62*:2584, 1938.
19. Ancel, P., and Bouin, P.: J. de physiol. et de path. gén. *13*:31, 1911.
20. Loeb, L.: Proc. Soc. Exper. Biol. & Med. *20*:441, 1923.
21. Hammond, J., and Asdell, S. A.: Am. J. Physiol. *103*:600, 1933.
22. Turner, C. W., and Gardner, W. U.: Missouri Agr. Sta. Res. Bull. No. 158, 1931.
23. Evans, H. M., and Simpson, M. E.: Proc. Soc. Exper. Biol. & Med. *26*:598, 1929.
24. Parkes, A. S.: Proc. Roy. Soc., London, s.B. *104*:189, 1929.
25. Jares, J. J.: Anat. Rec. *45*:264, 1930.
26. Stricker, P., and Grueter, F.: Presse méd. *37*:1268, 1929; Klin. Wchnschr. *8*:2322, 1929
27. Corner, G. W.: Am. J. Physiol. *95*:43, 1930.
28. Gardner, W. U., Diddle, A. W., Allen, E., and Strong, L. C.: Anat. Rec. *60*:457, 1934.
29. Gomez, E. T., Turner, C. W., and Reece, R. P.: Proc Soc. Exper Biol. & Med. *36*:286 287, 1937.

30. Gomez, E. T., and Turner, C. W.: Proc. Soc. Exper. Biol. & Med. *37*:607; ibid. *39*:140, 1938; Missouri Agr. Exper. Sta. Bull. No. 259, 1937.
31. Lewis, A. A., and Turner, C. W.: Proc. Soc. Exper. Biol. & Med. *39*:435, 1938; Missouri Agr. Exper. Sta. Bull. No. 319, 1939.
32. Nelson, W. O.: Anat. Rec. *72* (Suppl.) : 117, 1938.
33. Reece, R. P., and Leonard, S. L.: Proc. Soc. Exper. Biol. & Med. *42*:200, 1939.
34. Reece, R. P., Turner, C. W., and Hill, R. T.: Proc. Soc. Exper. Biol. & Med. *34*:204, 1936.
35. Lyons, W. R., and Pencharz, R. I.: Proc. Soc. Exper. Biol. & Med. *33*:589, 1936.
36. Desclin, L.: Compt. rend. Soc. de Biol. *131*:837, 1939.
37. Asdell, S. A., and Seidenstein, H. R.: Proc. Soc. Exper. Biol. & Med., *32*:931, 1935.
38. Gardner, W. U.: Proc. Soc. Exper. Biol. & Med. *45*:835, 1940.
39. Uyldert, I. E., David, K. J., and Freud, J.: Acta brev. Neerland. *10*:105, 1940.
40. Reece, R. P., and Leonard, S. L.: Endocrinol. *29*:297, 1941.
41. Astwood, E. B., Geschickter, C. F., and Rausch, E. O.: Am. J. Anat. *61*:373, 1937.
42. Samuels, L. T., Reinecke, R. M., and Petersen, W. E.: Proc. Soc. Exper. Biol. & Med. *46*:379, 1941.
43. Trentin, J. J., and Turner, C. W.: Endocrinol. *29*:984, 1941.
44. Lyons, W. R., and Sako, Y.: Proc. Soc. Exper. Biol. & Med. *44*:398, 1940.
45. Chamberlin, T. L., Gardner, W. U., and Allen, E.: Endocrinol. *28*:753, 1941.
46. Leonard, S. L., and Reece, R. P.: Endocrinol. *30*:32, 1942.
47. Lewis, A. A., Gomez, E. T., and Turner, C. W.: Endocrinol. *30*:37, 1942.
48. Greep, R. O., and Stavely, H. E.: Endocrinol. *29*:18, 1941.
49. Gardner, W. U., Gomez, E. T., and Turner, C. W.: Am. J. Physiol. *113*:673, 1935.
50. Riddle, O., Bates, R. W., and Dykshorn, S. W.: Am. J. Physiol. *105*:191, 1933.
51. Gomez, E. T., and Turner, C. W.: Proc. Soc. Exper. Biol. & Med *34*:404, 1936; ibid. *35*:59, 1936; Missouri Agr. Exper. Sta. Bull. No. 259, 1937.
52. Gomez, E. T., and Turner, C. W.: Proc. Soc. Exper. Biol. & Med. *35*:365, 1936.
53. Gomez, E. T., and Turner, C. W.: Proc. Soc. Exper. Biol. & Med. *36*:78, 1937.
54. Nelson, W. O., and Gaunt, R.: Proc. Soc. Exper. Biol. & Med. *34*:671, 1936; ibid. *36*: 136, 1937.
55. Pencharz, R. I., and Lyons, W. R.: Proc. Soc. Exper. Biol. & Med. *38*:388, 1938.
56. Folley, S. J., and Young, F. G.: Proc. Roy. Soc., London, s.B. *126*:45, 1938.
57. Meites, J., and Turner, C. W.: J. Clin. Endocrinol. *1*:918, 1941.
58. Bergman, A. J., and Turner, C. W.: J. Dairy Sci. *23*:1229, 1940.
59. Reece, R. P., and Turner, C. W.: Missouri Agr. Exper. Sta. Bull. No. 266, 1937.
60. Holst, S., and Turner, C. W.: Proc. Soc. Exper. Biol. & Med. *42*:479, 1939.
61. Lessman, F.: Ztschr. f. Geburtsh. u. Gynäk. *119*:271, 1939.
62. Ehrhardt, K.: Munch. med. Wchnschr. *29*:1163, 1936.
63. Leblond, C. P.: Compt. rend. Soc. de biol. *124*:1062, 1937.
64. Turner, C. W., and Gomez, E. T.: Missouri Agr. Exper. Sta. Bull. No. 207, 1934.
65. Langecker, H., and Schenk, F.: Med. Klin. *32*:1104, 1936.
66. Selye, H., Collip, J. B., and Thomson, D. L.: Proc. Soc. Exper. Biol. & Med. *30*:589, 1933.
67. Collip, J. B.: J. Mt. Sinai Hosp. *1*:28, 1934.
68. Turner, C. W., and Meites, J.: Endocrinol. *29*:165, 1941.
69. Reece, R. P., and Hathaway, I. R., and Davis, H. P.: J. Dairy Sci. *22*:1, 1939.
70. Meites, J., and Turner, C. W.: Endocrinol. *31*:341, 1942.
71. Halban, J.: Arch. f. Gynäk. *75*:353, 1905.
72. Frankl, O.: Am. J. Obst. & Gynec. *6*:394, 1923.
73. Smith, G. V., and Smith, O. W.: Am. J. Physiol. *103*:356, 1933.
74. Nelson, W. O.: Endocrinol. *18*:33, 1934.
75. Hammond, J.: Proc. Roy. Soc., London, s.B. *89*:534, 1917.
76. Drummond-Robinson, G., and Asdell, S. A.: J. Physiol. *61*:608, 1926.
77. Anselmino, K. J., Hoffmann, F., and Pencharz, R. I.: Zentralbl. f. Gynäk. *60*:7, 1936.
78. Anselmino, K. J., Herold, L., and Hoffmann, F.: Zentralbl. f. Gynäk. *60*:501, 1936.
79. Folley, S. J., and Kon, S. K.: Nature, London *139*:1107, 1937.

80. Selye, H.: Anat. Rec. 75:59, 1939.
81. Abarbanel, A. R.: Am. J. Obst. & Gynec. 42:110, 1941.
82. Bruhl, R.: Zentralbl. f. Gynäk. 54:192, 1930.
83. Loeb, L.: Special Cytology, ed. by E. V. Cowdry, New York, Paul B. Hoeber, Inc., 1932, vol. 3, sect. 41.
84. Selye, H., Collip, J. B., and Thomson, D. L.: Endocrinol. 18:237, 1934.
85. Reece, R. P., and Turner, C. W.: Proc. Soc. Exper. Biol. & Med. 34:402, 1936; ibid 36:283, 1937.
86. Lewis, A. A., and Turner, C. W.: Proc. Soc. Exper. Biol. & Med. 48:439, 1941.
87. Meites, J., and Turner, C. W.: Proc. Soc. Exper. Biol. & Med. 49:190, 1942.
88. Haterius, H. O.: Proc. Soc. Exper. Biol. & Med. 29:962, 1932.
89. Kraus, E. J.: Klin. Wchnschr. 14:1718, 1935.
90. De Jongh, S. E., and Laqueur, E.: Klin. Wchnschr. 9:2344, 1930.
91. Walker, S. M., and Stanley, A. J.: Proc. Soc. Exper. Biol. & Med. 48:50, 1941.
92. Folley, S. J., Watson, H. M. S., and Bottomley, A. C.: J. Physiol. 98:15P, 1940.
93. Meites, J., and Turner, C. W.: Endocrinol. 30:719, 1942.
94. Collip, J. B., Selye, H., and Thomson, D. L.: Nature, London 131:56, 1933.
95. Kuramitsu, C., and Loeb, L.: Am. J. Physiol. 56:40, 1921.
96. Hammond, J., and Marshall, F. H. A.: Reproduction in the Rabbit, Edinburgh, Oliver & Boyd, 1925.
97. Selye, H.: Am. J. Physiol. 107:535, 1934.
98. Selye, H., and McKeown, T.: Anat. Rec. 60:323, 1934.
99. Reece, R. P., and Turner, C. W.: Proc. Soc. Exper. Biol. & Med. 35:367, 621, 1937.
100. Eckhardt, C.: Beitr. z. Anat. Physiol., 1855.
101. Goltz, F., and Ewald, J. R.: Pflüger's Arch. f. d. ges. Physiol. 63:362, 1896.
102. Ingelbrecht, P.: Compt. rend. Soc. de biol. 120:1369, 1935.
103. Parkes, A. S.: Proc. Roy. Soc. London, s.B. 102:51, 1927.
104. Turner, C. W., and Reineke, E. P.: Missouri Agr. Exper. Sta. Bull. No. 235, 1936.
105. Grant, G. A.: Biochem. J. 31:1538, 1937.
106. Tobin, C. E.: Anat. Rec. 76 (Suppl.) : 55, 1940.
107. Nelson, W. O., and Gaunt, R.: Proc. Soc. Exper. Biol. & Med. 36:136, 1937.
108. Brownell, K. A., Lockwood, J. E., and Hartman, F. A.: Proc. Soc. Exper. Biol. & Med 30:783, 1933.
109. Spoor, H., Hartman, F. A., and Brownell, K. A.: Am. J. Physiol. 134:12, 1941.
110. Gaunt, R., and Tobin, C. E.: Am. J. Physiol. 115:588, 1936.
111. Levenstein, I.: Anat. Rec. 67:477, 1937.
112. Gaunt, R., Eversole, W. J., and Kendall, E. C.: Endocrinol. 31:84, 1942.
113. Nelson, W. O.: Anat. Rec. 77 (Suppl.) : 97, 1941.
114. Graham, W. R., Jr.: J. Nutrition 7:407, 1934.
115. Grueter, F.: Proc. Internat. Cong. Sex Res. (1930), Edinburgh, Oliver & Boyd, 1931, p. 443.
116. Houssay, B. A.: Compt. rend. Soc. de biol. 120:502, 1935.
117. Nelson, W. O., and Tobin, C. E.: Anat. Rec. 67 (Suppl.) : 110, 1936.
118. Herman, A., Graham, W. R., Jr., and Turner, C. W.: Missouri Agr. Exper. Sta. No. 275, 1928.
119. Ralston, N. P., Cowsert, W. C., Ragsdale, A. C., Herman, H. A., and Turner, C. W.: Missouri Agr. Exper. Sta. Bull. No. 317, 1940.
120. Siegert, F.: Zentralbl. f. Gynäk. 59:2530, 1935.
121. Ott, I., and Scott, J. C.: Proc. Soc. Exper. Biol. & Med. 8:48, 1940.
122. Gomez, E. T.: J. Dairy Sci. 22:488, 1939; ibid. 23:537, 1940.
123. Turner, C. W., and Cooper, W. D.: Endocrinol. 29:320, 1941.
124. Smith, P. E.: Am. J. Physiol. 99:345, 1932.
125. Chaikoff, I. L., and Lyons, W. R.: Am. J. Physiol. 106:716, 1933.
126. Nelson, W. O., Himwich, H. E., and Fazekas, J. F.: Anat. Rec. 66:201, 1936.
127. Kurzrok, R., Lass, P. M., and Smelser, J.: Proc. Soc. Exper. Biol. & Med. 36:356, 1937.
128. Selye, H., Harlow, C., and McKeown, T.: Proc. Soc. Exper. Biol. & Med. 32:1253, 1935.
129. Parkes, A. S.: Proc. Roy. Soc., London, s.B. 102:51, 1927.

130. Votquenne, M.: Compt. rend. Soc. de biol. *102*:51, 1927.
131. Selye, H., and McKeown, T.: Proc. *31*:683, 1934; Surg., Gynec. & Obst. *59*:886, 1934.
132. Desclin, L., and Gregoire, C.: Compt. rend. Soc. de Biol. *126*:250, 1937.
133. Nathanson, I. T., and Fevold, H. L.: Endocrinol. *22*:86, 1938.
134. Lyons, W. R., Simpson, M. E., and Evans, H. M.: Proc. Soc. Exper. Biol. & Med. *48*:
       634, 1941.
135. Tobin, C. E.: Endocrinol. *31*:197, 1942.
136. McKeown, T., and Zuckerman, S.: Proc. Roy. Soc., London, s.B. *124*:464, 1937.
137. Weichert, C. K.: Anat. Rec. *75* (Suppl.) : 72, 1939.
138. Bates, R. W., Lahr, E. L., and Riddle, O.: Am. J. Physiol. *111*:361, 1935.
139. Riddle, O., and Bates, R. W.: Endocrinol. *17*:689, 1933.
140. Riddle, O., Lahr, E. L., Bates, R. W., and Moran, C. S.: Proc. Soc. Exper. Biol. &
       Med. *32*:509, 1934.
141. Lahr, E. L., and Riddle, O.: Proc. Soc. Exper. Biol. & Med. *34*:880, 1936.
142. Allen, E., Gardner, W. U., and Diddle, A. W.: Endocrinol. *19*:305, 1935.
143. Moir, C.: Trans. Edinburgh Obst. Soc., 1933–34, p. 93.
144. Kuramitsu, C., and Loeb, L.: Am. J. Physiol. *55*:422, 443, 1921.
145. Speert, H.: Surg., Gynec. & Obst. *73*:388, 1941.
146. Folley, S. J.: Nature, London *150*:266, 1942.

CHAPTER XI

THE PHYSIOLOGY OF THE TESTIS

The male gonad, like the ovary, performs an excretory and incretory function. It is concerned primarily with production of male germ cells (spermatogenesis), and secondarily with secretion of the so-called "male sex hormones." The spermatozoa are produced by the seminiferous tubules, while the male hormones are secreted by the Leydig cells of the interstitial portion. Though the function of these two components of the testis normally runs parallel, instances of dissociation have been noted.

SPERMATOGENIC FUNCTION

In man, spermatogenesis normally begins during the puberal epoch, and is usually fully established by the fifteenth year. The age at which it declines and is fully extinguished varies widely. In the monkey, man, and such mammals as the rabbit, guinea pig, and rat, spermatogenesis once initiated is a continuous process. On the other hand, in most vertebrates and mammals, it is intermittent, occurring usually at intervals of one year and persisting for only a limited period, the so-called breeding season.

ENDOCRINE FUNCTION OF THE TESTIS

On the basis of changes noted following castration, and effects obtained with testicular implants or extracts in intact and castrate subjects, it is now generally agreed that the testis produces an internal secretion which (1) causes the secondary sexual characteristics to differentiate from the neuter to the mature male type; (2) causes descent of the testis into the scrotum; (3) maintains the secretory activity of the accessory sex organs; (4) activates the erectile and ejaculatory mechanism; (5) maintains the function of the epididymis and (6) influences the gonadotropic activity of the anterior hypophysis.

Studies in fish, amphibia, reptiles, birds, and mammals have uniformly shown that removal of the testes in the immature animal precludes development of the accessory sex organs and secondary sex characters. In the mature animal, this operation leads to involution of the sex organs and loss of sex drive. Proof that these changes are due to withdrawal of a testicular hormone was first provided by Berthold,[1] who demonstrated that the amputated comb and wattles of the capon can be regenerated by transplanting the extirpated testicular tissue to another part of the body. This was virtually the beginning of our knowledge of the internal secretion of the testis and showed that this organ produces a hormonal principle which controls the outward appearance of maleness.

Isolation of the Male Sex Hormone.—Brown-Séquard[2] first employed a testicular extract to replace deficient testicular function. He tried to rejuvenate himself with hypodermic injections of a testicular extract prepared by him, but though he claimed subjective improvement, his results were unconvincing. Pegard later prepared an extract of swine testes, which induced comb growth in capons. In 1927, McGee[3] prepared a potent lipoid extract of bull testes which produced marked growth of the comb, wattles, and ear lobes in capons, and restored the accessory genital organs of castrate rats to their precastration state. Gallagher and Koch[4] purified the crude lipoid extract and obtained a product with highly concentrated activity. David and associates,[5] in 1935, obtained the active principle of bull's testes in crystalline form. They named it *testosterone* and suggested $C_{19}H_{28}O_2$ as its empirical formula. This substance has been synthesized from cholesterol by Ruzicka[6] and Butenandt.[7]

An androgenic substance, differing chemically from that derived from testis tissue, was extracted from human male urine by Loewe and Voss,[8] and Funk and Harrow,[9] in 1929. Shortly after this, Butenandt[10, 11] prepared the active principle in crystalline form and named it *androsterone*. He found it to be a ketone-alcohol derivative, and suggested the empirical formula $C_{19}H_{30}O_2$, which he subsequently confirmed. This substance has been synthesized from cholesterol by Ruzicka and associates.[12] Butenandt[13] has also obtained from human male urine, a second crystalline hormone which he named *dehydroandrosterone*. This substance is an isomer of testosterone and has the empirical formula $C_{19}H_{28}O_2$.

To date, more than thirty androgenic compounds related to testosterone have been synthetically prepared from the sterols. The true testicular hormone has not been identified, but it is thought to be very close to testosterone.

The testicular extracts are much more potent than the androgens derived from the urine. Testosterone is six to ten times as potent as androsterone, depending on the biologic test used. Androsterone in turn is more potent than dehydroandrosterone. A large number of esters of the parent hormone have been prepared and shown to possess greater androgenic potency than the free hormone. The most active one, *testosterone propionate,* is now most widely used.

Site of Origin of the Testicular Hormone.—The interstitial cells of the testis are probably the main source of the male sex hormone. Bouin and Ancel,[14] in 1903, demonstrated that vasoligation in the rabbit leads to degeneration of the germinal epithelium and cessation of spermatogenesis, associated with marked proliferation of the interstitial cells. Since the structure and function of the accessory sex organs remained unaltered, they concluded that the interstitial cells are the source of the male sex hormone. This assumption finds support in the observation that in *cryptorchidism,* spermatogenesis is diminished or absent, but the accessory genitalia and secondary sex characters may nevertheless attain normal proportions.[15] Also significant is the observation[16, 17] that the hypophysectomized male rat responds to anterior pituitary follicle stimulating hormone with tubular growth, but the size of the accessory sex organs remains unchanged, indicating that growth of the tubules is unassociated with male sex hormone production. The luteinizing factor, on the other hand, elicits interstitial cell hypertrophy associated with a marked increase in the weight of the accessory genital organs. From this it would appear that the interstitial cells are the chief if not the sole source of male sex hormone in the rat and probably also in other species, including man. In birds, there is some evidence that androgen may be secreted by both the germinal epithelium and the interstitial cells.[88]

Time of Onset of Testicular Hormone Production.—In constant breeders, such as man, testicular hormone production coincides with full testicular development, normally achieved at puberty, and persists throughout reproductive life. The testicle, if properly stimulated, is apparently capable of producing male sex hormone during childhood, for development of the accessory genitalia and secondary sex characters has been observed in prepuberal animals following treatment with pituitary implants or potent gonadotropic extracts.

EFFECTS OF ANDROGENS IN THE MALE

Development of Accessory Genitalia.—The physiologic effects of androgenic substances in the male have not yet been fully explored. The available androgens vary considerably in their ability to produce the structural and functional alterations thought to be controlled by the testicular hormones. This is apparently due to differences in their chemical structure. Testosterone, believed to be closer chemically to the true testicular hormone than any other of the known androgens, is apparently capable of producing all the effects known to be dependent on testicular function. In the immature mammal, the androgens cause development of the accessory sex organs, and stimulate sexual behavior. In the adult castrate animal, they either prevent or repair the damage to the accessory sex organs. The effects of the crystalline androgens in man, as listed by Hamilton,[18] are as follows: (1) Increased frequency of erection; (2) establishment of ejaculates where such were previously lacking; (3) growth of the scrotum and penis; (4) prostatic enlargement; (5) changes in hair distribution, and (6) modifications of the voice.

Effect of the Androgens on the Testis.—The effect of the androgens on the testis is not clear, for both *inhibitory* and *stimulative* effects have been reported. Moore and Price[19] found that 6 bird units of testis extract, given daily for three weeks, inhibited testicular development in young growing rats. The testes of the treated animals were 80 per cent smaller than those of the controls and showed histologic evidence of severe damage and cessation of spermatozoon production. In the adult rat, on the other hand, as much as 21 bird units of bull testis extract or 6 mgm. of androsterone daily had no apparent deleterious effect.[20, 21] When testosterone propionate was used, the degree of retardation and injury to the testis was inversely proportional to the age of the animals, being most marked in young normal rats. Small doses were more effective than large ones in causing inhibition. Cutuly and Cutuly[22] found that in intact immature rats given testosterone propionate or dehydroandrosterone acetate, in doses

of 3 mg. daily for twenty-three or twenty-four days, spermatogenesis proceeded normally but the interstitial cells were atrophied. On the basis of
these and other observations, these investigators suggest that spermatogenesis falls into three stages, a premeiotic, reduction-division, and post-
meiotic phase. The first occurs in the untreated hypophysectomized animal
and is independent of hormonal stimulation. The second is apparently

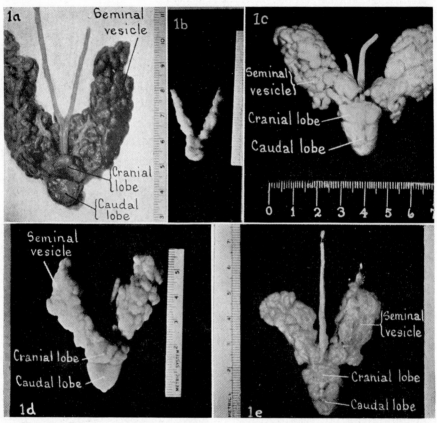

Fig. 35.—Effects of androgenic substance on prostate and seminal vesicles of the immature castrate monkey. 1a, After subcutaneous injections of testosterone proprionate in
oil. 1b, Untreated control. 1c, After subcutaneous injections of testosterone propionate in
oil. 1d, After implantations of pellets of crystalline testosterone. 1e, After implantations into
the omentum of pellets of crystalline testosterone. (Vest, S. A., Drew, J. E. and Langworthy,
O. R.: Endocrinol. Vol. 27.)

controlled by the pituitary gonadotropes, while the third is either independent of hormonal stimulation or progresses under the influence of
testicular hormone. Shay and associates[23] found that 3 mgm. of testosterone propionate weekly, administered to prepuberal rats (first to thirtieth day of life), decreased the weight of the testes and prevented sperm
formation. Similar treatment in postpuberal animals (thirtieth to sixtieth

day) had no apparent deleterious effect. Larger doses (30 mgm. weekly) given over a period of thirty days to either prepuberal or postpuberal animals, increased the weight of the testes and stimulated spermatogenic function. The same dose, given continuously from the first to the sixtieth day of life inhibited testicular function.

Selye and Friedman,[24] also working with the rat, obtained stimulative effects with large doses and inhibition of testicular function with small ones. Rubinstein and Kurland,[25] on the other hand, found that small doses administered to rats from the twenty-second to the thirty-second day of life increased the weight of the testes and stimulated proliferation of the germinal epithelium, but did not cause maturation of spermatozoa. An increase in the dosage resulted in inhibition, but doses large enough to inhibit testicular function in the prepuberal animal, did not have this effect when continued into postpuberal life. Wainman and associates[89] observed a marked reduction in the weight of the testes and injury to the testicular tubules in rats receiving testosterone propionate daily for twenty-five days, beginning on the sixtieth day of life. Testis weight reduction was greater where the daily dose was 0.2 mg. than when 0.5 mg. was given.

Studies in species other than the rat have been limited. Testicular damage has been noted in young growing dogs and guinea pigs receiving androgenic substance. In the annual breeding squirrel, Wells and Moore[26] found that androgens administered during the non-breeding season caused spermatozoa to appear earlier than in untreated controls. In man, Heckel,[27] McCullagh,[28] and others found that testosterone propionate therapy markedly reduced the number of spermatozoa.

Mechanism of Androgen Effects.—It is generally believed that the androgens cause inhibition by depressing the anterior hypophysis, thus indirectly depriving the testes of the hormonal stimuli on which their function primarily depends. The stimulating effects noted in androgen treated animals are difficult to explain. A possible clue is provided by recent observations in the hypophysectomized animal. Androgens administered to rats immediately after hypophysectomy prevent atrophy of the seminiferous tubules, but have no such protective action on the interstitial cells. If treatment is delayed until atrophy has set in, this protective action is no longer evident. In the hypophysectomized guinea pig,[29] androgens given immediately following operation maintain the weight of the testes for ten days but do not sustain spermatogenesis. After the tenth day, the weight of the testes drops rapidly despite continued treatment. These observations suggest that under certain conditions, the male sex hormones may affect the seminiferous tubules without the intervention of the adenohypophysis. Since they are effective only if given immediately after hypophysectomy, it would appear that their function is to enhance the action of the follicle stimulating factor on which tubular activity primarily depends. Some observers maintain that this so-called "protective" action is nonspecific since it may be duplicated with yeast extract[30] or progesterone.[31]

From the available data, it would appear that *dosage, length of treat-*

11

ment, and the *age* and *species* of the test animal play an important part in determining whether testicular inhibition or stimulation will follow. Differences in response are probably at least partly attributable to variations in the gonadotropic activity of the adenohypophysis and the functional status of the gonads. The *type of androgen* used and the *degree of its folliculoid (estrogenic) activity* may also be a determining factor. Selye[90] has recently presented evidence suggesting that the folliculoid action of testosterone is responsible for its anti-spermatogenic effect when given in small doses. With larger doses, this is apparently offset by the androgenic action of the testosterone molecule, which favors spermatogenesis. The precise circumstances under which stimulation or inhibition may be produced cannot be defined from the data at hand. Since there is no reliable method of predicting the response of the testis in a particular instance, and in view of the possibility that an inhibitory effect may be produced, the androgens should be used with caution in male hypogonadism (see Chap. XXXVI).

EFFECTS OF ANDROGENS IN THE FEMALE

Numerous effects, ranging from complete inhibition to stimulation of sex function have been obtained with the androgens in the female. This can perhaps be partly accounted for by the fact that the male sex hormones are closely related chemically to those of the female and can modify the gonadotropic activity of the anterior hypophysis. The nature of the androgen administered, the dose and duration of treatment, and the age and species of the test animal are apparently important factors in determining the reaction.

Effects on the Ovary.—Studies in the rat,[32] mouse,[33] rabbit,[34] monkey[35] and man[36, 37, 38] indicate that the androgens may cause atrophy of the ovary, inhibit ovulation, accelerate corpus luteum regression, stimulate follicular maturation and cystosis, or cause luteinization. These effects are generally believed to be mediated through the adenohypophysis,[39] the response apparently depending on the extent to which the gland is affected. The occurrence of ovarian atrophy would imply complete suppression of its gonadotropic activity. A milder degree of inhibition may account for suppression of ovulation, or rapid regression of corpora lutea. Follicular cystosis or formation of corpora lutea[40, 41] may be due to a disturbance in the balance of the follicle stimulating and luteinizing factors. Androgen treatment may conceivably lead to follicle cystosis either by suppressing the luteinizing factor and thus creating a relative excess of follicle stimulator, or by stimulating the production of follicle-stimulating hormone. Where luteinization follows androgen administration, it may be that the concentration of the androgens is such that they stimulate the hypophysis to release its luteinizer.

Effects on the Accessory Genitalia and Secondary Sex Characters.
—Large doses of androgen over a protracted period may stimulate the masculine rudiments or homologues of male structures in the female. Marked enlargement of the clitoris and Skene glands have been described

in various species following such treatment. In women, the androgens may cause deepening of the voice, hirsutism, enlargement of the clitoris and other signs of masculinization.[42, 43] Aside from their masculinizing action, they exert either an inhibitory or stimulative effect on the female accessory genitalia and mammae.

Antagonistic Effects.—Inhibition of estrus has been observed in the rat[32] and mouse[33] following androgen treatment. In the monkey and man, adequate doses inhibit the effect of endogenously supplied estrogen on the vaginal mucosa[44, 45] suppress menstruation[46, 47] for the duration of treatment, and cause endometrial atrophy.[36, 48] Since these effects are associated with suppression of follicular maturation and corpus luteum formation, they are probably mediated through the adenohypophysis and ovaries. The androgens apparently suppress the gonadotropic effect of the hypophysis with consequent cessation of cyclic ovarian activity, on which endometrial function and menstruation depend.

Stimulative Effects.—Certain androgens have been shown to evoke in the female accessory genitalia and mammae effects like those produced by estrogen, progestin, or a combination of both.

(a) *Estrogen-like Effects:* In the infantile rodent, testosterone causes estrus and vaginal opening,[49, 50, 51] even in the absence of the hypophysis.[39] The mature castrate rodent responds with vaginal cornification to androsterone and dehydroandrosterone, but not testosterone.[52] In the mature castrate rabbit, the androgens cause growth of the atrophic uterus. Protracted androgen treatment in the mature castrate guinea pig leads to cystic dilatation of the endometrial glands with moderate proliferation of the surface epithelium and stroma, modifications simulating those produced by protracted estrogen stimulation.[53] In the castrate rhesus monkey, testosterone postpones the bleeding which would otherwise follow estrogen withdrawal.[54] The interval between the last injection of testosterone and the onset of bleeding is approximately equal to that which follows estrogen withdrawal. In the lower mammal and man, testosterone, like estrogen, prevents breast engorgement and the onset of lactation.[55, 56]

(b) *Progesterone-like Effects:* Like progesterone, the androgens inhibit estrogen induced uterine motility and reactivity to pituitrin in the rabbit, postpone parturition in the rat, and prevent the abortion which would otherwise follow ovariectomy.[57, 58] Androgens induce progestational modifications in the estrogen-primed endometrium of the castrate cat[59] and rat.[60] In man, they inhibit the contractions of the Fallopian tubes, an effect not unlike that obtained with progesterone.[61] In the monkey,[91] the progesterone-like action of testosterone is evident in its ability to inhibit estrogen-withdrawal bleeding; precipitate bleeding in the presence of a maintenance dose of estrogen; prevent enlargement of the cervix and metaplasia of the cervical glands which would otherwise follow estrogen administration; decrease cornification of the vaginal mucosa, and cause loss of edema of the sexual skin.

Certain effects which normally depend on the combined action of estrogen and progestin have also been obtained with the androgens. When given in adequate doses over a sufficient length of time, androgenic substances, acting alone and without preliminary estrogen treatment, induce vaginal mucification in the castrate rat.[62] Under similar conditions, they produce, in the castrate rat and rabbit, proliferative and progestational modifications of the endometrium, and full development of the duct and alveolar systems of the breast.[63, 64]

These effects on the ovary and female accessory genitalia have formed the basis for the adoption of androgen therapy in menstrual and reproductive disorders.

THE TESTIS AND THE ANTERIOR HYPOPHYSIS

Anterior Hypophyseal Control of Testicular Function.—It is well established that the anterior hypophysis initiates and maintains testicular function. Hypophysectomy precludes spermatogenic function, while implants or potent extracts of anterior lobe tissue restore this function in the hypophysectomized animal.[65] In amphibia and birds, anterior pituitary implants or extracts given before maturity cause precocious spermatogenic function.[66, 67, 68] In mammals, on the other hand, attempts to hasten the initiation of spermatogenic function have thus far proved unsuccessful.[69]

Effects on Spermatogenesis.—Studies with fractioned extracts of anterior lobe tissue indicate that growth of the seminiferous tubules and spermatogenesis depend primarily on the follicle stimulating factor of the adenohypophysis. In the immature intact rat, Fevold[92] found that this factor stimulated tubular development and spermatogenesis but had no apparent effect on the interstitial tissue. When administered immediately after hypophysectomy, it maintained spermatogenic function. If treatment was delayed until two weeks after operation, it restored full spermatogenic function.

The cyclic rise and fall of spermatogenic activity in seasonal breeders apparently depends on variations in the level of anterior pituitary gonadotropic activity, for pregnancy urine gonadotropic extract, given during the nonbreeding season stimulates the dormant testis to produce spermatozoa.[70] This, coupled with the fact that the gonadotropic hormone content of the pituitary of seasonal breeders decreases during the period of sexual inactivity suggests that the absence of spermatogenic function at this time is due to a deficiency of the pituitary gonadotropes rather than unresponsiveness of the testes.

Nonendocrine causes, such as inanition, vitamin deficiency, and debilitating states, may materially depress spermatogenic function.[71] In certain species, this function may be influenced by changes in temperature or variations in the length of time that the animal is exposed to light each day.[72] The available evidence strongly suggests that these factors exert their effect on spermatogenesis through the mediation of the adenohypophysis.

Effects on Incretory Function.—The incretory function of the testis is likewise dependent primarily on the gonadotropic activity of the anterior hypophysis. Following hypophysectomy in the immature animal, the interstitial cells remain retarded, no male sex hormone is produced, and the accessory genitalia and secondary sex characters fail to develop. In the adult animal, this operation is followed within a short time by progressive involution of the accessory sex organs. Implantation of fresh hypophyseal tissue or potent gonadotropic extracts repairs the damage. In the intact immature animal such treatment causes precocious maturation of the accessory genitalia.

There is evidence that growth and function of the interstitial cells of the testis depends on the luteinizing factor (LH) of the anterior hypophysis. Fevold's group[73] found this hormone, when administered to the hypophysectomized rat, repaired the interstitial cell damage and indirectly restored the accessory genital organs to their pre-operative status, presumably by stimulating male sex hormone secretion. For a time, Evans and associates[74, 75] were convinced that the factor which stimulates the interstitial cells of the rat testis is not the luteinizing hormone but a separate principle which they named *interstitial-cell-stimulating hormone,* ICSH. Fevold could obtain no evidence pointing to the existence of a separate ICSH factor distinct from LH. More recently, Evans also reached the conclusion that the so-called ICSH and LH factors are identical (see Chap. XII).

Effect of the Testis on the Anterior Hypophysis.—While the anterior hypophysis dominates testicular function, studies in intact and castrate animals indicate that alterations in the sexual sphere may in turn materially affect the structure and function of the pituitary.

In the male, as in the female (see Chap. XII), *gonadectomy* is followed by enlargement of the hypophysis, due to the formation of so-called "castration" cells. This hypertrophy is accompanied by a rise in the gonadotropin content of the gland and the appearance of follicle-stimulating hormone (*prolan A*) in the urine.[76] These effects can be prevented or reversed by administering male sex hormone.[77] This suggests the existence of a reciprocal relationship between the adenohypophysis and testis, that is, the hypophyseal gonadotropes stimulate testicular function which in turn tends to reduce the level of pituitary activity.

The male hypophysis is more difficult to inhibit than the female gland, requiring five times as much estrogen or testosterone.[78] A mixture of the male and female sex hormone is more effective for this purpose than either alone. It has been suggested that this may be the function of the female sex hormone normally present in the male organism (see Chap. XL). While some workers believe that an estrogen-androgen combination regulates hypophyseal activity, others maintain that a specific hormone secreted by the germinal cells of the testicle performs this function. The latter view is based on the observation that destruction of the germinal epithelium in rats, by the x-rays or radium, is followed by the appearance of "castration cells" in the hypophysis and an increase in its gonadotropic hormone content, while the accessory genital organs show no castration changes. Further evidence is provided by the observation of Martins and Rocha[79] that an aqueous extract of testis tissue repaired the postcastration changes in the hypophysis of castrate male animals, without stimulating the accessory genitalia. The term *inhibin* has been applied by McCullagh[80] to the hypothetical principle responsible for this effect. The separate existence of this principle has been questioned on the ground that the ability of testis extracts to repair the castration changes in the hypophysis parallels their ability to stimulate the accessory genitalia. Moore[81] and others maintain that there is no need to postulate the existence of a second testicular hormone to account for the fact that castration changes may occur in the hypophysis of experimental cryptorchid animals while the accessory genitalia continue to show evidence of stimulation. This, they believe, may as reasonably be explained on the basis of differences in the concentration of testicular hormone required for these two effects. As Moore has recently pointed out, there is no known change dependent on the naturally secreted hormone, which cannot be repaired by a pure chemical compound such as testosterone propionate.

Clinical Application of the Androgens.—Androgen therapy has been recommended for a large variety of conditions in both the male and female. In the male, it is employed for the treatment of cryptorchidism, hypogonadism, sterility, impotence (see Chap. XXXV), the male climacteric,[82] and benign prostatic hypertrophy.[83] The androgens are apparently effective in initiating erections and sterile ejaculations, can cause considerable enlargement of the penis and prostate, stimulate growth of pubic and, occasionally, facial hair, and modify the pitch of the voice. In view of their unfavorable effect on spermatogenic function,[84] they are best reserved for cases where genital development is desired and the preservation of spermatogenic function is not a consideration. They should be used only where the gonads are absent or so retarded as to be incapable of responding to stimulation. In the prepuberal and postpuberal castrate or eunuchoid individual, they may not only stimulate development of the genitalia and secondary sex characters, but apparently also give relief from mental depression, general muscular weakness and fatigability.[85] Unfortunately, it would seem that these effects cannot be prolonged indefinitely. As treatment is continued, the patient may become increasingly refractory, requiring larger doses for an effect.[86, 87] This process may be slowed down to a certain extent but cannot be prevented by permitting intervening periods of rest.[86]

The androgens are used in the female because of their ability to inhibit anterior pituitary function and antagonize the effect of estrogen on the accessory genitalia.[37, 38] Their value in functional uterine bleeding, dysmenorrhea, chronic mastitis, premenstrual tension and the symptomatic menopause, and their use for the suppression of lactation is considered in detail in the chapters dealing with these conditions.

BIBLIOGRAPHY

1. Berthold, A. A.: Arch. f. Anat., Physiol., u. Wissensch. Med., 1849, p. 42.
2. Brown-Séquard, C. E.: Arch. de physiol. norm. et path. *21*:651, 1889.
3. McGee, L. C.: Proc. Inst. Med. Chicago *6*:242, 1927.
4. Gallagher, T. F., and Koch, F. C.: Endocrinol. *18*:107, 1934.

5. David, K., Dingemanse, E., Freud, J., and Laqueur, E.: Ztschr. f. physiol. Chem. *233:* 281, 1935.
6. Ruzicka, L., and Wettstein, A.: Helv. chim. Acta *18:*1264, 1935.
7. Butenandt, A., and Hanisch, G.: Ztschr. f. physiol. Chem. *237:*89, 1935.
8. Loewe, S., and Voss, H. E.: Sitz. Akad. Wiss. Wien. Math. Nature Klin. No. 20, 1929.
9. Funk, C., and Harrow, B.: Proc. Soc. Exper. Biol. & Med. *26:*325, 1929.
10. Butenandt, A.: Ztschr. f. angew. Chem. *44:*905, 1931; ibid. *45:*655, 1932.
11. Butenandt, A., and Tscherning, K.: Ztschr. f. physiol. Chem. *229:*167, 1934.
12. Ruzicka, L., Goldberg, M. W., Meyer, J., Brungger, H., and Eichenberger, E.: Helv. chim. Acta *17:*1395, 1934.
13. Butenandt, A., and Danenbaum, H.: Ztschr. f. physiol. Chem. *229:*192, 1934.
14. Bouin, P., and Ancel, P.: Arch. de zool. exper. et gén. *1:*437, 1903.
15. Moore, C. R.: Am. J. Anat. *34:*269, 1924.
16. Greep, R. O.: Anat. Rec. *67* (Suppl.) : 22, 1937.
17. Smith, P. E., Engle, E. T., and Tyndale, H. H.: Proc. Soc. Exper. Biol. & Med. *31:*745, 1934.
18. Hamilton, J. B.: Endocrinol. *21:*649, 1937.
19. Moore, C. R., and Price, D.: Am. J. Anat. *50:*13, 1932.
20. Moore, C. R., and Price, D.: Anat. Rec. *71:*59, 1938.
21. Moore, C. R., and Price, D.: Endocrinol. *21:*313, 1937.
22. Cutuly, E., and Cutuly, E. C.: Endocrinol. *26:*502, 1940.
23. Shay, H., Gershon-Cohen, J., Paschkis, K. E., and Fels, S. S.: Endocrinol. *28:*485, 1941.
24. Selye, H., and Friedman, S.: Endocrinol. *28:*129, 1941.
25. Rubinstein, H. S., and Kurland, A. A.: Endocrinol. *28:*495, 1941.
26. Wells, L. J., and Moore, C. R.: Anat. Rec. *66:*181, 1936.
27. Heckel, N. J.: Proc. Soc. Exper. Biol. & Med. *40:*658, 1939.
28. McCullagh, D. R.: J. Urol. *42:*1265, 1939.
29. Scowen, E.: Anat. Rec. *71* (Suppl.) : 178, 1938.
30. Hisaw, F. L., Greep, R. O., and Fevold, H. L.: Anat. Rec. *67* (Suppl.) : 50, 1936.
31. Nelson, W. O.: Anat. Rec. *67* (Suppl.) : 110, 1936.
32. Browman, L. G.: Proc. Soc. Exper. Biol. & Med. *36:*205, 1937.
33. Robson, J. M.: Proc. Soc. Exper. Biol. & Med. *35:*49, 1936.
34. Cotte, G., Martin, J. F., and Mankiewicz, E.: Gynecologie *86:*561, 1937.
35. Zuckerman, S.: Lancet *2:*676, 1937.
36. Gaines, J. A., Salmon, U. J., and Geist, S. H.: Proc. Soc. Exper. Biol. & Med. *38:*779, 1938.
37. Geist, S. H.: J. Clin. Endocrinol. *1:*154, 1941.
38. Salmon, U. J.: J. Clin. Endocrinol. *1:*162, 1941.
39. Nathanson, I. T., Franseen, C. C., and Sweeney, A. R., Jr.: Proc. Soc. Exper. Biol. & Med. *39:*385, 1938.
40. Selye, H., and Friedman, S. M.: Endocrinol. *27:*857, 1940.
41. Fluhmann, C. F.: Endocrinol. *28:*214, 1941.
42. Geist, S. H., Salmon, U. J., and Gaines, J. A.: Endocrinol. *23:*784, 1938.
43. Greenhill, J. P., and Freed, S. C.: J.A.M.A. *112:*1573, 1939.
44. Rothermich, N. O.: Endocrinol. *25:*520, 1939.
45. Papanicolaou, G. N., Ripley, H. S., and Shorr, E.: Endocrinol. *24:*339, 1939.
46. Hartman, C. G.: Proc. Soc. Exper. Biol. & Med. *37:*87, 1937.
47. Menninger-Lerchenthal, E.: Deut. med. Wchnschr. *62:*1132, 1936.
48. Geist, S. H.: J.A.M.A. *114:*1539, 1940.
49. Deanesly, R., and Parkes, A. S.: Brit. Med. J. *1:*257, 1936.
50. Korenchevsky, V., Dennison, M., and Simpson, S. L.: Biochem. J. *29:*2534, 1935.
51. Butenandt, A., and Kindzus, H.: Ztschr. f. physiol. Chem. *237:*75, 1935.
52. Wolff, E., and Ginglinger, A.: Compt. rend. Soc. de biol. *121:*1476, 1936.
53. Phelps, D., Burch, J. C., and Ellison, E. T.: Endocrinol. *23:*458, 1938.
54. Duncan, P. A., Allen, E., and Hamilton, J. B.: Endocrinol. *28:*107, 1941.
55. Kurzrok, R., and O'Connell, C. P.: Endocrinol. *23:*476, 1938.
56. Robson, J. M.: Proc. Soc. Exper. Biol. & Med. *36:*153, 1937.

57. Scipiades, E.: Proc. Soc. Exper. Biol. & Med. *37*:242, 1937.
58. Robson, J. M.: Quart. J. Exper. Physiol. *26*:355, 1937.
59. Courrier, R., and Gros, G.: Compt. rend. Soc. de biol. *127*:921, 1938; ibid. *128*:194, 1938.
60. Korenchevsky, V., and Hall, K.: J. Path. & Bact. *45*:681, 1937.
61. Geist, S. H., Salmon, U. J., and Mintz, M.: Proc. Soc. Exper. Biol. & Med. *39*:467, 1938.
62. Korenchevsky, V., Dennison, M., and Hall, K.: Biochem. J. *31*:780, 1937.
63. Cotte, G., Martin, J. F., and Mileff: Lyon Chir. *36*:372, 1939.
64. Selye, H., McEuen, C. S., and Collip, J. B.: Proc. Soc. Exper. Biol. & Med. *34*:201, 1936.
65. Smith, P. E.: Am. J. Anat. *45*:205, 1930.
66. Evans, L. T.: Anat. Rec. *62*:213, 1935.
67. Schockaert, J. A.: Anat. Rec. *50*:381, 1931.
68. Witschi, E., and Keck, W. N.: Proc. Soc. Exper. Biol. & Med. *32*:598, 1935.
69. Engle, E. T.: Endocrinol. *16*:513, 1932.
70. Baker, B. L., and Johnson, G. E.: Endocrinol. *20*:219, 1936.
71. Moore, C. R., and Samuels, L. T.: Am. J. Physiol. *96*:273, 1931.
72. Clark, L. B., Leonard, S. L., and Bump, G.: Science *83*:2150, 1936.
73. Greep, R. O., Fevold, H. L., and Hisaw, F. L.: Anat. Rec. *65*:261, 1936.
74. Evans, H. M., Korpi, K., Simpson, M. E., Pencharz, R. I., and Wonder, D L.: Univ. California Publ. in Anat. *1*:255, 1936.
75. Evans, H. M., Pencharz, R. I., and Simpson, M. E.: Science *80*:144, 1934.
76. Hamburger, C.: Ugesk. f. laeger *93*:27, 1931.
77. Reese, J. D., and McQueen-Williams, M.: Am. J. Physiol. *101*:239, 1932.
78. Schoeller, W., Dohrn, M., and Hohlweg, W.: Klin. Wchnschr. *15*:1907, 1936.
79. Martins, T., and Rocha, A.: Endocrinol. *15*:421, 1931.
80. McCullagh, D. R.: Science *76*:19, 1932.
81. Moore, C. R.: Bull. New York Acad. Med. *16*:135, 1940.
82. Werner, A. A.: J.A.M.A. *112*:1441, 1939.
83. Heckel, N. J.: J. Urol. *43*:286, 1940.
84. McCullagh, E. P., and Rossmiller, H. R.: J. Clin. Endocrinol. *1*:496, 1941.
85. Kearns, W. M.: J. Clin. Endocrinol. *1*:126, 1941.
86. Pratt, J. P.: J. Clin. Endocrinol. *2*:460, 1942.
87. Tager, B. N., and Shelton, E. K.: J. Clin. Endocrinol. *1*:131, 1941.
88. Pfeiffer, C. A., and Kirschbaum, A.: Anat. Rec. *85*:211, 1943.
89. Wainman, P., Reese, J. D., and Koneff, A. A.: Endocrinol. *31*:303, 1942.
90. Selye, H.: Endocrinol. *32*:116, 1943.
91. Hisaw, F. L.: Endocrinol. *33*:39, 1943.
92. Greep, R. O., and Fevold, H. L.: Endocrinol. *21*:611, 1937.

CHAPTER XII

THE PHYSIOLOGY OF THE ANTERIOR HYPOPHYSIS

The hypophysis is a composite organ which develops from two anlagen and consists of a larger anterior, and a smaller posterior portion. The anterior portion, which includes the pars distalis, anterior lobe proper and pars tuberalis, arises from Rathke's pouch, an extension of the ectoderm or primitive oral cavity. The posterior portion, made up of the pars nervosa

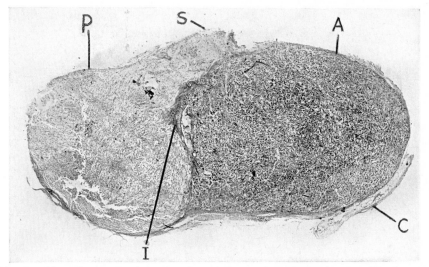

Fig. 36.—Microphotograph of section through human hypophysis (× 9). (P) Posterior lobe; (A) Anterior lobe; (I) Intermediate lobe; (S) Stalk; (C) Capsule.

or posterior lobe proper, and the pars intermedia, stems from the infundibular process of the diencephalon.

CYTOLOGY

The Chromophobes and the Chromophils.—The anterior lobe presents the histologic characteristics of an incretory organ. It is composed of two main groups of cells, the chromophobes or neutrophils, and the chromophils. The former constitute approximately one half of all the cells in the adult human hypophysis. They are smaller than the chromophils and contain a nongranular, poorly staining, homogenous cytoplasm, and a small round nucleus rich in chromatin. The chromophobes present no evidence of secretory activity.

The chromophils are of two types, named acidophils or eosinophils, and basophils, under the erroneous impression that the former stain only with acid, the latter only with basic dyes. The *acidophils* make up about 43 per cent of all the cells of the adenohypophysis in the nonpregnant woman. Polyhedral in shape, they contain a nearly homogeneous cytoplasm almost completely filled with coarse acidophilic granules, and have small spherical nuclei. The *basophils* comprise only 11 per cent of all the cells in the male and 7 per cent in the female. They are distributed in a haphazard fashion throughout the anterior lobe. Somewhat larger than the acidophils, they possess slightly eccentric nuclei, and a cytoplasm which harbors coarse basophilic granules.

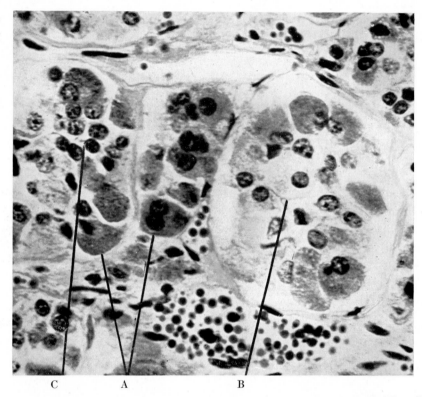

C   A   B

Fig. 37.—Microphotograph of human anterior pituitary gland ($\times$ 720). A, Acidophilic cells. B, Basophilic cells. C, Group of chromophobic cells. (Courtesy of Dr. N. W. Winkelman.)

Proportion of Cell Types.—The proportion of each cell type varies; the basophils show the greatest variability, the chromophobes the least. This cannot be attributed to cell division for fission does not occur in the mature gland. It is generally agreed that one cell type is transformed into another. The chromophobes, most observers believe, represent the "mother" or "reserve" cells from which the other two cell types spring. There has been considerable controversy as to whether the basophils and acidophils represent different phases of a single cell type or derive independently from the chromophobes. An outstanding protagonist of the latter view is

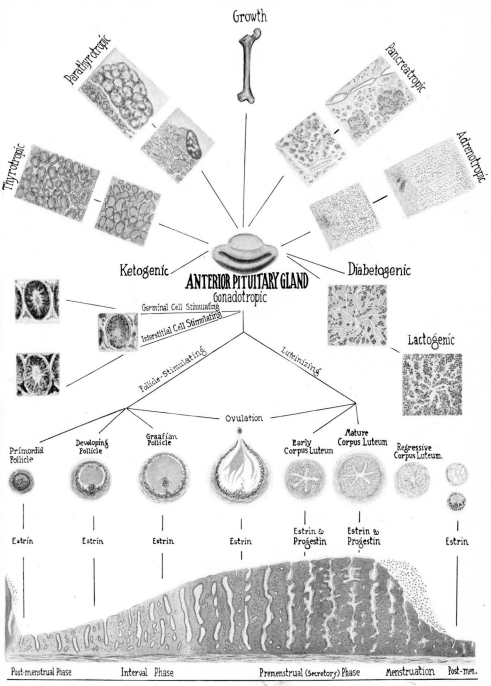

Growth

Parathyrotropic

Pancreatropic

Thyrotropic

Adrenotropic

Ketogenic

ANTERIOR PITUITARY GLAND

Diabetogenic

Gonadotropic

Germinal Cell Stimulating

Interstitial Cell Stimulating

Lactogenic

Follicle-Stimulating

Luteinizing

Ovulation

Primordial Follicle

Developing Follicle

Graafian Follicle

Early Corpus Luteum

Mature Corpus Luteum

Regressive Corpus Luteum

Estrin | Estrin | Estrin | Estrin | Estrin & Progestin | Estrin & Progestin | Estrin

Post-menstrual Phase | Interval Phase | Premenstrual (Secretory) Phase | Menstruation | Post-men.

Endometrium

Fig. 38.—Anterior pituitary hormones.

Severinghaus,[1] who points out that the human hypophysis contains chromophobic cells which are of definite basophilic and acidophilic lineage, respectively. As an additional argument he offers the fact that *chromophilic tumors* are composed exclusively of basophils or acidophils, and tend to remain so. He suggests that the specific granules of the acidophils and basophils are the precursors of endocrine secretion. These cells, he maintains, show cycles of secretion: they elaborate their incretory products, store them in gradually increasing amounts in the cytoplasm, discharge them, and then begin to elaborate and accumulate a new store of granules. On losing their granules, the chromophils become chromophobes, while chromophobes which accumulate specific granules become acidophils or basophils, as the case may be. Thus, according to Severinghaus, the changes in the proportion of each cell type may properly be interpreted as the result of the varying phases of secretory activity in which the cells are found at a given moment.

Function of the Anterior Hypophyseal Cells.—While it is generally agreed that the chromophils are secretory cells, their specific functions are still a matter of conjecture. Rapid advances in the physiology of this gland have given impetus to its histologic study, but progress has been considerably hampered by technical difficulties. While the acidophils are generally believed to secrete the growth-promoting principle it is still uncertain what cells elaborate the anterior hypophyseal hormones that control sexual function and general metabolic activity. Attempts to associate the basophils with sexual function have thus far yielded inconclusive results.

THE ANTERIOR HYPOPHYSIS AND THE GONADS

The anterior hypophysis is the dominant member of the endocrine system. Hypophysectomy experiments and studies with anterior lobe implants and extracts in hypophysectomized and normal animals suggest that this gland plays an important role in somatic growth, sexual function and the metabolic activities of the organism. Whether the varied effects produced with anterior lobe extracts are due to one or several distinct hormones is not known. While as many as sixteen anterior pituitary hormones have been postulated, their existence must remain uncertain until more is known of the chemistry of this gland.

Gonadal Effects of Hypophysectomy.—The anterior lobe initiates and maintains gonadal function and is vitally concerned with reproduction. Total ablation of this gland leads to profound involution and atrophy of the gonads and accessory genitalia. The regressive changes begin soon after operation and are progressive. Retention of even a small part of the gland will prevent these effects.

In the Female.—In the immature female animal, total ablation precludes ovarian development, while in the mature subject it causes a reduction in the size of the ovary and gradual extinction of its function. As the retrogressive process proceeds, the ovary becomes filled with interstitial tissue because of the incomplete development of follicles and atresia.

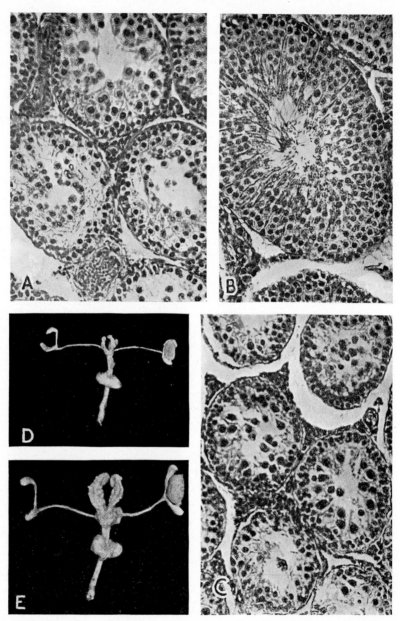

Fig. 39.—Hypophysectomy and replacement therapy in the male rat. A, Testis thirty-four days after hypophysectomy. B, Testis of hypophysectomized rat given daily anterior pituitary homeotransplants for thirty days. C, Testis of hypophysectomized rat thirty days after stopping anterior pituitary transplantations. D, Atrophied reproductive system of rat thirty-four days after hypophysectomy. E, Reproductive system of hypophysectomized rat given daily anterior pituitary transplants for thirty days. (Smith, P. E.: Am. J. Anat. Vol. 45.)

In the rat, a modified interstitial cell, known as "theca deficiency" or "wheel cell," appears within a short time after hypophysectomy. The regressive changes which follow operation apparently do not involve the oocytes and primordial follicles, which continue to develop to the stage of beginning antrum formation. It would thus appear that the anterior hypophysis is not essential for the early stages of germ cell development. The fate of corpora lutea formed shortly before or during hypophysectomy varies in different species. In most animals, they regress soon after operation, but in the rat they tend to persist or regress at a very slow rate.

In the pregnant animal, the effect of hypophysectomy varies according to the species of the test animal and the stage of gestation. In some species, abortion invariably occurs no matter when operation is performed. In

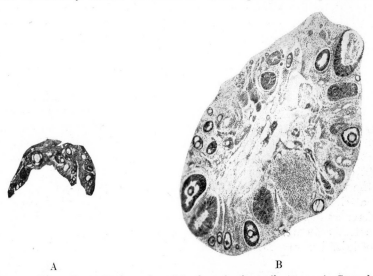

A   B

Fig. 40.—Effect of anterior hypophyseal implants in the senile mouse. A, Control ovary; B, ovary removed from senile mouse ninety-six hours after implantation of fresh bovine anterior hypophyseal tissue. Note presence of mature follicles and corpora lutea.

others, abortion ensues only if the hypophysis is removed during early gestation. If operation is performed during the latter half of pregnancy, the young may be born dead, or parturition may be postponed.

In the Male.—In the male as in the female animal hypophysectomy performed before puberty precludes subsequent gonadal development and function. In the mature male it leads to involution and atrophy of the testis. The epithelium of the seminiferous tubules undergoes marked regressive changes. Spermatogenesis ceases, but absence of the hypophysis does not seem to interfere with the early stages of germ cell development. The Leydig cells cease to secrete male sex hormone, as seen from the regressive modifications in the accessory genitalia. In the hypophysectomized monkey, the testes are retracted and may eventually become abdominal organs.

The gonadal atrophy noted in *hypophyseal cachexia* (see Chap. XXXV) clearly indicates that in man, as in the experimental animal, gonadal function is primarily dependent on the adenohypophysis. Of interest in this connection is a case, reported by Moricard,[146] in which removal of the pituitary because of tumor was followed by amenorrhea and complete genital atrophy although there was no evidence of abnormal gonadal function before the operation.

Effects of Implants and Extracts.—Smith and Engle,[2] and Aschheim and Zondek,[3] in 1927, first demonstrated that implants of fresh anterior pituitary tissue can restore the atrophied gonads of the hypophysectomized rodent and induce precocious sexual maturity in the intact immature animal. In the same year, the author,[4] working in Zondek's laboratory, showed that such implants are also capable of fully reactivating the ovaries of senile mice. The discovery of gonadotropic activity in anterior pituitary gland tissue initiated a series of chemical investigations aimed at extracting the active gonadotropic principles. In general, the effects originally reported with tissue implants have been duplicated with extracts.

SEX HORMONES OF THE ANTERIOR HYPOPHYSIS

In the course of the earlier studies observers were struck by the fact that their anterior pituitary gland extracts caused either maturation of follicles with ovulation and formation of true corpora lutea, atresia and cystic degeneration of follicles, or excessive luteinization with imprisonment of ova. The explanation of these divergent responses has been the subject of much controversy. Some believe the anterior hypophysis controls the various phases of gonadal function through a single sex principle. They attribute the varied effects elicited with anterior pituitary extracts to differences in the concentration of the active substance, in the reactivity of the test animal, mode of administration, state of the ovaries at the time of injection, and interval between administration of the hormone and inspection of the ovaries. Engle,[5] one of the early protagonists of this view, argued that the developing follicle, if properly stimulated, can do but one thing outside of becoming atretic, that is, it must inevitably be transformed into lutein tissue. Therefore any extract, no matter how pure, which causes proliferation of the granulosa, will hasten the normal maturation of the follicle and its luteal transformation. In other words, the anterior pituitary merely furnishes the motivating force which helps the follicle along its way, but the path that it shall take is determined within the follicle itself.

Others have maintained that the varied effects of anterior lobe extracts are due to two or more distinct sex principles. Thus far at least eight hypophyseal hormones capable of influencing gonadal function have been postulated. These include the (1) follicle-stimulating hormone (follicle stimulator, FSH, thylakentrin); (2) luteinizing hormone (luteinizer, LH); (3) interstitial-cell-stimulating hormone, ICSH, metakentrin; (4) ovulation hormone; (5) synergic factor (synergist, augmenting factor); (6) antagonistic factor (antagonist, atresin); (7) luteotrophin; and (8) anti-luteogenic hormone.

The Follicle-Stimulating and Luteinizing Hormones (FSH and LH).
—During the past decade, Fevold,[6] Wallen-Lawrence,[7] Evans,[8] and their
respective collaborators, claimed success in obtaining from whole anterior
pituitary gonadotropic extract two fractions, of which one is predominantly
follicle stimulating, the other predominantly luteinizing, when tested in
the intact or hypophysectomized rat or rabbit. At first the fractionation
methods used by these investigators failed to achieve complete separation
of these two hormones. This was evident in the fact that both follicle
stimulation and luteinization could be produced with either fraction alone
by increasing the dose or length of treatment. Improved extraction methods
have made further purification possible. Both Fevold's[9] and Evans' group[10]
have recently described fractionation procedures by which they claim to
have obtained highly purified extracts of the follicle stimulator and
luteinizer.

In Estrogen Secretion.—Those who believe that follicular maturation
and luteinization depend on two distinct anterior pituitary gonadotropic
principles, have generally assumed that growth of follicles and the accompanying secretion of estrogen are both dependent exclusively on the action
of FSH. Doubt has been cast on this assumption by the recent studies of
Fevold.[11] This worker found that purified FSH, when administered to immature rats over a period of forty-eight hours, increased the ovarian weight
200 per cent due to development of follicles, but induced only slight estrogen secretion, as judged by the weight of the uterus. When FSH and LH
were given simultaneously, pronounced uterine growth occurred, though
the dose of FSH was such that, when given alone, it could produce neither
ovarian nor uterine growth. The amount of LH required for this complementary effect was very small, 0.0008 mg. being sufficient to produce
a 90 per cent increase in uterine weight when combined with an amount
of FSH which alone could cause no uterine enlargement. Gross and microscopic examination of the ovaries revealed no significant difference between
those stimulated by FSH alone and those acted on by FSH plus a trace of
LH. When the two fractions were given in succession, this complementary
effect was not obtained. He concluded that both FSH and LH are concerned with estrogen secretion. FSH apparently plays the primary role in
that it is capable of initiating such secretion, while LH is only of secondary
importance, since it is unable to affect the secretory mechanism when
given alone. He suggests that the slight secretion of estrogen induced with
FSH alone is probably due to traces of LH present in the extract, and
that FSH, if completely free from LH, might possibly stimulate the development of follicles without initiating estrogen secretion.

Interstitial-Cell-Stimulating Hormone (ICSH).—On the basis of
studies carried out with various pituitary extracts in intact and hypophysectomized rats, Evans and his associates,[8] in 1936, proposed that the
anterior hypophysis elaborates a third factor distinct from its follicle-
stimulating and luteinizing principles. They designated it "interstitial-cell-
stimulating hormone," or ICSH, because it stimulates the interstitial tissue
of the rat ovary and prevents formation of theca deficiency cells in the

hypophysectomized rat. This has been questioned by Fevold's group,[9] who have presented evidence indicating that the hormone causing these effects is identical with the luteinizing factor. Evans and his coworkers[10] have recently arrived at the same conclusion on the basis of studies with their highly purified follicle stimulating and luteinizing fractions.

Ovulation-Inducing Factors.—The experiments of Smith and Engle,[2] and Zondek and Aschheim,[3] in 1927, clearly established the dependence of ovulation on the anterior hypophysis. Leonard,[12] in 1931, postulated the existence of an ovulation hormone distinct from the follicle-stimulating and luteinizing principles. This suggestion was challenged by Evans and his associates,[13] on the ground that ovulation can be induced with follicle-stimulating and luteinizing extracts if the dosage is properly adjusted.

FSH and LH.—An important step toward clarification of this problem was the preparation of the follicle-stimulating and luteinizing principles in relatively pure form. This enabled observers to ascertain the ovulation-inducing effect of the two factors when given singly and in combination. Hertz and Hisaw[14] induced follicular rupture in juvenile rabbits by administering their purified follicle-stimulating extract for three days followed by a luteinizing extract on the next three days. Ovulation did not occur when either fraction was given alone, or an unfractionated anterior pituitary preparation was used. Casida,[15] working with the immature rat, induced ovulation by first administering a follicle-stimulating extract, and then following with the same preparation plus a trace of luteinizing extract. When the amount of luteinizing substance added to the follicle-stimulating extract was increased, ovulation did not follow but instead corpora lutea atretica with entrapped ova were produced. Casida concluded that, in order to induce ovulation, the luteinizing principle must supplement the action of the follicle stimulator, but if the luteinizer is excessive, it may interfere with the ovulatory mechanism.

FSH and LH Balance.—The importance of maintaining the ratio of the follicle stimulator to the luteinizer within certain limits is emphasized by the observations of Foster and Hisaw in the anestrus cat[16] and juvenile rabbit.[17] These observers administered a follicle-stimulating extract subcutaneously for five days in order to cause maturation of follicles, and then followed this with a single intravenous injection of either follicle stimulating or luteinizing extract, or varying combinations of both fractions. In the anestrus cat, the largest number of ovulation points appeared after the intravenous injection of follicle stimulator and luteinizer in the ratio of 100 to 1. In the juvenile rabbit, a single intravenous injection of follicle stimulator plus luteinizer in the concentration of 100:1, 50:1, 25:1 and 15:1, resulted in an average of 75, 19, 15 and 0 ruptured follicles respectively. When the amount of luteinizer added to a constant quantity of follicle stimulating extract was increased, the number of ovulations likewise rapidly fell to zero. Though a single intravenous injection of either follicle-stimulating or luteinizing extract could induce ovulation, the minimal amount of each required for this effect could be reduced 50 to 85 per cent by adding a trace of the other. It would therefore appear that *ovulation depends on the synergistic interaction of the follicle-stimulating and luteinizing factors,* which must bear a definite quantitative relationship to each other in order to insure optimal conditions for follicular rupture. Should this relationship be disturbed, either by increasing the amount of luteinizer added to a constant quantity of follicle stimulator, or decreasing the amount of follicle stimulator combined with a constant quantity of luteinizer, the ovulation-inducing efficiency of the mixture is markedly diminished.

This balance must be maintained not only to insure ovulation, but also to avoid abnormal changes in the ovary. Foster and Hisaw found that when a single intravenous injection of follicle-stimulating extract was administered to properly prepared animals, only a few ovulations occurred and cystic follicles appeared in a considerable proportion of the treated animals. On the other hand, when the intravenously injected "ovulating mixture" contained a quantity of luteinizer in excess of that required for a maximum ovulation response, only a few follicles ovulated and luteinized follicles with entrapped ova appeared.

*Optimal Conditions for Ovulation.—Experimental Studies.—*To create optimal conditions for ovulation, it is not only necessary to supply the follicle stimulator and luteinizer in the proper proportion, but also at the proper point in the follicle's development. Foster and Fevold[17] found that an optimal ovulating mixture that proved ideal for inducing ovulation in the estrus rabbit, failed to cause follicular rupture in the juvenile animal which lacks mature follicles. When the latter received purified follicle-stimulating extract subcutaneously for five days, follicular maturation, without atresia, cystic degeneration or ovulation occurred, and the mature follicles thus produced invariably ovulated in response to a single intravenous injection of an optimal ovulating mixture. On the other hand, when growth of follicles was induced in juvenile rabbits by subcutaneous injections of follicle-stimulating extract combined with small amounts of luteinizer, some follicles ovulated in the course of treatment, but the subsequent intravenous injection of an ovulating mixture failed to elicit any further ovulations. On increasing the amount of luteinizer given subcutaneously with follicle-stimulating extract, luteinization with imprisonment of ova resulted. No follicles ovulated during the course of the subcutaneous injections or after the intravenous administration of an appropriate ovulating mixture. It would thus appear that only follicles matured by a relatively pure follicle-stimulating preparation are in a proper physiological state to respond to an optimal ovulating stimulus. The premature application of luteinizer apparently produces changes in the follicle which interfere with its ability to ovulate when an appropriate ovulating mixture is supplied.

The ovulating mechanism may also be disturbed when the luteinizer acts too late. This is implied in Casida's[15] observation that when maturation of follicles was induced in the immature sow by administering a follicle-stimulating extract, the subsequent injection of a luteinizing extract induced ovulation only in those follicles which approximated the preovulatory size of those normally present in the mature sow's ovary. Follicles which had passed this point at the time the luteinizer was administered, did not rupture. This would suggest that the follicle is ripe for rupture at

12

a particular point in its development, and that once this is passed, it can no longer respond to an ovulating stimulus.

Studies in the mature hypophysectomized rabbit have confirmed the findings in the intact animal. Foster and his associates[118] could not induce ovulation in the hypophysectomized animal with follicle stimulator or luteinizer alone, but rupture did occur when a follicle-stimulating extract was injected subcutaneously for five days followed by a single intravenous injection of follicle-stimulating extract combined with a trace of luteinizer. The response diminished as the interval between hypophysectomy and the first subcutaneous injection of follicle stimulator increased. When more than two or three weeks were allowed to elapse, no ovulations occurred though antra-bearing follicles were still present in the ovary.

In Man and Monkey.—Though the studies thus far carried out in the monkey[19] and man[20] are still too limited to permit any conclusions, they suggest that ovulation in the primate depends on the same factors that operate in the lower mammal.

Summary.—In summation, it may be stated that ovulation is not due to a distinct ovulation hormone but depends on the interaction of the follicle-stimulating and luteinizing hormones. To insure the occurrence of ovulation, the following requirements must be fulfilled:

(1) The ovary must contain antra-bearing follicles capable of responding normally to the follicle-stimulating principle.

(2) Follicle-stimulating extract, practically free from luteinizer, must be supplied in adequate amounts and long enough to develop the follicle to the preovulatory stage.

(3) Luteinizing hormone must be permitted to supplement the follicle stimulator at the moment when the follicle reaches this stage, and must be supplied in an amount which bears a certain relationship to the quantity of follicle stimulator available.

The Synergic Factor.—Evans,[21] in 1931, observed that a crude anterior pituitary extract containing minimal or subminimal amounts of gonadotropic substance, when given together with a human pregnancy urine gonadotropic extract, produced an increase in ovarian size and weight above a mere additive effect. This so-called "activation" or "augumentation" phenomenon has been variously interpreted. Evans thought at first that it might be due to a "synergic" principle distinct from the known pituitary sex hormones. Fevold and his group,[22] on the other hand, have always maintained that this phenomenon may reasonably be explained on the basis of the synergistic interaction of the follicle-stimulating and luteinizing factors. As proof they offered their observation that purified follicle stimulating and luteinizing extracts of anterior lobe tissue, when recombined, produced an ovarian weight increase far exceeding that which might be expected from the effects of the two factors given singly. They suggested that the hypothetical "synergist" allegedly present in Evans' crude anterior pituitary extract is in reality the follicle stimulator, whose effect is augmented by luteinizing substances present in pregnancy urine extract (see below). Saunders and Cole,[23] who question the existence of a luteinizing factor apart from the follicle-stimulating principle, attribute the augmentation obtained by combining a follicle-stimulating and luteinizing extract to a foreign protein present in the latter. This, they believe, augments the effect of the follicle-stimulating extract by delaying its absorption and thus minimizing waste. As proof, they point to reports that the effect of gonadotropic preparations can be appreciably enhanced by adding any one of a wide variety of nonspecific materials, as for example, tannic acid, copper, zinc sulphate, casein or egg albumen, extract of liver, milk, lemon juice or yeast. While this effect of nonspecific substances cannot be denied, it does not necessarily follow that the augmentation obtained by combining follicle-stimulating and luteinizing extracts is due to a foreign protein. That it is attributable rather to the hormonal content of such extracts is suggested by Lein's[24] observation that the augmentation which occurs on combining pituitary "synergist" with mare's serum gonadotropin (see below) is prevented if the pituitary extract is inactivated by heating or replaced by muscle extract having the same protein content.

Evans and his associates[10] have recently expressed the view that the assumption of a separate synergist, apart from the follicle stimulator, is not justified. This they base on their observation that augmentation can be obtained with certain combinations of highly purified follicle stimulating and luteinizing extract, given subcutaneously. Unlike Saunders and Cole, and in conformity with the view of Fevold and his associates, they maintain that the luteinizing factor exists as a distinct principle and "possesses specific physiological properties, namely to stimulate the interstitial tissue and to act as a specific augmenting agent when given in combination with the follicle-stimulating factor under certain conditions."

The Antagonistic Factor.—In the course of the earlier experiments, it was repeatedly observed that crude extracts of bovine pituitary inhibited gonadal function when administered by the intraperitoneal route. Evans,[25] in 1929, suggested that this is due to a hormone distinct from the growth factor, since destruction of the growth promoting activity of his extracts did not impair their inhibitory effect. Loeb, in 1935,[26] observed that certain anterior lobe extracts promoted follicular atresia and postulated the existence of a distinct principle which he named *atresin*. The following year, Evans reported[27] the isolation of an inhibitory principle which he named *antagonist*. In the immature rat, it prevented follicular maturation, caused atresia of follicles already present, and reduced the size of the ovary, while in the adult animal it caused excessive luteinization. The pregnant animal also responded with excessive luteinization and consequent prolongation of gestation. Evans concluded that the antagonistic principle inhibits follicular maturation but does not interfere with luteinization. He assumed that it is distinct from the luteinizing principle because he could separate the two types of activity by ammonium sulphate fractionation. Since the antagonist was effective in the absence of the adrenals, and was present only in traces in potent lactogenic extracts, he concluded that it is not identical with either the corticotropic or lactogenic factor.

Evans[10] was recently led to deny the existence of a distinct antagonistic principle, because of his observation that follicular development in the hypophysectomized rat can be inhibited by administering certain combinations of highly purified follicle stimulating and luteinizing extracts by the intraperitoneal route.

The Anti-Luteogenic Principle.—It has been generally assumed that regression of the corpus luteum, which normally occurs at the end of the infertile cycle, is a negative phenomenon due to withdrawal of the luteinizing stimulus. The observation that corpora lutea, which form during or shortly before hypophysectomy in the rat and guinea pig, tend to persist for some time after operation, has led some observers to interpret corpus luteum regression as a positive phenomenon dependent on an active principle secreted by the anterior hypophysis.

In an attempt to identify this principle, Bunde and Greep[28] tested the effect of estrogen, progestin, and purified follicle-stimulating and luteinizing extracts in hypophysectomized rats. Regression of the persisting corpora lutea occurred only when the luteinizer was employed. In a later communication, Greep[29] reported that regression ensued even more rapidly when a combination of follicle stimulator and luteinizer was administered. Foster[30] found that in the rabbit the corpora lutea of pseudopregnancy, which normally persist thirteen to fourteen days, regress after the ninth day when luteinizer is administered, and after the sixth day or sooner, if follicle stimulator is used.

In 1937, Freud[31] observed that the corpora lutea did not persist following hypophysectomy in rats receiving an extract of beef anterior pituitary shortly before operation. To determine whether such extract contains an "anti-luteogenic" factor, he investigated its effect when given alone, and together with a luteinizing extract of human pregnancy urine. Many corpora lutea formed when it was administered alone by the subcutaneous route, but not when the intraperitoneal route was used. When it was injected intraperitoneally, and a pregnancy urine luteinizing extract was given simultaneously by the subcutaneous route, no corpora lutea formed although many would have appeared had the pregnancy urine extract been given alone. Freud concluded that beef pituitary extract contains an anti-luteogenic principle which is effective intraperitoneally but not by the subcutaneous route. Whether such a principle exists or the anti-luteogenic effect, like the antagonistic and synergistic phenomena, is due to a particular combination of the follicle-stimulating and luteinizing hormones, cannot be decided from the available evidence.

Luteotrophin.—Though there is fairly convincing evidence indicating that conversion of the mature follicle into a corpus luteum is due to the concerted action of FSH and LH, the identity of the stimulus which sustains the function of formed corpora lutea is not certain. As noted above, Greep[28, 29] found that FSH and LH, given singly or in combination, did not sustain but actually accelerated the regression of persisting corpora lutea in hypophysectomized rats. This observation, coupled with the finding that progesterone inhibits the release of LH from the anterior hypophysis,[32] led Astwood and Fevold[33] to suspect that the function of formed corpora lutea depends on some anterior pituitary hormone, distinct from FSH and LH, to which they have applied the name "luteotrophin."

Rat Experiments.—To establish the validity of their hypothesis, they tested the ability of various sheep pituitary extracts to sustain luteal activity in hypophysectomized immature rats.[34] Before hypophysectomy, they injected chorionic gonadotropin for four days to induce corpus luteum formation. Estradiol dipropionate was then administered daily to insure sustained estrogen action. This, together with the progesterone secreted by the induced corpora lutea, evoked a mucification reaction in the vaginal mucosa. After hypophysectomy, the animals received repeated injections of various extracts of sheep pituitary gland. If vaginal mucification persisted, it was assumed that the extract was effective in maintaining the function of the corpora lutea present at the time of operation. On the other hand, if mucification was replaced by cornification, denoting an estrogen effect, it was taken to signify that progesterone production had ceased due to absence of luteotrophin in the extract. Luteotrophic activity could not be demonstrated in a purified extract of FSH, LH, and thyrotropic hormone, prepared by the method of Fevold and associates.[35] On the other hand, the residue left after removing all traces of FSH, LH, and thyrotropic hormone, was found to possess marked luteotrophic activity. Further investigation with anterior pituitary extract prepared by the method of Lyons,[36] yielded evidence indicating that the luteotrophic principle is closely associated chemically, but is nevertheless distinct from the growth, lactogenic and adrenotropic factors. Luteotrophic extracts proved ineffective for sustaining luteal function when more than twenty to thirty hours were allowed to elapse between hypophysectomy and the first injection. If injections were started immediately after operation, luteal activity persisted for ten to thirteen days, after which regression occurred despite continued treatment. Additional evidence that the luteotrophic factor is closely related to and possibly identical with the lactogenic factor has been provided by Evans' group.[148]

GONADOTROPES OF EXTRA-HYPOPHYSEAL ORIGIN

Aschheim and Zondek's[37] discovery of a gonad-stimulating substance *in the urine of pregnant women* provided the first evidence that gonadotropins may occur outside the hypophysis. Since then, such substances have been demonstrated in the blood and urine of women with *hydatid mole* and *chorionepithelioma*, and of men bearing certain types of *embryonic testicular neoplasm*. Small amounts of gonad-stimulating substance have also been detected in the blood and urine of castrate and menopausal women, and in the body fluids of children, mature nonpregnant women, and men. A potent gonadotrope has recently been demonstrated in the *blood of pregnant mares*. The origin, nature and functions of these extra-hypophyseal gonadotropes, and their relationship to those produced by the anterior pituitary gland have been the subject of extensive investigation.

Chorionic Gonadotropin.—The term chorionic gonadotropin describes the gonad-stimulating substances found in pregnancy and conditions associated with abnormal chorionic proliferation, such as hydatid mole or chorionepithelioma. Studies in the intact and hypophysectomized female animal indicate that the chorionic hormones are predominantly *luteinizing* and possess little or no *follicle stimulating activity*. In the immature female rodent, chorionic gonadotropin induces maturation of follicles followed by ovulation and corpus luteum formation.[37] In the hypophysectomized mature animal, it causes thecal luteinization with estrogen secretion, as shown by the occurrence of persistent estrus, but does not induce maturation of follicles or their conversion into true corpora lutea.[38] This would suggest that the follicle-stimulating effect obtained in the intact animal is not due to a follicle stimulator present in the extract, but to activation of the test animal's hypophysis with a resulting discharge of its follicle-stimulating principle. In the immature hypophysectomized animal which lacks mature follicles, the chorionic hormone cannot produce true corpora lutea. If the animal is mature so that ripe follicles are present at the time of hypophysectomy, chorionic hormone given immediately following operation leads to the formation of corpora lutea.[39]

Of interest is Greep's[40] observation that, when corpora lutea were induced by administering a luteinizing extract to normal adult rats, and the hypophysis was then removed, subsequent administration of chorionic gonadotropin caused no growth of follicles but produced a long continued estrus. This effect was apparently due to estrogens secreted by the persistent corpora lutea, for estrus did not occur if these structures were made to regress before the chorionic hormone was given. This, and a similar observation reported by Gaarenstroom and de Jongh,[41] would suggest that though chorionic gonadotropin is usually described as "luteinizing" and assumed to be primarily concerned with stimulating progestin secretion, it may, under certain conditions, stimulate estrogen production instead. This should be borne in mind when the use of this substance is contemplated for the correction of conditions associated with luteal deficiency and a relative or absolute excess of estrogen.

The follicle-stimulating and ovulation inducing effects elicited with the chorionic gonadotropins in the immature intact rodent have also been observed in the intact anestrus ferret[42] and cat.[16] On the other hand, the immature guinea pig ovary shows interstitial cell hypertrophy. Treatment in this species,[43] as well as in newborn rats[44] and mice,[45] leads to definite masculinization and sterility. In the intact mature rabbit in estrus, chorionic gonadotropin readily induces ovulation and corpus luteum formation.[46] This is to be expected since the ovaries of such animals contain many mature and growing follicles. This response is not prevented by hypophysectomy provided the chorionic hormone is administered immediately after operation and before the follicles have undergone regression, but the dose required tends to be somewhat larger than in the intact animal.[47]

In the immature and mature monkey, the chorionic hormones cause neither follicular maturation nor luteinization. If administered during the follicular phase of the cycle in the adult female monkey, atretic involution with suppression of estrogen secretion results. Occasional luteoid changes appear but no granulosa luteinization occurs.[48]

In the male rat and mouse, chorionic gonadotropin primarily affects the interstitial cells.[49] In the hypophysectomized male rat, it stimulates the interstitial cells but does not prevent degeneration of the germinal epithelium.[38] If administered immediately after hypophysectomy, it maintains the tubular structures and spermatogenic function for a limited period.[50] In the intact male monkey, an increase in the interstitial cells, tubular growth without differentiation, and descent of the testes have been recorded following use of this hormone.[51]

Comparison of Chorionic and Hypophyseal Gonadotropes.—The observation that pregnancy urine extract produces mature follicles, hemorrhagic follicles and true or false corpora lutea in the immature rodent, at first led observers to assume that the urinary and hypophyseal hormones are identical. That they differ biologically and may be regarded as distinct is indicated by a considerable body of evidence.[52, 149] It has been found that the chorionic hormones effect a much less marked ovarian weight increase than the hypophyseal gonadotropes.[53] In the immature rat receiving chorionic gonadotropin, a few follicles are converted into corpora lutea, while in the animal given hypophyseal gonadotropin, the follicles which reach the corpus luteum phase are smaller but much more numerous. Superovulation, which can readily be induced in the mature rodent with the hypophyseal hormones,[54] cannot be duplicated with the chorionic gonadotropes. The latter, if given over a protracted period, are more likely to produce abnormal ovaries containing luteinized follicles with imprisoned ova. In the very young rodent, before antra-bearing follicles appear, thecal luteinization is more marked with the chorionic hormones[55] than with those of hypophyseal origin. In the immature monkey, hypophyseal extract causes follicular maturation and estrogen production, as shown by reddening of the sex skin; chorionic gonadotropin has a depressant effect, causing atresia of the large follicles and hyalinization of the small ones.[51] In the hypophysectomized rodent, the hypophyseal hormones completely repair the gonadal atrophy, while the reparative effect of the chorionic hormones is limited to the interstitial tissue.

Castrate and Menopausal Urine Gonadotropes.—The presence of gonadotropic substances in the blood and urine of castrate and menopausal women was first demonstrated by Zondek[56] and Fluhmann,[57] in 1929. These hormones are believed to be of hypophyseal origin and are generally conceded to have a predominantly *follicle-stimulating effect.* Whether they also possess luteinizing activity has been the subject of some controversy.

Effects on the Ovaries.—In the earlier experiments in intact rodents, castrate and menopausal urine extracts were found to elicit follicular maturation without luteinization. It was therefore assumed that they contain only the follicle-stimulating principle. This was questioned by Frank[58] on the basis of his observation that corpora lutea could be produced with such extracts if the dose was adequate and sufficient time was permitted to elapse between the last injection and inspection of the ovaries. Since his studies were carried out in intact animals, they were open to the objection that the luteinization noted was due to luteinizer supplied by the animal's own hypophysis.

Studies in the hypophysectomized rodent indicate that castrate and menopausal urine extracts are not entirely free from luteinizing activity, though the amount present is probably much smaller than would appear from results obtained in the intact subject. Doses sufficient to induce corpus luteum formation in the intact rodent, produce only maturation of follicles in the hypophysectomized animal. To induce corpus luteum formation in the latter, it is necessary to administer up to twelve times the dose required in the intact animal.[59]

The observation that such extracts induce ovulation in the intact mature unmated rabbit in estrus,[60] is not inconsistent with the assumption that they possess only slight luteinizing activity. As shown elewhere, ovulation in this species requires a mixture of follicle stimulator and a trace of luteinizer, acting on a fully matured follicle, which is known to be present in the estrus rabbit.

The intact or hypophysectomized female monkey responds to these extracts with follicular maturation, but no luteinization occurs regardless of the dose used.[48]

Effects on the Testes.—In the immature male mouse, extracts of castrate or menopausal urine have no effect on the interstitial cells of the testis. The immature rat responds to such extracts with testicular descent. In both the mature and immature rat, they increase the weight of the testes and the amount of interstitial tissue. Germinal cell proliferation is accelerated but maturation is not hastened.

In the hypophysectomized male rat, small doses apparently have no effect on the interstitial cells, while large doses cause hypertrophy of these cells and secretion of male sex hormone, as indicated by the associated enlargement of the accessory genitalia. Extracts of castrate or menopausal urine are more effective than the chorionic hormones in stimulating spermatogenesis in the hypophysectomized test animal.[48]

In the immature male monkey, the doses used thus far increase the size of the tubules but have no apparent effect on spermatogenesis or the interstitial cells.

Pregnant Mare's Serum Gonadotropin.—Cole and Hart,[61] and Zondek,[62] in 1930, working independently, demonstrated the presence of considerable quantities of gonad-stimulating substance in the blood serum of pregnant mares. The hormone appeared with remarkable rapidity between the thirty-seventh and forty-second day after fertile coitus, and reached a concentration of 50,000 rat units per liter between the forty-second and eightieth day. After the eightieth day, its concentration declined, being reduced one half every eight to ten days. The hormone finally disappeared from the blood between the one hundred and thirtieth and one hundred and eightieth day.

Biologically, the equine hormones more closely simulate the action of hypophyseal gonadotropes than do the chorionic hormones. They differ from the other gonadotropes in that the ovarian weight increases with the dose over an extremely wide range. One peculiarity of these substances is their *nonexcretability.* Even when at their peak in the blood, they cannot be demonstrated in the urine. This has been attributed to their inability to pass the kidney. In this connection, Evans[63] demonstrated that if mare's serum hormone is injected into monkeys or rats, it does not appear in the urine, although these species excrete injected chorionic gonadotropin. Catchpole and associates,[64] who investigated the fate of injected equine hormone in the rabbit and gelding, found that its concentration in the blood was reduced one-half every twenty-six hours in the rabbit and every six days in the gelding. Finding no trace of the hormone in the urine, feces, uterus, lungs, kidneys, or liver, they concluded that it is probably destroyed within the body before reaching the liver and excretory organs. The gonads were apparently not implicated in this conversion and destruction, for the hormone disappeared at practically the same rate in the intact and castrate rabbit.

In contrast to the hypophyseal and chorionic hormones, equine gonadotropin is equally effective in single or divided doses. This may be due to its nonexcretability and slow destruction in the organism, as well as its high protein content, which delays absorption from the site of injection.

Source.—Whether the equine hormone is of hypophyseal or placental origin is not clear. Its production by the *anterior hypophysis* is suggested by its close biological similarity to the pituitary gonadotropes. Against this possibility, however, is the fact that its appearance in the blood is not accompanied by any changes in the histology or gonadotropic hormone content of the hypophysis which might indicate increased secretory activity.

Its origin in the *placenta* is suggested by the fact that it is peculiarly associated with chorionic tissue. Perhaps the most cogent argument is provided by Catchpole and Lyons'[65] observation that the hormone accumulates preferentially in the fertile horn of the uterus, and specifically at the site of the chorionic vesicles. Their study of the distribution of the hormone in the placenta, endometrium, blood, and hypophysis at various stages of pregnancy yielded values more consistent with a placental than a hypophyseal origin.

Biological Effects.—The equine hormones, like the hypophyseal gonadotropes, completely repair the gonadal atrophy in the hypophysectomized adult male and female rodent. They restore spermatogenesis in the hypophysectomized male rat, dog, and guinea pig, but even large doses fail to produce this effect in the hypophysectomized adult monkey.[141]

In the intact immature male rat, the equine hormones, like the human chorionic gonadotropes, induce interstitial cell hypertrophy, and cause an increase in the size of the testis and seminal vesicles, which far exceeds that obtained with other gonadotropic substances. In common with other gonadotropic agents, they fail to hasten spermatogenesis in the immature animal.[142] In the hypophysectomized immature rat, Sotiriadu[143] found horse pituitary extract more potent than either sheep pituitary extract or chorionic gonadotropin in increasing the size of the testis and seminal vesicles. None of these preparations induced the final stages of spermatogenesis prematurely (see Figs. 41, 42).

In the intact immature female rodent, mare's serum gonadotropin induces maturation of follicles and luteinization, associated with a marked increase in ovarian weight. It has proved effective in inducing ovulation

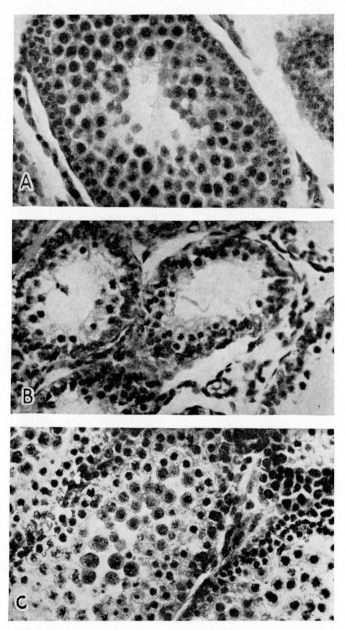

Fig. 41.—Effect of gonadotropes in hypophysectomized immature rat. A, Normal twenty-eight-day-old rat. Note spermatogonia with numerous mitoses, primary and secondary spermatocytes in the seminiferous tubules. B, Hypophysectomized twenty-eight-day-old rat. Smaller number of mitoses; spermatogonia irregularly arranged; spermatocytes scarce and small; C, Hypophysectomized immature rat treated with sheep pituitary extract. Size of tubules and spermatocytes almost normal, but spermatogonia remain small and irregular in some tubules. (Sotiriadou, E.: Acta brev. Neerland. Vol. 11.)

in the rat, ewe, sow, cow, and mare. In the juvenile rabbit, Foster and Fevold[17] found that it stimulated growth of only a small number of follicles when given subcutaneously, and, when administered intravenously as an ovulating stimulus, caused only a few follicles to rupture. In the guinea pig, Leonard and Leonard[66] found that the equine hormone caused

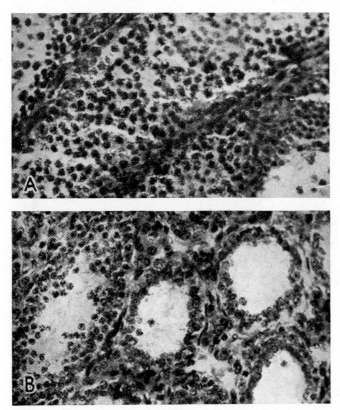

Fig. 42.—Effect of gonadotropes in hypophysectomized immature rat. A, After treatment with equine pituitary extract. Lumen of tubules packed with numerous small spermatocytes. Spermatogonia remain small and irregular; interstitial tissue strongly developed. B, After treatment with chorionic gonadotropin. Strongly developed interstitial tissue; tubules almost free from cells; spermatogonia irregularly arranged and a few spermatocytes present. (Sotiriadou, E.: Acta brev. Neerland. Vol. 11.)

interstitial cell hypertrophy, thecal luteinization and pseudo-lutein changes, and formation of large follicles and true corpora lutea.

In the intact immature monkey, Engle and Hamburger[67] elicited follicular maturation without luteinization. More recently, Hartman[68] reported that in adult rhesus monkeys, the equine hormone was without effect in some cases, while in others it caused follicular enlargement without ovulation, or diffuse over-stimulation of the ovaries with ovulation. He attributed these divergent responses to variations in dosage. Cartland and Nelson[69] likewise found that the effect of equine gonadotropin varies according to the dose used. In the immature rat, small doses produced corpora lutea of ovulation, intermediate doses had a purely follicle stimulating effect, while large doses caused the formation of corpora lutea atretica. The age of the test animal apparently also determines the response to mare's serum extract. Saunders and Cole[70] found that the extract produced only growth of interstitial tissue in ten day old intact female rats, a pure follicle stimulating effect in eighteen day old rats, ovulation in some animals at the

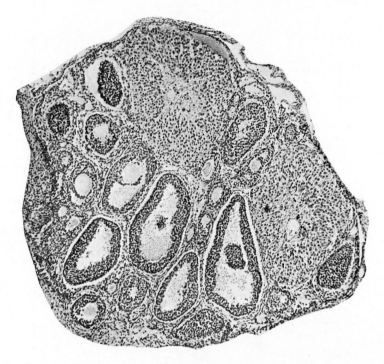

Fig. 43.—Ovary of immature mouse injected with pregnant mare's serum extract. Note mature follicles and corpora lutea.

nineteenth day, and follicular growth, ovulation and corpus luteum formation in twenty-one and twenty-five day old animals.

The foregoing evidence suggests that mare's serum extract possesses both *follicle-stimulating* and *luteinizing activity* and that the former predominates. This is borne out by the results of studies with fractioned extracts. Evans,[71] in 1936, reported the preparation of both a follicle-stimulating and interstitial-cell-stimulating extract from mare's serum. When tested in hypophysectomized female rats, the interstitial-cell-stimulating fraction evoked a response similar to that induced with human chorionic gonadotropin, while the follicle-stimulating fraction produced large follicles. Neither fraction, when given alone, induced corpus luteum formation.

RESPONSE OF THE HUMAN OVARY TO THE GONADOTROPES

Reliable information relating to the response of the human ovary to the available gonadotropes is limited. To estimate accurately the effect of a given preparation, it is essential to ascertain the status of ovarian function before and after treatment, and to exclude or at least take into account all extraneous influences which may conceivably alter gonadal activity. In no investigation thus far carried out have both these prerequisites been satisfactorily fulfilled.

Several observers have tested gonadotropic preparations in women about to undergo abdominal section for some pathology. Since examination of the ovaries after treatment can give no clue to their pre-treatment status, such studies are of little value. They are also open to the objection that the associated pelvic pathology may have a disturbing effect on ovarian function and thus obscure the response to treatment.

Recognizing the impracticability of performing laparotomy before and after treatment, some investigators have resorted to endometrial biopsy as a means of estimating gonadal function. It must be emphasized that, though the endometrial picture is valuable for detecting alterations of gonadal activity, minor changes may not be discernible by this method alone. Moreover, should the mucosa be refractory to the influence of the ovarian hormones, it cannot mirror ovarian function.

Evidence derived from quantitative determinations of the estrogen and gonadotropic hormone content of the blood and urine, and the pregnanediol level in the urine, may be helpful when combined with other evidence, but cannot per se serve as proof that a particular form of therapy has resulted in ovarian stimulation. Changes in the level of these substances are known to occur spontaneously in the absence of treatment. Until more is known of the laws governing the utilization, inactivation, destruction, and excretion of endogenously and exogenously supplied hormones, the significance of variations in their level must remain uncertain.

The clinical response of the patient, offered by some observers as proof of the efficacy of hormone therapy, is obviously unreliable. Subjective improvement may be due to the psychotherapeutic effect of the treatment. The correction of menstrual irregularity may occur in the absence of therapy, or in response to other influences operating concurrently, and therefore may not be ascribed with certainty to hormone therapy.

Gonadotropes from Anterior Hypophyseal Tissue.—The available glandular gonadotropes, because of their low unitage, are of little therapeutic value. While some observers claim to have induced corpus luteum formation, and enlargement of the uterus with progestational modification of the endometrium, other competent investigators could demonstrate no such effects in the human.

Human Chorionic Gonadotropin.—While there is no doubt that chorionic gonadotropin can induce follicular maturation, ovulation and corpus luteum formation in the rodent and rabbit, there is no convincing evidence that these effects can be duplicated in the human being. Some workers[72] have described mature follicles and corpora lutea in ovaries examined at laparotomy, following a series of chorionic hormone injections. Since no attempt was made to determine the condition of the ovaries before therapy was instituted, these reports do not constitute satisfactory proof of its efficacy.

Carefully controlled studies, particularly those of Geist's[73] and Hamblen's group,[74] have uniformly shown that chorionic gonadotropin does not stimulate ovarian function but tends rather to promote follicular atresia. Pratt,[75] who examined the ovaries of 100 women following treatment with a pregnancy urine extract, could find evidence of corpus luteum formation in only one case. The only appreciable modification noted was an increase in the number of atretic follicles. In fifty women observed by Geist,[73] treatment with pregnancy urine extract apparently resulted in an increase in the number of cystic follicles and perifollicular hemorrhage. Arrested ripe follicles could be seen with degenerating ova and theca cell hypertrophy. In some ovaries, the theca cells were prominent and increased in number.

In an extensive study, Hamblen and his coworkers[74] examined the ovaries and endometrium in fifty-seven cases, and the endometrium alone in twenty-eight, following the administration of from 8000 to 24,250 rat units of chorionic gonadotropin over a period of one to eighty-seven days. They found no evidence which would justify the assumption that ovulation and corpus luteum formation had resulted from the treatment. While conceding that the chorionic hormones cannot initiate ovulation and corpus luteum formation, Hamblen believes they are capable of augmenting the function of an existing corpus luteum. This he bases on his observation that chorionic hormone therapy was followed by a rise in pregnanediol excretion and prolongation of the luteal phase in normally menstruating women, and by an increase in the pregnanediol content of the urine in women with irregular bleeding associated with subnormal pregnanediol values.[74]

Of interest is the report of Brown and associates[76] that 500 R. U. of chorionic hormone daily for four to six weeks induced amenorrhea of one to five months duration, accompanied by progressive atrophy of the endometrium, in five out of twelve regularly menstruating women. In no case did the endometrium show secretory changes. They concluded that these substances are not gonadotropic in the human female and in sufficient dosage may be gonadotoxic.

Mare's Serum Gonadotropin.—Several investigators have reported *follicular stimulation* following treatment with equine gonadotropin in the human being. Kurzrok's group[77] found that young women with normal menstrual cycles responded to a total dose of 3600 mouse units, given during the first half of the cycle, with formation of numerous follicular cysts and a marked increase in the size and weight of the ovaries. Stimulation of follicles has also been described by Hamblen,[74] Siegmund,[78] Westman[79] and others.

The ability of the equine gonadotropes to induce *ovulation* in man has not been convincingly established. Davis and Koff,[20] in 1938, reported the successful induction of ovulation in approximately 50 per cent of a group of thirty-six women, following the intravenous injection of from 50 to 90 units of mare's serum hormone (*gonadogen*). In most of the cases, ovulation had apparently occurred between the fifth and twelfth, or between the seventeenth and twenty-third days of the cycle. In three patients with *hyperplastic endometria*, no corpora lutea could be found.

Attempts to duplicate these results *in women with hypofunctioning ovaries* have thus far proved disappointing. Huber and Davis,[80] and Gray[81] found that the equine gonadotropin had a beneficial effect in only a small percentage of patients with spontaneous ovarian failure. Erving and his associates[82] obtained completely negative results in forty-eight women with ovarian failure. Hamblen[83] has likewise found the "therapeutic results with the use of equine gonadotropins alone . . . extremely disappointing." Davis, in discussing Hamblen's report on the efficacy of the equine gonadotropins, stated that such therapy, though effective in secondary amenorrhea, is of only limited benefit in the primary form. In the same discussion, Koff acknowledged that his results have been inconsistent and disappointing. Greene's clinical experience likewise has been "uniformly unsuccessful." Brewer, Jones and Skiles administered from 600 to 5000 rat units or 1200 to 10,000 I. U. of equine gonadotropin to twenty-four women with normal menstrual cycles and presumably normal ovaries. Laparotomy performed one to five days after the last injection failed to yield conclusive evidence that the treatment had induced ovulation in a single instance.

On the whole it would appear that the equine hormones have not justified the expectations inspired by Davis and Koff's report.

Combined Equine and Human Chorionic Gonadotropin Therapy.— Since the equine hormones are primarily follicle stimulating and the human chorionic gonadotropes predominantly luteinizing in their effect, it would seem reasonable to expect that both preparations, given in succession, might more closely duplicate the action of the anterior pituitary gland than either hormone alone. Ovulation has been reported following this form of therapy in the monkey[67] and man.[20, 84] According to Hamblen,[74] the results are more satisfactory than those obtained with any other form of gonadotropic hormone therapy. In nineteen women between fourteen and thirty-one years of age, with menometrorrhagia from *estrogenic endometria*, the administration of equine gonadotropin for ten days and chorionic gonadotropin for the next ten days, was followed by the appearance of progestational changes of the endometrium in five cases. A similar effect was elicited in three out of nine women with *oligomenorrhea* and estrogenic endometria. He reports a favorable response in 50 per cent of his cases in a more recent study.[85] In evaluating these results, it should be borne in mind that spontaneous conversion of an estrogenic mucosa to the progestational phase is not uncommon.

Combined Therapy with Human Chorionic Gonadotropin and Anterior Hypophyseal Extract.—The clinical use of anterior pituitary gland extract together with chorionic gonadotropin is based on the observation that such combined treatment in the laboratory animal results in an ovarian weight increase exceeding that which might be expected from the two hormones given singly.[21] Mazer,[86] one of the chief protagonists of this form of therapy, has recently reported his experience with *synapoidin,* a combination of chorionic gonadotropin and a pituitary extract with only slight gonadotropic activity. In twenty-three women, aged twelve to forty-six years, examination of the ovaries following treatment with varying doses of this substance revealed over-sized ovaries, hemorrhagic follicles and in many instances multiple incompletely formed corpora lutea. Only one of sixteen patients whose ovaries were available for microscopic examination failed to show evidence of "intense stimulation." No information was given regarding the status of the ovaries before treatment nor was any attempt made to compare the ovaries with those of untreated controls with similar gynecologic conditions. In nineteen of twenty-three patients with *amenorrhea,* one or more menstrual flows followed treatment with this preparation. Control of abnormal uterine bleeding was observed in fourteen of eighteen patients. Conception occurred shortly after a course of treatment in two of eight women with sterility associated with anovular menstruation.

Geist and his associates[87] have recently reported the results of a carefully controlled study of ninety-one cases in which the ovaries were available for microscopic examination following treatment with hypophyseal, chorionic and equine gonadotropin and various combinations of these hormones. In no instance did they find evidence of ovulation which could be unquestionably attributed to the administered gonadotropins; nor were any synergistic effects observed with any of the gonadotropin combinations. From the histologic alterations noted, they concluded that, "while the available gonadotropins may stimulate those granulosa and theca interna cells, in follicles undergoing atresia, which are still capable of response, they apparently do not induce follicle maturation or stimulate the development of follicles containing normal ova to maturity and ovulation."

RESPONSE OF THE HUMAN TESTIS TO THE GONADOTROPES

Opportunities for microscopic examination of the human testis following treatment with gonadotropic substances have been limited. The effect of these substances on testicular development and function has been estimated largely from the clinical response in cryptorchidism, hypogenitalism, and male sterility due to spermatogenic deficiency.

Efficacy in Cryptorchidism.—The efficacy of the hypophyseal, chorionic and equine gonadotropes in cryptorchidism is not established. Some have reported spectacular cures, while others could see no improvement which might be definitely ascribed to the treatment. These divergent findings are probably attributable to differences in the type of case treated. In true cryptorchidism, due to some anatomic fault which precludes descent of the testes, it is doubtful whether organotherapy can be of any value. This type of case probably accounts for many of the failures reported with endocrine treatment. On the other hand, in pseudocryptorchidism, where there is no mechanical impediment to descent of the testes, the experience of competent observers indicates that spontaneous correction eventually occurs in the vast majority of the cases. It is not unlikely that most of the brilliant results reported in the literature were obtained in this type of cryptorchidism. At all events, we cannot be sure, in a specific instance, to what extent the organotherapy contributed to the improvement noted. (See Chap. XXXVI).

Efficacy in Hypogenitalism.—Enlargement of the testes, associated with development of the accessory genitalia and secondary sex characters, have been reported in cases of hypogonadism, following treatment with gonadotropic hormone, particularly that of chorionic origin. It is noteworthy, however, that most of the good results were obtained in young boys where the hypogenitalism was associated with adiposity of the *Fröhlich's type*, or emaciation suggesting *Simmonds' disease*. It should be emphasized that the large majority of fat boys with small genitalia are not cases of true Fröhlich's syndrome. Many of these individuals eventually attain sexual maturity without endocrine therapy or through weight reduction alone.[88] It is significant that older males presenting the Fröhlich's type of adiposity with genital hypoplasia do not respond to organotherapy. The improvement noted following gonadotropin therapy in cases diagnosed as Simmonds' disease is not convincing proof of the efficacy of such treatment. It is possible that such cases were actually instances of anorexia nervosa (see Chap. XXXV), which were benefited by the psychotherapeutic effect of the treatment, or were examples of emaciation due to nutritional faults, which improved because of dietary and supportive measures used concomitantly.

Efficacy in Spermatogenic Deficiency.—Improvement in the motility, morphology, quality, and number of sperm in males with spermatogenic deficiency has been reported by some observers following gonadotropin therapy. In the author's experience and that of others,[89] the results of such treatment have been too inconstant to be acceptable as evidence of stimulation. McCullagh and Ryan,[90] for example, could demonstrate no increase in spermatogenesis or rise in the urinary androgen level in the majority of their cases receiving chorionic, equine or hypophyseal gonadotropin. Improvement seemed to follow treatment in a few of their cases, but this may have been coincidental, for there is ample evidence that spontaneous variations in the number and quality of the sperm, and in the androgen level in the urine, may occur from time to time in the same individual. Davis and his associates[145] treated twenty males with seminal inadequacy with combined chorionic gonadotropin and pituitary "synergist," in doses of 30 to 45 "synergy" units daily for four to twelve weeks. The seminal values showed some increase in eight, decreased in five and remained the same in seven. The post-treatment values showed a definite trend toward lower than pre-treatment values. They suggest that antibody formation may be responsible. It is apparent, therefore, that convincing proof of the efficacy of the available gonadotropes in the male is still lacking.

THE AGE FACTOR IN THE GONADAL RESPONSE TO THE GONADOTROPES

The gonadal response to the gonadotropes depends not only on the adequacy of the stimulus, but also on the developmental status of the receptor organ. This in turn is apparently dependent upon the age and degree of somatic development.

13

Experiments carried out with gonadotropic extracts at different phases of life indicate that a response can be evoked only during, and shortly before and after the period of maturity. The gonads of the very young, and the senile subject are apparently refractory to gonadotropic stimuli. Some degree of response can be elicited in animals approaching maturity, and those which have recently completed this epoch. On the basis of the gonad's reactivity, we may speak of the following stages: (1) immaturity, (2) pre-maturity or juvenility, (3) maturity, (4) post-maturity, and (5) senility.

Immaturity.—Studies in fetuses and very young mammals indicate that the gonadotropes can evoke little or no response in the gonads. Evans and Swezy[91] could demonstrate no ovarian change whatsoever in the rat fetus, while Aron[92] found that, in guinea pig fetuses over 40 mm. long, the only apparent effect was development of the interstitial cells in the medulla and hilum of the ovary. This refractory state persists after birth for a period of time which varies in different species. In the rat, Smith and Engle[93] could not elicit a full gonadal response with anterior lobe implants before the twentieth day of life, while in the mouse, the ovaries remained refractory until the fifteenth day. When a follicle-stimulating extract was used in very young rats, no growth of follicles occurred, but when treatment was continued until the twenty-first day of life, marked stimulation of follicles resulted. They therefore concluded that the gametes and granulosa must undergo some maturation change before they can respond to an appropriate gonadotropic stimulus. On the basis of microscopic studies, it would appear that the refractory state persists until antra-bearing follicles appear. Evans and Swezy[94] observed that anterior pituitary extract evoked a response only in those follicles which had passed the primary stage and possessed more than one row of follicle cells.

Ripening of the gonads to a point where they can respond fully to the gonadotropes is apparently related to body *size* and general *somatic development*. Zondek[94] could not induce follicular maturation and corpus luteum formation in rabbits weighing 600 grams or less. Siegmund[95] also recognized that in order to insure a gonadal response to stimulation, the test animal must achieve a certain minimum weight which is greater in heavier than in lighter breeds. Of interest in this connection is Hertz's[96] observation that ovaries lacking antra-bearing follicles remain refractory to stimulation even after transplantation to an adult host. This would imply that, though maturation of the soma normally runs parallel to and may possibly assist in the maturation of the gonad, it cannot of itself compensate for incomplete ripening.

The studies of Selye,[55] Collip,[97] Aron,[98] and Bachman[99] in the rat, mouse, guinea pig and rabbit, tend to emphasize the fact that the gonad, in its progress towards full maturity, first passes through a stage of immaturity, when gonadotropic hormone evokes at best only a response in the interstitial tissue, and then through a phase of pre-maturity or juvenility, when the granulosa cells and ova show steadily increasing reactivity to gonadotropic stimulation.

Prematurity or Juvenility.—During this phase, follicular maturation, ovulation and corpus luteum formation can be induced with adequate doses of potent gonadotropes. As the animal more closely approaches the normal age for puberty, the response becomes more rapid, and the amount of hormone required for an effect steadily diminishes. This would indicate that the granulosa has finally achieved sufficient maturity to respond to stimulation and is gradually progressing towards the climax of its development which marks the fully mature gonad. Since the ovary, at this time, is capable of responding to exogenous gonadotropes, it seems likely that the absence of full ovarian function in the juvenile animal is due to an inadequate endogenous supply of gonadotropic hormone. As the age of maturity is reached, the available supply of gonad-stimulating hormone, which probably also increases as the organism matures, apparently becomes sufficient for the initiation and maintenance of full gonadal function.

Postmaturity and Senile Period.—At the end of the reproductive period, the ovary again gradually becomes refractory to hypophyseal stimulation. Histologic studies in the human and lower animals have shown that the ovary, at this time of life, gradually undergoes involutionary changes which begin in the ovarian tunic and work inward, affecting more and more of the ovarian parenchyma, until all function is extinguished.

The ova and granulosa cells are apparently first affected by this involutionary process, while the theca cells are last to suffer. This is suggested by the fact that, while ovulation and corpus luteum formation gradually ceases, incomplete maturation of follicles with proliferation of theca cells and estrogen production may continue for some time. Thus, it would appear that, in the life span of the ovary, the interstitial cells are the first to achieve function and the last to be deprived of it, while the granulosa cells and ova are the last to attain full maturity and function and the first to suffer from any regressive process which may affect the organ.

There is reason to believe that this involutionary process is not due to withdrawal of pituitary stimulation, but represents a local expression of the general involution which foreshadows senility and from which no part of the organism is exempt. Hormonal studies of the blood and urine of menopausal women (see Chap. XL) have shown that the quantity of gonad-stimulating hormone may actually be increased, and may remain relatively high for many years past the menopause. The hormonal content of the pituitary at this time may also be appreciably higher than during the reproductive period.[100] That the decline of ovarian function is partly due to diminishing anterior hypophyseal activity is suggested by Wolfe's[144] observation that the structural alterations characteristic of old age accumulate in the anterior hypophysis of the rat coincident with the appearance in the ovary of wheel cells, which he attributes to pituitary deficiency.

Degree of Reactivity.—That the ovaries of *old animals* retain some degree of reactivity to stimulation after estrus cycles have ceased, is indicated by the author's observation[4] in senile rats whose ovarian function, as evidenced by the vaginal smear, had long ceased. Implants of fresh anterior lobe tissue reactivated the ovaries and restored the estrus cycles. In some of the animals, coitus was followed by conception and the birth of normal young.

In the human being, Kurzrok[101] found that much larger doses of gonadotropic hormone are required to evoke a response in the ovary of women approaching the menopause than in younger women. In women in the third decade of life, 3600 m.u. of equine gonadotropin caused a marked increase in the size and weight of the ovaries and formation of large follicular cysts. In the fourth decade, the response was slight, only an occasional follicle being found. In the fifth decade as much as 9000 m.u. failed to evoke any response whatsoever. These findings clearly emphasize the increasing refractoriness of the ovaries with advancing age.

Whether more potent gonadotropes given in larger doses would elicit a response in the senile subject is a question for future investigation. It is likely that the involuting ovary passes through an intermediate stage, when it is relatively refractory to stimulation but can nevertheless be made to respond if an adequate stimulus is brought to bear. This assumption, if true, would reconcile the author's success in reactivating the ovaries of senile rats, with Kurzrok's negative results in postmenopausal women.

EFFECT OF THE GONADS ON THE ANTERIOR HYPOPHYSIS

Studies of the histology and hormonal content of the adenohypophysis during pregnancy, after the natural and artificial menopause, and following treatment with the male and female sex hormones, have shown that the gonads influence anterior pituitary function.

Hypophyseal Modifications during Pregnancy.—Comte,[102] in 1898, first pointed out that the human hypophysis increases in size and weight during pregnancy. Rasmussen's[103] recent studies indicate that the *hypertrophy* is confined to the anterior lobe. According to this observer, the average weight of the gland in the pregnant woman exceeds that of the nonpregnant subject by more than 100 mgms. The degree of enlargement, he found, depends on the duration of gestation and the number of previous pregnancies. This would imply that the hypophysis enlarges progressively during gestation, and retains part of the added weight for some time after parturition.

Cytologic Alterations.—This physiologic hypertrophy is associated with characteristic cytologic modifications. Erdheim and Stumme,[104] in 1909, described an acidophil-like cell, apparently derived from the chromophobes, which they interpreted as a specialized cell peculiar to the pregnant state, and accordingly named it *pregnancy cell*. While the so-called "pregnancy cell" has been repeatedly described both in man and other species, there has been considerable controversy as to its derivation and significance. Rasmussen[103] found that, except for a 2 per cent increase in chromophobes, and a corresponding decrease in acidophils, there is no statistically significant difference between the cells of pituitaries of pregnant and nonpregnant women. This observer points out that, though the chromophobes seem to contain more cytoplasm, the hypophysis of the pregnant subject contains no unusually large chromophobes which might be considered different from any that can be found in the gland of the nonpregnant woman. He concludes that the pituitary enlargement cannot be attributed to hyperplasia of any one cell type. Severinghaus[105] maintains that the so-called "pregnancy cell" is not a new cell type, but rather represents "some transitional aspect of the chromophobe-chromophile-chromophobe changes which occur in the secretory cycle of the cells, and which are accentuated in the secretory activity of the pituitary gland of pregnancy."

The functional significance of the cytologic modifications observed in the anterior hypophysis during pregnancy is not clear. Some interpret them as evidence of diminished function, while Severinghaus[105] believes they signify heightened secretory activity of both the basophils and acidophils, associated with a rapid discharge of their incretory products. On the basis of Rasmussen's and Severinghaus' findings, it would appear that pregnancy evokes in the anterior hypophysis a spurt of secretory activity which involves all its cellular constituents alike and is macroscopically evident in enlargement of the gland.

Hormonal Content during Pregnancy.—Philipp[106] and later Zondek[107] demonstrated that the adenohypophysis of the pregnant woman contains little or no gonadotropic hormone. This finding has since been amply confirmed, but its significance is not clear. According to one interpretation, the gonadotropic activity of the hypophysis ceases and is taken over by the placenta (see Chap. VIII). Another view holds that the pituitary gland is hyperactive but discharges its secretions so rapidly that no hormone can be demonstrated in the gland at a given moment. In support of the latter interpretation, Severinghaus[105] has pointed out that, in the pregnant woman, monkey and rat, the hypophysis contains actively secreting acidophils and basophils. He emphasizes the fact that, though many cells lose most of their granules, their Golgi apparatus remains large and their mitochondria abundant, the whole picture suggesting marked activity and speedy discharge.

Cause of the Modifications.—Attempts to induce changes like those seen during pregnancy by administering various hormonal extracts, have yielded conflicting results. Haterius and Charipper[108] produced a pregnancy type of hypophysis in the intact male and female animal by means of anterior pituitary implants. A similar effect was obtained in normal immature rats by administering human pregnancy urine gonadotropin. Such treatment was without effect in castrate animals. It would therefore appear that the modifications observed in the hypophysis during pregnancy are not due to a specific fetal or placental hormone, but to some substance secreted by the gonads in response to gonadotropic hormone. That *progestin* may contribute to this effect is suggested by the observation that characteristic pregnancy modifications appear in the adenohypophysis of the pseudopregnant guinea pig, rat and rabbit. Also significant is Wolfe's[109] observation that the administration of pregnancy urine gonadotropin to intact animals produced numerous corpora lutea, and changes in the pituitary described as an exaggeration of those seen in early gestation and pseudopregnancy. Charipper[110] demonstrated typical pregnancy changes in the hypophysis following progestin administration in both intact and castrate male and female rats. Since this effect could not be obtained with estrogen, he concluded that the essential factor for the pituitary modifications originates in the luteinized ovary and is not sex specific.

In contrast to these observations, several investigators have reported that characteristic pregnancy changes can be induced in the pituitary with *estrogen*. Siegmund[111] elicited this effect with estrogen but not with corpus luteum extract, while Wolfe[112] found that estrogen plus progestin had the same effect as estrogen alone.

The available evidence, though conflicting, suggests that both estrogen and progestin probably contribute toward the production of the characteristic pregnancy modifications in the adenohypophysis.

Hypophyseal Modifications following Castration.—*Cytologic Alterations.*—There is evidence that the hypophysis enlarges following castration. In most species, including man, the most conspicuous change is an increase in the number and size of the basophils. Many of these cells are granular and apparently actively secreting. Others are vacuolated and, due to displacement of their cytoplasm by accumulating colloid-like substance, assume a signet-ring-like appearance. These vacuolated cells, first described by Zacherl[113] in the hypophysis of the castrate rat, were identified as modified basophils by Addison.[114] Usually referred to as "signet ring" or "castration cells," they have been demonstrated in many species. In the human being, the basophils become more numerous and vacuolated following castration, but they do not acquire the signet-ring-like appearance described in other species. The status of the acidophils following castration is not clear; some workers report an increase, others a decrease in their number and size.

Whether the postcastration modifications in the hypophysis persist indefinitely or regress after a time is not certain. Schenk[115] observed a return to normal within two years after gonadectomy, while other observers[116] could demonstrate no such reversion.

The functional significance of the hypophyseal changes in the castrate has been the subject of much controversy. Some believe that the process of vacuolation signifies heightened secretory activity, due to removal of the inhibiting influence of the gonadal hormones. Severinghaus[105] construes the hypophyseal modifications as evidence of progressive atrophy, resulting possibly from interference with the release of the cell's secretory products. The increased granular content of the basophils he attributes to the slow rate of discharge rather than to heightened secretory activity. Nelson[117] believes that the gonadal hormones control the rate of differentiation and dedifferentiation of the basophils, and that when this control is removed by gonadectomy, there results not only a more rapid differentiation, but also a failure to dedifferentiate and a tendency to enlarge and vacuolate.

Hormonal Content.—Engle,[118] in 1929, called attention to a significant increase in the gonadotropic hormone content of the rat's hypophysis following castration. This has been confirmed[119] and shown to hold also for the guinea pig and rabbit. Since it may signify either increased production, or increased storage due to slow discharge, it is of little value in deciding whether anterior pituitary function is heightened or diminished following castration.

Cause of the Modifications.—Withdrawal of the ovarian secretions is apparently responsible for the postcastration changes in the hypophysis, for the administration of estrogenic substances can prevent or correct the cytologic modifications as well as the increase in the hormonal content of this gland. The amount of *estrogen* required for this effect is proportional to the interval between castration and the institution of therapy.

Whether *progestin* can likewise prevent postcastration changes in the hypophysis is not certain. Hohlweg and Dohrn[120] found that 1 rat unit of estrogen daily did not prevent castration changes, unless supplemented by ⅕ rabbit unit of progestin. On the other hand, progesterone alone, in doses of 540 gamma daily, proved ineffective for this purpose. Fels[121] likewise obtained negative results with progestin alone in the castrate female rat, but Clauberg and Breipohl,[122] and Brooksby[123] have noted a reversal of castration changes following progestin administration in this species. In a more recent study, Biddulph and associates[124] found progesterone effective in controlling increased gonadotropic hormone secretion in the castrate female rat. Male sex hormone, according to Nelson and Gallagher,[125] prevents the characteristic hypophyseal modifications in castrate rats regardless of sex, but Martins and Rocha,[126] and Migliavacca,[127] found testicular extract more effective in the male. Somewhat puzzling is the observation of Wolfe and Hamilton[128] that the simultaneous administration of estrone and testosterone acetate in the female rat did not prevent the castration increase in the basophiles, although each one was effected when injected alone.

Effect of Estrogen on Anterior Hypophyseal Function.—Studies in the experimental animal indicate that the estrogens may exert either an inhibitory or stimulative effect on anterior pituitary function, depending in part on the dosage and length of treatment. This apparent ability of the estrogens to modify pituitary activity has aroused considerable interest, for if shown to apply to the human being, it would provide an effective method of regulating abnormal hypophyseal function.

Estrogen as an Inhibitor of Hypophyseal Function.—Chronic estrogen treatment in the experimental animal may cause ovarian degeneration and atrophy. This effect was attributed at first to the direct action of the hormone on the ovary, but it is now generally believed that estrogen acts by suppressing the gonadotropic activity of the adenohypophysis. This view finds support in the following observations: (1) the gonadotropic potency of the human hypophysis decreases in the presence of a high concentration of estrogen, such as occurs during pregnancy or following the administration of estrogen, and increases when this hormone is present only in minute amounts, as in the castrate; (2) the regressive changes which appear in the gonads following chronic estrogen treatment are associated with a decrease in the gonadotropic hormone content of the anterior lobe; (3) the simultaneous administration of gonadotropic extract offsets the depressive effect of estrogenic substance on the ovary; (4) the degree of ovarian atrophy is not appreciably greater in estrogen treated hypophysectomized animals than in untreated hypophysectomized controls; (5) the gonadal hypertrophy which normally occurs in one partner of a parabiotic union when the other is castrated, can be prevented by administering estrogen to the castrate partner; (6) the gonadotropic substances that appear in the urine of castrate and menopausal women, and are presumably of hypophyseal origin, disappear when adequate doses of estrogen are administered.

Microscopic studies of the pituitary following chronic estrogen treatment likewise suggest an inhibitory effect. Some investigators, notably Zondek,[129] have reported enlargement of the hypophysis due mainly to hypertrophy and hyperplasia of the chromophobes. If treatment is sufficiently prolonged, the basophils become completely degranulated and the acidophils likewise show loss of granules. When this transformation from a chromophilic to a chromophobic state is carried to an extreme by very protracted treatment, large chromophobic adenomata may form. These pituitary modifications not only give rise to symptoms of hypogonadism but also other manifestations of pituitary insufficiency. If treatment is instituted early in life, it may cause dwarfism, while in the mature animal, it may lead to cachexia and regressive changes in the thyroid, adrenals and other glands dependent on pituitary function. In extreme cases, death may occur from intracranial pressure produced by the enlarging pituitary tumor. Inhibition of the lactogenic and diabetogenic activity of the adenohypophysis has also been reported following estrogen treatment.

Estrogen as a Stimulator of Hypophyseal Function.—Hohlweg,[130] in 1934, observed that a single dose of 500 rat units of estrogen produced corpora lutea and pituitary enlargement in immature rats. This has since been corroborated by several observers. Klaften[131] induced corpus luteum formation in immature rabbits weighing not less than 1800 gm., by administering 60,000 to 100,000 international benzoate units of estrogen over a four week period, or by giving somewhat smaller doses over a six week period. The corpora lutea thus induced were functional, as shown by their ability to inhibit uterine reactivity to pituitrin, and induce progestational modifications of the endometrium.

That this effect of estrogen is dependent upon the pituitary is indicated by Hohlweg and Chamorro's[132] observation that corpora lutea, which form in the intact animal within five days after estrogen treatment is begun, fail to appear if the hypophysis is removed on the second day of treatment, but not if operation is delayed until the fourth day. This would suggest that estrogen stimulates the rabbit hypophysis to release its luteinizing principle at some point between the second and fourth day of treatment.

To reconcile the apparently conflicting reports of depression and stimulation following estrogen administration, Halpern and D'Amour[133] have suggested that "the depression of the anterior lobe seen when estrin is administered, may be considered as one aspect of a reaction to intense stimulation. The demands of the stimulus having exceeded the secretory capacity of the gland, a period of hyperplasia follows. During this period, the secretion of the gonadotropic hormone is diminished because most of the energies of the gland are now consumed by the rapid cellular proliferation." A somewhat similar interpretation has been offered by Severinghaus.[105] Lane[134] likewise believes the initial effect of estrogen is stimulative but attributes the depression caused by prolonged treatment to inhibition rather than exhaustion. Clauberg and Breipohl[122] hold that massive doses of estrogen, acting over a short period, temporarily suppress pituitary activity, and that upon withdrawal of this inhibitory influence, the gland shows a marked spurt of activity with release of its luteinizing factor. Zondek's[135] studies led him to conclude that the effect of estrogen depends on the amount administered and the duration of treatment, small doses stimulating, while large doses depress hypophyseal function. Noting that prolonged estrogen administration in rats caused ovarian atrophy, although the gonadotropic hormone content of the pituitary remained equal to that of untreated controls, Zondek concluded that estrogen checks the delivery but not the production of gonadotropic hormone. Significant in this connection is Engle's[136] concept of a "releasing mechanism" over which estrogen exerts some control. According to this view, estrogen acts as a force which actively influences hypophyseal activity. More recently, Wolfe and Brown[147] pointed out that the cytological evidence indicates a stimulative effect of estrogen, whereas physiological findings suggest that it stimulates production and release of the luteinizing and luteotrophic factors, but suppresses the follicle-stimulating principle. To reconcile the conflict between the two types of evidence as regards FSH, they suggest that release of this factor after estrogen injections may be accompanied by discharge of a second substance which inhibits its action. A final solution awaits further investigation.

Whether estrogen exerts its effect on the adenohypophysis by nervous or humoral pathways is still uncertain. Hohlweg and his associates[137] have postulated the existence of a nervous center in the diencephalon through which variations in the estrogen level of the blood influence anterior hypophyseal function. As proof they offer their observation that the characteristic cytologic changes which appear in the hypophysis following castration, are not discernible in pituitary implants, and conversely, that the pituitaries of castrate animals, in which castration changes have already appeared, return to normal when transplanted to a castrate host. From this they conclude that the pituitary cannot respond to changes in the estrogen level when its nervous connections are severed.

Hohlweg's hypothesis has been criticized by Desclin and Gregoire[138] on the ground that it is based on inadequate evidence. These observers maintain that estrogen acts through humoral pathways on the basis of their observation that the intact pituitary and pituitary grafts react identically to estrogen treatment. They attribute the absence of castration changes in pituitary transplants to the fact that they do not function under strictly physiologic conditions. As a result, they may be unaffected by the relatively slight change in the hormonal environment incident to castration. Desclin's interpretation finds suport in Phelps's observation[139] that some if not all the effects of estrogen on the structure of the intact anterior lobe can be produced in pituitary grafts. Also significant is Uotila's report[140] that section of the pituitary stalk does not interfere with the ability of estrogen to cause hypertrophy and cytologic changes in the anterior lobe, or to suppress its secretion of gonadotropic hormone. He concludes that estrogen acts directly on the anterior hypophysis, and that "this action is part of the humoral control of the basic secretory rhythm of the gland."

BIBLIOGRAPHY

1. Severinghaus, A. E.: Anat. Rec. *61* (Suppl.): 61, 1935; Physiol. Rev. *17*:566, 1937.
2. Smith, P. E., and Engle, E. T.: Am. J. Anat. *40*:159, 1927.
3. Zondek, B., and Aschheim, S.: Arch. f. Gynäk. *130*:1, 1927; Klin. Wchnschr. *6*:248, 1927.
4. Hoffman, J.: Am. J. Obst. & Gynec. *22*:231, 1931.
5. Engle, E. T.: Sex and Internal Secretions, ed. by E. Allen. Baltimore, Williams & Wilkins Co., 1932, chap. 16, p. 794.
6. Fevold, H. L., Hisaw, F. L., Hellbaum, A., and Hertz, R.: Am. J. Physiol. *104*:710, 1933.
7. Wallen-Lawrence, Z.: J. Pharm. & Exper. Therap. *51*:263, 1934.
8. Evans, H. M., Korpi, K., Simpson, M. E., Pencharz, R. I., and Wonder, D. H.: Univ. of California Pub. in Anat. (No. 9) *1*:255, 1936.
9. Fevold, H. L.: Endocrinol. *24*:435, 1939; J. Biol. Chem. *128*:83, 1939.
   Fevold, H. L., Lee, M., Hisaw, F. L., and Cohn, E. J.: Endocrinol. *26*:999, 1940; ibid. *27*:781, 1940.
   Shedlovsky, T., Rothen, A., Greep, R. O., Van Dyke, H. B., and Chow, B. F.: Science *92*:178, 1940.
   Greep, R. O., Van Dyke, H. B., and Chow, B. F.: J. Biol. Chem. *133*:289, 1940; Endocrinol. *30*:635, 1942.
10. Evans, H. M., Simpson, M. E., Tolksdorf, S., and Jensen, H.: Endocrinol. *25*:529, 1939.
    Tolksdorf, S., and Jensen, H.: Proc. Soc. Exper. Biol. & Med. *42*:466, 1939.
    Jensen, H., Tolksdorf, S., and Bamman, F.: J. Biol. Chem. *135*:791, 1940.
    Li, C. H., Simpson, M. E., and Evans, H. M.: Endocrinol. *27*:803, 1940.
11. Fevold, H. L.: Endocrinol. *28*:33, 1941.
12. Leonard, S. L.: Am. J. Physiol. *98*:406, 1931.
13. Evans, H. M., Meyer, K., and Simpson, M. E.: Mem. Univ. Calif. 1933, sect. 111, pp. 151–206.
14. Hertz, R., and Hisaw, F. L.: Am. J. Physiol. *108*:1, 1934.
15. Casida, L. E.: Endocrinol. *18*:714, 1934.
16. Foster, M. A., and Hisaw, F. L.: Anat. Rec. *62*:75, 1935.
17. Foster, M. A., and Fevold, H. L.: Anat. Rec. *61*:18, 1935; Am. J. Physiol. *121*:625, 1938.
18. Foster, M. A., Foster, R. C., and Fevold, H. L.: Endocrinol. *21*:249, 1937.
19. Hisaw, F. L., Greep, R. O., and Fevold, H. L.: Anat. Rec. *61* (Suppl.): 24, 1935.
20. Davis, M. E., and Koff, A. K.: Am. J. Obst. & Gynec. *36*:183, 1938.
    Siegler, S. L., and Fein, M. J.: Am. J. Obst. & Gynec. *38*:1021, 1939.
    Brewer, J. I., Jones, H. O., and Skiles, J. H., Jr.: J.A.M.A. *118*:278, 1942.
21. Evans, H. M., Meyer, K., and Simpson, M. E.: Proc. Soc. Exper. Biol. & Med. *28*:845, 1931.
22. Fevold, H. L., Hisaw, F., Hellbaum, A., and Hertz, R.: Proc. Soc. Exper. Biol. & Med. *30*:914, 1933.
    Fevold, H. L., and Hisaw, F. L.: Am. J. Physiol. *190*:655, 1934.
23. Saunders, F. J., and Cole, H. H.: Endocrinol. *23*:302, 1938.
24. Lein, A.: Proc. Soc. Exper. Biol. & Med. *36*:609, 1937.
25. Evans, H. M., and Simpson, M. E.: Proc. Soc. Exper. Biol. & Med. *26*:595, 1929.
26. Loeb, L., Anderson, W. C., Saxton, J., Hayward, S. J., and Kippen, A. A.: California & West. Med. *43*:199, 1935.
27. Evans, H. M., Korpi, K., Pencharz, R. I., and Simpson, M. E.: Univ. of California Pub. in Anat. (No. 8) *1*:237, 1936.
28. Bunde, C. A., and Greep, R. O.: Proc. Soc. Exper. Biol. & Med. *35*:235, 1936.
29. Greep, R. O.: Anat. Rec. *70* (Suppl.): 32, 1938; Endocrinol. *23*:154, 1938.
30. Foster, M. A.: Am. J. Physiol. *121*:633, 1938.
31. Freud, J.: Nature, London *139*:880, 1937; Acta brev. Neerland. *8*:176, 1938.
32. Makepeace, A. W., Weinstein, G. L., and Friedman, M. H.: Am. J. Physiol. *119*:812, 1937.
33. Astwood, E. B., and Fevold, H. L.: Am. J. Physiol. *127*:192, 1939.
34. Astwood, E. B., and Fevold, H. L.: Endocrinol. *28*:309, 1941.
35. Fevold, H. L., Lee, M., Hisaw, F. L., and Cohn, E. J.: Endocrinol. *26*:999, 1940.

36. Lyons, W. R.: Cold Spring Harbor Symp. Quant. Biol. 5:93, 1937.
37. Aschheim, S., and Zondek, B.: Klin. Wchnschr. 6:1332, 1927.
38. Collip, J. B., Selye, H., and Thomson, D. L.: Nature, London 131:56, 1933.
39. Leonard, S. L., and Smith, P. E.: Anat. Rec. 58:175, 1934.
40. Greep, R. O.: Endocrinol. 23:154, 1938; Anat. Rec. 70 (Suppl.) : 32, 1938.
41. Gaarenstroom, J. H., and de Jongh, S. E.: Acta brev. Neerland. 10:202, 1940.
42. Hill, M., and Parkes, A. S.: J. Physiol. 69:Proc. XVIII, 1930.
43. Falk, E. A., and Papanicolaou, G. N.: Anat. Rec. 64 (Suppl.) : 16, 1935.
44. Bradbury, J. T.: Endocrinol. 28:101, 1941.
45. Pfeiffer, C. A.: Anat. Rec. 77 (Supp.) : 59, 1941.
46. Friedman, M. H.: Am. J. Physiol. 90:617, 1929.
47. White, W. E., and Leonard, S. L.: Am. J. Physiol. 104:44, 1933.
48. Engle, E. T.: Sex and Internal Secretions, ed. by E. Allen. Baltimore, Williams & Wilkins Co., 1939, chap. 18, p. 1014.
49. Engle, E. T.: Anat. Rec. 43:187, 1929.
50. Smith, P. E., and Leonard, S. L.: Anat. Rec. 58:145, 1934; Proc. Soc. Exper. Biol. & Med. 30:1246, 1934.
51. Engle, E. T.: Endocrinol. 16:513, 1932.
52. Orbin, F., and Watrin, J.: Compt. rend. Soc. de biol. 100:438, 1929.
Engle, E. T.: Am. J. Phys. 106:145, 1933.
Schockaert, J. A.: Am. J. Physiol. 105:497, 1933.
53. Fluhmann, C. F.: Endocrinol. 17:550, 1933; Am. J. Obst. & Gynec. 28:668, 1934.
54. Smith, P. E., and Engle, E. T.: Am. J. Anat. 40:159, 1927.
Evans, H. M., and Simpson, M. E.: Endocrinol. 27:305, 1940.
55. Selye, H., Collip, J. B., and Thomson, D. L.: Proc. Soc. Exper. Biol. & Med. 30:647, 780, 1933.
56. Zondek, B.: Klin. Wchnschr. 9:393, 1930.
57. Fluhmann, C. F.: J.A.M.A. 93:672, 1929.
58. Frank, R. T., and Goldberger, M. A.: Proc. Soc. Exper. Biol. & Med. 32:1663, 1935.
59. Levin, L., and Tyndale, H. H.: cited by Engle, E. T. (supra 48).
60. Friedman, M. H.: cited by Engle, E. T. (supra 48).
61. Cole, H. H., and Hart, G. H.: Am. J. Physiol. 93:57, 1930.
62. Zondek, B.: Klin. Wchnschr. 9:2285, 1930.
63. Evans, H. M., Simpson, M. E., and Austin, P. R.: J. Exper. Med. 58:561, 1933.
64. Catchpole, H. R., and Lyons, W. R.: Am. J. Physiol. 112:21, 1935.
65. Catchpole, H. R., and Lyons, W. R.: Am. J. Anat. 55:167, 1934.
66. Leonard, S. L., and Leonard, O. L.: Anat. Rec. 64 (Suppl.) : 51, 1935.
67. Engle, E. T., and Hamburger, C.: Proc. Soc. Exper. Biol. & Med. 32:1531, 1935.
68. Hartman, C. G.: Bull. Johns Hopkins Hosp. 63:351, 1938.
69. Cartland, G. F., and Nelson, J. W.: Am. J. Physiol. 122:201, 1938.
70. Saunders, F. J., and Cole, H. H.: Proc. Soc. Exper. Biol. & Med. 32:1476, 1935.
71. Evans, H. M., Korpi, K., Simpson, M. E., and Pencharz, R. I.: Univ. California Pub. Anat. 1:275, 1936.
72. Westman, A.: Zentralbl. f. Gynäk. 58:1090, 1934; ibid. 59:1090, 1935.
73. Geist, S. H.: Am. J. Obst. & Gynec. 26:588, 1933.
74. Hamblen, E. C.: Endocrine Gynecology. Springfield, Ill., Charles C. Thomas, 1939.
75. Pratt, J. P.: J.A.M.A. 101:Abst. p. 556, 1933.
76. Brown, W. E., Bradbury, J. T., and Metzger, I.: Am. J. Obst. & Gynec. 41:582, 1941.
77. Kurzrok, R.: The Endocrines in Obstetrics and Gynecology. Baltimore, Williams & Wilkins Co., 1937.
78. Siegmund, H.: Zentralbl. f. Gynäk. 62:2113, 1938.
79. Westman, A.: Zentralbl. f. Gynäk. 59:676, 1935.
80. Huber, C. P., and Davis, M. E.: Surg., Gynec. & Obst. 70:996, 1940.
81. Gray, L. A.: South. Med. J. 33:160, 1940; Am. J. Obst. & Gynec. 43:387, 1942.
82. Erving, H. W., Sears, C., and Rock, J.: Am. J. Obst. & Gynec. 40:695, 1940.
83. Hamblen, E. C.: Am. J. Obst. & Gynec. 41:495, 1941.
84. Büttner, W.: Arch. f. Gynäk. 163:487, 1937.

85. Hamblen, E. C.: J. Clin. Endocrinol. *1*:749, 1941.
86. Mazer, C., and Israel, S. L.: Diagnosis and Treatment of Menstrual Disorders and Sterility. New York, Paul B. Hoeber, Inc., 1941.
87. Geist, S. H., Gaines, J. A., and Salmon, U. J.: Am. J. Obst. & Gynec. *42*:619, 1941; New York State J. Med. *41*:2220, 1941.
88. Werner, S. C.: J. Clin. Endocrinol. *1*:134, 1941.
89. Eisenstaedt, J. S., Appel, M., and Fraenkel, M.: J.A.M.A. *115*:200, 1940.
90. McCullagh, E. P., and Ryan, E. J.: J. Clin. Endocrinol. *1*:728, 1941.
91. Evans, H. M., and Swezy, O.: Anat. Rec. *50*:189, 1931.
92. Aron, M.: Compt. rend. Soc. de biol. *108*:25, 1931.
93. Smith, P. E., and Engle, E. T.: Am. J. Anat. *40*:159, 1928; J. Pediat. *5*:163, 1934.
94. Zondek, B.: Klin. Wchnschr. *10*:1484, 1931.
95. Siegmund, H.: Arch. f. Gynäk. *142*:702, 1930.
96. Hertz, R., and Hisaw, F. L.: Am. J. Physiol. *108*:1, 1934.
97. Collip, J. B.: Proc. Soc. Exper. Biol. & Med. *30*:647, 1933; ibid. *32*:800, 1935.
98. Aron, M.: Rev. franc. de gynéc. et d'obst. *29*:295, 1934.
99. Bachman, C.: Proc. Soc. Exper. Biol. & Med. *34*:33, 1936.
100. Henderson, W. R., and Rowlands, I. W.: Brit. Med. J. *1*:1094, 1938.
101. Watson, B. P., Smith, P. E., and Kurzrok, R.: Am. J. Obst. & Gynec. *36*:562, 1938.
102. Comte, L.: Thése de doctorat, Lausanne, 1898, Beitr. z. path. Anat. u. z. allg. Path. *23*:90, 1898.
103. Rasmussen, A. T.: Am. J. Path. *9*:459, 1933.
104. Erdheim, J., and Stumme, E.: Ziegler's Beitr. z. path. Anat. u. z. allg. Path. *46*:1, 1909.
105. Severinghaus, A. E.: Anat. Rec. *60*:43, 1934; Anat. Rec. *61* (Suppl.):61, 1935; Physiol. Rev. *17*:566; 1937; Proc. A. Research Ment. & Nerv. Dis., 1938.
106. Philipp, E.: Zentralbl. f. Gynäk. *54*:1858, 1930.
107. Zondek, B.: Klin. Wchnschr. *10*:2121, 1931.
108. Charipper, H. A., and Haterius, H. O.: Anat. Rec. *54*:15, 1932.
109. Wolfe, J. M.: Anat. Rec. *63*:3, 1935.
110. Charipper, H. A.: Proc. Soc. Biol. & Med. *32*:402, 1934.
111. Siegmund, H.: Zentralbl. f. Gynäk. *56*:953, 1932.
112. Wolfe, J. M.: Anat. Rec. *68*:237, 1937.
113. Zacherl: cited by A. Biedl in, Innere Sekretion, *2*:107, 1913.
114. Addison, W. H. F.: J. Comp. Neur. *28*:441, 1917.
115. Schenk, F.: Monatschr. f. Geburtsh. u. Gynäk. *82*:424, 1929.
116. Ellison, E. T., and Wolfe, J. M.: Endocrinol. *18*:555, 1934.
117. Nelson, W. O.: Endocrinol. *19*:187, 1935.
118. Engle, E. T.: Am. J. Physiol. *88*:101, 1929.
119. Lauson, H. D., Golden, J. B., and Sevringhaus, E. L.: Endocrinol. *25*:47, 1939.
120. Hohlweg, W., and Dohrn, M.: Klin. Wchnschr. *11*:233, 1932.
     Hohlweg, W.: Klin. Wchnschr. *14*:1027, 1935.
121. Fels, E.: Compt. rend. Soc. de biol. *120*:730, 1935.
122. Clauberg, C., and Breipohl, W.: Klin. Wchnschr. *14*:119, 1935.
123. Brooksby, J. B.: Proc. Soc. Exper. Biol. & Med. *38*:832, 1938.
124. Biddulph, C., Meyer, R. K., and Gumbreck, L. G.: Endocrinol. *26*:280, 1940.
125. Nelson, W. O., and Gallagher, T. F.: Anat. Rec. *64*:129, 1935.
126. Martins, T., and Rocha, A.: Endocrinol. *15*:421, 1931.
127. Migliavacca, A.: Boll. d. Soc. ital. biol. Sper. *10*:105, 1935.
128. Wolfe, J. M., and Hamilton, J. B.: Endocrinol. *21*:603, 1937.
129. Zondek, B.: Am. J. Obst. & Gynec. *33*:979, 1937.
     Cramer, W., and Horning, E. S.: Lancet *1*:247, 1936; ibid. *1*:1056, 1937.
130. Hohlweg, W.: Klin. Wchnschr. *13*:92, 1934.
131. Klaften, E.: Ztschr. f. Geburtsh. u. Gynäk. *115*:64, 1937.
132. Hohlweg, W., and Chamorro, A.: Klin. Wchnschr. *16*:196, 1937.
133. Halpern, S., and D'Amour, F. E.: Am. J. Physiol. *115*:229, 1936.
134. Lane, C. E.: Am. J. Physiol. *110*:681, 1935.
135. Zondek, B.: Lancet *2*:842, 1936; Wien. klin. Wchnschr. *15*:455, 1936.

136. Engle, E. T.: Am. J. Physiol. *88*:101, 1929.
137. Hohlweg, W., and Junkmann, K.: Klin. Wchnschr. *11*:321, 1932.
138. Desclin, L., and Gregoire, C.: Compt. rend. Soc. de biol. *121*:1366, 1936.
139. Phelps, D., Ellison, E. T., and Burch, J. C.: Endocrinol. *25*:227, 1939.
140. Uotila, U. U.: Endocrinol. *26*:123, 1940.
141. Smith, P. E.: Endocrinol. *31*:1, 1942.
142. Moore, C. R.: Am. J. Anat. *59*:63, 1936.
143. Sotiriadu, E.: Acta brev. Neerland. *11*:1, 1941.
144. Wolfe, J. M.: Am. J. Anat. *72*:361, 1943.
145. Davis, C. D., Madden, J. H. M., and Hamblen, E. C.: J. Clin. Endocrinol. *3*:357, 1943.
146. Moricard, R.: Bull. Soc. d'obst. et de gynéc. *25*:777, 1936.
147. Wolfe, J. M., and Brown, A. D.: Endocrinol. *31*:467, 1942.
148. Lyons, W. R., Simpson, M. E., and Evans, H. M.: Proc. Soc. Exper. Biol. & Med. *52:*
    134, 1943.
149. Salter, W. T., Basset, M. A., and Sappington, T. S.: Am. J. Med. Sci., *202*:516, 1942.

CHAPTER XIII

THE ANTERIOR HYPOPHYSIS IN GROWTH AND METABOLISM

The Anterior Hypophysis and Body Growth.—The observation that *acromegaly* and *giantism* are associated with pituitary hyperactivity, and conversely that certain types of *dwarfism* accompany hypopituitarism, constituted the first evidence that the adenohypophysis is concerned with the regulation of body growth.

Experimental proof of this assumption was first provided by Aschner,[1] who induced dwarfism in young growing dogs by removing the hypophysis. In 1921, Evans and Long[2] reported that repeated injection of an alkaline extract of anterior lobe tissue accelerated the growth rate and produced giant rats. Subsequent studies amply confirmed these experiments and left little doubt that the anterior lobe is vitally concerned with body growth.

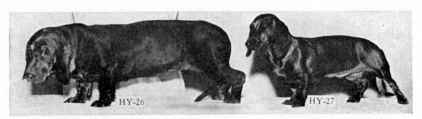

Fig. 44.—Effect of anterior hypophyseal growth-promoting extract in the dachshund. Female dogs from the same litter, aged eleven and a half months. Right, untreated dog. Left, dog injected with growth hormone for thirty-five weeks. (Evans, H. M. *et al.*, in Memoirs of the University of California, Vol. 2, sect. 14.)

The studies of Silberberg[4] and Freud[5] have directed attention to the fact that the growth defect which develops after hypophysectomy is localized in the growing epiphyseal cartilage. They observed that following hypophyseal ablation in the immature animal, bone tissue and desmal bone, such as the cranium, develops normally, but the *epiphyses* close and longitudinal growth ceases. These effects can be prevented by administering growth extract soon after operation but not if treatment is delayed until closure is complete. At first Freud and his associates were led to believe from these findings that the anterior pituitary growth hormone acts specifically on the proliferating zone of cartilage and suggested that the terms "growth hormone" and "chondrotrophic hormone" be considered synonymous. On further investigation, however, they became convinced that the growth hormone also has a general systemic effect. As emphasized by Collip,[6] the pituitary growth principle is concerned with growth in the sense that it increases body size, but apparently does not influence the differentiation of body tissue in general, since proliferation of cells and growth of individual organs and tissues continues in the absence of the adenohypophysis.

Whether the anterior lobe influences body growth through a specific growth-promoting principle or through the combined action of several hormones is not established. The latter possibility has been suggested by Riddle[7] on the basis of his observation that administration of lactogenic and thyrotropic extracts stimulated growth in a strain of hereditary dwarfed mice, and caused general body growth as well as splanchnomegaly in hypophysectomized pigeons. Pituitary extracts free from the lactogenic factor failed to stimulate growth. These findings, coupled with the fact that a pure growth-stimulating extract has not yet been prepared, led Riddle to conclude that body growth is due to the synergistic action of the lactogenic and thyrotropic factors. Evans[8] has criticized Riddle's conclusions on the ground that the lactogenic and thyrotropic extracts used were not shown to be entirely free from growth hormone, and were employed in animals whose hypophysis, though deficient, was nevertheless intact and might conceivably have been stimulated to produce its specific growth principle by the injected hormones. Evans found that in hypophysectomized animals, thyrotropic and lactogenic hormone, in the amounts present in impure but potent growth promoting preparations, produced little or no growth effect. He also demonstrated that the response of the hypophysectomized animal to a potent growth-promoting extract was not affected by removing the thyroid, from which it would appear that the thyrotropic principle is not implicated. While granting that a completely pure growth extract has not yet been prepared, he points out that preparations are available which possess a high growth-promoting potency and a very low thyrotropic and lactogenic hormone content. Evans' group[130] have recently prepared a relatively pure growth hormone extract of beef anterior lobe, containing approximately 130 growth hormone units per milligram and only minute amounts of follicle-stimulating, interstitial-cell-stimulating, lactogenic, thyrotropic and adrenocorticotropic activity.

THE ANTERIOR HYPOPHYSIS AND THE OTHER ENDOCRINE GLANDS

Anterior Hypophysis-Thyroid Relationship.—*The Thyrotropic Principle.*—A hypophyseal-thyroid relationship is suggested by an abundance of clinical and experimental evidence. Acromegaly is often accompanied by a high basal metabolic rate, while hypopituitarism, exemplified by *Simmonds' disease*, is characterized by a subnormal metabolism. Hypophysectomy in all species thus far studied leads to thyroid involution and marked depression of the basal metabolic rate. Anterior hypophyseal substance repairs the involuted thyroid of the hypophysectomized animal and raises the depressed basal metabolic rate to normal.

The anterior pituitary principle responsible for these reparative effects has been prepared in relatively pure form and named the *thyrotropic hormone*. In 1938, the Third International Conference on the Standardization of Hormones agreed that, in assaying extracts of this factor, comparison should be made with an international standard preparation, of which 250 micrograms is equivalent to 1 unit. It was further agreed that only those tests will be considered safe, which are based on actual observation of a stimulation of the thyroid, since other effects noted may be due to impurities in the extract.

Effects of Thyrotropic Extracts.—The effects reported following the administration of thyrotropic extract in experimental animals, include (1) enlargement and hyperplasia of the thyroid gland,[9] (2) a rise in the basal metabolic rate and increased oxygen consumption,[10] (3) exophthalmos,[11] an increase in the heart rate,[12] (4) loss of body weight,[13] (5) hyperirritability,[14] (6) reduction of the iodine content of the thyroid gland,[15] (7) an increase in the alcohol-insoluble iodine content of the blood,[16] (8) reduction of the liver glycogen,[17] (9) lowered sugar tolerance,[18] (10) elevation of the acetone bodies in the blood,[19] (11) increased excretion of creatine and a decrease in the serum cholesterol,[20] (12) and diuresis.[21] All of these, with the exception of exophthalmos,[22] are prevented by thyroidectomy.

Billingsley[23] has presented evidence suggesting that the anterior hypophysis exerts a dual action on the thyroid, influencing the rate of discharge of its secretions, and producing changes in its morphology. He believes that a different mechanism is involved in each of these effects. That the thyrotropic hormone acts directly on the thyroid is indicated by the observation that potent extracts produce hyperplasia of the guinea pig thyroid in vitro.[24] This, together with the observation that hyperplasia can be induced in homotransplants and autotransplants,[25] would seem to eliminate participation of the nervous system in this effect.

The action of the thyrotropic principle can be checked or nullified by simultaneously administering iodine, the iodides, thyroxine, or related substances. Estrogens, in large doses, have a similar inhibitory effect. Of interest in this connection is the observation of Reforzo-Membrives[129] that a thyroid-inhibiting substance is demonstrable in the anterior hypophysis of thyroid-fed rats.

Jensen and Tolksdorf[26] earlier suggested a possible identity of the thyrotropic and interstitial-cell-stimulating principles, but their recent success in separating these two principles[27] eliminates this possibility. The thyrotropic factor has also been shown to be distinct from the growth, gonadotropic[28] and corticotropic[29] factors.

Thyrotropic Substances in Blood and Urine.—Substances possessing thyrotropic activity have been demonstrated in the blood and urine of some lower mammals and occasionally in man. Of particular interest are the studies of the thyrotropic hormone content of the blood and urine in thyroid and pituitary disease. Low values have been obtained in hypophyseal cachexia and high ones in acromegaly and *Cushing's disease*. In *myxedema* and other forms of hypothyroidism, both high and low values have been reported. These divergent results may perhaps be explained by assuming that two types of hypothyroidism exist, namely *primary hypothyroidism* due to some fault inherent in the thyroid per se, and *secondary hypothyroidism* due to pituitary hypofunction. In the former, one would expect to find normal or high thyrotropic hormone values, since the defective thyroid gland is incapable of utilizing the available hormone. In hypothyroidism secondary to hypophyseal deficiency, on the other hand, low thyrotropic hormone values may be expected. If these assumptions are valid, it would follow, as Aron[30] has suggested, that the concentration of this hormone in the body fluids may serve as an aid in the differential diagnosis between primary hypothyroidism and secondary hypothyroidism due to hypopituitarism.

In *hyperthyroidism*, the thyrotropic hormone content of the blood and urine has likewise been found to vary. This may conceivably be due in large part to differences in the rate of production and utilization of the hormone. Low values may signify that all the available hormone is being utilized by the hyperactive thyroid, while high values may indicate that the hypophysis is secreting more than is required to maintain the thyroid in a hyperactive state. It has been suggested that the negative findings obtained in some cases may be accounted for by the presence, in the blood and urine, of some antagonistic substance which nullifies the effect of the thyrotropic hormone in the experimental animal.

Therapeutic Considerations.—Clinical reports relating to the efficacy of thyrotropic hormone therapy are still too limited to permit any conclusions.[31] Most observers agree that such therapy is of no value where the thyroid is primarily at fault and cannot respond to stimulation. On the other hand, thyrotropic hormone would seem to be rational therapy in hypothyroidism secondary to pituitary insufficiency. To distinguish between the two forms, Aron,[30] as already noted, determines the thyrotropic hormone content of the urine. In the absence of dependable data concerning the limits of normal thyrotropic hormone excretion, this method is not satisfactory. Harrison[32] distinguishes between primary and secondary hypothyroidism by administering a test dose of thyrotropic hormone and observing the effect on the basal metabolic rate. Wilkins and Fleischmann[20] note the effect of a test dose of thyrotropic hormone on the creatine level in the urine and the serum cholesterol. If no effect is noted, thyroid substance is then given to determine whether the negative reaction was due to the thyroid gland's inability to respond, or to the fact that the serum cholesterol and creatine excretion is unaffected by the thyroid hormone.

The importance of distinguishing between the primary and secondary forms of hypothyroidism is emphasized by recent reports that patients with hypothyroid manifestations secondary to pituitary insufficiency may die as the result of thyroid therapy.[33] This is due to the fact that the associated deficiency of the pituitary corticotropic factor results in *adrenal cortical insufficiency*, which is aggravated by the thyroid hormone. Unless supplemented by large amounts of salt and anterior pituitary corticotropic or adrenal cortical extract, the administration of thyroid substance[33] or thyrotropic hormone[34] may precipitate a crisis eventuating in death. It is therefore important to ascertain the functional status of the pituitary and adrenal cortex before instituting such therapy.

Recent evidence[35] that the thyrotropic principle acts synergistically with the growth hormone in promoting growth in hypophysectomized animals suggests that it may be of value, in a similar combination, for the treatment of pituitary dwarfism in man (see Chap. XXXV).

14

Anterior Hypophysis-Adrenal Relationship.—*Adrenocorticotropic Factor.*—Destruction or hypofunction of the anterior hypophysis, as in Simmonds' disease (see Chap. XXXV), is often associated with adrenal cortical atrophy. On the other hand, pituitary hyperactivity, such as occurs in acromegaly, is accompanied by hyperplasia and hypertrophy of the adrenal cortex. Smith,[36] in 1920, demonstrated that hypophyseal ablation in the tadpole leads to adrenal cortical atrophy, which can be prevented or repaired by administering anterior lobe substance. These findings have since been confirmed in the rat,[37] dog,[38] and cat.[39] In the intact animal, anterior lobe extract produces hypertrophy of the adrenal cortex and, if treatment is sufficiently prolonged, may lead to the development of *adrenal cortical adenomata.*[40]

The active principle, named *adrenocorticotropic or corticotropic hormone,* appears to have no effect other than that of stimulating the adrenal cortex, and has been shown to be distinct from the thyrotropic, growth-promoting, lactogenic and other hormones of the adenohypophysis. Its isolation from sheep anterior lobe tissue, in pure form free from other biologically active contaminants, has been reported by Evans' group.[131]

Crude anterior pituitary extract, or implants of anterior lobe tissue not only restore the atrophied adrenal cortex of the hypophysectomized animal, but can cause it to enlarge beyond normal limits. Purified corticotropic extracts, on the other hand, though effective in restoring the cortex to normal, cannot cause any further increase in size. This suggests that some anterior pituitary factor, distinct from the corticotropic principle, contributes to the adrenal cortical hypertrophy induced with crude extracts. That purified extracts are as effective as crude preparations in the intact animal, can probably be explained by assuming that the animal's own hypophysis supplies the synergistic substance.

The cells which secrete the corticotropic principle have not yet been identified. The observation that basophil cell adenomas are not infrequently encountered in patients with adrenal cortical hyperplasia or adenoma has led some observers to believe the basophils may be the source of this hormone.

Adrenomedullotropic Principle.—The relationship between the anterior hypophysis and adrenal medulla is not yet clearly defined. Hypophysectomy in the tadpole, according to Smith,[36] does not materially alter the medulla. Nor could Houssay[41] demonstrate any difference in the adrenalin content of the medulla in the intact and hypophysectomized toad. Negative findings have also been reported following hypophysectomy in the rat and dog. These observations suggest that the anterior hypophysis exerts no specific effect on the structure or function of the adrenal medulla.

Despite the negative findings in degenerative experiments, several investigators have postulated the existence of an hypophyseal *adrenomedullotropic principle.* Anselmino and his associates[42] have reported preparation of an extract which has a stimulative effect on the medulla. Emery and Atwell[43] elicited an increase in the size of the medulla with an anterior pituitary extract which induced marked adrenal cortical hypertrophy. In dogs receiving an anterior lobe extract, Houssay and his associates[44] observed a relative and absolute drop in the adrenalin content of the adrenals followed by a decrease in the concentration but not in the total quantity of adrenalin present. Of interest is Collip's report[45] that primary alcoholic extracts of prime gland tissue contain a medullotropic principle, which, when administered orally to hypophysectomized rats, exerts a tropic effect on the so-called *dark cells* of the adrenal medulla. While these findings are suggestive, further investigation is necessary to establish the existence of a specific pituitary principle capable of stimulating the medulla.

Anterior Hypophysis-Parathyroid Relationship.—*Parathyrotropic Principle.*—An anterior pituitary-parathyroid relationship is suggested by the occurrence of *parathyroid hyperplasia* in some cases of acromegaly, and the presence of *parathyroid enlargement, osteoporosis,* and other manifestations of parathyroid hyperactivity in some individuals with basophil cell adenomas.

Experimental evidence relating to a possible direct action of the anterior lobe on parathyroid function is vague and conflicting. Following ablation of the hypophysis in the tadpole, Smith[36] noted atrophy of the epithelial bodies, analogues of the mammalian parathyroids. In a later study, he demonstrated that parathyroid atrophy also follows hypophysectomy in the rat.[46] Collip and associates,[47] on the other hand, could demonstrate no constant degenerative changes in this species. The findings in hypophysectomized dogs have been equally contradictory. Collip[47] and Houssay[48] observed that parathyroid atrophy is not uncommon after removal of both the hypophysis and pancreas, but only occasionally follows ablation of the hypophysis alone.

The changes in the *blood calcium level* noted following hypophyseal ablation have likewise varied. In the hypophysectomized dog, Gerschman[49] could demonstrate no appreciable deviation from normal, but Geesink and Koster[50] noted a significant drop.

Anselmino and his associates,[51] in 1933, prepared an extract of anterior pituitary gland tissue which caused enlargement of the parathyroids and a rise in the serum calcium of the rat. Since it had no effect on the serum calcium of parathyroidectomized animals, they concluded that it acts through the parathyroids. Hertz and Kranes[52] later reported an increase in the size and vascularity of the parathyroids and a rise in the serum calcium of rabbits receiving an extract of beef pituitary. Attempts to corroborate these reports of a blood calcium raising effect of anterior lobe extracts have yielded conflicting results.

Though the foregoing evidence suggests that certain anterior pituitary extracts may elicit morphologic and possibly also functional alterations in the parathyroids, it does not warrant the conclusion that the hypophysis acts directly through a specific parathyrotropic principle. The possibility that it affects the parathyroids indirectly through the mediation of the gonads is suggested by Hertz and Krane's observation[52] that the changes produced with anterior lobe extract can be duplicated with chorionic gonadotropin or estrone. Also significant is Riddle and Dotti's report[53] that prolonged administration of adequate amounts of an anterior lobe gonadotropic extract increased the serum calcium of intact, hypophysectomized, or thyroidectomized pigeons, but not that of castrates.

In a recent study of the anatomy and histology of the parathyroids in the *Macaca mulatta* following hypophysectomy, Baker[54] could detect no change in the structure of the cells or distribution of cell types. He concluded that if a hypophyseal parathyrotropic factor does exist, it is not comparable in significance in the adult animal, to those principles governing thyroid, adrenal cortical and gonadal activity. The existence of a direct physiological regulation of the parathyroids by the hypophysis has also been questioned by Carnes and associates,[127] who found that parathyroid function in the hypophysectomized male rat remained unimpaired even under the stress of a low calcium diet.

Anterior Hypophysis-Pancreas Relationship: *Pancreatropic Principle.*—The existence of a "pancreatropic" principle was first postulated by Anselmino and Hoffman[55] on the basis of their observation that an extract of beef anterior pituitary gland caused *hyperemia* with hypertrophy and hyperplasia of the islet tissue of the pancreas, and a drop in the *blood sugar* and *hepatic glycogen*. Subsequent attempts to corroborate their findings yielded conflicting results.[56] Richardson and Young[57] could not confirm their observations under the conditions employed by them, but did show that daily injections of crude anterior pituitary extract for two weeks to rats approximately doubled the amount of pancreatic islet tissue. Later Marks and Young[58] showed that such treatment also increases the insulin content of the pancreas in the rat.

These and other recent studies[59] have established the existence in beef anterior pituitary of a substance which increases the insulin content of the rat pancreas. Some confusion has arisen from the fact that extracts which have a pancreatropic effect in the rat may lower the insulin content of the dog pancreas. Moreover, the observation[60] that hypophysectomy in the rat is not followed by an appreciable drop in the insulin content of the pancreas has led some observers to question the physiological role of the "pancreatropic" principle. An explanation favored by some investigators,[61, 62] is that the anterior lobe produces two principles with opposite effects, namely the pancreatropic and diabetogenic or blood-sugar-raising principle (see below). Whether one or the other will predominate depends on the relative amount of each present in the extract, and the reactivity of the pancreas of the test animal. If this is responsive, the increased production of insulin will mask the effect of the diabetogenic principle; but if it is defective or becomes exhausted following protracted stimulation by the pancreatropic principle, the diabetogenic factor gains the ascendancy. According to this explanation, hypophysectomy is not followed by an appreciable drop in the insulin content of the pancreas because the operation simultaneously removes both the diabetogenic and pancreatropic factors. Some workers deny the existence of a specific pancreatropic principle. They maintain that the hyperactivity followed by exhaustion of the pancreas in animals receiving anterior lobe extract over a protracted period represents the reaction of the gland to increased glucose in the blood brought about by the action of the diabetogenic factor.

A definite answer awaits the chemical separation of the diabetogenic and pancreatropic factors. The studies of Young and Marks[63] led them to conclude that the pancreatropic, diabetogenic and growth principles are closely associated chemically but are distinct factors. According to Mirsky,[64] the pancreatropic factor is at least partly responsible for the retention of nitrogen (see below) seen in animals receiving growth extract. Young[65] believes that the pancreatropic factor, which is probably not a hormone, is not identical with the lactogenic, gonadotropic, thyrotropic or glycotropic factors. Evans and his associates,[62] however, were able to demonstrate pancreatropic activity in pure lactogenic extract.

Relation of the Anterior Hypophysis to the Pineal and Thymus Glands.—Except for Aschner's early observation[66] that hypophysectomy in the dog is without effect on the *pineal,* studies relating to a possible pituitary-pineal relationship have been very limited. In the absence of evidence to the contrary, it may be assumed that the anterior hypophysis exerts no appreciable influence over the pineal body.

The relation of the adenohypophysis to the *thymus,* though more extensively investigated, is not clear because of the varied results reported. According to Smith,[67] hypophysectomy in the immature rat causes the thymus to undergo involution more rapidly than in the intact animal. In the adult rat, on the other hand, Richter and Wislocki[68] noted marked thymus hypertrophy following this operation. In the hypophysectomized dog, Koster[69] observed that the thymus enlarged and persisted longer than normal but Houssay and his associates[70] found that its involution was accelerated.

The effects obtained with anterior hypophyseal extracts have failed to clarify the pituitary-thymus relationship. In the rat[71] and guinea pig,[72] implants or extracts of anterior lobe tissue hasten involution of the thymus. In hereditary dwarf mice, on the other hand, marked proliferation of the thymus parenchyma has been described following the administration of an anterior lobe growth-promoting extract[73] (see Chap. XX).

Anterior Hypophysis in Mammary Growth and Function.—Recent studies have led observers to postulate the existence of a "mammogenic" and a "lactogenic" principle of the adenohypophysis, which stimulate mammary growth and secretory activity, respectively. The evidence relating to these hypothetical pituitary factors is presented in detail elsewhere (see Chap X).

ROLE OF THE ANTERIOR HYPOPHYSIS IN METABOLISM

Anterior Hypophysis and Carbohydrate Metabolism.—It is generally conceded that the adenohypophysis plays an important role in carbohydrate metabolism. Recent experiments indicate that hypophysectomy profoundly disturbs the mechanism which helps maintain the *blood sugar* and conserve the *glycogen stores.* In most species, if the food and fluid intake is adequate, the blood sugar level[74] and liver and glycogen reserves[75] may remain within normal limits despite hypophyseal ablation. In the fasting hypophysectomized animal, on the other hand, the blood sugar falls rapidly[77] and the glycogen stores are quickly depleted.[76] Such animals are subject to frequent hypoglycemic crises[78] which may eventuate in death. The hypophysectomized animal also shows a marked hypersensitivity to *insulin,*[79] and a

diminished response to subcutaneously administered *adrenalin*,[80] even in
the presence of adequate glycogen reserves.[81] The rate at which glucose is
absorbed from the intestines[82] and glycogen is stored in the liver and
muscle[83] is appreciably reduced. The tolerance to ingested sugar is increased,[82] while the tolerance to intravenously administered glucose is
normal or diminished.[84]

Hypophysectomy in Pancreatic Diabetes.—Much interest has been
aroused by the observation that hypophysectomy ameliorates experimental
pancreatic diabetes. This was first demonstrated in the dog by Houssay and
associates,[85] and has since been amply confirmed in many species, including
primates. The hypophysectomized, depancreatized animal is almost completely free from *ketonuria*,[78] has an almost normal *glucose tolerance
curve*,[86] and the *glycogen* content of its liver is within normal limits.[87]
Such animals respond to fasting with marked hypoglycemia. Their survival
period is prolonged beyond that of animals subjected to pancreatectomy
alone. Himwich[88] believes this is due not only to increased oxidation of
carbohydrate, but probably also to the diminished protein metabolism,
lessened ketosis, and lowered metabolic rate which follows hypophyseal
ablation.

Diabetogenic Extracts.—The important position of the hypophysis in
carbohydrate metabolism is further emphasized by the results of recent
studies with extracts of anterior lobe tissue. The available evidence indicates
that it not only affects sugar metabolism indirectly through its tropic effect
on the thyroid and adrenals, but probably also acts directly on the peripheral tissues. In the hypophysectomized animal, anterior pituitary extract
(1) corrects or prevents the increased sensitivity to insulin,[89] (2) checks
the drop in blood sugar, and (3) prevents depletion of liver and muscle
glycogen. If given in sufficient quantity, it may increase the muscle glycogen
above normal values.[90] It aggravates experimental pancreatic diabetes,[91]
and causes a recurrence of diabetes in the hypophysectomized, depancreatized subject.[92]

An immediate but transient *hyperglycemia* and *glycosuria* has been reported following the administration of certain anterior lobe extracts in the
intact animal. According to Lucke and associates,[93] this effect can be prevented by splanchnotomy or destruction of the adrenal medulla. From this
they infer that the active principle involved acts through a "sugar center,"
which in turn sends nervous impulses to the adrenal medulla, causing it to
release adrenalin. On the basis of more recent studies, it has been suggested[94] that this reaction is not due to an anterior lobe principle but
rather to some posterior lobe substance with which the extract is contaminated.

A delayed but prolonged hyperglycemia and glycosuria has likewise been
noted following the use of anterior pituitary extracts. This effect is associated with ketonuria, the whole picture closely simulating diabetes mellitus.
The term *diabetogenic* has accordingly been applied to extracts possessing
this type of activity. In the hypophysectomized or hypophysectomized,
depancreatized animal, such extracts produce hyperglycemia, glycosuria,
hyperlipemia, ketonuria, polyuria, and other symptoms of diabetes mellitus.

In the intact dog, the administration of progressively larger doses for a relatively short period may lead to the development of permanent diabetes.[95] The pancreas of such animals presents pathological changes of the islet tissue and a decreased insulin content.[96] Dogs rendered permanently diabetic by this means differ from the depancreatized diabetic animal in that they remain in good health and lose but little weight, though kept for long periods without insulin.[97] The injury to the pancreas is thought to be due to the strain imposed upon it by the need of counteracting the blood sugar-raising, anti-insulin action of the extract. The pig, mouse and rat do not develop permanent diabetes following similar treatment. This is thought to be due to the fact that their pancreas can withstand more strain. The observation that anterior pituitary extract induces permanent diabetes in these species if part of the pancreas is first removed, would seem to support this assumption.

The *nature and identity of the diabetogenic factor* is still uncertain. Some believe that a single hormone is responsible for both the hyperglycemia and ketonuria, while others hold that two distinct principles are involved. Riddle[98] has suggested that the diabetogenic factor may be identical with prolactin, but Houssay[99] has presented evidence which would seem to eliminate this possibility. According to the latter observer, it is distinct from the corticotropic principle,[100] but others[101] believe the latter principle is at least partly responsible for the diabetogenic effect. As proof they offer the observation that adrenalectomy, like hypophysectomy, ameliorates experimentally induced pancreatic diabetes, while adrenal cortical extract causes a recurrence of the diabetic state in the hypophysectomized, depancreatized subject.

Glycotropic Factor.—The term "glycotropic" has been applied by Young[102] to a hypothetical anterior pituitary principle which inhibits the hypoglycemic action of insulin in the hypophysectomized and intact animal. According to this investigator, it is distinct from the diabetogenic, lactogenic, thyrotropic and gonadotropic principles.[103] When administered to the hypophysectomized animal, it prevents insulin induced hypoglycemia, but not that elicited by fasting.[104] It also inhibits the peripheral effect of insulin in accelerating the removal of blood sugar in animals whose liver has been excluded from the circulation.[105]

Glycostatic Factor.—Russell and Bennett[94] have postulated the existence of a "glycostatic" principle to account for the observation that the fasting hypophysectomized animal shows a marked loss in muscle glycogen, which can be prevented by administering anterior pituitary extract. These observers believe that this principle inhibits the rate of muscle glycogen breakdown and carbohydrate utilization, and consider its loss responsible for the increased respiratory quotient and marked decrease in glycogen stores seen in fasting hypophysectomized animals. Russell attempts to explain the anti-insulin action of anterior pituitary extract on the basis of its glycostatic effect. She suggests that it checks the hypoglycemic action of insulin partly by preventing the withdrawal of glucose from the blood as muscle glycogen, and partly by its action in depressing carbohydrate oxidation.

Soskin and associates[106] have questioned Russell's assumptions on the basis of their observation in the eviscerated animal. These observers believe that the rapid disappearance of sugar in the fasting hypophysectomized animal is due not to loss of an hypophyseal "glycostatic" factor, but rather to markedly diminished *gluconeogenesis* in the liver, which permits depletion of the carbohydrate stores despite diminished utilization. The so-called "glycostatic" effect of anterior pituitary extract, they attribute to increased formation of carbohydrate in excess of the amount utilized, with a resulting rise in the carbohydrate stores.

The relation of the "glycostatic" factor to other known pituitary principles is not clear. It apparently does not act through the adrenal cortex, for adrenalectomy does not interfere with the ability of anterior pituitary extract to prevent loss of muscle glycogen in the fasting hypophysectomized animal.

Anterior Hypophysis and Fat Metabolism.—Raab[107] has prepared from anterior lobe tissue as well as from the posterior hypophysis and tuber cinereum, an extract which lowers the *blood fat* and increases *liver fat*. According to this observer, the active principle, which he has named *lipoitrin*, has a mesencephalic point of attack, and acts by stimulating the tuber, from which impulses travel by way of the spinal cord and splanchnic nerves to the liver. By causing mobilization of storage fat and its consumption by the liver, it increases the fat content of this organ. A disturbance of this mechanism, Raab believes, is responsible for increased fat storage in the periphery.

The Ketogenic Factor.—The terms *fat metabolism hormone, orophysin,* and *ketogenic hormone* have been applied to a hypothetical anterior pituitary principle which increases the ketone bodies in the blood and urine of the fasting or fat fed animal. This effect has been demonstrated in several species, including man, but the mechanism involved is not clear. Anselmino and Hoffmann[108] interpret the *ketonemia* and *ketonuria* as evidence of an increased rate of fat metabolism. Observing a substance with ketogenic properties in the blood of fat fed dogs, they suggest that the anterior hypophysis normally produces increased amounts of this hormone when the organism is forced to metabolize an excess amount of fat. That a deficiency of this principle may be an etiologic factor in so-called *pituitary obesity* is suggested by Goldzieher[109] on the basis of his observation that patients with this type of adiposity fail to excrete the ketogenic principle after a fat meal.

Blotner[110] suggests that the ketonemia and ketonuria produced with anterior lobe extracts may signify interference with normal or complete oxidation of fat, while Leiner[111] points out that it may constitute nothing more than the natural increase in ketogenesis from loss of liver fat. According to Shipley and Long,[112] anterior pituitary extract causes ketosis indirectly by inhibiting glycogen breakdown and carbohydrate oxidation, and by preventing the transformation of protein into carbohydrate. To meet the energy requirements, more fat is burned and ketosis results.

The ketogenic principle is apparently distinct from the growth factor for, as shown by Black and associates,[113] the two activities are not correlated in various fractionated extracts. Since the effect of the ketogenic factor is lessened but not completely abolished by adrenalectomy, it may not be considered identical with the adrenalotropic principle, though the latter would seem to contribute to the ketogenic effect.

Ketogenic and Diabetogenic Factors.—The relation of the ketogenic factor to the blood sugar-raising principle is not clear. Anselmino and Hoffmann[114] hold that the hyperglycemia and ketosis produced with anterior lobe extracts are caused by two distinct principles, because of their observation that the fat metabolism hormone is ultrafiltrable, while the blood sugar-raising principle is not. On the other hand, Shipley and Long,[112] among others, question the existence of a separate anterior hypophyseal hormone specifically concerned with the mobilization and metabolism of fatty acids, because of their inability to dissociate, by chemical means, the ketogenic and diabetogenic activities of anterior lobe extracts.

Anterior Hypophysis and Water Metabolism.—A diuretic action of the anterior hypophysis was earlier suggested by the observation[115] that marked *diuresis* occurs in animals receiving anterior pituitary growth-promoting extract. In a recent study, Chen and Geiling[128] found that water diuresis in rats was greatly decreased both in rate and quantity by removal of the anterior hypophysis. Fisher and Ingram[116] believe that the diuretic action of the anterior hypophysis is not due to a specific diuretic principle but is rather the result of this gland's general control of metabolism and activity.

Diabetes Insipidus.—The belief that diabetes insipidus follows destruction of the posterior lobe only if the anterior lobe is preserved in all or in part, was first expressed by von Hann[117] in 1918. This was based on his clinical observation that complete destruction of the hypophysis may exist without diabetes insipidus, whereas cases of diabetes insipidus show destruction of the posterior lobe while the anterior lobe is completely or partially intact. This view was more recently reiterated by Richter,[118] and by Fisher and his associates,[119] who offered as additional evidence their observation that an extract of beef anterior lobe had a diuretic effect in cats with a latent tendency to diabetes insipidus. This theory has been challenged by Heinbecker and White,[120] who succeeded in inducing in dogs a permanent and maximum diabetes insipidus despite complete destruction of the anterior lobe. They suggest that the failure of some observers to produce diabetes insipidus following destruction of the posterior lobe was not due to absence of anterior lobe tissue, but to failure to destroy the median eminence, which hypertrophies and secretes antidiuretic substance following removal of the posterior lobe.

"Specific Metabolic Principle" of the Adenohypophysis.—In the earlier experiments with anterior lobe extracts, it was noted that a rise in the basal metabolic rate may be induced in the absence of the thyroid gland.[121] This observation suggested that the anterior pituitary gland produces a principle capable of stimulating metabolic activity presumably by direct action on the periphery. Separation of the factor responsible for this effect has been reported by Collip and his associates.[122] Their extract possesses glycostatic, lactogenic and respiratory quotient-depressing activity, besides increasing the total metabolism. Feinstein and Gordon[123] tested this extract in human beings and rabbits. Though the response of the total metabolism and respiratory quotient was erratic, they nevertheless believe that their data supports the existence of a specific metabolic principle. More convincing evidence is necessary before we can be certain that the rise in the total metabolism is due to a specific metabolic principle or occurs by reason of the anterior lobe's general control of metabolism and activity.

Anterior Hypophysis and Protein Metabolism.—There is evidence that anterior pituitary extracts may cause decreased excretion of nitrogen. This effect is closely associated with the ability of such extracts to promote growth. Mirsky[64] has shown that nitrogen retention is brought about at least in part through the mediation of the pancreas, but the work of Gaebler and Galbraith[124] indicates that increased insulin output is not the immediate and only cause of nitrogen retention. Paschkis[125] found that anterior pituitary extract reduced the *blood urea nitrogen* in normal, adrenalectomized, and partially depancreatized fasted rats, the change occurring independently of any change in blood glucose. He concluded that the anterior pituitary acts independently on protein and carbohydrate metabolism. According to Long,[126] the growth promoting properties of anterior pituitary extracts are due to their ability to decrease nitrogen excretion.

Summary.—It is evident that many metabolic effects may be traced directly or indirectly to the adenohypophysis. Despite the many gaps in our knowledge of its physiology, and our uncertainty as to the actual number of specific hormones it secretes, its position as the "master gland" would seem to be well established.

BIBLIOGRAPHY

1. Aschner, B.: Wien. klin. Wchnschr. *22:*1730, 1909.
2. Evans, H. M., and Long, J. A.: Anat. Rec. *21:*62, 1921.
3. Smith, P. E.: J.A.M.A. *88:*158, 1927.
   Reichert, F. L., Simpson, M. E., Cornish, R. E., and Evans, H. M.: Mem. Univ. California *11:*409, 1933.
4. Silberberg, M., and Silberberg, R.: Endocrinol. *29:*475, 1941.
5. Freud, J., Levie, J. H., and Kroon, D. B.: J. Endocrinol. *1:*56, 1939; Ann. Rev. Biochem. *8:*301, 1939.
6. Collip, J. B.: Edinburgh Med. J. *45:*782, 1938.
7. Riddle, O.: Endocrinol. *19:*1, 1935.
   Bates, R. W., Laanes, T., and Riddle, O.: Proc. Soc. Exper. Biol. & Med. *33:*446, 1935.
   Schooley, J. P., Riddle, O., and Bates, R. W.: Anat. Rec. *72* (Suppl.): 90, 1939.
8. Evans, H. M.: J.A.M.A. *117:*287, 1941; A. Research Nerv. & Ment. Dis. Proc. (1936) *17:*175, 1938.
9. Loeb, L., and Bassett, R. B.: Proc. Soc. Exper. Biol. & Med. *26:*860, 1929.
10. Siebert, W. J., and Smith, R. S.: Am. J. Physiol. *95:*396, 1930.
11. Loeb, L., and Friedman, H.: Proc. Soc. Exper. Biol. & Med. *29:*648, 1932.
    Aird, R. B.: Ann. Int. Med. *15:*564, 1941.
12. Schittenhelm, A., and Eisler, B.: Klin. Wchnschr. *11:*1092, 1932.
13. Friedgood, H. B.: Bull. Johns Hopkins Hosp. *54:*48, 1934.
14. Hageman, P. O., and McCordock, H. A.: Proc. Soc. Exper. Biol. & Med. *30:*297, 1933.
15. Loeser, A.: Arch. f. exper. Path. u. Pharmakol. *167:*381, 1932.
    Hertz, S., and Roberts, A.: Endocrinol. *29:*82, 1932.

16. Closs, W., Loeb, L., and McKay, E. M.: J. Biol. Chem. *96*:585, 1932.
17. Eitel, W., and Loeser, A.: Arch. f. exper. Path. u. Pharmakol. *167*:381, 1932.
18. Jonáš, V.: Zeitschr. f. d. ges. exper. Med. *49*:495, 1934.
19. Eitel, W., Lohr, G., and Loeser, A.: Arch. f. exper. Path. u. Pharmakol. *173*:205, 1933.
20. Wilkins, L., and Fleischmann, W.: J.A.M.A. *116*:2459, 1941.
21. Biassotti, A.: Rev. Soc. argent. de biol. *9*:499, 1933.
22. Marine, D., and Rosen, S. H.: Am. J. Med. Sc. *188*:565, 1934.
23. Billingsley, L. W.: Thesis, McGill Univ. Grad. School, 1937, cited by J. B. Collip,
    J.A.M.A. *115*:2073, 1940.
24. Eitel, H., Krebs, H. A., and Loeser, A.: Klin. Wchnschr. *12*:615, 1933.
25. Marine, D., and Rosen, S. H.: Am. J. Physiol. *107*:677, 1934.
26. Jensen, H., and Tolksdorf, S.: Endocrinol. *25*:429, 1939.
27. Jensen, H., and Tolksdorf, S.: Proc. Soc. Exper. Biol. & Med. *47*:223, 1941.
28. Crew, F. A., and Wiesner, B. P.: Brit. Med. J. *1*:777, 1930.
29. Friedgood, H. B.: Endocrinol. *20*:159, 1936.
30. Aron, M., and Klein, M.: Compt. rend. Soc. de biol. *103*:702, 1933.
31. Scowen, E. F.: Lancet *2*:799, 1937.
    Wachstein, M.: Klin. Wchnschr. *13*:1434, 1934.
    Hoet, M.: Bull. Acad. roy. de méd. de Belgique *13*:445, 1933.
32. Harrison, K. S.: Med. J. Australia *1*:681, 1939.
33. Means, J. H., Hertz, S., and Lerman, J.: Tr. A. Am. Physicians *55*:32, 1940.
    Stephens, D. J.: J. Clin. Endocrinol. *1*:109, 1941.
    Lerman, J., and Stebbins, H. D.: J.A.M.A. *117*:391, 1942.
34. Bulger, J. A., and Barr, D. P.: Endocrinol. *1*:109, 1941.
35. Marx, W., Simpson, M. E., and Evans, H. M.: Proc. Soc. Exper. Biol. & Med. *49*:594,
    1942.
36. Smith, P. E.: Amer. Anat. Mem. 11, Philadelphia, 1920
37. Smith, P. E.: Am. J. Anat. *45*:205, 1930.
38. Houssay, B. A., Biasotti, A., and Mazzocco, P.: Compt. rend. Soc. de biol. *114*:714,
    1933.
39. McPhail, M. K.: Proc. Roy. Soc., London, s.B. *117*:45, 1935.
40. Putnam, T. J., Benedict, E. B., and Teel, H. M.: Arch. Surg. *18*:1708, 1929.
41. Houssay, B. A., and Mazzocco, P.: Compt. rend. Soc. de biol. *114*:722, 1933.
42. Anselmino, K. J., Herold, L., and Hoffmann, F.: Klin. Wchnschr. *13*:1724, 1934.
43. Emery, F. E., and Atwell, W. J.: Anat. Rec. *58*:17, 1933.
44. Houssay, B. A., Biasotti, A., Mazzocco, P., and Sammartino, R.: Compt. rend. Soc. de
    biol. *114*:737, 1933.
45. Collip, J. B.: Canad. M. A. J. *42*:2, 1940.
46. Smith, P. E.: J.A.M.A. *88*:158, 1927.
47. Collip, J. B.: J. Mt. Sinai Hosp. *1*:28, 1934.
48. Houssay, B. A., and Sammartino, R.: Compt. rend. Soc. de biol. *114*:729, 1933.
49. Gerschman, R.: Compt. rend. Soc. de biol. *108*:494, 1931.
50. Geesink, A., and Koster, S.: Arch. f. d. ges. Physiol. *222*:293, 1929.
51. Anselmino, K. J., Hoffmann, F., and Herold, L.: Klin. Wchnschr. *13*:45, 1934.
52. Hertz, S., and Kranes, A.: Endocrinol. *18*:350, 1934.
53. Riddle, O., and Dotti, L. B.: Science *84*:557, 1936.
54. Baker, B. L.: Anat. Rec. *83*:47, 1942.
55. Anselmino, K. J., and Hoffmann, F.: Klin. Wchnschr. *12*:1245, 1933.
56. Bierring, K.: Bull. d'histol. appliq. a la physiol. *11*:297, 1934.
    Fichera, G.: Pathologica *30*:286, 1938.
    Santo, E.: Zeitschr. f. d. ges. exper. Med. *102*:390, 1938.
57. Richardson, K. C., and Young, F. G.: Lancet *1*:1098, 1938.
58. Marks, H. P., and Young, F. G.: J. Soc. Chem. Industry (London) *58*:652, 1939.
59. Guthert, H.: Virchows Arch. f. path. Anat. *307*:175, 1940.
    Houssay, B. A.: Medicina *2*:2051, 1942.
60. Haist, R. E., and Best, C. H.: J. Physiol. *98*:419, 1940; Science *9*:410, 1940.
61. Young, F. G.: Brit. Med. J. *2*:897, 1941.

62. Fraenkel-Conrat, H. L., Herring, V. V., Simpson, M. E., and Evans, H. M.: Am. J. Physiol. *135*:404, 1942.
63. Marks, H. P., and Young, F. G.: J. Endocrinol. *1*:470, 1938; Lancet *1*:493, 1940.
64. Mirsky, I. A.: Endocrinol. *25*:52, 1939.
65. Marks, H. P., and Young, F. G.: Lancet *2*:710, 1940.
66. Aschner, B.: Pflüger's Arch. *146*:1, 1912.
67. Smith, P. E.: Anat. Rec. *47*:119, 1930.
68. Richter, C. P., and Wislocki, G. B.: Am. J. Physiol. *95*:481, 1930.
69. Koster, S.: Arch. f. d. ges. Physiol. *224*:212, 1930.
70. Houssay, B. A., and Lascano-Gonzalez: Compt. rend. Soc. de biol. *117*:463, 1934.
71. Tsunoda, T.: Trans. Jap. path. Soc. *24*:405, 1934.
72. Watrin, J., and Florentin, P.: Compt. rend. Soc. de biol. *110*:1161, 1932.
73. Kemp, T.: Klin. Wchnschr. *13*:1854, 1934.
74. Orias, O.: Biol. Bull. *63*:477, 1932.
75. Chaikoff, I. L., Holtom, G. F., and Reichert, F. L.: Am. J. Physiol. *114*:468, 1936. Russell, J. A., and Bennett, L. L.: Am. J. Physiol. *118*:196, 1937.
76. Fisher, R. E., Russell, J. A., and Cori, C. F.: J. Biol. Chem. *115*:627, 1936.
77. Biasotti, A., and Houssay, B. A.: J. Physiol. *77*:81, 1932.
78. Long, C. N. H., and Lukens, F. D. W.: J. Exper. Med. *63*:465, 1936.
79. Houssay, B. A., and Busso, R. R.: Compt. rend. Soc. de biol. *91*:1037, 1924.
80. Bachman, C., and Toby, G.: J. Physiol. *87*:1, 1936.
81. Chaikoff, I. L., Reichert, F. L., Read, L. S., and Mathes, M. E.: Am. J. Physiol. *113*: 306, 1935.
82. Samuels, L. T., and Ball, H. A.: J. Pharmacol & Exper. Therap. (Proceed.) *57*:140, 1936.
83. Phillips, R. A., and Robb, P.: Am. J. Physiol. *109*:82, 1934.
84. Ball, H. A., Samuels, L. T., and Schott, H. F.: Proc. Soc. Exper. Biol. & Med. *35*:633, 1937.
85. Houssay, B. A., and Biasotti, A.: Compt. rend. Soc. de biol. *105*:121, 1930.
86. Barnes, B. O., and Regan, J. F.: Endocrinol. *17*:522, 1933.
87. Houssay. B. A., and Biasotti, A.: Compt. rend. Soc. de biol. *113*:469, 1933.
88. Himwich, H. E.: Ann. Rev. Biochem. *7*:143, 1938.
89. Young, F. G.: J. Physiol. *87*:13P, 1936.
90. Dambrosi, R. G.: Compt. rend. Soc. de biol. *125*:539, 1937.
91. Houssay, B. A., and Biasotti, A.: Compt. rend. Soc. de biol. *107*:733, 1931.
92. Houssay, B. A.: Endokrinol. *5*:103, 1929.
93. Lucke, H., Heydemann, E. R., and Hechler, R.: Zeitschr. f. d. ges. exper. Med. *88*: 65, 1933.
94. Russell, J. A., and Bennett, L. L.: Physiol. Rev. *18*:1, 1938.
95. Young, F. G.: Lancet *2*:372, 1937.
96. Dohan, F. C., and Lukens, F. D. W.: Am. J. Physiol. *125*:188, 1939.
97. Young, F. G.: Biochem. J. *32*:524, 1938.
98. Riddle, O., cited by Houssay, B. A., and Biasotti, A.: Compt. rend. Soc. de biol. *129*: 1259, 1938.
99. Houssay, B. A.: Compt. rend. Soc. de biol. *129*:1259, 1938.
100. Houssay, B. A.: Compt. rend. Soc. de biol. *129*:1261, 1938.
101. Long, C. N. H., and Lukens, F. D. W.: Am. J. Physiol. *116*:96, 1936.
102. Young, F. G.: Biochem. J. *32*:513, 1938.
103. Young, F. G.: Biochem. J. *32*:524, 1521, 1938.
104. Russell, J. A.: Am. J. Physiol. *124*:774, 1938.
105. Himsworth, H. P., and Scott, D. D. M.: J. Physiol. *92*:183, 1938.
106. Soskin, S., Levine, R., and Lehmann, W.: Am. J. Physiol. *127*:463, 1939.
107. Raab, W.: Zeitschr. f. d. ges. exp. Med. *89*:588, 1933; ibid. *90*:729, 1933.
108. Anselmino, K. J., and Hoffmann, F.: Klin. Wchnschr. *10*:2380, 1931; Zeitschr. f. d. ges. exper. Med. *94*:305, 1934.
109. Goldzieher, M. A., Sherman, I., and Alperstein, B. B.: Endocrinol. *18*:505, 1934.
110. Blotner, H.: Endocrinol. *19*:587, 1935.
111. Leiner, G.: Zeitschr. f. d. ges. exper. Med. *94*:84, 1934.

112. Shipley, R. A., and Long, C. N. H.: Biochem. J. *32*:224, 1938.
113. Black, P. T., Collip, J. B., and Thomson, D. L.: J. Physiol. *82*:385, 1934.
114. Anselmino, K. J., and Hoffmann, F.: Klin. Wchnschr. *13*:1048, 1934.
115. Teel, H. M., and Cushing, H.: Endocrinol. *14*:157, 1930.
116. Fisher, C.: Proc. Inst. Med. Chicago *13*:117, 1940–41.
117. von Hann, F.: Frankfurt. zeitschr. f. Path. *21*:337, 1918.
118. Richter, C. P.: Am. J. Physiol. *110*:439, 1934; ibid. *113*:578, 1935.
119. Fisher, C., Ingram, W. R., and Ranson, S. W.: Diabetes Insipidus. Ann Arbor, Mich., Edwards, Inc., 1938.
120. Heinbecker, P., and White, H. L.: Am. J. Physiol. *133*:582, 1941.
121. Houssay, B. A., and Artundo, A.: Compt. rend. Soc. de biol. *114*:391, 1933.
   Gaebler, O. H.: Am. J. Physiol. *110*:584, 1935.
   Riddle, O., Smith, G. C., Bates, R. W., Moran, C. S., and Lahr, E. L.: Endocrinol. *23*:718, 1938.
122. O'Donovan, D. K., and Collip, J. B.: Endocrinol. *23*:718, 1938.
   Neufeld, A. H., and Collip, J. B.: Canad. M. A. J. *40*:535, 1939.
123. Feinstein, R. N., and Gordon, E. S.: Endocrinol. *27*:592, 1940.
124. Gaebler, O. H., and Galbraith, H. W.: Endocrinol. *28*:171, 1941.
125. Paschkis, K. E.: Am. J. Physiol. *133*:409 (Proc.), 1941.
126. Long, C. N. H.: Ann. Rev. Physiol. *4*:465, 1942.
127. Carnes, W. H., Osebold, J., and Stoerk, H. C.: Am. J. Physiol. *139*:188, 1943.
128. Chen, G., and Geiling, E. M. K.: Proc. Soc. Exper. Biol. & Med. *52*:152, 1943.
129. Reforzo-Membrives, J.: Endocrinol. *32*:263, 1943.
130. Marx, W., Simpson, M. E., and Evans, H. M.: J. Biol. Chem. *147*:77, 1943.
131. Li, C. H., Simpson, M. E., and Evans, H. M.: Science *96*:450, 1942.

CHAPTER XIV

THE PHYSIOLOGY OF THE POSTERIOR HYPOPHYSIS

The role of the posterior hypophysis in the body economy still awaits clarification. Substances possessing *pressor, oxytocic,* and *antidiuretic* properties have been extracted from it, but proof that they are secreted here and perform a physiologic function, has only recently begun to accumulate.

INCRETORY FUNCTION OF THE POSTERIOR HYPOPHYSIS

The suggestion that the posterior hypophysis has an incretory function has been resisted because of its neural origin and lack of true epithelial elements. The substances extractable from it have been interpreted as secretory products of basophilic cells, which have wandered from the anterior lobe into the substance of the pars nervosa, or as stored products conveyed here from the anterior lobe and its extensions, the pars intermedia and pars tuberalis. In line with this reasoning, the colloid masses observed in the pars nervosa by Herring,[1] were assumed to be secretion antecedents which arise in the pars intermedia and pass into the lumen of the third ventricle. This has been questioned by Tarr and Gersh,[2] who maintain that these masses are fixation artefacts.

Attempts to determine the source of the active substances present in posterior lobe tissue were hampered at first by the fact that the several components of the hypophysis, in the species selected for study, were too closely related anatomically to permit their complete physical separation for purposes of extraction. To avoid this difficulty, Geiling and his associates[3] employed pituitaries of the whale, porpoise, chicken, armadillo, and South American manatee, in which a distinct pars intermedia is lacking, and the anterior lobe is separated from the pars nervosa by a thick dural septum. They could demonstrate pressor, antidiuretic, and oxytocic substances only in the pars nervosa and therefore concluded that they originate here.

The Antidiuretic Factor.—Earlier studies of the effect of removal of the posterior lobe yielded inconstant results. Reports that this operation may be accomplished without any alteration in the blood pressure,[4] water exchange,[5] or mechanism of parturition,[6] seemed to justify the conclusion that the active substances found in the posterior lobe are mere pharmacologic artefacts and perform no physiologic function. That this is not true, at least so far as the *antidiuretic principle* is concerned, is indicated by recent studies. Fisher and his associates[7] have shown that diabetes insipidus can be induced in the monkey and cat by experimental lesions so placed as to interrupt the supraoptico-hypophyseal tract. Responsibility of the posterior lobe for this effect is indicated by the fact that animals which develop this condition invariably present an intact pars intermedia and a markedly degenerated pars nervosa, almost devoid of the pressor, antidiuretic, and oxytocic principles. To account for reports that destruction of the pars nervosa does not lead to diabetes insipidus, they suggested that an intact anterior lobe is essential for this effect and that the negative results were due to simultaneous destruction of this gland. According to Heinbecker and White,[8] however, diabetes insipidus may be induced in the absence of the anterior hypophysis, provided that all tissue capable of producing the antidiuretic principle is destroyed. Failure to induce diabetes insipidus, they believe, is due to retention of the median eminence (see Fig. 45), which is part of the neural lobe and not of the hypothalamus, as was previously thought. It would thus appear that the posterior hypophysis, through its antidiuretic principle, plays an important part in the regulation of water metabolism. Corey and Britton[9] have suggested that water and salt regulation may depend on a balanced relationship between the posterior pituitary and adrenal cortex. They base this on their observation that posterior pituitary extract in the rat greatly increased the output of *urinary sodium*, while *desoxycorticosterone* markedly reduced it. More recently, Anderson and Murlin[45] presented findings in a human subject with diabetes insipidus, which they believe confirm the physiologic antagonistic action of adrenal cortical extract and posterior lobe antidiuretic substance on the excretion of sodium, chloride and water.

The Oxytocic Factor.—The theory that the oxytocic substance found in the posterior lobe is essential for parturition has generally been considered untenable because of reports that parturition may proceed normally despite total hypophysectomy in the cat,[6] rat,[10] rabbit[11] and dog.[12] The question has recently been reopened by Fisher and his associates.[13] In the course of their studies of experimental diabetes insipidus in the cat, these observers noted that such animals may become pregnant and carry to term but develop a disturbance of the delivery mechanism. Labor is difficult or prolonged or they may fail to deliver part or all of their young. Since all of the animals had diabetes insipidus, they suggested that the disturbance in parturition was due to atrophy of the posterior lobe with consequent deficiency of the oxytocic principle. In a subsequent study in the guinea pig,[14] they found that among animals which received hypothalamic lesions while pregnant, or conceived after the operation, some aborted, while a few died shortly before, during, or after delivery. In others, pregnancy was prolonged or labor was long and difficult. Among those that delivered normally, some had diabetes insipidus. On the other hand, some of the animals with delayed or prolonged labor showed a normal water intake. They concede that their findings cannot be offered as conclusive proof that oxytocin is essential for parturition, but point out that the evidence which has led many investigators to reject this possibility is equally unconvincing. In none of the experiments purporting to prove that parturition may proceed normally in the absence of the posterior hypophysis, was it definitely established that all tissue capable of secreting oxytocin was destroyed. In view of the inconclusive nature of the evidence on both sides, this question must remain open.

Recent evidence suggesting that the oxytocic principle may play an essential role in facilitating the removal of *milk* during nursing is discussed elsewhere (see Chap. X).

Role in Metabolism.—Participation of the posterior lobe in the regulation of carbohydrate metabolism was suggested by Geiling's[15] observation that posterior lobe extract protected hypophysectomized dogs against the hypoglycemic action of insulin. The implication that insulin sensitivity of the hypophysectomized animal is at least partly due to loss of the posterior hypophysis has recently been questioned by Heinbecker and his associates.[16] These observers have presented evidence indicating that this effect is entirely due to the loss of the anterior lobe.

PHARMACOLOGIC EFFECTS OF POSTERIOR LOBE EXTRACTS

Pitressin and Oxytocin.—It is well established that posterior lobe extract can elicit a number of striking pharmacologic effects. That these are produced by at least two separable factors has been demonstrated by Kamm and associates,[17] and Stehle.[18] One of these, known as *pitressin* or *vasopressin*, produces cardiovascular, renal, respiratory, intestinal, and metabolic effects; the other, named *pitocin* or *oxytocin*, stimulates contractions of the uterine musculature. Complete chemical separation of these two factors has not yet been achieved. Evidence suggesting that the antidiuretic effect is due to a principle distinct from both the oxytocic and vasopressor fractions has recently been presented by Heller.[19] Van Dyke and his associates[46] have presented evidence suggesting that the oxytocic, vasopressor and antidiuretic activities are not distinct hormones but parts of a single protein molecule which are separable by drastic chemical procedures.

Cardiovascular Effects.—Therapeutic doses of pitressin, injected subcutaneously or intramuscularly in man, induce rapid blanching of the *skin* but no significant rise in blood pressure.[20] This is accompanied by a momentary fall succeeded by a more prolonged rise in the *pulse rate, oxygen consumption,* and *cardiac output.*[21] Repeated injections have a depressive effect, which is attributed by some observers to a hypothetical antipressor substance present in the vasopressor extracts. The pressor effects of posterior pituitary solution are apparently the direct result of action on the muscle fibers of the blood vessels, since they are not antagonized by nicotine. Posterior pituitary solution also causes constriction of the coronary arteries with changes in the electrocardiogram and cardiac output.

The vasopressor principle causes marked but transient impairment of cardiac efficiency, which may lead to dilatation and even asphyxia of the cardiac muscle. This is attributed to constriction of the coronaries.

Respiratory Effects.—Vasopressin, administered intravenously, produces immediate acceleration of the respiratory rate, alternating with periods of *apnea.* This effect has been attributed to local circulatory changes in the respiratory center.[22]

Renal Effects.—Herring,[23] in 1908, obtained from posterior lobe tissue a water soluble substance which produced dilatation of the renal blood vessels and diuresis. In addition, he noted a transient antidiuretic effect which he ascribed to vasoconstriction of the renal blood vessels. These opposite effects of posterior lobe extract apparently depend on the route of administration. If given intravenously, it produces immediate diuresis followed by a more prolonged antidiuretic effect, while subcutaneous injections produce antidiuresis followed by diuresis. According to Heller,[24] the diuretic effect is due to the pressor and not the antidiuretic principle. It has been suggested that the urinary effect of posterior lobe extract is due to its action on a water metabolism center at the base of the third ventricle, or its effect on the fluid interchange between the blood and tissues. Most workers, however, believe it acts directly on the kidney.[25]

Gastrointestinal Effects.—Pitressin, intramuscularly in small doses, stimulates the smooth musculature of the small and large intestines, setting up powerful and painful *peristalsis* accompanied by urgency to defecate and one or more copious bowel movements.[26] Opposite effects have been obtained with the oxytocic fraction. In the rabbit, massive doses of posterior lobe extract may produce *hemorrhagic necrosis* and *ulceration* of the gastric mucosa, which may lead to marked blood loss.[27] This is thought to be due to a local ischemic action of the pressor principle. Inhibition of the secretion of *gastric juice*, particularly hydrochloric acid, has also been observed following the administration of posterior lobe extract.[28, 29]

Metabolic Effects.—Glycosuria and *hyperglycemia* have been noted following injection of the whole extract.[30] That this effect is due to a direct action on the liver cells is suggested by the observation[31] that it does not occur if the liver is excluded from the circulation or its glycogen store is depleted. Though hyperglycemia can be induced with both pitressin and pitocin, the latter is more specifically antagonistic to insulin.[32] Griffiths[33] has presented evidence suggesting that posterior pituitary extract prevents the hypoglycemic response to insulin through its vasoconstrictor action, which delays absorption of the drug. Neufeld and Collip[34] postulate the existence of a posterior pituitary substance which inhibits adrenalin hyperglycemia and is distinct from the pressor and oxytocic principles.

There is some evidence that posterior lobe extract, in large doses, increases the concentration of fat in the liver. This is apparently due to the vasopressor substance. According to Raab,[35] the posterior lobe produces a hormone, *lipoitrin*, which acts on a fat metabolism center in the tuber cinereum, causing a reduction in the concentration of neutral fat in the blood.

Oxytocic Effects.—The oxytocic fraction stimulates *myometrial contractions* which vary in intensity according to the phase of the menstrual cycle, whether the uterus is nongravid or gravid and, where it is gravid, on the stage of pregnancy. Oxytocin produces its maximum effect during parturition, elicits only a slight response in early pregnancy, and a negligible one following labor and during lactation (see Chap. VI).

Clinical Uses.—Pitressin and pitocin are widely employed, both as prophylactic and therapeutic agents, in a number of conditions. *Pitressin* is used in some cases of *postoperative abdominal distention* and *paralytic ileus*, because of its ability to induce powerful peristalsis.[26, 39] The dose is

15

1 cc. intramuscularly every four hours until the condition is alleviated. It is obviously contraindicated in intestinal obstruction due to mechanical causes. Roentgenologists advocate its use to combat the intestinal gas shadows in *abdominal roentgenography*.[40] Use of pitressin in the treatment of *pyelitis* is based on its ability to stimulate peristalsis of the ureteral musculature, thus facilitating drainage.[41] The dose is 5 to 20 minims intramuscularly every four hours. Its ability to elevate the blood pressure and improve the peripheral circulation makes it valuable for combating *shock*. The dose depends on the gravity of the condition. Its antidiuretic action is utilized to control the polyuria and thirst of *diabetes insipidus*.[42] The dose is ½ to 1 cc. intramuscularly every four hours. Some observers[43, 44] utilize its antidiuretic effect in concentrating the urine for a test of renal function. Its use in the treatment of peptic ulcer is based on its ability to inhibit gastric secretion.

Pitocin is extensively used to stimulate contractions in primary or secondary *uterine inertia*, and prevent or control *postpartum hemorrhage*. In selected cases, the judicious use of small doses is indicated to induce *labor*, provided no mechanical impediment exists (see Chap. XXXI).

CLINICAL ASPECTS OF POSTERIOR PITUITARY DISEASE

It has been suggested that a deficiency or absence of the antidiuretic principle of the posterior hypophysis is an important etiologic factor in diabetes insipidus.[36] This would seem to be a reasonable conclusion from recent experiments demonstrating that only those lesions of the hypothalamus, which lead to posterior lobe atrophy, result in diabetes insipidus. The clinical observation that posterior lobe extracts are often efficacious in controlling the excessive thirst and polyuria which characterize this disease is significant but not conclusive. Attempts to demonstrate that the concentration of antidiuretic substances in the urine of such individuals is below normal, have yielded inconstant results.

Anselmino and his associates[37] have suggested that an excess of the posterior pituitary antidiuretic hormone may account for some cases of water retention associated with edema and hypertension. An excess of the vasopressor principle is believed by some observers to play an important part in *late toxemias of pregnancy* (see Chap. XXXI).

Jones[38] has called attention to a syndrome characterized by hypertension, hyperchromic anemia, achlorhydria, and abnormal carbohydrate tolerance, which he attributes to hyperfunction of the posterior hypophysis. According to this observer, such patients excrete a pituitrin-like substance which diminishes as the malady subsides.

BIBLIOGRAPHY

1. Herring, P. T., Quart. J. Med. *1*:121, 1908.
2. Gersh, I., and Tarr, A.: Anat. Rec. *63*:231, 1935.
3. Geiling, E. M. K., and Robbins, L. L.: Proc. A. Res. Ment. & Nerv. Dis. *17*:437, 1938.
4. Wyman, L. C., and Suden, C. T.: Am. J. Physiol. *109*:115, 1934.
5. Houssay, B. A., and Hug, E.: Compt. rend. Soc. de biol. *85*:315, 1921.
6. Allan, H., and Wiles, P.: J. Physiol. *99*:345, 1932.

7. Fisher, C., Ingram, W. R., and Ranson, S. W.: Diabetes Insipidus and the Neurohormonal Control of Water Balance. Ann. Arbor, Edwards Bros., 1938.
8. Heinbecker, P., and White, H. L.: Am. J. Physiol. *133:*582, 1941.
9. Corey, E. L., and Britton, S. W.: Am. J. Physiol. *133:*511, 1941.
10. Smith, P. E.: Am. J. Physiol. *99:*345, 1932.
11. Firor, W. M.: Am. J. Physiol. *104:*204, 1933.
12. Dott, N. M.: Quart. J. Exper. Physiol. *13:*241, 1923.
13. Fisher, C., Magoun, H. W., and Ranson, S. W.: Am. J. Obst. & Gynec. *36:*1, 1938.
14. Dey, F. L., Fisher, C., and Ranson, S. W.: Am. J. Obst. & Gynec. *42:*459, 1941.
15. Geiling, E. M. K., Campbell, D., and Ishikawa, Y.: J. Pharmacol. & Exper. Therap. *53:*377, 1935.
16. Heinbecker, P., White, H. L., and Rolf, D.: Am. J. Physiol. *136:*592, 1942.
17. Kamm, O., Aldrich, T. B., Grote, I. W., Rowe, L. W., and Bugbee, E. P.: J. Am. Chem. Soc. *50:*573, 1928.
18. Stehle, R. L.: J. Biol. Chem. *102:*573, 1933.
19. Heller, H.: J. Physiol. *96:*337, 1939.
20. Moffat, W. M.: Am. J. Med. Sci. *186:*854, 1933.
21. Grollman, A., and Geiling, E. M. K.: J. Pharmacol. & Exper. Therap. *46:*447, 1932.
22. Sharpey-Schafer, E., and MacDonald, A. D.: Quart. J. Exper. Physiol. *16:*251, 1926.
23. Herring, P. T.: Quart. J. Exper. Physiol. *1:*187, 1908.
24. Heller, H.: J. Physiol. *98:*405, 1940.
25. Silvette, H.: Am. J. Physiol. *128:*747, 1940.
26. Burnstein, C. L.: Am. J. Surg. *52:*455, 1941.
27. Berg, M.: Am. J. Digest. Dis. *7:*78, 1940.
28. Hess, W. R., and Grundlach, R.: Arch. f. d. ges. Physiol. *185:*137, 1920.
29. Gross, E. G., Ingram, W. R., and Fugo, N. F.: Am. J. Digest. Dis. *9:*234, 1942.
30. Borchardt, L.: Ztschr. f. klin. Med. *66:*322, 1908.
31. Clark, G. A.: J. Physiol. *64:*324, 1928.
32. Holman, D. V., and Ellsworth, H. C.: J. Pharmacol. & Exper. Therap. *53:*377, 1935.
33. Griffiths, M.: J. Physiol. *100:*112, 1941.
34. Neufeld, A. H., and Collip, J. B.: Canad. M. A. J. *40:*537, 1939; Endocrinol. *25:*775, 1939.
35. Raab, W.: Ztschr. f. d. ges. exper. Med. *89:*588, 1933.
36. Richter, C. P.: Proc. A. Ment. & Nerv. Dis. *17:*392, 1938.
37. Anselmino, K. J., Hoffmann, F., and Kennedy, W. P.: Edin. Med. J. *39:*376, 1932.
38. Jones, E. I.: Lancet *1:*11, 1938.
39. Potter, P. C., and Mueller, R. S.: Ann. Surg. *96:*364, 1932.
40. Kirklin, B. R., and Seedorf, E. E.: Proc. Staff Meet. Mayo Clin. *14:*502, 1939.
41. Draper, W. B., Darley, W., and Harvey, J. L.: J. Urol. *26:*1, 1931.
42. Hoskins, R. G.: Pennsylvania Med. J. *40:*167, 1936.
43. Paine, W. G., and Nelson, E. E.: Proc. Soc. Exper. Biol. & Med. *42:*729, 1939.
44. Sodeman, W. A., and Engelhardt, H. T.: Proc. Soc. Exper. Biol. & Med. *46:*688, 1941.
45. Anderson, J. A., and Murlin, W. R.: J. Pediat. *21:*326, 1942.
46. Van Dyke, H. B., Chow, B. F., Greep, R. O., and Rothen, A.: J. Pharm. & Exper. Therap. *74:*190, 1942.

CHAPTER XV

THE HYPOTHALAMICO-HYPOPHYSEAL SYSTEM

INTRODUCTION

Though the glands of internal secretion and vegetative nervous system are intimately connected, the nature of this relationship is still obscure. The adrenal medulla, for example, is derived from the neural crest along with the vertebral ganglionic chain. Vegetative nerve fibers have been

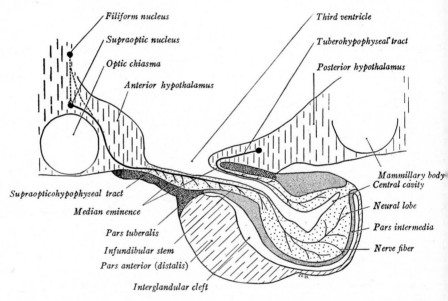

Fig. 45.—Diagram of a midsagittal section through the hypothalamus and hypophysis of the cat. (Ranson, S. W.: The Anatomy of the Nervous System, ed. 7, Philadelphia, W. B. Saunders Co., 1943.)

traced in the blood vessels which enter the endocrine glands, and in the thyroid actual innervation of the glandular tissue has been observed. A neuro-endocrine unit which has recently attracted much attention is the so-called *hypothalamico-hypophyseal system or neuro-hypophyseal mechanism*.[1] Accumulating data indicates that the hypophysis and hypothalamus are both anatomically and functionally related. Recognition of this close association has strengthened the realization that the regulation of metabolic and other important processes depends on the collaboration of the endocrine and neurovegetative systems. As Collin[2] has stated, "the physiology of the endocrines is at an impasse and will remain so until more is known of the mechanism by which they act. The notion that the hormones are chemical regulators has been adopted with such enthusiasm that we have come to think of organic functions on a physio-chemical model entirely too simple and narrow and have completely neglected nervous activity. This intellectual attitude is the consequence of technical specialization—Biology must view its problem in its completeness!"

A consideration of the anatomical and functional relationship between the hypophysis and hypothalamus is appropriate in a study of gynecic endocrinology, for not only does it appear that their combined activities affect important vital processes, which in turn may influence gonadal function, but lesions in either or both structures may lead to alterations in the sexual sphere.

ANATOMY

The pituitary is not an isolated organ. Its posterior lobe is continuous with the *diencephalon*, a very old portion of the brain which surrounds the third ventricle and includes the thalamus, hypothalamus and infundibulum. The hypothalamus lies ventral to the thalamus, and is situated medially at the base of the diencephalon, forming part of the lateral wall and floor of the *tuber cinereum* and its nuclei. The tuber is part of the third ventricle and extends from the optic chiasma anteriorly to the corpora mammillaria behind. In the center is the infundibulum, from which arises the stalk of the pituitary. Thus the hypophysis appears as an out-pocketing of the ventral wall of the diencephalon to which it is attached by the infundibulum.[3]

Throughout the hypothalamus are groups of *nerve cells* arranged in a more or less definite nuclear pattern. The fiber tracts which connect the hypothalamic nuclei with each other, and join the hypothalamus with other parts of the nervous system and with the hypophysis, have not yet been clearly defined. Cortico-hypothalamic pathways apparently enable the cortex to control hypothalamic function. That this control takes the form of inhibition is suggested by the observation that removal of the cerebral cortex or all the brain above the hypothalamus, permits unrestrained activity of the hypothalamic region, while stimulation of the tract connecting the cortex with the hypothalamus inhibits its activity. Cortico-hypothalamic paths which stimulate the hypothalamus are believed to exist but have not yet been traced. The hypothalamus is apparently connected with the *subthalamus* and *corpus striatum*, but the pathways which link them are still only vaguely understood. Efferent paths have been traced from the hypothalamus to the thalamus, brain stem spinal cord, and hypophysis.[4]

The Hypothalamico-Hypophyseal Tract.—Of particular interest is the so-called hypothalamico-hypophyseal tract, which joins the hypothalamus with the neural lobe of the hypophysis. In man, according to Rasmussen,[5] 50,000 fibers enter the pars nervosa from the infundibular stem. These separate into the *supraoptico-hypophyseal* and the *tubero-hypophyseal* tracts. The former is composed of unmyelinated fibers which arise mainly from the paired supraoptic nucleus in the floor of the third ventricle. They pass over the chiasm, course medially along the base of the anterior hypothalamus and enter the median eminence, a part of the neural lobe of the hypophysis. Large numbers, grouped together in dense bundles are found in the infundibulum. On reaching the infundibular process they spread out in fan-like fashion. Though still arranged in bundles, each aggregation is smaller and individual fibers separate from the rest to form a network about the cells of the pars nervosa. Many fibers pass through the entire pars nervosa, terminating in the connective tissue capsule. A few may reach and extend a short way into the pars intermedia. Often they terminate in large end-bulbs. The tubero-hypophyseal tract is a fairly thick bundle of unmyelinated fibers which pass through the dorsal wall of the infundibular stem. Their site of origin is uncertain, but it is believed to be some area close to the infundibulum.

It has been suggested that the nerve fibers leading to the neural hypophysis enact a secretion exciting role. In favor of this view is the observation[6] that injury to the tracts may be followed by a drop in the oxytocic, vasopressor and antidiuretic hormone content of the neural lobe, while stimulation of these fibers may increase the concentration of these substances. Roussy and Mosinger,[7] Collin[8] and others subscribe to this theory on histologic grounds.

Vascular Connections between Hypothalamus and Hypophysis.— There is evidence that the pituitary is connected with the diencephalon by a *portal circulation of veins.* The venous return from the hypophysis may be divided into two parts. Veins from the pars anterior and pars nervosa pass directly to the cavernous sinuses on either side. Other large veins arise separately from the pars anterior, pars intermedia, pars tuberalis and pars nervosa and ascend the stalk, where they have no branches or connections with each other. In the lower part of the stalk, they lie in the pars tuberalis but soon cross over to the infundibulum, where they are surrounded by a sheath of neuroglia. These veins ascend the infundibulum to the hypothalamus. There they break into a venous network beneath the infundibular recess, whence they seem to send branches toward the nuclei supraoptica and paraventricularis.

The existence of this system of portal veins, and the presence of *colloid droplets* in the blood passing through them, as well as in the supraoptic nucleus, led Popa and Fielding[9] to suggest that the active principles of the pituitary are borne through these veins to the hypothalamus, whose function they directly affect. This suggestion has been questioned by Bucy[10] on the ground that the appearance of colloid droplets is inconstant and that there is no proof that those in the hypophysis and hypothalamus are identical. Wislocki and King[11] maintain that the drainage is downward and not, as Popa believes, towards the hypothalamus. This they base on their observation that venules arise from the plexus and sinusoidal capillaries and penetrate the infundibular stem and median eminence, which is a part of the neural lobe of the hypophysis and not the hypothalamus, as was earlier believed. They then unite on the stem into veins which enter the pars anterior, there breaking up into sinusoids. They argue that since only threadlike capillaries can be found entering from the median eminence into the hypothalamus, it is unlikely that this system of veins constitutes an important pathway for the passage of the hypophyseal hormones into the hypothalamic region.

FUNCTIONS OF THE HYPOTHALAMUS

Numerous manifestations have been traced to lesions of the hypothalamus, but only recently, through the use of precise instruments for the localization of experimental lesions has it been possible to determine the sites of some of its functions. The available evidence suggests that some of the effects initiated in this region may be produced with the aid or through the mediation of the hypophysis, while others are produced independently of this gland. Conversely, some of the effects produced by the hypophysis apparently require the intervention of the hypothalamus, though the extent of its participation is still obscure. The uncertainty as to what functions each of these structures performs independently and conjointly with the other is not surprising in view of their close topographic relation which makes it difficult to produce lesions in one without involving the other.

Water Metabolism.—The observation that polyuria can be produced by injuring the tuber cinereum while the pituitary remains intact led many to believe that the hypothalamus plays an important part in maintaining the water balance. For a time, emphasis was shifted from this region to the posterior hypophysis as the controlling factor in water metabolism (see Chap. XIV). At present, the view favored by most observers holds that both the hypothalamus and posterior lobe participate in regulating the water exchange. It is now believed that diabetes insipidus is due to interruption of the supraoptico-hypophyseal tract by which they are connected. Of the recent studies dealing with this subject, those of Ranson and associates[12] in the cat are outstanding. These observers found that lesions so placed as to interrupt the supraoptico-hypophyseal tract, caused diabetes insipidus which varied in intensity according to the extent to which the supraoptico-hypophyseal tract was interrupted. The lesions were followed by striking degenerative changes in the hypothalamus and neural division of the hypophysis. Diabetes insipidus was also found to follow complete removal of the neural lobe or bilateral destruction of the supraoptic nuclei, provided enough anterior lobe tissue was retained to maintain the individual in a fairly normal state of metabolism and activity. In animals with supraoptico-hypophyseal lesions, the antidiuretic hormone content of the posterior lobe was found to be lowered. They therefore concluded that the supraoptico-hypohyseal system regulates the secretion of the antidiuretic hormone by the neural portion of the hypophysis. Interruption of the supraoptico-hypophyseal tract lowers production of this hormone, causing polyuria with secondary polydypsia. The polyuria represents the resultant of diuretic processes in the body unchecked by the antidiuretic mechanism.

Carbohydrate Metabolism.—It was recognized as early as 1912[13] that the hypothalamus influences carbohydrate metabolism. Transient *hyper-*

glycemia[14] and *glycosuria*[15] have been reported following hypothalamic lesions. Some[16] have reported a rise in the blood sugar following stimulation of this region. This effect is apparently mediated through the adrenal medulla for it is prevented by adrenalectomy.[17] Appropriately placed hypothalamic lesions have also been found to cause *hypoglycemia*,[18] increased sensitivity to *insulin*, and decreased sensitivity to the hyperglycemic action of *adrenalin*.[19] Such lesions prevent the hyperglycemia which would otherwise follow pancreatectomy in certain species.[20] These effects are similar to those seen following destruction of the anterior hypophysis (see Chap. XII) and suggest that the anterior lobe and hypothalamus may act together as a functional unit in regulating the metabolism of sugar. Convincing proof of such cooperation is still lacking.

Fat Metabolism.—Since adiposity is one of the cardinal manifestations of spontaneous or experimentally induced lesions of the hypothalamus, hypophysis, or both, it seems likely that the hypophyseal-hypothalamic mechanism plays an important role in regulating fat metabolism. Raab[21] has suggested that a hypophyseal hormone, "lipoitrin," stimulates a hypothetical fat metabolism center in the tuber cinereum, which sends nervous impulses by way of the cervical spinal cord and splanchnic nerves to the liver. Interruption of this pathway, he believes, interferes with the liver's ability to absorb fat, which is stored instead, making for obesity. His theory has not thus far been corroborated. That the hypothalamus harbors a center for the regulaton of fat metabolism is strongly indicated by the report of Hetherington and Ranson[22] that marked obesity can be induced in rats by symmetrical bilateral destruction of the ventral hypothalamus. Also significant are Heinbecker and White's[23] findings in dogs, from which they concluded that obesity results from partial destruction or retrograde degeneration of the paraventricular nuclei, particularly their caudal portions (see Chap. XXXIII).

Gonadal Function.—Pathologic processes or experimentally induced lesions at the base of the diencephalon are often associated with *genital atrophy*, even where the pituitary is morphologically intact. This may or may not be associated with obesity, just as obesity due to hypothalamic involvement may or may not be associated with genital atrophy. On the basis of these observations, it has frequently been suggested that the hypothalamus harbors a sex center distinct from but probably adjacent to its fat metabolism center.

Influence on Anterior Hypophysis.—That hypothalamic lesions lead to genital atrophy through the mediation of the hypophysis was suggested by Biedl [24] in 1916. His suggestion has been borne out by more recent evidence (see Chap. XII) establishing the anterior lobe as the source of the specific hormones on which gonadal function depends. Since these hormones act independently of nervous pathways, as shown by their ability to stimulate completely denervated ovarian transplants (see Chap. XII), it seems likely that hypothalamic lesions adversely affect gonadal function by suppressing the production of gonadotropic hormone by the hypophysis, and not by interrupting a pathway through which the hypophyseal gonadotropes exert their effect.

Proof that the hypothalamus regulates the gonadotropic function of the anterior hypophysis is still lacking. Anatomical studies in man[25] have failed to reveal a sufficient number of nerve fibers leading from the hypothalamus to the anterior lobe to support this assumption. Attempts to demonstrate that an intact hypothalamus is essential for estrogen-induced mating behavior have yielded conflicting results.[26] Genital atrophy only occasionally follows experimentally induced hypothalamic lesions.[27] It is significant, however, that in the rabbit, where ovulation depends on the stimulus of coitus, it can be prevented by section of the pituitary stalk[28] or decerebration within one hour after mating.[29] In this species, ovulation can be induced by pricking the tuber cinereum unless the anterior lobe is removed.[30] Since coitus-induced ovulation in the rabbit is presumably due to release of luteinizing hormone by the anterior lobe, it would follow that some impulse emanating from the hypothalamus is capable of causing such release. Whether this impulse is carried directly to the anterior pituitary by nervous pathways or a neuro-hormonal mechanism is involved, is a question for future investigation. Significant in this connection is the observation that an *acetylcholine-like substance* from the hypothalamus causes discharge of luteinizer by the anterior lobe.[31] In guinea pigs with lesions of the anterior hypothalamus, follicles mature but there is no ovulation or corpus luteum formation. This is apparently due to interference with production or release of luteinizer, for such animals ovulate and form corpora lutea if this hormone is supplied by injection.[40]

The evidence at hand suggests that the gonadotropic function of the anterior hypophysis is not dependent upon the presence of an intact hypothalamus, though it is apparently subject to the latter's control under certain circumstances. The functional and anatomic relationship between the two is apparently not so intimate that morphologic alterations in one inevitably lead to functional disturbances in the other. A connection undoubtedly exists however, and it is conceivable that hypothalamic lesions, if sufficiently extensive and appropriately located, may disturb the gonadotropic function of the anterior lobe, if not through nervous pathways, then by reason of vascular disturbances arising therefrom.

Regulation of Temperature.—It is generally believed that the hypothalamus plays an important role in the regulation of temperature. Some maintain that there is a single center for temperature control,[32] while others hold that different cell groups within the hypothalamus participate.[33] In man, hypothalamic lesions may disturb the temperature regulating mechanism of the body with resulting *hyperthermia*[34] or *hypothermia*.[35] In their studies of heat regulation in the cat and monkey Ranson and his associates[36] found that heat loss mechanisms, such as panting and sweating, and heat conserving mechanisms, such as vasoconstriction, fluffing of the hair, shivering and increased muscle tension, are apparently controlled by distinct areas in the hypothalamus.

Hypothalamus as a Sleep Center.—That the hypothalamus harbors a center for the control of sleep is suggested by the fact that somnolence is a common manifestation of hypothalamic involvement. Some observers hold that hypothalamic lesions induce sleep by stimulating a sleep center.[37]

Ranson and his associates[38] believe that this region may more accurately be designated a waking center, because the evidence suggests that its function is to promote wakefulness, somnolence resulting when its function is suppressed.

Hypothalamus as a Center for Emotional Expression.—Stimulation of appropriate parts of the hypothalamus produces the characteristic visceral responses seen in emotional excitement, suggesting that this part of the brain functions as a center for emotional expression.[39] The manifestations are suggestive of *rage* or *fear*. In the cat properly stimulated, there may occur a rise in blood pressure, increased pulse rate, increased rate and amplitude of respiration, inhibition of gastrointestinal motility, pupillar dilatation, protrusion of the eyes, retraction of the eyelids, erection of the hair, increased secretion of sweat, tears and saliva, retraction of the facial and masticator muscles, running movements, and struggling.[40]

BIBLIOGRAPHY

1. Cushing, H.: Papers Relating to the Pituitary Body, Hypothalamus, and Parasympathetic Nervous System. Springfield, Ill., Thomas, 1932.
2. Collin, R.: Ann. de méd. *33*:239, 1934.
3. Brain, W. R., and Straus, E. B.: Recent Advances in Neurology, ed. 3, Philadelphia, P. Blakiston's Son & Co., Inc., 1934, chap. 15, pp. 256–270.
4. Ranson, S. W., and Magoun, H. W.: Ergebn. d. Physiol. *41*:56, 1939.
   Roussy, G., and Mosinger, M.: Ann. de méd. *33*:301, 1933.
5. Rasmussen, A. T.: Anat. Rec. *70*:64, 1938; Endocrinol. *23*:263, 1938; A. Research Nerv. & Ment. Dis., Proc. 1938, p. 415.
6. Fisher, C., and Ingram, W. R.: Endocrinol. *20*:762, 1936.
7. Roussy, G., and Mosinger, M.: Compt. rend. Soc. de biol. *112*:557, 775, 1933; ibid. *122*:643, 1935; Rev. neurol. *63*:1, 1935.
8. Collin, R.: Arch. de morph. gén. et expér. *28*:1, 1928; Ann. de physiol. *10*:953, 1934; Compt. rend. Soc. de biol. *121*:81, 84, 1936; L'innervation de la glande pituitaire: anatomie et physiologie, Paris, Hermann, 1937.
9. Popa, G. L., and Fielding, U.: J. Anat. *65*:88, 1930; ibid. *67*:227, 1933; Lancet *2*:238, 1930. Popa, G. L.: Presse méd. *46*:663, 1938.
10. Bucy, P. C.: The Hypophysis Cerebri, in, Cytology and Cellular Pathology of the Nervous System, ed. by W. Penfield, New York, Paul B. Hoeber, Inc., 1932, vol. 2, p. 705.
11. Wislocki, G. B., and King, L. S.: Am. J. Anat. *58*:421, 1936.
12. Fisher, C., Ingram, W. R., Hare, W. K., and Ranson, S. W.: Anat. Rec. *63*:29, 1935.
13. Aschner, B.: Arch. f. d. ges. Physiol. *146*:1, 1912.
14. Karplus, I. P., and Peczenik, O.: Arch. f. d. ges. Physiol. *225*:654, 1930.
15. Weed, L., Cushing, H., and Jacobson, C.: Bull. Johns Hopkins Hosp. *24*:40, 1913. Davis, L., Cleveland, D., and Ingram, W. R.: Arch. Neurol. & Psychiat. *33*:592, 1935.
16. Himwich, H. E., and Keller, A. D.: Am. J. Physiol. *93*:658, 1930.
17. van Bogaert, A.: Arch. internat. de Pharmacodyn. et de thérap. *53*:137, 1936.
18. Barris, R. W., and Ingram, W. R.: Am. J. Physiol. *114*:555, 1936.
19. Ingram, W. R., and Barris, R. W.: Am. J. Physiol. *114*:562, 1936.
20. Davis, L., Cleveland, D., and Ingram, W. R.: Arch. Neurol. & Psychiat. *33*:592, 1935.
21. Raab, W.: Ztschr. f. d. ges. exper. Med. *49*:179, 1926; Klin. Wchnschr. *13*:281, 1934; Ergebn. d. inn. Med. *51*:125, 1936.
22. Hetherington, A. W., and Ranson, S. W.: Anat. Rec. *78*:149, 1941.
23. Heinbecker, P., and White, H. L.: Proc. Soc. Exper. Biol. & Med. *49*:324, 1942.
24. Biedl, A.: Innere Sekretion, Berlin, 1916, vol. 2, p. 176.
25. Rasmussen, A. T.: Anat. Rec. *70*:64, 1938.
26. Dempsey, E. W., and Rioch, D. M.: J. Neurophysiol. *2*:9, 1939.

Brookhart, J. M., Dey, F. L., and Ranson, S. W.: Proc. Soc. Exper. Biol. & Med. *44:* 61, 1940.

Dey, F. L., Leininger, C. R., and Ranson, S. W.: Endocrinol. *30:*323, 1942.

Bard, P.: Res. Publ. Assoc. Nerv. & Ment. Dis. *21:*551, 1940.

27. Smith, P. E.: J.A.M.A. *88:*158, 1927.

Ingram, W. R., and Fisher, C.: Endocrinol. *21:*273, 1937.

Westman, A.: Schweiz. med. Wchnschr. *72:*113, 1942.

Dey, F. L., Fisher, C., and Ranson, S. W.: Am. J. Obst. & Gynec. *42:*459, 1941.

Dey, F. L.: Am. J. Physiol. *133:*551, 1941; Am. J. Anat. *69:*61, 1941.

28. Westman, A., and Jacobsohn, D.: Acta obst. et gynec. Scandinav. *17:*235, 1937.

Brooks, C. M.: Res. Publ. Assoc. Nerv. & Ment. Dis. *20:*523, 1940.

29. Fee, A. R., and Parkes, A. S.: J. Physiol. *67:*383, 1929.

30. Houssay, B. A., and Giusti, L.: Rev. Soc. argent. de biol. *5:*47, 1929.

31. Taubenhaus, M., and Soskin, S.: Endocrinol. *29:*958, 1941.

32. Isenschmid, R.: Physiologie der Warmeregulation, in, Handb. d. norm. u. path. Physiol. Berlin, Springer, 1926, vol. 17, p. 1.

Gagel, O.: Handb. d. Neurologie (Bumke & Foerster). Berlin, Springer, 1936, vol. 483.

33. Meyer, H. H.: Verhandl. d. deutsch. Gesellsch. f. inn .Med. *30:*15, 1913.

Miller, H. R.: Central Autonomic Regulations in Health & Disease. New York, Grune & Stratton, 1942, chap. 2, p. 50.

34. Zimmerman, H. M.: Res. Publ. Assoc. Nerv. & Ment. Dis. *20:*824, 1940.

35. Davison, C., and Selby, N. E.: Arch. Neurol. & Psychiat. *33:*570, 1935.

36. Clark, G., Magoun, H. W., and Ranson, S. W.: J. Neurophysiol. *2:*202, 1939.

Ranson, S. W., Fisher, C., and Ingram, W. R.: Arch. Neurol. & Psychiat. *38:*445, 1937.

37. von Economo, E.: Rev. Neurol. *1:*837, 1927; J. Nerv. Dis. *71:*249, 1930.

38. Kabat, H., Anson, B. J.: Magoun, H. W., and Ranson, S. W.: Am. J. Physiol. *112:*214, 1935.

39. Ranson, S. W., Kabat, H., and Magoun, H. W.: Arch. Neurol. & Psychiat. *33:*467, 1935.

Kabat, H.: J. Comp. Neurol. *64:*187, 1936.

Crouch, R., and Elliott, W. H., Jr.: Am. J. Physiol. *115:*245, 1936.

40. Brookhart, J. M., Dey, F. L., and Ranson, S. W.: Endocrinol. *28:*561, 1941.

CHAPTER XVI

THE PHYSIOLOGY OF THE THYROID GLAND

Gull,[1] in 1874, first called attention to a symptom-complex characterized by a diminution of physical and mental power, a thick, dry skin, loss of hair, and atrophy of the thyroid gland. In 1878, Ord[2] applied the term *myxedema* to this syndrome, on the assumption that mucin formation is responsible for the peculiar swelling of the subcutaneous tissues seen in patients with this malady. Proof that the thyroid atrophy and the associated symptoms are causally related was furnished by Kocher's[3] observation that manifestations like those seen in cretinism and adult myxedema appear in goitrous patients subjected to total thyroidectomy. From this he inferred that *cretinism, adult myxedema,* and *cachexia strumipriva* are all due to thyroid insufficiency.

EXPERIMENTAL STUDIES OF THYROID FUNCTION

Thyroid Ablation Experiments.—The results of the early ablation experiments were confusing, largely because of failure to recognize the separate existence of the *parathyroids*. The *tetanic manifestations* which frequently followed such operations were erroneously attributed to loss of thyroid tissue. Gley,[4] in 1891, rediscovered the so-called "accessory thyroids," now known as the parathyroids, and showed that they are functionally and anatomically distinct from the thyroid gland. On the basis of his findings, he concluded that the *tetanic symptoms* noted in earlier thyroid ablation experiments were due to inclusion of the parathyroids with the extirpated thyroid tissue. By avoiding these structures in subsequent ablation experiments, more consistent results were obtained. It is now generally agreed that *total thyroidectomy* in the adult animal produces physical and mental sluggishness, lowering of the body temperature and basal metabolic rate, dryness and thickening of the skin, brittleness of the nails, loss of hair, gain in weight, and swelling of the extremities. In the young, growing animal, it causes besides the above symptomatology, a striking stunting of body growth and retardation of mental development, manifestations not unlike those seen in cretinism.

Replacement Experiments.—Earlier reports of beneficial effects with thyroid grafts in thyroidectomized animals led Murray[5] to employ a glycerol thyroid extract for human myxedema with startling success. Equally satisfactory results were subsequently reported by other observers,[6] who also demonstrated that myxedema can be controlled by administering thyroid substance by mouth. Oral administration of this substance for the treatment of *postoperative cachexia strumipriva* and *sporadic cretinism* soon followed.

Biochemical Investigations.—In 1896, Baumann[7] obtained from the thyroid by means of acid hydrolysis an amorphous substance containing 9.3 per cent of iodine, which he called *iodothyrin*. His discovery that iodine is a normal constituent of the thyroid marks the beginning of our knowledge of the chemistry of this gland. In 1899, Oswald[8] isolated *iodothyroglobulin*, an iodine bearing protein which seemed to possess all the properties of *globulin* and had the same pharmacological effect as thyroid substance. He also called attention to the fact that the iodine is contained in the *colloid*, which he demonstrated to be globulin, and that the iodine content of the thyroid gland varies in accordance with the amount of visible colloid. A few years later, Marine and Lenhart[9] demonstrated a close relationship between the histologic structure of the human thyroid and its iodine content.

In 1916, Kendall[10] isolated from the thyroid gland a crystalline compound containing 65 per cent of iodine. This preparation, which he named *thyroxin*, has since been shown to possess the same pharmacological properties as thyroid substance, and is now believed to be the hormone of the thyroid gland. In 1926, Harington[11] found its empiric formula to be $C_{15}H_{11}O_4NI_4$, and its structural formula, $3;5;3^1;5^1$ tetraiodothyronine. In the following year, Harington and Barger[12] produced synthetic *thyroxine*, a product physiologically as active as the naturally occurring hormone. For clinical use, desiccated thyroid, thyroxine and thyroid globulin are now available. The globulin form is claimed to be equal to the others in calorigenic activity but less likely to increase the heart rate.[60]

PRESENT CONCEPT OF THYROID FUNCTION

Probably the most important contribution to our present concept of thyroid function was Magnus-Levy's observation that thyroid feeding materially raises the basal rate of *oxygen* consumption. He further demonstrated that the basal rate is notably elevated in hyperthyroidism, whereas in myxedema it is markedly depressed, but can be restored to normal by thyroid feeding. On the basis of these findings, since fully corroborated, it is now generally conceded that *the essential function of the thyroid gland is to maintain the general metabolism of the body at its proper level*. The studies which have followed the publication of Magnus-Levy's[13] findings indicate that, besides its role in general metabolism, the thyroid is concerned with tissue growth and differentiation, the metabolism of carbohydrate, fat, and protein, and the excretion of calcium and magnesium. It apparently also influences the activity of the circulatory and nervous systems, the gonads, and other members of the endocrine system.

Growth and Differentiation of Tissue.—Participation of the thyroid in the regulation of *somatic growth* is implied in the observation that in cretinism, juvenile myxedema, and in animals thyroidectomized during the growth period, there is a marked stunting of body growth which can be prevented or corrected by thyroid feeding. Though the thyroid gland apparently promotes body growth under normal conditions, there is evidence that an *excess* of its active principle may have an inhibitory effect. In the tadpole, Gudernatsch[14] observed that thyroid feeding markedly increased the rate of metamorphosis but at the same time notably retarded somatic growth, thus producing dwarfed frogs. Similar effects have been noted in the rat and rabbit.[15, 16]

The thyroid hormone is apparently concerned with growth of hair, teeth, skin, and nails. This is implied in the observation that these structures undergo degenerative changes in hypothyroidism and can often be restored to normal by thyroid feeding.

Specific Dynamic Action.—The specific dynamic action of foodstuffs apparently depends to some extent on the thyroid hormone. This is indicated by Baumann and Hunt's[17] observation that this action completely disappears in the rabbit within sixty-five days after thyroid ablation, and can be restored by thyroid feeding.

Carbohydrate Metabolism.—There is evidence that the sugar tolerance is often low in *Graves' disease* and high in *myxedema*, and that hyperthyroidism or thyroid treatment tends to aggravate *diabetes mellitus*, while thyroidectomy ameliorates it. Experimentally, it has been shown that thyroid feeding increases the rate of absorption of carbohydrate from the intestine.[18] Excessive thyroid feeding depletes both the *liver* and *muscle glycogen*. The drop in hepatic glycogen is generally interpreted to signify increased utilization of carbohydrate rather than impairment of the liver's capacity for storing it.

The thyroid hormone apparently acts synergistically with *adrenalin*, for thyroidectomy decreases and thyroid feeding increases the hyperglycemic action of this hormone. Since the latter effect can be elicited only so long as glycogen is present in the liver, the thyroid hormone probably acts by sensitizing this organ to stimuli which cause it to discharge glycogen.

An antagonism between the thyroid and *pancreas*, originally postulated by Falta,[19] is implied in the observation that diabetes mellitus is sometimes relieved by thyroidectomy and aggravated by thyroid feeding. This finds support in the observation that thyroid ablation heightens, while thyroid treatment depresses the hypoglycemic action of insulin in the experimental animal.[20] Whether the thyroid hormone neutralizes the effect of insulin by stimulating glycogenolysis, or sensitizing the liver to stimuli which cause it to discharge glycogen, is not known.

Protein Metabolism.—The excretion of *nitrogen*, particularly *urea* and *creatine*, is often increased in Grave's disease and in the thyroid-fed animal, and is decreased in myxedema or experimentally induced hypothyroidism.[21] The administration of iodine in hyperthyroidism, and of thyroid substance in hypothyroidism is effective in maintaining the urea and creatine in the urine at a normal level. It is generally believed that the thyroid hormone raises the level of urea and creatine by promoting the breakdown of both exogenous and endogenous protein.

Fat Metabolism.—The tendency of some myxedematous patients to accumulate fat, and the progressive loss of adipose tissue in Graves' disease or following thyroid feeding, point to some connection between the thyroid and fat metabolism. The observation that the *blood fat* diminishes in spontaneous or experimentally induced hyperthyroidism and increases after thyroidectomy also suggests some relationship. How the thyroid hormone affects fat metabolism is not clear. Magnus-Levy[22] suggested that it indirectly accelerates fat consumption by stimulating muscular activity and thus increasing the total energy expenditure. Abelin and Kursteiner[23] believe it acts directly, on the basis of their observation that thyroid-fed animals show considerable loss of body fat within a short time after treatment is begun and before the general metabolic effect of the thyroid hormone is apparent.

Calcium Metabolism.—The *calcium* and *phosphorus* level in the urine falls in myxedema or following thyroid ablation.[24] On the other hand, a marked increase in calcium excretion, associated with a rise in the phosphorus content of the urine and feces, is a frequent finding in both spontaneous and experimentally induced hyperthyroidism. That the excreted minerals are at least partly derived from the bones is suggested by the frequent occurrence of *osteoporosis* in severe Graves' disease, and by the increase in the calcium and phosphorus deposits in the bones noted following thyroidectomy.

Whether the thyroid hormone influences calcium metabolism directly, or through the mediation of the parathyroids, is not clear. The first possibility is suggested by the observation that thyroid feeding raises the urine calcium without affecting that of the blood, while the parathyroid hormone increases the concentration of both.

Water Metabolism.—Participation of the thyroid in water metabolism is suggested by the frequent occurrence of *polyuria* in hyperthyroidism, and of *oliguria* in hypothyroidism. There are wide species differences in the extent to which this gland is involved in water metabolism. In dogs, thyroid feeding appreciably increases the urinary output, but in rats it has no effect on the fluid exchange unless salt is simultaneously administered.[25] That it has a diuretic effect in man may be inferred from reports of its efficacy in the treatment of certain forms of *edema*. The *mechanism* involved is not clear. The suggestion that it acts by stimulating the sympathetic nerves supplying the kidney and bladder seems untenable, since its diuretic action persists despite section of the cervical cord. A more plausible explanation is that it increases capillary permeability, permitting the water to pass from the tissues into the circulation, whence it is discharged through the kidney. It is noteworthy in this connection that hypothyroidism is characterized by retention of water in the tissues and a low plasma volume, and that both effects can be reversed by administering thyroid hormone. The action of the hormone on water elimination is apparently not limited to the kidney for in spontaneous and experimentally induced hyperthyroidism, water loss is effected at least partly through the bowel.

A thyroid-posterior lobe antagonism is suggested by reports[26] that thyroid ablation checks the diabetes insipidus which would otherwise follow injury to the posterior hypophysis. If thyroid substance is then administered, the polyuria returns.

Nervous and Cardiovascular Effects.—The thyroid profoundly affects both the central and vegetative nervous systems. *Nervous irritability* is markedly increased in spontaneous or experimentally induced hyperthyroidism, and appreciably diminished in myxedema or following thyroid ablation.

That the thyroid hormone influences the *cardiovascular system* is suggested by the observation that hyperthyroidism is associated with acceleration of the heart action, and hypothyroidism with a slow pulse rate. Whether these changes are effected through the sympathetics, or are a response to variations in the utilization of oxygen by the peripheral tissues, is not certain.

RELATION OF THE THYROID TO THE ANTERIOR HYPOPHYSIS

The thyroid apparently influences and is in turn influenced by the anterior hypophysis. *Pituitary hypertrophy* has been observed in such hypothyroid states as *parenchymatous goiter, cretinism, myxedema* and *cachexia thyropriva.*[27, 28] The earliest experimental evidence of a thyroid-anterior pituitary relationship was Rogowitsch's[29] observation that pituitary enlargement follows thyroid ablation in the rat and dog. Further light has been thrown on this relationship by recent studies of the effects of thyroid ablation and thyroid feeding on the size, cytologic appearance, and hormonal content of the anterior lobe.

Though some observers have confirmed Rogowitsch's original observation, others report no appreciable change in the size of the pituitary following thyroidectomy. As suggested by Marine,[30] negative findings may be due to the maturity of the test animals, for the degree of pituitary hypertrophy induced by thyroidectomy is proportional to the youth of the subject.

Anterior Lobe Effects of Thyroidectomy.—The most striking and constant *cytologic modification* noted in the adenohypophysis after thyroid ablation is a marked decrease or complete disappearance of *acidophiles* and the appearance of so-called *thyroidectomy cells.* The latter strongly resemble "castration cells" (see Chap. XII) and are believed to be of basophilic origin.[31, 32, 33]

Studies of the *gonadotropic hormone* content of the anterior lobe following thyroid ablation have yielded conflicting results. Some have reported an increase, others a decrease or no change whatsoever. A rise in the *thyrotropic hormone* content of the gland has also been noted following thyroidectomy.[33] This probably accounts for the appearance of thyrotropic substances in the blood of the thyroidectomized subject.[34] It has also been suggested that the thyrotropic hormone is derived from the "thyroidectomy cells," whose presence presumably signifies increased secretory activity or storage.

That *growth hormone* production by the adenohypophysis diminishes following thyroidectomy is suggested by the observation that the acidophiles, which are generally conceded to be the source of this hormone, regularly disappear after this operation. Moreover, their disappearance is associated with marked stunting of body growth when the operation is performed during the growth period.[35] This would seem to imply that the thyroid helps maintain the growth-promoting activity of the anterior hypophysis, and that the retardation of growth which follows its removal is at least partly due to the ensuing pituitary alterations. That the thyroid can also act on the skeleton independently of the anterior pituitary growth hormone was recently demonstrated by Evans' group[59] in the rat. Thyroxine and the growth hormone are apparently synergistic in their action on endochondral ossification. When acting in the absence of thyroxine, the growth hormone causes a somewhat disproportional growth. The addition of thyroxine results in a more normal, mature picture of endochrondral ossification.

The changes in the cytology of the hypophysis[31, 33] and the increase in its thyrotropic hormone content following thyroidectomy, can be prevented by thyroid feeding. This may explain why the thyrotropic hormone content of the blood is elevated in hypothyroidism, and diminished in hyperthyroidism.[36] Reports[37, 38] that thyroid feeding may increase the gonadotropic hormone content of the anterior hypophysis suggest a possible explanation of the favorable results obtained with small doses of thyroid in the treatment of menstrual and reproductive disorders.

Anterior Lobe Effects on Thyroid Function.—Not only do changes in thyroid function affect the adenohypophysis, but the thyroid is itself dominated by this master gland. The available evidence indicates that an increase in anterior hypophyseal function leads to thyroid hypertrophy with a corresponding rise in thyroid hormone production, and a decrease in anterior pituitary function leads to regressive changes in the thyroid gland and diminished secretion of its active principle. It is generally conceded that these effects are due to changes in the supply of a specific *thyrotropic* principle of the anterior lobe. (See Chap. XIII.)

RELATION OF THE THYROID TO THE GONADS

An intimate thyroid-gonadal interrelationship is suggested by the *transient thyroid enlargement* which frequently accompanies puberty, menstruation, sexual excitement, pregnancy, and lactation, and by the high incidence of thyroid disease during adolescence and particularly at the menopause. This association is further emphasized by the observation that menstrual and reproductive disorders are often encountered in thyroid disease, and are frequently benefited by thyroid therapy.

Effects of Thyroid Ablation.—The effects in the sexual sphere observed following thyroidectomy have been too varied to permit any conclusions. According to some workers, thyroid ablation in the immature animal usually delays the time of maturity and appreciably retards genital development. In the mature animal, lengthening or absence of the estrual cycles, involutionary changes in the secondary sex organs, retardation of follicular maturation, and marked depression of reproductive function have been reported following this operation. On the other hand, several competent investigators found that thyroid ablation did not delay the onset

16

of estrual cycles or appreciably disturb gonadal and reproductive function in the mature animal.

Effects of Thyroid Feeding.—The effects of thyroid feeding on gonadal and reproductive function have been inconstant, due possibly to individual variations in the susceptibility of the test animals, and differences in the intensity and duration of treatment. In general, it would appear that small doses stimulate, while larger ones or prolonged treatment have a depressive effect.

Ovulation.—Under certain conditions, thyroid substance apparently stimulates the rate of egg production. For example, Winchester[39] observed a 50 to 60 per cent increase in the rate of egg production in hens following the administration of small doses. Since there is no proof that thyroid extract contains a specific ovulation-inducing principle, its favorable effect is probably attributable to its ability to stimulate the local metabolism of the ovary, anterior pituitary, or both.

Reproductive Function.—There is evidence that thyroid feeding in large doses or for a protracted period, may retard sexual maturation in the immature animal. In the mature subject such treatment may inhibit or completely suppress the estrual cycles and cause regressive changes in the sex organs, which interfere with procreative activity. On discontinuing treatment, the reproductive organs return to normal and the estrual rhythm is reestablished.

Mechanism.—Though the available evidence leaves little doubt that alterations in the supply of thyroid hormone influence the function of the gonads, the mechanism involved is obscure. The action of the thyroid on the sex glands is probably neither direct nor specific, for the striking sexual precocity which can be elicited with anterior pituitary hormone (see Chap. XII), cannot be duplicated with thyroid substance. Nor is thyroid ablation followed by the complete suppression of gonadal function which is invariably a sequel of hypophysectomy. The heightened gonadal activity which may follow the administration of small doses of thyroid substance may reasonably be explained on the basis of its calorigenic action, by virtue of which it can accelerate the local metabolism of the adenohypophysis and gonads.

The gonadal depression which follows intensive or prolonged treatment with thyroid hormone may conceivably be due to the toxicity of the drug, or its ability to accelerate the destruction or elimination of the anterior pituitary and ovarian sex hormones. The latter possibility is suggested by the observation that more estrogen is required to induce estrus in the thyroid fed than in the untreated castrate. It is also significant that thyroid ablation increases and thyroid feeding decreases the gonadal response to a given quantity of gonadotropic extract.

Effect of the Gonads on Thyroid Function.—The relationship between the thyroid and gonads is apparently reciprocal. The effect of the ovary on this gland has been investigated by observing its histologic appearance and functional status during puberty, menstruation, pregnancy, the menopause, and also following castration or the administration of potent ovarian extracts.

Menstrual Cycle.—Attempts to correlate thyroid activity with the sexual cycle have yielded divergent results. In the human, Von Arvay and Meyer[40] noted that the basal metabolic rate rose at the premenstruum and dropped to its lowest level at the time of the flow. In the lower animal, some observers[41] have noted cyclic changes in the colloid or iodine content of the gland paralleling the estrual cycle, while others[42, 43] could see no significant alteration in its size, histologic appearance, or in its colloid and iodine content.

Estrogen Effects.—The effect of estrogen on thyroid function apparently depends on the *dosage.*[45, 46] In the lower animal, large doses or prolonged treatment depress the thyroid gland[47] and lower the basal metabolic rate.[48, 49] A similar effect has been observed in the human following administration of chorionic gonadotropin. Estrogen is apparently the immediate cause of the depression thus produced, for it occurs only in the presence of functioning ovaries.[50] A direct inhibitory effect of estrogen on the thyroid gland is implied in the observation[51] that it prevents the thyroid hyperplasia and hyperactivity which would otherwise follow the administration of anterior pituitary thyrotropic extract. That its effect on the basal metabolic rate is at least partly independent of the thyroid gland is suggested by the report that thyroidectomized animals receiving thyroid substance followed by estrogen, return more rapidly to their previous hypothyroid level than those given thyroid substance alone.[52]

Thyroid Gland in Pregnancy.—*Enlargement and Hyperactivity.*— Thyroid enlargement is a common manifestation of normal pregnancy. The basal metabolic rate rises to between 20 and 30 per cent during the last few months of gestation,[53] but following parturition, the thyroid as a rule undergoes involution and the basal rate returns to normal.[54] It has been suggested that the increased basal metabolic rate of late pregnancy represents the sum total of both the maternal and fetal metabolism. The thyroid enlargement and hyperactivity has been attributed to hyperplasia of the normally functioning tissue, which is part of a general acceleration of endocrine activity designed to meet the extraordinary demands of pregnancy. It seems reasonable to assume that pregnancy demands an increased secretion of the thyroid hormone to accommodate the growing mass of active protoplasm. In this connection, Enright and associates[55] found a close relationship between the change in *body weight* and the variations in *oxygen consumption.* This would suggest that the energy required in laying down the new tissue of the fetus and accessory structures is responsible for the increased heat production of advanced pregnancy.

Anselmino and Hoffmann[56] have suggested that an actual hyperthyroid state exists during pregnancy. This they base on their observation that the blood of pregnant women contains a thyroxine-like substance which reaches its maximum concentration at term, and disappears soon after delivery. Neuweiler[57] could not substantiate these findings and denies that a hyperthyroid or Basedow-like state exists during pregnancy. He argues that though the activity of the thyroid gland increases at this time, there is no absolute excess of the thyroid hormone for the additional supply is utilized. The acceleration of thyroid function, he believes, is within physiologic limits and therefore need not imply pathologic hyperfunction. Moreover, the histologic picture of the gland in normal pregnancy shows no alteration which might tbe taken to indicate hyperfunction in a pathologic sense.

Mechanism.—Whether the thyroid hypertrophy represents a compensatory response to the increased metabolic demands of pregnancy, or is induced by hormones present in the pregnant organism[44] is not known. That the thyroid hyperplasia and hyperfunction is secondary to increased production of the anterior pituitary thyrotropic hormone is suggested by reports of a rise in the level of this hormone in the urine of pregnant women.

It should be emphasized that enlargement of the thyroid during pregnancy does not always imply hyperfunction, for the gland frequently hypertrophies and tends toward the colloid type when its secretion is inadequate for the extraordinary demands of gestation. Marine[30] attributes this to a deficiency in iodine, on the basis of his observation that during pregnancy the thyroid constantly shows a decrease in iodine content, and undergoes hypertrophy or hyperplasia when its iodine content falls below 0.1 per cent of its dried weight. The mechanism involved has been explained by Mussey[58] as follows: "So-called simple or colloid goitre, then, is the result of the deposit of colloid substance in the thyroid gland. This occurs when a functioning gland is not furnished with sufficient iodine to enable it to discharge all the thyroxine it is stimulated to produce. In other words, the deposit of colloid substance is not an indication of lowered thyroid function but rather of a deficient supply of available iodine. The amount of ingested iodine may be barely sufficient to supply the thyroid gland under ordinary conditions and quite insufficient for the extraphysiologic demands of increased metabolism which occurs at puberty, during pregnancy and sometimes during menses and at the menopause; under such conditions this results in the commonly noted appearance of colloid or simple goitre. When the supply of iodine is particularly meager— there is commonly an especially noticeable enlargement of the thyroid during pregnancy."

BIBLIOGRAPHY

 1. Gull, W.: Tr. Clin. Soc. London *7:*180, 1874.
 2. Ord, W. M.: Med.-Chir. Tr. London *61:*57, 1878.
 3. Kocher, T.: Arch. f. klin. Chir. Berlin *29:*254, 1883.
 4. Gley, E.: Compt. rend. Soc. de biol. *43:*250, 366, 841, 1891.
 5. Murray, G. R.: Brit. J. Med. *2:*796, 1891.
 6. Howitz, F.: Ugesk. f. Laeger *26:*109, 1892.
 7. Baumann, E.: Ztschr. f. physiol. Chem. *21:*319, 1896; ibid. *22:*1, 1896.
 8. Oswald, A.: Ztschr. f. Physiol. Chem. *27:*14, 1899; ibid. *32:*121, 1901.
 9. Marine, D., and Lenhart, C. H.: Arch. Int. Med. *3:*66, 1909.
10. Kendall, E. C.: Collected Papers of the Mayo Clinic *8:*513, 1916.
11. Harington, C. R.: Biochem. J. *20:*393, 1926.
12. Harington, C. R., and Barger, G.: Biochem. J. *21:*169, 1927.
13. Magnus-Levy, A.: Ber. Klin. Wchnschr. *32:*650, 1895.
14. Gudernatsch, J. F.: Am. J. Anat. *15:*431, 1914.

15. Cameron, A. T., and Carmichael, J.: J. Biol. Chem. 45:69, 1920.
16. Cameron, A. T., and Carmichael, J.: J. Biol. Chem. 46:35, 1921.
17. Baumann, E., and Hunt, L.: J. Biol. Chem. 64:709, 1925.
18. Althausen, T. L., and Stockholm, M.: Am. J. Physiol. 123:577, 1938.
19. Falta, W.: Med. Klin. 6:40, 1910.
20. Bodansky, A.: Proc. Soc. Exper. Biol. & Med. 21:46, 1923.
21. Deuel, H. J., Jr., Sandiford, I., Sandiford, K., and Boothby, W. M.: J. Biol. Chem. 76: 391, 1928.
22. Magnus-Levy, A.: Ztschr. f. klin. Med. 33:269, 1907.
23. Abelin, I., and Kursteiner, P.: Biochem. Ztschr. 198:19, 1928.
24. Aub, J. C., Bauer, W., Ropes, M., and Heath, C.: Tr. A. Am. Physicians 42:344, 1927.
25. Swann, H. G., and Johnson, P. E.: Endocrinol. 24:397, 1939.
26. Mahoney, W., and Sheehan, D.: Am. J. Physiol. 112:250, 1935.
27. Schonemann, A.: Virchow's Arch. f. path. Anat. 129:310, 1892.
28. MacCallum, W. G., and Fabyan, M.: Bull. Johns Hopkins Hosp. 18:341, 1907.
29. Rogowitsch, N.: Beitr. z. path. Anat. u. z. allg. Path. 4:453, 1888.
30. Marine, D.: The Physiology and Principal Interrelations of the Thyroid, in, Glandular Physiology and Therapy. Chicago, American Medical Association, 1935, chap. 21, pp. 315–334.
31. Bryant, A. R.: Anat. Rec. 47:131, 1930.
32. Smelser, C. L.: Proc. Soc. Exper. Biol. & Med. 31:1127, 1934.
33. Hohlweg, W., and Junkmann, K.: Arch. f. d. ges. Physiol. 232:148, 1933.
34. Loeser, A.: Arch. f. exp. Path. u. Pharmakol. 176:697, 1934.
35. Zeckwer, I. T., Davidson, L. W., Keller, T. B., and Livingood, C. S.: Am. J. Med. Sc. 190:145, 1935.
36. Aron, M.: Compt. rend. Soc. de biol. 114:20, 1933.
37. Evans, H. M., and Simpson, M. E.: Anat. Rec. 45:215, 1930.
38. Van Horn, W. M.: Endocrinol. 17:152, 1933.
39. Winchester, C. F.: Endocrinol. 24:697, 1939.
40. von Arvay, A., and Meyer, H.: Zentralbl. f. Gynäk. 56:194, 1932.
41. Nakamura, U.: Jap. J. Obst. & Gynec. 16:246, 1933.
42. Anderson, D. H.: Proc. Soc. Exper. Biol. & Med. 30:657, 1933.
43. Geuer, C.: Ztschr. f. Anat. u. Entwcklgsgesch. 95:473, 1931.
44. Zalesky, M.: Anat. Rec. 62:109, 1935.
45. Sherwood, T. C., and Bowers, L. M.: Am. J. Physiol. 115:645, 1936.
46. Pincus, G., and Werthessen, N.: Am. J. Physiol. 103:631, 1933.
47. Laprida, E.: Universidad Nacional de Buenos Aires, Theses 4705, 1933, p. 91.
48. Kunde, M. M., D'Amour, F. E., Carlson, A. J., and Gustavson, R. G.: Am. J. Physiol. 95:630, 1930.
49. Sherwood, T. C., Savage, M., and Hall, J. F.: Am. J. Physiol. 105:241, 1933.
50. Starr, P., and Patton, H.: Endocrinol. 18:113, 1934.
51. Aron, M., and Benoit, J.: Compt. rend. Soc. de biol. 62:329, 1924.
52. Sherwood, T. C.: Am. J. Physiol. 124:114, 1938.
53. Sandiford, I., and Wheeler, T.: J. Biol. Chem. 62:329, 1924.
54. Dietel, F. G.: Ztschr. f. Geburtsh. u. Gynäk. 111:326, 1935.
55. Enright, L., Cole, V. V., and Hitchcock, F. A.: Am. J. Physiol. 113:221, 1935.
56. Anselmino, K. J., and Hoffmann, F.: Arch. f. Gynäk. 145:95, 1931.
57. Neuweiler, W.: Arch. f. Gynäk. 154:326, 1933.
58. Mussey, R. D.: Am. J. Obst. & Gynec. 36:529, 1938.
59. Becks, H., Roy, R. D., Simpson, M. E., and Evans, H. M.: Arch. Path. 34:334, 1942.
60. Kalb, S. W.: J. Clin. Endocrinol. 3:7, 1943.

CHAPTER XVII

THE PHYSIOLOGY OF THE SUPRARENAL GLANDS

PHYSIOLOGY OF THE ADRENAL MEDULLA

Epinephrine.—Oliver and Schäfer's[1] demonstration of a pressor substance in extracts of adrenal medulla initiated investigations which led to the isolation of epinephrine, its active principle. In 1901, Takamine[2] and Aldrich[3] working independently, obtained this principle in crystalline form, while Stolz,[4] in 1904, produced synthetic *adrenalin,* which differs from the natural product in that it is optically inactive. Adrenalin, also known as *adrenin* and *suprarenalin,* is a white, crystalline, hydroscopic substance which melts between 216° and 263°. Its chemical formula, as determined by Aldrich, is $C_9H_{13}O_3N$.

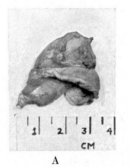 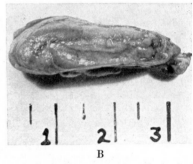

A   B

Fig. 46.—Adrenal gland. A, Gross appearance of gland; B, cross-section of gland, showing cortex and medulla.

Theories of Function.—Though its active principle is known to elicit definite pharmacologic reactions (see below), the adrenal medulla has not yet been assigned any specific function. It is apparently not indispensable to life, for ablation of one adrenal, and denervation of the other with destruction of its medullary component does not impair the health of experimental animals. Nor do any deficiency symptoms follow total destruction of the medulla, an observation which has led some observers to doubt whether it performs any functions whatsoever.

Of the many views advanced at one time or another to explain the role of the adrenal medulla in the body economy, Cannon's[5] so-called *emergency function* theory has probably enjoyed widest popularity. According to this view, epinephrine is not secreted under normal conditions, but is poured into the blood stream during emotional or physical stress, resulting from severe fright, danger, anger, pain, asphyxia, hemorrhage or other emergencies which threaten the organism. It is released under such conditions presumably to combat muscular fatigue, accelerate the coagulability of the blood, and otherwise help the organism to meet the emergency. This theory, though attractive, has not been substantiated by experimental evidence. Stewart and Rogoff[6] could demonstrate no significant alteration in the rate of epinephrine production during periods of stress, and found that adrenalectomized animals maintained on adequate doses of life-sustaining adrenal cortical hormone (see below) responded to emergencies as successfully as intact controls.

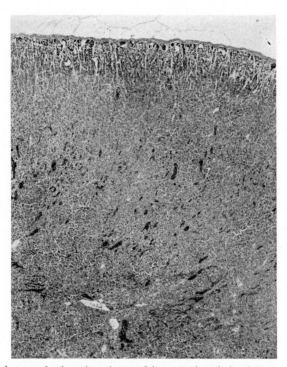

Fig. 47.—Microphotograph of section of normal human adrenal showing capsule, glomerulosa, fasciculata, reticularis and medulla.

Oliver and Schäfer's[1] observation that extracts of the adrenal medulla elevate the blood pressure suggested the possibility that it may be an important adjunct in maintaining the *blood pressure* at its normal level. Proceeding on this assumption, some observers suggested that the low blood pressure which characterizes adrenal insufficiency is due to a deficiency of epinephrine while hypertension is attributable to an excess of this hormone. Doubt is cast on this view by the observation of Hoskins and McClure[7] that suppression of the epinephrine supply, by ligating the adrenal vessels or severing the splanchnics, has no apparent effect on the blood pressure. It is also noteworthy that no increase in the epinephrine content of the blood is demonstrable in hypertensive patients.[8]

That the medulla may play a part in regulating *carbohydrate metabolism* is suggested by the observation that its extracts induce hyperglycemia and glycosuria in the experimental animal. Zuelzer[9] earlier suggested that the function of the adrenal medulla is to oppose the action of the pancreas, and that hyperactivity of the medulla may play a part in the etiology of diabetes mellitus. This appears doubtful, however, in view of the observation that suppression of epinephrine production neither hinders nor prevents experimentally induced pancreatic diabetes.[10]

PHARMACOLOGY OF EPINEPHRINE

Although the function of the adrenal medulla is obscure, it is generally recognized that its active principle, epinephrine, elicits definite reactions when given in pharmacologic doses. This substance acts on the sympathetic nervous system, and all organs and tissues innervated by it. Because of its powerful stimulating effect, it is sometimes referred to as a *sympathomimetic substance*. Its action is immediate, the nature and intensity of the response depending on the dosage, route of administration, status of the sympathetic nervous system, and type of tissue under its control. The effect is transient, ceasing as soon as the hormone is withdrawn from the site of action. Adrenalin apparently acts on the *myoneural junction*, for destruction of the nerves, or degeneration of the nerve endings exaggerate its effect on an organ.

Cardiovascular Effects.—Adrenalin in pharmacological doses produces an immediate acceleration of the pulse rate and minute volume. This is associated with a transient elevation of the arterial and venous pressure, an effect usually ascribed to its constrictor action on the peripheral blood vessels. Following the initial acceleration of the heart rate, some have noted a reflex bradycardia, which Stella[11] attributes to the effect of the elevated blood pressure on the sensitive region of the carotid sinus, the territory of distribution of the depressor nerves. Though adrenalin exerts a general constricting effect on the blood vessels, it causes dilatation of the cerebral, pulmonary, and coronary vessels, and those supplying the skeletal muscles.

Effects on Smooth Muscle.—Adrenalin increases the rate and amplitude of the heart muscle contractions. The bronchial musculature relaxes under its influence, the degree of relaxation being proportional to the muscle tonus at the time of injection. This accounts for the efficacy of adrenalin in relieving *bronchial spasm*.

In pharmacologic doses, adrenalin inhibits the *rhythmic movements* and lowers the *tonus* of the esophagus, stomach and intestines. On the other hand, the cardiac, pyloric, ileocecal and internal anal sphincters, which receive motor fibers from the sympathetics, contract tetanically under its influence. In large doses, it may cause paralysis of the bowel.

Its effect on the *uterine musculature* is identical with that produced by stimulating the hypogastric nerves. Muscle strips from the uteri of pregnant rabbits contract in vitro when adrenalin is added to the perfusing fluid. In vivo, adrenalin produces a continuous tonic contraction, powerful enough to express almost the entire blood content of the uterine wall. In the guinea pig and man,[12] on the other hand, moderate doses inhibit the myometrial contractions.

Adrenalin elicits a transient constriction of the *renal vessels* and a diminished urine output. This is soon followed by vasodilatation and marked diuresis. It causes dilatation of the pupil, elevation of the upper lid, and mild exophthalmos, but has no effect on the pupil, when applied locally to the conjunctival surface.

Effect on Striated Muscle.—Adrenalin stimulates striated muscle, though less markedly than smooth muscle. It decreases the fatigability and increases the work capacity of voluntary muscle strips in vitro. A stimulative effect has also been noted in vivo, due probably to the concomitant increase in circulation, and general elevation of the metabolic processes.

Effect on Metabolism.—Adrenalin causes a temporary rise in the basal metabolic rate of both the intact and thyroidectomized subject. *Heat production* is increased, due possibly to its constrictor effect on the peripheral blood vessels or, as some suggest, to its action on a heat center in the midbrain. Destruction of the medulla does not seem to interfere with oxygen consumption, indicating that it plays at best but a minor role in maintaining the normal basal metabolic rate.

Hyperglycemia and *glycosuria* may follow the parenteral administration of adrenalin, the effect lasting as long as the hormone is present in the blood. The liver is apparently the source of the additional sugar in the blood, for its ablation precludes this effect. In the fasting animal, the muscles also contribute. It is of interest that stimulation of the sympathetic nervous system elicits an identical hyperglycemic reaction, which apparently depends on adrenalin, since it does not occur if the adrenal medulla is removed, or the splanchnic nerves leading to it severed. It is unlikely that adrenalin increases the blood sugar by inhibiting insulin secretion for its hyperglycemic action persists despite pancreatectomy. The apparent antagonism between adrenalin and insulin may be explained by assuming that the mobilization of sugar effected by adrenalin, is counteracted by the increased utilization of sugar and inhibition of glycogenolysis in the liver, caused by insulin. Adrenalin's ability to stimulate glycogenolysis has led to its use as an antidote for *insulin poisoning* in cases where the glycogen store of the liver is not depleted.

The administration of adrenalin is followed by a rise in the excretion of urea, creatine and creatinine which is moderate in the fed animal and marked in the fasting subject. It also increases the excretion of sodium, potassium, and calcium.

Effect on the Skin and Mucous Membranes.—By stimulating the arrectores pilorum, adrenalin causes formation of "goose flesh." Its ability to cause contraction of the cutaneous arterioles is responsible for blanching of the skin which follows its administration. Its direct application to the mucous membranes is followed by blanching due to marked constriction of the blood vessels.

Toxic Effects.—Adrenalin in toxic doses may cause sweating, vomiting.

muscular tremors, marked asthenia, palpitation, paralytic ileus, cardiac failure and even death.

Therapeutic Application.—Because of its effect on the vascular apparatus, adrenalin, given parenterally, is often effective as an emergency measure in combatting *acute circulatory failure* incident to shock or anaesthetic accidents. It temporarily relieves *bronchial spasm*. It serves as a temporary *styptic* in nose and throat surgery, because of its vasoconstrictor action on the mucous membrane, and is valuable for shrinking nasal mucous membranes to facilitate inspection of the nasal passages. Adrenalin is also used as a *mydriatic*. When combined with local anaesthetics, it prolongs their action by constricting the arterioles and capillaries at the site of injection and thus retarding absorption.

PHYSIOLOGY OF THE ADRENAL CORTEX

Our present concept of the physiology of the adrenal cortex is based on effects observed in spontaneous and experimentally induced adrenal cortical insufficiency, and the response obtained in this condition with adrenal cortical extracts. That the adrenal cortex is indispensable to life is undisputed, for death invariably follows total bilateral adrenalectomy, and can be prevented by administering potent adrenal cortical extract. Much of the confusion which has surrounded the role of this gland in the body economy may perhaps soon be dispelled, thanks to the preparation of various biologically active crystalline compounds from adrenal cortical tissue. To date, more than twenty-five compounds have been isolated. Of these, seven have been found effective in replacing the functions of the cortex in one respect or another.[114] They include *corticosterone, 11-dehydrocorticosterone, 17-hydroxycorticosterone, 17-hydroxy-11-dehydrocorticosterone, 11-desoxycorticosterone, 11-desoxy-17-hydroxycorticosterone* and *progesterone* (see Fig. 48).

Maintenance of the Electrolytic Balance.—Probably the most important function of the adrenal cortex is to maintain the normal electrolytic balance. Suppression of its function is followed by increased excretion of *sodium* and a corresponding decrease in the concentration of this element in the blood. This is accompanied by a fall in the *serum chlorides* and *bicarbonates*, and a rise in *potassium* and most of the fixed elements. The loss of blood sodium, according to Loeb,[13] leads to an increased elimination of water, which depletes the circulating fluid volume and makes for shock. Many observers believe that this disturbance in the electrolytic balance is responsible for many of the manifestations of adrenal insufficiency. Support for this view is provided by the observation[14, 15, 16] that the administration of sodium chloride or sodium bicarbonate to adrenalectomized animals is life saving, and apparently restores them to normal for long periods of time without the aid of cortical hormone therapy. Grollman[17] and others argue that, since the adrenalectomized animal cannot be kept alive indefinitely with sodium chloride and other salts calculated to mimic the normal blood composition, the altered electrolytic balance is probably not the sole factor involved.

Circulation.—*Blood Volume.*—Swingle and associates[18] contend that the major role of the adrenal cortex is to regulate and maintain the normal volume of circulating fluid within the vascular apparatus. The adrenalectomized animal, they believe, ultimately dies from circulatory collapse induced by a deficiency of circulating fluid and a fall in blood pressure paralleled by a steady and progressive decline in blood volume. To account for the decrease in blood volume, they assume that the function of the adrenal cortex is to regulate capillary tone and maintain the normal fluid exchange between the vascular and extra-vascular tissue. Suppression of cortical function permits increased capillary permeability, thus permitting a shift of fluid from the blood to the tissue. Loeb,[13] on the other hand, argues that since large amounts of water and salt are known to be lost

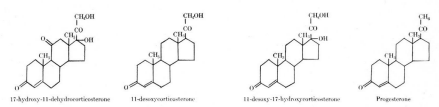

Corticosterone

11-dehydrocorticosterone

17-hydroxycorticosterone

17-hydroxy-11-dehydrocorticosterone

11-desoxycorticosterone

11-desoxy-17-hydroxycorticosterone

Progesterone

Fig. 48.—Compounds of adrenal cortical origin effective in replacing adrenal cortical functions in one respect or another.

from the body via the kidneys, it is unnecessary to assume a shift of fluid to the tissue spaces.

Arterial Tension.—Though hypotension is a cardinal manifestation of Addison's disease and experimentally induced adrenal insufficiency, it is not clear whether this is attributable to withdrawal of some adrenal cortical hormone which regulates the blood pressure, or depression of other vital processes incident to adrenal cortical insufficiency. Of interest are recent reports[19, 20] that adrenal cortical ablation prevents or corrects the hypertension which would otherwise follow constriction of the renal artery. On the basis of these observations, most workers conclude that the adrenal cortex maintains the body in such a state that it can respond to restriction of the renal artery with arterial hypertension.

Carbohydrate Metabolism.—Implication of the adrenal cortex in carbohydrate metabolism is suggested by the frequent occurrence of *hypoglycemia* in adrenal insufficiency, and of *hyperglycemia* and *glycosuria* in patients with adrenal cortical hyperplasia or neoplasms. In the laboratory animal, adrenalectomy markedly retards the rate at which glucose is absorbed from the intestines, and impairs the ability to form glycogen, with a resulting depletion of the glycogen stores of the liver and muscles, and a drop in the blood sugar. The depleted blood sugar, and liver and muscle glycogen can be restored to normal values by administering adrenal cortical extract. In the intact animal, adrenal cortical extract increases the liver and, to a lesser extent, the muscle glycogen, and may induce hyperglycemia[21] and glycosuria.[22] Long[23] suggests that the increase in liver glycogen following cortical extract administration may be due either to the production of glucose from protein, or a decrease in the rate of glucose utilization in the tissues.

Pancreas-Adrenal Cortex Relation.—An antagonism between the adrenal cortex and pancreas is suggested by the observation that diabetes induced by pancreatectomy can be ameliorated by adrenalectomy[24] or by ligating the lumbo-adrenal veins on both sides,[25] and can be made to reappear by administering adrenal cortical extract.[26] In the partially depancreatized rat, spontaneous glycosuria does not always occur, though it can be induced[27] or, if present, be aggravated[28] by administering cortical extract. In the animal deprived of the pancreas and adrenals, the administration of cortical extract aggravates the diabetes.[29]

Hypophysis-Adrenal Cortex Relation.—Several observers have attempted to ascertain what part, if any, the adrenal cortex plays in producing the changes in carbohydrate metabolism seen following hypophysectomy and the administration of anterior pituitary extracts. Britton and his associates[30] hold that the drop in the blood sugar and liver and muscle glycogen following hypophysectomy, is due to depression of adrenal cortical function caused by withdrawal of the hypophyseal corticotropic principle. This they base on their observation that adrenal cortical extract restores the blood sugar and muscle and liver glycogen of hypophysectomized animals to normal or nearly normal values. Support for this view is provided by the observations that adrenalectomy, like hypophysectomy, causes a drop in the blood sugar of the depancreatized animal;[26] that the same low level of carbohydrate metabolism occurs in the depancreatized dog after adrenalectomy, hypophysectomy or both,[31] and that adrenal cortical, like anterior pituitary extract, aggravates the glycosuria of the depancreatized animal.[26] On the other hand, this interpretation is not borne out by reports that cortical extract cannot restore to normal the muscle glycogen of the hypophysectomized animal;[32] that anterior pituitary extract can restore to normal or maintain at a normal level the liver and muscle glycogen of hypophysectomized animals, even in the absence of the adrenal cortex;[32, 33] that anterior pituitary extract can prevent the fall in the blood sugar induced with insulin in the adrenalectomized animal;[34] and that in the depancreatized, adrenalectomized rat, maintained at a constant level of glycosuria by daily administration of adrenal cortical extract, anterior pituitary extract further enhances the glycosuria.[28] These observations suggest that the anterior lobe influences carbohydrate metabolism not only through its corticotropic principle but also through some other hormone which acts directly on the tissues.

Hormonal Factors in Carbohydrate Metabolism.—Until recently, there was considerable controversy as to whether a single[35] or two distinct adrenal cortical principles influence electrolytic and carbohydrate metabolism. The latter possibility was suggested by Himwich's[25] observation that maintenance of a normal electrolytic balance was not related to the influence of the cortical extract on carbohydrate metabolism. Also significant was the observation of Loeb and associates[36] that there is no correlation between the occurrence of hypoglycemia and the electrolytic pattern of the blood of Addisonian patients. Recent studies with crystalline compounds from adrenal cortical gland tissue have provided further evidence that the hormone which influences carbohydrate metabolism is distinct from the water and salt hormone. Thorn and his associates[37] have shown that 17-hydroxycorticosterone and 11-dehydro-17-hydroxycorticosterone, which are the most active of all known adrenal cortical steroids in their effect on carbohydrate metabolism, have no effect on sodium retention in the dog.

Disturbances Following Adrenalectomy.—There is still uncertainty as to the part played by the disturbances in carbohydrate metabolism noted following adrenalectomy, in causing the death which eventually follows this operation. Hartman[38] found that dogs dying of adrenal insufficiency give normal or above normal blood sugar values, and are not relieved by glucose. On the other hand, Corey and Britton[30] observed that carbohydrate metabolism was profoundly disturbed in adrenalectomized monkeys: the liver lost its ability to form and furnish glycogen, and death resulted from depletion of the carbohydrate in the blood and hepatic tissues. This, coupled with the observation that glucose may help control the convulsions in patients with adrenal cortical insufficiency suggests that the adrenal cortex may play a more important role in carbohydrate metabolism in primates than in the lower mammals.

Fat Metabolism.—Adrenal cortical insufficiency is characterized by rapid loss of adipose tissue, which can be restored by administering maintenance doses of potent cortical extract. On the other hand, deposition of fat is a cardinal manifestation of *adrenal cortical hyperplasia* and certain *cortical neoplasms* (see Chap. XXXV). In the experimental animal, adrenal cortical ablation impairs absorption of fat from the intestines,[39] reduces the deposition of fat in the regenerating liver tissue of the fasting adrenalectomized rat, and interferes with the transport of fat to the liver.[40, 41] These effects can be corrected by giving cortical extract. Failure of fat absorption by the intestines can be corrected by administering saline solution to prevent dehydration.[42] Adrenalectomy reduces the *ketosis* in fasting animals and those receiving anterior pituitary ketogenic extract. Whether it does so by decreasing the rate at which ketone bodies are produced, or by increasing their rate of oxidation, or both, is not certain.[43] According to Goldzieher,[44] certain adrenal cortical extracts inhibit the mobilization of fat and fix it in the peripheral tissues.

Renal Function.—Retention of total nonprotein nitrogen is a common finding in the Addisonian patient and adrenalectomized animal. This is associated with diminished phenolsulphonphthalein excretion and a decrease in urea clearance. These alterations in renal function are apparently due to loss of the adrenal's cortical component, for adrenal cortical extract administered to such animals brings on diuresis and excretion of the retained substances.[45, 46]

Oxygen Consumption.—Though the thyroid gland plays the dominant role in maintaining the basal metabolic rate at its normal level, there is evidence that the adrenal cortex may exert some influence on the rate of oxygen consumption. The basal rate is characteristically low in both spontaneous and experimentally induced adrenal cortical insufficiency, and can be restored to normal by maintenance doses of potent adrenal cortical extract.[47] It is not certain whether depression of the basal rate following adrenal ablation is due to withdrawal of a specific principle which stimulates oxygen consumption, or is an expression of the general depression caused by adrenalectomy. The latter possibility seems more likely, for though adrenal cortical extract can restore the depressed rate of adrenalectomized animals to normal, it cannot further increase the basal rate of the intact animal. It is also significant that the basal rate does not drop immediately after the animal is deprived of the adrenal cortical secretions, but only after a latent period of several days. Marine and Baumann[48] have noted on initial rise in the basal metabolic rate following severe adrenal injury. This effect is apparently mediated through the thyroid gland for it does not occur in the thyroidectomized animal.

Miscellaneous Effects.—Detoxicating or *antidotal properties* were first ascribed to the adrenal cortical hormone on the basis of Meyer's[49] observation that cobra venom loses its toxicity when mixed with emulsions of cortical tissue. This assumption is supported by the fact that adrenalectomized animals are exceedingly sensitive to certain drugs, bacterial toxins, exposure to cold, and trauma; and that their resistance can be increased by administering maintenance doses of cortical hormone. It is likely, however, that the beneficial results thereby obtained are not due to the cortical hormone's antitoxic properties but to correction of a serious adrenal deficiency.

The adrenal cortex apparently plays some part in promoting *wound healing*. According to Hartman,[50] this function ceases in adrenal cortical insufficiency, and can be restored by administering maintenance doses of potent cortical extracts. Though the mechanism involved is not known, it seems likely that such extracts favor growth and healing of wounds in the adrenalectomized animal by raising the depressed vital processes rather than through any specific effect.

ADRENAL-ANTERIOR HYPOPHYSIS RELATIONSHIP

In Adrenal and Hypophyseal Diseases.—There is ample clinical and experimental evidence indicating an intimate functional relationship between the adrenal glands and anterior hypophysis. The similarity of the manifestations of both adrenal and pituitary disease is striking. In both

Simmonds' (*hypophyseal cachexia*) and *Addison's disease* (*adrenal cortical insufficiency*), emaciation, weakness and hypotension are cardinal manifestations. On the other hand, the symptomatology of *pituitary basophilism* so closely simulates that of *adrenal cortical hyperplasia* or *neoplasms*, that the two conditions may be clinically indistinguishable. A close relationship between the two glands is further emphasized by Anderson and Haymaker's[51] observation that the blood of patients with *Cushing's disease* contains excessive amounts of a substance which can prolong the life span of the adrenalectomized rat.

Adrenal cortical disease is associated with histologic and functional modifications in the adenohypophysis, and conversely pituitary disease leads to structural and functional alterations in the adrenal cortex. In Addison's disease the number of basophil cells of the anterior lobe may be markedly diminished.[52] Simmonds' disease, on the other hand, is often accompanied by adrenal cortical atrophy, while *basophilism*, or *acromegaly*, may be associated with adrenal cortical hyperplasia.

Adrenal Effects of Hypophysectomy.—Pituitary ablation in the laboratory animal is soon followed by atrophy of the zona fasciculata and reticularis, but not the zona glomerulosa or medulla. The gland can be restored to normal by administering anterior pituitary substance. The active principle responsible for this effect has been termed the *adrenocorticotropic or corticotropic hormone*[54, 55] (see Chap. XIII).

Hypophyseal Effects of Adrenalectomy.—That the adrenal cortex affects the anterior hypophysis is indicated by the observation[56] that adrenalectomy causes a drop in the gonadotropic hormone content of the adenohypophysis and a decrease in the size and number of acidophils and basophils. On the other hand, large doses of cortical extract cause hypertrophy of the anterior hypophysis. The existence of a specific adrenal cortical principle capable of influencing anterior hypophyseal function seems doubtful in view of Martin's[57] observation that sodium chloride restored normal hypophyseal-ovarian activity in over half their adrenalectomized animals.

In Gonad Stimulation.—The adrenal cortex may in some manner assist the anterior pituitary in performing its gonad-stimulating role. Friedgood[58] successfully prevented the ovulation which would otherwise follow coitus in rabbits, by removing the adrenals within one hour after mating. When operation was delayed until six hours post-coitum, ovulation occurred as it ordinarily would in animals with adrenals intact. The significance of this observation is not clear. Whether removal of the adrenals interferes with the production or release of gonadotropic hormone by the anterior hypophysis, raises the ovary's threshold of response to the pituitary hormones, or deprives the organism of a specific principle which augments the effect of the pituitary hormones on the ovaries, we cannot say.

ADRENAL-THYROID RELATIONSHIP

An antagonism between the adrenal cortex and thyroid is suggested by the observation[59] that thyroidectomy prolongs the survival period of adrenalectomized animals, while thyroid extract[60] aggravates the manifestations of adrenal insufficiency and unfavorably influences its course. Sub-lethal injury to the adrenals may lead to thyroid hyperactivity.[61] Whether this effect is specific or due to trauma, as Grollman[62] suggests, remains uncertain. According to Oehme,[63] cortical extract prevents the rise in the basal metabolic rate which would otherwise follow the administration of thyroid hormone or the hypophyseal thyrotropic principle. On the basis of these observations, some observers attribute Graves' disease to adrenal cortical insufficiency, and recommend cortical hormone therapy. Though a few workers have reported improvement following such treatment,[64] others[65] deny its efficacy and attribute the improvement to spontaneous remissions, which are concededly common in this malady.

Several investigators have demonstrated hyperplasia of the adrenal cortex following the administration of thyroid hormone.[66] Whether this is accompanied by an increase in the function of the gland has not been ascertained. Grollman[17] attributes the adrenal cortical hyperplasia as well as the reduction in the survival period of thyroid-fed, adrenalectomized animals, to the increase in metabolism rather than to any specific effect. He challenges Marine's suggestion that the adrenal gland controls the thyroid gland or directly controls metabolism in the same sense as the thyroid. While adrenal ablation, like thyroidectomy, lowers metabolic activity, the effect of thyroid ablation is chronic and not incompatible with life, while that of total adrenalectomy is acute and invariably fatal. Moreover, while thyroxin increases metabolism, cortical hormone even in large doses, does not have this effect.

RELATION OF THE ADRENAL CORTEX TO THE SEXUAL SPHERE

Embryologic and Cytologic Evidence.—An intimate adrenal cortical-gonadal relationship is suggested by embryologic, cytologic, clinical, and experimental evidence. It is noteworthy that both the adrenal cortex and gonad are derived from adjacent parts of the genital ridge. Moreover, the corpus luteum closely resembles the adrenal cortex not only in its histologic appearance but also in its high vitamin C content. A close relationship between the secretions of the adrenal cortex and the yellow body is implied in the observation that adrenalectomy is less likely to cause death if performed during pregnancy when a functioning corpus luteum is present.[67, 68] It is also significant that progesterone, like adrenal cortical extract, prolongs the survival period of adrenalectomized animals,[69] causes water and salt retention[70] and leads to adrenal cortical atrophy.[71] Recent studies of the chemistry of the adrenal cortical and gonadal hormones have revealed that all are derived from the sterols and are closely related chemically (see Chap. XLI).

Influence on Sex Characters.—Both clinical and experimental evidence indicates that the adrenal cortex exerts a profound influence on the genitalia and secondary sex characters. Chronic adrenal insufficiency, as manifested in Addison's disease, is associated, particularly in its terminal phases, with ovarian atrophy, amenorrhea and sterility. On the other hand, hyperfunction of the adrenal cortex due to hyperplasia or tumor, is associated with defeminization and development of male secondary sex characters in the female, and with the premature appearance of male secondary sex characters in the male. Certain rare carcinomatous lesions of the adrenal cortex may have a profound feminizing effect in the male, causing suppression of testicular function, loss of libido, retrogression of male secondary sex characters, and development of the breasts.

Experimental Evidence.—The explanation of the profound sexual alterations associated with adrenal cortical disease has been sought by observing the effects of adrenalectomy and the response to various adrenal cortical extracts, and by determining the androgen and estrogen content of the body fluids in patients bearing masculinizing or feminizing adrenal cortical neoplasms.

Ablation Experiments.—Adrenalectomy in the lower mammal may not suppress gonadal function immediately but as the insufficiency becomes acute the estrus cycles cease and regressive changes appear in the ovaries.[72] The effect of this operation in the pregnant animal varies. In some species, gestation continues normally and the appearance of signs of acute adrenal insufficiency is postponed until after the termination of pregnancy.[72, 73] In others,[74] adrenalectomy is followed by resorption or abortion of the fetuses and eventually by death of the mother. The prolonged survival of animals adrenalectomized during pregnancy is now generally believed to be due to the presence of *progesterone*, which is apparently capable of replacing the life-sustaining hormone of the adrenal cortex because of their close chemical relationship. The fetal adrenal cortex may also contribute.[73] Where pregnancy fails to postpone the acute stage of adrenal insufficiency, it may be supposed that the supply of progesterone and fetal adrenal cortical hormone is not sufficient to make up for the lack of the maternal adrenal cortex.

It is not definitely established whether the gonadal and reproductive disturbances which follow adrenalectomy are due to loss of a specific gonad-stimulating hormone, to depression of the gonadotropic activity of the anterior pituitary gland, or to the general debility and altered chemistry caused by loss of the metabolic principles of the adrenal cortex. The last-mentioned possibility finds support in the observation that gonadal function can be restored in the Addisonian patient and adrenalectomized animal by administering adrenal cortical extract or salt solution. That secondary changes in the adenohypophysis are at least partly responsible for the gonadal depression in adrenal insufficiency is suggested by the observation that the gonadotropic hormone content of the anterior lobe is materially reduced following adrenalectomy, and that anterior pituitary extract is effective in restoring the estrus cycles in the adrenalectomized animal.

Effects of Adrenal Cortical Implants and Extracts.—Experimental studies with adrenal cortical implants and extracts have yielded conflicting results. Nice and Schiffer[75] noted premature vaginal opening in rats receiving adrenal cortical implants. Chidester and his associates[76] observed a similar effect following the administration of adrenal cortical

17

extract. Atwell[77] found that potent cortical extracts, given over a period of two months to hypophysectomized animals, produced ovaries two and one-half times the size of the untreated hypophysectomized controls. Migliavacca[78] has described massive luteinization of follicles in mature mice receiving a cortical extract. Casida and Hellbaum[79] observed large follicles and corpora lutea in twenty-one to twenty-five day old rats receiving extracts prepared from the adrenal cortex of nonpregnant mares and geldings. Ovulation occurred in 50 per cent of the treated animals. Hall and his associates[80] found that adrenal cortical hormone, given to normal sexually mature rats prior to mating, materially increased the incidence of pregnancy and size of the litters. Allen and Bourne[81] have recently obtained an extract of whole adrenal gland, chemically distinct from the life-sustaining principle. They named it *adrenoluterin* because it induced luteinization and a considerable degree of endometrial hypertrophy.

Contrasting with these observations are reports that cortical extracts do not stimulate and may even depress gonadal function. Neumann[82] could observe no premature sexual ripening in mice receiving adrenal cortical extract. In mature animals, the extract arrested or slowed down the estrus cycles and caused a temporary sterility. Grollman[17] also failed to induce sexual precocity and suggested that the sexual alterations noted by other workers were probably due to the crudity of the extracts used. Eng[83] repeated Migliavacca's experiments in mature mice, but observed no luteinization and only such hyperemia and swelling of the uterus as may be produced with nonspecific extracts. Winter[84] observed no corpora lutea in rabbits receiving an adrenal cortical extract. The uterus was enlarged but neither the mucosa nor the musculature showed any significant changes. Hicks and Matters[85] found that the luteinizing action of human chorionic gonadotropin was not augmented when an adrenal cortical extract was simultaneously administered. Pottenger and Simonsen[86] prepared an adrenal cortical fraction which enhanced the size of the testes and promoted spermatogenesis in male rats, while in females it produced atrophy of the ovaries and accessory genitalia.

The explanation of these divergent findings is not clear. Further investigation with the various crystalline compounds thus far isolated from adrenal cortical extracts may eventually determine whether the gonadotropic effects obtained by some observers were due to a specific gonad-stimulating hormone of the adrenal cortex, to some by-product of adrenal cortical metabolism, or to its specific metabolic principles, which indirectly stimulate gonadal function through their effect on general metabolism.

Estrogenic and Progestational Activity of Adrenal Cortical Extracts.— Engelhart,[87] in 1930, obtained an extract of adrenal cortical tissue which induced *estrus* and *progestational changes* in the endometrium of immature rabbits. Callow and Parkes[88] subsequently confirmed his findings and separated the active estrogenic and progestational materials by the method of Allen and Meyer. The isolation of *progesterone* and a closely related compound, *allopregnanolone,* from the adrenals has been reported by Beall and Reichstein.[89] Beall[90] later isolated *estrone* from a concentrate of adrenal tissue, from which the greater part of the adrenalin and cortical hormone group of steroids had previously been removed.

That adrenal cortical tissue should yield estrogenic and progestational material is not surprising in view of the fact that there have been separated from adrenal cortical extracts a series of life-sustaining compounds which are steroid derivatives and closely related chemically to the hormones derived from the male and female gonads (see Chap. XLI). As Callow and Parkes[88] have suggested, it is entirely possible that compounds very similar to, if not identical with, the ovarian sex hormones are formed as by-products of the synthetic or degradative processes taking place in this gland. Significant in this connection are recent reports that *desoxy-corticosterone*, one of the active compounds isolated from adrenal cortical tissue, produces changes like those elicited by estrogen in the monkey[91] and human vagina,[92] and when given in sufficiently large doses, induces progestational changes in the endometrium of the rabbit[93] and monkey.[94] It is also noteworthy that *pregnanediol*, chief end-product of progesterone metabolism, appears in unusually large amounts in the urine of patients with *adrenal virilism*,[95, 96] and that some patients with *adrenal cortical neoplasms* excrete large quantities of estrogenic material. The ability of certain cortical neoplasms to produce large quantities of estrogenic substance may account for the feminization sometimes associated with adrenal cortical disease in the male. In one such case studied by Levy-Simpson and Joll,[97] as much as 5000 mouse units of estrogen per liter was demonstrated. Somewhat surprising is Frank's[98] report that large quantities of estrogenic substance were excreted by two female patients in which adrenal cortical carcinomas were associated with masculinization. This is difficult to explain unless it is assumed that the tumor simultaneously produced androgenic substances (see below) in even greater quantities.

Androgenic Activity of the Adrenal Cortex: Adrenal Virilism.—The secretion of an *androgenic principle* by the adrenal cortex, at least under certain pathological conditions, would seem to be an inescapable conclusion from the clinical observation that exaggerated virilism in the male, and masculinization in the female often accompany *adrenal cortical hyperplasia* or *tumors*, and that these manifestations regress upon extirpation of such lesions. Krabbe[99] has suggested that the androgens present under such conditions are secreted by reactivated testicular remnants which have become incorporated in the adrenal cortex during embryonic life. This suggestion is based on the fact that the adrenal cortex and gonads arise from closely adjacent sites in the genital ridge. Another interpretation, offered by Grollman,[17] assigns an androgenic function to the so-called "x-zone" which normally regresses during postnatal life but may, under abnormal conditions, become reactivated and give rise to hyperplasia or tumor formation. In a more recent study, Gersh and Grollman[100] found that the x-zone in male rats and mice exerts no demonstrable effect on the development of the male reproductive system. They concluded that the normal adrenal cortex is devoid of androgenic activity but pathological conditions may result in a metabolic disorder of the cell, with consequent formation of an androgen instead of the chemically related cortical hormone. That the production of androgens by the adrenal cortex is due to a perversion of its function would seem to be the most acceptable explanation, for it would also serve to explain why, under certain pathological conditions, the gland produces estrogenic substances.

Whatever the actual identity of the androgen secreting cells, recent studies with cortical extracts, and quantitative determinations of the androgen or *17-ketosteroid* content of the body fluids (see Chap. XXXIX) in virilism associated with adrenal cortical tumor or hyperplasia, leave no doubt that the masculinizing stimuli which are active in such individuals arise within the adrenal cortex. In 1936, Reichstein[101] obtained from the adrenal cortex a sterol with androgenic properties, which he named *adrenosterone* and declared to be distinct from other known androgens. In 1937, Broster and Vines[102] demonstrated an androgenic principle in the urine of patients with adrenal virilism. They isolated from such urines a new biochemical principle, which they believe to be specific to adrenal virilism, since they could not detect it in the urine of normal men or of normal pregnant and nonpregnant women. This substance, known as *pregnane-3 (alpha)*, *17, 20-triol,* is a saturated triol with the formula $C_{21}H_{33}(OH)_3$. The urine of women with adrenal virilism also yields isoandrosterone and transdehydroandrosterone, which possess weak androgenic activity. According to Callow,[103] the adrenal cortex is the source of the excessive amounts of androgen excreted by patients with adrenal cortical neoplasms, the smaller amounts (up to 10 mgm. daily) normally found in women and men, and the somewhat larger quantities (up to 35 mgm. daily) excreted by women with virilism but without adrenal cortical tumors. This he bases on his observation that androgen excretion is characteristically low in chronic adrenal insufficiency and is excessive only in adrenal cortical hyperplasia or tumor.[104] He argues that the adrenals are the source of most of the androgens found in the urine of normal women, for the level of these substances is not appreciably altered by ovariectomy (see Chap. XL).

Summary.—On the whole, it would appear that though the adrenal cortex plays an important part in gonadal and reproductive activity, a specific gonadotropic role may not be assigned to it on the basis of the available data. Moreover, as recently emphasized by Thaddea,[107] the evidence at hand fails to establish this gland as the normal site for the production of sex hormones, though it suggests a possible accessory role.

Effect of the Gonads on the Adrenal Cortex.—The adrenal cortex, like other members of the endocrine system, is apparently affected to a certain extent by alterations in the sexual sphere. Varying degrees of hypertrophy of this gland have been described during *estrus,*[105] *pseudopregnancy, pregnancy*[106] and *lactation.* Whether these alterations signify direct participation of the gland in gonadal and reproductive function, or merely represent its response to the increased metabolic demands of the organism during these physiologic states,[107] cannot be decided from the available evidence. The effect of *castration* on adrenal cortical function varies according to the age and species of the test animal. In some species hypertrophy has been described,[108] while in others atrophy is said to ensue after a latent period.[109] The explanation of these divergent findings is not clear. No characteristic modifications have been described in castrate or menopausal women. Quantitative studies of the urinary 17-ketosteroids (see Chap. XL) indicate that the extinction of ovarian function is followed by increased production of androgens by the adrenal cortex.[110] Whether this is due to removal of the antagonistic influence of the female sex hormones, which permits ascendancy of the adrenal cortex, or is attributable to increased production of adrenocorticotropic hormone[111] by the adenohypophysis, following its release from the inhibiting action of the ovarian hormones, we cannot say. Reports of the effect of estrogens on the adrenal cortex have failed to provide a definite answer.

The Adrenal Cortex and Lactation.—There is evidence that the adrenal cortex is essential for the maintenance of normal lactation. Some observers contend that it secretes a specific lactogenic hormone,[112] while others[113] believe it plays merely an accessory role, augmenting the action of the specific lactogenic hormone of the anterior pituitary gland through its effect on electrolyte and carbohydrate metabolism (see Chap. X).

BIBLIOGRAPHY

1. Oliver, G., and Schäfer, E. A.: J. Physiol. *18:*230, 1895.
2. Takamine, J.: Am. J. Pharm. *73:*528, 1901.
3. Aldrich, T. B.: Am. J. Physiol. *54:*57, 1901.
4. Stolz, F.: Ber. deutsch. chem. Ges. *37:*4149, 1904.
5. Cannon, W. B.: Endocrinol. & Metab. *2:*171, 1921; Am. J. Physiol. *98:*447, 1931.
6. Stewart, G. N., and Rogoff, J. M.: J. Exper. Med. *26:*637, 1927; Am. J. Physiol. *84:*660, 1928.
7. Hoskins, R. G., and McClure, C. W.: Arch. Int. Med. *10:*343, 1912.
8. Neulenberg, P.: Ergebn. d. Physiol. *21:*500, 1923.
   Rogoff, J. M., and Marcus, E.: J.A.M.A. *110:*2127, 1938.
9. Zuelzer, G.: Klin. Wchnschr. *38:*1209, 1901.
10. Stewart, G. N., and Rogoff, J. M.: Am. J. Physiol. *65:*319, 1933.
11. Stella, G.: J. Physiol. *77:*68, 1932.
12. Bourne, A., and Burn, J. H.: J. Obst. & Gynec. Brit. Emp. *34:*249, 1927.
13. Loeb, R. F.: Science *76:*420, 1932.
14. Harrop, G. A., Weinstein, A., Soffer, L. J., Threscher, J. H.: J. Exper. Med. *58:*17, 1933.
15. Loeb, R. F., Atchley, D. W., and Stahl, J.: J.A.M.A. *104:*2149, 1935.
16. Harrop, G. A., Soffer, L. J., Nicholson, W. M., and Strauss, M.: J. Exper. Med. *61:*839, 1935.
17. Grollman, A.: The Adrenals. Baltimore, Williams, Wilkins Co., 1936.
18. Swingle, W. W., and Pfiffner, J. J.: Science *77:*58, 1933; Am. J. Physiol. *123:*659, 1938.
19. Goldblatt, H.: Ann. Int. Med. *11:*69, 1937.
20. Collins, D. A., and Wood, E. H.: Am. J. Physiol. *123:*224, 1938.
21. Britton, S. W., and Silvette, H.: Science *75:*644, 1932; Am. J. Physiol. *107:*190, 1934; ibid. *118:*594, 1937.
22. Katzin, B., and Long, C. N. H.: Am. J. Physiol. *123:*725, 1938.
23. Long, C. N. H.: Sigma Xi Quart. *26:*175, 1938.
24. Long, C. N. H., and Lukens, F. D. W.: J. Exper. Med. *63:*465, 1936.
25. Himwich, H. E., Fazekas, J. F., and Martin, S. J.: Am. J. Physiol. *123:*725, 1938.
26. Long, C. N. H., Fry, E. G., and Thompson, K. W.: Am. J. Physiol. *123:*130, 1938.
27. Kendall, E. C.: Proc. Staff Meet. Mayo Clin. *13:*519, 1938.
28. Fry, E. G., Long, C. N. H., and Ritter, H. B.: Am. J. Physiol. *126:*497 (Proc.), 1939.
29. Lukens, F. D. W., and Dohan, F. C.: Endocrinol. *22:*51, 1938.
30. Corey, E. L., and Britton, S. W.: Am. J. Physiol. *126:*148, 1939.

31. Chambers, W. H., Sweet, J. E., and Chandler, J. P.: Am. J. Physiol. *126:*460 (Proc.), 1939.
32. Bennett, L. L.: Endocrinol. *22:*193, 1938.
33. Houssay, B. A.: Compt. rend. Soc. de biol. *129:*1261, 1938.
34. Himsworth, H. P., and Scott, D. B. M.: J. Physiol. *91:*447, 1938; ibid. *92:*183, 1938.
35. Kendall, E. C.: Endocrinol. *24:*798, 1939.
36. Loeb, R. F., Atchley, D. W., and Parson, W.: Tr. A. Am. Physicians *52:*228, 1937.
37. Thorn, G. W., Engel, L. L., and Lewis, R. A.: Science *94:*348, 1941.
38. Hartman, F. A.: Ann. Int. Med. *7:*1, 1933.
39. Verzar, F.: Ann. Rev. Biochem. *7:*178, 1938.
40. MacKay, E. M., and Carne, H. O.: Proc. Soc. Exper. Biol. & Med. *38:*131, 1938.
41. Verzar, F., and Laszt, L.: Biochem. Zeitschr. *285:*356, 1936; ibid. *288:*356, 1939.
42. Barnes, R. H., Wick, A. N., Miller, E. S., and MacKay, E. M.: Proc. Soc. Exper. Biol. & Med. *40:*651, 1939.
43. MacKay, E. M., and Barnes, R. H.: Am. J. Physiol. *123:*101, 1938.
44. Goldzieher, M. A.: Endocrinol. *18:*179, 1934.
45. Harrop, G. A., Pfiffner, J. J., Weinstein, A., and Swingle, W. W.: Science *73:*683, 1931.
46. Swingle, W. W., and Pfiffner, J. J.: Am. J. Physiol. *96:*186, 1931.
47. Webster, B., Pfiffner, W. W., and Swingle, J. J.: Am. J. Physiol. *99:*710, 1932.
48. Marine, D., and Baumann, E. J.: Am. J. Physiol. *57:*135, 1921.
49. Meyer, W.: Trans. Path. Soc. London *49:*368, 1898.
50. Hartman, F. A.: Am. J. Physiol. *86:*36, 1928.
51. Anderson, E., and Haymaker, W.: Proc. Soc. Exper. Biol. & Med. *38:*610, 1938.
52. Kraus, E. J.: Beitr. Path. Anat. *78:*283, 1927.
53. Crooke, A. C., and Russell, D. S.: J. Path. & Bact. *40:*255, 1935.
54. Anselmino, K. J., and Hoffmann, F. H.: Klin. Wchnschr. *13:*209, 1934.
55. Collip, J. B., Anderson, E. M., and Thomson, D. L.: Lancet *2:*347, 1933.
56. Lopez, F. S.: Frankfurt. Ztschr. f. Path. *46:*350, 1934.
57. Martin, S. J., and Fazekas, J. F.: Proc. Soc. Exper. Biol. & Med. *37:*369, 1937.
58. Friedgood, H.: Science *86:*84, 1937.
59. Carr, H. L., and Connor, L. C.: Ann. Int. Med. *6:*1225, 1933.
60. Thaddea, S.: Ztschr. f. Exper. Med. *95:*60, 1935.
61. Marine, D., and Baumann, E. J.: Am. J. Physiol. *59:*353, 1922.
62. Grollman, A.: Am. J. Physiol. *107:*480, 1934.
63. Oehme, C.: Klin. Wchnschr. *15:*512, 1936.
64. Richardson, J. S.: Acta med. Scandinav. *98:*583, 1939.
65. Weinstein, A., and Marlow, A.: Bull. Johns Hopkins Hosp. *52:*408, 1933.
66. Shapiro, S., and Marine, D.: Endocrinol. *5:*699, 1921.
67. Rogoff, J. M., and Stewart, G. N.: Am. J. Physiol. *79:*508, 1927.
68. Firor, W. M., and Grollman, A.: Am. J. Physiol. *103:*686, 1933.
69. Corey, E. L.: Proc. Soc. Exper. Biol. & Med. *41:*397, 1939.
70. Thorn, G. W., Nelson, K. R., and Thorn, D. W.: Endocrinol. *22:*155, 1938.
71. Clausen, H. J.: Anat. Rec. *76* (Suppl.) : 2, 14, 1940.
72. Tobin, C. E.: Endocrinol. *28:*419, 1941.
73. Rogoff, J. M., and Stewart, G. N.: Am. J. Physiol. *86:*20, 1928.
74. Gradinescu, A.: Compt. rend. Soc. de biol. *120:*356, 1935.
75. Nice, L. B., and Schiffer, A. L.: Endocrinol. *15:*205, 1931.
76. Chidester, F. E., Eaton, A. G., and Thompson, E. P.: Am. J. Physiol. *88:*191, 1929.
77. Atwell, W. J.: Endocrinol. *16:*639, 1932.
78. Migliavacca, A.: Zentralbl. f. Gynäk. *56:*1874, 1932.
79. Casida, L. E., and Hellbaum, A. A.: Endocrinol. *18:*245, 1934.
80. Hall, V. E., Chamberlin, P. E., and Muller, O. H.: Am. J. Physiol. *122:*16, 1938.
81. Allen, R., and Bourne, G.: Austral. J. Exper. Biol. & Med. Sci. *14:*45, 1936.
82. Neumann, H. O.: Arch. f. Gynäk. *160:*481, 1936; ibid. *162:*158, 1936.
83. Eng, H.: Zentralbl. f. Gynäk. *58:*2846, 1934.
84. Winter, E. W.: Ztschr. f. Geburtsh. u. Gynäk. *109:*273, 1934.
85. Hicks, C. S., and Matters, R. F.: Austral. J. Exp. Biol. & Med. Sci. *13:*27, 1935.

86. Pottenger, F. M., and Simonsen, D. G.: Endocrinol. *22*:197, 1937.
87. Engelhart, E.: Klin. Wchnschr. *9*:2114, 1930.
88. Callow, R. K., and Parkes, A. S.: J. Physiol. *87*:28P, 1936.
89. Beall, D., Reichstein, T.: Nature, London *142*:479, 1938.
    Beall, D.: J. Biol. Chem. *32*:1957, 1938.
90. Beall, D.: Nature, London *144*:76, 1939; J. Clin. Endocrinol. *2*:81, 1940.
91. Speert, H.: Bull. Johns Hopkins Hosp. *67*:189, 1940.
92. Salmon, U. J.: Proc. Soc. Exper. Biol. & Med. *41*:515, 1939.
93. Miescher, K., Fischer, W. H., and Tschopp, E.: Nature, London *142*:435, 1938.
94. Zuckerman, S.: J. Endocrinol. *2*:311, 1940.
95. Butler, G. C., and Marrian, G. F.: J. Biol. Chem. *119*:565, 1938.
96. Salmon, U. J., Geist, S. H., and Salmon, A. A.: Proc. Soc. Exper. Biol. & Med. *47*: 279, 1941.
97. Levy-Simpson, S., and Joll, C. A.: Endocrinol. *22*:595, 1938.
98. Frank, R. T.: Proc. Soc. Exper. Biol. & Med. *31*:1204, 1934; J. Mt. Sinai Hosp. *8*:514, 1942.
99. Krabbe, K. H.: New York Med. J. *114*:4, 1921.
100. Gersh, I., and Grollman, A.: Am. J. Physiol. *126*:368, 1939.
101. Reichstein, T.: Helvet. chim. acta *19*:223, 1936.
102. Broster, L. R., and Vines, H. W. C.: Brit. Med. J. *1*:662, 1937.
103. Callow, R. K.: Proc. Roy. Soc. Med. *31*:841, 1938.
104. Callow, N. H., Callow, R. K., and Emmens, C. W.: J. Endocrinol. *2*:88, 1940.
105. Swingle, W. W., Parkins, W. M., Taylor, A. R., Hays, H. W., and Morrell, J. A.: Am. J. Physiol. *119*:675, 1937.
106. Guthmann, H., and Voelcker, L.: Arch. f. Gynäk. *154*:591, 1933.
107. Thaddea, S.: Geburtsh. u. Frauenh. *3*:48, 1941.
108. Woolley, G., Fekete, E., and Little, C. C.: Endocrinol. *28*:341, 1941.
109. Blumenfeld, C. W.: Endocrinol. *24*:723, 1939.
110. Hamblen, E. C., Cuyler, W. K., and Baptist, M.: J. Clin. Endocrinol. *1*:763, 1941.
111. Nelson, W. O.: Anat. Rec. *77* (Suppl.) :97, 1941.
112. Hartman, F. A., Lockwood, J. E., and Brownell, K. A.: Proc. Soc. Exper. Biol. & Med. *30*:783, 1933.
     Spoor, H., Hartman, F. A., and Brownell, K. A.: Am. J. Physiol. *134*:12, 1941.
113. Gaunt, R., and Tobin, C. E.: Am. J. Physiol. *115*:588, 1936.
114. Ingle, D. J.: Endocrinol. *31*:419, 1942.

CHAPTER XVIII

THE PHYSIOLOGY OF THE PARATHYROIDS

Sandstrom,[1] in 1880, first described the external parathyroids, but it was not until 1891, when Gley[2] rediscovered them, that these tiny glands attracted general attention. In 1895, Kohn[3] discovered the internal parathyroids and pointed out that they are embryologically, anatomically, and functionally distinct from the thyroid gland.

EXPERIMENTAL STUDIES OF PARATHYROID FUNCTIONS

While much is known of the parathyroids' role in *calcium* and *phosphorus metabolism*, their relation to other metabolic processes, and to the various members of the endocrine system is not clear. Whether they are indispensable to life is likewise uncertain.

Effects of Parathyroidectomy.—Vassale and Generali,[4] in 1900, demonstrated that parathyroidectomy in dogs is followed by tetanic manifestations and often death. Since these effects did not ensue when pieces of thyroid tissue were removed and the parathyroids left intact, they concluded that *tetany* is a manifestation of parathyroid and not thyroid deficiency, as was earlier believed. Their findings have since been fully corroborated. It has been observed that the response to parathyroidectomy shows wide individual variations, some animals responding with striking tetanic manifestations, while others experience few or no ill effects. The presence of aberrant parathyroid tissue may account for some cases which remain unaffected. The response to parathyroid ablation is probably also determined by the supply of calcium and phosphorus through the diet, and the demands placed on the available reserves of these elements. Animals subsisting on a meat diet are much more prone to tetanic manifestations following parathyroidectomy than those on a vegetable diet. Parathyroidectomized animals survive for long periods of time if a normal serum calcium and phosphorus level is maintained by dietary means. Parathyroprivic tetany is less likely to develop in old animals than in younger ones whose calcium requirements are relatively greater. Pregnant and lactating animals, whose calcium reserves are subjected to extraordinary demands, are particularly prone to parathyroprivic tetany.

Effect of Parathyroidectomy on the Electrolytic Balance.—Mac-Callum and Voegtlin's[5] observation, in 1908, that the serum calcium is lowered in the parathyroprivic animal constituted a major advance in our knowledge of parathyroid function. It is now well established that parathyroid hormone deficiency is associated with a fall in the serum calcium and a rise in the serum phosphorus. This is accompanied by a decrease in the urinary calcium and inorganic phosphorus, and an accumulation of nitrogenous waste products in the body fluids. Some believe that the low concentration of "ionized calcium" is responsible for the increased excitability of the neuromuscular apparatus and impending tetany. On the other hand, the observation that the severity of the tetanic manifestations bear no constant relationship to the blood calcium level led Greenwald,[6] Rohmer[7] and Shelling[8] to suggest that the lowered serum calcium and tetany are both secondary to the retention of inorganic phosphorus. The view that the primary action of the parathyroid hormone is on *phosphorus metabolism* has recently been reiterated by Albright.[9] According to Neufeld and Collip,[10] the parathyroid hormone has no direct effect on bone, its primary action being on the excretion of phosphate by the kidneys.

Effects of Parathyroid Extracts.—In 1924 and 1925, Berman,[11] Hanson,[12] and Collip[13] independently obtained parathyroid extracts capable of raising the serum calcium in both the normal and parathyroidectomized animal. These extracts proved effective for the control of hypocalcemic tetany and, when administered to normal animals, induced a state of *hyperparathyroidism.* Collip's preparation, *parathormone,* apparently the most potent of these extracts, is not yet available in crystalline form. It is an albuminose, soluble in water and 80 per cent alcohol, but insoluble in acetone or pyridine. It is destroyed by boiling with acids and alkalies, and since it is digested by pepsin and trypsin, is not suitable for oral use. It was earlier standardized in terms of Collip units, defined as one-hundredth of the amount of the hormone required to cause, within fifteen hours, a 5 mg. per cent increase in the serum calcium of a dog weighing 20 kg. The recently adopted international unit represents one-fifth of the Collip unit.

It is now generally conceded that the parathyroid hormone regulates calcium and phosphorus metabolism, mobilizes calcium from the bones, and maintains the equilibrium between the diffusible and nondiffusible calcium of the blood. Its administration is followed by an increase in the excretion of inorganic phosphorus and calcium, a slight decrease in the serum phosphorus, a rise in the serum calcium and phosphatase, and a slight transitory increase in the serum manganese. Parathormone elicits a more rapid but less sustained hypercalcemia by the intravenous than the intramuscular or subcutaneous route. In the parathyroidectomized animal it causes phosphate diuresis, lowers the serum phosphorus, and raises the serum calcium. According to Albright and Ellsworth,[14] the blood calcium may attain a concentration of 8.5 mg. per 100 cc. or more before it appears in the urine.

Prolonged administration of the parathyroid hormone induces *hypercalcemia, hypophosphatemia,* and increased *excretion of calcium and phosphorus.* This eventuates in resorption of the spongy or cortical portions of the bone, which ultimately leads to softening, and bone neoplasm or cyst formation (*Von Recklinghausen's disease*). Some workers maintain that the phosphate diuresis which follows parathyroid administration is due to the direct action of the parathyroid hormone on the renal threshold for phosphates. Others deny this on the ground that the characteristic skeletal effects of parathyroid hormone are not prevented by bilateral nephrectomy. Prolonged treatment with parathyroid extract, after the serum calcium has reached 20 mg. per 100 cc., is followed by a further decrease in the blood calcium, an increase in the serum phosphorus, and by nausea, vomiting, diarrhea, anuria, uremic coma and other symptoms of parathyroid poisoning. According to Cantarow and associates,[15] death is due to loss of water and minerals through the kidney, a terminal rise in the blood non-protein nitrogen, and a fall in plasma carbon dioxide capacity.

PARATHYROID-GONADAL RELATIONSHIP

The available evidence relating to the parathyroid-gonadal relationship is not uniform. In general it would appear that, though not directly related, neither of these glands is entirely immune to disturbances in the other's function.

Genital Development and Function.—Hammett[16] observed retardation of ovarian and uterine development and decreased fertility following thyroid-parathyroidectomy in rats. Loss of the parathyroids could not be definitely blamed for these effects, because the thyroid was also removed and ablation of this gland alone is sufficient to cause disturbances of genital development and function. Removal of the parathyroids alone, according to Chandler,[17] does not interfere with the estrus cycles or conception in the rat, but others have reported disturbances of gonadal function following this operation. The disorders thus produced are probably due to the metabolic upset precipitated by withdrawal of the parathyroid hormone concerned with calcium metabolism, and not to loss of a specific gonad-stimulating factor. This interpretation finds support in the observation that menstruation and pregnancy may proceed normally in human hypoparathyroidism, provided the symptoms of hyperirritability are controlled by an adequate supply of calcium. Moreover, gonadal and reproductive function in the parathyroidectomized animal remains undisturbed so long as the calcium and phosphorus balance is maintained at a normal level.[18]

Menstruation.—The favorable effect of parathyroid extract in *excessive uterine bleeding* is probably due to its ability to increase the viscosity and coagulability of the blood rather than to a specific action on the ovaries or uterus.[19] Hartley[20] has reported that calcium gluconate relieves some cases of *dysmenorrhea* even when no hypocalcemia can be demonstrated. He was led to employ this form of therapy by his observation that menstrual cramps are common in women who suffer tetanoid symptoms when pregnant. Except for the possibility that the effect is purely psychic, it may be that in cases responding to calcium gluconate, the menstrual pain is a local manifestation of general neuromuscular irritability, due to calcium deficiency. Even if it is granted that some cases of painful menstruation are traceable to abnormal parathyroid function, the corrective effect of calcium therapy is proof that the fault is a deficiency of the specific principle regulating calcium metabolism, and not of some factor specifically concerned with ovarian or uterine function.

Hyperparathyroidism.—That the parathyroids exert no specific effect on the gonads may also be inferred from the observation that no constant alterations in the genital sphere accompany spontaneous or experimentally induced hyperparathyroidism. In human hyperparathyroidism, menstruation may either remain normal, become irregular, or cease abruptly. In the male, this malady is often accompanied by loss of libido and potentia, an effect generally attributed to the hypotonia and lassitude which characterizes this disease. Of interest is Neuweiler's[21] observation that, despite the hypercalcemia and osteoclasis induced in the rat by protracted parathyroid hormone treatment, the reproductive organs showed no significant alterations and the estrus cycles remained undisturbed.

Effect of the Gonads on the Parathyroids.—Activation of latent tetany has often been observed during menstruation, pregnancy, the puerperium, and lactation. Whether this is due to the strain on an already inadequate calcium reserve, or to some hormone emanating from the sexual sphere, which adversely affects parathyroid function or antagonizes its specific hormone, is not certain. Studies of parathyroid histology, the serum calcium level, and the condition of the skeletal system following castration or the administration of the ovarian sex hormones, have failed to provide a definite answer.

Sex Hormone and Castration Effects.—Ovarian ablation causes no significant change in the weight of the parathyroids in the rat;[22] nor is it followed by any perceptible change in the skeleton of the normal or rachitic rat. The effects noted following estrogen administration show considerable variation. Shapiro and Zwarenstein[23] found that estrogen restored to normal the lowered serum calcium of the castrate toad, and increased that of intact animals. Bach[24] observed a marked increase in the serum calcium and a decrease in the calcium content of the muscles, bones and skin in rats, following estrogen treatment. Riddle and Dotti[25] likewise detected a rise in the serum calcium level in estrogen treated rats, dogs, pigeons and doves. This rise was not prevented by hypophysectomy, thyroidectomy, or ovariectomy. On the other hand, Folley[26] found that estrogen administration in the lactating cow caused a drop in the serum calcium and a rise in the serum phosphatase. Mathieu[27] observed no change in the serum calcium level of intact dogs receiving estrogen, but parathyroidectomized animals responded with a drop in the blood calcium and tetanic manifestations.

There is evidence that in the chicken,[28, 29] duck[30] and pigeon,[31] estrogens lead to formation of medullary bone which is associated with a rise in serum calcium. According to Bloom and associates,[32] these two effects are probably not physiologically interdependent.

Clarification of the effect of the gonadal hormones on calcium metabolism and their relationship to parathyroid function awaits further investigation.

The Gonads and Osteomalacia.—Since osteomalacia is most apt to occur at puberty, or during pregnancy, and only rarely in males or postmenopausal women, earlier observers assumed that hyperovarianism is an etiologic factor and advocated bilateral ovariectomy for its control. This belief has since been discarded, and it is now generally agreed that osteomalacia is at least partly attributable to a deficiency of sunlight and vitamin D. The parathyroid hyperplasia which is a constant finding in this malady, is interpreted as a compensatory reaction to overcome the calcium deficiency resulting from this vitamin deficiency. The tendency to osteomalacia at puberty and during pregnancy is believed to be due to the drain on the calcium reserve, rather than to increased gonadal activity. The favorable effects earlier noted following ovarian ablation are attributed to relief from subsequent pregnancies rather than removal of some ovarian factor. It is significant in this connection that osteomalacia may be controlled by ligating the tubes and thus precluding subsequent pregnancies.[37]

Anterior Hypophysis-Parathyroid Interrelationship.—Some observers maintain that the anterior hypophysis stimulates parathyroid function (see Chap. XIII). Whether it acts directly through a specific "parathyrotropic" principle is not certain; nor is it known whether it in turn is influenced by the parathyroids.

Parathyroid-Thyroid Interrelationship.—Despite the close anatomic connection existing between the thyroid and parathyroids, there is no convincing proof that they are functionally related. Clinically, either tetany or hyperparathyroidism may occur in Graves' disease and conversely, myxedema or hyperthyroidism may accompany parathyroid tetany. It has been shown that removal of either gland is followed by hypertrophy of the other. Thyroid feeding relieves the tetanic manifestations of the parathyroidectomized dog[33] and augments the effect of parathyroid hormone in tetany.[34] It is also significant that thyroid feeding raises the serum calcium and increases the excretion of both calcium and phosphorus in the hypoparathyroid subject.[35] In general the evidence suggests that the thyroid acts synergistically with the parathyroids so far as calcium metabolism is concerned. Whether the parathyroids in turn assist the thyroid in performing its specific functions is not certain. The observation[36] that parathyroid extract is of no value in controlling myxedema argues against this possibility.

Parathyroids and Eclampsia.—The suggestion that the parathyroids are concerned in the etiology of eclampsia is based on the observation that this malady, like maternal tetany, occurs only during pregnancy. Some support for this assumption is provided by the observation that calcium gluconate may help control the hypoglycemia and relieve the symptoms of eclampsia. Brougher's[38] report that parathyroid hormone is a useful adjunct for the control of preeclamptic toxemia is of interest in this connection. Kehrer's[39] observation that eclampsia is often associated with a low serum calcium level would also seem to support this assumption, but his evidence has been questioned by Cantarow,[40] who could detect no significant lowering of the serum calcium in this malady.

BIBLIOGRAPHY

1. Sandstrom, I. V.: Upsala Läkaref. Förh. *15*:441, 1880.
2. Gley, E.: Compt. rend. Soc. de biol. *43*:841, 1891.
3. Kohn, A.: Arch. f. mikr. Anat. *44*:366, 1895.
4. Vassale, G., and Generali, F.: Arch. ital. di biol. *33*:154, 1900.
5. MacCallum, W. G., and Voegtlin, C.: J. Exper. Med. *11*:118, 1909.
6. Greenwald, I.: J. Biol. Chem. *67*:1, 1926.

7. Rohmer, P., and Woringer, P.: Compt. rend. Soc. de biol. *89:*575, 1923.
8. Shelling, D. H.: J. Biol. Chem. *56:*443, 1923.
9. Albright, F.: J.A.M.A. *117:*527, 1941.
10. Neufeld, A. H., and Collip, J. B.: Endocrinol. *30:*135, 1942.
11. Berman, L.: Proc. Soc. Exper. Biol. & Med. *21:*465, 1924.
12. Hanson, A. M.: Proc. Soc. Exper. Biol. & Med. *22:*560, 1925.
13. Collip, J. B.: J. Biol. Chem. *63:*395, 1925.
14. Albright, F., and Ellsworth, R.: J. Clin. Investigation *7:*183, 1929.
15. Cantarow, A., Brundage, J. T., and Housel, E. L.: Endocrinol. *21:*368, 1937.
16. Hammett, F. S.: Am. J. Anat. *32:*53, 1923.
17. Chandler, S. B.: Anat. Rec. *53:*105, 1932.
18. Kozelka, F. L., Hart, E. B., and Bohstedt, G.: J. Biol. Chem. *100:*715, 1928.
19. Gordon, B., and Cantarow, A.: J.A.M.A. *88:*1301, 1927.
20. Hartley, E. C.: Am. J. Obst. & Gynec. *21:*725, 1931; ibid. *27:*253, 1934.
21. Neuweiler, W.: Zentralbl. f. Gynäk. *57:*456, 1933.
22. Overholser, M. D.: Anat. Rec. *41:*303, 1929.
23. Shapiro, H. A., and Zwarenstein, H.: J. Exper. Biol. *10:*186, 1933; ibid. *11:*267, 1934.
24. Bach, E.: Klin. Wchnschr. *16:*280, 1937.
25. Riddle, O., and Dotti, L. B.: Science *84:*557, 1936.
26. Folley, S. J.: Biochem. J. *30:*2262, 1936; Lancet *2:*423, 1938.
27. Mathieu, F.: Arch. internat. de Physiol. *38:*365, 1934.
28. Zondek, B.: Folia Clin. Orient. *1:*1, 1937.
29. Landauer, W., Pfeiffer, C. A., Gardner, W. U., and Man, E. B.: Proc. Soc. Exper. Biol. & Med. *41:*80, 1939.
30. Landauer, W., Pfeiffer, C. A., Gardner, W. U., and Shaw, J. C.: Endocrinol. *28:*458, 1941
31. Pfeiffer, C. A., and Gardner, W. U.: Endocrinol. *23:*485, 1938.
32. Bloom, M. A., McLean, F. C., and Bloom, W.: Anat. Rec. *83:*99, 1942.
33. Kunde, M. M., Oslund, R., and Kern, R.: Am. J. Physiol. *85:*387, 1928.
34. Aub, J. C., Bauer, W., Heath, C., and Ropes, M.: J. Clin. Investigation *1:*97, 1929.
35. Albright, F., Aub, J. C., and Bauer, W.: J.A.M.A. *102:*1276, 1934.
36. Goldzieher, M. A.: The Endocrine Glands. New York, D. Appleton Century Co., 1939, p. 210.
37. Wyatt, H. G.: China Med. J. *44:*1168, 1930.
38. Brougher, J. C.: Am. J. Obst. & Gynec. *43:*710, 1942.
39. Kehrer, E.: Arch. f. Gynäk. *112:*487, 1920.
40. Cantarow, A.: Proc. Roy. Soc. Med. *37:*639, 1930.

CHAPTER XIX

THE PANCREAS AND THE GONADS

The role of the pancreas in the regulation of carbohydrate metabolism is well established and needs no comment here. Its relationship to the gonads is still obscure, though the available evidence suggests that, while not directly related, each is affected to some extent by functional alterations in the other.

EFFECT OF THE PANCREAS ON GONADAL AND REPRODUCTIVE FUNCTION

In Diabetes Mellitus.—Pancreatic deficiency apparently unfavorably affects sexual function. This is readily discernible on comparing the status of sexual and reproductive function of diabetic patients before and after the advent of insulin therapy.

Growth and Sexual Development.—In the pre-insulin era, stunting of growth and genital retardation were common manifestations in juvenile diabetics. This was at first blamed on nutritional deficiency incident to the diabetic state. Recognition of the importance of the adenohypophysis in the regulation of carbohydrate metabolism has led some observers to believe that some other factor in addition to insular deficiency may be responsible for these effects. Gibson and Fowler[1] suggest that the diabetes, growth stunting, and genital retardation are independent manifestations of anterior pituitary deficiency, involving its pancreatropic, growth, and gonadotropic principles. White and her associates[2] observed that juvenile diabetics show an acceleration of growth and sexual development at the onset of the disease but later show retardation. From this they concluded that the growth stunting and genital retardation are due to exhaustion of the adenohypophysis following a period of hyperactivity, involving its growth, gonadotropic, pancreatropic, and diabetogenic factors. Persistence of the diabetes, beyond the hyperactive stage, is presumably due to secondary changes in the pancreatic islets, the situation being analogous to that seen in dogs rendered permanently diabetic by chronic treatment with anterior lobe extract (see Chap XIII).

While this interpretation may apply to some cases, the good effect of insulin in the majority of juvenile diabetics suggests that in such cases insular deficiency is responsible for the statural and genital retardation as well as the diabetes.[3] Improvement in growth and sexual development has been repeatedly achieved with insulin therapy in young diabetics.[4, 5] Among a group of treated diabetic girls observed by White and her associates,[2] all those over sixteen years of age showed complete sexual development. Were anterior pituitary exhaustion a factor, insulin therapy alone could hardly be expected to suffice. The importance of the nutritional factor in the causation of dwarfism associated with diabetes is emphasized by the observation that growth stunting was more common in the earlier days when insulin therapy was combined with a limited diet, than now when a diet adequate in all respects is prescribed.[3]

Sexual Disturbances in the Adult.—Observations in adult diabetics during the pre-insulin and post-insulin era provide a striking contrast. Menstrual disturbances and sterility in the female, and spermatogenic faults and impotence in the male were commonly encountered before the advent of insulin. With the introduction of this drug, marked improvement was soon apparent. The efficacy of insulin therapy in restoring normal menstrual function and fertility in diabetic women has been repeatedly demonstrated.[8, 9, 10] Mengert and Laughlin,[12] in their study of thirty-three pregnancies in twenty-eight diabetic women, concluded that a controlled diabetic who becomes pregnant is, obstetrically speaking, a normal woman.

Maternal and Fetal Mortality.—Aside from the high incidence of sterility,[6] the maternal and fetal mortality was previously high. Brandstrup and Okkels,[7] who reviewed the literature on diabetes and pregnancy in pre-insulin days, found a maternal mortality of 30 per cent. Abortion, or fetal death shortly before, during, or within twenty-four to forty-eight hours after delivery, exceeded 60 per cent. The maternal mortality of diabetics, in the words of Lawrence and Oakley,[11] has been reduced to an almost negligible figure. Despite the availability of insulin, the fetal mortality is still estimated to be about 45 per cent.[6] As White[13] has pointed out, insulin therapy has lowered the incidence of fetal death in early but not in late pregnancy. Some attribute this to inadequate control of the diabetes, due to failure to recognize all the variables which come into play during the latter months of gestation. Others suggest that some extra-diabetic factor, beyond the control of insulin, may be operating. Fetal anomalies, excessive size of the fetus, and a marked tendency to toxemia have been blamed for the high fetal mortality.[11] Some blame the large amount of available carbohydrate,[11] others an excess of anterior pituitary growth hormone, for the oversized fetuses. The *toxemia* in the pregnant diabetic, according to Smith and Smith,[14] and White,[13, 15] is preceded and accompanied by high gonadotropin and low estrogen and pregnanediol titers in the urine. These observers postulate the existence of an extra-diabetic factor and claim to have controlled the toxemic manifestations with massive doses of estrogen. Their findings await confirmation. The death of infants of diabetic mothers within a short time after birth is attributed by some to hypoglycemia,[11] by others to cerebral anoxia with involvement of the respiratory centers.[15]

Experimental Evidence.—Experimental evidence relating to the effect of *hypo- or hyperinsulinism* on gonadal and reproductive function is limited and inconclusive. Liegner[10] noted numerous atretic follicles, follicular cysts, but no fresh corpora lutea following partial destruction of the insular apparatus in experimental animals. Crainicianu[16] found that puberal rats given 1 to 4 units of insulin daily for twenty days, showed continuous estrus, enlargement of the uterus, and congestion and marked vascularization of the ovaries, with hemorrhagic points and massive luteinization of the follicles. Klaften[17] observed that small doses of insulin hastened follicular maturation, increased the number of mature and growing follicles, and lengthened estrus. Medium doses caused moderate luteinization and large ones produced marked luteinization, slowed up follicular maturation, and favored follicular atresia. Inhibition of ovulation with insulin has been observed in the pigeon,[18] mouse,[19] and rat[20] but Del Castillo and Calatroni[21] were unable to duplicate this effect.

Though incomplete, the evidence at hand suggests that gonadal and reproductive function may be altered by either an excess or deficiency of insulin. Whether the effect is direct or mediated through the adeno-hypophysis is not clear. Also to be considered is the possibility that changes in the sexual sphere are due to the unfavorable systemic effect of hypo- and hyperinsulinism.

Clinically, it has often been noted that improvement in menstrual function, in the thin, asthenic, nondiabetic woman, may follow insulin therapy supplemented by a high carbohydrate diet. This cannot be construed as signifying that insulin stimulates gonadal function, for the improvement in such cases coincides with a material gain in weight, induced by such therapy, and may reasonably be attributed to the improved nutritional status of the individual.

EFFECT OF THE GONADS ON THE PANCREAS

Menstruation and Pregnancy.—There is some indirect evidence that pancreatic function may be influenced by alterations in the sexual sphere. Peperkorn[22] observed a diabetic who suffered exacerbations at the time of the flow, and on one occasion went into a coma. A patient observed by Weil[23] presented recurrent manifestations suggestive of hypoglycemia dur-in menstruation. During pregnancy, the diabetic is apparently influenced by factors connected with reproduction, as shown by changing insulin requirements in the course of gestation.[11, 24] It is significant that the incidence of diabetes is highest at or shortly after the menopause. In view of recent evidence that other glands besides the pancreas play an important role in carbohydrate metabolism, there are several possible explanations of the mechanism whereby events in the sexual sphere influence this process. Stimuli emanating from the gonads may conceivably affect carbohydrate metabolism through a direct action on the periphery, or indirectly through the mediation of the pancreas, anterior pituitary, or adrenal cortex.

Effects of Estrogen.—Studies of the effect of estrogen on the blood and liver glycogen have failed to provide a definite solution. Some observers report increased sugar tolerance and decreased insulin requirements,[24, 25, 26, 27] while others observed a rise in blood sugar and liver glycogen,[28, 29, 30, 31] or no effect whatsoever.[32, 33] The explanation of these divergent results is not clear. It is conceivable that estrogen influences carbohydrate metabolism through several routes, the response varying according to the state of the various organs and tissues involved. Henley[24] has presented evidence suggesting that this hormone may increase the sugar tolerance by lowering the renal threshold for glucose. It has been suggested that estrogen inhibits the diabetogenic activity of the anterior pituitary and may thus increase the sugar tolerance and reduce the insulin requirements. This explanation would seem applicable where an excess of the diabetogenic factor is an etiologic factor. On the other hand, where the diabetes is primarily due to a deficiency or permanent damage to the insular apparatus, estrogen would be expected to have no effect, or to influence the sugar level only to the extent that the diabetogenic hormone contributes to the hyperglycemia. Of interest in this connection is Spiegelman's[27] observation that estrogen therapy caused a more marked drop in the insulin requirements of premenopausal than of postmenopausal women.

The hyperglycemic effect of estrogen, reported by some investigators, may perhaps be attributable to its close chemical relationship to the adrenal steroids (see Chap. XLI). It is possible that variations in dosage, the type of estrogen used, and the species of the test animal are among the factors which determine whether its hyperglycemic or anti-diabetogenic action will predominate.

BIBLIOGRAPHY

1. Gibson, R. B., and Fowler, W. M.: Arch. Int. Med. *57:*695, 1936.
2. Wagner, R., White, P., and Bogan, I. K.: Am. J. Dis. Child. *63:*667, 1942.
3. Rynearson, E. H., and Hildebrand, A. G.: Arch. Int. Med. *18:*134, 1941.
4. Joslin, E. P., Root, H. F., White, P., and Marble, A.: Boston M. & S. J. *193:*1092, 1925.
5. Gardiner-Hill, H.: Practitioner *125:*97, 1930.
6. Nothmann, M.: New England J. Med. *64:*275, 1941.
7. Brandstrup, E., and Okkels, H.: Acta obst. & gynec. Scandinav. *18:*136, 1938.
8. Witherius, E. P.: Lancet *2:*858, 1933.
9. Duncan, G. G., and Fetter, F.: Am. J. Med. Sci. *18:*347, 1934.
10. Liegner, B.: Zentralbl. f. Gynäk. *59:*2883, 1935.
11. Lawrence, R. D., and Oakley, W.: Quart. J. Med. *11:*45, 1942.
12. Mengert, W. F., and Laughlin, K. A.: Surg., Gynec. & Obst. *69:*615, 1939.
13. White, P., Titus, R. S., Joslin, E. P., and Hunt, H.: Am. J. Med. Sci. *198:*482, 1939.
14. Smith, G. V., and Smith, O. W.: Am. J. Obst. & Gynec. *38:*618, 1939.
15. White, P., and Hunt, H.: J.A.M.A. *115:*2039, 1940.
16. Crainicianu, A., and Copelman, L.: Compt. rend. Soc. de biol. *121:*1303, 1936.
17. Klaften, E.: Zentralbl. f. Gynäk. *59:*1512, 1935.
18. Riddle, O.: Proc. Soc. Exper. Biol. & Med. *20:*244, 1922.
19. Vogt, E.: Med. Klin. *23:*557, 1927; ibid. *25:*1163, 1929.
20. Migliavacca, A.: Compt. rend. Soc. de biol. *104:*1266, 1930.
21. Del Castillo, E. B., and Calatroni, C.: Compt. rend. Soc. de biol. *102:*454, 1929.
22. Peperkorn, R.: München. med. Wchnschr. *79:*1748, 1932.
23. Weil, A., cited by Harris, S., Endocrinol. *16:*29, 1932.
24. Henley, W.: New Zealand Med. J. *39:*308, 1940.
25. Barnes, B. O., Regan, J. F., and Nelson, W. O.: J.A.M.A. *101:*926, 1933.
26. Kurzrok, R.: The Endocrines in Obstetrics and Gynecology. Baltimore, Williams & Wilkins Co., 1937.
27. Spiegelman, A. R.: Proc. Soc. Exper. Biol. & Med. *43:*307, 1940.
28. Gulick, M., Samuels, L. T., and Deuel, H. J., Jr.: J. Biol Chem. *105:*29, 1934.
29. Zunz, E., and LaBarre, J.: Arch. internat. Physiol. *48:*287, 1939.
30. Griffiths, M., Marks, H. P., and Young, F. C.: Nature *147:*359, 1941.
31. Ingle, D. J.: Endocrinol. *29:*838, 1941.
32. Collens, W. S., Slo-Bodkin, S. G., Rosenbliett, S., and Boas, L. C.: J.A.M.A. *106:*678, 1936.
33. Lawrence, R. D., and Madders, K.: Lancet *1:*601, 1941.

18

CHAPTER XX

THE PHYSIOLOGY OF THE THYMUS GLAND

The role of the thymus in the body economy is not established. It is generally agreed that it is not essential to life, but whether it functions as a gland of internal secretion is still the subject of controversy. Histologic and morphologic studies, as well as thymectomy and thymus feeding

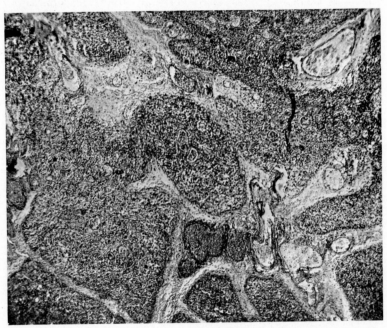

Fig. 49.—Microphotograph of normal thymus of newborn.

experiments have failed to resolve this conflict. Whether this structure secretes hormonal substances which influence somatic growth and genital development is still an open question.

THE THYMUS AND GROWTH

Effects of Thymectomy.—The somatic alterations described following thymectomy have varied considerably even where it was reasonably certain that the entire organ had been removed. Basch[1] observed that following thymectomy in the dog, the bones became soft and pliable, the epiphyses of the radiuses enlarged, and growth was retarded. Klose and Vogt,[2] working independently, also demonstrated osseous disturbances and growth retardation a few months after thymus ablation in this species. These changes were progressive, and were associated with cachexia which terminated in death. Einhorn and Rowntree[3] have more recently reported that thymectomy in successive generations of rats was followed by progressive retardation of growth beginning with the second generation. This effect was transient, for the animals eventually attained the size of unoperated controls. Shay and his associates[4] found that intense x-ray irradiation of the thymus region caused stunting of growth in rats. Young dogs similarly treated, according to Bentivoglio and associates,[5] responded with general nutritional and somatic disturbances and bone changes not unlike those seen in rickets. In contrast to these reports, several competent observers could demonstrate no alteration in somatic growth in thymectomized animals. Nordmann[6] observed neither nutritional nor skeletal modi-

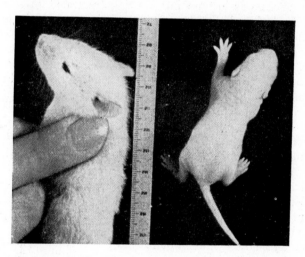

Fig. 50.—Effect of continuous treatment of successive generations of rats with thymus extract (Hanson). Right, untreated control rat seven days old; left, fourth generation thymus test rat, six days old, the eyes open. (Rowntree, L. G., Clark, J. H., Hanson, A. M. and Sternberg, A.: J.A.M.A. Vol. 103.)

fications following thymus ablation in the dog. In carefully controlled studies of thymectomized dogs, Park and McClure[7] could demonstrate none of the rachitic manifestations described by Klose and Vogt.[2] Calling attention to the fact that Klose's animals were kept in sunless quarters on an inadequate diet, while their own dogs were well fed and kept out of doors, they attribute the changes described by Klose to dietary and vitamin deficiency and not to loss of some specific thymus growth-promoting hormone. More recently, Hashimoto and Freudenberger,[8] working with male rats, and Chiodi[9] and Segaloff and Nelson,[10] who studied the effect of thymectomy in successive generations of rats, found this operation compatible with normal growth.

Effects of Implants and Extracts.—The results obtained with thymus implants and extracts have been as contradictory as those following thymectomy. In the tadpole, Gudernatsch[11] and Romeis[12] observed marked acceleration of growth after the oral administration of calves' thymus tissue. In mammals similarly treated, some workers have noted acceleration, while others report retardation of the growth rate, or no effect whatsoever. Striking effects have been noted by some investigators following the administration of thymus extracts. Asher[13] prepared an extract, *thymocrescin*, which accelerated the growth rate in rats. Rowntree and his coworkers[14] reported startling effects in successive generations of rats treated with a thymus extract prepared by Hanson. Somatic precocity was apparent as early as the second generation, and became more and more accentuated with each succeeding one. Though the growth rate at first appreciably exceeded that of the controls, the maximum size achieved was not significantly greater than that of the untreated adult animal. This growth-accelerating effect was lost on interrupting treatment in any generation. Burrill and Ivy[15] found that fresh thymus substance fed to pregnant rats through four generations caused no significant acceleration of growth, and had no effect on the developmental rate in the offspring. Unlike Rowntree's experiment, the treatment did not extend beyond the period of pregnancy. Negative results with extracts prepared by Hanson's and Asher's methods have been reported by Segaloff and Nelson,[64] who suggest that dietary deficiencies may account for the slower development of Rowntree's controls.

It has been suggested that the accelerated growth and development obtained with Asher's and Hanson's extracts is a *nutritional* rather than an endocrine phenomenon. It is noteworthy that the growth-stimulating activity of Asher's extract is demonstrable only in vitamin deficient animals[16] and has no additional effect in subjects whose diet contains all essential elements. It is also significant that acceleration of growth and development in successive generations of animals can be produced by means of vitamins.[17]

Since the effect of thymus implants is qualitatively though not quantitatively equal to that of thymus extracts,[18] it would seem reasonable to suppose that the growth-stimulating substance is a normal constituent of thymus tissue and not merely a by-product formed in the process of extraction. Gudernatsch[19] has suggested that the active substance is probably *glutathione*, which is apparently present in both Asher's and Hanson's extract, and was shown by Hoffman and Gudernatsch[20] to have growth-stimulating properties. His suggestion is borne out by the studies of Rowntree's group[21, 22, 23] who also demonstrated the growth-stimulating activity of glutathione and found that all biologically potent thymus extracts contain this substance. On the other hand, others[64, 65] obtained negative results in successive generations of rats, even with large doses of glutathione.

THYMUS-GONADAL RELATION

The Thymus in Gonadal Function.—*Stimulating Effects.*—A gonad stimulating effect of the thymus was first suggested by reports that thymectomy delays testicular development and causes atrophy of sperm forming cells. Apparent support for this supposition has been more recently provided by the observation of Shay and his associates[4] that x-ray irradiation of the thymus in young male rats was followed by an arrest in the development of the spermatogenic portion of the testes, and castration changes in the anterior hypophysis. These changes were progressive until the one hundredth day, when reparative processes set in and the testes and hypophysis returned to normal. Similar treatment in the female animal had no apparent effect on gonadal function. These findings have been criticized[8] on the ground that no effort was made to exclude injury to the thyroid, whose ablation has been shown to elicit pituitary modifications and clinical manifestations not unlike those observed in the thymus irradiated rats.

That the thymus stimulates gonadal development and function seems questionable in view of the well controlled experiments of Park and Mc-Clure,[7] Chiodi,[9] and others who showed that complete extirpation of the thymus in rats did not affect the size of the gonads, or delay the onset of puberty. Anderson[24] has suggested that the regressive changes in the sexual sphere noted by some observers following thymectomy, were probably due to trauma and infection incident to the operation. The observation that x-ray irradiation of an enlarged thymus in infants has no apparent effect on subsequent sexual development also casts doubt on the view that the thymus stimulates gonadal function.

Effects of Thymus Extracts.—Experiments with thymus substance or extract have yielded conflicting results. Groebbels[25] noted an increase in the number and size of the litters in certain species of fish. A stimulative effect is likewise suggested by Asher's[13] observation that thymus extract caused an appreciable increase in the weight of the gonads in rats, and by reports of precocious genital development following administration of thymus extract. Rowntree and his associates[14] found that injection of thymus extract into successive generations of rats caused marked growth of the genitalia and sexual precocity in the offspring of the treated animals. The precocious offspring breeded earlier and cast their litters at an earlier date than untreated controls. It is likely that the sexual precocity, like the accelerated somatic development with which it is associated, is due to a nutritional factor rather than a specific thymus hormone.

Effect of the Gonads on the Thymus.—The observation that the thymus undergoes involution during the puberal period, when the gonads are in the ascendancy, suggests that the sex glands exert an *inhibitory effect* on thymus function. This antagonism is also implied in the fact that thymus involution begins prematurely in the sexually precocious individual, while hyperplasia and persistence of this structure is not uncommon in young castrates and individuals with retarded sexual development. *Status thymicolymphaticus*, which is characterized by enlargement of the thymus, is usually associated with genital hypoplasia. In the adult male and female rat, thymus hypertrophy follows gonadectomy,[31, 32, 33] while involution of this gland can be induced by administering estrogen.[34, 35] Estrogen also prevents the thymus hyperplasia which would otherwise follow ovariectomy in the adult female rat. Chiodi[36] observed thymus atrophy in intact and castrate rats of both sexes following treatment with testosterone propionate, estrone or estradiol benzoate. Schacher and his associates[37] found that sterols which are closely related chemically to estrone, estradiol, and testosterone, but possess no estrogenic activity, exert no apparent inhibitory effect on the thymus. This would suggest that the thymus involution induced with the estrogens is related to their physiologic effect in the sexual sphere.

The inhibitory effect of the gonadal sex hormones may account for the observation that thymus involution is accelerated during pregnancy, while regeneration occurs soon after parturition. Thymus involution has been observed in laboratory animals following treatment with extracts of human pregnancy urine and pregnant mare's serum gonadotropin.[38, 39] This is apparently mediated through the gonads, for it can be prevented by gonadectomy.[40]

THE RELATION OF THE THYMUS TO OTHER GLANDS

Thymus-Anterior Hypophysis Relationship.—*The Thymus in Hypophyseal Function.*—It is not clear whether the thymus influences anterior pituitary function. Park and McClure[7] could see no significant change in the morphology or histology of the hypophysis following thymectomy. Clark and his associates,[41] on the other hand, noted pituitary enlargement and an increase in the number of acidophils in thymus fed rats.

The Anterior Hypophysis in Thymus Function.—That the anterior hypophysis exerts some influence over the thymus is suggested by the occurrence of thymus involution in Simmonds' disease[42] and following hypophysectomy in the rat[43] and dog,[44] and by the association of thymus hyperplasia with acromegaly.[45] The effects thus far obtained with anterior lobe extracts have varied. Evans and his associates[46] observed marked thymus involution following the administration of large doses of adrenocorticotropic hormone, but not after treatment with mammotropic extract. This effect was not prevented by gonadectomy or hypophysectomy. Watrin and Florentin[47] noted thymus involution in infantile guinea pigs bearing anterior lobe implants. They suggested that it was secondary to the thyroid hyperactivity caused by the implants. Kemp[48] found that in mice an anterior pituitary growth extract caused parallel growth of all organs except the thymus, which enlarged more than the rest. Uyldert and Freud,[43] who employed an anterior pituitary growth extract practically free of thyrotropic and gonadotropic activity, observed that the thymus doubled in size.

The Thymotropic Hormone.—The hope that the role of the thymus in growth and gonadal function may be clarified has been raised by the recent findings of Bomskov and associates.[26, 49] These observers claim to have isolated the specific thymus hormone, which is lipoid soluble and was therefore lacking in the earlier water soluble thymus extracts. According to these investigators, the thymus is the gland through which the anterior pituitary growth hormone produces its effect. They maintain that both the growth promoting and diabetogenic effects of anterior pituitary extracts are produced by a single hormone which acts by way of the thymus and may therefore appropriately be named *thymotropic* hormone. They report that destruction of the thymus by irradiation prevents the sharp fall in liver glycogen which would otherwise follow injection of the diabetogenic factor. On the other hand, their thymus hormone causes a drop in liver glycogen and also stimulates growth in thymus irradiated animals. In mature male rats, this extract reduced the size of the testes and accessory genitalia.[27] Confirmation of their findings is still lacking. According to Reinhardt and his associates,[28] anterior pituitary growth extract is effective in thymectomized animals. Since thymus hypertrophy is always seen in animals which respond to growth hormone,[29] it would seem that the "thymotropic" and growth principles are separate but closely associated chemically, or alternatively, that both stimulation of the thymus and of skeletal growth are independent effects of a single pituitary factor. Riddle's group[30] have tried to repeat part of Bomskov's experiment with a lipoid soluble extract of thymus tissue. Since world conditions prevented them from obtaining precise details as to the method of extraction employed by Bomskov, Riddle followed the brief description given in Bomskov's reports. The extract thus obtained produced no significant effect on growth in the young rat, chick, or pigeon, and no effect on liver glycogen or blood sugar in the rat or pigeon. No attempt was made to ascertain its effect on the gonads.

It is noteworthy that the thymus involution, produced by Evans[46] with adrenocorticotropic extract, was usually though not invariably associated with growth stunting or loss of body weight. From the available data, it would appear that anterior lobe extracts are capable of either stimulating or suppressing thymus function. The growth factor, or some principle closely associated with it, apparently stimulates, while the gonadotropic,[39] adrenocorticotropic,[46] and possibly also the thyrotropic factor[47] indirectly suppress thymus function.

Thymus-Thyroid Relationship.—The uncertainty regarding the role of the thymus also exists with respect to its relationship to the thyroid gland. It has been observed that thymus hypertrophy and *struma* are common in the new born in goitrous regions; that thymus hyperplasia and *goiter* are frequently associated in adults; that the thymus is often atrophic in *congenital myxedema*, and that thymus hyperplasia is not uncommon in Basedow's disease. It has been suggested that the lymphocytosis of Basedow's disease is related somehow to thymus enlargement. Hansmann[50] found that suppression of thymus function by the x-rays relieves the symptoms of *hyperthyroidism*, the results being more pronounced than might be expected with similar doses directed to the thyroid region.

Experimental Evidence.—Following thyroidectomy, some have observed thymus hyperplasia, others accelerated thymus involution. On the other hand, thyroid enlargement has been reported following thymectomy. In animals receiving thymus substance or implants, both stimulation and depression of thyroid function have been described. On the basis of the available evidence, Crotti[51] was led to conclude that the two glands are antagonistic. This view is borne out by Bomskov's[52] observation that a lipoid soluble extract of calves' thymus prevented the structural changes in the thyroid and the increase in the basal metabolic rate which would otherwise follow thyrotropic hormone administration in the guinea pig. As further proof of their antagonism, he points to the fact that the weight of the thyroid is low at the time of life when that of the thymus reaches its peak, and begins to increase when thymus involution begins. He concludes that the thymus hyperplasia noted in Basedow's disease is a compensatory reaction. Bomskov attributes the lymphocytosis of Basedow's disease to an excess of thymus hormone, on the basis of his observation[26] that his thymus extract could increase the number of lymphocytes in the blood of rats. He attributes the tendency to sudden heart failure in such

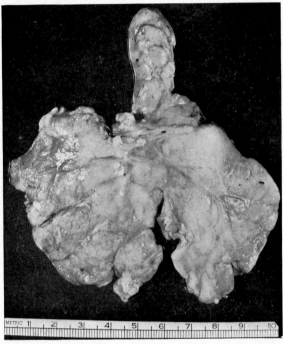

Fig. 51.—Thymus gland obtained from ten-year-old boy dying from hemorrhage and shock.

patients to the ability of the thymus hormone to cause loss of heart muscle glycogen. The relief which follows thyroidectomy, he believes, is partly due to slackening of thymus function following this operation.

Thymus-Adrenal Relationship.—An inhibitory effect of the adrenals on the thymus is suggested by the observation that the thymus enlarges following adrenalectomy,[53] or if already involuted, regenerates.[54] The rapid thymus involution, which is part of the so-called *alarm reaction* evoked by serious injury,[55] can be prevented by removing both adrenals. On the other hand, some degree of thymus involution can be induced in the adrenalectomized animal by administering adrenal cortical extract.[56] Kemp[57] observed that adrenal cortical extract had a beneficial effect on *status thymicolymphaticus* in children. Also noteworthy is Evans'[46] observation that anterior pituitary adrenocorticotropic extract caused a prompt reduction in size and complete regression of the thymus. Since this effect was like that obtained by Ingle[58] with adrenal cortical extract, Evans concluded that it was mediated through the adrenal cortex.

Whether the thymus in turn influences the adrenals is not certain. Following thymus feeding, some have observed a decrease in the size of the adrenals,[59] while others have described changes suggesting a stimulating effect.[60] Of interest is Segaloff's[61] observation that the growth curve and survival period of the bilaterally adrenalectomized rat was not influenced by thymectomy. He concludes that if the thymus is in any sense antagonistic to the adrenals, the antagonism is not such as to enable it to contribute towards producing the ill effects which follow adrenalectomy.

Thymus-Parathyroid Relationship.—A thymus-parathyroid antagonism is implied in the observation that salamander larvae which have no parathyroids, respond to thymus feeding with tetanic manifestations not unlike those exhibited by the parathyroidectomized mammal,[62] while tadpoles which develop parathyroids a few days after hatching, are unaffected by such treatment. On the basis of these observations, it has been suggested that the thymus produces tetany inducing substances whose removal or inactivation is a function of the parathyroids. This finds some support in Nitschke's[63] observation that thymus tissue yields an extract capable of lowering the serum calcium. On the other hand, it is apparently contradicted by reports that thymectomy does not significantly alter the morphology and histology of the parathyroids or appreciably affect calcium metabolism; and further, that parathyroid hormone administration is without effect on the histology of the thymus.

Thymus-Pancreas Relations.—A thymus-pancreas antagonism is suggested by Bentivoglio's[5] observation that irradiation of the thymus in dogs led to hypertrophy and hyperplasia of the islet tissue of the pancreas. The extent of the pancreatic modifications was directly proportional to the degree of thymic atrophy induced by the rays. If Bomskov[26, 52] is correct in assuming that the diabetogenic and thymotropic effects of anterior lobe extracts are due to a single hormone, and that the thymus hormone is immediately responsible for the loss of liver glycogen, hyperglycemia and glycosuria induced with diabetogenic extracts, it would follow that the function of the thymus and pancreatic islets are antagonistic. In view of Riddle's[30] negative findings, a definite conclusion on this point must await further investigation.

BIBLIOGRAPHY

1. Basch, K.: Wien. klin. Wchnschr. *16*:893, 1903; Jahrb. f. Kinderh. *64*:289, 1908.
2. Klose, H., and Vogt, H.: Beitr. z. klin. Chir., Tübingen *69*:1, 1910.
3. Einhorn, N. H., and Rowntree, L. G.: Science *83*:443, 1936; Endocrinol. *21*:659, 1937.
4. Shay, H., Gershon-Cohen, J., Fels, S. S., Meranze, D. R., and Meranze, T.: J.A.M.A. *112*:290, 1939.
5. Bentivoglio, G. C., and Fumi, C.: Sperimentale. Arch. di biol. *9*:219, 1937.
6. Nordmann, O.: Deut. med. Wchnschr. *40*:1702, 1914.
7. Park, E. A., and McClure, R. D.: Am. J. Dis. Child. *68*:317, 1919.

8. Hashimoto, E. I., and Freudenberger, C. B.: J.A.M.A. *112*:1680, 1939.
9. Chiodi, H.: Compt. rend. Soc. de biol. *130*:298, 1939.
10. Segaloff, A., and Nelson, W. O.: Am. J. Physiol. *130*:671, 1940.
11. Gudernatsch, J. F.: Am. J. Anat. *15*:431, 1914.
12. Romeis, B.: Arch. f. Entwcklngsmechn. d. Organ. *37*:571, 1914.
13. Asher, L.: Endokrinol. *7*:321, 1930; Wien. med. Wchnschr. *84*:565, 1934.
14. Rowntree, L. G., Clark, J. H., Hanson, A. M., and Steinberg, A.: J.A.M.A. *103*:1425, 1934; Arch. Int. Med. *56*:1, 1935.
15. Burrill, M. W., and Ivy, A. C.: Endocrinol. *28*:94, 1941.
16. Glanzmann, E.: Jahrb. f. Kinderh. *101*:1, 1923.
17. Marangoni, P.: Boll. d. Soc. med.-chir., Pavia *48*:41, 1934.
18. Einhorn, N. H., and Rowntree, L. G.: Science *84*:23, 1936.
19. Gudernatsch, J. F.: Med. Rec. *146*:101, 1937.
20. Hoffman, O., and Gudernatsch, J. F.: Am. J. Physiol. *97*:527, 1931; Proc. Soc. Exper. Biol. & Med. *28*:731, 1931; Am. J. Physiol. *113*:67 (Proc.) 1935.
21. Rowntree, L. G., Clark, J. H., Steinberg, A., and Einhorn, N. H.: New York State Med. J. *36*:1277, 1936.
22. Rowntree, L. G., Steinberg, A., Einhorn, N. H., and Schaffer, N. K.: Endocrinol. *23*:584, 1938.
23. Schaffer, N. K., Ziegler, W. M., and Rowntree, L. G.: Endocrinol. *23*:593, 1938.
24. Andersen, D. H.: Physiol. Rev. *12*:1, 1932.
25. Groebbels, F.: Arch. f. d. ges. Physiol. *235*:26, 1934.
26. Bomskov, C., and Sladovic, L.: Deutsche Ztschr. f. Chir. *253*:563, 1940.
27. Bomskov, C., and Lipps, H. G.: Endokrinol. *23*:239, 1941.
28. Reinhardt, W. O., Marx, W., and Evans, H. M.: Proc. Soc. Exper. Biol. & Med. *49*:473, 1942.
29. Evans, H. M.: J.A.M.A. *117*:287, 1941.
30. Wells, B. B., Riddle, O., and Marvin, H. N.: Proc. Soc. Exper. Biol. & Med. *49*:473, 1942.
31. Chiodi, H.: Compt. rend. Soc. de biol. *130*:457, 1939.
32. Moore, C. R.: Am. J. Anat. *59*:63, 1936.
33. Lauson, H., Heller, C. G., and Sevringhaus, E. L.: Endocrinol. *21*:735, 1937.
34. Selye, H., Harlow, C. M., and Collip, J. B.: Endokrinol. *18*:81, 1936.
35. Bühler, F.: Ztschr. f. d. ges. exper. Med. *98*:151, 1936.
36. Chiodi, H.: Compt. rend. Soc. de biol. *129*:1258, 1938.
37. Schacher, J., Browne, J. S. L., and Selye, H.: Proc. Soc. Exper. Biol. & Med. *36*:488, 1936.
38. Klein, F.: Klin. Wchnschr. *15*:371, 1936.
39. Evans, H. M., and Simpson, M. E.: Anat. Rec. *60*:423, 1934.
40. Butcher, E. O., and Persike, E. C.: Endocrinol. *23*:501, 1938.
41. Clark, J. H., Steinberg, A., and Rowntree, L. G.; Proc. Soc. Exper. Biol. & Med. *35*:239, 1936.
42. Altman, F.: Ztschr. f. Path. *36*:393, 1928.
43. Uyldert, I. E., and Freud, J.: Acta brev. Neerland. *8*:188, 1938.
44. Houssay, B. A., and Lascano-Gonzalez, J. M.: Compt. rend. Soc. de biol. *117*:463, 1934.
45. Hammar, J. A.: Die Menschenthymus in Gesundheit und Krankheit. Leipzig, Akademische Verlagsgesellschaft M. B. H., 1926–29.
46. Evans, H. M., Moon, H., Simpson, M. E., and Lyons, W. R.: Proc. Soc. Exper. Biol. & Med. *38*:419, 1938.
47. Watrin, J., and Florentin, P.: Compt. rend. Soc. de biol. *110*:1161, 1932.
48. Kemp, T.: Klin. Wchnschr. *13*:1854, 1934.
49. Bomskov, C., and Holscher, B.: Ztschr. f. klin. Med. *137*:745, 1940.
50. Hansmann, F. S.: Med. J. Australia *2*:402, 1939.
51. Crotti, A.: Diseases of the Thyroid, Parathyroids, and Thymus. Philadelphia, Lea & Febiger, 1938, chap. 48, pp. 978–1040.
52. Bomskov, C., and Spiegel, R.: Endokrinol. *23*:225, 1941.
53. Auld, A. G.: Brit. Med. J. *1*:1327, 1899.
54. Marine, D., Manley, O. T., and Baumann, E. J.: J. Exper. Med. *40*:429, 1924.
55. Selye, H.: Nature, London *138*:32, 1936.
56. Selye, H.: Brit. J. Exper. Path. *17*:234, 1936.

57. Kemp, W. N.: Brit. Med. J. *1*:1194, 1937.
58. Ingle, D. J.: Unpublished, cited by Evans et al. (*supra* 44).
59. Clark, J. H., Steinberg, A., and Rowntree, L. G.: Proc. Soc. Exper. Biol. & Med. *35*: 143, 1936.
60. Tislowitz, R., and Chodkowska, S.: Compt. rend. Soc. de biol. *122*:841, 1936.
61. Segaloff, A., and Nelson, W. O.: Am. J. Physiol. *128*:475, 1940.
62. Uhlenhuth, E.: Proc. Soc. Exper. Biol. & Med. *16*:70, 1918.
63. Nitschke, A.: Ztschr. f. d. ges. exper. Med. *65*:637, 1929.
64. Segaloff, A., and Nelson, W. O.: Endocrinol. *29*:483, 1941.
65. Sherrod, T. R., and Struck, H. C.: Growth *7*:11, 1943.

CHAPTER XXI

THE PHYSIOLOGY OF THE PINEAL BODY

Despite the mass of experimental data relating to the function of the pineal body, our knowledge on this point is vague. Some observers consider this structure a vestigial organ analogous to the median or parietal eye of some of the lower vertebrates. Cowdry[1] calls attention to the fact that the pineal body is not associated with the alimentary tract at any stage of its development, and is derived from ectoderm which possesses sensory rather than incretory potentialities. On the other hand, there are competent investigators[2] who believe that the pineal region is "preponderately glandiferous" in its derivatives. According to Calvet,[3] the pineal represents a fusion of an ancestral photoreceptor apparatus and a hormonal apparatus, one of which has regressed while the other progressed. He believes that the hormonal part performs a gonadotropic function. Horrax,[4] who has done considerable research on the function of this structure, is of the opinion that an endocrine function may not yet be definitely ascribed to it. The existing confusion arises partly from the fact that, at one point in the course of its embryonic development, the pineal body apparently assumes the form of a gland, but loses its glandular structure very early in postnatal life.

Our present concept of pineal physiology rests largely upon the results of ablation experiments, the effects obtained with pineal implants and extracts, and the symptomatology associated with pineal neoplasms.

EXPERIMENTAL STUDIES OF PINEAL FUNCTION

Effects of Pinealectomy.—The evidence provided by earlier ablation experiments was unsatisfactory because of the high mortality rate incident to this operation. Though some reported negative results, many of the earlier investigators described acceleration of body growth, adiposity, and precocious development of the secondary sex characters following surgical removal of the pineal body. In more recent experiments with an improved pinealectomy technique, which has helped to minimize the injury to important adjacent areas in the midbrain, the results have for the most part been negative. Thus Dandy[5] found that young as well as mature dogs, who survived the operation three to fifteen months, showed no apparent alterations in the endocrine glands, or in somatic or genital growth. He concluded that the pineal is not indispensable to life and is not essential to the general well-being of the individual. D'Amour and D'Amour,[6] who performed pinealectomy in successive generations of rats, observed no appreciable change in the first and second generation. In the third and fourth generations, they noted a significant weight gain, but no acceleration of sexual development. In a similar experiment carried out by Rowntree and his associates,[7] retardation of growth and acceleration of sexual development was observed.

These divergent results may perhaps best be explained by assuming that positive effects, where noted, were due to concomitant injury to some midbrain center or centers which regulate the rate of sexual and somatic maturation and not to loss of some pineal hormone.

Effects of Pineal Feeding and Implants.—The effects noted following pineal feeding have likewise been inconstant and contradictory. Dana and Berkeley[8] found that young guinea pigs, cats and rabbits which were fed calf's pineal, responded with an appreciable gain in weight and size. McCord and Allen[9] observed that tadpoles so treated grew to twice the size of the controls. Adair and Chidester,[10] also working with tadpoles, found that pineal feeding hastened metamorphosis, though not to the degree obtained with thyroid substance. When treatment was discontinued, development proceeded at a slower rate, but was once more abruptly accelerated on resumption of pineal feeding. In contrast to these reports, Hoskins,[11] Kozelka,[12] and others could observe no appreciable effect on growth following pineal feeding. Goddard,[13] who fed pineal substance to dwarfed children, failed to note any improvement.

The reported effects of pineal implants have likewise been highly divergent, some describing an increased rate of growth and others no effect, or a definite inhibition of sexual development associated with normal somatic growth. Engel[14] observed that pineal implants delayed the appearance of estrus following administration of estrogen. Fleischmann and Goldhammer[15] could inhibit the estrus cycles of adult female rodents with implants of pineal tissue from immature but not from mature animals.

Effects of Pineal Extracts.—Anti-growth, anti-gonadotropic, estrogenic and anti-estrogenic effects have been described following the administration of pineal extracts.

Somatic Growth.—Engel,[14] employing *Epiphysan*, an extract of pineal tissue, observed inhibition of growth in his test animals. Rowntree and associates,[7] who administered an extract prepared by Hanson, to successive generations of rats, found that growth was retarded and differentiation accelerated in the offspring of treated animals. Fourteen day old rats of the fifth generation weighed only 8 gm. as compared with 20 gm. for the controls. In animals of the sixth generation, eruption of teeth and opening of the eyes occurred on the fifth day of life, when their weight was under 5 gm.

Gonadal Function.—An anti-gonadotropic effect has been reported by Engel,[16] who inhibited the action of 10 rat units of gonadotropic hormone with one-fourth to one-half of a human pineal. Both the follicle-stimulating and luteinizing effects were suppressed, though inhibition of the latter was more pronounced. Fleischmann and Goldhammer,[17] and Wade,[18] employing Engel's extract, were unable to confirm his findings. Wade found that extracts representing one to four beef pineals had no anti-gonadotropic effect in the infantile rat.

A stimulative effect of the pineal body on the gonads is implied in

Vinal's[19] observation that macerated pineal tissue augmented the action of pregnancy urine extract in the rabbit. A gonad-stimulating effect has also been reported by Rowntree and associates,[20] who found that the administration of Hanson's pineal extract to successive generations of rats caused precocious sexual development.

Silberstein and Engel[21] induced estrus in spayed mice with implants or extracts of pineal tissue from steers or calves. Saphir[22] obtained a similar effect with human pineal implants. The estrus-inducing substance present in pineal extracts differs from the estrogen derived from the ovary and placenta in that it is not soluble in alcohol, ethyl ether, or acetone. Silberstein and Engel[21] obtained 16 mouse units of estrogenic substance from a steer's pineal weighing 640 mg., while Saphir[22] demonstrated 2 to 3 mouse units in 150 mg. of human pineal tissue. On the other hand, calf pineals have been used by Tarkham[23] with negative results, and Wade[18] has reported that extracts made from 4 to 9.5 beef pineals failed to induce estrus in adult spayed rats.

PINEAL TUMORS

Clinical evidence suggesting that the pineal body plays an important part in the regulation of somatic and sexual development is provided by a small group of cases of pineal tumor associated with somatic and sexual precocity. This syndrome, which occurs almost exclusively in males and is usually referred to as *macrogenitosomia praecox*, is characterized by an astonishing physical, mental, and sexual precocity, associated with neurologic and metabolic disturbances. The observation that somatic and sexual precocity may arise in the absence of pineal pathology, while conversely pineal tumors may arise during the prepuberal years without evidence of precocity[24, 25, 26] has led some observers to deny that the precocity sometimes associated with pineal tumor is attributable to a disturbance in the incretory function of this structure (see Chap. XXXV).

In view of the confused state of the available evidence, an endocrine function may not yet be ascribed to the pineal body.

BIBLIOGRAPHY

1. Cowdry, E. V.: The Anatomy, Embryology, Comparative Anatomy and Histology of the Pineal, in, Endocrinology and Metabolism. New York, Appleton & Co., 1922, vol. 5, p. 3.
2. Tilney, F., and Warren, L. F.: Am. Anat. Mem. Wistar Inst. Anat. No. 9, 1922.
3. Calvet, J.: L'Epiphyse. Paris, J. B. Baillière et fils, 1934.
4. Horrax, G.: Arch. Int. Med. *17*:627, 1916.
5. Dandy, W. E.: Surg., Gynec. & Obst. *33*:113, 1921.
6. D'Amour, M. C., and D'Amour, F. E.: Proc. Soc. Exper. Biol. & Med. *37*:244, 1937.
7. Rowntree, L. G., Clark, J. H., Steinberg, A., and Hanson, A. M.: J.A.M.A. *106*:370, 1936.
8. Dana, C. L., and Berkeley, W. N.: Med. Rec. *83*:835, 1913.
9. McCord, C. P., and Allen, M.: J. Exper. Zool. *23*:207, 1917.
10. Adair, J., and Chidester, F. E.: Endocrinol. *12*:791, 1928.
11. Hoskins, R. G.: The Tides of Life. New York, W. W. Norton & Co., 1933.
12. Kozelka, A. W.: Proc. Soc. Exper. Biol. & Med. *30*:842, 1933.
13. Goddard, H. H.: J.A.M.A., *68*:1340, 1917.

14. Engel, P.: Wien. klin. Wchnschr. *16:*481, 1935.
15. Fleischmann, W., and Goldhammer, H.: Klin. Wchnschr. *14:*415, 1935.
16. Engel, P.: Ztschr. f. d. ges. exper. Med. *95:*149, 441, 1935.
17. Fleischmann, W., and Goldhammer, H.: Klin. Wchnschr. *15:*1047, 1936.
18. Wade, N. J.: Endocrinol. *21:*681, 1937.
19. Vinals, E.: Compt. rend. Soc. de biol. *119:*259, 1935.
20. Rowntree, L. G., Clark, J. H., Steinberg, A., Hanson, A. M., Einhorn, N. J., and Shannon, W. A.: Ann. Int. Med. *9:*359, 1935.
21. Silberstein, F., and Engel, P.: Klin. Wchnschr. *12:*908, 1933.
22. Saphir, W.: Endocrinol. *18:*625, 1934.
23. Tarkham, A. A.: Endokrinol. *18:*234, 1937.
24. Wirth, W.: Zentralbl. f. Konstlehre *15:*477, 1930.
25. Krabbe, K. H.: Pineal Body, in, Cyclopedia of Medicine. Philadelphia, F. A. Davis Co., 1934, vol. 9, pp. 861–868.
26. Dandy, W. E.: Arch. Surg. *33:*19, 1936.

CHAPTER XXII

THE ANTI-HORMONES

Definition.—The term *anti-hormones* is applied to inhibitory substances of obscure origin which appear in the blood serum of animals subjected to prolonged treatment with certain hormonal preparations. The existence of these substances was first suspected when Loeb[1] and Collip[2] observed that chronic treatment with anterior pituitary thyrotropic extract resulted in a state of refractoriness to the effects of the injected substance. Collip and Anderson[3] demonstrated that the refractory state thus induced is associated with, and apparently due to the formation of inhibitory substances. They showed that blood serum of rats rendered refractory to thyrotropic hormone, when injected into untreated, nonresistant rats, prevented their response to simultaneously administered thyrotropic extract. Antihormone sera have since been produced in the guinea pig, rabbit, goat, horse, dog, monkey and man, and have been shown to form against the growth,[3] gonadotropic,[4] lactogenic,[5] ketogenic,[6] and diabetogenic[7] principle of the anterior pituitary. Blood-borne inhibitory substances have also been demonstrated following chronic treatment with adrenal cortical[8] and thymus[9] extracts, and with gonadotropic substances from the blood and urine of pregnant women,[10] urine of males with teratoma testis,[11] and blood of pregnant mares.[12]

THE NATURE OF THE ANTI-HORMONES

Theory of Inhibitory Substances.—The nature of these hormone-inhibiting substances has been the subject of considerable speculation. According to Collip and his associates,[3] there is, for each hormone, an opposite, antagonistic principle, or anti-hormone. These, they believe, are normal constituents of the blood and tissues, and serve as buffers against the positively acting hormones. They assume that in the normal individual the inhibitory substances are so balanced against the hormones as to make for normal endocrine function. Under such conditions, their presence is masked, but where the balance between hormones and anti-hormones is upset in favor of the latter, they become demonstrable in the blood and give rise to a hypofunctional state. This theory immediately aroused considerable interest and a large body of evidence, of a conflicting nature, has accumulated since its announcement. Space permits mention of only a few of the arguments thus far presented for and against this hypothesis.

Collip's theory finds support in reports than anti-thyrotropic[13, 14] and anti-gonadotropic[15, 16] substances are demonstrable in the blood of some normal, untreated animals, as well as in some castrate[15] and amenorrheic women.[17] This would seem to imply that hormone inhibiting substances may appear spontaneously and tends to substantiate Collip's suggestion that they are normal constituents of the blood. It should be emphasized, however, that there is no proof that these spontaneously occurring inhibitory substances are identical with those which form in response to chronically administered hormonal extracts, or that their presence is constantly associated with hypofunctional states. A few investigators have reported negative findings in patients with hypogonadism.[18, 19]

In support of Collip's theory, several observers have presented evidence indicating that anti-hormone sera are specific neither for species nor source.[4, 20, 21, 22] In view of the fact that other competent observers[23, 24] have reported diametrically opposite results, this evidence is inconclusive. Perhaps the most cogent argument in favor of Collip's interpretation is provided by reports that anti-hormone sera are apparently effective against endogenous hormones. Collip[25] found that serum of horses refractory to thyrotropic hormone lowered the basal metabolic rate of untreated nonresistant animals. In a later study,[20] they noted that normal cyclic rats, receiving anti-serum to sheep pituitary gonadotropic extract, became acyclic and did not conceive when mated. Parkes and Rowlands[26] and Thompson and Cushing[22] have reported that anti-sera to ox pituitary extract depressed the gonads of normal guinea pigs, producing changes not unlike those seen after hypophysectomy. In the pregnant animal, similar treatment was found to interrupt gestation.[27, 28] Severinghaus and Thompson[29] observed atrophy of the thyroid and gonads in dogs chronically treated with anterior lobe extract. On the basis of the cytologic appearance of the pituitary of their test animals, they attributed the thyroid and gonadal atrophy to "physiological hypophysectomy," resulting from neutralization of the hypophyseal hormones by antagonistic substances which form against the chronically administered extract.

In contrast to these reports, Van Wagenen and Cole[30] have observed that, in monkeys receiving mare's serum hormone, the gonads were activated at first, regressed and remained quiescent for two to six months, but then resumed their function despite continued treatment. Kraatz and Nice[9] found that anti-thymus serum, when administered to juvenile animals, did not delay sexual maturation or interfere with subsequent reproductive function, though such serum could completely inhibit the maturity-accelerating effect of thymus extract.

Immunologic Theory.—Some investigators maintain that the so-called anti-hormone phenomenon is a purely immunological reaction, in which the chronically administered extract acts as an antigen, and the inhibitory substances are detectable as antibodies. As proof, they point out that the anterior pituitary preparations, which so readily elicit the formation of hormone-inhibiting substances, are contaminated by the protein of the species from which they are obtained. On the other hand, insulin, thyroid extract, as well as crystalline estrogen, progesterone, and androgens, against which serologically transferable antagonistic substances apparently do not form,[31, 32, 33] are free from such impurities. Significant

19

in this connection is the observation[34] that a refractory state can be induced with crude adrenal cortical extracts but not with chemically pure preparations, such as corticosterone.

As additional arguments in favor of this interpretation, it has been pointed out that (1) sub-threshold quantities of hormone are as efficient as large doses in producing a refractory state;[35] (2) refractoriness develops against crude pituitary extracts but not against relatively pure extracts or those from which the antigenic complex has been removed;[36, 37] (3) anti-serum against pregnancy urine gonadotropin can be produced by protracted administration of male urine extract prepared by the same method used to concentrate pregnancy urine gonadotropic extract;[38] (4) the level of precipitins parallels the anti-gonadotropic activity of the blood in animals chronically treated with gonadotropic extract;[39] (5) anti-gonadotropic substances are not demonstrable in the blood of puerperal women despite the presence of large amounts of gonadotropic hormone throughout gestation;[23, 40] and (6) pregnancy urine gonadotropic extracts cause anti-serum formation despite destruction of most of their gonadotropic activity by boiling or other means.[35]

Evidence favoring the immunologic theory has also been provided by *parabiotic experiments.*[41, 42] It has been shown that when one partner to a parabiotic union is ovariectomized, the gonads of the other are thereafter subjected to stimulation by gonadotropic hormones from the hypophysis of both animals. A situation is thus created in which endogenously supplied hormones, free of contaminating impurities, can act over a protracted period of time. It is significant that the ovaries of the intact partner do not develop a state of refractoriness even after being exposed for a year or more to hormones from the castrate partner's pituitary.

From the foregoing discussion, it is apparent that the existence of anti-hormones, as defined by Collip, is still questionable. The confused and conflicting state of the available evidence makes it difficult to reach a final decision as to the true nature of the inhibitory substances which form against certain hormonal extracts. Whether they are immune bodies in the ordinary sense, or a new type of blood substance closely related to the immune bodies, as Zondek and Sulman[19] believe, is a question which must remain open for the present.

Source of Anti-Hormones.—The source of the inhibitory substances in anti-hormone sera is likewise uncertain. Anti-thyrotropic substances apparently do not originate in the hypophysis[43, 44] or thyroid,[45] since they form in the absence of these glands. Scowen and Spence[14] have suggested the adrenal cortex as a possible source, but the evidence on which they base their assumption is unconvincing. The anti-gonadotropic substances apparently are not derived from the ovary, for they can be produced in the gonadectomized animal.[46] Engel[47] has suggested that they may form in the pineal, on the basis of his failure to demonstrate them in the blood of pinealectomized animals chronically treated with gonadotropic extract. The studies of Gordon and his associates[48, 49] strongly indicate that the reticulo-endothelial system is the probable source of the anti-hormones.

Mode of Action.—Obscurity also surrounds the mode of action of these hormone-antagonizing substances. Conceivably they may either act on the receptor organ, or directly neutralize the positively acting hormones in the body tissues and fluids. Okkels[50] believes that the inhibitory effect of anti-thyrotropic serum is not a simple matter of neutralization, and suggests that some as yet undefined extra-thyroid mechanism is involved. Until more is known of the nature of these substances, the question of their mode of action must remain unanswered.

Clinical Significance.—From the clinical standpoint, the existence of hormone-inhibiting substances is significant. Since they form in response to prolonged treatment with certain hormone preparations, particularly against mare's serum gonadotropin,[51, 52] and gonadotropic[53] and other[54] extracts of animal pituitary, it is obvious that such preparations can have only a limited therapeutic value. If used for long periods, they may tend to aggravate the deficiency which they are intended to correct. On the other hand, the fact that such inhibitory substances can be produced at will in experimental animals has raised the hope that they may prove useful for the control of certain hyperfunctional states. Whether this expectation is justified cannot be decided from the limited clinical evidence at hand. Recognition of the "anti-hormone phenomenon" serves to emphasize the desirability of correcting hypofunctional states by non-endocrine measures, calculated to improve the general condition of the individual and thus increase the endogenous supply of hormone, against which no inhibitory substances are known to form.

BIBLIOGRAPHY

1. Loeb, L., and Friedman, H.: Proc. Soc. Exper. Biol. & Med. *29*:172, 1931.
2. Collip, J. B.: Ann. Int. Med. *8*:10, 1934.
3. Collip, J. B., and Anderson, E. M.: Lancet *1*:76, 1934.
4. Gegerson, H. B., Clark, A. R., and Kurzrok, R.: Proc. Soc. Exper. Biol. & Med. *32*: 193, 1936.
5. Young, F. G.: J. Physiol. *92*:4P, 1938.
6. Black, P. T., Collip, J. B., and Thomson, D. L.: J. Physiol. *82*:385, 1934; ibid. *84*:15, 1935.
7. Dohan, F. C., and Lukens, F. D. W.: Proc Soc. Exper. Biol. & Med. *42*:167, 1939.
8. Toby, C. G., and Lewis, L. A.: Proc. Soc. Exper. Biol. & Med. *37*:352, 1937.
9. Kraatz, C. P., and Nice, L. B.: Am. J. Physiol. *123*:123 (Proc.), 1938.
10. Harington, C. R., and Rowlands, I. W.: Biochem. J. *31*:2049, 1937.
11. Twombly, G. H., and Ferguson, R. S.: Proc. Soc. Exper. Biol. & Med. *32*:69, 1934.
12. Meyer, R. K., and Gustus, E. L.: Science *81*:208, 1935.
13. Eisenhardt, L., and Thompson, K. W.: Yale J. Biol. & Med. *5*:507, 1939.
14. Scowen, E. F., and Spence, A. W.: J. Physiol. *86*:109, 1936.
15. Laroche, G., and Simmonet, H.: Compt. rend. Soc. de biol. *121*:416, 1936.
16. Engel, P.: Wien. klin. Wchnschr. *1*:481, 1935.
17. Takahashi, K.: Ztschr. f. Geburtsh. u. Gynäk. *118*:391, 1939.
18. Fellows, M. D.: Endocrinol. *26*:369, 1940.
19. Zondek, B., and Sulman, F.: The Antigonadotropic Factor. Baltimore, Williams & Wilkins Co., 1942.
20. Collip, J. B.: Canad. M. A. J. *36*:99, 1937.
21. Rowlands, I. W.: Proc. Roy. Soc. London, s.B. *121*:517, 1937.
22. Thompson, K. W., and Cushing, H.: Proc. Roy. Soc. London, s.B. *121*:501, 1937.
23. Fluhmann, C. F.: Proc. Soc. Exper. Biol. & Med. *32*:1595, 1935; Am. J. Obst. & Gynec. *30*:584, 1935.

24. Kupperman, H. S., Mellish, C. H., and McShan, W. H.: Proc. Soc. Exper. Biol. & Med. *48*:79, 1941.
25. Collip, J. B., and Anderson, E. M.: Lancet *1*:784, 1934.
26. Parkes, A. S., and Rowlands, I. W.: J. Physiol. *88*:305, 1936.
27. Thompson, K. W., and Cushing, H.: Proc. Roy. Soc. London, s.B. *115*:88, 1934.
28. Thompson, K. W.: Endocrinol. *24*:613, 1939.
29. Severinghaus, A. E., and Thompson, K. W.: Am. J. Path. *15*:391, 1939.
30. Van Wagenen, G., and Cole, H. H.: Am. J. Physiol. *123*:208 (Proc.), 1938.
31. Black, P. T.: Brit. J. Exper. Path. *14*:318, 1935.
32. Selye, H.: Am. J. Physiol. *130*:358, 1940.
33. D'Amour, F. E., Dumont, C., and Gustavson, R. G.: Proc. Soc. Exper. Biol. & Med. *32*:192, 1934.
34. Hartman, F. A., Lewis, L. A., and Gabriel, J. E.: Endocrinol. *24*:197, 1940.
35. Twombly, G. H.: Endocrinol. *20*:311, 1936.
36. Werner, S. C.: Proc. Soc. Exper. Biol. & Med. *34*:390, 1936.
37. Rowlands, I. W., and Young, F. G.: J. Physiol. *95*:410, 1939.
38. Fremery, P. de, and Scheygrond, B.: Nature, London *139*:1015, 1937.
39. Wolfe, H. R., and Meyer, R. K.: Anat. Rec. *70*(Suppl.):46, 1937.
40. Zondek, B., and Sulman, F.: Proc. Soc. Exper. Biol. & Med. *42*:342, 1939.
41. DuShane, G. P., Levine, W. T., Pfeiffer, C. A., and Witschi, E.: Proc. Soc. Exper. Biol. & Med. *33*:339, 1935.
42. McCahey, J. F., Soloway, D., and Hansen, L. P.: Penna. M. A. J. *39*:228, 1936.
43. Collip, J. B., and Anderson, E. M.: J.A.M.A. *104*:965, 1935.
44. Bachman, C., Collip, J. B., and Selye, H.: Proc. Soc. Exper. Biol. & Med. *32*:544, 1934.
45. Oudet, P.: Compt. rend. Soc. de biol. *123*:1180, 1937.
46. Honda, K.: Jap. J. Obst. & Gynec. *24*:19, 1941.
47. Engel, P.: Klin. Wchnschr. *14*:970, 1935.
48. Gordon, A. S., Kleinberg, W., and Charipper, H. A.: Anat. Rec. *70*(Suppl.):49, 1937; Proc. Soc. Exper. Biol. & Med. *36*:484, 1937; J. Exper. Med. *70*:333, 1939.
49. Gordon, A. S., Levenstein, I., and Charipper, H. A.: Am. J. Physiol. *129*:364, 1940.
50. Okkels, H.: J. Exper. Med. *66*:305, 1937.
51. Rowlands, I. W., and Spence, A. W.: Brit. Med. J. *2*:947, 1939.
52. Jailer, W., and Leathem, J. H.: Proc. Soc. Exper. Biol. & Med. *45*:506, 1940.
53. Meyer, R. K., and Severinghaus, E. L., cited by R. K. Meyer, and H. R. Wolfe, in, J. Immun. *37*:91, 1939.
54. Boom, H.: Nederland. tijdschr. v. Geneesk. *80*:3336, 1936; ibid. *82*:5731, 1938.

PART II

CLINIC

CHAPTER XXIII

ADOLESCENCE

Definition.—Adolescence describes the transitional period between childhood and adulthood. Puberty is that phase in the maturation process during which sex characters and functions make their appearance.[1] Under normal conditions, adolescence begins shortly before or after the end of the first decade of life and is completed during the early part of the third decade. Some observers divide it into three stages: (1) beginning of pubescence; (2) height of pubescence or adolescence; and (3) completion of adolescence, or maturity.

This epoch is of great physiologic significance, for its course determines to a large extent the subsequent physical and mental status of the individual. It is characterized by alterations in which the entire organism participates, and as a result of which the child gradually attains somatic and sexual maturity. Zeller[2] distinguishes between "qualitative" and "quantitative" sex ripening. The former, usually achieved by the eighteenth year, involves the appearance of all sex characters which distinguish the female from the male. "Quantitative" sex ripening, on the other hand, implies the full somatic and sexual development which characterizes the mature woman and is normally attained between the twentieth and thirtieth year.

SEXUAL ALTERATIONS

Secondary Sex Characters.—The changes in the gonads and accessory genitalia between childhood and maturity are described in detail elsewhere (see Chap. I), and only the external manifestations of puberal sex ripening will be considered here. In the average normal girl, development of the secondary sex characters begins after the eighth or ninth year. The angular, boyish figure of the prepuberal child is gradually transformed into the more rounded, soft and undulating contours characteristic of the postadolescent young woman. Differences between male and female, already noticeable at the age of eight, become more accentuated by the eleventh or twelfth year, when the female pelvis widens and there is a marked increase in adipose tissue, particularly about the shoulders, thorax, breasts, hips, buttocks and mons veneris. The calves become heavier than those of the male. In contrast to the male, whose thighs are columnar in shape, those of the female suggest an inverted cone and show a tendency to obliquity which, if exaggerated, may result in knock-knees and a peculiar way of running.

The breasts gradually develop and assume the firm, full, hemispherical contour which characterizes those of the normal mature woman. Pubic hair usually appears after the breast changes and before the first menstrual flow, while axillary hair as a rule makes its appearance at a later date. At the same time, structural modifications in the larynx raise the pitch of the voice. As Pryor[3] has recently emphasized, the "interrelationships among certain secondary sex characters suggest themselves as criteria of a physiologic age which is much more constant than chronological age for predicting the onset of the catamenia."

Menarche.—In the female, the initial appearance of the menstrual flow, usually referred to as the *menarche*, is the most conspicuous event of the puberal epoch. The terms "menarche" and *puberty* are often considered synonymous and used interchangeably, but this practice is erroneous, since the phenomena they describe are not identical. Menarche, it must be emphasized, is merely one of many manifestations of the puberal period, and does not necessarily mark either its inception or completion. In the words of Engle,[4] "in relation to time, puberty is an area in the life of an individual in which menarche is only a readily determinable point."

Factors Controlling Age of Onset.—The age at which the menstrual flow first appears varies widely and apparently depends upon racial, constitutional, and environmental factors. Thus the menses appear earlier in the Semitic and Oriental than in the Aryan and Slavic races. The importance of *climatic* and *racial factors* is implied in the observation[5] that Hindu and Mohammedan girls of India begin to menstruate several years earlier than English girls born and raised in India; and that the latter menstruate earlier than English girls living in England. Ito[28] recently compared the average menarcheal age of Japanese, Chinese, Mexican, Negro and white women residing in Southern California, with that of the same races residing elsewhere. He found the average age for each race earlier than for its respective race elsewhere, "the degree of difference depending on its racial characteristic constitutionality."

The impression that menstrual function is achieved at an earlier age in warmer climates has been contradicted by Mills,[6] who found that individuals inhabiting the stimulating temperate regions menstruate two years earlier than those residing in the tropical zones. Of interest in this connection is Engle and Schlesnyak's[7] observation that, among girls living in temperate climates, the first flow appears less often during the hot summer months than during the cooler seasons of the year. Also significant is Mills'[8] recent report that the trend toward earlier menarcheal age and greater height, observed during the past half century, has shown a reversal in recent years in the lower latitudes, where a general trend towards higher temperatures has especially made itself felt.

Constitutional factors also influence the age of the menarche. The individual of broad, rugged build tends to menstruate earlier than the tall, slender girl.[9, 10, 11, 12] Observers[13, 14] differ as to whether blondes or brunettes menstruate earlier. Environment is apparently likewise a determining factor. In countries where the population is sharply divided into an upper and lower class, the menarche occurs earlier in the former, due probably to better hygiene and nutrition.[15]

The average age of the menarche in women residing in the United States is between the thirteenth and fourteenth year. In a series of 250 cases collected by Engle and Shelesnyak,[7] the age of the first flow varied from 11 to 16 years, the average being 13.5 years. This figure is close to the 13.9 years obtained by Engelmann[16] in a series of 10,000 cases. In European women, the menarche occurs from one to two years later. Recent studies have tended to emphasize the fact that the first menstrual flow is not necessarily followed by regular periods. On the contrary, the succeeding periods usually occur at fairly long and irregular intervals, and a considerable time may elapse before normal periodicity is established.

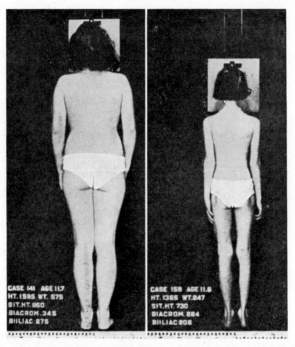

Fig. 52.—Standardized photographs of a linear and a lateral girl matched for chronological age. Girl on the right lagged behind one on the left two and a half years in ossification, and four years in the establishment of the catamenia. (Pryor, H. B., and Carter, H. D.: California & West. Med. Vol. 48.)

In Engle and Shelesnyak's[7] series of 250 cases, an average of 40 cycles intervened between the first flow and establishment of a normal menstrual rhythm.

Adolescent Sterility.—The appearance of the menses does not necessarily imply that the individual has acquired the ability to conceive. Mills and Ogle,[17] on the basis of statistics on menarche, marriage and first delivery ages, concluded that adolescent sterility is a very real phenomenon. Ashley-Montagu,[18] who reviewed the literature on human fertility, observed that females under twenty conceive much less readily and frequently than those between 20 and 30 years of age, and that optimal conditions for reproduction exist at 23 ± 2 years. He concluded that "menarche and the attainment of the capacity to reproduce are distinctly separable phenomena, both in time and in character." This would help to explain why, among races which practice child marriage or indulge in sexual intercourse at an early age, conception as a rule does not occur until three or more years after the menarche.

The duration of this period of relative sterility is variable and probably depends on genetic and environmental factors. Ashley-Montagu estimates that the average interval between the first flow and the achievement of procreative function is about three years. Mikulicz-Radecki and Kausch,[19] who studied a group of ten to twenty year old girls, found that the majority first conceived several years after the onset of menstruation. Not until the twentieth year were all the members of the group capable of conceiving.

This physiologic sterility may perhaps best be explained by assuming that the early menstrual periods are anovulatory, the condition being analogous to that seen in the adolescent monkey.[20] Convincing proof is necessarily limited because of the impracticability of employing endometrial biopsy in the young unmarried girl as a means of ascertaining the occurrence of ovulation. Systematic studies of pregnanediol excretion during this epoch are still lacking (see Chap. XL).

SOMATIC ALTERATIONS

Statural growth from childhood to maturity does not follow a steady course, but occurs in spurts. Stratz[21] speaks of alternating periods of lengthening (increase in height) and broadening (increase in weight) as follows:

> 1 to 4 years—broadening
> 5 to 7 years—lengthening
> 8 to 10 years—broadening
> 11 to 15 years—lengthening
> 15 to 20 years—broadening

The growth curve is closely related to sexual development. The rate of growth in boys and girls tends to equalize itself by the eighth or ninth year. After this, there is a slump in the growth rate for boys, while girls show a marked spurt. The age at which girls begin to take the lead, and the extent to which their height and weight exceed that of males of the same chronological age, apparently depend on racial, climatic, and environmental factors. A comparable acceleration of growth does not become apparent in the male until two or three years later. It is noteworthy that the period of most vigorous growth is usually followed within a short time by the appearance of the menarche and the secondary sex characters.[3, 22, 23]

After the initiation of menstrual function, somatic growth proceeds at a slower rate for one to three years, when epiphyseal union is completed and longitudinal growth ceases. There is evidence that the earlier the menarche, the sooner epiphyseal closure occurs. Girls whose sexual development is delayed tend to be taller as adults than those who mature early,[24] due presumably to the ability of the gonadal hormones to accelerate maturation and closure of the epiphyses. Of interest is Mills'[25] observation that, during the last half century, there has been a tendency to increased statural growth associated with an earlier onset of sexual development. This is not necessarily inconsistent with the rule stated above, for it may reasonably be taken to signify that both somatic and sexual development have been simultaneously accelerated. As a result, though sexual maturity is achieved at an earlier age and epiphyseal closure follows soon afterward, the amount of statural growth achieved by the time of closure is greater than previously, when both somatic and sexual development proceeded at a slower rate.

The pronounced increase in stature and weight, incident to the puberal epoch, is associated with enlargement of the viscera, and different parts of the body. This growth process does not affect all regions alike. In the female, development of the pelvis is greater than that of the chest and upper girdle, and growth of the trunk exceeds that of the long bones. In the male, the situation is reversed. These regional variations in the growth impulse probably explain the lack of body symmetry and general awkwardness of the rapidly growing adolescent.

TROUBLESOME PUBERAL MANIFESTATIONS

Incidence.—According to Schacher,[26] 20 per cent of all puberal girls are free from annoying symptomatology, 70 per cent experience mild symptoms requiring no treatment, and 10 per cent are subject to severe and annoying manifestations. The symptoms are varied in nature and may be referable to the cardiovascular, nervous, and digestive systems. Fortunately, in the vast majority of cases, they are transient and self-limited.

Psychic Manifestations.—Psychic manifestations are common and likely to be severe in girls whose nervous system is unstable. Changes in behavior, moodiness, secretiveness, reclusiveness, irresponsibility, stubbornness, and fits of laughter or crying are not uncommon. Erotic and heterosexual tendencies, and awakening of the sex desire may or may not occur during the puberal era. The nervous irritability, insomnia, restlessness, and emotional dreams of the pubescent girl are in sharp contrast with the undisturbed, carefree days of childhood. Abnormalities of speech, such as stammering and stuttering and ocular disorders are often encountered in the pubescent individual.

Physical Manifestations.—The marked *vasomotor lability* which characterizes the puberal girl is responsible for such manifestation as blushing, pallor, sweats, and tachycardia.[27] Migraine, asthma, headaches, and epilepsy may have their inception during this phase of life.

The rapid enlargement of the *heart*, which occurs at this time, may be associated with a transient dilatation and give rise to dyspnea, palpitation, feeble pulse, and general languor. Irregularities and alterations in the cardiac rhythm are not uncommon, particularly in the anemic, rapidly growing pubescent. Loss or perversion of appetite, flatulence, nausea, vomiting, colic, and other *digestive symptoms,* as well as acne, herpes, urticaria and other *skin diseases* have been observed.

Etiology.—Since the entire organism is undergoing radical changes at this time, it is difficult to determine to what extent the rising tide of gonadal activity contributes to the annoying symptomatology. It seems likely that during puberty, as at the climacteric, the varied manifestations are due to the interaction of many factors of an endocrine and non-endocrine nature. The nature and severity of the symptoms probably depends on the status of the various systems of the body, which is in turn determined by hereditary and environmental influences. As puberty proceeds and the body achieves maturity, the harmonious interplay of the various systems becomes possible and the annoying manifestations may subside.

Treatment.—To ease the patient through this transitional period, the physician should use all measures designed to put her into the best possible physical condition. Mental, physical and nervous strain should be avoided. A tendency to obesity should be controlled by appropriate measures (see Chap. XXXIII), and a condition of underweight corrected by prescribing a high caloric diet which provides all necessary minerals and vitamins. In the adolescent with an unstable nervous system, reassurance that the symptoms are of a transient nature is often beneficial. The cooperation of understanding parents is particularly helpful.

BIBLIOGRAPHY

1. Bruch, H.: J. Pediat. *19:*365, 1941.
2. Zeller, W.: Gesundhfurs. f. d. Kindesalt. *8:*79, 1933.
3. Pryor, H. B.: J. Pediat. *8:*52, 1936.
4. Engle, E. T.: Human Biol. *9:*564, 1937.
5. Das, K.: Handbook of Obstetrics. Calcutta, Butterworth & Co., 1914.
6. Mills, C. A.: Am. J. Hygiene *15:*593, 1932; Medical Climatology, Springfield, Ill., Chas. C. Thomas, 1939.
7. Engle, E. T., and Shelesnyak, M. C.: Human Biol. *6:*431, 1934.
8. Mills, A. C.: Human Biol. *13:*363, 1941.
9. Pryor, H. B., and Carter, H. D.: Calif. & West. Med. *48:*89, 1938.
10. Pryor, H. B., and Smith, R. T.: J. Pediat. *14:*610, 1939.
11. Gordon, F. F.: Am. J. Pub. Health *20:*963, 1930.
12. Scheyer, H. E.: Ztschr. f. Geburtsh. u. Gynäk. *102:*579, 1932.
13. Bolk, L.: Ztschr. f. Geburtsh. u. Gynäk. *89:*364, 1925.
14. Breipohl, W.: Zentralbl. f. Gynäk. *61:*1335, 1937.
15. Schaeffer, R.: Arch. f. Gynäk. *84:*657, 1908.
16. Engelmann, G. J.: New York Med. J. *75:*221, 1902.
17. Mills, C. A., and Ogle, C.: Human Biol. *8:*607, 1936.
18. Ashley-Montagu, M. F.: Quart. Rev. Biol. *14:*13, 192, 1939.
19. Mikulicz-Radecki, F. von, and Kausch, E.: Zentralbl. f. Gynäk. *59:*2290, 1935.
20. Hartman, C. G.: Science *74:*226, 1931; Carnegie Inst. Wash. Publ. Anat. No. 433, 1932, p. 1.
21. Stratz, C. H.: Der Körper des Kindes und Seine Pflege. Stuttgart, F. Enke, 1922.
22. Boas, F.: Human Biol. *5:*429, 1933.
23. Stone, C. P., and Barker, R. G.: Human Biol. *9:*1, 1937.
24. Barker, R. G., and Stone, C. P.: Human Biol. *8:*198, 1936.
25. Mills, C. A.: Human Biol. *9:*43, 1937.
26. Schachter, M.: Med. inf. *40:*90, 1933.
27. Leschke, E.: Ztschr. f. artzl. Fortb. *31:*365, 398, 430, 1934.
28. Ito, P. K.: Human Biol. *14:*279, 1942.

CHAPTER XXIV

AMENORRHEA, OLIGOMENORRHEA, AND HYPOMENORRHEA

INTRODUCTION

Absence or deficiency of the menstrual flow, though likely to have an unfavorable psychologic effect, entails no danger to the general health. It merits serious attention, however, since it may be an expression of endocrinopathic disease, (see Chap. XXXV) or occur in association with genital hypoplasia, sterility, or troublesome subjective manifestations.

Definition and Terminology.—The term *amenorrhea* denotes absence of the flow. It is considered abnormal when it occurs within the limits of the reproductive period, in the absence of pregnancy or lactation. *Primary amenorrhea* describes cases in which menstruation has never occurred, although the normal time for the menarche has long passed. The condition is described as *secondary amenorrhea* if the menses cease at some time after menstrual function is established. *Oligomenorrhea* signifies cyclic bleeding at abnormally long intervals, and *hypomenorrhea* a reduction in the amount and duration of the monthly flow.

The terms *organic* and *functional* are used to distinguish between amenorrhea due to organic lesions of the generative organs, and that which arises in the absence of such abnormalities. The "functional" type is also described as *endocrine* or *hormonal* amenorrhea, on the assumption that some derangement of the endocrine glands which control menstrual function is at fault.

Physiologic Amenorrhea.—*Prepuberty and the Menopause.*—The average individual in temperate climates does not begin to menstruate until the age of thirteen, and loses this function some time between the fortieth and fiftieth year. The menses may begin later (*pubertas tarda*), or cease earlier (*climax praecox*), without exceeding physiologic limits, but if they do not appear by the eighteenth, or cease before the thirty-fifth year, the condition may be considered pathologic. Recent findings indicate that the physiologic amenorrhea of prepuberty and the menopause is due in large part to the ovaries' inability to respond to the anterior pituitary sex hormones (see Chap. XII), in one case because of immaturity, in the other because of involutionary changes incident to approaching senility.

During Pregnancy.—The absence of menstrual bleeding during gestation is probably due to the fact that the decidua vera is supported by a continuous supply of the estrogenic and progestational hormones essential for its maintenance. Occasionally periodic staining or bleeding may occur during the first few months and, in rare cases, throughout gestation. Such bleeding probably occurs by diapedesis, and stems either from the decidua vera, cervix, or some other part of the lower genital tract. The cause is obscure, though some attribute this to cyclic fluctuations in the estrogen level.

Postpartum.—Following parturition, and in the absence of suckling, the menstrual flow usually remains in abeyance for about six weeks. In the nursing mother, on the other hand, periodic bleeding may begin as early as the second month or as late as one year or more after delivery. Of interest is Kurzrok's[1, 2] observation that a large proportion of the cycles which occur during lactation are of the anovulatory type, as indicated by the finding of an estrogenic type of endometrium shortly before the onset of bleeding. This would imply that in the lactating woman reestablishment of ovarian function is a gradual process, which is not necessarily completed with the first postpartum flow.

During Lactation.—The cause of lactational amenorrhea is uncertain. One view postulates a mutual antagonism between the ovaries and mammae, but the evidence adduced in its support is unconvincing. It has been suggested that the lactogenic principle of the adenohypophysis inhibits ovarian function either directly or by suppressing the gonadotropic activity of this gland.[3, 4] Though there is some evidence that such a mechanism may operate in birds and to a limited extent in the lower mammals, inhibition of gonadal function by the lactogenic hormone in man has not been demonstrated. Recent evidence that the lactogenic principle may be identical with the luteotrophic factor[85] suggests that lactation prevents the return of ovarian cycles by causing persistence of the corpus luteum. The absence of progestational modifications in the endometrium of most women with lactational amenorrhea[86] argues against this possibility. Since lactation and gonadal function constitute a drain upon the nutritional resources of the organism, and both require the hormonal support of the anterior pituitary and other endocrine glands (see Chap. X), it is possible that lactational amenorrhea represents an effort of the organism as a whole, and the endocrine system in particular, to conserve their resources for purposes of milk production. The breasts are the dominant organs at this time and consequently, in the competition for the hormonal and nutritional resources of the organism, take precedence over the ovaries, which require some time to recover from the relative quiescence seen during gestation.

ETIOLOGY OF PATHOLOGIC AMENORRHEA

For a clear understanding of the etiology, a brief review of the salient features of true ovulatory menstruation is essential. This phenomenon, it will be recalled, is the end result of an intricate chain of events in which the anterior hypophysis, ovary, and uterus participate. Under the influence of the follicle stimulating principle of the anterior lobe, supplemented by minute quantities of its luteinizing factor, the follicle matures and elaborates estrogen, which elicits proliferative changes in the uterine mucosa. At approximately the mid-point of the cycle, the mature graafian follicle ruptures as a result of the combined action of the follicle stimulating and luteinizing principles. Following extrusion of the ovum, the collapsed follicle, under the influence of the luteinizer, is transformed into a corpus luteum. This structure produces the second ovarian hormone, progestin, which, with the support of small quantities of estrogen, converts the estrogen-primed endometrium to the pregravid, secretory phase. Failing conception, the yellow body regresses, to be followed by desquamation of the pregravid mucosa and bleeding.

It follows that any condition which acts directly on the uterus, or indirectly by way of the ovary to hinder or preclude endometrial growth,

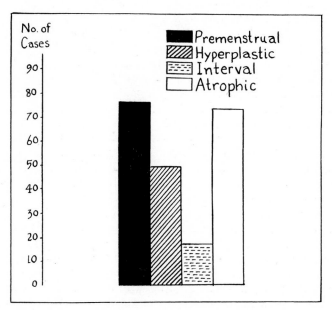

Fig. 53.—Graph showing distribution of various types of endometria in 218 cases of amenorrhea, oligomenorrhea, and hypomenorrhea. Note that all types of endometria are present. The premenstrual (pregravid) and atrophic forms predominate, each comprising about one-third of the entire group.

or prevent normal disintegration of the uterine mucosa, is a potential cause of amenorrhea. The fault may lie in the uterus, whose response to the ovarian sex hormones determines whether bleeding shall occur; in the ovary, whose sex hormones stimulate endometrial growth and function; or in the anterior pituitary gland, on which ovarian function depends.

UTERINE CAUSES

Developmental Anomalies.—Severe developmental anomalies, such as absence of the uterus, uterus rudimentarus solidus, or marked degrees of uterine infantilism, will obviously preclude endometrial growth and periodic menstrual bleeding, causing primary and permanent amenorrhea. Fortunately, these conditions are rare. Much more common are the mild forms of *uterine hypoplasia*, which may result from unfavorable influences operating during prepuberal life. The developmental status of the uterus in such cases may be only slightly below the minimum requirements for normal menstrual function. As a result, the menarche is usually delayed and the menses, once they appear, tend to be scanty or occur at long intervals. This condition is usually encountered in the constitutionally inferior woman with ill-developed secondary sex characters.

Injuries.—Extirpation of the uterus obviously precludes menstrual function. Injury to the endometrium by excessive curettage, radium, destructive neoplasms, caseous tuberculous endometritis,[5] actinomycosis, and puerperal infections, may result in permanent or temporary amenorrhea, depending on the nature and extent of the damage to the bleeding surface. If the destruction is complete, permanent amenorrhea will follow; but where part of the mucosa escapes unharmed or healing is possible, the loss of menstrual function may be temporary.

Functional Amenorrhea.—In some women, the flow may be absent for a long period of time despite normal ovarian and endometrial function, as indicated by the cyclic excretion of normal amounts of estrogen and pregnanediol, and the demonstration of pregravid mucosal modifications at monthly intervals. The cause of the amenorrhea is obscure. Schröder[6] believes that desquamation and bleeding take place, but, due to a deficient uterine blood supply, or excessive myometrial contractions, the blood loss is so minute as to pass unnoticed. His theory finds support in the author's observation that vaginal washings, taken coincident with the appearance of menstrual molimina in such patients, sometimes contain red blood cells. That underdevelopment of the uterine vascular apparatus is a cause of the amenorrhea is borne out by the observation that a full term pregnancy, with its marked vascularizing effect on the uterus, may correct the condition. It seems likely that *hypomenorrhea* associated with normal endometrial and hormonal findings, may likewise be explained on this basis.

The absence of periodic bleeding, despite normal ovarian and endometrial function, may conceivably represent a reversion to the nonhemorrhagic type of desquamation peculiar to nonprimates. As pointed out by Bartelmez,[7] the tissue loss in the menstruating human uterus varies widely, and in some cases may be almost negligible. Normally, regression and shrinkage of the mucosa is accomplished, in part at least, by resorption of the accumulated endometrial secretions. It may be that in some women the menstrual secretions are completely resorbed and regression and shrinkage occurs without loss of tissue or blood. Though the role of the endometrial blood vessels in menstruation has been greatly clarified by the studies of Bartelmez,[7] Daron,[8] and Markee[9] in the human being and monkey, further investigation is necessary before a satisfactory solution of this problem can be reached (see Chap. V).

Ovarian Causes

Disturbances in the production of the ovarian sex hormones are responsible for a large percentage of amenorrheic cases. The primary cause may reside in the ovary (*primary ovarian amenorrhea*), or may arise elsewhere in the organism (*secondary ovarian amenorrhea*). Interference with normal cyclic ovarian activity may cause either hypohormonal or hyperhormonal amenorrhea, depending on the nature and severity of the disturbance.

Hypohormonal Amenorrhea.—In the hypohormonal amenorrheas, the ovary does not produce its hormones in quantities sufficient to bring the endometrium to a point where its disintegration, on withdrawal of hormonal support, will result in manifest bleeding. This type of amenorrhea may result from congenital or developmental anomalies of the ovary, or be due to acquired faults, involving partial or total destruction of the follicular apparatus. Surgery, irradiation, inflammatory disease or de-

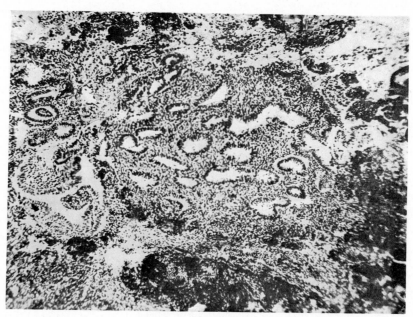

Fig. 54.—Atrophic type of endometrium. Microphotograph of tissue obtained from thirty-one-year-old woman with amenorrhea for three years.

structive neoplasms of the ovary are frequent causes of hypohormonal amenorrhea. In rare cases it may be caused by a masculinizing arrhenoblastoma, which neutralizes the feminizing influence of the ovary (see Chap. XXXV).

The duration of the amenorrheic state, and the nature of the associated endometrial and hormonal findings will depend on the extent to which ovarian function is suppressed. In the severe ovarian hypoplasias, or where the follicular apparatus has been completely destroyed, neither estrogen nor progestin is produced and both the anabolic and catabolic phase of the endometrial cycle are therefore precluded. As may be expected, neither estrogen nor pregnanediol is demonstrable in the body fluids and the mucosa presents atrophic changes. In the mild ovarian hypoplasias, or where the ovarian parenchyma has escaped complete destruction, the follicles achieve some degree of maturity, but undergo atresia at an early stage of their development. Here only small amounts of estrogen are present in the blood and urine (subthreshold cycle), and the endometrium presents slight proliferative changes. If the amount of estrogen secreted is very small, the endometrium may not attain the threshold for bleeding for long periods of time and the amenorrhea will be correspondingly prolonged. Where larger quantities are elaborated, the minimal requirements for bleeding may be achieved within a shorter period of time, and the amenorrhea may be interrupted by occasional bleeding episodes of varying amount and duration.

Hyperhormonal Amenorrhea.—The results of recent endometrial and hormonal studies[10, 11] indicate that some cases of amenorrhea, particularly those of short duration, may be due to excessive or prolonged secretion of estrogen or progestin. This condition is sometimes termed "hyperhormonal amenorrhea." In contrast to the hypohormonal amenorrheas, the absence of bleeding in the hyperhormonal type is attributable to a persistence of endometrial growth and corresponding delay in the onset of bleeding. The condition might more accurately be described as a postponement of the flow. The term *polyfolliculin* amenorrhea is used where nonappearance of the flow is attributable to excessive or prolonged estrogen secretion, while *polylutein* amenorrhea is applied where prolonged secretion of progestin is apparently responsible.

Polyfolliculin Amenorrhea.—The ovarian, endometrial, and hormonal findings in polyfolliculin amenorrhea are like those in hyperplastic bleeding (see Chap. XXV). The follicles do not rupture and form corpora lutea, but undergo atresia or persist as *cysts* of varying size. The successive crops of growing and cystic follicles provide a continuous supply of *estrogen* which causes the endometrium to proliferate and eventually become hyperplastic. Estrogen may be excreted in excessive amounts[10] or be within normal limits but appear continuously instead of showing the cyclic rise and fall which characterizes the normal menstrual cycle. Absence of bleeding under these conditions may be due to the fact that the estrogen level is adequate to maintain the proliferated mucosa and prevent breakdown and bleeding. Some condition within the uterus which raises the threshold for bleeding may conceivably account for some cases. This type of amenorrhea is of particular interest because it emphasizes the fact that, under certain conditions, amenorrhea and excessive uterine bleeding may have the same genesis, each representing a different phase of the same fundamental disturbance.

While polyfolliculin amenorrhea is usually of short *duration*, the author has occasionally encountered cases in which amenorrhea of more than one year's duration was associated with endometrial hyperplasia and high estrogen titers in the blood and urine. In one patient, who had not menstruated for fourteen years, repeated curettage over a period of several months revealed on each occasion marked hyperplastic modifications. The prolonged absence of bleeding is difficult to explain. Some vascular anomaly of the uterus which precludes manifest bleeding may possibly be responsible.

Local ovarian faults, such as circulatory disturbances, or capsular adhesions which prevent rupture of follicles and cause follicular cystosis, may lead to polyfolliculin amenorrhea. *Reduction of the ovarian parenchyma* by destructive neoplasms, surgery, or x-ray irradiation may have the same effect. Occasionally an estrogen-secreting *granulosa cell tumor* is responsible. Where the condition develops at the beginning of menstrual life, immaturity of the ovary may be at fault. As shown elsewhere (see Chap. XII), the immature ovary can respond only partially to the gonadotropic hormones. The theca cells are apparently capable of a response at an early age, but the granulosa cells react normally, achieving

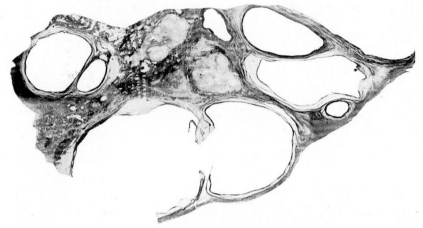

Fig. 55.—Microphotograph of ovary removed from a thirty-two-year-old woman with amenorrhea for three years. Endometrium atrophic. Estrogen findings negative; gonadotropin test (Fluhmann) positive.

luteinization and progestin production, only as the ovary approaches maturity.

Follicular Cysts with Uterine Hypoplasia.—Attention should be called to a group of cases in which amenorrhea is associated with multiple simple follicle cysts and uterine hypoplasia.[12, 13, 14] A thick fibrous capsule is characteristic of the ovaries in such cases and is associated with increased fibrosis of the ovary and hyperplasia of the theca layers. The absence of any estrogen effect in the uterus is apparently due to the fact that the cysts are not functioning, as a consequence of attenuation and compression within the overcrowded ovary. Such cases may possibly represent the end result of protracted follicular activity uninterrupted by ovulation and corpus luteum formation. This is suggested by the fact that such women usually give a history of originally normal periods, followed by some irregularity accompanied by excessive bleeding. Later the flow appears at increasingly extended intervals, eventuating in amenorrhea.[13] It is possible that examination in the earlier stages of the development of

20

the condition might have revealed proliferative or hyperplastic endometrial changes and high or persistent estrogen excretion.

Polylutein Amenorrhea.—A functioning corpus luteum cyst may postpone endometrial desquamation and bleeding by providing a continuous supply of progestin. Here the endometrial mucosa presents pregravid changes and the amenorrhea is usually of short duration, being terminated by bleeding when the persistent yellow body regresses or is removed. The cause of a functioning corpus luteum cyst is not clear. Some observers maintain that it is possible only in the presence of viable chorionic villi. That it may arise from some other cause than pregnancy is suggested by reports of amenorrhea associated with a corpus luteum cyst in cases where pregnancy

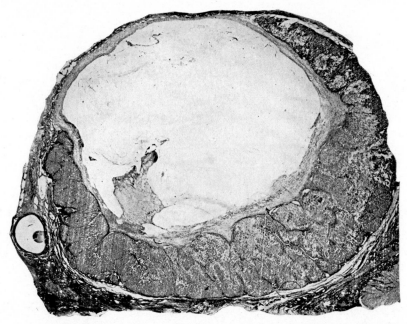

Fig. 56.—Cystic corpus luteum from a thirty-three-year-old woman with amenorrhea for nine weeks. Endometrial tissue removed simultaneously showed pregravid changes.

was definitely excluded.[15, 16, 87] Conceivably, persistence of the yellow body may result from disordered function of the anterior pituitary gland, or from some ovarian disturbance, possibly vascular, which delays corpus luteum regression.

Oligomenorrhea.—In oligomenorrhea, bleeding occurs from a pregravid, secretory type of endometrium, but the intervals between the flows are appreciably lengthened. Whether these "long cycles" are due to lengthening of the follicular or luteal phase or a slowing down of the cycle as a whole, is not certain. Schröder[17] suggests that lengthening of the interval between the flows may be attributable to slow maturation of the follicle. Frankl[18] believes that a delay in the initiation of each new cycle, following regression of the corpus luteum, may be responsible.

Studies of the length of the pre-ovulatory and post-ovulatory phase in cycles of varying length have yielded conflicting results. On the basis of observations in the monkey, Hartman[19] concluded that variations in the length of the cycle are due to changes in the length of the luteal phase, while the follicular phase remains fairly constant. On the other hand, observations in women led Vollmann,[20] and Rock and Bartlett[21] to conclude that the follicular phase is more variable.

The *underlying cause* of long cycles is likewise obscure. Whether they are due to mechanical or circulatory factors within the ovary, or are traceable to a disturbance of anterior pituitary function, has not been determined.

ROLE OF THE ANTERIOR HYPOPHYSIS

Since the adenohypophysis initiates and maintains gonadal function, it follows that malfunction of this dominant gland is of primary importance in the etiology of amenorrhea. Hypopituitarism, exemplified by *Simmonds' disease* and *Fröhlich's syndrome*, is almost always associated with amenorrhea, which may be primary or secondary, depending on whether the malady has its inception before or after puberty. In hyperpituitarism, as manifested in *giantism* or *acromegaly*, the later stages are associated with amenorrhea, due possibly to ovarian exhaustion following a period of hyperactivity, or to pressure atrophy of the anterior pituitary cells which secrete its gonadotropic hormone (see Chap. XXXV).

Functional disturbances of the adenohypophysis probably account for many cases of amenorrhea. Definite information relating to the precise state of pituitary function in the various types of amenorrhea is not yet available. In the light of our present understanding of the hypophyseal-ovarian relationship (see Chap. XII), deficiencies of menstruation which arise in the absence of ovarian or uterine faults may conceivably be explained as follows:

1. Suppression of both the follicle-stimulating and luteinizing hormones of the anterior lobe, which would preclude follicular maturation, ovulation and corpus luteum formation, may account for amenorrhea of long duration, associated with negative estrogen and gonadotropin findings, and an atrophic type of endometrium.

2. Partial suppression of the anterior pituitary sex principles may be responsible for the amenorrheas of long or short duration, associated with negative gonadotropin findings, a subthreshold level of estrogen in the blood and urine, and mild proliferative changes in the uterine mucosa.

3. A relative or absolute excess of the follicle-stimulating principle, which might cause follicular cystosis and a state of hyperestrinism, may account for some cases of amenorrhea associated with endometrial hyperplasia and a high estrogen level in the body fluids.

4. Overproduction of the luteotrophic factor may explain some cases of amenorrhea associated with persistence of the corpus luteum and pregravid changes of the endometrium.

5. A slowing down in the production of one or both pituitary sex

principles, which might cause lengthening of the ovarian cycle, may account for some cases of oligomenorrhea.

ROLE OF OTHER ENDOCRINE GLANDS

Structural or functional alterations in the thyroid,[22, 23, 24] adrenals,[25] and other incretory glands may disturb ovarian function and lead to amenorrhea. Though primarily concerned with metabolic activities, these glands are functionally related to the anterior hypophysis, and through it, dis-

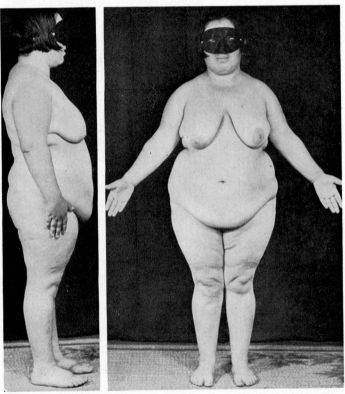

Fig. 57.—Single girl aged eighteen, weight 160 pounds, height 56 inches. Primary amenorrhea; hypoplastic genitalia; negative estrogen tests. B.M.R. —25. Scanty pubic hair. Dull mentality. Menses established following thyroid medication.

turbances in their function may conceivably be reflected in the gonads. The extent to which menstrual function is affected will depend on the time of onset, severity and duration of the glandular disturbance, and the degree of ovarian damage incurred (see Chap. XXXV).

NONENDOCRINE CAUSES OF AMENORRHEA

Amenorrhea may result from unfavorable endogenous or exogenous influences which depress the organism. These remote but important factors are too often overlooked, because recent spectacular revelations in the field of endocrinology have focused attention on the gonads and their endocrine regulators.

Infectious Diseases.—Amenorrhea is a frequent accompaniment of acute and chronic infectious diseases. Here absence of the flow apparently represents an effort of the depressed organism to conserve its resources. *Acute infections* of short duration may have little effect on the menstrual rhythm, but chronic infections often depress the organism so profoundly that protracted amenorrhea results. As the disease subsides, the menstrual flow usually returns to normal unless the general depression has been so severe and protracted that irreversible changes are induced in the gonads or their endocrine regulators.

Tuberculosis is of particular importance in the etiology. Amenorrhea is often a very early, and at times the only symptom of incipient tuberculosis; hence the gynecologist may be the first to suspect the malady. Its far-reaching effect is evident in the observation that approximately 50 per cent of all patients in the early stages of tuberculosis are amenorrheic.[26, 27, 28] According to some investigators, the incidence of amenorrhea increases in proportion to the severity of the disease. An arrest of the lesion may be followed by a return of normal menstruation.

Amenorrhea is often encountered in empyema, postappendiceal abscess, ulcerative colitis, and other *chronic and prolonged purulent infections,* and usually persists throughout the active stage of the disease. The gonadal depression is probably secondary to the cachexia caused by the toxins elaborated. Chronic parenchymatous nephritis, diabetes, malignancy, prolonged cardiac decompensation, and other *debilitating diseases* often lead to amenorrhea of long duration. *Intoxications* due to chronic alcoholism, morphinism, and other poisons may likewise depress the gonads and cause amenorrhea. The anemias, leukemias, and other *blood dyscrasias* may account for some cases of amenorrhea. Simple achlorhydric anemia, a chronic blood disorder of cryptic origin, is stressed by some observers[29] as a possible cause of amenorrhea in young girls.

Nutritional Faults.—*Malnutrition.*—Malnutrition, whether due to inadequate food and vitamin intake, or faulty assimilation, may cause amenorrhea, probably by depressing the endocrine glands, or depriving them of the basic materials from which they manufacture their specific hormones. A striking example of *famine amenorrhea* was seen in the blockaded countries during the World War.[30, 31] According to Kloppner,[32] the incidence of genital hypoplasia and menstrual deficiencies in the post-war period (1929–1933) was twice that in the pre-war period (1907–1918). This would imply that malnutrition during the war years not only depressed menstrual function in those who had already reached adulthood, but retarded genital development in young girls who were then approaching puberty. In recent years, there have been an increasing number of cases of amenorrhea in young women subject to injudicious *reducing diets.* Following a material reduction in weight, these individuals experience a marked loss of strength and vitality, become subject to depressive nervous manifestations, and develop an aversion for food. Secondary anemia, a low

basal metabolic rate, and low blood pressure are common associated findings. A large percentage present proliferative changes of the endometrium
and a subthreshold estrogen cycle. Institution of a well balanced diet is
usually followed by the return of normal menstrual periods and improvement in the symptomatology. It should be emphasized that the associated
low basal metabolic rate is part of the general depression brought on by
the nutritional deficiency. A similar drop has been observed in experimental

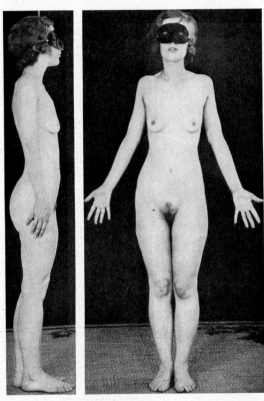

Fig. 58.—Hypogonadism. Patient aged twenty-six, weight 110 pounds. Amenorrhea for
five years. Poorly developed secondary sex characters; hypoplastic genitalia; atrophic changes
in endometrium; negative estrogen tests. B.M.R. —22. Transient edema of face and extremities. Asthenia. With high caloric diet and small doses of thyroid, symptoms controlled
and regular menses established. Case exemplifies amenorrhea due to mild hypothyroidism.

animals on a starvation diet, and is apparently a protective mechanism
by which the organism conserves its declining resources. It is obvious that
treatment with thyroid substance or any other metabolic stimulant is
contraindicated in this type of amenorrhea.

A state of malnutrition, despite adequate food intake, may result from
chronic gastro-intestinal disturbances which interfere with normal assimilation. The resulting suppression of gonadal and menstrual function is sometimes referred to as "alimentary castration."

Obesity.—Obesity and amenorrhea are very frequently associated.[43] They may appear simultaneously or one may precede the other. Whether they are causally related or merely dissociated manifestations of a common cause is not certain. The available evidence suggests that the midbrain harbors distinct but closely situated centers for the regulation of gonadal function and fat metabolism. It is conceivable that both centers may be disturbed simultaneously, or that a disturbance in one may be reflected in the other. On the other hand, it is possible that excess weight leads to

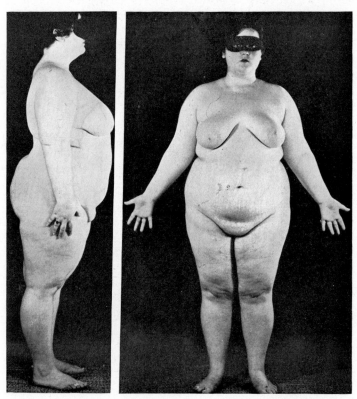

Fig. 59.—Fröhlich's type of adiposity associated with primary amenorrhea. Girl aged eighteen, weight 237 pounds. Hypoplastic genitalia; low estrogen values. X-ray of sella turcica negative.

gonadal depression by overburdening the endocrine system. The improvement in gonadal function which often follows mere reduction in weight may be due to removal of this burden with a resulting increase in the efficiency of the incretory glands (see Chap. XXXIII).

Nervous and Psychic Factors.—Unfavorable nervous and psychic influences may sometimes lead to suppression of menstrual function, particularly in women with an inherently defective nervous system.[33, 34, 35] Strong emotional upsets such as great fright, worry, surprise, or joy, may frequently cause abrupt cessation of the flow. Fear of, or desire for, pregnancy may have a similar effect producing the condition known as *pseudocyesis*. The menstrual rhythm is sometimes disturbed by a change of environment, which may bring with it an element of nervous excitement. Tietze[36] found that initiation of a group of students into their new activities coincided with a disturbance of their menstrual periodicity, which took the form of amenorrhea in many instances. How psychic stimuli elicit functional alterations in the sexual sphere is not known. It has been suggested that they pass from the cortex to the hypothalamus and thence to the closely adjacent hypophysis, suppressing its gonadotropic activity. The importance of psychic factors should always be borne in mind when

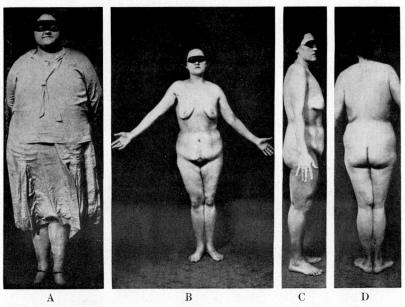

A   B   C   D

Fig. 60.—Generalized obesity. A, Married woman aged twenty-six, weight 238 pounds, with amenorrhea for one year. B, C and D, Same patient one year later following loss of 97 pounds as result of dietotherapy comb.ned with thyroid extract. Loss of weight coincided with return of normal menses.

evaluating the efficacy of treatment. The brilliant results reported with the various sex hormone preparations may, at least in some cases, be due to the psychotherapeutic effect of the injections.

Amenorrhea is known to be a frequent accompaniment of epilepsy, chorea, progressive paralysis, anorexia nervosa, and especially the depressive types of psychoses.[37, 38, 39] Whether the nervous and sexual abnormalities are causally related, or are independent manifestations of constitutional inferiority is not certain.

SYMPTOMATOLOGY AND DIAGNOSIS

Symptoms.—While absence of the flow may be the sole symptom, it is often associated with troublesome subjective and objective manifestations. Where the loss of menstrual function is due to systemic disease, the associated symptomatology will obviously be related to the malady. The amenorrheas incident to endocrinopathic disease are associated with a varied symptomatology, which depends on the time of onset of the endocrinopathy and the gland primarily affected (see Chap. XXV).

Absence of the flow due to primary ovarian failure is sometimes accompanied by flushes, sweats, tachycardia, vertigo, psychoneurotic instability, and other manifestations reminiscent of the natural or artificial menopause (see Chap. XXIX).

In some cases, epileptiform seizures, migraine, vicarious menstruation, mastalgia, or galactorrhea may occur, particularly at the time when men-

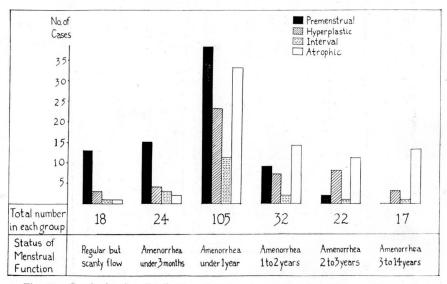

Fig. 61.—Graph showing distribution of various types of endometria according to duration of the amenorrhea in a group of 218 cases. Note that the incidence of premenstrual (pregravid) endometria decreases, while that of atrophic endometria increases with the length of the amenorrhea. It is noteworthy that a pregravid mucosa occurred in no case of amenorrhea for three or more years, but was encountered in 11 of 54 cases of amenorrhea lasting one to three years.

struation would normally be expected. In the hyperhormonal amenorrheas, the symptomatology may suggest premenstrual tension (see Chap. XXX) or early gestation. Since any one of a number of general or local causes may give rise to amenorrhea, a careful, painstaking investigation is essential.

History.—The anamnesis should aim to elicit all past events which may have caused ovarian or uterine damage. Of particular significance is a history of pelvic operations, irradiation of the reproductive organs, or endocrinopathic disease. The menstrual history is often a valuable aid in estimating the status of ovarian function. Primary amenorrhea suggests congenital or developmental anomalies of the generative organs or some deep seated endocrinopathy, having its inception during the prepuberal period. **Secondary amenorrhea,** on the other hand, points to some acquired fault which has disturbed an originally normal reproductive apparatus. A clue to the degree of ovarian depression may be obtained from the duration of the amenorrhea. In an analysis of 218 cases (see Fig. 61), the author found that the proportion of cases presenting an atrophic type of endometrium, usually indicative of marked gonadal depression, increased with the duration of the amenorrhea. Where the menses cease abruptly, especially in a woman whose periods were previously regular, pregnancy, psychic shock, or some physical injury to the generative organs may be suspected.

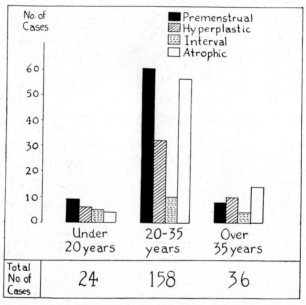

Fig. 62.—Graph showing distribution of various types of endometria, according to age, in a group of 218 cases of amenorrhea, oligomenorrhea and hypomenorrhea. The oldest patient was forty-one, the youngest sixteen years of age. Note that the proportion of atrophic endometria is highest in the group over thirty-five years of age.

Physical Examination.—A careful search should be made for all faults, endocrine or otherwise, which are intimately or remotely connected with the sexual sphere. The physician should be on the lookout for evidence of incipient tuberculosis, blood dyscrasias and other systemic diseases. Particular attention should be directed to the constitutional makeup of the individual and endocrinopathic stigmata, which may serve as valuable clues in the search for the primary cause. Anthropometric measurements may disclose statural abnormalities, an important sign of disordered endocrine function. The developmental status of the secondary sex characters may suggest the degree of ovarian retardation.

Pelvic Examination.—Besides eliminating mechanical obstruction to the egress of the menstrual fluid (cryptomenorrhea), pelvic examination may disclose congenital anomalies or genital hypoplasia. The developmental status of the external genitalia, vagina, cervix and fundus, and the size and consistency of the adnexa are useful in determining the gravity of the condition. The degree of sexual retardation may also be judged by the length of the uterine cavity, as determined by sounding. Zondek[40] divides the amenorrheas into three groups: *Grade I*, or amenorrhea of less than one year's duration, in which the uterine cavity measures from 5½ to 6½ cm.; *Grade II*, or amenorrhea of one to two years' duration, in which

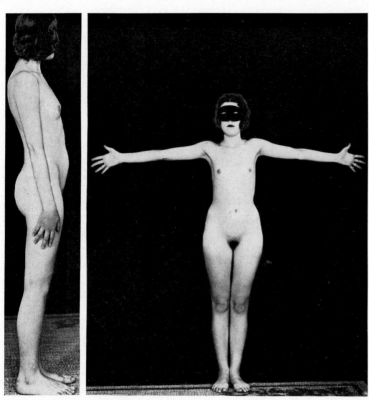

Fig. 62a.—Female eunuchoidism. Single girl aged twenty-two with primary amenorrhea and marked retardation of primary and secondary sex characters. Atrophic changes in endometrium; negative estrogen and gonadotropin tests. Note tall stature. Lower exceeds upper measurement and span exceeds height.

the cavity measures 3½ to 5 cm., and *Grade III*, or amenorrhea of two to ten years' duration, in which it measures less than 3½ cm.

Routine Laboratory Studies.—Routine laboratory examinations, the basal metabolism and sugar tolerance tests, and eye ground examination, may prove of value in disclosing endocrinopathic disease. The x-rays may be used not only to ascertain the presence of systemic disease, but also to determine the state of the epiphyses, which may reveal some abnormality in the growth impulse. X-ray of the sella turcica is of limited value, for in the large majority of cases no significant deviation from normal can be detected by this means. Definite evidence of pituitary disease is demonstrable only where a pituitary neoplasm has distended the sella or eroded the clinoids or floor.

Endometrial Findings.—Histologic evaluation of endometrial tissue obtained by the curette or suction pipette (for technique, see Chap. XXXIX), is a direct, practical, and accurate method of evaluating gonadal function. This diagnostic procedure will help differentiate the hypohormonal amenorrheas, associated with an atrophic or proliferative type of endometrium, from the hyperhormonal forms, in which the mucosa presents hyperplastic or pregravid secretory changes. It should be emphasized that the endometrial picture, though usually a reliable mirror of ovarian function, may be misleading where the uterine mucosa is refractory to the ovarian sex hormones. If the mucosa shows full pregravid changes, it may be assumed that the ovary secretes adequate amounts of estrogen and progestin. On the other hand, if the mucosa is atrophic, it may signify either uterine refractoriness or absence of the ovarian sex hormones. The two conditions may be differentiated by quantitative sex hormone studies of the blood and urine (see below).

Vaginal Smear Findings.—According to Papanicolaou,[41] the vaginal smear is a reliable index of ovarian function. He classifies the amenorrheas on the basis of the associated vaginal smear findings, as follows: (1) Amenorrhea associated with the constant presence of an atrophic smear, indicating absence of ovarian activity. Most primary and many secondary amenorrheas fall into this group. (2) Amenorrhea associated with a constant estrogenic smear, indicating subnormal but uniform ovarian activity. This group includes most of the secondary amenorrheas. (3) Amenorrheas associated with irregular cyclic smear changes, simulating those of the normal cycle, but insufficient to produce overt menstruation. In this group fall some secondary amenorrheas and cases of delayed puberty. In the author's experience, this method has proved much less reliable as an index of ovarian function than endometrial curettage.

TABLE 2

CLASSIFICATION OF AMENORRHEAS ACCORDING TO ASSOCIATED ENDOMETRIAL, VAGINAL AND HORMONAL FINDINGS*

Type of Amenorrhea		Endometrial Findings	Vaginal Smear	Estrogen Test	Gonadotropin Test	Pregnanediol Test
Primary Uterine		Atrophic changes	Estrogenic	Positive	Negative	Positive
Hypo-hormonal	Primary Ovarian	Atrophic or Proliferative	Atrophic or weak estrogenic	Negative or sub-threshold	Positive or negative	Negative
	Secondary Ovarian	Atrophic or Proliferative	Atrophic or weak estrogenic	Negative or sub-threshold	Negative	Negative
Hyper-hormonal	Polyfolliculin	Hyperplastic	Estrogenic	Positive	Negative	Negative
	Polylutein	Pregravid	Luteal	Positive	Negative	Positive

*This classification is suggested by the author's experience, coupled with endometrial, vaginal and hormonal findings reported in the literature. It does not intend to imply that such findings will invariably be encountered, but merely indicates what may usually be expected. Exceptions, due to variations in technique or interpretation, or to other variable factors, are not uncommon. The gonadotropin test referred to is that of Fluhmann.

Sex Hormone Findings.—*Estrogen.*—In the normally menstruating woman, according to Frank,[42] 1 mouse unit of estrogen can be demonstrated in 10 to 20 cc. of vein blood, obtained just before the expected flow. The total quantity of estrogen excreted in the urine in the course of the normal menstrual cycle ranges from 1300 to 1700 mouse units (for technique, see Chap. XXXIX). In the amenorrheas, the estrogen content of the blood and urine varies according to the degree of follicular function present. The estrogen tests may serve as a basis for differentiating the hypohormonal from the hyperhormonal (polyfolliculin) amenorrheas. In the former, vein blood taken at weekly intervals for five weeks is as a rule uniformly negative, and the total amount of estrogen excreted in the urine over a period of thirty days may range from 500 to 800 mouse units (subthreshold estrin cycle) in the mild cases, and from 200 to 50 mouse units or less, in severe hypogonadism. In the polyfolliculin amenorrheas, on the other hand, the blood may contain excessive amounts of estrogen, and the total quantity excreted in the course of a thirty day period may exceed 2000 mouse units.

The estrogen tests may not only serve as an index of follicular activity, but may also help differentiate between primary ovarian and primary uterine amenorrhea. Where curettage reveals an atrophic type of endometrium, a positive estrogen test absolves the ovary of responsibility and points to some inherent fault in the uterus, which makes it refractory to the ovarian sex hormones.

It should be emphasized that the estrogen level of the blood and urine is not a reliable criterion of ovulatory or luteal function. In the author's experience,[44] a pregravid type of mucosa, which implies the presence of functioning luteal tissue, was not constantly associated with any one type of estrogen level.

Pregnanediol.—Quantitative tests of pregnanediol in the urine may be useful in establishing the presence of functioning luteal tissue.[45] These tests are particularly valuable in the unmarried woman, where curettage is undesirable. Where the endometrium is atrophic or hyperplastic, pregnanediol studies may help in deciding whether the absence of secretory activity is due to lack of progestin, or refractoriness of the mucosa. In hypomenorrhea and oligomenorrhea, the tests may be carried out daily during the second half of the cycle, while in amenorrhea of long duration where cyclic phenomena are absent, they may be performed daily over a period of thirty days or longer. In hypomenorrhea, the excretion of 1 to 10 or more mg. of pregnanediol daily during the latter half of the cycle suggests that ovarian function is normal and that some uterine defect may be responsible for the scanty flow. In amenorrhea of long duration, care must be taken in interpreting the results. If the excretion of pregnanediol is cyclic, approximating the values in the normally menstruating woman, and the associated estrogen findings are within normal limits, it may be assumed that ovarian function is normal and that the cause of the amenorrhea may reside in the uterus. On the other hand, where pregnanediol appears persistently or irregularly, and is associated with low estrogen and high androgen values, an adrenal cortical rather than a luteal origin may be suspected (see Chap. XL), particularly if there is evidence of virilism. Negative findings suggest the absence of functioning luteal tissue but are not conclusive.

Androgen.—The normal cyclically menstruating woman excretes up to 50 I.U. of androgen daily. Recent studies (see Chap. XL) indicate that suppression of ovarian function is associated with a rise in androgen excretion which is roughly proportional to the degree of ovarian failure. In amenorrhea associated with virilism, arrhenoblastoma of the ovary, or adrenal cortical hyperplasia or tumor, values up to 500 I.U. daily have been reported.

Gonadotropin.—Barring pregnancy, the finding of 1 mouse unit of follicle stimulating hormone in 15 to 20 cc. of vein blood,[46] or 110 mouse units per liter of morning urine,[47] in association with negative estrogen tests is generally interpreted as pointing to primary ovarian failure. This assumption is based on the observation that comparable amounts of this hormone can be demonstrated in a large percentage of cases following the

TABLE 3

ASSOCIATION BETWEEN ENDOMETRIAL AND HORMONAL FINDINGS IN 218 CASES OF AMENORRHEA, OLIGOMENORRHEA, AND HYPOMENORRHEA

State of Endometrium	Blood Estrogen Test			Blood Gonadotropin Test			Total Number of Cases
	Positive	Threshold	Negative	APR I	APR II–III	Negative	
Premenstrual.................	31	18	15	0	0	64	64
Early Premenstrual...........	7	5	1	0	0	13	13
Hyperplasia..................	16	10	5	0	0	31	31
Local Hyperplasia............	3	6	8	1	0	16	17
Interval.....................	4	8	7	0	0	19	19
Atrophic....................	5	27	42	27	3	44	74
Total number of tests.........	66	74	78	28	3	187	218

natural or artificial menopause, but only rarely in the normal mature non-pregnant woman. In the author's experience,[44] a positive test was frequently obtained in amenorrhea of long duration associated with negative estrogen findings and an atrophic endometrium (see Table 3). That a positive reaction is reliable evidence of ovarian damage and a poor prognostic sign, is borne out by the fact that, with few exceptions, such cases fail to respond to any form of treatment. Fluhmann and Murphy[43] found positive gonadotropin tests more common in primary than in secondary amenorrhea. Where a positive reaction was encountered in secondary amenorrhea, the condition was invariably of long duration. They conclude that this finding points to a serious or prolonged ovarian disturbance.

Differential Diagnosis.—Pathologic amenorrhea must be distinguished from cryptomenorrhea, and absence of the flow incident to gestation. Retention of the menstrual secretions, because of some mechanical obstruction, may readily be excluded by pelvic examination. The hyperhormonal amenorrheas, particularly the polylutein type, may often simulate early intra- or extra-uterine pregnancy.[87] Absence of the flow, the cyanotic appearance of the cervix, and unilateral adnexal enlargement due to the presence of a follicular or corpus luteum cyst may suggest tubal gestation. The biologic tests for pregnancy (see Chap. XXXIX) may differentiate the two conditions. In the differential diagnosis between ectopic pregnancy and amenorrhea due to a corpus luteum cyst, the gonadotropin tests for pregnancy are conclusive only when strongly positive. A mild positive or negative reaction is not altogether reliable, for it may be encountered in both conditions.[87] These tests are also of value in distinguishing between pseudo-cyesis and true pregnancy, and are useful in the obesity amenorrheas, where the abdominal adiposity makes uterine palpation difficult.

PROGNOSIS

Where the structural alterations in the genitalia are still reversible, and the primary cause can be remedied or eliminated, a return to normal gonadal and menstrual function may be expected. On the other hand, if the amenorrhea is due to some irreparable injury to the uterus or ovary, or some deep seated and progressive endocrinopathy, the outlook is obviously poor.

The type and duration of the amenorrhea, and the state of somatic and sexual development, have an important bearing on the prognosis. It is usually poor in the primary amenorrheas associated with marked retardation of the primary and secondary sex characters, for here congenital or developmental defects, or some prepuberal endocrinopathy is often at fault. Where the amenorrhea is associated with some degree of secondary sex character development, menstrual function may be established sooner or later. The secondary amenorrheas, due to acquired endocrine disease, are likely to persist, unless the malady is corrected before irreversible gonadal changes occur.

In the amenorrheas due to systemic disease or depressive states, the prognosis is good provided the cause can be found and eliminated. The outlook in amenorrhea resulting from x-ray or radium irradiation will depend on the degree of ovarian or uterine damage incurred. A rise in the gonadotropin level in the blood and urine, especially when associated with negative estrogen findings and an atrophic type of endometrium, is a poor prognostic sign.

TREATMENT

Since amenorrhea is merely a symptom, its treatment necessarily entails the correction of its underlying cause. In a large proportion of the cases, particularly those of short duration, the condition is often transient and self-limited, and entirely compatible with good health. General medical measures and watchful waiting are often all that is required. On the other hand, primary amenorrhea or secondary amenorrhea of long duration demand the serious attention of the physician, especially when associated with genital hypoplasia, sterility, or a troublesome symptomatology.

The therapeutic measures adopted should have a rational basis, entail no danger to gonadal function and aim to eradicate the primary cause. Mere induction of bleeding without removing the cause is useless and may prove harmful, particularly when the amenorrhea represents an effort of the depressed organism to conserve its waning resources.

Early recognition of developmental faults, endocrinopathic disease, and depressive states in young girls approaching the menarche is of the utmost importance. The parent should be instructed to be on the watch for statural aberrations, retardation of the secondary sex characters, obesity, hirsutism, or other endocrinopathic stigmata.

Medical Measures.—General medical measures (see Chap. XXV) directed toward the elimination of all subnormal manifestations, whether intimately or remotely connected with gonadal function, are often effective in initiating or reestablishing normal menstrual rhythmicity. Correction of nutritional faults is of prime importance. In both the underweight and overweight amenorrheic patient, dietary and other measures calculated to bring the weight to normal, are often followed by normal menstrual periods (see Chap. XXXIII).

Gynecologic Measures.—Pelvic faults conducive to amenorrhea should be corrected where possible. *Dilatation* and *curettage* is sometimes followed by a return to normal menstrual rhythmicity. Whether this sequence of events indicates a causal relationship or is purely coincidental, we cannot say. Conceivably, this procedure may terminate an amenorrheic career by stimulating the anterior hypophysis through nervous pathways, as in the rabbit, though this is by no means proved. On the other hand, it may act by removing unresponsive mucosal tissue and thus clearing the way for a normal endometrial response to the ovarian sex hormones.

The amenorrheas associated with cystic follicles or persistent corpora lutea are sometimes benefited by removal of the abnormal structures. In some cases, this may be accomplished by *manual expression* (bimanual pelvic massage per vaginam or rectum), a method employed by the author and advocated by Zondek,[10] Wagner,[48] and others.[49] The aim of this procedure is to express the fluid from the larger cysts and improve the circulation of the ovary. *Aspiration* of retention cysts per vaginam,[10] or *ovarian resection*[13, 50, 51, 52] is recommended by some observers for the larger cysts associated with lower abdominal pain. Even here, the author believes surgery should be entertained only as a last resort, care being taken to conserve as much healthy tissue as possible. The improvement noted following these procedures is generally assumed to be due to removal of a mechanical obstacle to the development of new crops of follicles. An increased blood supply may also contribute to this effect. As pointed out by Brewer,[53] puncture of cysts, vaginal massage of the ovaries, and resection have one feature in common, namely trauma. This is certain to increase the blood supply, "which physiologically any organ needs for increased function." Surgery should be avoided for the small simple cysts, which are characteristically evanescent. Surgical intervention in such cases is not only unnecessary but may lead to more serious disturbances of ovarian function.[88]

Organotherapy.—Endocrine preparations are used with the aim of stimulating the depressed gonads or supplying deficient sex hormones.

Estrogenic Substances.—Use of the estrogens in the treatment of amenorrhea is based on the clinical observation that adequate doses induce
proliferative changes in the endometrium, and cessation of treatment is
followed by uterine bleeding clinically resembling menstruation. The *dose*
is 10,000 to 50,000 I.U. of estradiol benzoate or dipropionate given intramuscularly two or three times a week, or 1 mg. of stilbestrol daily by
mouth for three weeks. Cyclic bleeding may be induced by repeating the
treatment after each induced flow. The bleeding is analogous to pseudomenstruation, since it occurs from an estrogenic type of endometrium.

Aside from its favorable psychological effect on the patient, such treatment accomplishes nothing, for the induced flow is unaccompanied by any
improvement in gonadal function. Though studies in the lower mammal
suggest that, under certain conditions, the estrogens may stimulate ovarian
function, possibly by augmenting the action of the endogenous gonadotropins, or stimulating their production or release by the adenohypophysis
(see Chap. XII), there is as yet no convincing evidence that this can
be duplicated in man. In view of the evidence that their protracted
administration may inhibit the gonadotropic activity of the pituitary,
these substances should be used with caution. It is noteworthy that most
of the cures attributed to estrogen therapy occurred in young women
with secondary amenorrhea of short duration, which has a marked tendency
to self-correction. Of interest in this connection is the observation of Fluhmann and Murphy[43] that uterine bleeding occurred before treatment had
been instituted in 33 per cent of a group of twenty-two amenorrheic
patients.

The estrogens have been advocated[54, 55, 56] for *amenorrhea associated
with uterine hypoplasia.* The aim here is to increase the size and vascularity
of the uterus to the point where it can respond to the hormones supplied
by the patient's own ovary. Such therapy is valueless where the sexual
retardation involves the ovary as well as the uterus. Where the ovary is
apparently functioning normally, it may be assumed that the hypoplastic
condition of the uterus is due to some inherent defect which makes it
refractory to stimulation. In this connection, Kaufmann[57] observed that
some of his cases failed to show uterine growth after as much as 15,000,000
I.U. of estrogenic hormone. Similarly, Hamblen[58] found that as much as
15,000 R.U. of estradiol benzoate or dipropionate daily for as long as three
months, failed to cause uterine enlargement in women who exhibited no
evidence of ovarian deficiency except rudimentary uteri. Even where some
uterine growth can be achieved by such therapy, this can only be accomplished at the expense of ovarian function, which is likely to be suppressed
by the large doses required for this purpose.

The estrogens are obviously *contraindicated* in polyfolliculin amenorrhea. They should also be avoided where the amenorrhea is due to systemic disease, particularly anemia and incipient tuberculosis, for here the
induced bleeding would constitute an added drain on the depressed
organism.

Estrogen and Progesterone.—Cyclic treatment with estrogen followed

21

by progesterone or *pregneninolone* is employed by some observers for the *hypohormonal amenorrheas*.[59, 60, 61] In determining the *dosage* in a given case, they are guided by the observation[57] that a total of 1,000,000 I.U. of estrogen injected over a period of two weeks, followed by 35 to 90 rabbit units of progesterone for five to seven days, are required to develop the atrophic endometrium of the castrate woman to the pregravid phase. Pregneninolone, an orally active compound with progestational properties has only recently been employed for this purpose. Salmon and his associates[63] induced a progestational type of endometrium with 120,000 to 655,000 R.U. of estradiol benzoate intramuscularly followed by 105 to 540 mg. of pregneninolone by mouth. Weber and his associates[64] found 45 to 60 mg. of estradiol by inunction followed by 1000 to 1200 mg. of pregneninolone by mouth effective for this purpose. Though such treatment may be followed by cyclic uterine bleeding from a pregravid mucosa, it is purely substitutive and consequently of little practical value, offering no advantage over estrogen alone.

A "simplified" form of treatment has been described by Zondek.[65] In *secondary amenorrhea* of over two years' duration he could induce bleeding by administering a total of 50 mg. of progesterone over a period of two to five days. For secondary amenorrhea of less than two years' duration he recommends the same dosage of progesterone, or a combination of 25 mg. of progesterone and 2.5 to 5 mg. of estradiol benzoate over a period of two days. In *primary* and *castration amenorrhea*, he employs 50 mg. of progesterone plus 2.5 to 5 mg. of estradiol benzoate over two days. Though this form of treatment reduces the expense and number of injections, it does as little to correct the underlying cause as estrogen alone, or estrogen followed by progestin. It takes advantage of the fact that the small quantities of estrogen secreted by some amenorrheic women may cause some degree of endometrial growth. No bleeding occurs, possibly because growth of the mucosa is not sufficient to permit bleeding on withdrawal of estrogen, or because estrogen is continuously supplied in sufficient quantities to maintain the integrity of the mucosa. Bleeding follows the administration of progesterone alone, or of progesterone plus estrogen, because the mucosa is thereby rendered resistant to the hemorrhage-inhibiting action of the endogenously supplied estrogens. On withdrawal of progesterone, the endometrium disintegrates for lack of adequate hormonal support and bleeding follows (see Chap. V).

Gonadotropic Hormone Therapy.—Potent follicle-stimulating and luteinizing preparations, capable of eliciting a response in the depressed human ovary, would seem to be ideal therapy for the *amenorrheas due to pituitary insufficiency*. While the hypophyseal and equine gonadotropes completely repair the gonadal atrophy in the hypophysectomized laboratory animal, it is doubtful whether they are equally effective in man. Gonadotropic extracts of anterior lobe tissue are too low in unitage to exert any appreciable effect on the human ovary. Though the equine hormones are highly active in the laboratory animal, and some observers have found them capable of inducing ovulation and corpus luteum formation in the normal human ovary,[66, 67] their value where the ovary is depressed has not been convincingly demonstrated.[68, 69, 70, 71] At best, they may induce growth of follicles. The chorionic gonadotropes, which have a predominantly luteinizing effect in the lower animal, apparently promote follicular atresia in man. There is no convincing evidence that they can induce ovulation or corpus luteum formation in the human ovary,[72] though they may possibly augment the activity of existing luteal structures.[73]

Despite their limitations, the available gonadotropins deserve a trial in functional amenorrhea due to depressed hypophyseal function. When resorting to their use, the physician should bear in mind the physiological action of the preparation under consideration, and the type of amenorrhea he is seeking to remedy. The dosage and duration of treatment will depend largely on the severity of the gonadal depression. The primary hypohormonal amenorrheas, associated with genital retardation, are likely to require prolonged treatment. In the secondary amenorrheas associated with normal genital development, smaller doses over a shorter period of time may suffice.

In the *hypohormonal amenorrheas*, where both follicular and luteal activity is depressed, it would seem rational to administer a follicle-stimulating preparation (hypophyseal or equine gonadotropin) followed by a luteinizer (chorionic gonadotropin).[63, 89] The equine hormones are administered in doses of 500 to 750 I.U. daily for two weeks, the chorionic hormones, in doses of 300 to 500 I.U. daily for an equal period. Several courses of treatment may be tried, with intervening rest periods to prevent antihormone formation (see Chap. XXII). As Hamblen[73] has emphasized, it is advisable, before resorting to combined therapy, to determine what response is evoked by the equine hormone alone. Endometrial biopsy, vaginal smears, and quantitative estrogen tests may be used for this purpose. The finding of estrogen in the body fluids, proliferative changes in the endometrium, and an estrogenic type of vaginal smear indicate that maturation of follicles has been induced. Unless this is accomplished, nothing can be gained by following up with a luteinizing preparation. Use of equine followed by human chorionic gonadotropin is also advocated by Rydberg and Pedersen-Bjergaard,[89] who employ much larger doses, namely, five injections of 2000 to 3000 I.U. of the equine hormone at three-day intervals, followed by five injections of 6000 I.U. of human chorionic gonadotropin at three-day intervals. Trial of such therapy should be undertaken with caution, in view of reports of allergic shock and ovarian hemorrhage[90] observed after equine hormone administration.

A form of *combination therapy* recommended by Mazer and Ravetz[74] involves the use of *synapoidin*, a preparation composed of chorionic gonadotropin and an anterior pituitary preparation which presumably contains the so-called "synergist" (see Chap. XII). This preparation, they claim, produces numerous hemorrhagic follicles and corpora lutea in the normally menstruating woman. In a series of twenty-three cases of amenorrhea, 30 "synergy" units of their preparation, or the equivalent of 30 Cartland-Nelson rat units, were given every other day over a period of twenty days, and repeated after a rest period of two weeks. Uterine bleeding occurred in 19 cases, but only two of the twenty-three patients continued to menstruate after treatment was stopped. Though a few observers[69, 75, 76] have reported evidence of stimulation following such therapy, the number of cases are too limited and the observations not sufficiently well controlled to permit any judgment as to its efficacy. The author's experience with this preparation, like that of Geist and associates,[77] has been disappointing.

In the *polyfolliculin amenorrheas*, a follicle-stimulating preparation would obviously be superfluous and might even do harm by exaggerating the tendency to follicular cystosis. Here, a potent luteinizer would appear to be rational therapy. For this purpose, some observers use *chorionic gonadotropin*. The *dose* is 300 to 500 I.U. daily for two weeks, to be repeated after a two weeks' rest period. Treatment is discontinued if, after several courses, the endometrial picture and pregnanediol determinations fail to show evidence that luteinization has occurred. Such therapy would seem to be of questionable value in cystic degeneration of the ovary due to some inherent defect, such as immaturity or circulatory disturbances which cause it to respond abnormally to otherwise normal gonadotropic stimuli. Observations in the lower mammal suggest that, when acting on such ovaries, chorionic gonadotropin may induce luteinization of the theca cells with estrogen production, but cannot cause ovulation and granulosa luteinization with progestin production, which is desirable in these cases. Consequently, its use may tend to aggravate rather than to ameliorate the condition (see Chap. XII).

In the author's experience, the gonadotropins, either singly or in combination, have been unsatisfactory in the amenorrheas of long duration. In the secondary amenorrheas of short duration, a return of normal periods sometimes follows their use, but since the condition in such cases is often self-limited,[43] we cannot be certain that the return of menstrual function was due to the treatment.

Thyroid Substance.—Thyroid substance is conceded by competent observers to be of distinct value in the *functional amenorrheas*, particularly when associated with obesity and a depressed basal metabolic rate.[24, 43, 78, 79] Such therapy is necessarily empirical, for its mode of action is still obscure. The most likely explanation is that it acts by increasing the metabolic activity of the organism as a whole, and with it that of the ovary and its endocrine regulators. The dose is ½ to 1 grain three times a day. Larger doses are indicated in the amenorrheas associated with hypothyroid manifestations. To avoid untoward effects, the pulse and metabolic rate should be checked at frequent intervals.

In amenorrhea associated with a high basal metabolic rate and other symptoms of hyperthyroidism, iodine therapy may be of value.

X-ray Therapy.—Low dosage x-ray radiation of the ovary and pituitary gland has been recommended by some observers for the treatment of *functional amenorrhea of pituitary and ovarian origin*.[80, 81, 82, 83] (For technique and dosage, see Chap. XXV.) It is difficult to evaluate this form of therapy, since in most of the studies, no systematic attempt was made to determine the status of ovarian function, before and after treatment, from the endometrial picture or other reliable objective criteria. Moreover, most reports fail to state the type and duration of the amenorrhea, and do not take into consideration the possible beneficial effect of other therapeutic measures previously or concomitantly employed. It is significant that the severe primary amenorrheas, which are only rarely corrected spontaneously, do not respond to x-ray treatment, even in the hands of its most enthusiastic proponents. On the other hand, the highest percentage of "cures" are reported in the secondary amenorrheas of short duration, which are known to terminate spontaneously in a large proportion of the cases.

Radiation of the Ovaries.—Those who champion radiation of the ovaries have offered various explanations to account for the good results which seem to follow its use. Some maintain that, though large doses of the x-rays have a destructive action on living cells, small doses stimulate cellular function. Others believe that the rays promote ovarian function indirectly by causing hyperemia, or by destroying inhibitory structures which interfere with its cyclic activity. The latter explanation might reasonably account for the good results reported in the hyperhormonal amenorrheas, where destruction of cystic follicles or a persistent corpus luteum would clear the way for a new crop of follicles and thus facilitate a return of normal ovarian cycles. In the hypohormonal amenorrheas, where the follicular apparatus is depressed, radiation would seem hazardous, for there is always the danger that even a small dose may destroy the last vestige of follicular function. The author has encountered cases in which permanent amenorrhea followed the application of small doses of x-ray for stimulative purposes. Such cases serve to emphasize the fact that individual variations in susceptibility to the x-rays make it impossible to predict their effect in a specific instance. Some observers deny that there is any element of danger, on the basis of their observation that no harmful effects follow low dosage radiation of the ovaries in normally menstruating women. Granting that this is true, there is no assurance that the hypofunctioning gonad will react in the same manner. Even if its stimulating effect were certain, low dosage radiation of the ovary could hardly be expected to benefit the amenorrheas of primary uterine origin, and those due to general depressive states or systemic disease. If employed at all, it should be reserved for the *hyperhormonal amenorrheas* associated with persistent follicular or corpus luteum cysts which fail to respond to conservative measures. The possibility of an early gestation should always be ruled out before the rays are applied.

Radiation of the Anterior Hypophysis.—Low dosage radiation of the adenohypophysis (for technique and dosage see Chap. XXV) with the hope of stimulating its gonadotropic activity, is advocated for the *amenorrheas due to pituitary insufficiency.*[83] The author does not recommend this form of therapy, for even if its stimulating effect is conceded, there is no assurance that the action of the rays will affect only the gonadotropic activity of this gland and leave its other important functions undisturbed. Nor is it certain that important adjacent nerve centers in the midbrain will not be adversely affected. It is argued that the brain and hypophysis are resistant to the rays and therefore not likely to be injured by the small doses used for stimulative purposes. While there is some evidence that small doses of x-ray produce no demonstrable structural modifications in the hypophysis of experimental animals, the possibility that they may nevertheless cause significant functional alterations is not thereby eliminated. As recently emphasized by Aub and Karnofsky,[84] "until more is known about the effect of x-ray treatment on the pituitary gland, its general use cannot be advocated. The pituitary functions are too vital for this gland to be indiscriminately exposed to irradiation."

X-ray radiation of the hypophysis should therefore be avoided in the amenorrheas of short duration, or those of primary ovarian or uterine origin. However, a trial of this form of therapy may be justified in the amenorrheas of long duration which prove resistant to all other forms of treatment.

BIBLIOGRAPHY

1. Kurzrok, R., Lass, P. M., and Smelser, J.: Proc. Soc. Exper. Biol. & Med. *36:*356, 1937.
2. Lass, P. M., Smelser, J., and Kurzrok, R.: Endocrinol. *23:*39, 1938.
3. Weichert, C. K.: Anat. Rec. *75* (Suppl.) : 86, 1939.
4. Kyriakis, L.: Zentralbl. f. Gynäk. *65:*1268, 1941.
5. Walter, R. I., Salmon, U. J., and Geist, S. H.: Am. J. Obst. & Gynec. *42:*505, 1941.
6. Schröder, R.: Der mensuellen Genitalzyklus u. seine Störungen, in Veit-Stoeckel's Handb. d. Gynäk., Munich, J. F. Bergmann, vol. 1, pt. 2, 1928.
7. Bartelmez, G. W.: Carnegie Inst. Wash. Publ. No. 443, Contrib. Embryol. No. 142, 1933, vol. 24, p. 143.
8. Daron, G. H.: Am. J. Anat. *58:*349, 1936; Anat. Rec. *67* (Suppl.) : 13, 1937.
9. Markee, J. E.: Carnegie Inst. Wash. Publ. No. 518, Contrib. Embryol. No. 177, 1940, vol. 28, p. 219.
10. Zondek, B.: Acta obst. & gynec. Scandinav. *12:*309, 1934; Harefuah *14:*12, 1938.
11. Anspach, B. M., and Hoffman, J.: Am. J. Obst. & Gynec. *28:*473, 1934.
12. Stein, I. F., and Leventhal, M.: Am. J. Obst. & Gynec. *29:*181, 1935.
13. Stein, I. F., and Cohen, M. R.: Am. J. Obst. & Gynec. *38:*465, 1939.
14. Leventhal, M.: Am. J. Obst. & Gynec. *41:*516, 1941.
15. Ochsner, E. H.: Surg., Gynec. & Obst. *31:*496, 1920.
16. von Probstner, A.: Endokrinol. *16:*174, 1935.
17. Schröder, R., Kessler, R., and Tietze, K.: Zentralbl. f. Gynäk. *57:*11, 1933.
18. Frankl, O.: Wien. med. Wchnschr. *84:*570, 1934.
19. Hartman, C. G.: Am. J. Obst. & Gynec. *26:*600, 1933.
20. Vollmann, R.: Monatschr. f. Geburtsh. u. Gynäk. *110:*193, 1939.
21. Rock, J., and Bartlett, M. K.: J.A.M.A. *108:*1022, 1937.
22. Litzenberg, J. C., and Carey, J. B.: Am. J. Obst & Gynec. *17:*550, 1929.
23. Gardiner-Hill, H., and Smith, J. F.: J. Obst. & Gynec. Brit. Emp. *34:*701, 1927.
24. Dodds, E. C., and Robertson, J. D.: J. Obst. & Gynec. Brit. Emp. *46:*213, 1939.
25. Adler, E. H., and Abrams, S. B.: Am. J. Obst. & Gynec. *45:*213, 1939.
26. Jamenson, E. M.: Am. J. Obst. & Gynec. *25:*22, 1933.
27. Hesseltine, H. C., and Spear, W. M.: Am. J. Obst. & Gynec. *27:*32, 1934.
28. Pedrini, I.: Gior. med. d. Alto Alige *11:*332, 1939.
29. Haden, R. L., and Singleton, J. M. S.: Am. J. Obst. & Gynec. *26:*330, 1933.
30. Fraenkel, L.: Zentralbl. f. Gynäk. *41:*1033, 1917.
31. Wehefritz, E., and Gierhake, E.: Zentralbl. f. Gynäk. *60:*2711, 1936.
32. Kloppner, K.: Munch. med. Wchnschr. *85:*1060, 1938.
33. Chadwick, M.: Nerv. & Ment. Dis. Mono. No. 56, 1932.
34. Aich, J.: Allg. Ztschr. f. Psychiat. *96:*325, 1932.
35. Allen, E. B., and Henry, G. W.: Am. J. Psychiat. *13:*239, 1933.
36. Tietze, K.: Arch. f. Gynäk. *156:*35, 1933.

37. Rochat, R. L.: Schweiz. med. Wchnschr. *66:*53, 1936.
38. Sheldon, J. H.: Lancet *1:*369, 1937.
39. Farquharson, R. F., and Hyland, H. H.: J.A.M.A. *111:*1085, 1938.
40. Zondek, B.: Die Hormone des Ovariums u. des Hypophysenvorderlappens, ed. 2. Vienna, J. Springer, 1935.
41. Papanicolaou, G. N.: Proc. Soc. Exper. Biol. & Med. *41:*629, 1939.
42. Frank, R. T., Goldberger, M. A., Salmon, U. J., and Felshin, G.: J.A.M.A. *109:*1863, 1937.
43. Fluhmann, C. F., and Murphy, K. M.: Am. J. Obst. & Gynec. *42:*656, 1941.
44. Anspach, B. M., and Hoffman, J.: Am. J. Obst. & Gynec. *26:*147, 1933.
45. Venning, E. H., and Browne, J. S. L.: Endocrinol. *21:*711, 1937.
46. Fluhmann, C. F.: Am. J. Obst. & Gynec. *20:*1, 1930.
47. Osterreicher, W.: Klin. Wchnschr. *12:*538, 1933.
48. Wagner, G. A.: Zentralbl. f. Gynäk. *52:*10, 1928.
49. Lehmann, P.: Rev. franç. de gynéc. et d'obst. *29:*573, 1934.
50. Robinson, M. R.: Am. J. Obst. & Gynec. *30:*18, 1935.
51. Bailey, K. V.: J. Obst. & Gynec. Brit. Emp. *44:*637, 1937.
52. Reycraft, J. L.: Am. J. Obst. & Gynec. *35:*505, 1938.
53. Brewer, J. I.: Discussion of Stein, I. F., and Cohen, M. (*supra* 14).
54. Mazer, C., and Israel, S. L.: J.A.M.A. *108:*163, 1937.
55. Kleegman, J. S.: Med. Woman's J. *46:*1, 1939.
56. Livingston, S. H., Birnberg, C. H., and Kurzrok, L.: Am. J. Surg. *44:*409, 1939.
57. Kaufmann, C.: J. Obst. & Gynec. Brit. Emp. *41:*409, 1935.
58. Hamblen, E. C.: J.A.M.A. *117:*2205, 1941.
59. Loeser, A.: J. Obst. & Gynec. Brit. Emp. *41:*86, 1934.
60. Kaufmann, C.: Geburtsh. u. Frauenh. *1:*313, 1939.
61. Neustaedter, T.: Am. J. Obst. & Gynec. *38:*609, 1939.
62. Kaufmann, C.: Klin. Wchnschr. *12:*1557, 1933.
63. Salmon, U. J., Walter, R. I., and Geist, S. H.: Proc. Soc. Exper. Biol. & Med. *40:*252, 1939.
64. Weber, H. W., Kurzrok, L., and Birnberg, C. H.: J. Clin. Endocrinol. *2:*392, 1942.
65. Zondek, B.: J.A.M.A. *118:*705, 1942.
66. Davis, M. E., and Koff, A. K.: Am. J. Obst. & Gynec. *36:*183, 1938.
67. Siegler, S. L., and Fein, M. J.: Am. J. Obst. & Gynec. *38:*1021, 1939.
68. Gray, L. A.: Am. J. Obst. & Gynec. *43:*387, 1942.
69. Buxton, C. L.: Am. J. Obst. & Gynec. *42:*236, 1941.
70. Vogt, W. H., and Sexton, D. L.: Am. J. Obst. & Gynec. *42:*81, 1941.
71. Bonime, R. G.: J. Clin. Endocrinol. *2:*254, 1942.
72. Report of Council on Pharmacy and Chemistry A. M. A., J.A.M.A. *114:*487, 1940.
73. Hamblen, E. C.: Endocrine Gynecology. Springfield, Ill., Charles C. Thomas, 1939.
74. Mazer, C., and Ravetz, E.: Am. J. Obst. & Gynec. *41:*474, 1941.
75. Greenblatt, R. B., and Pund, E. R.: South. M. J. *34:*730, 1941.
76. Goldzieher, M. A.: Practical Endocrinology. Appleton-Century Co., 1935.
77. Geist, S. H., Gaines, J. A., and Salmon, U. J.: Am. J. Obst. & Gynec. *42:*619, 1941.
78. Haines, S. F., and Mussey, R. D.: J.A.M.A. *105:*557, 1935.
79. Collins, R. M.: Iowa State Med. J. *31:*576, 1941.
80. Mazer, C., and Spitz, L., Jr.: Am. J. Obst. & Gynec. *31:*576, 1941.
81. Tamis, A. B.: Am. J. Obst. & Gynec. *32:*845, 1936.
82. Kaplan, I. I.: Am. J. Obst. & Gynec. *34:*420, 1937.
83. Friedman, A. B., and Seligman, B.: Radiology *29:*99, 1937.
84. Aub, J. C., and Karnofsky, D.: New England J. Med. *226:*759, 1942.
85. Lyons, W. R., Simpson, M. E., and Evans, H. M.: Proc. Soc. Exper. Biol. & Med. *52:*134, 1943.
86. Topkins, P.: Am. J. Obst. & Gynec. *45:*48, 1943.
87. Cotte, G.: Gynéc. et Obstét. *41:*5, 1941.
88. Miller, N. F., and Willson, J. R.: New York State J. Med. *42:*1851, 1942.
89. Rydberg, E., and Pedersen-Bjergaard, K.: J.A.M.A. *121:*1117, 1943.
90. Castallo, M. A.: M. Rec. *154:*56, 1941.

CHAPTER XXV

FUNCTIONAL UTERINE BLEEDING

INTRODUCTION

Abnormal uterine bleeding may be a signal of organic disease or indicate some disturbance of the endocrine glands upon which normal menstrual function depends. Bleeding unassociated with demonstrable pathology has long taxed the diagnostic acumen and therapeutic resources of the clinician.

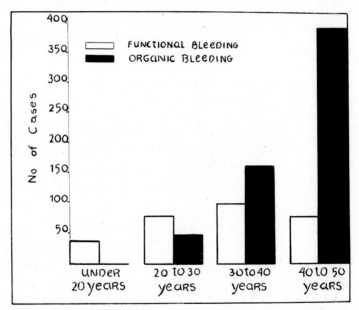

Fig. 63.—Graph showing distribution of functional and organic uterine bleeding, according to age, in a group of 886 cases admitted to the Gynecologic Clinic of the Jefferson Hospital over a ten-year period. Note that functional cases are more common during the earlier years, while those of organic origin predominate in later life.

Recent studies relating to the hormonal control of menstrual function have greatly clarified its etiology and suggested a logical approach for its recognition and treatment.

Incidence.—Uterine bleeding is one of the most common and important gynecologic complaints. Of 4185 patients admitted to the gynecologic wards of the Jefferson Hospital over a ten-year period, 886 or 21 per cent complained of abnormal uterine hemorrhage. Of these, 296 or about 33 per

326

cent presented no evident local or general organic disease. Among a series of 500 cases studied by Fluhmann and Morse,[1] 25 per cent were free from demonstrable pathology.

Definition and Nomenclature.—The term *functional* is applied to abnormal uterine bleeding which occurs in the absence of organic disease. Bleeding from the uterus is considered abnormal when it occurs independently of menstruation, exceeds the normal flow in frequency, duration or amount, or is so irregular that it cannot be considered a periodic phenomenon. The term *menorrhagia* describes profuse or prolonged bleeding which appears cyclically at intervals of approximately twenty-eight days. *Metrorrhagia*, on the other hand, is applied to acyclic

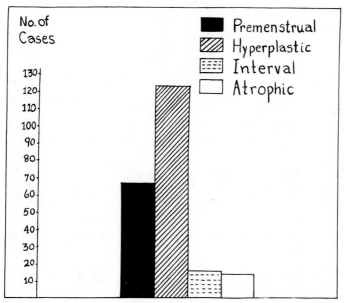

Fig. 64.—Graph showing endometrial findings in 225 cases of uterine bleeding without demonstrable pathology. All types of bleeding were represented and all forms of endometria encountered, but no correlation could be observed between the endometrial picture and the type of bleeding, whether regular and profuse, frequent, continuous, etc.

bleeding not related to the menstrual flow. *Polymenorrhea* describes normal or profuse bleeding at regular intervals of twenty-one days or less.

Functional uterine bleeding has been variously classified. In the present writing, the status of ovarian function has been adopted as the basis for classification. Abnormal bleeding preceded by ovulation and corpus luteum formation is described as *ovulatory* to distinguish it from *anovulatory* bleeding which occurs in the absence of these events. Other terms currently employed stress the status of endometrial function. For example, *hyperplastic bleeding* is applied to abnormal bleeding from a hyperplastic endometrium. Hamblen[2] has introduced descriptive terms suggesting the identity of the hormonal stimuli responsible for the various types of endometria with which abnormal bleeding may be associated. He speaks of abnormal bleeding from a (1) hypo-estrogenic, (2) normal estrogenic,

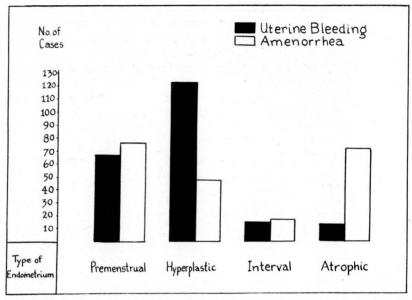

Fig. 65.—Graph comparing distribution of various types of endometria in functional uterine bleeding (225 cases) and amenorrhea, hypomenorrhea, and oligomenorrhea (218 cases). The proportion of premenstrual (pregravid) and interval (proliferative) endometria in the two groups does not differ significantly. On the other hand, hyperplastic endometria are more common in the bleeding group (31 against 12), atrophic endometria in the group with amenorrhea (18 against 3). These findings demonstrate that any type of menstrual disturbance may occur from any type of endometrium.[79]

(3) persistent estrogenic, (4) hyperestrogenic, (5) mixed, (6) progestational and (7) menstrual endometrium.

ANOVULATORY BLEEDING

Anovulatory bleeding is much more common than the ovulatory form. It usually occurs from a hyperplastic type of endometrium, though the uterine mucosa not infrequently presents interval (proliferative, normal estrogenic) or atrophic (hypoestrogenic) changes. This type of bleeding is also known as *metropathia haemorrhagica* or *hyperplastic bleeding*.

ANATOMICAL AND HISTOLOGICAL CHARACTERISTICS

Striking alterations have been observed in the ovaries and uterus in hyperplastic bleeding. Though not always perceptible on gross examination, they can readily be recognized microscopically.

Ovarian Changes.—The ovaries may be normal in size, but frequently one or both are cystically enlarged. Occasionally, a cyst the size of a pigeon's egg may be palpated. In the severe case of long duration, the ovarian parenchyma may be largely replaced by cystic follicles of varying size (see Fig. 66).

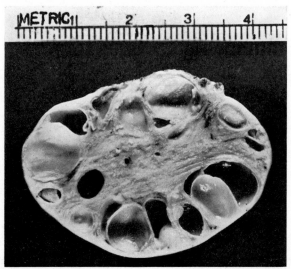

Fig. 66.—Small cystic degeneration of the ovary. Cross section of ovary removed from thirty-two-year-old woman with irregular uterine bleeding for eighteen months, associated with endometrial hyperplasia.

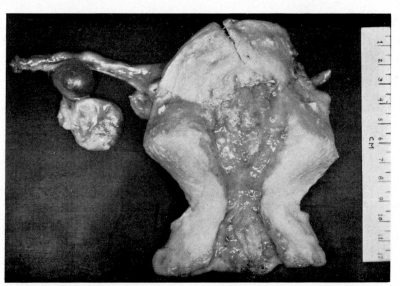

Fig. 67.—Cystic degeneration of the ovary associated with hyperplasia of the endometrium. Photograph of specimen obtained from thirty-five-year-old female with excessive uterine bleeding for eighteen months.

Histologically, numerous ripening, cystic or atretic follicles are observed. These may be lined by one or more layers of granulosa cells which

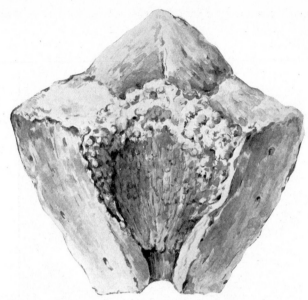

Fig. 68.—Drawing of uterus with marked hyperplasia of the endometrium. Note sharp line of demarcation between mucosa and myometrium. Endocervix is characteristically uninvolved.

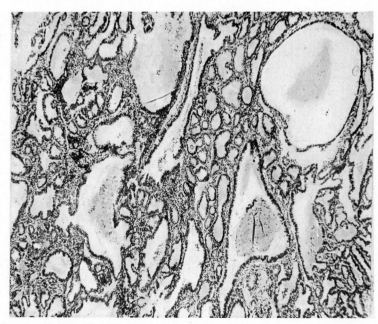

Fig. 69.—Marked glandular hyperplasia of the endometrium. Microphotograph of tissue obtained from twenty-eight-year-old woman complaining of excessive uterine bleeding alternating with periods of amenorrhea.

at times show degenerative changes. Ova may or may not be present but recent corpora lutea are characteristically absent.

Uterine Changes.—The uterus may be normal in size or symmetrically enlarged, especially in the parous patient or where the condition has persisted for some time. The consistency of this organ likewise varies. It tends to be soft and boggy during active reproductive life, and firm and fibrotic at the menopause. The cervix is often soft, faintly discolored, and patulous during the bleeding phase. The endometrium is either partially or wholly thickened and may be thrown into folds or fungous projections. In some instances, the mucosa is so enormously thickened as to almost completely occlude the uterine cavity. Regardless of the degree of pro-

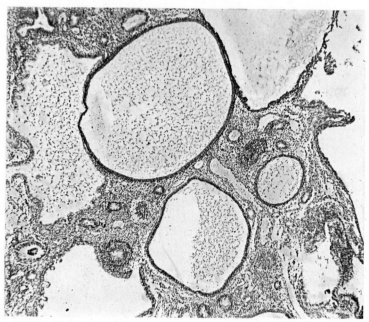

Fig. 70.—Cystic glandular hyperplasia of the endometrium. Microphotograph of tissue obtained from a forty-five-year-old woman with irregular uterine bleeding for eight months.

liferation, the endometrium remains sharply demarcated from the myometrium and cervical mucosa.

Large irregular fragments or masses of pinkish-red, soft tissue may be obtained by the curette. Occasionally, polypoid and vesicular formations are apparent. The abundance of the tissue in some instances may suggest malignancy, particularly if the patient is at the cancer age. At times, especially following a long bleeding phase, or in old women, only a small amount of tissue can be detached by the curette. Regardless of the amount of tissue obtained, its histologic appearance is always characteristic (see Figs. 69, 70).

Microscopic Appearance of the Hyperplastic Endometrium.—The hyperplastic proliferation may involve the entire mucosa (see Fig. 70), or be confined to local areas (see Fig. 71). The glandular elements, stroma, and blood vessels are all implicated in this process.

Glandular Changes.—The glands are greatly increased in number, cystically dilated, and show a marked disparity in size, the whole picture suggesting a swiss-cheese pattern. They are usually scattered throughout the mucosa in haphazard fashion, making the compacta, spongiosa, and basalis indistinguishable. Their disorderly arrangement and irregular pattern contrasts sharply with the orderly appearance of the glands during the proliferative phase of the normal menstrual cycle.

The glands are lined by one or more rows of cells containing centrally situated, darkly staining, round or oval shaped nuclei, which may or may

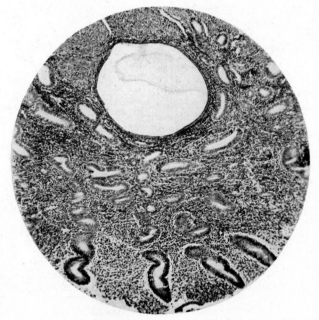

Fig. 71.—Interval endometrium with local areas of hyperplasia. Microphotograph of tissue obtained from a twenty-four-year-old woman with irregular uterine bleeding for one year.

not show mitotic activity. The protoplasmic zone is always sharply demarcated in contrast to the wavy protoplasmic contours seen during the pregravid secretory phase of the normal endometrial cycle. The lumina of the glands, though usually empty, may contain a homogeneous material or cellular debris. Their epithelial lining varies considerably, not only in different endometria but in different regions of the same mucosa. At one extreme are the cystically dilated glands which, as a rule, are lined by a single layer of flattened cuboidal epithelium. Nearby may appear glands lined by many rows of cells with polypoid or fungous projections extending into the lumen. At times, the epithelial proliferation may be so marked and of such bizarre appearance as to suggest malignancy. Regardless of the type of epithelial proliferation, evidence of secretory activity and glycogen formation is never seen in true hyperplasia. In the very severe case, the number of glands is so great that very little interglandular stroma is apparent. Such cases are not infrequently confused with fundal cancer. This condition, sometimes termed "polypoid" or "carcinoid" hyperplasia, was encountered by the author in four cases (see Fig. 72).

Stromal Changes.—The endometrial stroma is usually increased, though at times it may be almost entirely replaced by the glandular elements. In the typical case, the stroma is very cellular and closely packed, and

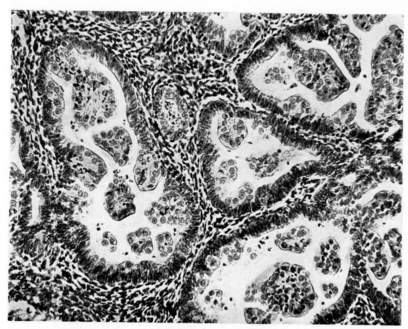

Fig. 72.—Polypoid hyperplasia of endometrium ("carcinoid" hyperplasia). Microphotograph of tissue obtained from twenty-eight-year-old sterile woman with amenorrhea alternating with uterine bleeding. Note intraglandular polypoid formations due to marked proliferation of the glandular epithelium. Such cases may sometimes be confused with adenocarcinoma.

mitosis is frequently observed. General or local edema, probably the result of circulatory stasis, is not uncommon, especially where the glands are not very numerous.

Vascular Changes.—The blood vessels are increased in number and very prominent. Because of the disparity in their size and shape, and their disorderly course and distribution, they have been aptly described as in a state of "histologic unrest." Numerous dilated, elongated, and often thick walled vessels appear throughout the depth of the mucosa. Markedly dilated veins are apparent beneath the surface epithelium, and numerous punctate intra- and extrastromal hemorrhages are often observed in the vicinity of apparently intact blood vessels. Thrombosis of large and small vessels is not uncommon and is especially evident near necrotic areas.

CLINICAL CHARACTERISTICS

Age Incidence.—Hyperplastic bleeding may occur at any time during the reproductive period. It has been estimated to occur in from 5 to 10 per cent of puberal girls, but is probably more common at this period of life than these figures would imply. Spontaneous adjustment before medical aid is sought, and the limited use of curettage to establish the

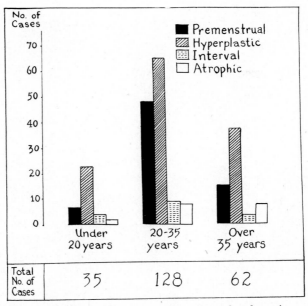

Fig. 73.—Graph showing distribution of various types of endometria according to age in a group of 225 cases of functional uterine bleeding. The oldest patient was fifty-five, the youngest fourteen years of age. Note that hyperplasia predominates in all age groups. The proportion of pregravid endometria is highest between twenty and thirty-five years, lowest before twenty years. On the other hand, the proportion of atrophic endometria is highest after thirty-five and lowest before twenty years

diagnosis in the young, unmarried individual, may account for the paucity of cases reported.

Cyclic and Acyclic Bleeding.—The bleeding may be cyclic or acyclic, though the latter form is much more common. Some women experience excessive bleeding for the first time following a period of amenorrhea. In others, it may begin as a profuse and prolonged, cyclically recurring flow, which later becomes irregular and continuous. In the severe case, bleeding may persist for months. Pain and menstrual molimina are as a rule absent.

Parous women are most apt to be affected. A history of one or more full term pregnancies or abortions, prior to the onset of the abnormal bleeding, was elicited in 65 per cent of the author's series. While the condition is often preceded by a period of fertility, sterility is the rule while the abnormality persists. This is readily accounted for by the fact that ovulation is usually absent and that, even in the event of a chance ovulation followed by conception, the abnormal state of the endometrium may interfere with implantation or retention of the fertilized ovum. With correction of the anomaly, fertility is usually restored.

ETIOLOGY

This clinicopathological entity is now generally conceded to be due to a disturbance of the hormonal stimuli on which normal menstrual function depends. A consideration of the etiology must include the role of the ovary, the anterior hypophysis, other incretory glands, and the uterus, site of the abnormal bleeding.

Role of the Ovary.—*Protracted Follicular Activity.*—Schröder,[3] in 1915, published his findings in a series of cases of endometrial hyperplasia, where the ovaries were available for histologic examination. He observed in each case a single large cystic follicle lined by several layers of well preserved granulosa cells indistinguishable from those of the normal ripening follicle. In a few instances, the follicle contained an intact ovum. No functioning corpora lutea were present. He concluded that ovulation and corpus luteum formation does not occur. The ovum remains alive in the persistent, unruptured follicle, which continues to function, elaborating substances which induce the associated endometrial modifications.

Shortly after Schröder's report, Robert Meyer[4] described his findings in a similar study. He likewise stressed the absence of functioning corpora lutea, but found numerous atretic follicles instead of a single large persistent follicle. He therefore concluded that the ovum does not persist but dies prematurely and the follicle undergoes atresia. Another soon develops, which in turn likewise becomes atretic. The continuous action of substances secreted by these successive crops of developing and atretic follicles is responsible for the associated endometrial hyperplasia.

Schröder's and Meyer's assumption that endometrial hyperplasia is due to protracted follicular activity in the absence of corpus luteum formation has been amply confirmed. Recent clinical and experimental findings indicate that both were correct in their deductions as to how such protracted follicular activity may arise. Cases may be encountered in which endometrial hyperplasia is associated with either a single large persistent follicle or numerous small developing and atretic follicles. The two conditions apparently represent different degrees of ovarian malfunction, the arrest of follicular development occurring later in one than the other.

Prolonged Estrogen Stimulation.—That the active principle of the follicle is responsible for endometrial hyperplasia was established when the follicular hormone, estrogen, was isolated and prepared in relatively pure form. It has been repeatedly demonstrated that large doses of this hormone given over a protracted period of time elicit hyperplastic endometrial

22

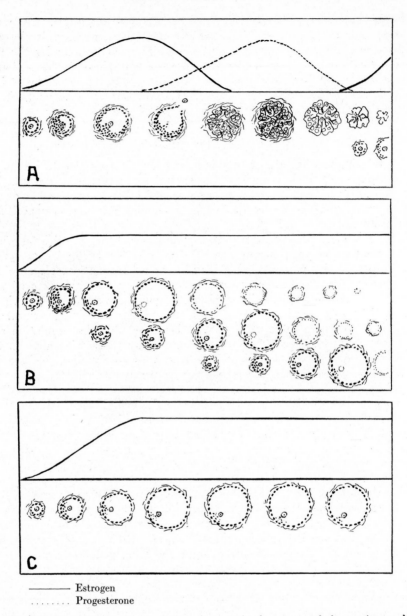

——————— Estrogen
· · · · · · · · Progesterone

Fig. 74.—Diagrammatic representation of events in the ovary and the ovarian sex hormone level in (A) the normal menstrual cycle; (B) uterine bleeding associated with endometrial hyperplasia and successive crops of developing and atretic follicles (R. Meyer); and
(C) uterine bleeding associated with endometrial hyperplasia and a single persistent follicle
(R. Schröder).

modifications in the castrate guinea pig,[5] rat,[6] mouse,[7] rabbit,[8] monkey,[9, 10]
and woman.[11, 12, 13] There is evidence that the experimental production of

endometrial hyperplasia depends not so much on the dosage but rather on the duration of its action. The reactivity of the mucosa to this hormone is apparently also a determining factor. This would also seem to apply in spontaneously occurring hyperplasia in man, for an absolute increase

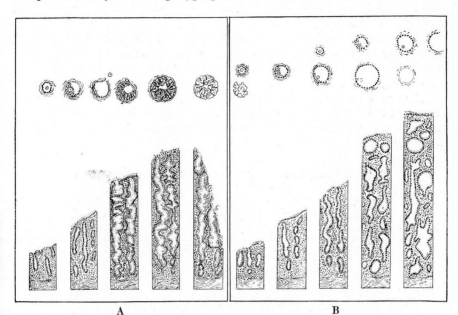

| | A | B |

Fig. 75.—Correlation of events in the ovary and endometrium in (A) normal menstrual cycle and (B) hyperplastic bleeding.

in the estrogen level is not a constant associated finding[14, 15] (Table 4). It would appear that, in the receptive endometrium, hyperplasia may arise whether the estrogen level is excessive or within normal limits. The essen-

TABLE 4

ASSOCIATION BETWEEN ENDOMETRIAL AND HORMONAL FINDINGS IN 225 CASES OF FUNCTIONAL UTERINE BLEEDING

State of Endometrium	Blood Estrogen Test			Blood Gonadotropin Test			Total Number of Cases
	Positive	Threshold	Negative	APR I	APR II–III	Negative	
Premenstrual	17	13	23	0	0	53	53
Early Premenstrual	2	3	10	0	0	15	15
Hyperplasia	21	39	22	9	2	71	82
Local Hyperplasia	5	13	23	7	3	31	41
Interval	3	5	10	0	0	18	18
Atrophic	1	7	8	9	1	6	16
Total number of cases	49	80	96	25	6	194	

tial prerequisite for its development would seem to be prolonged estrogen stimulation, unrelieved by any interruption due to the intervention of progestin, or to removal of the proliferating endometrial tissue through spontaneous breakdown or curettage. Undue reactivity of the receptor organ, rather than an inherent disturbance in estrogen metabolism within the uterus, as some[15] suggest, would seem to be an important factor in the etiology.

Corpora Lutea.—It is generally agreed that the absence of ovulation and corpus luteum formation, originally stressed by both Schröder and Meyer, contributes to the development of endometrial hyperplasia by permitting uninterrupted follicular activity. Rare instances[16, 17, 18] in which apparently functioning corpora lutea have been found associated with a hyperplastic endometrium would appear to challenge this view. This inconsistency may possibly be explained by assuming that they were nonfunctioning bodies, or at least not true luteal structures. This possibility is suggested by Corner's[19] observation that there sometimes appear, in the monkey ovary, atypical bodies, which resemble fresh corpora lutea, show none of the usual signs of regression, but are not associated with pregravid

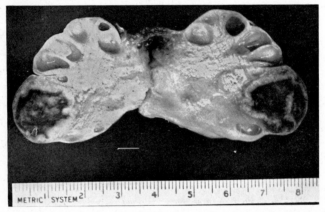

Fig. 76.—Fresh corpus luteum associated with small cystic degeneration of the ovary. Endometrial tissue obtained simultaneously showed partial hyperplasia in a pregravid mucosa (see Fig. 77).

mucosal modifications. Corner concluded that these so-called *corpora aberrantia* are nonfunctioning bodies, or at least secrete no progestin. In a more recent study,[20] he found that corpus luteum regression may take one of two forms: the standard form in which it is transformed into a corpus atreticum, and a second form in which it is converted into a corpus aberrantium. In the latter case, it may persist for a considerable period but apparently no longer functions as a corpus luteum. Whether this holds for man has not been determined.

Endometrial Resistance to Progesterone.—Another possibility is that corpora lutea associated with endometrial hyperplasia are true luteal bodies formed as the result of a recent chance ovulation. This finds support in the clinical observation that a spontaneous return to normal ovarian and menstrual function is not uncommon in metropathia haemorrhagica, particularly in young subjects. Some of the cases in which pregravid mucosal modifications were absent despite the presence of a functioning corpus luteum may possibly be explained by assuming that the hyperplastic mucosa is refractory to progestin. In this connection, we may recall the principle, alluded to elsewhere (see Chap. X), that excessive tissue growth is incompatible with secretory function. If this is true, it would follow that the excessively proliferated tissue, which composes the hyperplastic mucosa, would be more or less resistant to the secretory stimulus, progestin. Proof of such resistance is provided by the finding of endometria in which areas fully converted to the secretory phase occur beside hyperplastic areas (see Fig. 77). Here progestin is undoubtedly available, but apparently can elicit a response only in those

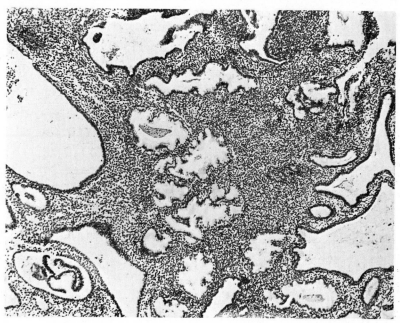

Fig. 77.—Local hyperplasia in a pregravid endometrium. Note serrated glands showing secretory activity, lying side by side with cystically dilated hyperplastic glands. Microphotograph of tissue obtained from twenty-six-year-old woman with irregular bleeding for six months.

areas where the hyperplastic tissue has been thrown off and replaced by tissue stimulated by estrogen but not to the point where secretory activity is no longer possible.

Of interest in this connection is Frankl's[21] observation that luteal hormone was effective in inducing secretory activity in the glands of a hyperplastic mucosa. It is noteworthy that the responsive glands presented the form of hyperplasia in which the proliferating glandular epithelium is thrown into folds (see Fig. 72). These contrast with the glands observed in localized areas of hyperplasia in a pregravid endometrium (see Fig. 77). Here, the lining epithelium of the cystically dilated glands has atrophied. It is of interest that the same type of hyperplasia was present in a case reported by Seegar[22] as refractory to large doses of progesterone. This would suggest that the ability of progestin to evoke a response in an endometrium which has been overstimulated by estrogen depends on the form the overgrowth has taken and the stage it has reached. If the epithelial lining of the glands is still intact, conversion to secretory activity may still be possible, but if it has reached the stage of exhaustion and atrophy, no response will be elicited.

Role of the Anterior Hypophysis.—Experiments carried out with anterior pituitary follicle stimulating and lutenizing extracts (see Chap. XII) indicate that the former causes follicular maturation, the latter lutein transformation, while the combined action of both is necessary to induce ovulation. A disturbance in the production of one or both pituitary sex principles may therefore interfere with ovulation and lead to the formation of unruptured atretic and cystic follicles. Conceivably a relative or absolute excess of the follicle stimulating principle may be responsible for the characteristic ovarian modifications in cases of endometrial hyperplasia. Quantitative studies of the gonadotropic hormone content of the blood and urine have been of little help in determining the validity of this assumption. While an increase in the follicle stimulating hormone content of the body fluids has been demonstrated in a small percentage of the cases, this is not significant, since similar findings have been obtained in other conditions.

Refractoriness of the ovary to the hypophyseal gonadotropes may account for some cases of protracted follicular activity and failure of corpus luteum formation. This is suggested by evidence (see Chap. XII) that the response of the ovary to the gonadotropic hormones is determined not only by the nature of the stimulus, but also by the reactivity of the gonad. The immature and senile, regressing ovary is apparently incapable of responding to the gonadotropic hormones with granulosa luteinization and progestin production, and at best only thecal proliferation and estrogen secretion can be elicited. It seems likely that some cases of hyperplastic bleeding at puberty and the menopause may be explained on this basis.

Role of Other Endocrine Glands.—Hyperplastic bleeding is rarely associated with severe endocrinopathic stigmata, though evidence of mild endocrine disturbance is fairly common. Only two of the author's 225 cases, and three of Hamblen's[2] 700 cases presented stigmata of severe endocrinopathic disease. On the other hand, over half of Hamblen's series presented one or more signs of mild endocrine disorders. The *thyroid gland* is apparently most often affected, especially in younger women. In the author's series, the *basal metabolic rate* was appreciably depressed in twenty one and elevated in fourteen cases. An association between hyperplastic bleeding and mild disturbances of the adrenals, parathyroids and pancreas has also been noted, though less frequently. It is possible that, while these glands are not directly concerned with gonadal activity they may, if disturbed, unfavorably affect the adenohypophysis and thus indirectly lead to disordered ovarian function and hyperplastic bleeding.

Nonendocrine Factors.—Poor hygiene, nutritional faults, undue physical and mental stress, and systemic disease may depress the organism and with it the gonads. These factors play an especially important role in the adolescent group, where ovarian function has not yet achieved a secure footing. The observation that correction of hygienic and nutritional faults alone is often followed by a return of normal menstrual periodicity, would seem to leave little doubt concerning their importance in the etiology.

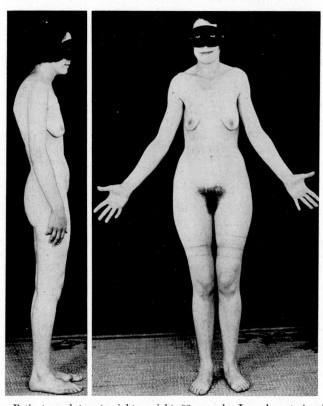

Fig. 78.—Patient aged twenty-eight, weight 98 pounds. Irregular uterine bleeding for one year associated with endometrial hyperplasia. Gain in weight, through diet rich in carbohydrates and vitamins, followed by return of normal periods.

Role of the Uterus.—While the underlying cause of endometrial hyperplasia is fairly clear, there is disagreement as to the immediate cause of the abnormal bleeding. Earlier observers attributed it to myometrial or vascular faults. Schröder[23] proposed that the hemorrhage ensues from localized necrotic areas due to thrombosis of the endometrial blood vessels. This has been questioned on the ground that necrotic areas are not a constant finding in endometrial hyperplasia and, where present, may reasonably be interpreted as the result rather than the cause of the bleeding.[24] In answer to this argument, Fluhmann[25] has suggested that failure to demonstrate necrotic areas may be due to the fact that the endometrium was not examined during the bleeding phase, or that the necrotic areas were washed away when the specimen was prepared for histologic examination. Ehrlich,[26] who studied the endometrial mucosa in a group of abnormally bleeding cases, observed what he terms "thrombotic plaques" in hyperplastic endometria obtained during the bleeding phase. On the basis of his histologic findings, he suggests that what have hitherto been described as "localized areas of necrosis" are actually "areas of capillary thrombosis, with partial or complete loss of the vessel walls, with progressive hyaline-like change of the thrombi, and a mechanical disintegration of the stroma." He could find no evidence of necrosis, nor any of the accepted criteria for infarction which might bear out Schröder's suggestion that localized "necrosis" represents infarction due to thrombosis. Ehrlich suggests that thrombosis is probably the result rather than the cause of the profuse bleeding in such cases, for it was never seen in the absence of hemorrhage, though the reverse was often the case.

On the basis of recent studies, two theories have been advanced to explain hyperplastic bleeding. One, the so-called *estrinpriva hypothesis*, interprets normal and abnormal uterine bleeding as a negative phenomenon precipitated by the partial or complete withdrawal of estrogen. This has been challenged on the ground that bleeding may occur without apparent relationship to the estrogen level. The second theory holds that bleeding from the uterus is a positive phenomenon induced by a hypothetical *bleeding factor* of undetermined origin. Abnormal bleeding is assumed to be caused by an excess of this substance.[27] The lack of unanimity as to the immediate cause of hyperplastic bleeding is probably due to the fact that more than one factor is involved. It may be recalled (see Chap. V) that normal menstruation is the result of a complex interplay between the ovarian sex hormones, on the one hand, and the uterine blood vessels, neuromuscular system, and endometrium, on the other. In hyperplastic bleeding, both hormonal and local uterine factors are apparently operating abnormally. Not only is there a disturbance in the production of estrogen and progestin, but excessive or protracted stimulation by the former induces abnormal changes in the uterus, which are conducive to hemorrhage independent of variations in the estrogen level. Consequently, bleeding at one time may result from variations in the estrogen level, while at another, the abnormal state of the endometrium may be at fault. Comparison of events in the uterus during hyperplastic bleeding and normal menstruation (Table 5) reveals certain differences which suggest a possible explanation of the abnormal bleeding. Especially noteworthy are (1) the vascular modifications, (2) the nature of the desquamative process, and (3) the activity of the myometrium.

Vascular Changes.—Preceding normal menstruation, the vascular tree presents an orderly arrangement. With the onset of the flow, the arterioles become constricted basally, thus hindering the entrance of blood to the endometrium. These slough off along with the rest of the functional layer, leaving the stumps of the blood vessels in the basalis. In the hyperplastic mucosa, on the other hand, the vascular apparatus is disorganized.[26, 28, 29] The blood vessels are increased in number, widely dilated, and follow an irregular course throughout the depth of the mucosa. Turning and twisting, they crowd on each other, making for rhexis or thrombosis. According to Ehrlich,[26] necrosis occurs during menstruation, but thrombosis apparently does not, whereas in the hyperplastic endometrium, thrombosis is a prominent feature but no evidence of necrosis can be found. During the bleeding phase in the hyperplastic endometrium, the blood vessels do not slough off but persist as ready avenues for the escape of blood.

Desquamation.—During normal menstruation, tissue disintegration, though local at first, soon becomes general. A sharp line of cleavage is perceptible, and in the course of a day or so, the entire upper functional

TABLE 5

COMPARISON OF NORMAL MENSTRUATION AND HYPERPLASTIC BLEEDING

	Normal Menstruation	Hyperplastic Bleeding
Nature of Bleeding	Cyclic, recurring about every 28 days; not exceeding 8 days in duration; bleeding controlled.	Usually acyclic, intermittent or continuous; often preceded by period of amenorrhea; bleeding usually uncontrolled.
Subjective Symptoms	Molimina or pain sometimes present. Fullness of breasts and nervous irritability not uncommon.	No molimina; pain rarely present. Fullness of breasts and nervous irritability usually absent.
Pelvic Findings	Uterus and adnexa normal.	Uterus often symmetrically enlarged, boggy. Cervix during bleeding phase softened, discolored, and patulous. One or both ovaries may be palpable or cystic.
Status of Ovaries	Pass through complete cycles, including follicular maturation, ovulation, and corpus luteum formation.	Ovulation and corpus luteum formation absent; persistent follicular activity due to cystic and atretic follicles.
Status of Endometrium	Glands and blood vessels show orderly arrangement. Secretory activity and glycogen present.	Glands, stroma, and blood vessels show marked proliferation. Glands cystically dilated; thrombosis of blood vessels and necrosis common. Secretory activity and glycogen absent.
Myometrial Activity	Powerful contractions begin shortly before onset of bleeding.	Contractions apparently mild or absent.
Desquamative Process	Compacta and spongiosa layers completely disintegrated within a few days. Basalis with stumps of glands and blood vessels remain.	Patchy, irregular; desquamation markedly prolonged, usually incomplete; only superficial parts of blood vessels removed.
Estrogen and Pregnanediol Excretion	Normal estrogen level in urine; pregnanediol usually demonstrable during second half of cycle.	Estrogen level often elevated; pregnanediol rarely demonstrable.

layer of the mucosa sloughs off, leaving the basal layer denuded, with the stumps of the glands and blood vessels exposed at the surface. Coincident with this process, a new growth of epithelium, stroma, and blood vessels begins from the basalis, closing the uterine blood circuit and checking the further influx of blood to the uterine cavity. In hyperplastic bleeding,[26, 28, 29] tissue disintegration and regeneration is patchy and irregular, occurring in widely separated areas and proceeding slowly. As each local area is bared, the blood vessels are opened and bleeding occurs, to be checked sooner or later by regeneration of tissue in the denuded region. As a result, successive hemorrhages occur from different parts of the mucosa. In some cases, the bleeding may appear almost continuous because of the rapidity with which hemorrhage in one area follows that in another.

In the light of recent evidence[30] (see Chap. V), it seems likely that the incomplete and patchy type of desquamation which characterizes hyperplastic bleeding is at least partly attributable to the fact that the hyperplastic tissue has not completed its life cycle by undergoing conversion to the secretory phase. It therefore tends to persist instead of being shed, as in the pregravid mucosa during menstruation. It is possible that the hyperplastic tissue breaks down in scattered areas because, as it grows, the available estrogen supply becomes inadequate to maintain it in its entirety. The fact that the estrogen level rises and falls but at no time is completely withdrawn may also help to explain the patchy type of desquamation. Trauma due to overcrowding of the pathologically overgrown mucosa may be a contributory factor.[31] That exhaustion of the overstimulated tissue may play a part is suggested by observations in monkeys receiving chronic estrogen treatment.[32] Such animals bleed irregularly during treatment, despite the fact that the dose is maintained at a constant level. The bleeding is apparently associated with loss of tissue, for the mucosa is seen to become thinner after each bleeding episode. It does not again attain the thickness achieved before bleeding, despite continued estrogen administration. This would suggest that the endometrium's capacity for growth is limited and that tissue subjected to a continuous growth stimulus must sooner or later cease to respond and disintegrate. The disorganized state of the blood vessels may also contribute to the abnormal type of disintegration which characterizes the hyperplastic mucosa. Ehrlich's observation that menstruation is characterized by necrosis without thrombosis, hyperplastic bleeding by thrombosis without necrosis, suggests that the cause as well as the mechanism of tissue disintegration in the two types of uterine bleeding are different.

Myometrial Activity.—There is evidence (see Chap. VI) that normal menstruation coincides with increasingly powerful myometrial contractions. These apparently play a part in expelling the menstrual decidua and probably also help to check the blood loss (see Chap. V). Not infrequently, these powerful contractions may give rise to a sensation of pain. The motility of the uterus in hyperplastic bleeding has received only scant attention, but the limited evidence at hand suggests that reactivity to oxytocin, which is present to a marked degree during normal menstruation, is absent during the early stages of hyperplastic bleeding.[33, 34] This, coupled with the fact that such bleeding is rarely associated with pain, suggests that powerful contractions are not a usual accompaniment of hemorrhage from a hyperplastic endometrium. This may partly account for the relatively greater loss of blood, as compared with normal menstruation.

Summary.—In summation, it may be stated that the immediate cause of excessive bleeding from a hyperplastic mucosa may be found in the abnormal state of the endometrial blood vessels, the irregular and patchy type of desquamation, and possibly also the absence of powerful myometrial contractions, conditions which in turn are traceable to protracted stimulation by estrogen unrelieved by progestin.

<h2 style="text-align:center">DIAGNOSIS AND DIFFERENTIAL DIAGNOSIS</h2>

The diagnosis of endometrial hyperplasia is readily established by histologic examination of *uterine curettings*. Where possible, curettage should be performed during the early phase of the bleeding, for where the bleeding is prolonged the hyperplastic tissue may be gradually cast off, leaving areas presenting interval or atrophic changes. Thorough curettage of the entire uterine cavity is preferable to use of the suction curette, which may miss local areas of hyperplasia. Local hyperplasia, associated with an atrophic, proliferative or pregravid, secretory type of endometrium is a not uncommon cause of abnormal uterine bleeding[35] and occurred in 13 per cent of the author's series.[36] It is possible that these circumscribed areas of hyperplasia are remnants of a preexisting hyperplastic mucosa which has not yet been completely shed.

Abnormal bleeding at any age may be an expression of pelvic pathology, systemic disease, or disordered endocrine function. *Differential diagnosis* is often difficult, for the character of the bleeding, pelvic findings and endometrial picture may be identical. It is obvious, therefore, that the diagnosis cannot stop with the demonstration of a hyperplastic endometrium. The history, general physical and bimanual pelvic examination, curettage, and quantitative sex hormone studies of the blood and urine (see Table 4) are all essential for the evaluation of a given case. The importance of a thorough investigation increases in proportion to the age of the patient. In the young unmarried girl, curettage is obviously undesirable, and the diagnosis must be made on the basis of the menstrual history, hormone studies, and rectal findings. During the child-bearing period, and particularly in the older woman, curettage and a complete painstaking investigation is imperative. Only after all possible organic causes of hyperplastic bleeding have been excluded may the condition be considered functional and treated as such.

Exclusion of Pelvic Pathology.—Organic lesions of the pelvic organs are not infrequently associated with abnormal bleeding from a hyperplastic mucosa. *Capsular adhesions* secondary to pelvic inflammatory disease may cause such bleeding by impeding ovulation and thus leading to follicular cystosis. A history of repeated attacks of lower abdominal pain, criminal abortion, puerperal infection, and the presence of Neisserian stigmata are important clues in the differential diagnosis.

In some cases, cystic degeneration of the ovary and hyperplastic bleeding may be traceable to *reduction of the ovarian parenchyma* by destructive neoplasms, surgery, or by x-ray or radium irradiation. A history of ovarian resection or exposure to irradiation is significant.

A state of hyperestrinism and excessive uterine bleeding may be due to a *granulosa cell tumor* of the ovary (see Chap. XXXV). In some cases, the neoplasm may be so small that it cannot be detected by pelvic examination. Resumption of uterine bleeding after the menopause, coupled with the finding of a hyperplastic mucosa and large quantities of estrogen in the body fluids, strongly suggests granulosa-cell tumor. Abdominal section and histologic examination of the ovary is the only means of confirming the diagnosis.

Hyperplastic bleeding during the childbearing age may be confused with *abortion, ectopic pregnancy,* or *chorionepithelioma.* It may be recalled that in hyperplasia, the uterus may be somewhat symmetrically enlarged, the cervix patent and slightly discolored. Not infrequently one adnexa may be palpable and tender. These findings, together with a history of amenorrhea preceding the bleeding, may suggest some abnormality of pregnancy. The biologic tests for pregnancy will differentiate the two conditions (see Chap. XXXIX).

Uterine hemorrhage due to small or inaccessible organic lesions of the generative tract may be mistaken for functional hyperplastic bleeding. The author has repeatedly encountered older women, treated with sex hormones for supposed functional bleeding, in whom diagnostic curettage and biopsy revealed fundal or cervical malignancy. The danger of such neglect in women of the cancer age is self-evident.

Clinical Course and Prognosis.—Hyperplastic bleeding may persist for weeks or months. It may cease spontaneously, only to recur after a period of amenorrhea of varying duration. In some instances, the cessation of bleeding may be followed by apparently normal periods. In the married woman, a chance ovulation followed by conception and full term pregnancy may permanently correct the condition. In the preclimacteric woman, the condition may persist but, with extinction of ovarian function, the abnormal bleeding passes into the permanent amenorrhea of the menopause. In the puberal group, spontaneous correction is estimated to occur in from 30 to 80 per cent[37] of the cases. Whether endometrial hyperplasia predisposes to cancer is not established. An association between the two conditions is not uncommon, but this does not necessarily bespeak a causal relationship.

TREATMENT

The aim of the treatment is to control the abnormal bleeding and prevent its recurrence. Choice of therapy depends on the age of the patient and the severity of the condition.

Menopausal Bleeding.—In the premenopausal and older patient, treatment is comparatively simple. *Curettage* should precede any form of treatment. Aside from its diagnostic value, it checks the bleeding temporarily, providing a breathing spell during which a decision may be made as to the best means of preventing a recurrence.

X-ray and Radium Therapy.—Since the preservation of reproductive function is of little moment at this time of life, and the chief object is to effectively and, if need be, permanently stop the bleeding, x-ray radiation of the ovaries, or the intra-uterine application of *radium* is ideally adapted for this type of case. By depressing ovarian function and, where radium is used, endometrial function as well, the uterine hemorrhage is effectively controlled. A so-called *castration dose of x-rays* is usually very effective. For this purpose, the following factors may be employed: 200

KV., 50 cm. STD., 8 MA., 0.5 mm. cu., 1.0 mm. al., 15 x 20 cm. field. Two fields anteriorly and two fields posteriorly over the pelvis are used. 600 r. is given over one field daily until the four fields are treated. In the preclimacteric woman, a so-called *subcastration dose of x-rays* may check the bleeding without precipitating an abrupt menopause. The same factors are used as in the castration dose; 200 r. is given over each of two fields, one anterior and the other posterior, over an area large enough to cover the pelvis. Where radium is to be used, our practice at the Jefferson Hospital is as follows: After diagnostic curettage, 50 mg. of radium in a single capsule or 100 mg. in two capsules in tandem (platinum 1.5 mm. filtration) is placed in the uterine cavity pending histologic examination of four-hour paraffine sections. After the diagnosis is made, the duration of the application is settled: for malignancy, a minimum of 3600 mg. hours; for benign conditions, from 300 to 1800 mg. hours depending on the urgency of the symptoms, age of the patient and her desire for children.

The choice between x-ray and radium radiation depends on the circumstances of the case under consideration. The dose of radium can be more accurately gauged; it can be applied at the same time that curettage is performed, and checks the bleeding more quickly because of its direct action on the bleeding surface. X-ray radiation, on the other hand, avoids undesirable local changes and does not necessitate hospitalization.

Hysterectomy.—Hysterectomy may be preferable to radiotherapy where abdominal section is indicated for some other condition. It may also be desirable where the patient is so constituted that she is likely to suffer severely in the event of an abrupt menopause.

Organotherapy is of little value in functional bleeding at the menopause and should never be used without preliminary curettage.

Puberty and Maturity Bleeding.—The treatment of functional bleeding during adolescence and the childbearing period is difficult and often unsatisfactory. Since the preservation of gonadal and reproductive function is of prime importance, radical procedures which are so effective in the menopausal case, must be avoided except as a last resort.

Endometrial Curettage.—In the mature, married woman, curettage should constitute the first step in the treatment. In the author's experience and that of others, [38], [39], [89] this procedure alone was followed by reestablishment of normal menstrual function in from 25 to 50 per cent of the cases. Curettage not only gives a respite from the bleeding, but also removes the pathologically proliferated mucosa, clearing the way for a normal endometrial response in the event that normal ovarian function is established spontaneously, or as the result of treatment. During reproductive life, especially where pregnancy is desired, the author prefers repeated curettage to radiotherapy. In some cases so treated, conception and pregnancy followed, with resumption of normal menstrual function postpartum. Curettage is undesirable in the young, unmarried girl and should be avoided unless the bleeding is uncontrollable and resists conservative treatment.

Hemostatic Measures.—For the immediate control of the bleeding, chorionic gonadotropin, progestational and androgenic substances have been advocated (see below). In addition, a number of nonspecific agents, such as blood transfusions, calcium, parathormone, ergotine, pituitrin, and vitamins C and K,[40] have been used. These are believed to control the uterine hemorrhage by increasing the coagulability of the blood, decreasing the permeability of the uterine blood vessels, or causing the myometrium to contract upon them. Moccasin snake venom in high dilution may be tried in the young subject.[41, 42] The initial dose is 0.5 cc. of a 1:3000 fresh solution given subcutaneously. This dose is gradually stepped up to 1 cc. by the third day and administered daily or every other day for three weeks or longer, as required.

After the bleeding is checked, attention should be directed to correction of the underlying cause with the view of preventing a recurrence and establishing normal menstrual function. For this purpose, general medical measures, organotherapy and, in the individual case, conservative pelvic surgery, and low dosage irradiation of the ovary and pituitary may be employed.

General Medical Measures.—All *depressive states* which may adversely affect gonadal function should receive attention. Foci of infection, systemic disease, blood dyscrasias,[43] and metabolic disturbances should be eradicated where possible. General hygienic measures are often effective, particularly in the puberal case. Undue physical exertion and mental stress should be avoided. Faults conducive to pelvic congestion should be eliminated. Where anemia is an associated finding, blood transfusions, liver extract and iron are indicated. Some observers[44, 45] recommend the use of from 300 to 500 cc. of whole blood, preferably from a pregnant donor, on the ground that, besides replacing the blood loss and exerting a hemostatic effect, its high luteinizing hormone content may favorably influence gonadal function. In view, however, of recent evidence of the inefficiency of the pregnancy gonadotropes for the stimulation of the hypofunctioning human ovary, the latter hope would seem to be unfounded.

Correction of *nutritional faults* is of the utmost importance. In the thin, undernourished, asthenic type of individual, a high caloric diet, rich in carbohydrate, fat and the essential vitamins, may effect a considerable gain in weight and incidentally correct the menstrual disturbance. In the obese patient, an appreciable reduction in weight (see Chap. XXXIII) is often followed by a return of normal menstrual periodicity.

General medical treatment alone proved effective in correcting the menstrual irregularity in 25 per cent of the author's cases. This approach is preferable to organotherapy because, instead of merely providing a temporary substitute, it seeks indirectly to improve the efficiency of the individual's endocrine apparatus and thus insure an adequate and continued endogenous supply. The response to medical treatment is especially good at puberty and the early part of the reproductive period, when all that is required in most instances is to fortify the tendency to spontaneous adjustment. A number of competent observers[46, 47, 48, 49] have attested to the efficacy of this approach.

Organotherapy.—All the known sex hormones, either singly or in various combinations, have been recommended for the control of the excessive bleeding or correction of the underlying cause. Opinions regarding their efficacy are too conflicting to permit any conclusions. They are nevertheless worth a trial, particularly in the young woman, where radical measures are to be avoided. Sex hormone therapy is indicated only in the functional case and never where there is reason to suspect some organic lesion of the pelvic organs, or systemic disease. There must be a rational basis for their use, and the preparation selected should be administered in a potent form, in adequate dosage, and at the proper time.

Gonadotropes.—Since hyperplastic bleeding would appear to be due to persistent follicular activity uninterrupted by ovulation and corpus luteum formation, a potent luteinizing hormone would appear to be rational therapy. *Human chorionic gonadotropin* has been widely employed for this purpose. [50, 51, 52] The *dose* is 100 to 500 I.U. daily during the bleeding phase. To prevent a recurrence of the bleeding, 100 to 200 I.U. twice weekly for several months is recommended. While many reports laud this preparation, critical observers agree that the results are inconstant and unsatisfactory. This has been the author's experience. The favorable effects sometimes noted following the use of chorionic gonadotropin have been variously explained. Some attribute the cessation of bleeding to its direct action on the myometrial elements, or its inhibitory effect on a hypothetical bleeding factor. Others believe that control of the bleeding is a nonspecific effect due to a foreign protein present in the extract. It is unlikely that it acts by causing luteinization with consequent progestin production, for in many of the cases, the bleeding stopped after only one or two injections and before any structural modifications in the ovary could have been induced. Moreover, there is no convincing proof that the chorionic gonadotropes have any appreciable stimulating effect on the hypofunctioning ovary. On the contrary, there is some evidence that their effect may be depressive (see Chap. XII).

Equine gonadotropin is recommended[53, 54] in *doses* of 100 to 1200 I.U. weekly, or 200 to 1200 I.U. three times a week for one or two weeks, to be repeated after a two week rest period. Since the equine hormone is predominantly a follicle stimulator, and of questionable value for the induction of ovulation and corpus luteum formation in the depressed human ovary (see Chap. XII), it may aggravate rather than minimize the tendency to follicular cystosis and estrogenic bleeding.

The inefficiency of chorionic and equine gonadotropin, when given alone, has led some observers[55] to employ both hormones in succession, with the hope of stimulating maturation of follicles followed by ovulation and corpus luteum formation. There is no convincing evidence that the improvement noted following such treatment significantly exceeded that known to occur spontaneously in the absence of treatment.

A combination of *chorionic gonadotropin and anterior pituitary "synergist"* (synapoidin) has been employed by Mazer.[56] Cessation of the bleeding for several months was noted following the administration of 1 cc. daily for 5 to 20 doses. Their findings await confirmation. This therapy should be used with caution, for overdosage may cause extreme ovarian enlargement, associated with lower abdominal pain, nausea, vomiting, chills, and even fever. This may possibly be due to intraperitoneal hemorrhage from the large hemorrhagic follicles found in such overstimulated ovaries. Allergic shock has also been reported[86] following treatment with synapoidin. When resorting to this form of therapy it should be borne in mind that there is at present no means of predicting what will constitute a safe dose in a specific instance.

Progesterone.—Progesterone[57, 58, 59] or *pregneninolone*[60, 61, 62] is employed by many observers with the hope that it will override the effect of estrogen on the mucosa and thus prevent further excessive proliferation and bleeding. Others believe that it helps to minimize the blood loss by inhibiting myometrial contractions and thus reducing the rate of blood flow to the endometrium. It should be emphasized that this is at best merely substitutive therapy and cannot be expected to correct the underlying disturbance. Since the hyperplastic mucosa is apparently relatively refractory to the action of progestin, the abnormally proliferated mucosa should be removed by curettage, where this is feasible, before administering this hormone. *Treatment* is best instituted about two weeks after curettage to give the endogenous estrogen ample time to prime the mucosa so that it may respond with progestational modifications when progesterone or pregneninolone is supplied. Where curettage is undesirable, as in the young girl or unmarried woman, some observers[59] administer as much as 25 mg. of progesterone daily for five days to check the bleeding. After a few days, progesterone bleeding occurs with disintegration of a progestational type of endometrium. Counting from the onset of such bleeding, three weeks are permitted to elapse to permit the endogenous estrogen to prime the mucosa. Progesterone is then administered intramuscularly in doses of 10 mg. daily for five days. Repetition of this treatment after the induced flow may result in cyclic bleeding from a secretory type of endometrium. The dosage of pregneninolone by mouth required to convert an estrogenic endometrium to the secretory phase is from 280 to 350 mg. in daily doses of 50 mg.[60] Seegar Jones and TeLinde[89] claim good results with an initial dose of 10 mg. of pregneninolone three times a day for seven days before the expected onset of bleeding. In successive months, the daily dose is reduced to 20 mg. They find that cyclic treatment for at least four months is usually necessary.

The favorable results reported with such therapy are difficult to evaluate, particularly where it is preceded by curettage, for mere removal of the hyperplastic mucosa is often followed by a return of normal menstrual periodicity.

Estrogen and Progesterone.—Hamblen and his associates[63] recommend estrogen, followed by progesterone or a combination of both hormones, given at periodic intervals. Such therapy, they maintain, effectively controls menometrorrhagia from an estrogenic endometrium and is followed by a return of normal menstrual periodicity in almost 50 per cent of the cases. On the basis of their results with cyclic estrogen therapy, they suggest that this hormone, possibly by altering the functional capacity of the endometrial vessels, is responsible for the shorter interval between flows and shorter bleeding phase observed during combined estrogen and progesterone therapy. The high percentage of recovery after such treatment they attribute to progesterone, which they believe prevents the progress of ovarian failure.

In the author's opinion, there would seem to be no justification for the use of estrogen in a condition where this hormone is apparently being supplied endogenously in adequate and sometimes excessive amounts. Shortening of the flow and of the interval between flows, observed during estrogen therapy does not necessarily imply a favorable influence on the function of the endometrial vessels. This may as reasonably be attributed to the fact that the threshold for bleeding is reached sooner, since larger amounts of estrogen are available, and the drop in the estrogen level, when a series of injections is completed, is more precipitous. Shortening of the bleeding phase may be due to the fact that endometrial breakdown occurs more rapidly after a steep drop in the estrogen level.[64] Estrogen therapy may improve the condition of the endometrial blood vessels to the extent that it promotes endometrial breakdown and removal of abnormal tissue, and clears the way for a new growth of blood vessels. This may be accomplished with progesterone alone, which has the added advantage that it is less likely to depress ovarian function.

Androgens.—The recent literature contains numerous reports[65, 66, 67] of the excellent effect of androgenic substances for the control of functional uterine bleeding. Estimates as to the total *dosage* required to check the bleeding vary from 300 to 1000 mg. of *testosterone propionate* intramuscularly per cycle. The prophylactic dose ranges from 75 to 200 mg., to be given in divided doses during the last two weeks of the cycle. Some observers claim that the bleeding may be checked within 48 hours after instituting therapy. It is not known whether the androgens act by inhibiting the anterior pituitary and indirectly suppressing estrogen secretion, by overriding the effect of this hormone on the endometrium, or by inhibiting uterine contractility and thus diminishing the influx of blood to the uterine cavity. The possibility that they are converted to progesterone in the organism and thus supply the deficiency of this hormone, has also been considered. Their use in the young woman would appear hazardous in view of the fact that they may exert a depressive effect on ovarian function, or cause uterine atrophy. Moreover, if given in large doses over a protracted period, hirsutism, deepening of the voice, and other signs of masculinization may appear.

Thyroid Substance.—Thyroid substance is often effective,[68, 69] particularly where the abnormal bleeding is associated with obesity or hypothyroidism. The *dose* is ½ to 1 grain three times a day. Larger doses are indicated where the bleeding is associated with hypothyroidism. While such therapy may prove of value at any age, it is especially efficacious in the puberal case. It is contraindicated in the thin, undernourished, nervous individual, or where the associated symptomatology suggests hyperthyroidism.

Whether thyroid substance corrects the underlying ovarian disturbance by supplying a deficiency and thus restoring the endocrine equilibrium, or increases the cellular activity of the organism as a whole, inci-

23

dentally activating the ovary and its endocrine regulators, is not certain. That it may promote luteinization is suggested by van der Hoeven's[70] observation that corpora lutea form following thyroid feeding in the laboratory animal. Van Horn's[71] observation that thyroid feeding triples the amount of estrogen required to induce estrus in the castrate rat suggests that thyroid therapy may control hyperplastic bleeding by accelerating the inactivation or excretion of estrogen.

Surgical Treatment.—*Hysterectomy* is only rarely indicated for abnormal bleeding during the childbearing period, and should be considered only where the alternative is castration. Ovarian resection[72, 73] and aspiration of large cystic follicles per vaginam[74] are recommended by some gynecologists on the assumption that persistent follicles mechanically interfere with maturation of new crops of follicles and subsequent ovulation and corpus luteum formation. When resorting to *ovarian resection,* it is of the utmost importance to conserve as much healthy tissue as possible, since retention of too little ovarian parenchyma makes for a recurrence of follicular cystosis, possibly by creating a relative excess of the anterior pituitary follicle stimulating hormone. This operation should therefore be reserved for cases where the ovaries are appreciably enlarged and there is reason to suspect an ovarian neoplasm, or where pelvic pain is an associated finding. The author has encountered several instances in which ovarian resection was followed after a year or more by a recurrence of the bleeding and cystic enlargement of both the traumatized and intact ovary.

Radiotherapy.—Low dosage x-ray *radiation of the ovary* has been recommended[75] for the control and treatment of functional uterine bleeding in young women, on the theory that such treatment stimulates ovarian function by inducing hyperemia and thus increasing the ovarian blood supply. Others speak of a selective destructive action, made possible by the fact that large graafian follicles are much more radiosensitive than primary follicles and corpora lutea. Small doses of x-ray presumably destroy the large cystic or persistent follicles, removing a mechanical obstacle to development of new crops of follicles.

Dangers.—It should be emphasized that while radiotherapy is ideally adapted for the preclimacteric woman, where the risk to gonadal function is of little concern, it may prove hazardous in the young patient. Individual variations in response to a given dose are so great that the outcome in a given case cannot be predicted with any degree of certainty. A dose that may benefit one individual, may cause permanent amenorrhea and sterility in another. For this reason, such therapy should be employed with due caution and only as a last resort in the young woman. The patient should be warned of the possible danger to gonadal and reproductive function and there should be close cooperation between the gynecologist and roentgenologist. The status of ovarian function before and after treatment should be ascertained by means of endometrial biopsy, the vaginal smear, and quantitative sex hormone studies of the blood and urine. A marked drop in the blood estrogen level, a rise in the gonadotropin content of the urine, or the appearance of retrogressive modifications of the endometrium or vaginal mucosa call for discontinuance of treatment.

It should be emphasized that failure to demonstrate structural changes in the ovaries following radiation does not necessarily rule out the possibility that damage to gonadal function has been incurred.

Low dosage x-ray *radiation of the adenohypophysis*[76, 91] is advocated by some investigators as a means of restoring normal ovarian function. Edeiken[77] recommends the following *routine*: Two x-ray treatments are given weekly at intervals of three days. The first is directed over the anterior pelvis through a field adequate to include both ovaries. The second is given over the pituitary body, the central rays being directed just above and posterior to the mid-point between the outer canthus and external auditory canal. These treatments are continued for three weeks. The following technical factors are used: 127 kilovolts, 14 inch distance, 5 millimeter aluminum filter for three to five minutes. This is equivalent to 50 to 80 R units, or $7\frac{1}{2}$ to $12\frac{1}{2}$ per cent S.E.D.

Recent surveys of both the experimental and clinical evidence relating to pituitary radiation have yielded no convincing proof that the gonadotropic activity of the anterior hypophysis can be stimulated by this means. Warren[87] concludes that "only heavy radiation has a very disturbing effect on the normal pituitary gland and there is little chance that therapeutic irradiation affects it at all." Denniston[88] states that "in view of the profound effects obtained through large doses of x-ray and the apparent lack of effect of doses, such as are used medically, on the inactive pituitary, a note of caution is sounded concerning the indiscriminate use of the therapy in question, and doubt is thrown on its usefulness to stimulate an inactive gland."

ABNORMAL BLEEDING FROM AN ATROPHIC ENDOMETRIUM

Incidence.—Excessive, prolonged or irregular bleeding from an atrophic endometrium occurred in eighteen cases, or 8 per cent of the author's series of 225 cases of functional uterine bleeding. According to Hamblen,[78] atrophic endometria were encountered in all the reported cases of fatal functional uterine hemorrhage, including two contributed by him.

Etiology.—The etiology is not clear. The atrophic mucosa may represent the end result of disintegration of a hyperplastic endometrium. In this connection, the author has not infrequently encountered cases in which the uterine curettings showed hyperplasia at one time and atrophy at another, particularly after a prolonged bleeding spell. Also significant is the observation that monkeys receiving estrogen over a protracted period of time bleed repeatedly during the course of treatment, while the proliferated endometrium shows progressive thinning or attenuation and, despite continued estrogen stimulation, does not again attain the thickness achieved before the occurrence of bleeding. If this assumption is correct, it would follow that excessive bleeding from an atrophic mucosa is due to the abnormal state of the vascular apparatus, which is apparently still responsive to estrogen stimulation though the glandular and stromal elements no longer react to this hormone.

In some instances, particularly in young girls, the atrophic state of the mucosa may possibly be explained on the basis of refractoriness, due to immaturity. The uncontrollable nature of the hemorrhage, which in some cases may prove fatal, may be partly due to myometrial atony. Inability of the refractory endometrium to respond with sufficient growth to provide an adequate covering for the uterine blood vessels may perhaps also be a contributing factor. Hamblen,[78] among others, has suggested that the condition may be due to hypoestrinism. This is unconvincing, for a deficiency of estrogen, sufficiently marked to account for complete absence of glandular and stromal proliferation, should also be associated with absence of vascular growth, resulting in amenorrhea rather than excessive uterine bleeding. It is obvious that a decision as to the etiology must await further investigation.

Diagnosis.—The diagnosis of bleeding associated with mucosal atrophy is readily made by histological examination of the endometrial curettings. Quantitative estrogen and pregnanediol studies may help distinguish between mucosal atrophy due to refractoriness and that attributable to deficiency of the ovarian sex hormones. Whether the atrophy is the end result of endometrial hyperplasia can be determined with certainty only if a previous curettage revealed hyperplastic modifications.

Treatment.—The immediate aim of the treatment is to control the hemorrhage. Where the bleeding is so severe and uncontrollable as to threaten the patient's life, heroic measures are justified. Organotherapy, in the author's experience, has proved ineffective in this type of uterine bleeding.

OVULATORY BLEEDING

Incidence.—Excessive uterine bleeding from a pregravid secretory type of endometrium has, until recently[79, 80, 81] received scant attention in the literature. It was encountered in sixty-eight patients or 30 per cent of the author's series of 225 cases. Usually cyclic in nature, it differs from normal menstruation in that it is more profuse, prolonged (*menorrhagia*), or occurs at shorter intervals (*polymenorrhea*).

Etiology.—*Menorrhagia.*—The etiology is obscure. Some observers blame a defective corpus luteum, while others believe the fault resides in the uterus per se. It has been suggested that some cases are due to myometrial insufficiency, resulting in weak uterine contractions and improper closure of the uterine blood vessels. This explanation would seem to be particularly applicable to cases of profuse, or prolonged bleeding at approximately twenty-eight day intervals from a mucosa, which has been fully converted to the pregravid phase and is apparently undergoing normal desquamation and regeneration. The menorrhagia sometimes encountered in young women with hypoplastic uteri may possibly be accounted for on this basis. A similar condition in the mature parous woman may be traceable to subinvolution of the uterus following too frequent gestations, while in the menopausal woman, it may be due to fibrosis of the uterus.

Recent studies, particularly those of Traut and Kuder,[82] stress the fact that profuse or prolonged cyclic bleeding may often occur from endometria which show evidence of luteal influence, but differ from the normal menstruating mucosa in that conversion to the secretory phase occurs only in scattered areas, or that shedding is irregular so that desquamation and regeneration of the mucosa is not completed within the normal time. Traut and Kuder describe these conditions as "irregular ripening" and "irregular shedding" respectively, and blame them for the excessive bleeding. The association of irregular ripening with subnormal pregnanediol values suggests that it may be due to a defective corpus luteum which secretes subnormal quantities of progestin. On the other hand, the observation that curettage alone may sometimes correct the abnormal bleeding, points to some fault in the mucosa which makes it respond irregularly to a

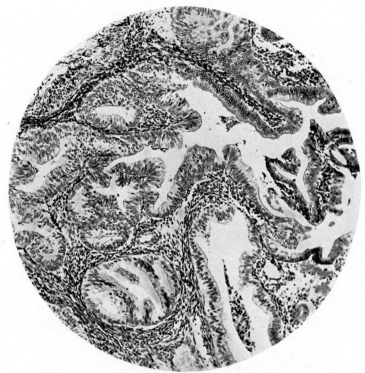

Fig. 79.—"Irregular ripening" of the endometrium. Note large stellate glands showing secretory activity lying adjacent to glands of the proliferative type.

normal supply of progestin. The cause of irregular shedding of the pregravid mucosa is likewise uncertain. Whether the cystic corpora lutea sometimes found in this condition[35] play a part in the etiology, we cannot say. It is conceivable that these structures regress so slowly that progestin is withdrawn less rapidly than in the normal case and mucosal desquamation and regeneration are correspondingly delayed. According to Rockstroh,[83] the endometrium shows no pathologic change to which the irregular and prolonged desquamation and regeneration might be ascribed. He suggests that the cause is not prolonged regression of the corpus luteum, but rather inadequate production of estrogen by the developing follicle of the succeeding cycle. As proof he offers his observation that the estrogen level in the blood of such patients is below normal. On the other hand, Samuels[90] found the estrogen and androgen values within normal limits in such cases, while pregnanediol continued to be excreted after the onset of menstruation. That an endometrial defect is responsible for some of the cases is suggested by reports of cure following curettage.[90]

Polymenorrhea.—The etiology of normal or profuse uterine bleeding, which occurs from a pregravid mucosa, at intervals of twenty-one days or less, is likewise obscure. This type of bleeding is usually encountered in the parous woman, especially between the thirty-fifth and forty-fifth year.

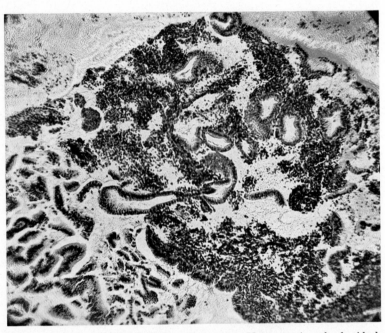

Fig. 80.—"Irregular shedding" of the endometrium. Note secreting glands side by side with glands showing proliferative changes. Some of the glands are collapsed and the stroma is dense. Endometrial tissue obtained on the eighth day of a prolonged flow. Process of disintegration and regeneration, which is normally completed by the second or third day of the flow, is apparently still in progress.

The ovaries may contain numerous cystic and atretic follicles, as well as one or more functioning corpora lutea of approximately the same age. The uterus may be normal in size, or symmetrically enlarged. In some instances, marked edema and hyperemia of the endometrial stroma has been observed. Schröder[84] attributes abbreviation of the menstrual cycle to premature regression of the corpus luteum. He bases this on his observation that, in short as in normal cycles, the transition from the proliferative to the secretory phase occurs about the fourteenth day, indicating that the follicular phase is of normal length, and the luteal phase shortened. Acceleration of the ovarian cycle as a whole, with abbreviation of both the follicular and luteal phase, may account for some cases. This is suggested by the finding of a fresh corpus luteum on the eleventh day of a fourteen day cycle in one instance. Short cycles may also conceivably be due to a tendency for one ovarian cycle to begin before the preceding one is completed. Cases have been recorded in which the corpus luteum of the preceding cycle had not regressed to the degree normally seen when a new cycle is on its way. Hamblen's[2] report of high pregnanediol values in some of his patients with polymenorrhea is significant in this connection.

Whether the *cause* of these temporal anomalies resides in the ovary, anterior pituitary gland, or elsewhere is not known. Hyperactivity of the adenohypophysis, with consequent speeding up of the cyclic activity of the ovary, has been suggested as a cause. A deficiency of anterior pituitary luteinizing hormone may account for shortening of the cycle due to premature regression of the corpus luteum. Proof of either possibility is still wanting.

The frequent association of polymenorrhea with *hypothyroidism* suggests a causal relationship. Conceivably thyroid hypofunction may adversely affect the adenohypophysis, ovary, or both, resulting in a deficient luteinizing impulse or defective corpus luteum. *Constitutional faults,* such as malnutrition and asthenia, have been stressed by Schröder[84] as possible causes of polymenorrhea. Some observers ascribe an important role to *psychic factors* on the ground that psychotherapy often corrects this condition. In addition, it has been pointed out that polymenorrhea is often encountered in mentally diseased, and sexually perverted women. Whether this association implies a causal relationship between the psychic and menstrual aberrations, or they are independent manifestations of constitutional inferiority, we cannot say.

Diagnosis and Differential Diagnosis.—Bleeding from a pregravid mucosa at approximately twenty-eight day intervals may be considered abnormal if the blood loss appreciably exceeds the limits of normal, or the bleeding persists more than seven days. Where the interval between the onset of each bleeding phase is twenty-one days or less, the condition may be tentatively diagnosed as polymenorrhea, pending the demonstration of pregravid mucosal modifications preceding each flow. These findings will help distinguish between ovulatory and anovulatory bleeding, which occurs from an atrophic, proliferative, or hyperplastic type of mucosa. Polymenorrhea may be differentiated from normal periods alternating with intermenstrual bleeding by the character of the endometrial curettings obtained before each of two successive flows. If both specimens present pregravid changes, the condition may be diagnosed as polymenorrhea, since intermenstrual bleeding occurs from a proliferative type of endometrium.

The bleeding may be considered functional if no local or general pathology is demonstrable.

Treatment.—Since the etiology is obscure, the treatment is necessarily empirical. *Curettage* is sometimes effective in menorrhagia associated with irregular ripening or shedding of the endometrium.[90] Where myometrial insufficiency is suspected, the oxytocics are worth a trial. The correction of faulty posture, visceroptosis, and other faults conducive to pelvic congestion may minimize the rate of blood flow to the uterus.

Estrogen, in doses of 10,000 to 20,000 I.U. intramuscularly twice weekly, is recommended for bleeding associated with uterine hypoplasia. Convincing evidence of the efficacy of such treatment is still lacking. Since the endogenous hormones have failed to elicit adequate development of the uterus, it is unlikely that exogenous estrogen will be more effective. Aside from the uncertainty of its effect on the uterus, such therapy may depress ovarian function.

In menorrhagia associated with irregular ripening of the endometrium, use of *progestin* would appear rational therapy, the aim being to complete the conversion of the mucosa to the pregravid phase and thus speed up the process of desquamation and regeneration. For this purpose, 1 to 2 mg. of progesterone daily by injection, or 10 to 25 mg. of pregneninolone by mouth, for seven days beginning on the fourteenth day of the cycle, may be tried.

Rockstroh[83] has reported good results in menorrhagia due to irregular shedding of the endometrium, following the injection of 1000 mouse units of estrogenic substance daily for four days, beginning on the second day of the flow. This may conceivably act by speeding up the process of regeneration.

Chorionic gonadotropin has been employed for the treatment of polymenorrhea on the assumption that it is due to premature regression of the corpus luteum. The dose is 500 I.U. daily or every other day, beginning two weeks after the onset of the preceding flow. Though the evidence is too limited to permit any conclusion as to its efficacy, chorionic gonadotropin merits a trial in view of evidence that it may augment existing luteal function in the human being (see Chap. XII). Use of equine or hypophyseal gonadotropin in this condition is of questionable value since they are predominantly follicle stimulating.

In view of recent evidence (see Chap. XII) that the luteotrophic and lactogenic factors of the anterior hypophysis are identical, use of a potent lactogenic preparation would seem to be rational therapy. Clinical evidence regarding the efficacy of this form of therapy is still lacking.

Thyroid substance, in doses of 1 grain three times daily is indicated where the menstrual anomaly is associated with a low basal metabolic rate and other signs of hypothyroidism.

INTERMENSTRUAL BLEEDING

Definition.—The term cyclic intermenstrual bleeding describes periodic staining or bleeding from the uterus, occurring approximately midway between the flows. Fortunately, the condition is relatively uncommon and the blood loss as a rule is too small to be a matter for concern.

The bleeding usually occurs at some time between the twelfth and sixteenth days of the menstrual cycle, and may last from a few hours to one or two days. It is often so slight as to be detectable only by microscopic examination of the vaginal washings, but at times is sufficiently free to require use of a napkin. Only rarely is the blood loss comparable to that of the normal menstrual flow. Lower abdominal pain (mittelschmerz) is frequently an associated symptom.

Etiology.—The etiology is obscure. Most investigators believe it is related in some way to follicular rupture, because it occurs at the supposed time of ovulation (see Chap. IV). The fact that mittelschmerz (see Chap. XXX) is often an associated symptom lends some support to this assumption. The occurrence of bleeding immediately before ovulation in the dog, and coincident with this phenomenon in the cow, is significant in this connection. Of interest also is Hartman's[85] observation that intermenstrual bleeding in the macaque occurs in the course of ovulatory but not of anovulatory cycles.

Though the available evidence suggests that intermenstrual bleeding is causally related to the ovulatory process, there is no definite information as to how the bleeding is produced, or why it occurs in some women and not in others. Some observers believe the immediate cause of the bleeding is an abrupt increase in the level of estrogen, which exerts a hyperemic and vascularizing effect on the uterus, causing diapedetic bleeding. This view is based on reports that the cycle of estrogen excretion reaches a peak at the time of ovulation, and the observation that intermenstrual bleeding occurs by diapedesis from a late proliferative or early secretory type of endometrium, which shows no evidence of regression or tissue disintegration.

To account for the fact that intermenstrual bleeding occurs in some women and not in others, it must be assumed that the rise in estrogen, incident to ovulation, is not the only factor involved. Since curettage sometimes corrects the condition, it is possible that some endometrial defect is at fault. Abnormal sensitivity of the endometrial blood vessels to the hyperemic action of estrogen may explain some cases of intermenstrual bleeding. Conditions making for pelvic congestion and overfilling of the uterine blood vessels may conceivably be a contributory cause.

Diagnosis and Differential Diagnosis.—Intermenstrual bleeding may be readily recognized by its periodicity and tendency to occur midway between the flows. It may be differentiated from polymenorrhea by microscopic examination of curettings obtained before each of two successive flows. If one occurs from a late proliferative mucosa and the other from a pregravid endometrium, a diagnosis of intermenstrual bleeding is justified. It is important to exclude, by curettage and a careful pelvic examination, any local organic disease which may give rise to intermenstrual bleeding.

Treatment.—Because of its obscure origin, treatment is necessarily empirical. Fortunately, the blood loss is usually too slight to cause concern, and once its functional character has been established, the patient may be assured that it is of little significance. Curettage is sometimes effective in correcting the condition, and elimination of local faults conducive to pelvic congestion may prove beneficial. There is no convincing evidence that any benefit may be expected from the available sex hormones. Androgen therapy, advocated by some observers because of its ability to antagonize the action of estrogen on the endometrium, should be avoided because of its possible inhibitory effect on the ovary.

BIBLIOGRAPHY

1. Fluhmann, C. F., and Morse, D. L.: Am. J. Obst. & Gynec. *21:*455, 1931.
2. Hamblen, E. C.: Endocrine Gynecology. Springfield, Ill., Charles C. Thomas, 1939, pp. 296–307.
3. Schröder, R.: Arch. f. Gynäk. *110:*633, 1919.
4. Meyer, R.: Arch. f. Gynäk. *113:*259, 1920.
5. Burch, J. C., Wolfe, J. M., and Cunningham, R. S.: Endocrinol. *16:*541, 1932.
6. Zondek, B.: J. Exper. Med. *63:*789, 1936.
7. Parkes, A. S.: Lancet *1:*485, 1935.
8. Reynolds, S. R. M.: Anat. Rec. *62:*269, 1935.
9. Zuckerman, S., and Morse, A. H.: Surg., Gynec. & Obst. *61:*15, 1935.
10. Tietze, K.: Ztschr. f. Geburtsh. u. Gynäk. *108:*79, 1934.
11. Kaufmann, C.: Proc. Roy. Soc. Med. *27:*849, 1934.
12. Damm, P. N.: Acta obst. & gynec. Scandinav. *15:*58, 1935.
13. Zondek, B.: Wien. klin. Wchnschr. *49:*455, 1936.
14. Hamblen, E. C.: J. Clin. Endocrinol. *1:*180, 1941.
15. Kurzrok, R.: J. Clin. Endocrinol. *1:*199, 1941.
16. Babes, A. A.: Arch. f. Gynäk. *122:*448, 1924.
17. Novak, E., and Martzloff, K. H.: Am. J. Obst. & Gynec. *8:*385, 1924.
18. Beckman, M.: Arch. f. Gynäk. *136:*519, 1929.
19. Corner, G. W., Bartelmez, G. W., and Hartman, C. G.: Am. J. Anat. *59:*433, 1936.
20. Corner, G. W.: Carnegie Inst. Wash. Publ. No. 541, Contrib. Embryol. No. 192, 1942, vol. 30, p. 85.
21. Frankl, O.: Arch. f. Gynäk. *165:*295, 1937.
22. Seegar, G. E.: Am. J. Obst. & Gynec. *39:*469, 1941.
23. Schröder, R.: Arch. f. Gynäk. *104:*27, 1915.
24. Novak, E.: South. M. J. *25:*261, 1932.
25. Fluhmann, C. F.: J.A.M.A. *93:*1136, 1929; Surg., Gynec. & Obst. *52:*1051, 1931.
26. Ehrlich, H. E.: Am. J. Obst. & Gynec. *42:*484, 1941.
27. Wilson, L., and Kurzrok, R.: Am. J. Obst. & Gynec. *31:*911, 1936.
28. Schröder, R.: Die mensuellen Genitalzyklus u. seine Störungen, in, Veit-Stoeckel's Handb. f. Gynäk., Munich, J. F. Bergmann, 1928, vol. 1, part 2.
29. Frankl, O.: Wien. klin. Wchnschr. *47:*839, 1934.
30. Watson, M. C., and McHenry, E. W.: Am. J. Obst. & Gynec. *35:*316, 1937.
31. Klinkenberg, H.: Klin. Wchnschr. *14:*1057, 1925.
32. Hisaw, F. L.: Am. J. Obst. & Gynec. *29:*638, 1935.
33. Junghans, E.: Zentralbl. f. Gynäk. *59:*1760, 1935.
34. Kneer, M.: Arch. f. Gynäk. *170:*483, 1940.
35. Pallos, K., and Treite, P.: Ztschr. f. Geburtsh. u. Gynäk. *122:*28, 1941.
36. Anspach, B. M., and Hoffman, J.: Am. J. Obst. & Gynec. *26:*147, 1933.
37. Klingelhofer, W.: Zentralbl. f. Gynäk. *65:*743, 1941.
38. Burch, L. E.: J. Indiana Med. A. *27:*560, 1934.
39. Heynemann, T.: Zentralbl. f. Gynäk. *57:*2055, 1933.
40. Dietz, R.: München. med. Wchnschr. *88:*1009, 1941.
41. Watkins, C. H.: Proc. Staff Meet., Mayo Clin. *11:*261, 1936.
42. Goldberger, M. A., and Peck, S. M.: Am. J. Obst. & Gynec. *33:*469, 1937.
43. Buxton, C. L.: Am. J. Obst. & Gynec. *42:*502, 1941.
44. Clauberg, C.: Zentralbl. f. Gynäk. *57:*47, 1933.
45. Engelhart, E., and Petzal, E.: Arch. f. Gynäk. *169:*347, 1939.
46. Frank, R. T.: J.A.M.A. *104:*1991, 1935.
47. Aschner, B.: Endocrinol., gynec. si obst. *1:*97, 1936.
48. Bauer, J.: Harvey Lectures. Baltimore, Williams & Wilkins Co., 1934, pp. 37–55.
49. Shorr, E.: J. Pediat. *19:*327, 1941.

50. Novak, E., and Hurd, G. B.: Am. J. Obst. & Gynec. *22*:501, 1931.
51. Clauberg, C.: Med. Welt *9*:367, 1933.
52. Jeffcoate, T. N. A.: J. Obst. & Gynec. Brit. Emp. *44*:31, 1937.
53. Kennedy, R. B., and Shelton, C. F.: J. Michigan M. Soc. *38*:209, 1939.
54. Gray, L. A.: South. M. J. *33*:160, 1940.
55. Hamblen, E. C.: Am. J. Obst. & Gynec. *40*:615, 1941.
56. Mazer, C., and Ravetz, E.: Am. J. Obst. & Gynec. *41*:474, 1941.
57. MacGregor, T. N.: Brit. Med. J. *2*:116, 1938.
58. Seegar, G. E.: Am. J. Obst. & Gynec. *39*:469, 1940.
59. Allen, W. M., and Heckel, G. P.: Am. J. Obst. & Gynec. *44*:984, 1942.
60. Wiesbader, H.: Am. J. Obst. & Gynec. *42*:1013, 1941.
61. Wenner, R.: Schweiz. med. Wchnschr. *71*:1334, 1941.
62. Gaines, J. A., Geist, S. H., and Salmon, U. J.: J. Clin. Endocrinol. *1*:554, 1941.
63. Hamblen, E. C., Hirst, D. V., and Cuyler, W. K.: Am. J. Obst. & Gynec. *45*:513, 1943.
64. Markee, J. E.: Carnegie Inst. Wash. No. 518, Contrib. Embryol. No. 177, 1940, vol. 28, p. 219.
65. Loeser, A. A.: Lancet *1*:373, 1938.
66. Abarbanel, A. R.: Am. J. Obst. & Gynec. *39*:243, 1940.
67. Geist, S. H., Salmon, U. J., and Gaines, J. A.: Endocrinol. *23*:784, 1938.
68. King, J. E.: Am. J. Obst. & Gynec. *26*:582, 1933.
69. Mussey, R. D., and Haines, S. F.: Am. J. Obst. & Gynec. *27*:404, 1934.
70. van der Hoeven, H.: Zentralbl. f. Gynäk. *58*:1405, 1934.
71. van Horn, W. M.: Endocrinol. *17*:152, 1933.
72. Robinson, M. R.: Am. J. Obst. & Gynec. *30*:18, 1935.
73. Bennett, M. J., and Russell, P. B., Jr.: South. Surg. *10*:154, 1941.
74. Zondek, B.: Harefuah *14*:12, 1938.
75. Kaplan, I. I.: Am. J. Obst. & Gynec. *34*:420, 1937.
76. King, J. C.: South. M. J. *35*:616, 1942.
77. Edeiken, L.: Am. J. Obst. & Gynec. *25*:511, 1933.
78. Hamblen, E. C., and Sprunt, D. H.: Endocrinol. *21*:553, 1937.
79. Anspach, B. M., and Hoffman, J.: Am. J. Obst. & Gynec. *28*:473, 1934.
80. Kurzrok, R., and Wilson, L.: Am. J. Obst. & Gynec. *31*:911, 1936.
81. Jones, H. W.: Am. J. Obst. & Gynec. *35*:64, 1938.
82. Traut, H. F., and Kuder, A.: Surg., Gynec. & Obst. *61*:145, 1935.
83. Rockstroh, H.: Ztschr. f. Geburtsh. u. Gynäk. *116*:232, 1937.
84. Schröder, R., Kessler, R., and Tietze, K.: Zentralbl. f. Gynäk. *57*:11, 1933.
85. Hartman, C. G.: Carnegie Inst. Wash. Publ. No. 433, Contrib. Embryol. No. 134, 1932, vol. 23, pp. 1–161.
86. Phillips, E. W.: Am. J. Obst. & Gynec. *44*:706, 1942.
87. Warren, S.: Arch. Path. *35*:304, 1943.
88. Denniston, R. H., II.: J. Exper. Zool. *91*:237, 1942.
89. Jones, G. E. S., and TeLinde, R. W.: Bull. J. Hopkins Hosp. *71*:282, 1942.
90. Samuels, L. T., cited by McKelvey, J. L.: Journal-Lancet *62*:434, 1942.
91. Kaplan, I. I.: J.A.M.A. *121*:1199, 1943.

CHAPTER XXVI

DYSMENORRHEA

INTRODUCTION

Incidence.—Menstrual pain is estimated to occur in over one half of all menstruating women.[1] Though often an expression of some local organic lesion, it frequently appears in the absence of pelvic pathology and may be entirely compatible with normal gonadal function and fertility. Unfortunately, the periodic attacks of pain tend to undermine the general health, especially in women with a poor nervous system. The loss of working time during attacks is a distinct social and economic handicap, a factor of importance since an increasing number of women are being thrown on their own resources for a livelihood. Obviously, these distressed individuals urgently need relief. Some progress in this direction has been made, but much has yet to be accomplished.

Definition and Nomenclature.—Dysmenorrhea literally signifies "difficult monthly flow." The term is applied to all cases in which lower abdominal pain is experienced just before and during the flow. Menstrual pain without demonstrable pathology is designated "primary," "essential," "idiopathic," "spasmodic" or *functional*, while that due to some local organic lesion is described as "secondary," "acquired," "congestive" or *organic*.

Symptomatology.—(Table 6) Dysmenorrhea is not a disease but a syndrome in which lower abdominal pain is the most prominent symptom. In the functional case, the pain usually begins shortly before or coincident with the onset of the flow, and subsides when it becomes free. It is intermittent, cramp-like and colicky in character, and varies in intensity from a mere exaggeration of the usual menstrual molimina to severe labor-like pain, which may incapacitate the patient for the duration of the attack. In dysmenorrhea of organic origin, the pain tends to begin at or shortly after the onset of the flow and persists throughout the bleeding phase or even beyond. Exceptions are not uncommon, however, and consequently the clinical symptomatology is not altogether reliable as an aid in distinguishing between functional and organic dysmenorrhea.

While lower abdominal pain may be the sole complaint, aching sensations in the lower back and thighs, and vesicle and rectal tenesmus are not uncommon. These are often accompanied by headache, nausea, vomiting, lassitude, fatigue, melancholia, extreme emotionalism, and other expressions of psychoneurotic hyperirritability.

ETIOLOGY

The uterus, like all other smooth muscle organs, may be the seat of two types of pain: one, purely visceral in character, which originates from

TABLE 6

Analysis of Clinical Findings in 124 Cases of Dysmenorrhea

Initiation of Dysmenorrheic Career...	a. With first flow	83
	b. After menstrual habit established	15
	c. During adult life	26
	Events immediately preceding onset:	
	1. Marriage	7
	2. Pregnancy	5
	3. Abortion	3
	4. Cold or infection	2
	5. Operation	2
	6. Constitutional disease	2
	7. Psychic shock	5
Nature of Pain	a. Steady dull feeling of fullness	5
	b. Cramps of rhythmic nature	38
	c. Severe paroxysmal pain	81
When Pain Begins	a. Before onset of flow	77
	b. With onset of flow	42
	c. After onset of flow	5
When Pain Ceases	a. With onset of flow	25
	b. After a day or two	70
	c. Persists throughout flow	29
Periodicity of Pain	a. Invariably accompanies flow	99
	b. Sometimes absent	25
Location of Pain	a. Always the same... 108 b. Varies	16
Passage of Fragments	a. Fragments passed.. 28 b. Not passed	96
Amount of Flow	a. Normal	59
	b. Profuse	41
	c. Scanty	24
Frequency of Flow	a. Normal	58
	b. Too frequent	33
	c. Infrequent	33
Condition of Genitalia	a. Normal	76
	b. Uterine hypoplasia	9
	c. Acute anteflexion	10
	d. Pin-point cervical os	14
	e. Adnexal masses	15
Constitutional Type	a. Normal	36
	b. Obese	43
	c. Asthenic	45
Nervous Status	a. Stable........... 71 b. Unstable	53
Allergic Diathesis	a. Present........... 12 b. Absent	112
Associated Symptoms	a. Headache......... 42 e. Fainting	2
	b. Nausea........... 29 f. Epilepsy	4
	c. Vomiting......... 21 g. Diarrhea	2
	d. Breast pain....... 10	

some cause outside the uterus and sets up paroxysmal myometrial contractions, and a second, somatic type of pain which is constant and more

definitely localized, and arises from some local organic lesion. The intensity of the visceral pain is determined by the force of the stimulus and the reactivity of the uterus, while the severity of the somatic pain is contingent upon the nature, location and extent of the lesion.

Organic Causes.—Pain at the flow may be due to fibromyomata, adenomata, endometriomata, acquired malpositions, endocervicitis, or cervical occlusions. It may also result from lesions of the adnexa and surrounding structures, particularly chronic pelvic inflammatory disease, ovarian neoplasms, endometriosis of the adnexa and retrovaginal septum, ureteral stricture, and chronic appendicitis. Endometriomata of the uterus or adnexa may account for cases of obscure origin. Such lesions are often overlooked, particularly when small or situated within the uterine wall. These endometrium-like growths undergo cyclic changes like those in the uterine mucosa. During the catabolic phase, the accumulated menstrual secretions, lacking an outlet, may give rise to pressure pain.

Fortunately, the diagnosis of dysmenorrhea of organic origin offers little difficulty. The cause can usually be ascertained by pelvic examination, or deduced from the past history and associated clinical findings. Moreover, the treatment is self-evident, and involves removal or correction of the underlying cause. A far more difficult problem is presented by the functional dysmenorrheas, where no gross pathology can be found to account for the pain.

Etiology of Functional Dysmenorrhea

This type of dysmenorrhea has long been the bugbear of gynecology. Because of its obscure etiology, many theories have been proposed at one time or another to explain its cause and the mechanism of the pain. Earlier observers stressed uterine faults, but emphasis has recently shifted to hormonal factors which influence uterine motility.

Uterine Causes.—Uterine hypoplasia, pathologic anteflexion and cervical stenosis, as well as myometrial, mucosal and vascular defects have all been suspected at one time or another as possible causes of functional dysmenorrhea.

Obstructive Theory.—The frequent association of dysmenorrhea with uterine hypoplasia, acute anteflexion and cervical stenosis formed the basis of Mackintosh's[2] so-called "obstructive theory." According to this observer, these uterine anomalies cause pain by mechanically obstructing the exit of the menstrual fluid. The retained blood, acting as a foreign body, sets up powerful uterine contractions which are experienced as pain. In support of this theory it has been pointed out that menstrual pain tends to subside when the flow becomes free; that pregnancy, which often corrects these anomalies, may terminate a dysmenorrheic career and that relief sometimes follows cervical dilatation or application of a stem pessary. Opponents of this view argue that such uteri offer no real obstruction since a sound can readily be passed, at least during the bleeding phase. They deny that mechanical obstruction to the flow is responsible for the pain, on the ground that a hematometra may be unassociated with pain, or at most cause discomfort which in no way resembles the spasmodic, colicky pain generally attributed to obstruction. The observation that dysmenorrhea may often occur in the absence of acute anteflexion and cervical stenosis, and conversely, that the flow may be painless despite the presence of these anomalies, would seem to detract from their importance as etiologic factors.[3] The fact that pain does not occur at every period and varies in severity from time to time in the same individual, suggests that the anatomical type of uterus, which is necessarily constant, is not the sole factor concerned. This is further emphasized by the observation that many adolescent girls bleed periodically without discomfort for several months or years before the periods become painful.[4, 5] Were the dysmenorrhea attributable to uterine hypoplasia, which is an expression of immaturity, one would expect the sequence of events to be reversed, pain accompanying the earlier periods and disappearing as the individual matures.

While the evidence would seem to justify a negation of the obstructive theory, it does not necessarily eliminate acute anteflexion and cervical stenosis as contributory causes of menstrual pain. Their association with dysmenorrhea is too frequent to be merely casual. It is possible that the uterine anomalies and the dysmenorrhea are independent manifestations of general inferiority, or that this type of uterus causes painful periods in some other way than by obstructing the flow. It may be, as Blair-Bell[6] has suggested, that the pain is due to interference with the normal peristaltic wave of contraction at the point of flexion, giving rise to irregular paroxysmal contractions. The relief which often follows correction of malpositions may be due to improved alignment of the uterus, which permits the waves of contraction to proceed unimpeded.

Myometrial Insufficiency.—Some investigators believe that an ill-developed uterine musculature is of considerable importance in the etiology. Reasoning from the fact that the hypoplastic uterus shows a preponderance of connective tissue over muscle fibers, Schultz[7] suggested that when the uterine blood vessels become engorged as a result of the normal hyperemia of menstruation, the myometrium is incapable of completely emptying the uterine veins. The resulting venous stasis elicits pressure stimulation of the uterine nerves, giving rise to powerful contractions and pain. Schröder[8] has suggested that the menstrual pain associated with uterine hypoplasia is due to the myometrium's inability to adapt itself to the monthly congestive process. He reasons that, in a small ill-developed uterus, with a narrow lumen and supported by short inelastic ligaments, pain results from distention of the serosa by the premenstrual swelling and hyperemia, and stretching of the inadequate musculature by the uterine contractions which occur during the period of desquamation. Protagonists of this view attribute the relief, which often follows pregnancy, to its growth-promoting effect on the uterine musculature.

Granting that myometrial insufficiency plays a part in producing pain at the flow, it is probably not the sole factor concerned, for many women with a poorly developed uterus have painless periods, while others with a well developed organ may suffer severely.[9] Moreover, histologic studies of extirpated uteri have revealed no correlation between the degree of fibrosis and the occurrence of pain.[10]

Mucosal Faults: Membranous Dysmenorrhea.—Abnormal separation of the menstrual mucosa has been proposed as a possible cause of dysmenorrhea. The condition known as "membranous dysmenorrhea" provides the most striking example of menstrual pain thus produced. In its most pronounced form, it is characterized by the passage of an organized material resembling the decidua of early pregnancy. With the onset of the flow, dehiscence of the membranous deposit occurs and it is ejected in shreds, patches or in its entirety. This is accompanied by severe expulsive pains and often by profuse bleeding. When intact, the cast assumes the

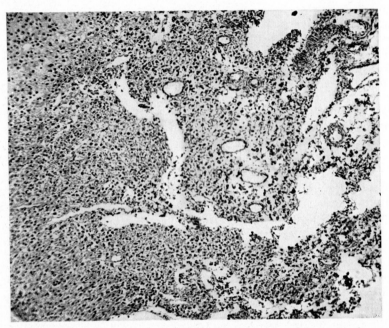

Fig. 81.—Dysmenorrheic membrane. Microphotograph of cast passed by twenty-five-year-old woman with severe dysmenorrhea.

shape of the uterine cavity. Microscopically, the tissue consists of an edematous, decidua-like stroma and dilated uterine glands.

While the severe forms of membranous dysmenorrhea are readily recognized, the *atypical case* may often be overlooked because the fragments passed are too small to attract the patient's attention. Whitehouse[3] believes the mild form is more common than is generally believed. This type of dysmenorrhea is often found in association with a well developed uterus. The pain, which is usually severe, begins after the onset of the flow and persists for a day or more, ceasing only with the passage of the mucosal fragments. This condition is usually resistant to pregnancy, cervical dilatation, or other measures which may relieve "simple" dysmenorrhea.

Abnormal separation of the menstrual mucosa may possibly account for pain at the flow in women with apparently normal uteri. Unfortunately, this theory merely replaces one unknown with another, for the cause of abnormal desquamation is obscure. It has been suggested[3, 9, 11] that both the mild and severe forms of membranous dysmenorrhea are due to an *overactive corpus luteum.* This suggestion finds some support in the observation that the cycles in dysmenorrhea are often slightly prolonged, while in the true membranous forms, the period associated with passage of a cast tends to be delayed for several days, suggesting persistence of the yellow body. On the other hand, reports of cases with persistent corpus luteum cysts do not mention pain as a prominent or frequent complaint during the bleeding phase. According to Fluhmann,[12] the administration of progestin in large amounts does not lead to abnormal desquamation or pain. The recent practice of administering progesterone for the relief of dysmenorrhea sometimes seems to benefit, while at other times it is without effect, but there is no evidence that it aggravates the pain.

Vascular Faults.—Relative impermeability of the uterine blood vessels, undue clotting of the menstrual blood, and ischemia of the myometrium have also been considered as possible causes of dysmenorrhea.

Novak[13] has suggested that *undue impermeability of the endometrial blood vessels,* due to a deficiency of some hypothetical substance produced by the uterus, may account for the menstrual pain in some cases. He based this suggestion on his observation that uterine hypoplasia and a scanty flow may be associated with a marked menstrual reaction of the endometrium, which appears unusually early in the cycle. He proposed that the hyperemia of the endometrium is equal to that in the normal uterus but, since the blood cannot pass freely through the impermeable blood vessels, only a small amount is lost. The uterine blood vessels consequently become engorged, giving rise to pain.

Blair-Bell[14] has advanced the theory that some cases of dysmenorrhea may be due to passage of *blood clots* through the cervical canal. According to this view, a deficiency or absence of some hypothetical anti-clotting substance permits the formation of clots within the uterine cavity. Some support is provided by the observation that initiation of a dysmenorrheic career often coincides with the passage of clots for the first time. On the other hand, the fact that the menstrual coagula is usually too friable to offer enough resistance to cause painful myometrial contractions would seem to detract from this theory.

A theory more recently advanced by Moir[15] is based on his studies of the motility of the human uterus during the various phases of the menstrual cycle. He found that just before and during the flow, the force of the *myometrial contractions* increases markedly, creating an intrauterine pressure exceeding that of the second stage of labor. During a painful period in one patient, he simultaneously recorded the myometrial contractions and pulsations of the uterine arteries (see Fig. 82). The latter disappeared as the contractions neared a point corresponding to an estimated pressure of 120 mm. of mercury, and reappeared when the pressure fell below this level. Comparison of the patient's subjective symptoms during the recording revealed that the greatest discomfort coincided with a point just after the summit of each uterine contraction and disappeared only after the

24

pressure fell to its lowest level. On the basis of these findings, Moir suggested that menstrual pain may be due to *ischemia of the uterine musculature* caused by temporary obliteration of the myometrial blood supply, a condition analogous to the pain of angina pectoris or intermittent claudication.

The significance of these findings can best be appreciated by recalling the role of ischemia in smooth muscle pain. To quote Lewis,[16] "a product of muscular contractions is directly or indirectly responsible for pain; .... where successive muscular contractions occur in the absence of the blood flow, the state of the muscle alters progressively and the products accumulate in the tissue space. Two factors are concerned in the production of pain; namely, the rate of energy expenditure on the one hand, and the quantity of fresh blood passing to the muscle on the other. It is the lack of balance between these two which ultimately causes pain to occur; the lack of balance is embodied in the term 'relative ischemia.' It is also known that pain that has once come will not disappear so long as blood supply

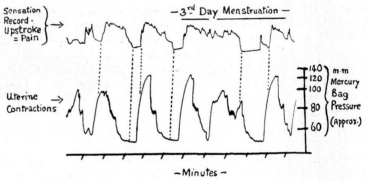

Fig. 82.—Contractions of human uterus during painful menstruation. A simultaneous pain-sensation record was made. (Moir, C.: Proc. Roy. Soc. Med. Vol. 29.)

is suppressed, but that with full blood supply, it will disappear quickly and with poor blood supply in time."

It would seem reasonable to suppose that any condition which produces uterine ischemia, either by increasing the intensity of the myometrial contractions, or by reducing the blood flow through the uterine blood vessels, is a potential cause of dysmenorrhea. In some cases excessive contractions, in others, some vascular condition which reduces the blood flow may be chiefly at fault. At times, both factors may contribute. Of interest in this connection is Brewer's[17] observation that the *vascular spasm*, which normally occurs at the onset of the flow, and is demonstrable in both the peripheral and endometrial blood vessels, was more prolonged during a painful, profuse period than during painless periods in the same individual. Such prolonged spasm may conceivably be due either to an excess of the hypothetical substance on which this phenomenon depends (see Chap. V), or to undue reactivity of the blood vessels to a normal supply. The role of a reduced circulation in the production of menstrual pain is also suggested by the observation that this symptom is often encountered in the thin hypotonic individual, whose blood pressure is characteristically low. It is also significant that measures calculated to improve the blood supply to the uterus often relieve menstrual pain and that pregnancy, which markedly increases the vascularity of this organ, may terminate a dysmenorrheic career in many cases.

Several observers[18, 19] have challenged Moir's explanation of menstrual pain on the ground that they could not demonstrate suppression of the arterial circulation during the pain in their cases. In addition, they point out that women free from pain may show contractions equivalent in all respects to those observed in dysmenorrheic women (Fig. 83). These observations do not necessarily discredit Moir's suggestion, but may only be taken to signify that compression of the arteries is not the sole factor involved. In a normally menstruating woman observed by Wilson and Kurzrok,[19] the administration of *pituitrin* increased the intrauterine pressure above the level of the systolic pressure without causing pain. On the other hand,

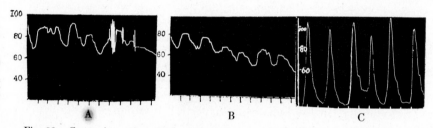

Fig. 83.—Comparison of motility of human uterus during painful and painless menses. A, Kymographic record made on second day of the flow during a spontaneous attack of dysmenorrhea. Vertical lines caused by vomiting and retching. B, Contractions recorded shortly after dysmenorrhea symptoms disappeared, showing little change to account for relief. C, Unusually large contractions recorded on first day of flow in patient with painless periods. (Wilson, L., and Kurzrok, R.: Endocrinol. Vol. 23.)

similar treatment during a painful period in another patient, increased the discomfort. This would suggest that suppression of the arterial circulation, though not of itself sufficient to cause pain, may contribute to this result when operating with some other factor or factors capable of producing this symptom.

Role of the Cervix.—That the cervix may be the site of menstrual pain is suggested by anatomic and clinical evidence. Larkin[20] elicited pain like that of dysmenorrhea by cervical dilatation in both normal women and those previously subjected to supravaginal hysterectomy. He concluded that the pain thus produced is not due to uterine contractions evoked by dilating the os, but is primarily and entirely within the cervix. Keiffer,[21] in a histologic study of the neurovegetative system of the human uterus, observed that the cervix, especially the sphincter and connective tissue surrounding it, is endowed with a special nervous system, independent of ganglions and composed mainly of minute terminal sensory bodies. The richness of this innervation makes this a veritable nodal reflex center for the entire organ. The rest of the organ is less well supplied and indeed almost devoid of nervous apparatus. He also called attention to nervous receptors in the musculature of the corpus which apparently play a part in the physiology of the myometrium. Theobald[22] found that insertion of a stick of silver nitrate into the endocervix, for the treatment of an erosion, evoked pain in dysmenorrheic but not in normally menstruating women. He concluded that though the cervix is relatively insensitive, the autonomic nerves supplying it are stimulated by silver nitrate, and the pain thus produced is referred to the area of the skin supplied by branches of the first lumbar nerve. The pain could be abolished by anesthetizing the nerve endings. In the author's experience, a sensitive cervical mucosa is frequently associated with painful menses, and cauterization of an erosion sometimes relieves a long-standing dysmenorrhea.

Extra-Uterine Causes of Dysmenorrhea.—Recent findings suggest that under certain conditions, endocrine, nervous, and metabolic disturbances may contribute to the production of menstrual pain.

Role of the Ovary.—Participation of the ovary in the etiology was suspected long before its endocrine function was established. Its role was somewhat clarified when its estrogenic and progestational principles were isolated and their effect on uterine motility determined (see Chap. VI). In the lower mammal, estrogen increases the motility of the uterus, while progestin exerts a quiescent effect which varies in degree in different species. Small amounts of estrogen, acting with progestin, support its quieting effect, but large quantities may override it and increase myometrial motility. In the human uterus, estrogen apparently induces small, rapid contractions, while progestin causes slower and more ample contractions of lower tonus.

On the basis of these findings, Novak and Reynolds[5] advanced the theory that dysmenorrhea in some cases may be traceable to a disturbance in the *temporal or quantitative relationship of estrogen and progestin.* According to this view, premature regression of the corpus luteum, with consequent withdrawal of progestin, permits renewed ascendancy of estrogen, which induces heightened uterine contractions and pain. While this hypothesis has aroused considerable interest, and forms the basis for the use of progesterone in the treatment, its validity has not been established. Hormonal and endometrial studies in normal and dysmenorrheic women have failed to demonstrate that a relative or absolute estrogen excess is a constant or even a more common finding in the latter.[18, 19, 23] On the contrary, normal progestational modifications, pointing to a normal estrogen-progestin balance, have been observed before the flow in many dysmenorrheic women. Moreover, the infrequency of pain in hyperplastic bleeding, which is conceded to be due to estrogen acting in the absence of progestin (see Chap. XXV), cannot be reconciled with this hypothesis.

In the search for evidence to substantiate this theory, several observers[24, 25, 26, 27] were impressed by the fact that the situation was actually opposite to what might be expected if it were correct. Not only was pain found associated in most cases with pregravid modifications, but when these were absent for some reason, or their appearance was prevented by administering estrogen, the flow which followed was painless. On the basis of this observation, it has been suggested that essential dysmenorrhea can only occur in the presence of a corpus luteum. This would imply that wherever pain is experienced during bleeding from an estrogenic type of endometrium, a functional basis is excluded. This implication is not borne out by the findings of other workers. Though endometrial studies indicate that *in the large majority of cases, pain in the absence of evident pathology accompanies bleeding from a secretory type of endometrium,* exceptions have been noted (see Fig. 84). Moreover, the functional nature of the dysmenorrhea in these exceptional cases is suggested by their response to therapy. In one patient observed by Lackner and his associates,[18] pain was associated with bleeding from an estrogenic type of endometrium.

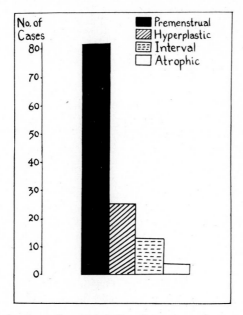

Fig. 84.—Graph showing endometrial findings in a group of 124 cases of dysmenorrhea. Note that premenstrual endometria predominate, being present in two-thirds of the entire group.

A course of estrogen therapy improved the scanty nature of the bleeding and increased the activity of the myometrium, and the flow which then ensued was painless. The frequent association of essential dysmenorrhea and ovulatory bleeding can only justify the conclusion that this symptom is far more likely to accompany ovulatory than anovulatory bleeding. Recognition of this association constitutes an important step toward the clarification of the etiology. It suggests a possible explanation of the fact that pain is often experienced for the first time several months or years after the menarche. Recent evidence (see Chap. XXIII) that the cycles are often anovulatory at the beginning of menstrual life is significant in this connection. It also helps to explain why some dysmenorrheic women may occasionally have a period free from pain. That mature women with normal ovulatory cycles may experience an occasional anovulatory cycle seems to be fairly well established.

Since the essential differences between true menstruation and pseudo-menstrual or hyperplastic bleeding are not yet fully understood, the *pain producing factor* or factors, which are operating frequently in the one and only infrequently in the other, cannot be identified with certainty. On the basis of the available evidence, several possibilities suggest themselves. As shown elsewhere (see Chap. V), pseudomenstrual bleeding occurs from an endometrium stimulated by estrogen alone and is precipitated by its partial or complete withdrawal. True menstruation, on the other hand, occurs from an endometrium stimulated by both estrogen and progestin, and is precipitated primarily by progestin withdrawal. Conceivably, the pain producing factor may be some *product of progestin metabolism* which does not form at all or only to a limited extent when estrogen is metabolized. It is also possible, in view of progestin's influence on *estrogen metabolism* (see Chap. III), that some substance is formed when both hormones are present, which is deficient or absent when only estrogen is available. In this connection, Smith and Smith[28] observed that the start of menstruation is associated with a sudden shift in the partition of urinary estrogens, which they interpret as evidence of increased estrogen destruction and attribute to withdrawal of progestin's protective influence. They suggest that a sudden concentration of estrogen breakdown products in the endometrium may result in the formation of a local "toxin" whose action is indirectly responsible for menstruation. In a patient with painful menses from a pregravid mucosa, their studies yielded evidence which they interpret as indicative of increased production and destruction of estrogen throughout the cycle.[29] The onset of bleeding coincided with a shift similar to, but less pronounced than, that observed during normal menstruation. They attribute this to luteal deficiency and suggest that it may be causally related to the dysmenorrhea. The significance of their findings and the validity of their conclusions cannot be decided without further evidence. So far as they go, their findings would seem to exclude the possibility that menstrual pain is due to an excessive concentration of estrogen breakdown products in the endometrium.

That the pain producing factor may be found in the uterus is suggested by Markee's[30] observations in ocular endometrial transplants in the monkey. This observer noted that periodic bleeding, whether ovulatory or anovulatory, is always preceded by constriction of the spiral arterioles in the basal zone and consequently occurs from an *anemic endometrium*. He suggests that the consequent anoxemia of the nerve endings may render them hyperesthetic. To account for reports that relief of menstrual pain may follow both estrogen and progestin, he suggests that they may have a common effect which is not on the uterine contractions but on the blood flow. On the basis of his observation that both hormones increase the blood flow through the basal and middle third of endometrial transplants, he reasons that these hormones relieve menstrual pain through reduction of the anemia. Markee offers no explanation of why anemia, which is a constant accompaniment of both ovulatory and anovulatory bleeding causes pain in some cases and not in others. If his theory is correct, it must be assumed that pain arises either because the nerve endings are unusually sensitive to a normal degree of anoxemia, or because the anemia is unduly prolonged due to an excess of the hypothetical substance which causes vaso-constriction in the menstruating endometrium. The observation of Brewer,[17] mentioned above, is significant in this connection. The identity and source of this substance has not been established. Markee suggests that it may be a *product of endometrial degeneration.* If this is true, it might be expected that its quantity would be roughly proportional to the amount of dis-integrating tissue. Significant in this connection is Markee's observation that the amount of tissue desquamated during ovulatory bleeding is sig-nificantly greater than during anovulatory bleeding. It is possible then, that the greater tendency to pain during ovulatory bleeding is indirectly related to the greater tissue destruction which characterizes such bleeding.

Yet another possibility merits consideration. Recent studies have shown that the large, slow contractions of the luteal phase of the menstrual cycle become increasingly powerful with the approach of the flow, reaching their climax on the first and second day of bleeding. Some observers[19] attribute their heightened activity at this time to the action of the luteal hormone. As shown elsewhere, however, this may more reasonably be attributed to regression of the corpus luteum which is known to occur at this point. It is conceivable that the endometrial degeneration which fol-lows progestin withdrawal results in the production of an *oxytocic sub-stance* which may either be identical with the hypothetical vasoconstrictor substance postulated by Markee, or closely related to it. Of interest in this connection is the observation of Phelps[31] that the urine of menstruating women possesses oxytocic activity which is directly proportional to the presence and severity of pain. It is possible then that the greater frequency of pain in ovulatory bleeding is due to the greater amounts of vasocon-strictor and oxytocic substance produced by the degenerating endometrium.

Moir[32] has suggested that the *strong contractions* of true menstruation may be attributable to the effort involved in shedding and expelling the menstrual decidua, which does not occur in pseudomenstrual bleeding.

Even if it is granted that anemia and increased myometrial activity play a part in the production of pain, they may hardly be considered the sole factors for they are presumably a constant feature of true menstrua-tion, whereas pain is not. In addition there is probably operating some factor, possibly vascular, nervous, mechanical, or chemical, which is capable of causing pain to arise in an actively contracting uterus with an anemic endometrium.

Kennedy[33] has suggested that a deficiency of estrogen may lead to dysmenorrhea by disturbing the sympathetic supply of the uterus. This he bases on Blotevogel and Poll's[34] report that castration produced de-generative changes in the ganglia of Frankenhauser, which can be cor-rected by administering estrogen. Fluhmann[12] criticizes this suggestion on the ground that an estrogen deficiency is not demonstrable in dysmen-orrhea, and that uterine hypoplasia and other evidence of ovarian defi-ciency is present in only some of the cases.

Role of the Anterior Hypophysis.—Disturbances of anterior pituitary function may conceivably lead to dysmenorrhea in one of two ways. A deficiency of its gonadotropic hormones before puberty may result in ovarian deficiency and inadequate development of the uterus. On the other hand, a disturbance in the production of its follicle-stimulating and luteinizing hormones may upset the balance of estrogen and progestin, leading to powerful uterine contractions and pain. Novak and Reynolds[5] have suggested that the anterior hypophysis may affect uterine motility through the mediation of the ovaries, or by directly stimulating the uterus. The latter possibility is based on their observation that human pregnancy urine gonadotropic extract inhibited uterine contractions in ovariectomized rabbits. A deficiency or absence of this motility-inhibiting principle, they believe, may account for some cases of menstrual pain. This has been questioned by Morgan,[35] who could inhibit uterine motility in rabbits with pregnancy urine gonadotropic extract only where the ovaries were intact and responded to the extract with formation of corpora lutea. He concluded that the gonadotropes do not act directly and can inhibit uterine motility only by stimulating progestin production.

Role of the Thyroid.—While there is no experimental evidence directly linking the thyroid with dysmenorrhea, a number of clinical observations suggest that hyperactivity of this gland may indirectly contribute to the pain, possibly through its action on the nervous system. According to Hertzler[36] and Wendell,[37] menstrual pain is a prominent symptom of *interstitial thyrotoxicosis* and may be relieved by correcting the thyroid disorder. The author has encountered a number of dysmenorrheic women who, though symptomless during the interval, complain of tachycardia, tremors, nervous instability, crying spells, and other manifestations reminiscent of *hyperthyroidism*, shortly before and during menstruation. It is possible that such individuals harbor a mild form of hyperthyroidism, which is exacerbated during the flow and heightens the sensitivity of the nervous system to the point where sensations, which would normally pass unnoticed, are experienced as pain.

Davis[38] denies that the thyroid gland has any part in the etiology of dysmenorrhea on the ground that a significant deviation from a normal basal metabolic rate is not demonstrable in the typical spasmodic type of dysmenorrhea. While conceding that interstitial thyrotoxicosis and dysmenorrhea are often associated, he interprets them as independent manifestations with a common neurological origin. In his own series of dysmenorrheic women, a moderate, diffuse enlargement of the thyroid was a feature in many of the cases, but he regards this as physiological and of little significance in the etiology. In a series of 129 untreated cases of thyrotoxicosis, Russell and Dean[76] found dysmenorrhea no more common than is usual among women without this condition.

Psychic and Nervous Factors.—It is generally recognized that menstrual pain is often a relative symptom dependent on the *psychic pattern* of the individual. Uterine contractions, which pass unnoticed in the normal woman, may become exaggerated into pain in those with a poor nervous organization. A psychic trauma, which leaves the normal woman undisturbed, may profoundly affect the neurotic individual. In the dysmenorrheic woman with a stable nervous system, psychoneurosis, if present, is likely to be the effect rather than the cause of menstrual pain, having been acquired as a result of repeated insults to the nervous system and increasing dread of the impending attack. In the neurotic individual, on the other hand, nervous instability may be the cause of her dysmenorrheic career. The precipitating factor may be a psychic shock of a sexual nature, or repugnance for the menstrual phenomenon. The pain may recur because of fear or disgust subconsciously associated with menstrual function. Nervous instability may contribute to the production of dysmenorrhea by lowering the pain threshold or increasing the irritability of the uterine neuromuscular system. The latter possibility is suggested by the observation that esophageal spasm, pylorospasm, rectal or vesicle tenesmus, and other manifestations of smooth muscle hypermotility, are often associated with dysmenorrhea.

Observers differ as to the importance of the psychic factor in the etiology. Some[39, 40] maintain that a careful search will almost always disclose psychic shock behind the first attack of menstrual pain. Others[3, 9] argue that nervous factors play only a negligible role, since menstrual pain occurs as often in the stolid, apathetic individual as in the high-strung, neurotic one. The importance of the psychic factor has more recently been emphasized by Wilson and Kurzok,[41] whose studies of myometrial activity during painful and painless periods revealed no appreciable difference (see Fig. 83). They therefore concluded that "functional dysmenorrhea appears to be a psychogenic disorder in which a reduced pain threshold or a disturbed pelvic autonomic nervous system permits uterine contractions during the phase of maximum amplitude to reach consciousness." The role of the psyche has been strikingly demonstrated by Boynton and Winther.[42] In a group of 50 women receiving placeboes under the impression that a potent hormone was being administered, all experienced relief from pain throughout the period of treatment. The author's experience suggests that the truth lies somewhere between these two extremes. While we cannot deny the importance of psychic factors, neither are we justified in tagging all dysmenorrheic women as psychoneurotic, for many are normal to all appearances and enjoy good health between periods.

A *neurogenic theory* of dysmenorrhea has recently been advanced by Davis.[38] According to this observer, in the majority of cases of severe dysmenorrhea, the peripheral sympathetic nerves of the uterus, as represented by the presacral nerve, are pathologically altered in some degree, in the direction of subacute or chronic neuritis. This manifests itself in widespread degeneration of the ganglion cells and interstitial infiltration. He concludes that "whatever the cause of the abnormal impulses which cause dysmenorrhea, they are initiated or at least exaggerated, in their passage, through sympathetic nerves rendered abnormally sensitive by previous inflammation." Similar changes have been described by Browne and Torrens,[43] who admit that the cause of these changes and their relation to the associated dysmenorrhea must remain unanswered for the present. Whether they may be considered the primary cause or are actually secondary to some other condition is a question for further investigation. It is conceivable that they represent a reaction to repeated attacks of severe uterine spasm.[77] They may in turn aggravate the discomfort, thus providing an explanation for the fact that the pain in some women may become increasingly severe with each period.

Allergy and Dysmenorrhea.—The recognition that allergens may affect the generative organs, particularly the uterus, is comparatively recent. The terms "generallergy" and "metrallergy" have been coined by Goodall[44] to denote, respectively, allergy of the genital system as a whole and of the uterus in particular. It is of interest that Campbell,[9] with no thought of an allergic basis, described dysmenorrhea as a "symptom-complex commonly involving nausea or other gastrointestinal symptoms and occasionally with shock, the whole picture simulating an allergic phenomenon." That some cases of dysmenorrhea may have an allergic basis is indicated by reports that relief may sometimes be secured by eliminating the offending food from the diet, by desensitization with the specific antigen, or administration of adrenalin. Dale[45] and Weinstein[46] have demonstrated that if the guinea pig is sensitized to various antigens, the uterine muscle responds with powerful contractions to minute amounts of such substances, acting in vitro or in vivo. The muscle can be desensitized by the specific antigen. Whether this phenomenon can be duplicated in man is not certain. Tuft[47] has reported negative results, but since only a single case was investigated, his findings are inconclusive.

That the uterus should be the site of allergic reactions is not surprising, since it is composed of smooth muscle fibers and supplied by two antagonistic nervous systems. Allergy may express itself not only as an extravasatory disease, as in hay fever, but also as an irritant to smooth muscle, causing spasm, as in asthma. Assuming that it may affect the uterine muscle in much the same way as the bronchi, it may be asked why the painful contractions occur only during menstruation. It has been suggested that the increased tendency to such manifestations during the flow is due to some end product of disturbed metabolism present in the menstrual blood, which creates a state of auto-intoxication. In a small series of cases studied by Salen,[48] desensitization with an extract of the patient's menstrual blood partially or completely relieved the dysmenorrhea. In a group of patients, who experienced allergic manifestations during the flow but were symptom-free during the interval, Geber[49] and Lichter[50] found that blood serum, obtained during menstruation, elicited allergic manifestations when administered during the interval. Urbach[78] found that skin eruptions associated with the flow could be cured by desensitizing the patient through repeated injections of serum taken during an attack. Such treatment was also effective in relieving an associated dysmenorrhea.

The Nasal Mucosa and Dysmenorrhea.—An intimate relationship between the nasal mucosa and the generative organs was originally postulated by Fliess[51] on the basis of his observation that certain areas, which he designated "genital spots," become congested and hypersensitive just before or during menstruation. By cocainizing or cauterizing these spots he was able to relieve an associated dysmenorrhea. While a few investigators have corroborated his findings, most competent authorities question his theory. It is possible that the relief obtained by Fliess was due to the psychotherapeutic effect of the treatment or, where cocaine was used, to its analgesic action.

Constitutional Factors.—Illness, poor hygiene, undue physical and mental stress, nutritional faults, visceroptosis, faulty posture, obstinate consti-

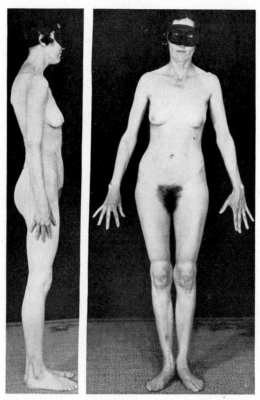

Fig. 85.—Female aged thirty-five, weight 100 pounds. Dysmenorrhea and irregular uterine bleeding. Note angular body, long bony fingers, poor posture, and spacing between thighs.

pation, and unfavorable occupation or environmental conditions may contribute to the production of menstrual pain. This is borne out by the fact that their correction often terminates a dysmenorrheic career.[52]

Summary.—In summation, it may be stated that no single cause can account for all cases of menstrual pain, and that usually several factors, of uterine and extra-uterine origin, probably combine to produce this symptom.

DIAGNOSIS AND DIFFERENTIAL DIAGNOSIS

The diagnosis of functional dysmenorrhea is one of exclusion. It is of prime importance to eliminate local organic conditions which may give rise to menstrual pain. Pelvic lesions which cause pain irrespective of the flow present no difficulty in the differential diagnosis. There are, however, lesions which remain quiescent during the interval but cause pain just before or during menstruation, due possibly to the congestion which usually ac-

TABLE 7

COMPARISON OF FUNCTIONAL, ORGANIC, AND MEMBRANOUS DYSMENORRHEA

	Functional	Organic	Membranous*
Time of Onset	With first flow or with establishment of menstrual habit.	At any time during the reproductive period.	At any time during the reproductive period.
Nature of Pain	Usually spasmodic; intensity varies.	Usually dull, steady, bearing down sensation.	Severe and labor-like.
Location of Pain	Lower abdomen, back, and thighs; may shift.	Lower abdomen; sometimes unilateral.	Lower abdomen, back and thighs.
Relation of Pain to Flow	Usually precedes flow and tends to subside as flow becomes free.	Begins before or with onset of bleeding; may persist throughout flow and even beyond.	Precedes flow and subsides with passage of fragments or cast.
Parity	Usually encountered in nulliparae; often disappears after pregnancy.	Encountered in both nulliparae and multiparae; not relieved by pregnancy.	Encountered in both nulliparae and multiparae; usually not relieved by pregnancy.
Constitutional Type	Any type may be affected, but asthenic type predominates.	Any type may be affected.	Any type may be affected.
General Symptoms	Often present.	Usually absent unless condition is superimposed on nervous background.	May or may not be present.
Pelvic Findings	Uterus may be normal, but hypoplasia, acute anteflexion, and cervical stenosis not uncommon.	Adnexal enlargement, pelvic fixation, and adnexal tenderness may be found.	Negative.
Endometrial Status	Curettings obtained before expected flow usually show pregravid changes.	Any type of endometrium may be encountered.	Marked pregravid changes.
Hormone Findings	No evidence of significant deviation from normal.	Vary according to status of ovarian function.	No evidence of significant deviation from normal.

* Not classified as either functional or organic because of its obscure etiology.

companies this physiologic process. While most pelvic lesions can be detected by a routine pelvic examination and laboratory studies, the minute size and obscure location of some may make their detection extremely difficult.

Among the conditions which may be confused with functional dysmenorrhea are endometriosis, chronic pelvic inflammatory disease, ureteral stricture, and chronic appendicitis.

Endometriosis may present considerable difficulty in the diagnosis, particularly where the endometrial implants are small. It may be suspected in acquired dysmenorrhea, where the pain is very severe and progressive, begins shortly before and persists throughout the flow, is exaggerated by physical exertion, and resists every form of treatment short of hysterec-

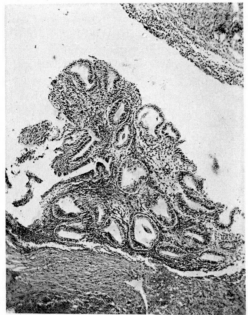

Fig. 86.—Endometriosis of the ovary. Tissue removed from thirty-two-year-old patient with severe dysmenorrhea of ten years' duration and resistant to all conservative therapy.

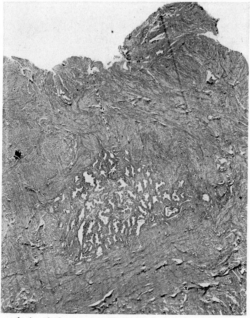

Fig. 87.—Endometriosis of the uterus. Note that ectopic glands show pregravid changes. Tissue obtained from twenty-four-year-old patient with severe and intractable dysmenorrhea.

tomy. Where the rectovaginal septum is involved, the pain is referred to the rectum and may be accompanied by rectal bleeding. If the adnexa are affected on only one side, the pain is unilateral and the periods are invariably painful, differing in this respect from the functional cases, where painless flows may sometimes intervene.

Endometrial implants situated within a viscus, can only be demonstrated by microscopic examination of the suspected tissue. The author has encountered three such cases. In one, suspension of the uterus and removal of a cystic ovary had been performed, while in the other two, one adnexa had been removed but the true nature of the condition was overlooked. Suspecting endometriosis from the severe and intractable nature of the pain, the author advised hysterectomy. Microscopic examination of the extirpated tissue established the diagnosis.

Ureteral stricture or spasm may remain symptomless during the interval, but the congestion incident to menstruation may cause narrowing of the ureter and colicky pain simulating that of spasmodic dysmenorrhea. A history of urinary frequency, and pain radiating over the course of the ureter, is significant. Passage of a ureteral sound and pyelographic studies will help in the differential diagnosis. Urologic studies are indicated in any case of intractable dysmenorrhea, particularly when operative procedures are contemplated.

Chronic pelvic inflammatory disease, particularly in its incipient stages, may cause pain at the flow. It should be suspected where there is a history of gonorrhea, criminal abortion, or puerperal infection. The cervical smear, the presence of external stigmata of gonorrhea, temperature records, sedimentation tests, and leukocyte counts are valuable adjuncts in the differential diagnosis, especially where the adnexa cannot be palpated because of abdominal adiposity.

Chronic appendicitis is not infrequently mistaken for dysmenorrhea, especially in the afebrile case, or where the leukocyte count is not materially altered. A careful history, x-ray visualization of the appendix, repeated blood studies and temperature records may differentiate the two conditions.

TREATMENT

The evasive and often complex nature of the etiology makes treatment empiric and often unsatisfactory. The therapeutic measures advocated are as manifold and varied as the supposed causes of dysmenorrhea. While some cases respond to conservative treatment, others resist all measures short of hysterectomy.

TREATMENT OF THE IMMEDIATE ATTACK

To relieve the immediate attack of pain, measures should be instituted to quiet the nervous system, improve the pelvic circulation, and subdue the myometrial contractions.

General Therapeutic Measures.—Avoidance of physical and mental exertion and, in severe cases, rest in bed are advisable. Hot stimulating drinks, local heat by means of the electric pad, diathermy to the pelvis, warm enemas or hot sitz baths, may give temporary relief by improving the pelvic circulation or exerting a sedative effect on the sensory nerve endings of the skin, to which visceral pain is referred. Proper evacuation of the bowels is important, for constipation may materially add to the premenstrual pelvic congestion. Catharsis preceding and during the attack has long been used empirically to alleviate the pain. The relief which sometimes follows such treatment may possibly be due to the fact that it depletes the blood of some hormone, allergen, or other substance capable of eliciting painful uterine contractions.

Drugs.—Sedatives, analgesics, and antispasmodics are extensively employed for the relief of menstrual pain. The coal tar derivatives, such as pyramidon, papaverin, peralga, antipyrine, aspirin and the barbiturates, may ease the pain. In the severe case, these may be combined with codeine. A combination of codeine sulphate gr. ½, aspirin gr. x, and sodium phenobarbital gr. ½, is effective in a fair number of cases. This may be repeated every few hours until the pain is relieved. Hypodermic injections of codeine sulphate gr. ¼ to ½ may be tried where the pain is accompanied by nausea and persistent vomiting. In the very severe case, morphine gr. ⅛ to ¼ combined with atropine sulphate gr. $\frac{1}{150}$ or elixir paregoric, one dram every four hours, may be given. The opiates are obviously undesirable and should only be given where the pain is excruciating and resists all other measures.

Antispasmodics are used with the hope of inhibiting the uterine contractions. As a rule they are poorly tolerated and cause gastro-intestinal disturbances. Atropine sulfate gr. $\frac{1}{120}$ or tincture of belladonna 10 minims t.i.d. may be given one or two days before, and on the first and second days of the flow. Benzyl benzoate 10 to 30 minims in alcohol solution every 4 hours is preferable to atropine because it is less toxic. Some observers[53] report that benzedrine sulfate, in doses of 5 to 20 mg. daily for two days before the expected flow, often gives relief, though occasionally it may aggravate the symptoms.

TREATMENT OF THE UNDERLYING CAUSE

Sex Hygiene.—The prepuberal and adolescent girl should receive instruction in sex hygiene in order to prevent any unfavorable effect which may arise from a misconception of the menstrual phenomenon. The nervous individual should be reassured that the monthly attacks of pain may be at least partly an expression of her subconscious reflexes, and are not due to disease of the pelvic organs. Occasionally, psychoanalysis is beneficial.

General Medical Measures.—An appreciable gain in weight is desirable in the thin, asthenic, visceroptotic individual. This may be accomplished by prescribing a well balanced, high caloric, vitamin rich diet, supplemented by supportive tonics. The cures so affected may be ascribed to the improvement in general health, or to deposition of intra-abdominal fat, which may help correct an associated visceroptosis. Faulty posture, which may be a contributory cause of the dysmenorrhea, may be improved by corrective exercise and the use of appropriate supports. The efficacy of such measures has been demonstrated recently by Goldwasser[53] in a series of 673 adolescent girls. Of these, 68 per cent recovered completely, while 20 per cent improved appreciably.

In dysmenorrhea of allergic origin, the patient should be removed from any undesirable occupational or environmental influence, and desensitized to the offending allergen. If some food is at fault, it should be excluded from the diet. Preceding the attack, two ounces of castor oil may be given and a milk diet prescribed. The administration of small doses of adrenalin, two to five minims of $\frac{1}{1000}$ solution, repeated if necessary, may give temporary relief.

Since pregnancy often cures functional dysmenorrhea, it should be advocated wherever circumstances permit. Whether it acts by promoting the growth and vascularity of the uterus, or in some other way, is not certain.

Organotherapy.—Estrogen, progesterone or pregneninolone, androgen, the gonadotropins, insulin, and thyroid substance[54] have all been advocated for the relief of functional dysmenorrhea. The results of controlled studies suggest that the benefits attributed to these substances were probably due to their psychotherapeutic effect or to measures concomitantly employed. The author has obtained results comparable to those claimed for organotherapy by giving injections of saline solution. It is a good plan to ascertain the patient's reaction to placeboes, given by the hypodermic route, to determine to what extent the pain is mental.

Progesterone.—Progesterone[55, 56, 57] and, more recently, orally active pregneninolone[23, 58] have been used in spasmodic dysmenorrhea with the aim of inhibiting the uterine contractions and promoting the excretion of the motility-stimulating hormone, estrogen. The results reported thus far have been inconstant and unconvincing. At best, this is substitutive therapy and can have no permanent beneficial effect. The *dose* varies from 0.25 to 2 I.U. of progesterone 2 to 3 times daily, beginning a few days before the expected flow and continuing until the pain subsides. The dose of pregneninolone by mouth, as recommended by Soule,[58] is 60 mg. daily for 5 to 6 days. In the author's experience, this form of therapy has proved disappointing.

Estrogenic Substances.—Some observers report relief of menstrual pain with estrogen. The average *dose* is 10,000 to 50,000 I.U. given intramuscularly daily or every other day, or 2 to 3 mg. of stilbestrol by mouth daily. The time when the hormone is given varies according to the particular view taken regarding its mode of action. Some administer it only during the first half of the cycle, while others give it during the premenstruum[18] or throughout the cycle.[59] Advocates of estrogen therapy have offered various explanations to account for the good results which seem to follow its use. It has been suggested that it develops or vascularizes a hypoplastic uterus or dilates the endometrial blood vessels. The possibility that its repeated administration during successive cycles causes endometrial refractoriness with consequent diminution of motility has also been considered. The observation that its administration, beginning early in the cycle, may be followed by painless bleeding from a proliferative type of endometrium, has been interpreted[59] as evidence that it suppresses anterior pituitary function, with consequent failure of ovulation and corpus luteum formation. This in turn precludes pregravid modifications of the endometrium, which are presumably a prerequisite for functional dysmenorrhea. If this is its mode of action, this form of therapy is obviously undesirable since it may endanger fertility. In the author's experience, as in that of Boynton and Winther,[42] the response to the estrogens has not differed significantly from that obtained with placeboes.

Androgenic Substances.—The androgens have only recently been introduced for the relief of menstrual pain.[60, 61, 62] According to Geist,[61] the effective *dose* varies from 500 to 900 mg. of testosterone propionate intramuscularly in divided doses during the course of the cycle, beginning not later than the sixth day. Fluhmann[12] recommends 10 to 25 mg. two to three times a week, no more than 200 mg. being given during any one cycle.

Observers are not agreed as to its mode of action. It has been suggested that the androgens may lessen vascular engorgement or neutralize the circulating estrogens and thus minimize the strength of the uterine contractions. Some observers believe that they inhibit the adenohypophysis and, by thus suppressing ovulation and corpus luteum formation, prevent conversion of the endometrium to the pregravid phase. Another possibility is that the androgens prevent pregravid modifications through a direct action on the uterine mucosa. In either case, their use would seem undesirable since they can only relieve at the expense of ovarian and endometrial function. Besides, there is the danger of inducing hirsutism and other masculine manifestations.

Gonadotropic Substances.—The equine[63, 64, 65] and chorionic[5, 57, 65] gonadotropes have been used with the aim of directly inhibiting myometrial activity, or stimulating luteal function and thus increasing the available supply of the motility-inhibiting hormone, progestin. The *dose* is 500 rat units intramuscularly every other day during the latter half of the cycle. The earlier enthusiastic reports have recently given way to scepticism.

On the whole, use of the ovarian and gonadotropic hormones has proved disappointing in the treatment of functional dysmenorrhea. This is not surprising in view of the fact that ovarian function, as judged by the endometrial picture and sex hormone content of the body fluids, is normal in the majority of the cases.

Gynecologic Measures.—Cervical dilatation, the stem pessary and, in individual cases, cervicoplasty, suspension of the uterus, presacral sympathectomy, and hysterectomy are advocated for the treatment of dysmenorrhea.

Cervical Dilatation.—Cervical dilatation, with or without curettage, is one of the oldest and most widely used methods for the relief of menstrual pain. It was originally recommended on the assumption that it corrects an obstruction to the egress of the menstrual blood, which is presumably responsible for the pain. Though the obstructive theory has been questioned, this procedure is still employed empirically because it temporarily relieves or permanently cures the dysmenorrhea in a fair percentage of the cases. Since it can do no harm, cervical dilatation should be tried in functional dysmenorrhea associated with uterine hypoplasia and a nar-

25

row unyielding cervix. According to some observers, it is useful only in the spasmodic type of dysmenorrhea. It has been suggested that cervical dilatation may bring relief by injuring some of the sensory nerves of the isthmus of the cervix. Cannon[66] believes it is effective where spasm of the circular muscle fibers surrounding the os is responsible for the pain. Cervical dilatation is obviously contraindicated in the presence of pelvic inflammatory disease, and in the young unmarried girl, unless the condition is very severe and resists other measures.

The Stem Pessary.—The stem pessary has long been advocated by protagonists of the obstructive theory.[67, 68, 69] While beneficial results may occasionally follow its use, irritation and infection may result from its improper application.

Cervicoplastomy.—Plastic cervical operations have been employed to straighten or widen the cervical canal, or to sever the circular muscle fibers at the internal os, thought by some to be the site of the pain. Aside from the uncertainty of their effect, they may do much harm. Endocervicitis or interference with subsequent parturition are possible untoward effects.

Suspension of the Uterus.—Suspension of the uterus is frequently advised for the parous woman in dysmenorrhea associated with malposition of the uterus. The value of this operation is often difficult to estimate, for cervical dilatation is usually simultaneously performed. In many of the reported cases, a questionable appendix or some other pelvic lesion was removed at the same time. Because of its doubtful therapeutic value, it is not advocated by the author. In any event, suspension should not be undertaken unless replacement by means of a pessary has first been tried. It is obvious that if the latter gives no relief, suspension will do no good.

Cures in a large percentage of cases have been reported following the *injection of 80 per cent alcohol* into the ganglia of Frankenhauser.[70] The object of this procedure is to cause degeneration of the nerve cells and thus prevent the transmission of sensory impulses from the uterus. The author has had no experience with this method.

Presacral Sympathectomy.—Presacral sympathectomy involves severance of the superior hypogastric plexus in order to interrupt the nervous pathways which conduct pain stimuli from the uterus to the brain centers. First recommended by Jaboulay,[71] in 1899, for the relief of intractable dysmenorrhea, this operation has recently aroused renewed interest. Cotte,[72] its chief protagonist, and a number of other investigators[73, 74, 75] have reported favorable results, but there is some difference of opinion as to whether it interferes with uterine motility and subsequent labors. Some observers maintain that menstruation, conception, gestation and labor are normal following this operation, but others contend that it may endanger gonadal activity and adversely affect vesicle and rectal function. Presacral sympathectomy should be reserved for cases which resist every form of therapy short of hysterectomy. It should be emphasized that the beneficial effects reported with this operation cannot be accepted at face value. In many of the reported cases, suspension of the uterus, removal of an ovarian tumor or some other lesion was performed simultaneously, the double operation thus obscuring the effect of presacral sympathectomy alone.

Hysterectomy.—Hysterectomy should be considered as a last resort, and reserved for cases where the pain is so severe and intractable as to incapacitate the patient or seriously threaten her health or nervous stability, or where there is good reason to suspect endometriosis. This formidable operation should not be undertaken unless all other measures have been tried over an extended period of time. It is ill adapted for individuals with an inferior constitution, for in such cases disturbance of the utero-ovarian complex (see Chap. VII) may precipitate an early and troublesome symptomatology like that encountered during the climacteric.

BIBLIOGRAPHY

1. Pullen, R. L., and Hamblen, E. C.: Virginia Med. Monthly *69*:19, 1942.
2. Mackintosh, J.: Principles of Pathology and Practice of Physic. Washington, D. Green, 1834, p. 652.
3. Whitehouse, B.: J. Obst. & Gynec. Brit. Emp. *33*:607, 1926.
4. Tobler, M.: Monatschr. f. Geburtsh. u. Gynäk. *26*:801, 1907.
5. Novak, E., and Reynolds, S. R. M.: J.A.M.A. *99*:1466, 1932.
6. Blair-Bell, W., Datnow, M. M., and Jeffcoate, T. N. A.: J. Obst. & Gynec. Brit. Emp. *40*:541, 1933.
7. Schultz, V.: Monatschr. f. Geburtsh. u. Gynäk. *18*:854, 1903.
8. Schröder, R.: Die mensuellen Genitalzyklus u. seine Störungen, in, Veit-Stoeckel's Handb. d. Gynäk. 1928, vol. 1, part 2.
9. Campbell, A. D.: Ann. Int. Med. *7*:330, 1933.
10. Schickele, G., and Keller, R.: Arch. f. Gynäk. *95*:609, 1912.
11. Cannon, D. J.: J. Obst. & Gynec. Brit. Emp. *43*:492, 1936.
12. Fluhmann, C. F.: Endocrinol. *23*:393, 1938.
13. Novak, E.: Menstruation and Its Disorders. New York and London, D. Appleton & Co., 1921.
14. Blair-Bell, W.: J. Obst. & Gynec. Brit. Emp. *30*:119, 1923.
15. Moir, C.: Trans. Edin. Obst. Soc. *41*:93, 1934.
16. Lewis, T.: Clinical Science. London, Shaw, 1934.
17. Brewer, J. I.: Am. J. Obst. & Gynec. *36*:597, 1938.
18. Lackner, J. E., Krohn, L., and Soskin, S.: Am. J. Obst. & Gynec. *34*:248, 1937.
19. Wilson, L., and Kurzrok, R.: Endocrinol. *27*:23, 1940.
20. Larkin, W. L.: Pennsylvania M. J. *41*:348, 1938.
21. Keiffer, H.: Bull. Acad. roy. de méd. de Belgique *1*:508, 1936.
22. Theobald, G. W.: Brit. Med. J. *2*:1307, 1936.
23. Greenblatt, R. B., McCall, E., and Torpin, R.: Am. J. Obst. & Gynec. *42*:50, 1941.
24. Kurzrok, R., Wiesbader, H., and Mulinos, M. G.: Endocrinol. *21*:335, 1937.
25. Sturgis, S. H., and Albright, F.: Endocrinol. *26*:684, 1940.
26. Bickers, W.: Am. J. Obst. & Gynec. *42*:1023, 1941.
27. Gillman, J.: J. Clin. Endocrinol. *2*:157, 1942.
28. Smith, G. V., and Smith, O. W.: Am. J. Obst. & Gynec. *36*:769, 1938.
29. Smith, O. W., Smith, G. V., and Schiller, S.: Am. J. Obst. & Gynec. *45*:15, 1943.
30. Markee, J. E.: Carnegie Inst. Wash. Publ. No. 518, Contrib. Embryol. No. 177, 1940, vol. 28, p. 219.
31. Phelps, D.: Am. J. Obst. & Gynec. *33*:750, 1937.
32. Moir, C.: Proc. Roy. Soc. Med. *29*:950, 1936.
33. Kennedy, W. P.: J. Obst. & Gynec. Brit. Emp. *40*:792, 1933.
34. Blotevogel, W., and Poll, H.: Med. Klin. *23*:1503, 1927.
35. Morgan, T. N. A.: J. Obst. & Gynec. Brit. Emp. *42*:79, 84, 1935.
36. Hertzler, A. E.: Am. J. Obst. & Gynec. *9*:783, 1925.
37. Wendell, A.: Am. J. Obst. & Gynec. *20*:633, 1930.
38. Davis, A. A.: Dysmenorrhea: Its Aetiology and Treatment. London, Oxford Univ. Press, 1938.

39. Novak, J., and Harnik, M.: Med. Klin. *25*:251, 1929.
40. Horney, K.: Am. J. Obst. & Gynec. *25*:694, 1933.
41. Wilson, L., and Kurzrok, R.: Endocrinol. *23*:79, 1938.
42. Boynton, R. E., and Winther, N.: J.A.M.A. *119*:122, 1942.
43. Browne, O., and Torrens, D. S.: Irish J. Med. Sci., pp. 7–13, 1941.
44. Goodall, J. R., and Power, R. M. H.: Am. J. Obst. & Gynec. *33*:194, 1937.
45. Dale, H. H., cited by Bray, G. W., in, Recent Advances in Allergy, ed. 2. Philadelphia, P. Blakiston's Son & Co., Inc., 1934, p. 112.
46. Weinstein, G. L., Reynolds, S. R. M., and Friedman, M. H.: Am. J. Obst. & Gynec. *29*:93, 1931.
47. Tuft, L.: J. Allergy *9*:390, 1938.
48. Salen, E. B.: Acta med. Scandinav. Suppl. *59*:463, 494, 1934.
49. Geber, H.: Med. Klin. *31*:1203, 1935.
50. Lichter, cited by Salen, E. B. (*supra* 48).
51. Fliess, W.: Beziehungen zwischen Nasa und Weiblichen Geschlechtsorganen, Leipzig, 1897.
52. Goldwasser, M.: Woman's Med. J. *47*:229, 1940.
53. Taylor, Z. E.: New England J. Med. *224*:197, 1941.
54. Gray, H.: Endocrinol. *26*:536, 1940.
55. Elden, C. A., and Wilson, K. M.: Am. J. Obst. & Gynec. *32*:91, 1936.
56. Campbell, R. E., and Hisaw, F. L.: Am. J. Obst. & Gynec. *31*:508, 1936.
57. Kurzrok, L., Birnberg, C. H., and Livingston, S.: Am. J. Surg. *46*:353, 1939.
58. Soule, S. D.: J. Clin. Endocrinol. *1*:567, 1941.
59. Sturgis, S. H., and Meigs, J. V.: Surg., Gynec. & Obst. *75*:87, 1942.
60. Abarbanel, A. R.: Endocrinol. *26*:140, 765, 1940.
61. Geist, S. H.: J. Clin. Endocrinol. *1*:154, 1941.
62. Cinberg, B. L.: New York State J. Med. *42*:2138, 1942.
63. Gray, L. A.: Am. J. Obst. & Gynec. *43*:387, 1942.
64. Gray, L. A., and Manly, W. F.: Internat. Clin. *4*:191, 1940.
65. Shute, E. V.: Can. M. A. J. *42*:145, 1940.
66. Cannon, D. J.: J. Obst. & Gynec. Brit. Emp. *44*:13, 1937.
67. Shaw, W.: Lancet *2*:143, 1933.
68. Crossen, H. S., and Crossen, R. G.: Operative Gynecology. St. Louis, C. V. Mosby & Co., 1938.
69. Weir, W. H.: Am. J. Obst. & Gynec. *33*:291, 1937
70. Davis, A. A.: Lancet *1*:80, 1936.
71. Jaboulay, M.: Lyon méd. *90*:102, 1899.
72. Cotte, G.: Lyon méd. *135*:153, 1925.
73. Meigs, J. V.: Surg., Gynec. & Obst. *68*:723, 1939
74. Henriksen, E.: West. J. Surg. *49*:1, 1941.
75. Colcock, B. P.: S. Clin. N. Am. *21*:855, 1941.
76. Russell, P. M. G., and Dean, E. M.: Lancet *2*:66, 1942.
77. Taylor, H. M.: J. Obst. & Gynec. Brit. Emp. *49*:341, 1942.
78. Urbach, E.: Allergy. New York, Grune & Stratton, 1943.

CHAPTER XXVII

STERILITY

Incidence.—Sterility has long been a source of concern because of its profound psychologic and sociologic implications. Unfortunately, the number of sterile couples has tended to increase partly because of late marriages, prolonged use of contraceptives, and the stress and strain of modern life. It is estimated that more than 12 per cent of all marriages are involuntarily childless.[1] Recent advances in reproductive physiology and pathology have at once considerably clarified the sterile problem and made available valuable aids for its diagnosis and treatment.

Definition and Nomenclature.—The term sterility is sometimes employed to denote inability to conceive and bear viable young. A narrower definition, which will be used here, limits this term to inability to conceive. Failure to carry the fertilized ovum to the age of viability will be considered separately under "Spontaneous and Habitual Abortion" (see Chap. XXVIII).

Primary sterility describes cases in which conception has never occurred, while the terms *secondary* or *acquired* are applied where the inability to conceive follows a period of fertility. The sterile state which normally accompanies prepuberty, gestation, lactation, the menopause, and certain phases of the menstrual cycle, is referred to as *physiologic sterility*. The terms *functional* or *endocrine* describe sterility due to some disturbance in the endocrine glands governing reproductive function.

ETIOLOGY

From earliest recorded history, the female partner has almost invariably borne the entire responsibility for a sterile union. Blame was erroneously fixed on her because of the widespread belief that potency is positive proof of male fertility. Fortunately, this misconception has been discarded and it is now customary to speak of a sterile couple, in recognition of the fact that one and often several defects in either or both partners may be responsible for the failure to conceive. The complexity of the sterile problem can best be appreciated by recalling the long and intricate chain of events which must precede conception.

Prerequisites for Conception.

1. The male must produce normal spermatozoa, capable of fertilizing the ovum.

2. The male genitalia should offer the semen a free passage from the testicle to the outside world, and the mechanism by which the sperm are deposited in the female genital tract should operate normally. (This is not an absolute prerequisite because of the possibility of artificial insemination.)

3. In the female, the vaginal flora and endocervical secretions must not impair the viability and fertilizing potentiality of the deposited sperm.

4. The vagina, cervix, fundus and tubes must offer a free and ample passage for the ascending spermatozoa.

5. The ovaries must produce healthy ova.

6. The mechanism of ovulation must function properly and there should be no mechanical barrier to extrusion of the ripe ovum.

7. The tubes must receive the ovum and be of ample calibre to permit union with the ascending sperm, and transport of the fertilized egg to the uterine cavity.

A deviation from normal in one or more of these requirements may

TABLE 8

MALE AND FEMALE FACTORS IN STERILITY

Male Factors	Female Factors

Faulty Spermatogenesis
1. Azoospermia resulting from
   a. Congenital abnormalities of the testes.
   b. Destruction of testes by disease, neoplasms, or physical injury.
   c. Marked testicular hypoplasia due to anterior pituitary hypofunction or severe systemic depression.
 	
2. Oligospermia resulting from
   a. Partial destruction of the testes.
   b. Mild hypofunction of anterior pituitary, thyroid, or other glands.
   c. Mild systemic depression.
 	
3. Necrospermia resulting from
   a. Lethal gene.
   b. Depressive states.
	Faulty Oogenesis
	1. Complete failure of oogenesis resulting from
	   a. Congenital abnormalities of the ovaries.
	   b. Destruction of the ovaries by disease, neoplasms, surgery, or x-ray radiation.
	   c. Marked ovarian hypoplasia due to anterior pituitary hypofunction or severe systemic depression.
	2. Partial suppression of oogenesis due to
	   a. Partial destruction of the ovaries by disease, neoplasms, surgery, or radiation.
	   b. Mild ovarian hypofunction secondary to deficiency of anterior pituitary or other glands, or to mild systemic depression.
	3. Defective ova resulting from
	   a. Lethal gene.
	   b. Depressive states.

Obstacles to Transmission of Sperm to Female Genitalia (Not absolute bar to fertility because of possibility of artificial insemination) 1. Impotence. 2. Penile lesions or anomalies. 3. Obstructive lesions of vas deferens, epididymis, or urethra.	Obstacles to Union of Ovum and Sperm 1. Obstructive lesions of vulva, vagina, cervix, uterus or tubes. 2. Thick cervical mucus plug impermeable to sperm, due to poor drainage or infection. 3. Adhesions or thick ovarian capsule which bars exit of mature ovum from ripe follicle.
	Inadequate Nidatory Bed due to 1. Destruction of endometrium by disease or physical injury. 2. Improper preparation of nidatory bed—excessive estrogen effect resulting in general or local hyperplasia. 3. Atrophic changes of endometrium due to refractoriness to ovarian sex hormones.

result in lowered reproductive capacity, ranging from mild self-limited infertility to permanent irremediable sterility. Since both partners may be implicated, consideration of both male and female faults is essential for an adequate understanding of human sterility.

Role of the Male in Sterility.—Meaker, in 1934,[2] estimated that the male partner is directly or indirectly responsible for two-thirds of all barren unions. In one-third of the cases, he indirectly causes sterility by transmitting gonorrheal infection which may cause tubal occlusion. Another third is attributable to his inability to deliver an adequate supply of normal spermatozoa, because of faulty spermatogenesis, or conditions that hinder or preclude transmission of the semen from the testicle to the female genitalia. In a more recent communication,[1] this observer reported that of 100 barren marriages, the male was solely responsible in 8, chiefly at fault in 12, shared the responsibility equally with the female in 51, and played a minor role in 15.

Spermatogenic Faults.—Conception may be hindered or precluded by absence or deficiency of sperm, or qualitative alterations in the male germ cell. Complete failure of spermatogenesis (*azoospermia*) may be due to severe congenital anomalies of the testicle, or may develop as the result of operative or radiation castration, bilateral destructive testicular neoplasms, pyogenic infections, or other conditions capable of destroying the testicular secretory structures. Partial suppression of sperm production (*oligospermia*) may be attributable to testicular hypoplasia, or partial destruction of the testicle by organic disease, surgery or radiation. Too frequent emissions which exhaust the testicular apparatus, and general depressive states or senility may likewise materially reduce the number of sperm.

Morphologic and biologic abnormalities in the sperm (*necrospermia*) may result from prostatic and testicular disease, or general debilitating conditions such as acute and chronic infectious diseases and intoxications, metabolic disturbances, lues, endocrine disorders, poor general hygiene and nutritional faults.

Faults in the Transmission of the Sperm.—Complete or partial *occlusion of the vas deferens or ejaculatory ducts,* and *urethral stricture* interfere with fertility by partially or totally blocking the egress of the semen. These genital defects may result from inflammatory disease of the seminal vesicles, epididymis, prostate, or urethra. Severance of the ejaculatory ducts, whether by operation or injury, has the same effect.

Impotence per se is not an insurmountable obstacle to conception. Where the cause is mechanical, as in deformity of the external genitalia which prevents intromission, or where it is psychic, arising from fear or disgust for the coital act, the difficulty may be overcome by testicular aspiration and artificial insemination. On the other hand, if it is an expression of some deep seated endocrinopathy or constitutional depressive state, which threatens spermatogenic function, the prognosis is obviously much less favorable.

Role of the Female in Sterility.—In the female, as in the male, sterility can be traced to two main faults: (1) impaired oogenesis, and (2) defects which bar union of the ovum and male germ cell.

Faults in Oogenesis and Ovulation.—Fertility may be precluded or seriously threatened by complete or partial suppression of egg building, production of defective nonfertilizable ova, or interference with the mechanism of ovulation. These abnormalities may arise from congenital or acquired faults of the ovary proper (primary ovarian sterility), disturbances in the endocrine glands which directly or indirectly control ovarian function, or nonendocrine faults which depress the organism as a whole and with it the gonads (secondary ovarian sterility).

The Ovary.—Severe congenital or developmental anomalies, such as marked degrees of *ovarian hypoplasia*, obviously entail complete and permanent suppression of oogenesis. The mild hypoplasias, on the other hand, are compatible with limited oogenic function. In such cases normal ova may be produced at infrequent intervals, and the probability of conception is correspondingly diminished, though union with a male of vigorous fertility may compensate for the deficiency.

Ovarian faults acquired as a result of organic disease, surgery, or radiation, may partly or totally suppress egg building, depending on the extent of the damage inflicted. It is well established that the *x-rays* have a sterilizing effect on the human ovary, the extent of the injury being determined by the dosage and the susceptibility of the ovary. A dose which in one woman may merely destroy the more susceptible follicles and temporarily suppress ovulation, in another may destroy the entire follicular apparatus, causing permanent amenorrhea and absolute sterility. The apparent ovarian regeneration and return of normal menstrual function and fertility, occasionally seen following intensive radiation, is probably due to the fact that some of the follicles escaped the destructive action of the rays.

A thick, unyielding tunica albuginea, or dense pericapsular adhesions may bar the exit of the ripe egg. The unruptured follicles may become atretic or cystic and mechanically interfere with the maturation of new crops of follicles.[3]

Barring congenital or acquired defects of the ovary, abnormalities in oogenic function or ovulation may result from *disturbances in its endocrine regulators,* particularly the anterior pituitary gland.

The Anterior Hypophysis.—That the anterior pituitary gland plays an important role in fertility is suggested by the high incidence of *sterility in hypophyseal endocrinopathies,* such as Simmonds' disease, giantism, acromegaly, dwarfism, and pituitary basophilism (see Chap. XXXV). Recent experimental studies (see Chap. XII) have thrown considerable light on the *mechanism* by which disorders of this gland hinder fertility. There is evidence that the anterior pituitary controls cyclic changes in the ovary through its follicle-stimulating, luteinizing and possibly also its luteotrophic principle. The FSH factor stimulates follicular maturation and egg-ripening, but the synergistic action of FSH and LH is necessary to induce follicular rupture and extrusion of the ovum (see Chap. XII). To insure ovulation, a delicate balance between these principles must be maintained. Disturbance of their temporal or quantitative relations may interfere with egg-ripening and ovulation. It would therefore follow that the conceptional potentiality of the individual may be adversely affected by either a deficiency or excess of the pituitary sex hormones. Absence of both sex principles will obviously preclude all cyclic ovarian activity. If only the luteinizing factor is absent, follicular development and maturation of ova may proceed normally, but ovulation cannot occur. If both hormones are produced but there is a relative or absolute excess of follicle stimulator, it may cause the formation of large cystic follicles, which do not rupture but confine the ripe ovum within their walls where it eventually dies. On the other hand, a relative or absolute excess of the luteinizing fraction may induce luteinization of the follicle before rupture can occur, thus entrapping the ovum. The luteinized structures thus formed may interfere with the maturation of new crops of follicles, either mechanically or through the hormones they elaborate.

Other Endocrine Glands.—On the basis of clinical and experimental evidence, it would appear that malfunction of the thyroid, adrenals, and other glands may hinder fertility by adversely affecting oogenic function. Because of their reciprocal relationship with the anterior hypophysis, they may, if disturbed, unfavorably influence its gonadotropic function and thus indirectly disturb ovarian activity. It is also conceivable that disorders of these glands may directly impair oogenesis and the quality of the germ cell by upsetting the normal metabolic equilibrium with which they are primarily concerned. In the severe endocrinopathies, whether due to marked hypofunction or hyperfunction of one or more of these glands, the damage to the organism in general and to the ovaries in particular is considerable and often irreversible. Maturation of ova is almost invariably suppressed and sterility is the rule. Because of the accompanying severe constitutional depression, fertility is rarely desired and these cases are therefore of little concern in the sterile problem. On the other hand, mild disturbances deserve particular emphasis because they may account for many unexplained cases of sterility. Since definite stigmata of glandular disease are usually absent in such cases, the condition may often be overlooked. The importance of mild endocrine disturbances should not be underestimated, and the possibility that they may be operating should always be considered, especially where no other cause for the sterility can be found.

Nonendocrine Causes.—A sound constitution is the foundation on which endocrine and, ultimately, oogenic function must depend. *Poor health* is quickly reflected in the ovaries, and the delicate germ cells are the first to suffer. Temporary or permanent suppression of oogenesis may result from systemic disease, blood dyscrasias, metabolic disorders, chronic infections and intoxications, lues, occupational disease, particularly in x-ray and lead workers, or any other condition which causes general debility. Fertility may likewise be lowered by poor hygiene, undue physical or mental stress, too little or too much exercise, lack of sleep, and nutritional faults. Undernutrition, because of dietary fads or a poorly balanced diet deficient in protein, mineral salts and the essential vitamins, may lead to general cellular malnutrition and gonadal inanition. Overnutrition, on the other hand, may unduly burden the metabolic and endocrine apparatus and thus indirectly lead to gonadal depression and infertility.

Nervous and psychic disturbances may conceivably depress oogenic function by way of the vegetative nervous system, which is intimately related to the endocrine glands. Sterile women have been known to conceive for the first time shortly after adopting a child, due possibly to relief from nervous tension on becoming resigned to the prospect of never conceiving.

Factors Responsible for Nonunion of the Gametes.—While the functional causes of sterility primarily concern us here, faults which hinder or preclude union of the gametes deserve brief mention since they are responsible for a large proportion of all cases. Union of the male and female germ cells may be barred by faults in the reception or retention of the semen, improper cervical insemination, or impediments to the transport of the gametes through the vagina, uterus and tubes.

Reception and Retention of the Semen.—Defects of the vulva, hymen, or vagina may mechanically obstruct the deposition of the semen. *Occlusion of the vulva* may be due to congenital atresia, as is pseudohermaphroditism, persistence of the sinus urogenitalis, gynatresia, infantilism, burns or acute and chronic infections, particularly gonorrheal vulvovaginitis. Large condylomata, fibroids, cysts and vulvar hypertrophies (elephantiasis), may also bar the entrance of the semen.

Hymenal atresias are of minor importance, for they usually become apparent soon after the onset of menstrual function, when retention of the menstrual blood leads to their detection and early correction. *Hymenal septa* are not necessarily a barrier to fertility, inasmuch as conception has been known to follow external coitus without penetration. An abnormally thick hymen, which resists penetration by the male organ, or a flexible one that permits intercourse without allowing the sperm to enter, are likewise of little significance, since they are readily recognized and easily corrected.

Vaginal defects, such as partial or total aplasia, failure of canalization, vaginal infantilism, or annular membranous occlusions, may likewise hinder the reception of the semen. Acquired occlusions may follow inflammatory processes, and thermic or chemical burns, with their resultant agglutinations and cicatrizations. Large solid or cystic neoplasms may obstruct the entrance of the spermatozoa. Effusion seminis or failure to retain the deposited semen, may result from anomalies of the perineum, a shallow vagina as seen in vaginal infantilism, lacerations, or an abnormally wide vagina due to marked relaxation of the musculature.

Painful coitus (*dyspareunia*) and sexual anesthesia (*frigidity*) may interfere with the proper performance of the sex act and lead to infrequent coitus, lessening the chances for conception. Dyspareunia, though often of psychoneurotic origin, is sometimes traceable to tender hymenal rests, painful urethral caruncles, inflammation or irritation of the vulva or vagina, uterine or ovarian displacements, and pelvic inflammatory disease.

Cervical Insemination.—Sterility may not infrequently be traceable to mechanical, bacterial, or chemical barriers which prevent the deposited sperm from reaching or passing the cervical canal in a viable state. Ascent of the sperm may be obstructed by congenital or acquired *defects* of the vagina or cervix, or thick *endocervical secretions.* The latter, by reason of their colloidal nature, may offer an impregnable barrier to the male germ cell. Such secretions are most apt to form in the narrow, elongated, stenotic cervix, where drainage is poor. That it is the mucus plug and not the narrow cervical canal that prevents ascent of the sperm can hardly be doubted in view of the fact that the lumen of the uterus and tubes, which is of comparatively smaller calibre, but contains serous secretions, offers no such barrier. The beneficial effect of cervical dilatation is presumably due to improved drainage.

Bacterial invasion of the vaginal pool, particularly that resulting from cervical infections, is an important cause of faulty insemination.[4, 5] The altered vaginal flora, and bacterial toxins elaborated by the alien bacteria, may inactivate or destroy the deposited sperm and thus prevent their further progress through the cervix. It is significant that a negative Hühner test often becomes positive following cauterization of an infected cervix, and that this procedure alone may sometimes correct a long standing sterile state. The importance of bacterial hostility has been questioned by Meaker on the ground that women with endocervical infections can conceive, and that sperm mixed with cervical secretion containing bacteria and leucocytes, are not impaired. This divergence of opinion may perhaps be accounted for by differences in the type of invading bacteria. It is likely that some organisms destroy the germ cells while others have little or no deleterious effect.

Abnormal chemistry of the genital secretions is considered by some observers[6] to be an obstacle to insemination. The assumption that undue acidity of the vaginal pool is inimical to the life of the deposited spermatozoa, has been invalidated by the demonstration that sperm can live in high acid titers.[7] It is noteworthy, however, that in a group of sterile women observed by Laffont and Bourgarel,[8] there was too much rather than too little acidity in the majority of the cases. Most workers now concede that the endocervical environment never vitiates the spermatozoa on a strictly chemical basis.

Transport through the Uterus and Tubes.—Uterine faults, which may bar ascent of the sperm, include severe genital anomalies, uterine infantilism, neoplasms and inflammatory processes of the endometrium.

Tubal occlusion, whether congenital or acquired, is perhaps the most frequent cause of female sterility. The acquired closures most often follow gonorrheal and puerperal infections, or inflammatory processes of the peritoneum, particularly suppurative appendicitis. Occasionally, neoplasms, endometriosis, or malposition due to displacement of the tubes by large uterine tumors, may occlude the tubal lumen.

Miscellaneous Causes of Nonunion.—Failure to conceive, despite normal gametes and no demonstrable obstacles to their union, has long perplexed observers. *Inherent incompatibility of the male and female germ cells* has been offered as a possible explanation. This theory is based on the clinical observation that partners of a sterile marriage often prove fertile on union with another mate. It has been challenged by competent observers[9] who suggest that such cases may as reasonably be explained by assuming that each partner of the sterile union has a low fertility index and that union with another mate with greater fertility potentialities, compensates for the deficiency. Another theory proposes that the female genitalia acquire *immunity to the spermatozoa* as a result of excessive intercourse.[10] It assumes that after the male germ cells are deposited in the female genitalia, they degenerate and produce a spermatoxin. To combat this, the female elaborates spermatocidal anti-bodies which inactivate the sperm, precluding conception. In support of this suggestion, it has been pointed out that spermatogenic function may be temporarily suppressed in some animals by injecting them with their own sperm;[11] and that women injected with human spermatozoa may be rendered sterile for as long as one year.[12, 13] The observation that a sterile state may be terminated following a period of abstinence is offered as additional support for this theory. This is not entirely convincing since abstinence may favorably influence fertility by giving the male a much needed rest and thus increasing the quantity or improving the quality of the seminal secretions. Evidence invalidating this theory has been provided by Henle and his associates.[14, 15] These observers found that active immunization of female guinea pigs with guinea pig spermatozoa led to antibody response in the large majority of the animals. Despite the antibody content of the sera, no decrease in fertility or delay in conception was observed.

DIAGNOSIS

Since inability to conceive may be traceable to one or more faults in either or both partners, the fertility index of each must be estimated in order to arrive at an accurate evaluation. This requires the complete cooperation of both members of the barren union, who should be impressed with the complex nature of the problem, and the necessity for a thorough investigation. Examination of the female partner should begin only after excluding irremediable faults in the male, since these would make study and treatment of the female futile.

INVESTIGATION OF THE MALE PARTNER

It is of prime importance to determine the extent of the husband's responsibility. This requires a careful history, complete physical and urologic examination, and routine laboratory studies. Appraisal of the semen constitutes the chief and final index of male fertility. To insure the greatest possible accuracy in the diagnosis, it is necessary to follow certain rules in collecting and examining the ejaculate.

Collection of the Semen.—Following sexual abstinence for a few days, the semen is obtained manually or by means of a condom. While the total volume and number of spermatozoa are practically the same in both the manual and condom specimen, their life span, as gauged by their motility may differ appreciably. Belding,[16] found that spermatozoa obtained by the manual method remained motile for 105 hours at 8° C., those in the condom specimen only 35 hours. This may be attributable to the action of talc and other chemicals used to preserve the condom. The author prefers the manual or withdrawal method and employs a wide mouthed sterile glass container for the collection of the ejaculate. Where a condom is used, it should be washed and dried beforehand, and the semen emptied into the glass container immediately after ejaculation.

Temperature of the Collected Semen.—The prevailing practice of keeping the semen at body temperature prior to examination, has been discredited by the demonstration that spermatozoa retain their motility much longer when kept cool. There is evidence that motility persists for over 23 hours at 37.5°C., and for 96 hours at 8°. Since the testicles are external organs, the spermatozoa in their natural environment are exposed to less than body temperature. For this reason, the semen is best maintained at room temperature.

Estimation of Fertility.—Standards based on normal variations in the fertile male have not yet been perfected and there is no unanimity of opinion as to what constitutes a fertile male. The number, motility, and morphology of the spermatozoa determine the fertility index.

Number of Spermatozoa.—Under normal conditions, the total volume of the ejaculate averages about 4 cc. Some workers consider less than 0.5 cc. an inadequate seminal pool. A small ejaculate is not per se an absolute bar to fertility for if the female is very fertile, she may compensate for this deficiency. It is estimated that each cubic centimeter of seminal fluid normally contains approximately 100,000,000 spermatozoa.[17] The belief that less than 60,000,000 is inadequate for normal fertility has been disproved by Hotchkiss and his associates,[18] who found less than this number in 25 per cent of a group of 200 fertile males. On the other hand, a high sperm count does not necessarily signify fertility. In one case reported by Seymour,[19] 94,000,000 spermatozoa per cc. of seminal fluid was found. When employed for artificial insemination of a group of 16 women, no conception followed, although all of the group as well as the patient's wife were subsequently impregnated by spermatozoa from another male.

It is erroneous to evaluate spermatogenic function on the basis of a single count, for the number of spermatozoa varies from time to time in the same individual. This is partly due to fluctuations in the proportion between the prostatic and testicular fluids and the interval between coital acts. Where repeated counts consistently show a deficiency or absence of spermatozoa, partial or complete suppression of spermatogenesis, or some bar to their exit may be suspected. Testicular aspiration will differentiate the two conditions. Some investigators[20, 21] recommend testicular biopsy for this purpose, on the ground that it may not only help exclude occlusion but also disclose the degree of testicular depression, thus serving as a prognostic aid and guide to therapy. The danger of injuring an already deficient testicular apparatus should be seriously considered before undertaking this procedure.

Motility of Spermatozoa.—Motility is a fairly reliable criterion of sperm vitality. It varies at different times in the same individual and is influenced by the temperature and menstruum of the spermatozoa. The motility index may be determined from the type of activity, number of sperm crossing a microscopic field, percentage of inactive cells, and duration of motility as revealed by repeated examinations at room temperature. At least 50 per cent should be actively motile and show some motility for at least eight hours. It must be emphasized that fertilizing power is not synonymous with motility, which may persist long after fertilizing power is lost.[22] For this reason, an absence of motility may be taken to signify lack of fertilizing power, but the reverse is not necessarily the case.

Morphology of Spermatozoa.—Abnormal sperm morphology, according to Moench[7, 9] and other competent investigators, has a distinct bearing on the fertility of the male and his fitness for procreation. Moench considers very long, tapering and narrow sperm heads of especially sinister import. It is generally conceded that a certain percentage of abnormal forms

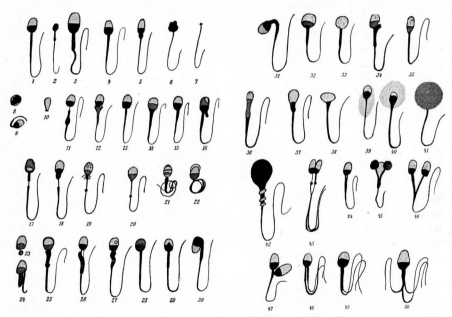

Fig. 88.—Sperm morphology in relation to fertility. 1. Normal spermatozoon. 2–50. Deviations from normal. Abnormalities of sperm head are most significant. Narrow cells and rounded cells tapering at the base represent the most sinister morphologic change of sperm head so far as fertilizing power is concerned (Moench).

may be found in fertile males, and if this is exceeded, the probability of conception diminishes accordingly. Some consider the presence of 10 per cent of abnormal forms within normal limits. According to Moench, sterility or abortion will result if the proportion exceeds 20 per cent. McClellan[23] states that more than 25 to 30 per cent of abnormal forms indicate at least temporary sterility in the male. Since the margin between fertile and infertile males with respect to the total number of abnormal forms is rather narrow, this criterion of male fertility is not infallible. To facilitate examination of the sperm, various staining methods have been devised, among them a differential stain recently recommended by Greenberg and his associates.[68]

INVESTIGATION OF THE FEMALE PARTNER

Investigation of the female partner should include a careful history, general physical and pelvic examination, and endocrinologic and other special studies pertinent to the solution of the sterile problem.

History.—*General.*—The *family history* may provide valuable information. Lues or endocrinopathic disease, which may unfavorably affect fertility in the second generation, are particularly significant. In the patient's past *medical history,* mumps, which may cause ovarian atrophy, and gonorrheal vulvovaginitis, which may produce vulvar or vaginal agglutinations and contractures, or render the vaginal flora inimical to the deposited semen, are noteworthy. Tuberculous or pneumoperitonitis, appendiceal abscess, colitis or sigmoiditis, are important antecedents for they may lead to perisalpingitis with subsequent stenosis, or cause ovarian adhesions which mechanically impede ovulation. In acquired sterility, a history of criminal abortion, puerperal infection, or chronic pelvic inflammatory disease is of the utmost importance, since these are often precursors of tubal sterility. Antecedent pelvic operations, systemic disease, chronic intoxications, poor general and sex hygiene, dietary faults, and exposure to x-rays may provide important clues.

The *age* of the female partner is important, for fertility is often below par toward the end of the reproductive period and during the early years of menstrual life, when anovulatory cycles are not uncommon. The age of the male partner is equally significant, since spermatogenic function tends to diminish with advancing years. The *duration of normal conjugal relations* must also be taken into consideration, for a couple should not be judged sterile unless given ample time to conceive. Opinions differ as to how many years must elapse before a union may be considered barren. Some require a lapse of three years, while others regard a period of five years a fair limit. Statistical studies[24] reveal that by far the largest number of married women conceive for the first time during the first two years of normal conjugal life. The percentage of conceptions after this time falls rapidly, less than five per cent conceiving after the fifth year. For practical purposes, a fixed time limit should be avoided in favor of a flexible one based on the age of the partners, presence or absence of apparent reproductive defects, and time consumed in the use of contraceptives. In the average case, if no contraceptives have been employed, three years is ample time to test fertility. In older couples, one year is sufficient. If some obvious defect is present, it is advisable to investigate the couple and institute appropriate therapy without further delay. Information relating to fertility in a previous marriage is of distinct value in absolving one or the other partner from responsibility for the fruitless union, but the possibility of an acquired defect should not be overlooked.

Menstrual History.—The *age of the menarche* may offer a clue to the degree of genital development, late onset of menstrual function suggesting retarded progress. A history of late onset of menstrual function was elicited in about 35 per cent of the author's series. Even more important is the character of the *menstrual habit.* This has long been considered a reliable index of ovarian function. Until recently, periodic bleeding of normal amount, duration and frequency, was accepted as proof of normal gonadal activity. That this assumption is not entirely justified is indicated by evidence that uterine bleeding clinically indistinguishable from true menstruation (see Chap V) may occur in the absence of ovulation and corpus luteum formation. Such bleeding, commonly referred to as "pseudomenstruation," occurred in 25 per cent of a group of sterile women studied by the author.[25] Jeffcoate,[26] Novak[27] and others[28, 29, 30] have likewise found it more common than has generally been supposed. Recognition of this entity constitutes an important advance in the diagnosis and treatment of sterility. That the menstrual habit is not a reliable index of ovarian function is also emphasized by the occurrence of conception and normal gestation in some women with long standing amenorrhea. At best, the character of the flow may be taken only as presumptive evidence, and deviations from the normal menstrual rhythm tentatively interpreted as follows: Amenorrhea, hypomenorrhea, and oligomenorrhea may signify gonadal depression. Here ovulation may be absent or occur at infrequent intervals, thus lessening the chances for conception. Excessive or irregular uterine bleeding may be an expression of pelvic pathology which impairs oogenic function or bars union of the gametes. In the absence of demonstrable pathology, such bleeding may signify disordered ovarian function involving suppression of ovulatory function. The final decision must depend on other evidence, particularly that provided by endometrial biopsy and quantitative hormone studies (see below). Dysmenorrhea, unless associated with genital hypoplasia or pelvic pathology is entirely compatible with fertility.

Physical Examination.—A thorough physical examination is important. Particular attention should be directed to the development of the secondary sex characters and the presence of endocrinopathic stigmata, such as statural anomalies, obesity, and hirsutism. Systemic disease and depressive states should be excluded, since any deviation from normal may contribute to the sterile state.

Pelvic Examination.—A careful bimanual pelvic examination will disclose the developmental status of the external and internal genitalia, and may reveal congenital or acquired defects which may hinder fertility.

Special Studies.—The occurrence of ovulation may be determined fairly accurately by premenstrual endometrial biopsy and quantitative sex hormone studies of the blood and urine (see chapter IV). Faults in cervical insemination may be disclosed by examining the post-coital secretions (Hühner test) or testing the ability of the sperm to penetrate the cervical mucus (Miller-Kurzrok test). Tubal insufflation (Rubin test) is of value for the detection of mechanical impediments to the transit of the gametes through the uterus and tubes.

Hühner Test.[31]—Primarily designed to determine the compatibility of the deposited spermatozoa with the vaginal pool and endocervical secretions, this test also furnishes a clue to the status of spermatogenic function, and establishes the mechanical potency of the male (see Table 9). It is particularly useful where the husband refuses to submit to examination.

Technique.—Following sexual abstinence for about one week, the wife is instructed to come to the office within an hour or two after coitus. To insure retention of as much of the deposited semen as possible, she should be instructed to empty her bladder and bowels before coitus, lie in bed for a half hour afterward, and wear a pad on her way to the office. Krigbaum[32] recommends the use of a bell-shaped rubber container which can be inserted into the vagina. This device creates an effective seal by suction and insures intimate contact between the semen and the genital secretions; hence its use is particularly indicated in effusion seminis. At the office, the rubber container is removed and its contents examined. Where it is not

TABLE 9

INTERPRETATION OF HÜHNER TEST

Vaginal Pool		Endocervical Secretions		Diagnosis
No. of Sperm	Motility of Sperm	No. of Sperm	Motility of Sperm	
Normal	Normal	Normal	Normal	Normal production and delivery by male. Sperm compatible with genital secretions.
Normal	Normal	Diminished or Absent		Incomplete penetration due to imperfect intromission or mechanical obstruction between vagina and cervix.
Normal	Normal	Normal	Dead	Hostile cervical secretions.
Normal	Dead	Normal	Dead	Production of amotile sperm by male or hostile vaginal pool and cervical secretions.
Diminished or Absent		Diminished or Absent		Deficiency or absence of spermatogenesis; failure of, or incomplete intromission, or partial or complete loss of deposited sperm.

employed, a sample of the vaginal pool may be obtained by means of a long bulb syringe. In obtaining a sample of the endocervical secretions, the cervix should first be dabbed with a cotton sponge, a fresh pipette used, and its contents placed on a separate slide. This test will provide important information (see Table 9). Where the test is negative, it should be repeated, for not infrequently a negative test may be followed later by a positive one.[33]

Miller-Kurzrok Test.[34]—The object of this procedure is to test the sperm's ability to penetrate the cervical mucus plug. It is particularly indicated where a large number of motile sperm are found in the vagina but not in the endocervical secretions.

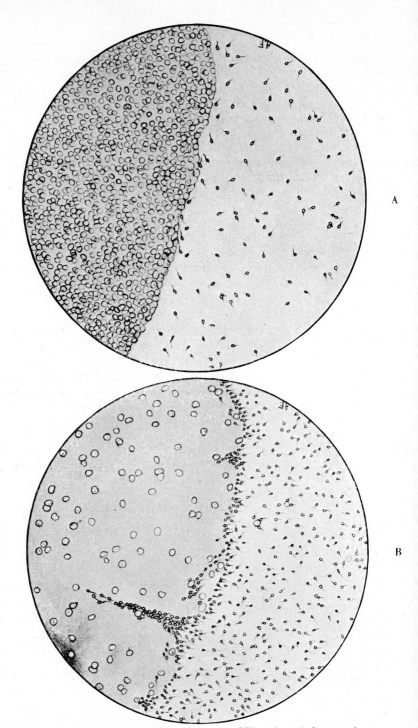

Fig. 89.—Miller-Kurzrok test to determine permeability of cervical mucus by spermatozoa. A, Contact between semen and infected mucus. B, Contact between semen and normal mucus. Orientation and beginning penetration. (Kurzrok, R.: Endocrines in Obstetrics, Baltimore, Williams and Wilkins Co.)

Technique.—1. Place a small drop of semen, about 3 to 5 mm. in diameter, in the center of a clean, dry glass slide.

2. Wipe the cervix clean, remove a small fragment of mucus, 3 to 5 mm. in diameter, from the cervical canal, and place it on the slide about 3 mm. away from the drop of semen. The space between the two drops must be completely dry and uncontaminated by either semen or mucus.

3. Drop a cover glass squarely on the drops so that its weight may bring their margins into contact and thus set up an immiscible phase boundary. If a small space intervenes, gentle pressure on the glass will help bridge the gap.

4. Examine the contact zone under low and then under high dry power.

Interpretation.—The test is negative if no penetration occurs and the sperm swims past the mucus plug without making the slightest effort to enter. According to Miller and Kurzrok, this usually occurs when the mucus is infected, although specimens from hypoplastic uteri may also offer definite resistance. Of particular interest are cases where the spermatozoa cannot penetrate apparently normal mucus, though capable of doing so when tested against cervical mucus from another patient.

Modified Miller-Kurzrok Test.—A modification of this procedure has recently been described by Lamar and associates,[35] who claim the following advantages over that of Miller and Kurzrok: it eliminates the possibility of undiscoverable mechanical mixing; it prevents drying of the preparation, with the attendant evils of currents in the mucus; and it makes possible a quantitative measure of penetration when this occurs.

Technique.—1. Prepare capillary tubing of 0.10 to 0.40 mm. inside diameter.

2. Draw a small amount of mucus into a length of tubing and observe the relative viscosity.

3. After the mucus, draw up a small bubble of air, then a column of fresh semen, and record the time when this is done. The purpose of the bubble is to prevent mechanical mixing of semen and mucus during their arrangement in the capillary tube. If the bubble is of correct size, this is accomplished and yet enough mucus adheres to the tube walls to furnish a medium through which the spermatozoa can pass the bubble and begin attacking the mucus.

4. Seal the tube with mineral oil and watch through a microscope. If penetration occurs, the bubble forms a landmark. By using a stop watch and a calibrated mechanical stage, the rate of penetration of a single spermatozoon can be measured accurately.

Tubal Insufflation (Rubin Test).[36]—This test is designed to determine tubal patency. Carbon dioxide gas, under manometric and volumetric control, is passed slowly into the uterine cavity by means of a long narrow cannula. The pressure fluctuations of the gas are registered by a pen attached to a recording kymograph.

Technique and Interpretation.—Tubal patency is established when the intrauterine pressure rises to 100 or 120 mm. of mercury and, as the gas begins to pass into the peritoneal cavity, falls sharply to 40 mm. or less. Pressure fluctuations between high and low points are recorded on the kymograph, and express the normal tubal contractions. The passage of the gas into the peritoneal cavity gives rise to a pneumoperitoneum, which is readily observed by the x-rays. Pressure of the gas on the subphrenic nerves causes pain, which is usually referred to the right shoulder when the patient assumes a sitting posture. Where anesthesia is used, auscultation will determine the course of the gas as it passes from the tubes into the abdominal cavity.

Tubal closure is indicated when there is a progressive rise in the pressure and introduction of the gas produces neither a pneumoperitoneum nor shoulder pain. Where the obstruction is unilateral, auscultation

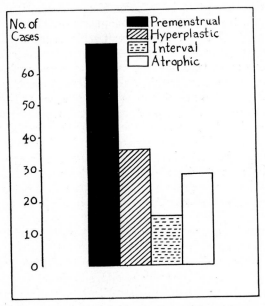

Fig. 90.—Graph showing endometrial findings in a group of 148 cases of sterility. Note that all types of endometria were encountered, the premenstrual type predominating. The sterility was associated with irregular uterine bleeding in fourteen cases, with amenorrhea or oligomenorrhea in seventy-three, and with apparently normal menses in sixty-one. Of these sixty-one cases, eleven or about 18 per cent had hyperplastic, interval or atrophic endometria, suggesting failure of ovulation.

is of value in locating it, for passage of the gas will be audible on the patent side. A high pressure is not per se conclusive evidence that organic obstruction exists, since it may also result from tubal spasm or the presence of inspissated mucus. In such cases, on reinsufflation during the same sitting, a sudden drop may follow the initial elevation. An antispasmodic given before the test may eliminate tubal spasm. If a normal pressure is recorded, but fluctuations are slight or absent, peritubal adhesions, which restrain tubal motility, may be suspected.

Where tubal surgery is contemplated, the site of the obstruction may be ascertained by salpingography.

Tubal insufflation should be performed postmenstrually and never just before or during the flow, because of the danger of retrograde dissemination of viable endometrial fragments which may become imbedded in the pelvic organs or cul de sac and constitute a potential cause for endometriosis. It is *contraindicated* in the presence of acute purulent infections of the vagina or cervix, or acute pelvic inflammatory disease. It is obviously of no avail where either partner has some other irremediable fault which precludes fertility.

Endometrial Biopsy and Curettage.—An indirect and fairly reliable method of ascertaining the status of ovarian function and establishing the occurrence of ovulation is the histologic evaluation of endometrial tissue obtained by biopsy or curettage. Where the periods are regular, this procedure may be carried out shortly before the expected flow. Some observers prefer to wait until after its onset in order not to miss a late ovulation or disturb an early pregnancy. Where the patient is amenorrheic, biopsy may be performed at weekly intervals for four weeks with the hope of detecting an endometrial cycle. The presence of secretory modifications may be taken as presumptive evidence of ovulation and corpus luteum formation. It has been pointed out that secretory changes cannot be taken as positive proof of ovulation because of the possibility of granulosa luteinization without rupture of the follicle. Since this is a rare occurrence in the human being, it does not constitute a serious source of error. If the mucosa presents evidence of only an estrogenic effect, it is likely that the current cycle is anovulatory. Studies of the estrogen and pregnanediol content of the urine (see below) are of value in determining whether the absence of luteal effect is due to failure of ovulation and corpus luteum formation, or is attributable to refractoriness of the uterine mucosa. While the absence of ovulation in one cycle does not necessarily imply that all cycles are anovulatory, it would seem to justify the conclusion that ovulatory function is subnormal.

Vaginal Smear.—Observers differ as to the value of the vaginal smear as a means of establishing the occurrence of ovulation (see Chap. XXXIX). Since the changes in the smear during the course of the menstrual cycle are not clearcut, and the sources of error are numerous, this method is a useful adjunct only in the hands of the experienced investigator. As emphasized by Krohn and his associates,[37] even the expert observer must analyze smears throughout the cycle to avoid error. For these reasons, its value as a practical diagnostic aid for general use is still limited.

Sex Hormone Studies.—Qualitative and quantitative determinations of the estrogen, pregnanediol, and gonadotropin content of the body fluids are a useful adjunct in the diagnosis only when combined with endometrial biopsy. These tests may provide a clue to the level of hormone production, while the endometrial picture indicates to what extent the hormones are being utilized (see Table 10). Together they permit a fairly accurate estimate of the functional status of the uterus, ovary, and anterior pituitary gland.

Estrogen Findings.—Because of variations in the kidney threshold, tests of the blood and urine estrogen should be carried out simultaneously.

A positive blood estrogen test obtained premenstrually in an individual with **regular** periods usually denotes normal ovarian function. A single negative test is inconclusive since it may represent a transient drop in the concentration of the hormone. If a second test is negative, depression of ovarian function may be suspected. In the amenorrheic patient, the blood estrogen tests should be performed at weekly intervals for four or five weeks to detect a possible blood estrogen cycle. More reliable information may be obtained by measuring the quantity of estrogen excreted in the urine over a period of thirty days, for error due to transient fluctuations in the estrogen level is thus avoided. According to Frank,[38] from 1300 to 1700 mouse

TABLE 10

ASSOCIATION OF ENDOMETRIAL AND HORMONAL FINDINGS IN 148 CASES OF STERILITY

State of Endometrium	Blood Estrogen Test			Blood Gonadotropin Test			Total Number of Cases
	Positive	Threshold	Negative	APR. I	APR. II–III	Negative	
Premenstrual..................	21	8	28	0	0	57	57
Early Premenstrual...........	4	6	2	0	0	12	12
Hyperplasia..................	15	10	7	2	0	30	32
Local Hyperplasia............	2	1	1	0	0	4	4
Interval.....................	9	5	1	0	0	15	15
Atrophic....................	0	3	25	9	6	13	28
Total number of cases........	51	33	64	11	6	131	148

units are normally excreted during an entire menstrual cycle; 500 to 800 is subthreshold, and under 200 units is acyclic, suggesting a low level of ovarian function.

The estrogen tests are particularly valuable in differentiating between primary uterine amenorrhea and that due to ovarian hypofunction (see Chap. XXIV). They may also serve as a guide in the treatment, for if normal or excessive amounts of estrogen are found, its administration is obviously superfluous.

Pregnanediol Findings.—In the normally menstruating woman, pregnanediol may be demonstrable in the urine during the latter half of the cycle.[39] This biologically inactive substance is believed to be an excretion product of progestin and its presence may be taken as presumptive evidence that ovulation and corpus luteum formation have occurred. On the other hand, negative findings are inconclusive. These studies may aid in differentiating between ovulatory and anovulatory cycles. It should be emphasized that pregnanediol is not associated exclusively with luteal function, but may also be demonstrable in the urine of patients with virilism, adrenal cortical hyperplasia or tumor, and arrhenoblastoma of the ovary. In these conditions, it is associated with amenorrhea and shows no cyclic pattern.

Androgen Findings.—Where the clinical findings point to ovarian hypofunction, quantitative studies of the androgen content of the urine may give some clue to the degree of ovarian depression (see Chap. XL).

Gonadotropin Findings.—Since the presence of excessive amounts of follicle-stimulating hormone in the blood, as shown by a positive Fluhmann test (see Chap. **XXXIX**), is generally considered a fairly reliable index of primary ovarian failure, this test may be employed to differentiate between primary and secondary ovarian sterility. In the patient with regular periods, urine gonadotropin tests may reveal a midcycle peak, interpreted by some as evidence of ovulation. (For evaluation of this and other methods of detecting ovulation, see Chap. **IV**.)

TREATMENT

It should be emphasized that in sterility, perhaps more than in any other functional disorder, the evaluation of therapy is difficult. The conscientious physician rarely stops with any single measure, but approaches his problem from every possible angle. The possible curative effect of tubal insufflation and curettage, routinely employed as diagnostic procedures in the female partner, further confuses the picture. Moreover, since the success of treatment is hardly ever established before several months or even years have elapsed, one cannot be certain whether the cure in a particular instance was attributable to the form of treatment last used, to previous measures, or a combination of all.

The treatment, in the male as in the female partner, resolves itself into the correction of gametogenic faults and eradication of all obstacles to union of the gametes.

TREATMENT OF THE MALE PARTNER

Obstacles to the deposition of the semen in the female genitalia should be removed where possible. If this is not possible, testicular aspiration and artificial insemination offers a ready solution of the difficulty. Where spermatogenic function is deficient or absent, the problem is much more difficult. The conditions under which such abnormalities may arise and measures available for their correction are discussed in detail elsewhere (see Chap. **XXXVI**).

TREATMENT OF THE FEMALE PARTNER

The varied nature of the etiology makes it necessary to treat each case as an individual problem. Often a multiple therapeutic approach is called for, because the sterility may be traceable to more than one cause. Selection of therapy obviously depends on the apparent causative factors. Needless delay, particularly in older couples, should be avoided lest the underlying cause become aggravated and more resistant to treatment. While simple measures may suffice in some cases, others require intensive and prolonged treatment, for which the close cooperation of the gynecologist, internist, endocrinologist and roentgenologist may be necessary. Conservative measures should always be tried first for a reasonable length of time. Radical methods, such as x-ray treatment and ovarian surgery, which may possibly endanger gonadal function, should be considered as a last resort and only where a definite indication exists.

Correction of Oogenic Faults.—The management of oogenic faults in the female may entail medical, gynecologic, endocrine and x-ray treatment.

Medical Treatment.—Early recognition and correction of potential causes of sterility in young girls may be of inestimable value in reducing the incidence of infertility later in life. The parent and physician should be on the lookout for developmental and menstrual aberrations. A delayed menarche, scanty periods or amenorrhea, poorly developed primary and secondary sex characters, or other endocrinopathic stigmata are danger signals pointing to some disorder which, if neglected, may seriously jeopardize the chances for conception later in life. Of interest is Mujuda and Horie's[40] observation that the rate of sterility increases as the menarche is delayed, and is especially high in women who first menstruate after the seventeenth year.

Existing nonendocrine faults which directly or indirectly depress ovarian function should be eradicated. Since constitutional factors have an important bearing on oogenic function, the patient should be put into the best possible physical condition. Systemic disease, metabolic disturbances, and all other debilitating conditions should be remedied where possible. A healthy regimen should be instituted, particular emphasis being placed on nutrition. The diet should be well balanced and rich in animal proteins, mineral salts and essential vitamins, particularly vitamin E.[41, 42] Measures should be instituted to normalize the patient's weight. In the thin, undernourished woman, a material gain in weight is always desirable, for this may improve the general health and indirectly raise the fertility level. In the obese, especially when amenorrhea is an associated finding, a reduction in weight will often re-establish normal menstrual function and terminate a sterile state (see Chap. XXIV). Undue physical and mental stress should be avoided. Sunlight and fresh air, judicious exercise, proper elimination and adequate rest are important.

Gynecologic Treatment.—Mechanical impediments to normal follicular maturation and ovulation may be eradicated by minor surgery. Aspiration of large retention cysts per vaginam, or their surgical removal is advocated by some gynecologists, on the ground that they interfere with normal follicular maturation and ovulation. The author does not favor these procedures since they cannot correct the underlying cause. Dilatation and curettage may exert a stimulating effect on oogenic function, possibly through nervous pathways leading to the adenohypophysis (see Chap. IV).

Organotherapy.—Endocrine products are recommended as a means of stimulating ovulatory function and promoting growth of a hypoplastic uterus. They are obviously of no avail where the sterile state is due to nonendocrine faults, or in the presence of some impediment to union of the gametes. Where deficient ovulatory function and sterility are associated with menstrual disorders, and both are apparently due to the same basic cause, measures calculated to correct the menstrual anomaly may also help terminate the sterile state. In such cases, the treatment is as outlined for amenorrhea and functional uterine bleeding (see Chaps. XXIV, XXV).

Gonadotropin therapy is advocated for sterility due to ovarian depression, secondary to anterior hypophyseal deficiency. The aim is to induce maturation of follicles, with ovulation and corpus luteum formation. Equine gonadotropin (see Chap. XII) has been hailed by some as effective therapy for inducing ovulation in the human.[29, 30, 43, 44] Their reports have raised the hope that it may be used with good effect in sterility associated with anovulatory cycles. Unfortunately there is no valid evidence that this hormone can induce ovulation in the depressed human ovary. On the contrary, several competent observers[45, 46, 47] could see no evidence of stimulation in women with anovulatory bleeding, amenorrhea, or oogenic sterility. Where a trial of the equine hormone is contemplated, due caution should be exercised to avoid overdosage and the danger of causing follicular cystosis should always be borne in mind. In anovulatory sterility, some recommend a total *dosage* of 1500 to 3500 I.U. per cycle to be given as follows: 500 I.U. intramuscularly on the sixth, eighth and tenth days of the cycle, and 2000 units on the twelfth day. A few observers favor a single large dose of 2000 I.U. 24 to 48 hours before the expected time of ovulation. The timing and dosage may be varied each month. Chorionic gonadotropin is generally conceded to be of no value for inducing ovulation, when given alone.[48] Some observers[49, 50] claim good results in anovulatory sterility with a combination of this hormone and anterior pituitary "synergist," available commercially in the form of *synapoidin*. Their claims await confirmation. Where a trial is made of this therapy, care must be taken to avoid overdosage, which may disrupt the follicular apparatus. The *dose* for which Mazer and Ravetz[49] claim good results is five injections of 1 cc. of synapoidin during the first half of the menstrual cycle. As emphasized by Hartman,[67] the perfect gonadotrope, with which ovulation might be induced in the human ovary, has not yet been prepared.

The *estrogens* are favored by some investigators for sterility due to primary uterine hypoplasia. The *dose* is 10,000 to 100,000 I.U. weekly until appreciable uterine growth has been obtained. Granting that such therapy is effective in increasing the size of the uterus, there is the danger that protracted estrogen treatment in such high dosage may depress the anterior hypophysis, thus indirectly inhibiting ovulatory function.

Thyroid substance is generally conceded to be beneficial in oogenic sterility associated with obesity and a low basal metabolic rate.[51, 52, 53] Many observers believe it is worth a trial even where the basal metabolic rate is normal. The *dose* is ½ to 1 grain three times daily, larger amounts being indicated in the presence of clinical hypothyroidism. The good results obtained with thyroid substance have been variously explained. Some believe it acts by accelerating general metabolism, thus indirectly improving gonadal function, while others believe it may improve a defective germ plasm. Where the basal metabolic rate is elevated, iodine may be of value.

Radiotherapy.—Low dosage *x-ray radiation of the ovary and hypophysis* is held by some[54, 55, 56] to be beneficial in sterility, particularly when associated with amenorrhea (for dosage see Chap. XXV). The mode of action of "stimulating" doses of the x-rays is obscure and attempts at a plausible explanation have thus far been unconvincing. The possibility that such treatment may further depress a hypofunctioning ovary should always be borne in mind. Since it is impossible to predict the ovarian response in a specific instance, radiotherapy should be considered only after all other measures have failed. Close cooperation of the roentgenologist and gynecologist is of the utmost importance. The author is in accord with the view recently expressed by Traut,[57] who states that "this is not a form of therapy which in its present state can be more than very sceptically accepted by a wise profession."

Correction of Obstacles to Union of the Gametes.—Elimination of impediments to union of the germ cells calls for (1) correction of errors in the performance of the sex act; (2) removal of mechanical barriers in the reproductive tract, and (3) restoration of the normal relationship of the reproductive apparatus.

Instruction in Sex Hygiene.—Instruction in sex hygiene, valuable in any case of sterility, is particularly indicated where no apparent cause for the sterility can be found. The couple should be warned against excessive coitus, since this may lower the male potentialities. Under such circumstances, the use of twin beds or separate vacations may be recommended. Infrequent coitus, which may lessen the chances for conception, may be corrected by relieving the couple from undue physical and mental strain, improving the diet, and instituting hygienic measures calculated to correct a depressed libido. If these measures fail, coitus should be limited to the fertile part of the cycle, approximately between the eleventh and sixteenth days (see Chap. IV). Where infrequent coitus is due to dyspareunia, arising from fear or disgust for the sex act, the patient should be reassured as to its normality. In the severe case, psychoanalysis may prove of value.

In *effusion seminis,* loss of the deposited semen may be minimized by emptying the bladder just before coitus, placing a pillow beneath the buttocks to elevate the hips and avoiding post-coital cleansing douches, sometimes used for esthetic purposes without thought of their contraceptive effect.

Patients under treatment should be warned that if a period is missed, especially where the menses were previously regular, they should avoid coitus, undue physical exertion, and purgatives. Under such circumstances, the physician should employ the biologic tests for pregnancy and refrain from pelvic examination, lest he interrupt an existing gestation.

Correction of Vaginal and Cervical Faults.—Minor pelvic surgery may be necessary to correct defects which interfere with reception or retention of the semen, or prevent proper cervical insemination. Mild *developmental anomalies* or acquired faults of the vulva, hymen or vagina, call for plastic surgery. Unfortunately, the more severe anomalies of the external genitalia are frequently associated with imperfections of the internal reproductive organs. Where this is the case, correction of the external defects will obviously be of no avail.

Vaginal surgery may be useful where a widely relaxed or *lacerated vagina* permits undue loss of the deposited semen. *Dyspareunia,* traceable to tender hymenal rests, fissures, or inflammatory lesions of the vulva or vagina, may benefit from sexual rest, hot soothing douches, and analgesic lubricating jellies. An imperforate hymen, tender urethral caruncles, narrow introitus, or large Bartholin's cyst may be corrected by minor surgery. Dyspareunia attributable to chronic pelvic inflammatory disease, adnexal prolapse, or uterine displacements, may be remedied by accepted gynecologic procedures. Plastic surgery and cervical dilatation is indicated for *membranous occlusions of the vagina* or a *stenotic cervical canal.* Undue viscosity of the endocervical secretions, incident to infection or erosion, calls for hot alkaline douches or cauterization of the cervix. A thick mucus plug, often the result of a stenotic cervix, may be remedied by ample dilatation or a small median discission.

Estrogen has been found effective in changing a thick, acid, and impenetrable mucus to one that is less viscous, alkaline, and readily penetrated by the spermatozoa. Guttmacher and Shettles[58] found that 1 mg. of stilbestrol by mouth daily for sixteen days was required for this purpose. As a result of the treatment, however, ovulation was suppressed. This form of therapy is therefore obviously contraindicated. Whether local application of a smaller quantity of estrogen, in the form of a vaginal suppository, would accomplish the same purpose without endangering ovarian function, has not been determined. On the assumption that excessive acidity of the vaginal and cervical secretions is a cause of sterility, some observers[59] advocate the use of alkaline douches, but competent workers, notably Meaker,[2] question their value on the ground that vaginal acidity is not an etiologic factor.

Should these measures fail and the Huhner test remain persistently negative, artificial insemination may be tried. This procedure is harmless provided that aseptic precautions are taken and the seminal fluid is free from bacteria.

Correction of Tubal Faults.—Repeated *tubal insufflation* is often effective in correcting tubal occlusions. According to reliable reports,[60, 61, 62] this procedure alone is followed by pregnancy in 10 to 25 per cent of cases of tubal sterility. The good results may be attributable to dislodgment of inspissated mucus, correction of tortuosities, separation of loose agglutinations of tubal plicae, or breaking up of fine fimbrial adhesions. To guard against the possibility of tubal pregnancy, attempts at conception should be postponed until ample dilatation has been effected. Unless the occlusion is fully relieved, the opening created, though sufficient to permit meeting of the gametes, may be inadequate for passage of the steadily enlarging fertilized ovum in its journey to the uterine cavity. This probably accounts for the tubal pregnancy sometimes seen following insufflation for the correction of tubal agglutinations. Diagnostic curettage and other pelvic manipulations should be avoided for at least two months after insufflation, lest they disturb an early gestation. In the event that a period is missed, a biologic test for pregnancy (see Chap. XXXIX) should precede further local diagnostic or therapeutic measures.

Plastic surgery for the correction of tubal occlusions is generally conceded to be of little value. As pointed out by Greenhill,[63] salpingostomy and tubal implantation are followed by a disproportionately high number of ectopics and other complications, and relatively few live babies are secured by this means. *Tubal surgery* is best adapted for occlusions produced by severe peritubal adhesions incident to postabortal or appendiceal infection, where the mucosa as a rule is unaffected. It is of little value where the occlusion is due to mucosal agglutinations or fimbrial adhesions, for here the mucosa is diseased and the condition tends to recur. In the fimbrial occlusions, the sealed ostium may be opened and gently dilated by means of a hemostat, provided the rest of the tubal lumen is patent. Titus[64] favors the "circumcision cuff" operation for clubbed tubes resulting from perisalpingitis. In cornual occlusions, the closed portion may be excised and the healthy part implanted into the uterus. A technique for this operation developed by Holden[65] is said to give good results. The poor results of salpingostomy are probably due to the fact that it is usually performed in cases of occlusion resulting from inflammatory processes of the mucosa, where the prognosis is generally poor. If plastic surgery is undertaken, it should be followed by repeated tubal insufflation to keep the lumen patent. In conditions necessitating removal of the tubes, implantation of the ovary in the uterine wall, by the modified Estes and Heitmeyer[66] operation, may be entertained.

Dense, capsular adhesions, which mechanically bar exit of the egg from the ovary, may be removed by surgery. Unfortunately, the chronic pelvic inflammatory disease which is usually responsible for such adhesions, may also involve the tubes, and unless the latter can be opened, correction of the ovarian adhesions will be of no avail.

BIBLIOGRAPHY

1. Meaker, S. R., and Vose, S. N.: J.A.M.A. *115*:1426, 1940.
2. Meaker, S. R.: Human Sterility. Baltimore, Williams, Wilkins Co., 1934.
3. Stein, I. F., and Cohen, M.: Am. J. Obst. & Gynec. *38*:465, 1939.
4. Meaker, S. R.: J.A.M.A. *107*:1847, 1936.
5. Laffont, A., and Bourgarel, R.: Bull. Soc. d'obst. & de gynéc. *28*:337, 1939.
6. Grafenberg, E.: Arch. f. Gynäk. *108*:628, 1918.
7. Moench, G. L.: Am. J. Obst. & Gynec. *33*:406, 1936.
8. Laffont, A., and Bourgarel, R.: Bull. Soc. d'obst. et de gynéc. *27*:221, 1938.
9. Moench, G. L.: Am. J. Surg. *47*:586, 1940; ibid. *48*:311, 1940.
10. Vogt, E.: Klin. Wchnschr. *23*:1144, 1922.
11. Schteingart, M., and Ramos, A. G. P.: Prensa méd. Argent. *21*:2087, 1934.
12. Baskin, M. J.: Am. J. Obst. & Gynec. *24*:892, 1932.
13. Gamarra, N., and Schouten, G. B.: Rev. de gynéc. et d'obst. *2*:445, 1939.
14. Henle, G., Church, C. F., and Foster, C.: J. Immunol. *38*:97, 1940.
15. Henle, W., and Henle, G.: J. Immunol. *38*:105, 1940.
16. Belding, D. L.: Am. J. Obst. & Gynec. *27*:25, 1934.
17. Hotchkiss, R. S.: J.A.M.A. *107*:1849, 1936.
18. Hotchkiss, R. S., Brunner, E. K., and Grenley, P.: Am. J. Med. Sci. *196*:362, 1938.
19. Seymour, F. I.: J.A.M.A. *112*:1817, 1939.
20. Charny, C. W., and Meranze, D. R.: Surg., Gynec. & Obst. *74*:836, 1942.
21. Hotchkiss, R. S.: Bull. New York Acad. Med. *18*:600, 1942.
22. Williams, W. W.: Urol. & Cutan. Rev. *43*:587, 1939.
23. McClellan, R. H.: Pennsylvania M. J. *43*:1582, 1940.
24. Koloth, J., and Kleefisch, J.: Arch. f. Gynäk. *133*:70, 1928.
25. Anspach, B. M., and Hoffman, J.: Am. J. Obst. & Gynec. *26*:473, 1934.
26. Jeffcoate, T. N. A.: J. Obst. & Gynec. Brit. Emp. *44*:31, 1937.
27. Novak, E.: Am. J. Obst. & Gynec. *37*:605, 1939.
28. Rock, J., Bartlett, M. K., and Matson, D.: Am. J. Obst. & Gynec. *37*:3, 1939.
29. Siegler, S. L.: Endocrinol. *27*:384, 1940.
30. Griffith, L. S., and McBride, W. P. L.: Am. J. Obst. & Gynec. *43*:1012, 1942.
31. Hühner, M.: Sterility in the Male and Female. New York, Rebman Co., 1913.
32. Krigbaum, R. E.: Am. J. Obst. & Gynec. *34*:1046, 1937

33. Williams, W. W., and Simmons, F. A.: Am. J. Obst. & Gynec. *43*:652, 1942.
34. Kurzrok, R.: Endocrines in Obstetrics and Gynecology. Baltimore, Williams, Wilkins Co., 1937.
35. Lamar, J. K., Shettles, L. B., and Delfs, E.: Am. J. Physiol. *129*:234, 1940.
36. Rubin, I. C.: J.A.M.A. *75*:661, 1920.
37. Krohn, L., Harris, J., and Hechter, O.: Am. J. Obst. & Gynec. *44*:213, 1942.
38. Frank, R. T.: J.A.M.A. *104*:1991, 1935.
39. Venning, E. H., and Browne, J. S. L.: Proc. Soc. Exper. Biol. & Med. *37*:792, 1936.
40. Mujuda, T., and Horie, K.: Jap. J. Obst. & Gynec. *22*:190, 1939.
41. Evans, H. M., and Bishop, K. S.: J. Metab. Research *1*:319, 1922.
42. Shute, E.: J. Obst. & Gynec. Brit. Emp. *44*:121, 1937.
43. Davis, M. E., and Koff, A. K.: Am. J. Obst. & Gynec. *36*:183, 1938.
44. Siegler, S. L., and Fein, M. J.: Am. J. Obst. & Gynec. *38*:1021, 1939.
45. Hamblen, E. C.: Am. J. Surg. *41*:35, 1938.
46. Erving, H. W., Sears, C., and Rock, J.: Am. J. Obst. & Gynec. *40*:695, 1940.
47. Brewer, J. I., Jones, H. O., and Skiles, J. H., Jr.: J.A.M.A. *118*:278, 1942.
48. Report of Council on Pharmacy and Chemistry. J.A.M.A. *114*:487, 1940.
49. Mazer, C., and Ravetz, E.: Am. J. Obst. & Gynec. *41*:474, 1941.
50. Gusman, H., and Goldzieher, M. A.: J. Clin. Endocrinol. *2*:468, 1942.
51. Litzenberg, J. C., and Carey, J. B.: Am. J. Obst. & Gynec. *17*:550, 1929.
52. Anspach, B. M., and Hoffman, J.: Am. J. Obst. & Gynec. *26*:147, 1933.
53. Winkelstein, L. B.: Am. J. Obst. & Gynec. *40*:1, 1940.
54. Kaplan, I. I.: New York State J. Med. *39*:1380, 1939.
55. Rock, J., Bartlett, M. K., Gauld, A. G., and Rutherford, R. N.: Surg., Gynec. & Obst. *70*:903, 1940.
56. Friedman, M., and Finkler, R. S.: Am. J. Obst. & Gynec. *43*:852, 1942.
57. Traut, H. F.: Am. J. Obst. & Gynec. *44*:638, 1942.
58. Guttmacher, A. F., and Shettles, L. B.: Human Fertility *5*:4, 1940.
59. Singleton, J. M., and Hunter, J. L.: Am. J. Obst. & Gynec. *37*:856, 1939.
60. Rubin, I. C.: Am. J. Obst. & Gynec. *24*:561, 1932; ibid. *28*:698, 1934.
61. Mazer, C., and Hoffman, J.: Med. J. & Rec. *129*:90, 1929.
62. Mintz, M. E.: Am. J. Obst. & Gynec. *34*:93, 1937.
63. Greenhill, J. P.: Am. J. Obst. & Gynec. *33*:39, 1937.
64. Titus, P.: Management of Obstetric Difficulties. St. Louis, C. V. Mosby Co., 1937.
65. Holden, F. C., and Sovak, F. W.: Am. J. Obst. & Gynec. *24*:684, 1932.
66. Estes, W. L., Jr., and Heitmeyer, P. L.: Am. J. Surg. *24*:563, 1934.
67. Hartman, C. G.: West. J. Surg. *50*:344, 1942.
68. Greenberg, B. E., Berman, S., Gargill, S. L., and Griffin, R. C.: J. Clin. Endocrinol. *3*: 179, 1943.

CHAPTER XXVIII

SPONTANEOUS AND HABITUAL ABORTION

Incidence.—Spontaneous or habitual abortion, without apparent organic cause, presents one of the most disheartening problems in gynecology. It is estimated that 10 to 20 per cent of all pregnancies terminate prematurely, usually between the second and third month.[1-3] The available estimates are not altogether reliable, since many early abortions probably fail to come to the attention of the physician or are erroneously diagnosed as irregularities of the menstrual flow. Recent advances in reproductive physiology have thrown some light on this evasive problem, and suggest a therapeutic approach which may prove of value in at least some of the cases.

Definition and Nomenclature.—The term *spontaneous abortion* describes expulsion of the fetus at some time before the twenty-eighth week. It is termed *habitual* when it occurs more than once, and *idiopathic* if there is no demonstrable cause.

ETIOLOGY

For a proper understanding of the etiology, it is necessary to review the prerequisites for the successful completion of gestation.

1. The male and female germ cells must be normal, and possess ample vitality to insure development of the fertilized ovum to the age of viability.

2. The endometrium, which forms the fetal bed, must be properly sensitized by the ovarian sex hormones, estrogen and progestin, to insure reception and retention of the egg until placentation occurs.

3. Normal placentation must take place and the placenta must secrete estrogen, progestin and gonadotropic hormones in normal amounts and at the proper time.

4. The uterus must be anatomically and physiologically adapted to accommodate the growing embryo.

5. The myometrium must remain in a relatively quiescent state so that the fetus may remain undisturbed, at least to the point of viability.

Any deviation from normal, in the fetus or its environment, is a potential cause of abortion.

FETAL FAULTS

The available data concerning the role of the fetus in the etiology of spontaneous abortion is limited and vague, due to technical difficulties inherent in a study of the germ plasm. For want of direct evidence, several theories based on the behavior of the developing embryo have been evolved. Inherent defects in the germ plasm, incompatibility of the male

412

and female germ cells, and abnormal activity of the fetal trophoblast have been considered as possible causes.

Defective Germ Plasm.—The observation that embryological abnormalities are frequent findings where abortion has occurred,[4, 5] forms the basis for the theory that an inherent defect in the sperm, ovum, or both may be an etiologic factor. In support of this view, it has been pointed out that in the lower mammal fertilized ova differ considerably in their ability to survive. A certain proportion are blighted before implantation. This phenomenon is so common in certain species that it is considered physiologic. Following implantation, some embryos die while others develop to term. To account for these wide variations, despite exposure to identical maternal influences, it seems reasonable to assume that the blighted ovum has some intrinsic fault which may manifest itself in lowered vitality or an obvious embryologic abnormality, which precludes the successful termination of pregnancy. Conceivably, a diminished capacity for survival may be inherited, or acquired as the result of debilitating states existing in either or both partners during the period of egg or sperm production. It is possible that depressive states which are potent causes of sterility (see Chap. XXVII) may, if less severe, result in the production of gametes which are capable of union but cannot survive to term.

Incompatibility of the Germ Cells.—Incompatibility of the male and female germ cells, according to Henkel,[6] may be responsible for faulty development of the fertilized ovum and abortion. This is based on the observation that women who prematurely abort defective young, may bear normal offspring in a subsequent marriage with another partner. It has been suggested that the explanation of such cases is not incompatibility but low vitality of the gametes. According to this view, the success of the second union is due to the superior vitality of the sperm in the new mate, which compensates for the deficiency in the female partner.

Abnormal Trophoblastic Activity.—Anomalies of the cord, amnion, chorion, or placenta are encountered in a large percentage of abortions.[7, 8] While some of these may be secondary to unfavorable maternal influences, it is likely that many are primary developmental defects.

Inability of the trophoblast to penetrate the nidatory bed and make contact with the maternal circulation, may cause early death of the fertilized ovum by depriving it of adequate nourishment. Undue trophoblastic activity, on the other hand, may erode large blood vessels and cause excessive hemorrhage which may wash away the early products of conception.

MATERNAL FAULTS

Organic or functional abnormalities in the host may prevent nidation or interfere with retention of the developing embryo. The cause may reside in the uterus proper, or elsewhere in the organism.

Uterine Abnormalities.—The uterine mucosa, which constitutes the fetal bed, may be partly or wholly destroyed by disease, destructive neoplasms, excessive curettage, or the intra-uterine application of radium. Tuberculosis, actinomycosis, and postabortal endometritis, particularly following criminal abortion or puerperal infection, may so distort the fetal bed or uterine lumen, as to make nidation or retention of the fertilized ovum unlikely or difficult. Myometrial abnormalities may permit nidation, but often interfere with the normal continuance of gestation. Submucous fibroids, for example, may dislodge the implanted ovum through mechanical pressure or hemorrhage.

Unfavorable extra-uterine influences, of endocrine or nonendocrine origin, may directly injure the fetus or so disturb its nutrition as to make the continuance of pregnancy impossible.

Debilitating Conditions.—Abortion may result from systemic disease, chronic intoxications, metabolic disturbances, or other debilitating conditions. Lues, though very rarely responsible for early abortion, is estimated to be the most common single cause of the late interruption of pregnancy.

Nutritional Deficiencies.—Nutritional deficiency has received special emphasis. This may be the immediate or remote cause of abortion. In this connection, Enneper[9] observed that among ninety-two aborting women, twenty showed a hypogenital constitution, partly inherited and partly due to poor environmental influences during the first World War. Experimental and clinical studies indicate that a deficiency of essential foodstuffs, particularly protein and minerals (iron, phosphorus, calcium) may be an etiologic factor.

Vitamin Deficiency.—Though an ample supply of all the vitamins is conceded to be desirable, there is evidence that some may play a more important part than others. Evans and Bishop[10] observed that pregnant rats on a *vitamin E deficient diet* showed a progressive disturbance in the nutrition of the fetal placenta with maceration and absorption of the fetus in utero. A similar deficiency in nonpregnant animals failed to disturb their general health and vigor, estrus cycles, or ability to conceive. Fetal destruction in vitamin E deficient rats could be prevented by vitamin E therapy, provided it was instituted before the critical phase of implantation. The mechanism of its action is not certain. That a lack of vitamin E depresses luteal function indirectly by way of the anterior hypophysis is suggested by the observation[11] that this gland shows an appreciable loss of luteinizing potency in vitamin E deficient animals. Also significant is the observation of Stahler and his associates[12, 13] that vitamin E administration to such animals augments luteal function and appreciably decreases the amount of progesterone required to elicit a progestational reaction in the uterine mucosa. According to Shute,[14] vitamin E prevents abortion by neutralizing an anti-tryptic substance, similar to or identical with estrogen, which increases the resistance of the blood to invasion of the fetal trophoblast, and thus prevents adequate attachment. He bases this on his observation that the administration of vitamin E to spontaneously aborting women simultaneously decreased this resistance of the blood and caused the symptoms of impending abortion to subside. His theory finds some support in the observation[15] that the chorionic villi of vitamin E deficient rats present degenerative changes identical with those seen in the guinea pig following the administration of large amounts of estrogenic substance. On the other hand, doubt is cast on his hypothesis by the report of Cuthbertson and Drummond[16] that no anti-tryptic activity is demonstrable in the serum of vitamin E deficient rats.

Vitamin C deficiency has likewise received attention as a contributory factor in abortion.[17] Of interest is the observation of Hosemann[18] that in normal pregnant women, the vitamin C content of the placenta increased while that of the circulating blood decreased with advancing gestation. In spontaneously aborting women, on the other hand, the concentration of this substance in both the placenta and blood dropped significantly. The presence of large amounts of vitamin C in the corpus luteum suggests that it may be a precursor of the progestational principle, which is apparently essential for the maintenance of pregnancy, at least in its early stages (see Chap. III). It is noteworthy in this connection that Israel and Meranze[19] found that ascorbic acid (vitamin C) feeding in rabbits produced endometrial modifications similar to, though less marked than those elicited by progesterone. Their findings have recently been questioned by Pratt,[20] who repeated their experiment with negative results.

That *vitamin K* is also essential for normal gestation is indicated by the observation of Moore and his associates[21] that retroplacental hemorrhage and abortion occurred during the late first and early second trimester in rabbits on a diet deficient in this vitamin.

While vitamin deficiency may account for some cases of spontaneous abortion, it is probably not an important etiologic factor in the United States, where the average diet is well balanced and contains adequate amounts of all essential vitamins.

Trauma.—Trauma as a cause of abortion is a matter of considerable importance from the medico-legal standpoint. Some observers maintain that physical injury is of little significance in the etiology and may be blamed for abortion only if it causes rupture of the membranes. In support of this contention, it is pointed out that women may be subjected to the grossest kind of manipulation, including abdominal section and curettage, without interrupting pregnancy. On the other hand, it may be argued that abortion follows trauma too often to be merely coincidental. It seems reasonable to suppose that a causal relationship exists, but that the trauma is not the sole factor involved. Whether it will lead to abortion apparently depends not only on the severity of the physical shock, but also on the stability of the pregnancy in the particular case.

Psychic Factors.—Unfavorable psychic influences may sometimes be responsible for premature expulsion of the fetus, particularly in individuals with an unstable nervous system. The incidence of spontaneous abortion is known to rise under circumstances conducive to psychic upheaval, such as war, flood, fire, or earthquake. Since nutritional and other unfavorable influences which operate at such times may play a part, this evidence is not conclusive. More convincing proof is provided by cases in which bleeding and other symptoms of impending abortion begin shortly after a severe emotional upset. Whether the nervous impulse thus initiated causes abortion directly by inducing expulsive contractions of the uterus, or acts indirectly by passing through the hypothalamus to the hypophysis and thus

27

disturbing the endocrine equilibrium essential for the maintenance of pregnancy, we cannot say.

Endocrine Factors.—An unfavorable hormonal environment probably accounts for some cases of spontaneous abortion. There is ample experimental evidence that the incretory glands are either directly or indirectly concerned with reproductive function and, if disturbed, may unfavorably affect the course of pregnancy. The successful continuance of gestation apparently depends in part at least on a normal balance of estrogen and progestin (see Chap. III). The available evidence indicates that before and during the attachment phase, these hormones are supplied by the ovary, and later chiefly by the placenta (see Chap. VIII). The combined action of estrogen and progestin is essential not only to prepare and maintain the nidatory bed, but also to preserve myometrial quiescence throughout gestation. A significant deviation from normal in the production of either hormone may seriously threaten pregnancy.

Role of Progestin.—Observations in the lower mammal[22, 23] indicate that a progestin deficiency, originating prior to implantation, may be responsible for inadequate preparation of the endometrium. In the event of conception, the fertilized ovum finds the mucosa unsuitable for implantation and its early death and resorption follow. Where progestin deficiency arises after the ovum has successfully embedded itself, the resulting impairment of the fetal bed and increased myometrial activity may lead to death of the embryo and its resorption or abortion depending on the stage of gestation when the deficiency develops. Progestin deficiency, as a cause of spontaneous abortion, has recently been stressed by Browne and associates,[24] on the basis of their studies of pregnanediol excretion in normal pregnancy and spontaneous abortion. These observers found that only relatively small amounts of this degradation product of progestin were demonstrable in the urine during the second and third months of normal gestation. Between the seventieth and ninetieth day, a rise occurred which they believe marks the transfer of progestin production from the ovary to the placenta. In spontaneously aborting women, the rise either failed to occur or was delayed. They therefore concluded that spontaneous abortion, which is especially apt to occur during this transitional period, may be due to a hiatus between the cessation of progestin secretion by the corpus luteum and the assumption of this function by the placenta. This may conceivably arise because the yellow body prematurely ceases to secrete this hormone, or the placenta is late in taking over this function.

Role of Estrogen.—There is evidence that a deficiency or excess of estrogen may be the remote or immediate cause of abortion. A *deficiency* of this hormone may conceivably preclude normal uterine development. Under such conditions, even should conception and nidation occur, the poor uterine musculature and deficient blood supply may be inadequate for the needs of the steadily enlarging embryo. Noteworthy in this connection is Brunner's[2] observation that the incidence of spontaneous abortions in a group of 979 women was over 20 per cent in those under 21 years of age, as compared with 12 per cent in those between 21 and 35. He suggests that the relative immaturity of the adolescent group, which makes for a limited number of conceptions (see Chap. XXIII), probably also accounts for the high incidence of abortions. Women with *uterine hypoplasia* frequently abort several times before successfully carrying to term. It is likely that the vascularizing and growth-promoting effect of the large quantities of estrogen produced during each abortive pregnancy develop the uterus to the point where it can retain the fetus to term.

Persistent follicular activity with a consequent *excess of estrogen*, arising prior to conception, may endanger a subsequent pregnancy by inducing hyperplastic modifications of the endometrium. Though follicular rupture usually does not occur in such cases (see Chap. XXV), chance ovulation may sometimes take place. Should conception follow while the endometrium is still hyperplastic, proper nidation may be precluded because the hyperplastic mucosa is relatively refractory to the action of the luteal hormone and may therefore be only partially converted to the pregravid phase (see Chap. XXV). Under these conditions, the hyperplastic, glycogen-poor, infarcted endometrium, with its tendency to repeated hemorrhages, offers a poor nidatory bed for the reception and retention of the ovum. Where the major part of the hyperplastic mucosa has been shed and all but a few local areas have been converted to the pregravid phase, the fertilized ovum may successfully attach itself to a normal portion of the endometrium, but under such conditions, the early products of conception may sooner or later be undermined or washed away by hemorrhages from the hyperplastic areas.

The observation[25] that some cases of inevitable abortion may be associated with excessive quantities of estrogen in the body fluids suggests that an estrogen excess may be an etiologic factor. This may conceivably lead to interruption of pregnancy by disturbing the fetal bed and increasing the motility of the uterine musculature. According to Shute,[14] an excess of this hormone, arising before implantation, may prevent embedding of the ovum by increasing the maternal resistance to the invasion of the fetal trophoblast. Assuming that the excessive amounts of estrogen observed in some aborting women are causally related to the symptoms, this explanation may hardly be considered adequate so long as the cause of the excess remains obscure.

Role of the Anterior Hypophysis.—That the anterior hypophysis is essential for the maintenance of pregnancy, at least in its early stages, is suggested by the observation that in some species, hypophysectomy is followed by regression of the corpora lutea and abortion, no matter when it is performed.[26] In others, it may have this effect only if performed during the early part of gestation.[27] Whether this signifies that the hypophyseal hormones cease to be essential for the continuance of gestation at this time, or that their production is taken over by the placenta, is not certain. The assumption that the anterior hypophysis is an indispensable source of gonadotropin, at least until placentation is complete, is apparently contradicted by the observation that little or no gonadotropin is detectable in the hypophysis during pregnancy.[28] According to some observers, the chorion is the source of the gonadotropins which appear in abundance in the body fluids almost immediately after implantation. Others believe the adenohypophysis produces these substances until the placenta takes over, but that they cannot be demonstrated in the gland because of their rapid discharge into the circulation.

The function of the *gonadotropes* produced during gestation is not established. Browne and associates,[24] on the basis of estrogen, pregnanediol, and gonadotropic hormone studies of the body fluids in normal pregnancy and spontaneous abortion, concluded that the gonadotropes are essential for the maintenance of pregnancy. They found that normally these substances are excreted in large amounts during early gestation, reaching a peak between the twentieth and fiftieth day. After this, the concentration gradually decreases and is maintained at a relatively low level until the end of gestation. In early spontaneous abortion they obtained low gonadotropin levels, while in late abortion, normal gonadotropin values were associated with low estrogen and pregnanediol levels. They suggest that the gonadotropes secreted by the placenta during early gestation maintain the corpus luteum. After the placenta assumes the task of estrogen and progestin production, the excretion of the gonadotropes drops, either because less is produced or more is utilized for the purpose of stimulating the placenta to secrete estrogen and progestin. Early abortion, they suggest, may be due to a defective placenta incapable of producing sufficient gonadotropin to maintain the corpus luteum. Late abortion, on the other hand, may occur despite the presence of normal amounts of gonadotropin and is probably due to failure of the placenta to secrete adequate amounts of estrogen and progestin.

Role of the Thyroid Gland.—Clinical and experimental evidence suggests that disturbances in thyroid function may be a cause of abortion. A tendency to abortion is frequently encountered in women with a low basal metabolic rate and other signs of thyroid deficiency.[29, 30] Hyperthyroidism, experimentally induced by thyroid feeding, and hypothyroidism following partial or total ablation of the gland in the pregnant animal often leads to premature fetal expulsion. According to Hunt and associates,[31] hypothyroidism leads to cholesteremia and the appearance of marked infarcts in the placenta, which they attribute to endarteritis possibly caused by the high cholesterol content of the blood. Thyroid substance is often efficacious in the treatment of habitual abortion. Some believe it supplies a deficiency and thus helps to re-establish a normal metabolic and hormonal environment. Others maintain that it improves the germ plasm. More recently, it has been suggested that thyroid substance decreases uterine irritability by increasing the elimination of the motility promoting hormone, estrogen,[32] or by neutralizing an excess of the posterior lobe hormones. Of particular significance in the etiology of idiopathic abortion are the mild or frustrated forms of thyroid disease, which may be overlooked because of the absence of definite stigmata.

Other members of the endocrine system, though less conspicuously implicated in the maintenance of gestation, should not be overlooked as possible factors in the etiology. Since the adrenals, parathyroids, and pancreas are intimately concerned with metabolic activity, disturbances of their function may cause metabolic disorders which may interfere with the normal continuance of pregnancy. Mild forms of endocrine disturbance are most likely to operate in such cases, for severe endocrinopathic disease is more apt to depress ovarian function so profoundly as to preclude conception.

TREATMENT

The treatment of idiopathic abortion is often extremely discouraging. In some patients, one or more abortions may be followed by a normal pregnancy without any treatment whatsoever, while in others every known aid may be of no avail. Recent emphasis on endocrine factors, and the increased availability of potent sex hormones has aroused new hope that something may be done for such stubborn cases.

PRECONCEPTIONAL TREATMENT

The best results obviously may be expected where therapy is instituted prior to conception, for then all necessary local measures may be employed without fear of disturbing an existing pregnancy. Moreover, it may be possible to correct or remove potential causes of a weak or defective germ plasm before union takes place and it is too late.

General Health.—Since the health of the partners may be reflected in the vitality of the germ cell, both should be put into the best possible physical condition. Besides eradicating systemic disease, syphilis and other depressive states, a healthy regimen should be prescribed, with particular emphasis on a well balanced vitamin-rich diet, particularly vitamin E. Contraception should be advised for a few months, until appreciable improvement is achieved.

Correction of Genital Anomalies.—Faults in the reproductive tract, which may disturb a future pregnancy, should be removed or corrected. Curettage is valuable, for it may at once disclose and remove a hyperplastic mucosa or some other endometrial anomaly likely to disturb the fetal bed, should conception occur. Malpositions, submucous myomata, and other anatomical defects of the genital organs which may interfere with retention of the implanted ovum, should be corrected by accepted gynecologic methods. Menstrual irregularities should receive appropriate treatment (see Chaps. XXIV, XXV) and seminal faults should receive the attention of a competent urologist.

Organotherapy.—*Thyroid substance* is indicated in both partners, particularly when the basal metabolic rate is low or the case clinically suggests thyroid hypofunction. The *dosage* varies with the degree of thyroid depression. Where the rate is only slightly lowered, ½ grain of thyroid substance, three times a day, may suffice; but the severe case may require as much as 3 to 8 grains daily, depending on the patient's tolerance. It may supplement dietary measures, where obesity is an associated finding, even though the metabolic rate is normal, but is contraindicated in thin individuals or those subject to nervous instability.

The *estrogens* have been recommended for habitual abortion associated with uterine hypoplasia. To develop the uterus, some observers recommend a total dosage of 1,000,000 international units, in five divided doses during the first two weeks of the cycle, to be repeated until sufficient growth is achieved.[33] While an increase in the size of the uterus has been observed following such therapy, its use would seem undesirable in view of evidence that large doses may depress ovarian function by inhibiting the hypophysis. A physiologic and far more effective method of developing a hypoplastic uterus is through repeated pregnancies. The cumulative effect of the hormonal stimuli brought to bear in each succeeding abortive gestation may eventually bring the uterus to the point where it can successfully carry an embryo to term.

Progesterone or *pregneninolone* may be tried as a preconceptional measure where premenstrual curettage reveals only mild secretory changes, suggesting a deficiency of this hormone. The *dose* is 1 to 5 I.U. of progesterone intramuscularly twice weekly, or 10 mg. of pregneninolone by mouth daily, during the second half of the cycle.

POSTCONCEPTIONAL TREATMENT

General Medical Measures.—Avoidance of unfavorable influences is far more important than the institution of positive therapy. When a period is missed and pregnancy suspected, the biologic tests should be employed and pelvic examination absolutely avoided lest it stimulate an irritable uterus. The patient should be emphatically cautioned against coitus, undue physical exertion, and use of purgatives. To avoid constipation and straining at the stool, the diet should be bland, and mineral oil or enemas may be advised. These precautions are indicated during the early stages of gestation and especially at the time when the menses would normally occur. At such times, it may be desirable to order the patient to bed for a few days and resort to mild sedatives.

Nutritional Measures.—General hygienic measures and the correction of nutritional faults is of the utmost importance. A diet rich in calcium, iron and vitamins, particularly D,[34] E,[35] C and K, should be prescribed. According to Singleton,[36] vitamin K inhibits decidual hemorrhage in threatened abortion. The *dosage for vitamin E* is not established. Some recommend 3 mg. of the synthetic product per os daily, beginning as soon as the diagnosis of pregnancy is made and continued to the thirty-second week of gestation. The value of vitamin E therapy cannot be decided from the available clinical evidence because it is rarely the sole measure employed.

Organotherapy.—*Thyroid Substance.*—Authorities are unanimous in their opinion of the value of thyroid therapy in habitually aborting women who show evidence of thyroid deficiency.[29, 37] The administration of thyroid substance is indicated where the basal metabolic rate is low at the outset, or fails to show the usual rise with advancing gestation.

Progesterone.—Progesterone and pregneninolone, the orally active progestogen, have found increasing favor during the past few years.[38-42] These substances are used by some observers on the assumption that some cases of spontaneous abortion are due to a deficiency of the progestational principle. Others employ them because of their supposed ability to inhibit uterine motility. The *value* of this form of therapy is not yet established. In a recent communication,[43] the Council on Pharmacy and Chemistry of the American Medical Association announced its conclusion that there is still no adequate evidence that progesterone therapy is of value in any of the clinical conditions for which it has been recommended. As Browne and his associates[24] have pointed out, evaluation of progesterone therapy is difficult because in most cases the pregnancy is abnormal, or the fetus is dead when symptoms first appear. Moreover, it is difficult to ascertain in what percentage of the cases the fetus would have survived without the aid of progesterone. Difficulty also arises from the fact that the conscientious physician employs other measures, such as bed rest and mild sedation, which are known to be adequate in many cases of threatened abortion.

Many clinicians employ progesterone, despite the absence of convincing proof of its efficacy, because of their desire to leave no stone unturned in their effort to prevent abortion. This attitude is justifiable provided that they can be certain no harm will result from its use. Hamblen[44] warns that large doses may hinder the intrinsic metabolism of progesterone, on the basis of his observation that the pregnanediol level may fall during progesterone therapy. The objection has been raised that such treatment may prevent abortion of a pathologic ovum. Though abnormalities have been encountered in the young of mothers carried to term on progesterone therapy,[45] there is as yet no proof that the incidence of such cases is greater than where progesterone is omitted. The value of this hormone has also been questioned on the ground that its ability to quiet the human uterus is not established. The confused state of the evidence on this point is apparent in the fact that some report inhibition, others stimulation, or no effect whatsoever. These divergent findings are probably due to technical difficulties involved in determining the response of the human uterus in vivo (see Chap. VI). In view of the fact that, in nature, the presence of a functioning corpus luteum and production of progestin by the placenta (see Chap. VIII) is compatible with relative myometrial quiescence, the suggestion that this hormone may stimulate expulsive uterine contractions seems questionable. Several observers[46, 47, 48] have reported that patients receiving progesterone during the proliferative phase of the cycle may experience cramping in the lower abdomen. This is apparently not due to increased uterine motility, for it occurs in the absence of any appreciable change in the movements of the uterus.[46] The explanation of this phenomenon is not clear. It is noteworthy that no cramping is felt if the hormone is given during the luteal phase, when endogenous progestin is present. That a similar immunity exists during pregnancy is suggested by the absence of reports of cramping during progesterone therapy in pregnant women with a history of habitual abortion.

It is obvious that further critical investigation is necessary before the advantages and disadvantages of progesterone therapy can be clearly defined. If used at all, it should be reserved for cases where the pregnanediol

level is subnormal. Repeated pregnanediol determinations during the course
of therapy may be of value in determining whether it should be continued.
A further drop in the pregnanediol level may signify that the dose is excessive[44] or that the defect in the particular case is beyond the power of
progesterone to control. On the other hand, a rise to normal values suggests
that the therapy is appropriate and adequate, or at least is doing no harm.

Opinion as to the *optimal dose* is still in a state of flux. In the earlier
trials with such therapy, small doses ranging from 0.5 to 5.0 mg. by injection two to three times weekly, were recommended as a prophylactic
measure in patients with a history of habitual abortion. The recent trend
has been toward larger doses. Browne and associates[24] recommend 5 mg.
daily. Larger doses are usually prescribed during the time when the menses
would otherwise be expected. Reports of the use of orally active *pregneninolone* are still limited. This compound is estimated to be from one-sixth
to one-tenth as effective by mouth as an equal weight of progesterone by
intramuscular injection. Krohn and Harris[49] employ 10 mg. twice weekly
as a prophylactic measure, while Soule[50] prescribes 10 to 30 mg. daily
for this purpose. In view of reports[51] that this substance may have toxic
effects, it should be used with caution.

Gonadotropic Hormone.—Chorionic gonadotropin, in doses of 100 to
200 I.U., two to three times a week during the first four to five months,
has been employed to a limited extent[52, 53, 54] in cases where the gonadotropic hormone level is low. The clinical evidence at hand is hardly adequate to establish the efficacy of such therapy.

TREATMENT OF IMPENDING ABORTION

With the onset of prodromal symptoms, such as backache, cramps,
and spotting, complete rest in bed, with no bathroom privileges, should
be ordered and continued for at least two weeks after all symptoms subside. Pelvic examination is definitely contraindicated, since it may convert
a threatened abortion into an inevitable one. Though some observers ad-
vise against the use of *morphine* and its derivatives, on the ground that
it stimulates uterine contractions,[53] the author's experience with this drug
has been entirely satisfactory. Morphine sulphate gr. 1/4, with or without
atropine gr. 1/150, should be administered and supplemented where necessary by an opium suppository. A capsule, containing codeine sulphate gr.
½, phenobarbital gr. ½ and atropine sulphate gr. ⅟₁₅₀, t.i.d., is often effective. Some observers employ *progesterone* as a physiologic anti-spasmodic,
in doses of 5 to 10 mg. daily until the symptoms subside. After this, 5 mg.
are given twice weekly until the normal continuance of pregnancy is no
longer in doubt. Others warn against the use of this hormone on the ground
that it appears to aggravate the symptoms in some cases. Whether this
was due to the hormone or merely coincidental is difficult to decide. Should
the symptoms persist despite these measures, evacuation of the uterus
should not be undertaken until death of the fetus is established. Persistence of the bleeding is not conclusive proof of fetal death, for pregnancy

may often continue to a successful conclusion despite protracted bleeding. For this reason, unless the hemorrhage is so profuse as to threaten the health of the patient, conservative treatment may be continued for a period of weeks. The viability of the fetus may be ascertained by following the estrogen or gonadotropin level of the blood and urine (see Chap. XXXIX).

BIBLIOGRAPHY

1. Taussig, E. J.: Abortion. St. Louis, C. V. Mosby Co., 1936.
2. Brunner, E. K.: Human Biol. *13*:159, 1941.
3. Stander, H. J.: Am. J. Obst. & Gynec. *44*:531, 1942.
4. Hertig, A. T., and Edmonds, E. W.: Arch. Path. *30*:260, 1940.
5. Schultze, K. W.: Zentralbl. f. Gynäk. *65*:161, 1941.
6. Henkel, M.: Gynaekologische Diagnostik. Berlin, S. Karger, 1905.
7. Bayer, R.: Geburtsh. u. Frauenh. *2*:641, 1940.
8. O'Connor, F. E., and Taylor, J. S.: Am. J. Obst. & Gynec. *38*:693, 1939.
9. Enneper, F.: Monatschr. f. Geburtsh. u. Gynäk. *105*:347, 1937.
10. Evans, H. M., and Bishop, K. S.: J. Metab. Research *1*:319, 1922.
11. Rowlands, I. W., and Singer, E.: J. Physiol. *86*:323, 1936.
12. Stähler, F., and Kaiser, W.: Arch. f. Gynäk. *171*:118, 1941.
13. Stähler, F., and Pehl, B.: Arch. f. Gynäk. *171*:134, 1941.
14. Shute, E.: J. Obst. & Gynec. Brit. Emp. *42*:1071, 1935.
15. Urner, J. A.: Tr. Sect. Obst., Gynec. & Abdom. Surg. A. M. A. 1930, p. 34.
16. Cuthbertson, W. F. J., and Drummond, J. C.: Biochem. J. *33*:1621, 1939.
17. Rodecurt, M.: Deutsche med. Wchnschr. *62*:1880, 1936.
18. Hosemann, H.: Zentralbl. f. Gynäk. *63*:1784, 1838, 1939.
19. Israel, S. L., and Meranze, D. R.: Endocrinol. *29*:210, 1941.
20. Pratt, P. C.: Endocrinol. *32*:92, 1943.
21. Moore, R. A., Bittenger, I., Miller, M. L., and Hellman, L. M.: Am. J. Obst. & Gynec. *44*:1007, 1942.
22. Corner, G. W., and Allen, W. M.: Am. J. Physiol. *88*:326, 1929.
23. Weichert, C. K.: Proc. Soc. Exper. Biol. & Med. *25*:490, 1928.
24. Browne, J. S. L., Henry, J. S., and Venning, E. H.: Am. J. Obst. & Gynec. *38*:927, 1939.
25. Jeffcoate, T. N. A.: J. Obst. & Gynec. Brit. Emp. *39*:67, 1932.
26. McPhail, M. K.: Proc. Roy. Soc. London, s.B. *117*:34, 1935.
27. Pencharz, R. I., and Lyon, W. R.: Proc. Soc. Exper. Biol. & Med. *31*:1131, 1934.
28. Philipp, E.: Zentralbl. f. Gynäk. *54*:15, 1932.
29. Litzenberg, J. C.: Tr. Am. A. Obst., Gynec. & Abdom. Surg. *41*:159, 1938.
30. King, E. L., and Herring, J. S.: J.A.M.A. *113*:1300, 1939.
31. Hunt and associates, cited in discussion of King and Herring (*supra* 30).
32. Van Horn, H. W.: Anat. Rec. *51* (Supp.) : 38, 1941.
33. Clauberg, C.: Deutsche med. Wchnschr. *63*:307, 1937.
34. Weysser, C.: Deutsche med. Wchnschr. *63*:307, 1937.
35. Lubin, S., and Waltman, R.: Am. J. Obst. & Gynec. *41*:960, 1941.
36. Singleton, J. M., discussion of Campbell and Sevringhaus (*infra* 38).
37. Bloss, J. R.: South. M. J. *30*:637, 1937.
38. Campbell, R. E., and Sevringhaus, E. L.: Am. J. Obst. & Gynec. *39*:573, 1940.
39. Wenner, R.: Schweiz. med. Wchnschr. *71*:873, 1941.
40. Falls, F. H., Rezek, G. H., and Benensohn, S. J.: Surg., Gynec. & Obst. *75*:289, 1942.
41. Mason, L. W.: Am. J. Obst. & Gynec. *44*:630, 1942.
42. Davis, C. D., Hamblen, E. C., Cuyler, W. K., and Baptist, M.: J. Clin. Endocrinol. *2*: 377, 1942.
43. Council on Pharmacy and Chemistry A. M. A.: J.A.M.A. *118*:1216, 1942.
44. Hamblen, E. C.: Am. J. Obst. & Gynec. *32*:110, 1936.
45. Kane, H. F.: Am. J. Obst. & Gynec. *32*:110, 1936.

46. Kurzrok, R., Wiesbader, H., Mulinos, M. G., and Watson, B. P.: Endocrinol. *21*:335, 1937.
47. Hamblen, E. C., Cuyler, W. K., Pattee, C. J., and Axelson, G. J.: J. Clin. Endocrinol. *1*:211, 1941.
48. Gillman, J.: J. Clin. Endocrinol. *2*:157, 1942.
49. Krohn, L., and Harris, J. M.: Am. J. Obst. & Gynec. *41*:95, 1941.
50. Soule, S. D.: Am. J. Obst. & Gynec. *44*:1009, 1942.
51. Cohen, M. R., and Stein, I. F.: Am. J. Obst. & Gynec. *40*:713, 1940.
52. Johnstone, R. W., Wiesner, B. P., and Marshall, P. G.: Lancet *2*:509, 1932.
53. Young, J.: Brit. Med. J. *1*:953, 1937.
54. Frazier, W. R.: Northwest Med. *37*:324, 1938.
55. Falls, F. H., Lackner, J. E., and Krohn, L.: J.A.M.A. *106*:271, 1936.

CHAPTER XXIX

THE CLIMACTERIC

Termination of the reproductive period is often associated with a general upheaval involving every system of the body. This transitional period of life, which normally extends through the fifth decade, represents the acme of endocrine and nervous instability. The organism at this time may become so highly sensitized that the slightest stimulus is likely to provoke troublesome subjective manifestations. The multiplicity of the complaints, absence of demonstrable pathology, and unequal response to therapy, often bewilder the physician. Fortunately, recent advances in the field of endocrinology have done much to dispel this confusion and put the treatment on a sounder basis.

Definition.—The terms *menopause* and *climacteric* are often used interchangeably, but though the phenomena they describe are usually synchronous, they are by no means synonymous. "Menopause" literally denotes cessation of menstrual function, while "climacteric" describes a transitional phase of which the extinction of menstrual function is but one manifestation.[1]

SYMPTOMATOLOGY

Incidence.—The climacteric may be symptom-free, or be attended by a long train of diversified complaints of varying intensity, which may persist for months or years. Estimates of the incidence of symptoms vary widely, due probably to differences of opinion as to what manifestations are causally related to the physiologic changes incident to this epoch. An analysis of 1000 menopausal women by the Council of the Medical Women's Federation in England[2] revealed troublesome manifestations in 84.2 per cent. In only 10 per cent were the symptoms incapacitating.

SEXUAL SYMPTOMATOLOGY

Menstrual Function.—The end of the reproductive period is heralded by a disturbance of ovulatory function and the menstrual rhythm. The transition from normal menstrual function to complete amenorrhea may occupy a period of months or years. In the majority of cases, loss of menstrual function is gradual: the intervals become longer, the flow more scanty until it ceases altogether. In some women, the flow may become irregular, excessive, or prolonged, before complete amenorrhea is established. Less often, the previously regular periods cease abruptly and remain absent thereafter.

Ovulation.—Ovulation is either abruptly suppressed or occurs at longer intervals until it ceases completely. Some women show a temporary spurt of ovulatory activity, so that two or more eggs mature and are extruded

425

at the same time. This may explain why some women conceive for the first time just before the menopause.[3]

Genital Structural Changes.—Structural alterations of the *ovarian capsule and parenchyma* are apparent during this epoch. Due to an increase in fibrous connective tissue, the tunica albuginea becomes thickened and fibrotic, constituting an effective barrier to ovulation. Failing rupture, the maturing follicles undergo atresia or form cysts of varying size. The granulosa, and later the theca interna are gradually absorbed and replaced by fibrous connective tissue. These regressive changes are reflected in the müllerian apparatus. During the earlier stages of this period, when

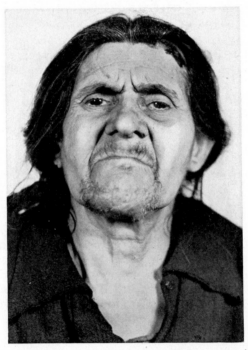

Fig. 91.—Hirsutism in a postmenopausal woman, aged fifty-two, excreting up to 85 I.U. of androgen daily.

the successive crops of unruptured cystic or atretic follicles continuously elaborate estrogen, the chronically stimulated *uterus* may become symmetrically enlarged and the endometrium hyperplastic. As follicular activity gradually ceases, estrogen is no longer produced and regressive changes become apparent in the uterine mucosa, myometrium and blood vessels. Involutionary modifications also appear in the *tubes, vagina, external genitalia,* and other structures dependent on the ovarian sex hormones. Recent studies[4-7] indicate that atrophy of the accessory genitalia may be postponed, despite the extinction of ovarian function, because of the presence of estrogenic substances derived from some extra-ovarian source, probably the adrenal cortex. Frank and his associates detected appreciable amounts of estrogenic substance in the urine of castrate[4, 5] and menopausal women.[6] Novak and Richardson[7] found that less than half of a group of postmenopausal women presented atrophic endometria. In the rest of the series, varying degrees of proliferative activity were observed.

Retrogression of Secondary Sex Characters.—The secondary sex characters likewise undergo varying degrees of retrogression. The epithelial elements of the *breast* are gradually replaced by fibrous tissue. In the thin individual, this is associated with loss of adipose tissue and shrinkage of the gland. In the obese subject, the regressive process is often masked by a marked increase in fat. The characteristic *feminine fat distribution* is altered. The fat pads in some women disappear early and the body reverts to the neuter or male type. In others, there is a rapid and marked accumulation of adipose tissue, particularly about the lower girdle and abdomen. The *hair* may change in quality, quantity, and distribution. Loss of pubic and axillary hair is not uncommon. In women with heterosexual tendencies, hair growth may be exaggerated to the point of beard and mustache formation, while some who were previously free from hirsutism, may show the male type of hair distribution for the first time. The *libido* may remain unaltered, diminish, or actually increase despite the loss of ovarian function. Occasionally homosexual tendencies are encountered.

NONSEXUAL SYMPTOMATOLOGY

Nonsexual manifestations usually appear with or soon after the cessation of menstrual function, but not infrequently, they may precede or follow it by several months or years.

Circulatory Symptoms.—The phenomenon known as the *hot flush* is the most constant and characteristic manifestation of the climacteric. During a seizure, the patient experiences a sudden wave of heat to the head and neck, and the face becomes intensely flushed. This is soon followed by a profuse sweat, pallor and a cold shivering sensation. These paroxysms are often accompanied by a sense of weakness, anguish, oppression, vertigo, and occasionally nausea and vomiting. The attack may last from a few seconds to several minutes. In the mild case, the flushes and sweats are infrequent and occur only as the result of undue excitement, but in the more severe forms, they recur at very short intervals both day and night. The seizures may precede, accompany, or follow the extinction of menstrual function, and may persist longer than any other climacteric symptom.

Alterations in the *cardiac rhythm* and *blood pressure* are common. Cardiac arrhythmias, such as simple or paroxysmal tachycardia and bradycardia, without any apparent anatomic basis, may occur alone or with other vasomotor phenomena. The irregularities may be mild, or so severe as to profoundly concern both patient and physician. The blood pressure frequently shows marked instability and variability. It may change from time to time and is often affected by muscular effort, emotion, or digestion, differing in this respect from hypertension due to cardiovascular-renal disease.

Paroxysms of pain over small and large arteries and veins are early and frequent complaints. These so-called *vasalgias* are apparently the result of vascular spasm elicited by stimuli which affect the vasomotor mechanism of the blood vessels. When the aorta or femorals are implicated, the pain may mimic angina pectoris or intermittent claudication, while splanchnic involvement may simulate the pain of a surgical abdomen.

Nervous and Psychic Manifestations.—Among the more frequent and troublesome climacteric symptoms are the neuralgias, anesthesias, paresthesias, and hyperesthesias of the skin and mucous membranes, painful sensations of the muscles, joints and bones, spasm of the sphincters, general and local pruritus, formications, insomnia, somnolence, sensorial and other nervous phenomena. *Joint pains* affecting the legs, arms, shoulders, sacral and lumbar regions, without anatomic alteration or interference with mobility, are of interest especially in the differential diagnosis. The *paresthesias* and *hyperesthesias* may be of a local or general nature. The local forms may involve any part of the body, though most frequently confined to the extremities, particularly the fingers and toes. In the extreme case, the slightest pressure, such as that exerted by the weight of the bed covers, may elicit painful sensations. Local and general *itching* of the skin and mucous membranes, particularly the vulva, vagina, rectum, hands, soles of the feet and scalp, is common. Scratching often leads to skin infections so prevalent at this time.

Headaches may appear for the first time, or be exaggerated with the onset of the climacteric. They are sometimes associated with a transient elevation of the blood pressure, vertigo, nausea, and occasionally vomiting. Some women complain of an indurated form of headache, characterized by painful swelling of the cranial points at the insertion of the muscles at the nape of the neck.

Vertigo may occur alone or with hot flushes, and is apt to appear on waking or after a sudden shift of position. It is often accompanied by visual disturbances, tachycardia, nausea, and buzzing in the ears. The attack may be mild, causing merely a feeling of uncertainty on walking or climbing stairs, or so severe that it throws the patient off balance.

Insomnia is a common climacteric complaint. The patient may have difficulty in falling asleep, or be awakened during the early hours of the morning. This is often provoked by formication, pruritus and hyperesthesia, which tend to become exaggerated at night. Restless nights and lack of sleep are probably at least partly responsible for the nervous exhaustion and hyperirritability of the climacteric woman.

Nervous fatigue is a prominent manifestation and is often accompanied by mental depression, melancholy and sensorial disturbances. Psychic manifestations, such as crying spells, mental depression (*involutionary melancholia*), and impaired memory are typical expressions of the critical epoch. Though often mild and self-limited, they may sometimes be so severe as to culminate in some form of functional psychosis. The severe forms are usually encountered in individuals with a previous tendency to psychic instability. As Young[8] has rightly emphasized, it is important to distinguish between nervousness due to the vegetative changes associated with the menopause, and pre-existing psychoneuroses which are exacerbated at this time.

Metabolic and Digestive Disturbances.—Alterations in fat and carbohydrate metabolism, often manifested in alimentary glycosuria, fatty stools, pancreatic diarrhea, diabetes mellitus, and obesity, are part of the climacteric symptom-complex. Loss of appetite or perversion of taste, intestinal colic, obstinate constipation, diarrhea and other gastro-intestinal disturbances are common. The diarrhea is of a serous nature, is unassociated with any apparent anatomic alterations, and seems wholly independent of the type of food ingested. It may appear at approximately four week intervals, or be precipitated by nervous or psychic stress, and often affects women previously subject to constipation. Abnormal gaseous formation, apparently unrelated to the food intake, may give rise to a sense of abdominal fullness, flatulence, dyspepsia, meteorism and eructations. This may be accompanied by colicky pain referable to the stomach and large intestines, and often presents a problem in differential diagnosis. In some women, the gaseous distention may be so marked that the resulting pressure on the diaphragm embarrasses respiration. Pharyngeal and esophageal spasm may cause difficulties in swallowing and arouse much concern. These digestive manifestations are usually encountered in individuals with an unstable nervous system. The absence of demonstrable lesions and their spontaneous disappearance at the end of the climacteric point to their functional nature.

Skin Changes.—Pigmentation, dermatosis, papilloma, fibroma, hemangioma, xanthoma, scleroderma and myxedema are not uncommon. Localized edema, acne rosacea, and urticaria are among the more common skin diseases that trouble the climacteric woman. Circumscribed or diffuse edemas of a transitory nature may appear in some cases.[9] The former may affect the face or, less often, the mucous membranes and cutaneous tissue of the limbs. The diffuse form may involve the hands, lower part of the arms, and occasionally the legs below the knees. The cutaneous swellings may appear and disappear many times during the day, and are usually associated with psychoneural and vasomotor phenomena.

ETIOLOGY

Though the initiation and maintenance of *sexual function* depends on the anterior pituitary sex hormones, regression of the ovary at the end of reproductive life cannot be attributed to a diminishing supply of these hormones, for the gonadotropic hormone content of the hypophysis[10, 11] and body fluids[12, 13, 14] is increased at this time (see Chap. XII). That it is due to progressive refractoriness of the ovaries to pituitary stimulation is suggested by the observation[15] that gonadotropic substances, which elicit a response in the younger individual, are without effect in the climacteric woman, even when administered in large doses. It would thus appear that the extinction of ovarian function is a local expression of the general regression which heralds the approach of senility, and is in large part determined by genetic and somatic factors beyond the control of the hypophysis.

Regression of the accessory genitalia and secondary sex characters, though largely due to the decline in estrogen and progestin production, is probably also partly the result of somatic influences, independent of the ovarian sex hormones. This is suggested by the fact that the atrophy of the müllerian organs is much more marked in the menopausal woman than in the young castrate. It is also significant that estrogen, in amounts sufficient to induce proliferative activity and withdrawal bleeding in the uterus of the young castrate, may fail to produce this effect in the menopausal woman.[16] The situation is apparently the reverse of what occurs at puberty, when the accessory genitalia show a progressive increase in their reactivity to the gonadal sex hormones.[17]

The mechanism involved in the production of the *nonsexual manifestations* of the climacteric is still obscure. The view that withdrawal of the ovarian secretions is at least partly responsible, particularly for the flushings encountered during this epoch, is based on the fact that extinction of gonadal function is a constant occurrence at this period of life, and that similar symptoms often follow the suppression of ovarian function by surgery or radiation in young women. How a decline in ovarian sex hormone production leads to disturbances in systems outside the sexual sphere, or why the manifestations are severe in some women and mild or absent in others, has not yet been satisfactorily explained. Nor is there yet a satisfactory explanation of the fact that some women may experience symptoms many months or even years before or after menstrual function ceases. Some light has been thrown on these problems by recent studies demonstrating a close functional relationship between the ovary and other incretory glands, and also between the endocrine and vegetative nervous systems (see Chap. XV). The evidence at hand strongly suggests that ovarian regression may help to precipitate the climacteric symptom-complex, but is by no means the sole factor involved.

The Ovary in the Climacteric.—Zondek[18] first called attention to the fact that the transition from full ovarian function to its complete extinction is associated at first with an excess of *estrogen* in the body fluids (*polyfolliculin phase*), then with a deficiency of this hormone (*oligofolliculin phase*), and finally with an excess of the follicle-stimulating hormone, prolan A (*polyprolan phase*). These findings, since amply confirmed, have formed the basis of two diametrically opposed views, one blaming an excess, the other a deficiency of estrogen, for the vasomotor and other nonsexual climacteric manifestations. Whitehouse,[19] chief protagonist of the *hyperestrogen theory,* points out that the vasomotor symptoms show a definite rhythm, and are relieved when the estrogen store of the body is depleted by an occasional hemorrhage from the uterus. As further proof, he offers the observation that estrogen therapy may sometimes aggravate the symptoms, and suggests that the relief attributed to this hormone may be due to the uterine bleeding which follows its withdrawal. It is significant that a vasomotor symptomatology, reminiscent of the climacteric, often accompanies premenstrual tension (see Chap. XXX) and polyfolliculin amenorrhea, conditions associated with a high blood estrogen level. The occurrence of uterine bleeding in such cases usually coincides with a drop in the estrogen content of the blood and relief from the annoying symptomatology.

The *estrogen-deprivation theory* finds support in the fact that a symptomatology, not unlike that seen at the climacteric, often follows castration in young women, and is sometimes relieved by estrogen therapy. Protagonists of this view point out that climacteric symptoms are more apt to appear during the oligofolliculin phase. The observation that annoying symptoms may appear for the first time in postmenopausal women, following removal of an estrogen-secreting granulosa cell tumor,[20] would also seem to favor this interpretation.

Studies of the estrogen content of the body fluids in climacteric women have failed to yield clear cut evidence supporting either view. Typical manifestations have been observed coincident with either high or low estrogen levels.[21, 22] Kurzrok[21] found that estrogen therapy relieved patients excreting subnormal amounts of this hormone, but aggravated the symptomatology where the estrogen content of the urine was within normal limits. A few investigators[23, 24, 25] have reported that estrogen is effective where a deficiency exists, but if the amount required to control the symptoms is exceeded, they may recur in their original or in an exaggerated form.

These conflicting observations may perhaps best be reconciled by assuming that, in some women, the mechanism immediately concerned in producing the symptoms is sensitive to fluctuations in the estrogen level, being upset by either an excess or a deficiency of this hormone.

The Anterior Hypophysis in the Climacteric.—The available evidence strongly suggests that the climacteric symptom-complex is attributable, in part at least, to functional alterations in the adenohypophysis, evoked by the gradual decline in ovarian function. Withdrawal of the ovarian secretions incident to the artificial or natural menopause is followed by cytologic modifications of the anterior lobe, associated with a rise in its gonadotropic hormone content,[10, 11] and the appearance of increased amounts of gonadotropin in the body fluids[12, 13, 14] (see Chap. XL). These findings form the basis for the view[26, 27] that anterior pituitary hyperactivity, secondary to ovarian hypofunction, plays an important part in producing the symptomatology of the climacteric.

The fact that typical vasomotor symptoms follow castration only after a lapse of weeks or months would seem to favor the assumption that they are contingent on secondary alterations in the anterior hypophysis. The absence of such symptoms in hypogonadism, secondary to hypofunction of the pituitary, also suggests that it is not the deficiency of ovarian sex hormones but the consequent hyperactivity of the adenohypophysis and glands dependent on it, which is responsible for the manifestations of the natural and artificial menopause. It is also noteworthy that, in a series of menopausal women observed by Murphy and Fluhmann,[28] the onset of symptoms was related to the appearance of gonadotropin and not to the disappearance of estrogen from the circulating blood. Perhaps the most cogent argument in favor of this interpretation is provided by reports[26, 29] that relief of symptoms following estrogen therapy coincides with a drop in the gonadotropic hormone level of the body fluids.

28

On the other hand, there is evidence[30, 31] that symptoms may appear where no excess of gonadotropic hormone is demonstrable, or be absent despite such excess. Moreover, a few observers[32, 33, 34] have noted that relief may follow estrogen administration long before a drop in the gonadotropin level occurs. These observations would seem to cast doubt on the importance of the anterior pituitary gland in the etiology. Participation of this gland cannot be excluded on the strength of this evidence alone. It is possible that the anterior lobe contributes to the climacteric symp-

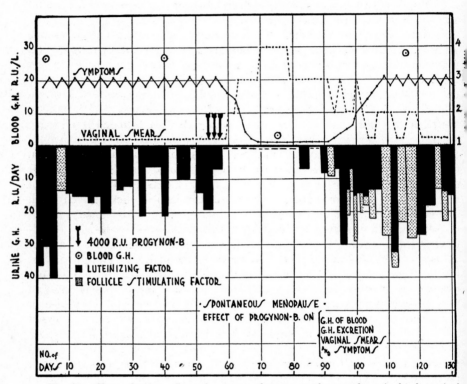

Fig. 92.—Chart showing effect of estrogen therapy on the gonadotropin level, vaginal smear and severity of symptoms in spontaneous menopause. Note estrogen administration followed by positive vaginal spreads, disappearance of symptoms and of gonadotropic factors in blood and urine. After lapse of twenty-five days, gradual return to pretreatment condition. (Frank, R. T., and Salmon, U. J.: New York State J. Med. Vol. 36.)

tom-complex through factors other than its gonadotropic hormones. The heterogeneous nature of the symptoms, and the high incidence of disorders of other incretory glands at the climacteric, suggests that the manifestations of this epoch may be related to a rise in its thyrotropic, adrenocorticotropic and other principles. This assumption, if true, would provide a clue to the mechanism through which gonadal regression leads to disturbances in systems outside the sexual sphere. That the symptoms are severe in some cases and mild or absent in others, becomes understandable if it is assumed that they not only depend on increased anterior pituitary function but also on the reactivity of the organs and tissues subject to its influence. A recent statement by Allen[35] is significant in this connection. To quote: "Interrelations of endocrine glands seem best interpreted by inclusion of a concept of balance through competitive utilization of certain limited vital necessities by successively dominant tissues and organs." It must be emphasized that extinction of ovarian function in the natural and artificial menopause not only removes the ovarian sex hormones, with their regulatory effect on pituitary function (see Chap. XII), but also deprives this gland of one of its principal points of attack. The glands and tissues which have shared the hypophyseal secretions with the gonads, now find themselves relieved of this competition. Which of these will become dominant depends on the inherent capacity of each to utilize the additional anterior pituitary secretions now available.

Since many as yet undetermined variables control the level of the anterior pituitary principles in the body fluids, the results of quantitative hormone determinations can hardly serve as a reliable index of the functional status of this gland. An excess of its thyrotropic or adrenocorticotropic factors may exist and yet neither may be demonstrable in the blood or urine because it is completely utilized by a responsive thyroid or adrenal gland. Failure to demonstrate an excess of gonadotropin in the body fluids does not necessarily exclude anterior pituitary hyperactivity. It may signify that other incretory glands, now dominant, have completely diverted the surplus energies of this gland to their own use. Absence of symptoms despite a rise in gonadotropin excretion may possibly be explained by assuming that the pituitary is hyperactive but the excess is not utilized because conditions inherent in the glands dependent on it limit their ability to respond to stimulation. It is possible that there is no absolute increase in anterior pituitary activity, the gonadotropin present in the urine representing a relative excess due to loss of its point of attack. It is conceivable, especially where gonadal extinction proceeds very gradually, that the general regression incident to approaching senility simultaneously affects the anterior pituitary and its dependent glands. The consequent decrease in their functional capacity would not only tend to minimize the surplus created by diminishing ovarian function, but would also minimize the reaction to it. This may account for the absence of symptoms in some menopausal women, and also suggests a possible explanation for the relatively greater severity of the symptoms which follow castration in young women. It is of interest in this connection that Rasmussen[36] observed shrinkage of the pituitaries of women in the fifth decade of life, and could demonstrate no increase in acidophils such as is seen in the enlarged pituitaries of young castrates.

The Thyroid Gland in the Climacteric.—It is significant that some of the most conspicuous climacteric manifestations, such as psychic and nervous instability, extreme emotionalism, tachycardia, tremors, and other vasomotor phenomena, are reminiscent of hyperthyroidism. Whether the sympathetic excitation, which is the immediate cause of these symptoms, is due to increased secretion of thyroxin is not certain. There is evidence that thyroxin stimulates the sympathetic nervous system, though it is still uncertain whether it directly affects the sympathetics or sensitizes the tissues innervated by them to other stimuli, particularly adrenalin.[37, 38] Manifestations of sympathetic excitation, like those encountered at the climacteric accompany hyperthyroidism, regardless of the age or sex of the patient. Such symptoms are especially apt to appear at the climacteric in women harboring a latent tendency to hyperthyroidism, and are absent as a rule in those with frank hypothyroidism. That the transient vaso-motor symptomatology observed in some climacteric women is at least partly due to thyroid hyperactivity secondary to increased thyrotropic hormone production is suggested by Grumbrecht's[39] observations in a group of climacteric patients. Demonstrable amounts of a substance pos-sessing thyrotropic properties appeared in the urine coincident with the periodic appearance of symptoms. A negative reaction was invariably ob-tained during the symptom-free intervals, and also in women who were free from symptoms at all times.

Symptoms suggesting hypothyroidism, such as sluggishness, mental torpor, loss of hair, undue sensitivity to cold, and in severe cases, myx-edema, may sometimes be encountered during the late stages of the climac-teric. These may conceivably be due to exhaustion of the gland following an initial period of hyperactivity, or aggravation of a latent deficiency by regressive changes in the thyroid, incident to approaching senility.

Role of the Adrenal Gland in the Climacteric.—The view that hyper-activity of the adrenal medulla contributes to the climacteric symptoma-tology is based on the observation that paroxysms of flushes and sweats may be induced at will in the climacteric woman with adrenalin, particu-larly if she is subject to these manifestations.[40, 41] It is noteworthy that paroxysmal tachycardia, choking sensations, headaches and hypertension, all reminiscent of the climacteric symptomatology, may occur in young individuals with chromaffin cell tumors of the adrenal gland. It is possible that adrenalin is an adjutant to the action of the sympathetic nerves, sensi-tizing them to other stimuli more directly concerned in the production of many of the climacteric nervous manifestations.

Hyperactivity of the adrenal cortex, secondary to increased adreno-corticotropic hormone production, may account for the hirsutism and other signs of masculinization encountered in some climacteric women. It seems likely that not only an absolute increase in androgen produc-tion by the adrenal cortex, but a relative excess created by withdrawal of the ovarian sex hormones with their opposite feminizing influence, plays a part. Of interest in this connection are recent reports of increased androgen excretion following the natural and artificial menopause.[42] What factors determine that the androgens will predominate over the estrogens, which are apparently also produced by the adrenal cortex following the extinction of ovarian function,[4-7] is not known.

Role of the Pancreas in the Climacteric.—The high incidence of dis-turbances of carbohydrate metabolism during the climacteric suggests that the pancreas may be involved in the general endocrine upheaval. Though the diabetes mellitus prevalent at this time may be traceable in many cases to exhaustion of the islets following dietary abuse, increased production of the anterior pituitary diabetogenic and pancreatropic principles is probably a contributory factor in some instances (see Chap. XIII). This finds support in reports[43, 44, 45] that the glycosuria of some climacteric women may be partially controlled by administering estrogen, which presumably acts by inhibiting the hyperactive hypophysis. Whether the glycosuria will be transient, or pass into permanent diabetes probably depends on the ability of the pancreas to withstand the added strain.

Nervous and Psychic Factors.—Participation of the nervous system in the etiology is suggested by the prevalence of nervous and psychic symptoms, and the favorable response to reassurance and psychotherapy. It is noteworthy that psychic shock may precipitate vasomotor symptoms in cases where adjustment has occurred spontaneously or as the result of treatment.[46] Of interest also is Reynolds'[47] recent study of the peripheral vascular response to estrogen in twenty-four menopausal women, whose vasomotor symptomatology was favorably affected by treatment with this hormone. He speaks of a negative, plateau, and flush type of response. The plateau type is characterized by a gradual but progressive increase in finger volume with no rise in skin temperature. In the flush type of response, the rate of increase in finger volume is suddenly accelerated and is accompanied by a rise in skin temperature of which the patient is aware. This response, according to Reynolds, is qualitatively similar to the spontaneous menopausal flush, differing only in degree. At times sweating occurred, but seldom a chill. Reynolds attributes the plateau type of response to the action of skin capillaries whose function is not appreciably altered by denervation. The flush type, on the other hand, he believes is due to dilatation of arterioles which are under the control of central autonomic centers. This response was frequently encountered in women tested before relief of symptoms had been achieved by estrogen therapy. Negative or plateau responses predominated where relief had already been obtained, either through suggestion, estrogen therapy, or other medication. On the basis of these findings, Reynolds concludes that "the basic physiological mechanism of the spontaneous menopausal flush and that induced by estrogen is heightened sensitivity of centers in the nervous system to otherwise inadequate stimuli. . . . It follows . . . that the essential physiological disturbance in the menopausal flush involves a primary endocrine dyscrasia coupled with psychic and somatic factors playing upon the peripheral vascular tree, affecting the innervation of the smaller arterioles of the skin on one hand and the irritability of the contractile elements of the blood capillaries themselves on the other."

This study is of interest because it establishes *neurovegetative hypersensitivity* as a factor in the etiology. Moreover, it demonstrates that this hypersensitivity may be controlled by either psychic or hormonal means. It seems paradoxical that a substance which is capable of inducing flushes should prove effective for their control. This property of estrogen would seem to be much more in harmony with reports that its use may aggravate the vasomotor symptomatology. Whether the relief noted following estrogen therapy is attributable to its ability to desensitize the vasomotor mechanism, or inhibit the production of some substance, possibly thyroxin or adrenalin, which is capable of exciting this mechanism, we cannot say. It is also conceivable that this hormone may correct a disturbance in the hypophyseal-hypothalamic system to which some observers attribute menopausal flushing,[48, 49, 50] or that the psychotherapeutic effect of its administration is responsible for the relief obtained.

Summary.—On the whole, it would appear that the climacteric symptom-complex is an expression of a general nervous and endocrine upheaval, possibly precipitated by the decline of ovarian function. The nature, intensity, and duration of the symptoms apparently depend on the severity of this disturbance and the response of the organism to the altered nervous and hormonal environment. This in turn depends to some extent on the previous status of each system and the extent to which it is implicated in the general regression which heralds the approaching senium.

DIAGNOSIS

The climacteric, more than any other period of life, offers problems in differential diagnosis which tax the diagnostic acumen of the most careful observer. Much confusion arises from the fact that many of the manifestations closely mimic the symptomatology of organic disease. Indeed, in many cases the only proof of the functional nature of the symptoms is their spontaneous disappearance with the completion of the climacteric. It is therefore of the utmost importance to rule out organic disease before instituting treatment. This calls for a complete physical and pelvic examination, and the use of appropriate laboratory procedures. All systems to which the symptoms are referable should be thoroughly investigated. The problem may be so complicated at times as to require the cooperation of the gynecologist, internist, neurologist, and endocrinologist. Endometrial curettage is important to determine the status of ovarian function and eliminate organic disease of the uterus, particularly where irregular uterine bleeding is an associated finding. Quantitative determinations of the estrogen, pregnanediol, androgen, and gonadotropin content of the body fluids, and the vaginal smear[51] (see Chap. XXXIX) may serve as a guide in the treatment.

TREATMENT

The object of the treatment is to relieve the troublesome symptoms and, where possible, correct any abnormalities which seem to be contributing to their causation. The physician must be fully aware of his limitations, always bearing in mind that advancing age and ovarian regression, the principal precipitating factors, cannot be stayed. At best, he may only hope to ease the patient through this critical epoch by employing general medical measures to improve her physical and nervous status, and organotherapy to supply existing hormone deficiencies.

MEDICAL TREATMENT

Emphasis should be placed on prophylactic as well as active medical treatment. The value of *prophylaxis* is readily appreciated when it is recalled that the nature and severity of the climacteric symptomatology depends to a large extent on the individual's previous constitutional, endocrine, and nervous status. Since this is largely determined by the stress and strain imposed on the patient earlier in life, it is important to correct or eradicate all depressive states encountered prior to the menopause. Endocrine disorders should receive particular attention, and appropriate measures taken to remedy them. Women of inferior constitution are especially in need of prophylactic treatment, for it is these unfortunates who are subject to endocrine and nervous instability and exhaustion, and

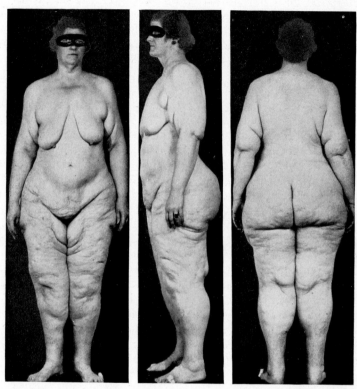

Fig. 93.—Menopausal obesity. Female aged forty-five, weight 258 pounds. Irregular uterine bleeding. Hyperplastic endometrium and above normal estrogen values. Note relative thinness of face and upper torso contrasting with lumpy fat deposits in lower half of body.

react so poorly to the physiologic burdens of reproductive life. In such cases the best procedure is to build up the general health as far as possible, and guard against all undue physical and nervous exertion. An early tendency to adiposity should be controlled (see Chap. XXXIII) in order to avoid the enormous obesities so often seen at the climacteric. Regulation of weight may do much to forestall an undue burden on the endocrine system, particularly the thyroid and pancreas.

Radical pelvic surgery or x-ray radiation of the ovaries during the reproductive period should be avoided except as a last resort. It is desirable to preserve ovarian function as long as possible, in order to avoid an abrupt break in the ovarian-pituitary complex. If the decline in ovarian function is gradual, the endocrine system may be better able to adapt itself to the altered hormonal conditions.

On reaching the climacteric, the patient should be reassured as to the transient and harmless nature of her symptoms. Environmental and social conflicts should be resolved where possible. These measures, supplemented by sedatives, control the vasomotor manifestations in a large proportion of the cases.[50] It must be emphasized that at the climacteric, more than at any other period of life, it is necessary to relieve the organism of its excess burdens and reinforce its physical reserves. The climacteric woman may be compared to a machine that has been worked hard and long, but may continue to perform tolerably well if handled with care and not overtaxed.

ORGANOTHERAPY

Evaluation.—Sex hormones, particularly the estrogens, are widely used to relieve the symptomatic menopause. The subjective nature of the symptoms, and marked psychoneurotic instability make it extremely difficult to evaluate the efficacy of organotherapy. Judging from the medical literature of a few decades ago, the older ovarian preparations, now conceded to be physiologically inert, were credited with effects comparable to those now claimed for the potent sex hormones. The problem is further complicated by the fact that the duration of the symptoms varies widely so that one cannot be certain whether the relief noted was due to a spontaneous remission and would have occurred in the absence of treatment. As Davis[52] points out, "in evaluating the results of any therapeutic regime in the treatment of the menopause, criteria are exceedingly difficult to select. The climacteric presents such a bizarre picture that few symptoms occur with sufficient regularity to be useful in evaluating results."

Estrogenic Substances.—While many clinicians have hailed the sex hormones, particularly the estrogens, as an outstanding therapeutic triumph, others are less enthusiastic. Novak[50] has found the results of estrogen therapy "variable, rarely brilliant, but often satisfactory." According to Davis,[52] such treatment gives moderate relief to the majority, and no relief to a considerable number. In the author's experience, general medical measures, reassurance, sedation, and sterile saline injections, used for their psychotherapeutic effect, have proved more efficacious than the estrogens or other hormonal preparations in the vast majority of his cases. This has also been the experience of Stolkind,[53] and of Pratt and Thomas,[54, 55] who could see no appreciable difference between the response of patients receiving estrogens, and those given phenobarbital and injections of sterile oil solution.

Those who favor estrogen therapy for the climacteric symptomatology are at variance as to what this hormone can accomplish. Some find the estrogens effective only for the control of the flushes. Others recommend them for kraurosis vulvae,[56] arthritic pains and intestinal symptoms,[57] hypertension,[58] edema,[59] a low basal metabolic rate,[60] hyperglycemia and glycosuria,[43, 44, 45] respiratory and circulatory disturbances,[61] dysuria and incontinence,[62] involutional melancholia,[63] and numerous other manifestations.

Indications and Contraindications.—Estrogen therapy should be tried only where a deficiency has been demonstrated. It is obviously superfluous during the polyfolliculin phase.[57] The aim is not to supply an estrogen deficiency indefinitely, but rather to avoid an abrupt withdrawal of the endogenous estrogens, so that the organism may adjust itself to the changing hormonal conditions with a minimum of discomfort. Protracted administration of large doses is to be avoided because of the possibility of stimulating a latent tendency to malignancy. Though many consider this unlikely with the doses generally employed, it must nevertheless be considered, especially since these patients are at the *cancer age*. It is often argued that there is no conclusive proof that estrogen therapy will cause cancer in the human being. The burden of proof should rest on those who insist on the harmlessness of such therapy. In the author's opinion, it should be used with caution, particularly in the presence of benign lesions of the breast or genitalia, or where there is a history of familial cancer. It is also *contraindicated in kraurosis vulvae* which eventuates in carcinoma in 50 per cent of the cases.[57]

Aside from its possible carcinogenic effect, estrogen therapy may cause the patient to be subjected to unnecessary curettage, because of the uterine bleeding which often follows such treatment. With the appearance of bleeding, the conscientious clinician may feel himself compelled to perform a diagnostic curettage to make certain that the hemorrhage is due to the therapy and not to some lesion which has developed during its course.

Administration.—The dosage and duration of treatment is entirely an individual problem and varies widely. The effective dose has been variously defined as the amount required to produce an estrogenic vaginal smear,[64] or the amount needed to cause a drop in the gonadotropin level of the body fluids.[65] Since relief may often be obtained before these effects are demonstrable,[34, 66] these criteria would appear to be unsatisfactory. As stated by Shorr,[46] "wide variations in the subjective and biological response to estrogens make attempts to standardize dosage futile."

The estrogens may be administered by mouth, subcutaneous injection, or in the form of pellets of crystalline hormone implanted beneath the skin. For control of the symptoms, it is preferable to employ the natural estrogens, because stilbestrol, in the large doses required for this purpose, is not likely to be well tolerated. In the average case, the *dose* recommended is 10,000 I.U. of estradiol benzoate or dipropionate given subcutaneously three times a week. The stubborn case may require doses up to 100,000 I.U. If relief is obtained, the dose should be gradually reduced to the lowest level compatible with the continued comfort of the patient. For maintenance purposes, stilbestrol may be given orally in doses of 0.5 to 1.0 mgm. daily.

Some workers[67, 68, 69] advocate the *subcutaneous implantation* of pellets of crystalline estrogen in order to insure a steady supply of hormone over a period of weeks or even months. Salmon and his associates[77] implant pellets at the time of bilateral ovariectomy as a prophylactic measure. The techniques employed for this purpose differ in detail. That recommended by Bennett and his associates[69] is as follows: From 3 to 10 pellets, each weighing 5 to 6 mgm. are used. These are first sterilized in a dry steam autoclave at 250° F., under 15 pounds pressure for 30 minutes. Implantation is made through a 12 gauge hollow needle fitted with a stylette. The pellets are loaded into the pointed end of the needle, which is pushed through the skin after procaine infiltration. Pressure on the stylette as the needle is withdrawn deposits the pellets in the subcutaneous tissue.

The availability of orally active estrogen would seem to make pellet implantation unnecessary, while the possibility that it may induce persistent uterine bleeding makes its use undesirable. Continuity of effect may be an advantage from the standpoint of controlling the symptoms, but it should be remembered that it is also an important factor in the production of experimental genital and mammary cancer.

Androgenic Substances.—The androgens are advocated by some observers[70, 71, 72, 73] because of their supposed ability to inhibit the hyperactive adenohypophysis, which is presumably contributing to the symptomatology. The *doses* employed range from 5 to 15 mgm. of testosterone propionate by subcutaneous injection two or three times a week until a total of 300 mgm. has been given. Since large doses may cause hirsutism, deepening of the voice, and other manifestations of masculinization, it would appear unwise to resort to such therapy, particularly at a time of life when a tendency to hirsutism is not uncommon.

Kurzrok and Rothbart[74] recommend combined *estrogen and androgen therapy*, on the assumption that they act synergistically in inhibiting the anterior hypophysis, but are antagonistic in their effect on the uterus. By combining them, it is hoped to inhibit the hyperactive pituitary without inducing bleeding from the uterus. The dose is 5 to 25 mgm. of methyl testosterone, an orally active androgen, and 2 to 3 mgm. of stilbestrol daily by mouth.

X-ray Therapy.—Depressive doses of x-ray *to the hypophysis* have been tried on the assumption that the climacteric symptomatology is either directly or indirectly traceable to anterior pituitary hyperactivity.[75, 76, 77] The *dosage* recommended by Geist and his associates[77] is 150 "R" units, 180 K.V., 4 M.A. filter—½ Cu. 1 Al., 40 mm. focal distance, 15 minutes, 6 x 8—size of field. Three treatments are given, one left temporal, one right temporal, and one frontal.

Evaluation.—The paucity of cases so treated, and the failure to employ objective criteria of the physiologic effect of the treatment, makes evaluation difficult. The uncertainty of its action and the possibility of injury to the hypophysis and adjacent nerve centers make such therapy undesirable and hazardous. If used at all, it should be reserved for cases where excessive amounts of gonadotropin or other hypophyseal principles are demonstrable in the body fluids, and the symptoms are severe and have resisted other more conservative measures.

BIBLIOGRAPHY

1. Marañón, G.: The Climacteric, trans. by K. S. Stevens, ed. by C. Culbertson. St. Louis, The C. V. Mosby Co., 1929.
2. Council of the Medical Women's Federation in England. Lancet *1*:106, 1933.
3. Kloppner, K.: Geburtsh. u. Frauenh. *1*:709, 1939.
4. Salmon, U. J., and Frank, R. T.: Proc. Soc. Exper. Biol. & Med. *33*:612, 1936.
5. Geist, S. H., and Salmon, U. J.: Am. J. Obst. & Gynec. *38*:392, 1939.
6. Frank, R. T., Goldberger, M. A., and Salmon, U. J.: Proc. Soc. Exper. Biol. & Med. *33*: 615, 1939.
7. Novak, E., and Richardson, E. H., Jr.: Am. J. Obst. & Gynec. *42*:564, 1941.
8. Young, R. H.: Am. J. Obst. & Gynec. *38*:111, 1939.
9. Curschmann, H.: Med. Klin. *29*:1265, 1933.
10. Henderson, W. R., and Rowlands, I. W.: Brit. Med. J. *1*:1094, 1938.
11. Witschi, E., and Riley, G. M.: Endocrinol. *26*:565, 1940.
12. Fluhmann, C. F.: Am. J. Obst. & Gynec. *20*:1, 1930.
13. Anspach, B. M., and Hoffman, J.: Am. J. Obst. & Gynec. *26*:147, 1933.
14. Walter, R. I., Geist, S. H., and Salmon, U. J.: Endocrinol. *27*:154, 1940.
15. Watson, B. P., Smith, P. E., and Kurzrok, R.: Am. J. Obst. & Gynec. *36*:562, 1938.
16. Frank, R. T., Goldberger, M. A., Salmon, U. J., and Felshin, G.: J.A.M.A. *109*:1863, 1937
17. Wilson, J. G., and Young, W. C.: Anat. Rec. *76* (Suppl.): 58, 1940.
18. Zondek, B.: Klin. Wchnschr. *20*:2121, 1929.
19. Whitehouse, B.: Canad. M. A. J. *29*:585, 1933.
20. Novak, E.: Am. J. Surg. *24*:595, 1934.
21. Kurzrok, R.: Endocrinol. *16*:366, 1932.
22. Tamis, A. B.: Am. J. Obst. & Gynec. *28*:48, 1934.
23. Sevringhaus, E. L.: Am. J. Obst. & Gynec. *25*:261, 1933.
24. Schneider, P. F.: Am. J. Obst. & Gynec. *37*:861, 1939.
25. Huberman, J., and Colmer, M. J.: Am. J. Obst. & Gynec. *39*:783, 1940.
26. Albright, F.: Endocrinol. *20*:24, 1936.
27. Engelhart, E., and Tscherne, E.: Zentralbl. f. Gynäk. *60*:790, 1936.
28. Murphy, K. M., and Fluhmann, C. F.: West. J. Surg., Gynec. & Obst. *46*:451, 1938.
29. Frank, R. T., and Salmon, U. J.: Proc. Soc. Exper. Biol. & Med. *33*:311, 1935.
30. Winter, E. W.: Schweiz. med. Wchnschr. *65*:1121, 1935.
31. Shorr, E., Stimmel, B. F., and Papanicolaou, G. N., cited by E. Shorr, in Bull. New York Acad. Med. *16*:453, 1940.
32. Damm, P. N.: Acta obst. & gynec. Scandinav. *14*:115, 1934.
33. Heller, C. G., and Heller, E. J.: J. Clin. Investigation *18*:171, 1939.
34. Heller, C. G., Heller, E. J., and Sevringhaus, E. L.: Endocrinol. *30*:309, 1942.
35. Allen, E.: J.A.M.A. *116*:405, 1941.
36. Rasmussen, A. T.: Am. J. Anat. *55*:253, 1934; Am. J. Path. *9*:459, 1933.
37. Blau, N. F., and McNamara, H.: Proc. Soc. Exper. Biol. & Med. *27*:997, 1930.
38. Bergwall, A., and Kuschinsky, G.: Arch. f. exp. Path. u. Pharm. *162*:169, 1931.
39. Grumbrecht, P.: Zentralbl. f. Gynäk. *59*:1331, 1936.
40. Hannan, J. H.: Brit. Med. J. *2*:14, 1927; Flushings of the Menopause, London, Bailliere, 1927.
41. Myers, W. K., and King, J. T.: Bull. Johns Hopkins Hosp. *47*:22, 1930.
42. Hamblen, E. C., Cuyler, W. K., and Baptist, M.: J. Clin. Endocrinol. *1*:777, 1941.
43. Gessler, C. J., Halsted, J. A., and Stetson, R. P.: J. Clin. Investigation *18*:715, 1939.
44. Cantilo, E.: Endocrinol. *28*:20, 1941.
45. Lawrence, R. D., and Madders, K.: Lancet *1*:601, 1941.
46. Shorr, E.: Bull. New York Acad. Med. *16*:453, 1940.
47. Reynolds, S. R. M., Kaminester, S., Foster, F. I., and Schloss, S.: Surg., Gynec. & Obst. *73*:206, 1941.
48. Brown, W. L., Thomson, A. P., Bishop, P. M. F., and Stolkind, E.: Proc. Roy. Soc. London, s.B. *29*:1085, 1936.
49. Crisler, G. R., and Allen, E. V.: Proc. Staff Meet., Mayo Clin. *12*:218, 1937.
50. Novak, E.: Am. J. Obst. & Gynec. *40*:589, 1940.

51. Papanicolaou, G. N., and Shorr, E.: Proc. Soc. Exper. Biol. & Med. *32*:585, 1934.
52. Davis, M. E.: Am. J. Obst. & Gynec. *39*:938, 1940.
53. Stolkind, E.: Proc. Roy. Soc London, s.B. *29*:1094, 1936.
54. Pratt, J. P., and Thomas, W. L.: J.A.M.A. *109*:1875, 1937.
55. Pratt, J. P.: South. M. J. *31*:562, 1938.
56. Finkler, R. S., and Antopol, W.: Endocrinol. *25*:925, 1939.
57. Frank, R. T.: Bull. New York Acad. Med. *17*:854, 1941.
58. Schaefer, R. L.: Endocrinol. *19*:705, 1935.
59. von Farkas, G.: Zentralbl. f. Gynäk. *61*:582, 1937.
60. Collett, M. E., Smith, J. T., and Wertenberger, G. E.: Am. J. Obst. & Gynec. *34*:639, 1937.
61. Scherf, D.: Ann. Int. Med. *13*:1414, 1940.
62. Salmon, U. J., Walter, R. I., and Geist, S. H.: Am. J. Obst. & Gynec. *42*:845, 1941.
63. Ault, C. C., Hoctor, E. F., and Werner, A. A.: J.A.M.A. *109*:1786, 1937.
64. Papanicolaou, G. N., and Shorr, E.: Am. J. Obst. & Gynec. *31*:806, 1936.
65. Geist, S. H., and Salmon, U. J.: New York State J. Med. *39*:1759, 1939.
66. Bennett, H. G., and TeLinde, R. W.: J.A.M.A. *118*:1341, 1942.
67. Twombly, G. H., and Millen, R. S.: Surg., Gynec. & Obst. *72*:610, 1941.
68. Mishell, D. R.: Am. J. Obst. & Gynec. *41*:1009, 1941.
69. Bennett, H. G., Jr., Biskind, G., and Mark, J.: Am. J. Obst. & Gynec. *39*:504, 1940.
70. Shorr, E., Papanicolaou, G. N., and Stimmel, B. F.: Proc. Soc. Exper. Biol. & Med. *38*:759, 1938.
71. Kurzrok, L., Birnberg, C. H., and Livingston, S.: Endocrinol. *24*:347, 1939.
72. Salmon, U. J.: J. Clin. Endocrinol. *1*:162, 1941.
73. Kurzrok, R., and Rothbart, H.: Am. J. Surg. *56*:636, 1942.
74. Collins, C. G., Menville, L. J., and Thomas, E. P.: Radiology *26*:682, 1936.
75. Lollinger, R., and Vaughan, W. W.: New England J. Med. *217*:219, 1937.
76. Geist, S. H., and Mintz, M.: Am. J. Obst. & Gynec. *33*:643, 1937.
77. Geist, S. H., Walter, R. I., and Salmon, U. J.: J. Mt. Sinai Hosp. *8*:543, 1942.

CHAPTER XXX

TROUBLESOME MANIFESTATIONS ASSOCIATED WITH THE MENSTRUAL CYCLE

INTERMENSTRUAL PAIN

Definition.—The term "intermenstrual pain" or "mittelschmerz" describes periodic lower abdominal discomfort or pain experienced during the midphase of the menstrual cycle. While only a comparatively small number of cases have been recorded, intermenstrual pain, especially in its milder forms, is probably relatively common, though often overlooked or confused with some other condition. In this connection, McSweeney and Wood[1] found that 21 of 134 patients with regular menstrual cycles experienced abdominal pain of a minor degree midway between the periods.

Symptomatology.—The pain is intermittent in character and may vary in intensity from a mild cramplike sensation to severe attacks simulating some abdominal catastrophe. It is most frequently confined to the right lower abdomen, but may alternate from one side to the other on each recurring attack. Though it usually begins approximately midway between the flows, it may be experienced as early as the seventh or as late as the twenty-fourth day of the menstrual cycle. The attack may last a few hours or persist for several days, and in some instances is terminated only with the onset of the flow.

Intermenstrual pain is sometimes accompanied by visible uterine bleeding or microscopic hemorrhage detectable only by examination of vaginal washings. At times there may be a slight mucoid discharge. Pelvic examination may be entirely negative, or one of the ovaries may be palpable and tender during the attack. Nervous hyperirritability, tachycardia, dizziness, sweating, and nausea without vomiting may accompany a severe attack.

Etiology.—*Relation to Ovulation.*—Despite the numerous theories advanced from time to time to explain intermenstrual pain, its cause is still uncertain. That it is related in some way to ovulation was first suggested by Priestley[2] in 1872. This possibility finds support in the fact that pain occurs only during menstrual life and appears at the midphase of the cycle, when ovulation usually takes place (see Chap. IV). Moreover, it tends to disappear with the advent of pregnancy, when ovulatory function is normally in abeyance, and is not infrequently absent at the beginning and end of the reproductive period, when the cycles tend to be of the anovulatory type.

Mechanism.—Though most observers believe that the pain is related to the ovulatory act, there is considerable uncertainty as to the mechanism immediately concerned in its production. Is it caused by the act of rupture, bleeding from the follicle incident to rupture, some alteration in the ovary which precedes or follows rupture, or some change in the accessory genitalia which is synchronous with ovulation? That the pain in at least some of the cases is due to some *alteration in the ovary* proper is suggested by reports of relief following unilateral ovariectomy where the pain was one-sided, or bilateral ovariectomy, where both sides were affected alternately. It is also significant that the pain may persist despite hysterectomy,[3] appendicectomy, or pelvic sympathectomy,[4, 5] but is often though not invariably relieved by ovarian neurectomy.[5]

Reynolds[6] has suggested that the pain in some cases may be due to exaggeration of the *uterine contractions* which, according to Dickinson,[7] normally accompany ovulation, or may be caused by *movements of the ovaries and tubes*, analogous to those observed by Westman[8] in the monkey. The latter observer noted that, at the time of ovulation, the ovary is pulled backward and forward with a partial rotary motion and at the same time is pulled in and out of the bursa ovarica, being massaged as it moves, by the tubal fimbriae. Assuming that the same type of activity occurs in the human being, it is conceivable that pain may arise when the ovary pulls and tugs on its ligaments.

Seguy,[9] who found that some cases of intermenstrual pain may show no evidence of follicular rupture at laparotomy performed shortly after an attack, attributes the pain to congestion of the ovary and tubes, preparatory to ovulation. He suggests that *preovulatory congestion* is due to a rise in estrogen, and may or may not be followed by ovulation, depending on whether a mature follicle, ripe for rupture, is present in the ovary. This congestion, he believes, may give rise to clinical symptoms if it is especially intense, or the ovarian sympathetic is particularly sensitive.

Though the evidence permits no definite conclusions, it seems likely that intermenstrual pain may be traceable to one or more of the various alterations in the ovary and accessory genitalia, which precede, accompany, and immediately follow follicular rupture. The immediate cause probably varies in different cases and no single explanation is universally applicable. Since the mechanism of ovulation is presumably the same in all women, it is necessary to look for some additional factor to account for the fact that this phenomenon passes unnoticed in some women, while others experience varying degrees of discomfort or pain. A low pain threshold, some abnormality in the innervation of the ovary, abnormal local blood vessel changes, pelvic inflammatory disease,[10] developmental or acquired abnormalities of the ovarian tunic which make rupture difficult, and adhesions between the point of rupture and the uterus or broad ligament, have all been considered as possible factors in the etiology. The suggestion that an excess of estrogen may be at fault has not thus far been substantiated.[11]

Diagnosis and Differential Diagnosis.—*Mild Form.*—In its mild forms, periodic intermenstrual pain offers little difficulty in the diagnosis, particularly when associated with slight spotting. In the absence of pelvic pathology, the condition need not concern the patient. Its recognition is important because of its possible confusion with chronic appendicitis. Intermenstrual pain may be distinguished from *chronic appendicitis* by the regularity of the attacks at the midphase of the cycle, shifting of the pain to alternate sides, the presence of a palpable tender ovary, and the occasional appearance of vaginal staining or bleeding. In some cases, the differential diagnosis may be possible only through laparotomy and inspection of the ovaries and appendix. This calls for a mid-line incision, since a small right rectus incision does not permit inspection of the ovaries.

Follicular Rupture and Hemorrhage.—Of greater concern from both the diagnostic and therapeutic standpoint are the rare cases of severe intermenstrual pain due to follicular rupture with intra-abdominal hemorrhage. The pain in such cases may sometimes be confused with *acute appendicitis* or ruptured tubal pregnancy. The differential diagnosis between pain due to follicular rupture and acute appendicitis is often very difficult. In both conditions, the pain may be confined to the right lower quadrant and be accompanied by nausea, vomiting, a moderate rise in temperature, leucocytosis, and tenderness at McBurney's point. A history of repeated short attacks at the midphase of the cycle, the presence of a palpable tender ovary, and the appearance of a brown or bloody discharge suggests that the ovary rather than the appendix is the site of the pain. According to some observers, the blood sedimentation rate is increased in follicular rupture, especially when it is accompanied by hemorrhage, whereas in acute appendicitis, the rate is usually normal. The temperature, pulse rate, and white cell count are nearer normal in follicular rupture.

In follicular rupture associated with intraperitoneal hemorrhage, the symptomatology may be identical with that in *ruptured tubal pregnancy.* In both, there may be shock and a bulging cul de sac. A history of a missed period, spotting, early symptoms and signs of pregnancy, and a decidual reaction of the uterine mucosa speak for ectopic pregnancy. In either event, surgery is urgent. If the symptoms are mild and there is no immediate danger in a brief delay, operation may be postponed so that a biologic test for pregnancy may help differentiate the two conditions (see Chap. XXXIX).

Treatment.—*Mild Attack.*—Because of its obscure etiology, the treatment of periodic intermenstrual pain is necessarily empirical. The mild case, free from demonstrable pathology, requires no treatment. Where the attacks are more severe, relief may be achieved by rest in bed and the use of codeine and the salicylates. Attempts to inhibit ovulation by means of large doses of estrogen or androgen, or by radiation of the ovaries, are unwarranted in young women during the childbearing age.

Severe Attack with Hemorrhage.—Where the attack is very severe and accompanied by signs of massive intra-abdominal hemorrhage and shock, immediate laparotomy is indicated. The abdomen should be opened by a midline incision so that both adnexa and appendix may be viewed. In the event that surgery is undertaken for a supposed appendicitis and slight follicular bleeding is encountered, the hemorrhage may be controlled by a lock-stitch suture at the same time that the appendix is removed. Where the follicular laceration is extensive and the bleeding severe, resection or removal of the ovary may be necessary.

PREMENSTRUAL TENSION

Definition.—The term "premenstrual tension," coined by Frank,[1] describes a syndrome characterized chiefly by an exaggeration of the usual menstrual molimina to the point where they become distressing or incapacitating. For milder forms of this syndrome, Greenhill and Freed[2] have proposed the term "premenstrual distress." The condition is relatively uncommon, though perhaps not so rare as the paucity of cases in the literature would suggest. It may occur at any time during the reproductive period, but is most apt to affect women approaching the climacteric.

Symptomatology.—The symptomatology is subjective in nature and in large part resembles that of the symptomatic menopause, except that it is experienced only during the premenstruum and disappears within a few hours after the onset of the flow. The most prominent symptom is a sensation of unbearable tension, which may be accompanied by marked hyperirritability, physical unrest, crying spells, emotional outbursts, insomnia, depression, vertigo, headache, fatigue, transient edema, painful swelling of the breast, and occasionally nymphomania.

Etiology.—*Role of Ovarian Sex Hormones.*—The etiology is obscure. Since the symptoms precede the menstrual flow and are relieved after its onset, it is not surprising that attention has been directed to the ovarian sex hormones in the search for the cause of this syndrome. An excess of *estrogen* in the blood was blamed by Frank.[1] This observer obtained high blood estrogen and low urine estrogen values in fifteen women with premenstrual tension. He inferred from this that such individuals have a high kidney threshold, which interferes with estrogen excretion. The hormone consequently accumulates in the circulating blood and produces the typical symptoms of premenstrual tension. This explanation was subsequently judged to be inadequate by Israel,[3] who could demonstrate a high renal threshold for estrogen in only four out of seven cases. Since premenstrual curettage revealed interval or hyperplastic changes in three out of four of his patients, he concluded that the symptoms are caused "not by an excess of circulating estrogen but rather by the presence of unantagonized estrogen," the primary cause being inadequate luteinization with consequent deficiency of progestin. Doubt has been cast on this hypothesis by reports of premenstrual tension in the presence of normal luteal activity, as shown by the presence of full secretory changes in the endometrium and normal pregnanediol values.[4] The fact that premenstrual tension is not a frequent accompaniment of pseudomenstrual or hyperplastic bleeding (see Chap. XXV) would also seem to argue against his theory. That an excess rather than a deficiency of *progestin* may account for some cases is suggested by the finding of excessive amounts of pregnanediol in the urine of one case observed by Hamblen,[5] and the appearance of symptoms like those of premenstrual tension following a single injection of progesterone, in several patients observed by Gillman.[6]

In view of the varied hormonal and endometrial findings, a definite conclusion as to the identity of the substance or substances responsible for the symptomatology is hardly justified. Whether it is estrogen, estrogen and progesterone, or some degradation product of the metabolism of estrogen or progesterone, is a problem for future investigation. Markee's suggestion that the cause may be some product of the regressing endometrium (see Chap. V), also awaits confirmation.

Edema.—An attempt to define the mechanism immediately concerned in the production of the symptoms has recently been made by Greenhill and Freed.[2, 7] These observers point to the well known clinical observation that women frequently gain weight during the premenstrual phase and lose a corresponding amount after the flow. This gain, according to Thorn and his coworkers,[8] is due to sodium retention with consequent retention of water. They attribute this tendency to the influence of the ovarian sterols. Greenhill and Freed[2] believe that the disposition to retain sodium and water may not only affect the subcutaneous tissues, resulting in visible edema, but may also involve internal tissues, causing hidden edema, which gives rise to the symptoms of premenstrual tension. In support of this interpretation, they offer their observation that relief uniformly follows the oral administration of ammonium chloride and curtailment of the salt intake during the second half of the cycle. It is noteworthy that Frank[1] also noted improvement following the oral administration of magnesium sulfate, employed by him to increase elimination and thereby deplete the excessive estrogen store. It is conceivable that such therapy relieves through a two-fold action, at once removing retained water and facilitating the elimination of some substance or substances which promote such retention. A fact which seems to weaken Greenhill and Freed's[2] explanation is that increased body weight and diminished sodium and water excretion, pointing to sodium and water retention, may persist throughout the menstrual period,[9] whereas the symptoms of premenstrual tension subside within a few hours after the onset of the flow. An explanation which avoids this objection has been offered by Brewer,[10] who suggests that menstrual edema may be due to increased capillary permeability, resulting from the prolonged vasospasm which occurs shortly before the flow and ceases with its onset. This vasospasm is demonstrable at the same time in both the endometrial and extragenital blood vessels. Brewer believes that the same cause is operating in both cases but fails to identify it. Whether it is one of the ovarian sterols or some extra-ovarian factor is not known. Reynolds and di Palma[11] have recently reported their failure to demonstrate cyclic alterations in the skin capillaries, to which somatic physiological changes, such as premenstrual tension, might be attributed. Their negative findings do not necessarily discredit those of Brewer, but may merely indicate that there exist wide individual variations in the response of extra-genital tissues to stimuli arising in the sexual sphere. That such variations exist is also evident in the fact that premenstrual tension, periodic extragenital hemorrhage and other annoying premenstrual manifestations are experienced by only a small proportion of all menstruating women.

Nervous Instability.—Though the identity of the substance responsible for the symptoms, and the mechanism immediately concerned in their

29

production are still a matter of speculation, most observers agree that this syndrome is most apt to occur in women with an unstable nervous system. Here again, the observation of Reynolds and his associates[12] that the stability of the nervous system influences the response of peripheral blood vessels to hormonal stimuli (estrogen), is significant. Frank[1] pointed out that premenstrual tension tends to arise in "labile" individuals. Gillman[6] found that the ability of progesterone to elicit symptoms suggestive of premenstrual tension varied according to the sensitivity of the nervous system. Some women experienced severe symptoms following a small dose, while others remained symptom-free despite a large dose of the hormone. It seems likely that an unstable nervous system plays an important and, in some cases, perhaps a primary role in the etiology.

Diagnosis.—The characteristic symptomatology and the time of its appearance makes the diagnosis relatively simple. To determine the underlying cause, investigation of the physical, hormonal and nervous status of the individual may be of value.

Treatment.—*Medical Measures.*—Since the etiology is obscure, treatment is necessarily empirical. On the assumption that the condition is due to hyperestrinemia, Frank[1] recommends saline cathartics, diuretics and venesection, with the view of depleting the estrogen store of the body. He also advocates roentgen castration for women in the late stages of the reproductive epoch. Protagonists of the view that defective luteinization is the primary cause, advocate luteinizing preparations of hypophyseal or chorionic origin.[13] Others[3, 14] prefer progesterone on the ground that the available gonadotropes cannot stimulate corpus luteum function in the human being. Israel[3] reports relief following the intramuscular injection of 2 I.U. of progesterone daily or every other day during the second half of the cycle. For permanent relief, he recommends low-dosage radiation of the pituitary and ovaries. In the author's opinion, this form of treatment should be used only where the symptoms are very severe and the patient is approaching the menopause.

Greenhill and Freed[2, 7] recommend 10 grains of ammonium chloride three times a day by mouth, and curtailment of table salt during the latter half of the cycle. The chloride of the ammonium salt, they believe, combines with the sodium ion in the extracellular fluid to form sodium chloride, which is excreted, thus precluding retention of the sodium ion and fluid in the tissues. This therapy is worth a trial since it can do no harm and may give relief by helping to rid the body of an excess of fluid and the "ovarian sterols" or other factors causing the symptoms. Good results have been reported with testosterone propionate, which is believed to act by neutralizing estrogen.[4, 15]

Hygienic Measures.—It should be emphasized that it is very difficult to evaluate any form of therapy in a condition where the symptomatology is purely subjective and the etiology obscure. In the author's experience, improvement has followed the use of sedatives and general hygienic measures aimed at improving the general health of the patient and stabilizing her nervous system. The value of this approach is borne out by Israel's[3] experience with one patient who, being markedly underweight, received a high caloric diet together with daily injections of insulin. The resulting gain in weight coincided with disappearance of the premenstrual tension.

MIGRAINE

Definition.—The term migraine describes a syndrome of obscure origin, characterized by recurrent headache, which is usually unilateral and often accompanied by scintillating scotomas, nausea, vomiting, and other psychoneurotic manifestations. The syndrome is much more common in women. It often appears shortly before the onset of the menstrual flow, but may also occur at other times. It tends to disappear during gestation and following the completion of the climacteric.

Etiology.—The cause of the migrainous syndrome is obscure. The available evidence suggests that more than one factor contributes to its causation. That *allergy* plays an important part, at least in some of the cases, is suggested by its frequent association with urticaria, hay fever and asthma. *Vasomotor instability*, which characterizes the migrainous patient, may also play a part.

The growing interest in the glands of internal secretion is responsible for attempts to explain migraine on a *hormonal basis*. Timme[1] has proposed that it may be caused by intermittent and recurrent swelling of the pituitary gland, the pain being due to pressure of the gland on the optic nerves and adjacent structures. As proof he offers his observation that x-ray of the sella turcica revealed evidence of gradual erosion and excavation in many of his migrainous patients. Goldzieher[2] questions this theory on the ground that such changes are relatively uncommon, and that migraine is more often found in women with a bridged-over, practically enclosed, or small and abnormally shaped sella.

Riley and his associates[3] have suggested that migraine may be due to a disturbance in the *anterior pituitary-ovarian relationship*. This they base on their observation that twenty of twenty-nine headaches experienced by eleven migrainous patients were preceded by a rise in the gonadotropin content of the urine, followed by a drop on the first day of the seizure. Little or no estrogen was demonstrable. Injection of human chorionic gonadotropin precipitated an attack in seven of nine cases. These observers concluded that migraine may be due to pituitary hyperfunction or ovarian hypofunction, and that the gonadotropic hormones probably play an important role. Since a rise in the gonadotropin level of the urine was not invariably followed by an attack, and some attacks were not preceded by such a rise, they suggested that an additional unidentified factor is probably involved in the etiology.

Goldzieher[2] points out that migraine is associated with a tendency to retain *water and salt in the tissues*. He suggests that the nervous instability which characterizes most of these patients, together with the increase in capillary permeability which normally precedes menstruation, may conceivably result in an exaggeration of this tendency near the period. The resulting swelling of the tissues within the enclosed cranial cavity causes increased intracranial pressure, experienced as pain. The increased intracranial pressure stimulates the function of the anterior hypophysis, causing it to elaborate more gonadotropic hormone, which consequently appears in the urine. Goldzieher's conclusion that "the appearance of gonadotropic hormones in the urine signifies the increase in intracranial pressure, the subsidence of which is followed by disappearance of hormone excretion" is not borne out by Riley's findings, for the increased gonadotropin excretion preceded the attack by one to six days, and disappearance of the hormone from the urine coincided with its onset.

It is obvious that little is known of the etiology or the immediate cause of the headache. It seems likely that the mechanism involved is complex, and that nervous, vascular, endocrine, and possibly other factors are implicated. The prevailing lack of agreement may arise out of the fact that the part played by each of these factors varies in different individuals.

Diagnosis.—The diagnosis of migraine is necessarily one of exclusion. Diseases of the brain and nervous system, sinusitis, and ocular disorders should be ruled out. This may be accomplished by a general physical and neurologic examination, roentgenograms of the skull, and ophthalmologic studies. It is also necessary to exclude cephalgias incident to diseases of the endocrine glands, as well as those which are merely an accompaniment of menstrual disorders of the climacteric.

Treatment.—*Immediate Seizure.*—*Ergotamine tartate,* according to competent observers,[4] is effective for the control of the migrainous seizure, but is of little value for the prevention of further attacks. The *dose* is 1 to 5 mg. by mouth followed by 1 to 2 mg. at hourly intervals until a total of 12 mg. is given. For a more rapid effect, a single dose of 0.25 to 0.5 mg. may be administered subcutaneously.

Control of Attacks.—Several observers[5,6,7] have reported improvement following *estrogen, androgen* or a combination of both. Crichlow[5] administered 2000 I.U. of estrone twice weekly by the parenteral route, with apparently good effect. Whether the relief which seems to follow such therapy is due to suppression of a hyperactive pituitary, to capillary dilatation with improvement in the circulation of the brain, as Bühler[6] suggests, or was merely coincidental or due to the psychotherapeutic effect of the treatment, cannot be decided from the evidence at hand. If migraine is due to pituitary hyperactivity secondary to ovarian hypofunction, estrogen would seem to be rational therapy; but if the condition is due to an exaggerated tendency to retain fluid and sodium chloride, this hormone would seem to be contraindicated in view of its apparent ability to promote water and salt retention.[8]

The author has had no success with estrogen or any other form of organotherapy in this condition. *Hygienic measures* supplemented by sedatives may give relief, especially where the sufferer is of the asthenic type, endowed with an inferior constitution and labile nervous system. Freedom from physical, mental and nervous strain is essential to calm the unstable nervous system. A diet of high caloric value, but low in fluid and salt content, may improve the general health of the patient and at the same time minimize any tendency to retain fluids.

The hope that *castration* may relieve some cases has been raised by the observation that migraine sometimes disappears with the onset of the menopause. Alvarez[9] recently concluded that this hope is unfounded. Of thirty-four cases subjected to x-ray or radium castration for reasons other than migraine, a few cases improved, but most remained unchanged, and in a few the condition was aggravated.

PERIODIC EXTRAGENITAL HEMORRHAGE ("VICARIOUS MENSTRUATION")

Definition.—*Vicarious menstruation* describes the periodic extragenital hemorrhage experienced by some women during the reproductive period. It is described as *supplementary* when it occurs shortly before or during the flow, and as *substitutional* when it appears in the amenorrheic woman at the time when the menses would normally be expected. The term "vicarious menstruation" is a misnomer for, except for its periodicity, cyclic extragenital hemorrhage in no way resembles true menstruation. Unlike the latter, it occurs by diapedesis, is unaccompanied by disintegration and desquamation of the affected tissues, and is not preceded by tissue modifications like those of the pregravid endometrium. Moreover, there is no evidence that it replaces or supplements the normal menstrual flow.

Clinical Characteristics.—Cyclic extragenital hemorrhage is very rare. The large majority of the cases are of the supplementary type. Though the condition may arise at any time during the reproductive period, it is most often encountered at the beginning or end of this epoch. It may occur in apparently normal women, but is more apt to affect those with an inherently unstable vascular and nervous system.[1] Such bleeding may follow hysterectomy, and is not uncommon in women with hypoplastic genitalia, or in young amenorrheic girls, particularly those of the asthenic type. It is usually, though not invariably absent during gestation, and ceases at or shortly after the menopause.

The hemorrhage as a rule is slight and of short duration, though in the severe case it may be so profuse as to threaten the health of the individual. It may occur from the inner or outer surfaces of the body, particularly from tissues rich in blood vessels. The most common *site* is the nasal mucous membrane. Less often affected are the stomach, intestines, lungs, nipples, skin, lips, eyes and eyelids, nevi, kidneys, cicatrices, abdominal fistulae, umbilicus, gums, varicose ulcers, and rarely, amputation stumps, the external auditory meatus, nails, and hemorrhoids.

Etiology.—The cause is obscure. Since the bleeding occurs only during menstrual life at the time of the flow, and ceases during pregnancy and after the menopause, it is generally believed to be related in some way to the menstrual process. The precise nature of this relationship is not clear. With increasing knowledge of the endocrine control of the menstrual cycle, attempts have been made to explain this phenomenon on a hormonal basis.

Role of Estrogen.—Some observers attribute vicarious menstruation to a deficiency, others to an excess of estrogen. No systematic attempt has been made to determine whether the estrogen content of the body fluids is consistently high or low in such cases. Those who blame an *estrogen deficiency* point to the fact that extragenital hemorrhage tends to occur in women with amenorrhea or hypomenorrhea, is absent at the mid-cycle when the estrogen level is high, and ceases during pregnancy, when large amounts of this hormone are present in the body fluids. Reports that estrogen therapy helps to control vicarious menstruation, improves gums which bleed easily,[2] and is useful in controlling hemorrhage from the nasal passages following nose and throat surgery,[3] would seem to support this theory and rule out the possibility that an excess of this hormone is responsible.

Indirect support for the view that an *excess of estrogen* is at fault is provided by the observation that cyclic extragenital hemorrhage may begin for the first time following hysterectomy or the suppression of menstruation. It is possible that in both the amenorrheic and hysterectomized woman with extragenital bleeding, estrogen is produced in normal amounts but is not utilized, in one case because the uterus is hypoplastic and therefore unresponsive, in the other because this organ has been removed. As a result, the concentration of estrogen in the circulating blood reaches a point where it can induce bleeding from extragenital tissues which would otherwise remain unaffected. That this hormone is capable of causing dilatation and increasing the permeability of the small blood vessels in the skin and other extragenital tissues such as the nasal mucosa, has been demonstrated by several observers.[4-8] It is noteworthy, however, that in none of the experiments thus far described, did the blood vessel changes thus induced culminate in bleeding. Whether this is attributable to inadequate dosage or the resistant state of the tissues in the experimental animals, or should be taken to signify that estrogen is not the hemorrhage inducing factor, we cannot say.

Role of Progesterone.—Since extragenital bleeding follows the height of the corpus luteum phase, it might be supposed that the luteal hormone is implicated in some way in the etiology. It is noteworthy that the progestational phase of the endometrial cycle is characterized by edema, congestion, and marked dilatation of the endometrial arteries. Progesterone, like estrogen, has been shown to increase the permeability of the capillaries in extragenital tissues.[7] Whether adequate doses of progesterone, acting alone or together with estrogen, can elicit vascular modifications culminating in hemorrhage from such tissues, has not thus far been demonstrated.

Changes in Skin Capillaries.—Though the cause of vicarious menstruation is still a matter of conjecture, recent studies correlating the changes in the skin capillaries and endometrial blood vessels during the menstrual cycle have tended to strengthen the belief that menstruation and periodic extragenital hemorrhage are closely related, and that the same factors may control both. Hagen,[9] who microscopically examined the skin capillaries of normally menstruating women, found that they became increasingly spastic as the time of menstruation approached, but dilated rapidly soon after the onset of the flow. His findings have since been confirmed by Gebert,[10] who demonstrated that the *dermographic latent period*, that is, the time required for the skin capillaries to dilate in response to a given stimulus, rapidly increases during the two days preceding the onset of the flow, reaching its height at the moment menstrual bleeding begins. After this point it decreases rapidly, but once again returns to normal after the second day of the flow. Brewer[11] tested the resistance of the skin capillaries by determining how much suction must be exerted on a given area to cause capillary hemorrhage. He found that in the normally menstruating women, capillary resistance decreased to a varying degree during the premenstruum, dropping rapidly on the first or second day of menstruation. After this it gradually increased again and returned to normal by the second or third day after the flow. He attributes the increased fragility to vascular spasm. These fluctuations in capillary resistance occurred at the expected time of menstruation, despite slight variations in the length of the cycle or the duration of the flow. In irregularly menstruating women, on the other hand, there was no correlation between the capillary alterations and the occurrence of uterine bleeding. In some instances, at the expected time of menstruation, the usual alterations in capillary fragility occurred in association with menstrual molimina but without bleeding from the uterus. Calling attention to Markee's[12] observation that in the monkey recurrent spasms of the uterine vessels begin on the nineteenth day of the ovulatory cycle and become increasingly frequent and prolonged as menstruation approaches, Brewer suggests that the vascular changes in the uterus and those in the skin are closely related. To quote: "Menstruation which is evidenced as a local vascular phenomenon, is in reality a part of a demonstrable generalized vascular phenomenon present in the entire body." His observation that the vascular alterations could be correlated with regular bleeding from a pregravid mucosa but not with irregular bleeding from an estrogenic type of endometrium suggests that their cause is some factor peculiarly associated with the presence of a corpus luteum. Further studies correlating changes in the peripheral blood vessels with the endometrial picture may throw some light on this problem. In view of the negative results recently reported by Reynolds and di Palma,[13] additional evidence corroborating Brewer's findings is desirable.

Granting that vasospasm with consequent increased permeability of the blood vessels of the uterus and extragenital tissues precedes menstruation, and is at least partly responsible for the extragenital hemorrhage which occurs in some women at this time, the cause of these vascular alterations has yet to be identified. The suggestion that it is some substance formed within the regressing endometrium (see Chap. V) cannot be reconciled with the fact that periodic extragenital hemorrhage may begin for the first time following hysterectomy. Whatever the cause, be it estrogen, progesterone, or some as yet unidentified by-product of estrogen and progesterone metabolism, it is conceivable that these vascular changes may lead to diapedetic bleeding from extragenital tissues, which are predisposed to hemorrhage because they are highly vascular, delicately supported, and thinly covered, or are endowed with inherently abnormal blood vessels.

Psychogenic Factors.—Psychogenic factors may also be at least partly responsible for the abnormal response of extragenital blood vessels to otherwise normal stimuli arising premenstrually. This is suggested by the fact that periodic extragenital hemorrhage is particularly apt to occur in women with psychoneurotic instability, and that such women may experience extragenital bleeding at other times than during the premenstruum, if subjected to undue emotional strain. Noteworthy in this connection is the observation of Reynolds and his associates[6] that the ability of estrogen to cause dilatation of the smallest capillaries of the skin, varies with the nervous stability of the individual, and may be improved by psychotherapy and upset by psychic shock.

Overfilling of the Blood Vessels.—Overfilling of the blood vessels, due to failure to discharge the usual amount of blood by way of the uterus, may conceivably be a contributory factor in some cases. This possibility is suggested by the fact that extragenital hemorrhage tends to affect amenorrheic, hypomenorrheic, and hysterectomized women, may sometimes be controlled by venesection, and often ceases following reestablishment of the menses.

Diagnosis.—A history of periodic extragenital hemorrhage at the time of the flow, or at the expected time for menstruation in the amenorrheic woman, is significant, particularly if the patient is free from such bleeding at all other times. Vicarious menstruation may be confused with hemorrhage incident to hemophilia, hemorrhagic purpura, trauma, or other organic causes. The diagnosis is therefore necessarily one of exclusion. A careful history, physical examination, and complete blood studies will usually establish the diagnosis.

Treatment.—The treatment is necessarily empirical. If the bleeding is slight and organic disease has been excluded, no treatment may be necessary. The severe case, on the other hand, may call for various hemostatic measures. The vitamins, particularly C and K, calcium, the ultraviolet rays, viosterol, snake venom, and numerous other agents have been advocated. The estrogens have been employed by some observers with apparently good effect, but others could see no improvement following their use. Where the bleeding point is accessible, cauterization may be tried. In the severe case, venesection may sometimes control the hemorrhage. Whether the favorable effect of this procedure is due to relief of overfilled blood vessels, or removal of an excess of estrogen, progesterone, or some other as yet unidentified hemorrhage inducing substance, we cannot say.

Medical and *general hygienic measures* designed to improve the health of the individual are indicated in any case. In the amenorrheic woman, reestablishment of menstrual function by appropriate means (see Chap. XXIV) may effect a cure of the extragenital bleeding. Reassurance and other measures calculated to quiet an unstable nervous system may also be of value.

BIBLIOGRAPHY

INTERMENSTRUAL PAIN

1. McSweeney, D. J., and Wood, F. O.: New England J. Med. *222*:174, 1940.
2. Priestley, W. O.: Brit. Med. J. *2*:431, 1872.
3. Wharton, L. R., and Henriksen, E.: J.A.M.A. *107*:1425, 1936.
4. Cotte, G.: La Chirurgie du sympathique pelvien en gynecologie. Paris, Masson, 1932.

5. Henriksen, E.: West. J. Surg., Gynec. & Obst. *49*:1, 1941.
6. Reynolds, S. R. M., discussion of C. G. Hartman, in J. Contracep. *2*:51, 1937.
7. Dickinson, R. L.: Am. J. Obst. & Gynec. *32*:828, 1936.
8. Westman, A.: Acta obst. & gynec. Scandinav. *8*:307, 1929.
9. Seguy, J.: Presse Med. *49*:660, 1941.
10. Gueissaz, M. E.: Gynéc. et Obst. *40*:223, 1939.
11. Beclere, in discussion of Gueissaz (*supra* 10).

PREMENSTRUAL TENSION

1. Frank, R. T.: Arch. Neurol. & Psychiat. *26*:1053, 1931.
2. Greenhill, J. P., and Freed, S. C.: J.A.M.A. *117*:504, 1941.
3. Israel, S. L.: J.A.M.A. *110*:1721, 1938.
4. Greenblatt, R. B.: J.A.M.A. *115*:120, 1940.
5. Hamblen, E. C.: Endocrinol. *24*:269, 1939.
6. Gillman, J.: J. Clin. Endocrinol. *2*:157, 1942.
7. Greenhill, J. P., and Freed, S. C.: Endocrinol. *26*:529, 1940.
8. Thorn, G. W., Nelson, K. R., and Thorn, D. W.: Endocrinol. *22*:155, 1938.
9. Pucher, G. W., Griffith, F. R., Jr., Brownell, K. A., Klein, J. D., and Carmer, M. E.: J. Nutrition *7*:131, 1934.
10. Brewer, J. I.: Am. J. Obst. & Gynec. *36*:597, 1938.
11. Reynolds, S. R. M., and di Palma, J. R.: J. Clin. Endocrinol. *2*:226, 1942.
12. Reynolds, S. R. M., Kaminester, S., Foster, F. I., and Schloss, S.: Surg., Gynec. & Obst. *73*:206, 1941.
13. Janeway, M. M.: Med. Woman's J. *46*:597, 1938.
14. Gray, L. A.: South. M. J. *34*:1004, 1941.
15. Geist, S. H.: J. Clin. Endocrinol. *1*:154, 1941.

MIGRAINE

1. Timme, W.: Bull. Neurol. Inst. New York *5*:437, 1936; Proc. A. Res. Nerv. & Ment. Dis. *17*:572, 1938.
2. Goldzieher, M. A.: The Endocrine Glands. New York and London, D. Appleton-Century Co., 1939, p. 480.
3. Riley, H. A., Brickner, R. M., and Kurzrok, R.: J. Nerv. & Ment. Dis. *77*:516, 1933.
4. von Storch, T. J. C.: New England J. Med. *217*:247, 1937.
5. Cricklow, R. S.: New Orleans Med. & Surg. J. *91*:490, 1939.
6. Bühler, F.: Deutsche med. Wchnschr. *65*:1739, 1939.
7. Lange, F.: München. med. Wchnschr. *88*:246, 1940.
8. Thorn, G. W., Nelson, K. R., and Thorn, D. W.: Endocrinol. *22*:155, 1938.
9. Alvarez, W. C.: Proc. Staff Meet., Mayo Clin. *15*:380, 1940.

PERIODIC EXTRAGENITAL HEMORRHAGE ("VICARIOUS MENSTRUATION")

1. Gossip, W. H.: Brit. Med. J. *1*:69, 1937.
2. Ziskin, D. E.: J. Dent. Research *16*:367, 1937.
3. Heinberg, C. J.: Arch. Otolaryngol. *24*:758, 1936.
4. Mortimer, H., Wright, R. P., Bachman, C., and Collip, J. B.: Proc. Soc. Exper. Biol. & Med. *34*:535, 1936; Canad. M. A. J. *35*:503, 1936.
5. Reynolds, S. R. M., and Foster, F. I.: J. Pharmacol. & Exper. Therap. *68*:173, 1940.
6. Reynolds, S. R. M., Kaminester, S., Foster, F. I., and Schloss, S.: Surg., Gynec. & Obst. *73*:206, 1941.
7. Werner, S. C., and Lindner, E.: Am. J. Physiol. *134*:258, 1941.
8. Rupp, H.: Zentralbl. f. Gynäk. *65*:1893, 1941.
9. Hagen, W.: Virch. Arch. f. path. Anat. *239*:504, 1922.
10. Gebert, W.: Klin. Wchnschr. *15*:828, 1936.
11. Brewer, J. I.: Am. J. Obst. & Gynec. *36*:597, 1938.
12. Markee, J. E., 1933, cited by Brewer (*supra* 11).
13. Reynolds, S. R. M., and di Palma, J. R.: J. Clin. Endocrinol. *2*:226, 1942.

CHAPTER XXXI

ABNORMAL MANIFESTATIONS ARISING DURING GESTATION

HYPEREMESIS GRAVIDARUM

Definition.—The term *hyperemesis gravidarum* describes nausea and vomiting of varying intensity experienced by a large percentage of women during the first trimester of gestation.

Etiology.—*Hyperemesis and Eclampsia.*—The etiology is obscure. Observers differ as to whether the early and late toxemias of pregnancy have a common origin. Ewing[1] stresses the similarity of the pathologic lesions in hyperemesis and eclamptic toxemia and maintains that the fundamental lesion in both is necrosis of the liver cells. Others argue that the two conditions are etiologically distinct, because in hyperemesis the necrotic process involves the central lobule, while in eclamptic toxemia it is confined to the peripheral zone. It has been pointed out, however, that eclampsia is not invariably associated with necrosis of the peripheral zone, for at times the central lobule may be involved, or small areas of focal necrosis may be the predominant lesion. Rakoff[2] believes hyperemesis and eclamptic toxemia are etiologically distinct, on the basis of his observation that in late toxemia the gonadotropin content of the blood is above, the estrogen content below normal values. An etiological difference has also been postulated by Hughes,[3] on the ground that the sodium chloride level in the blood and urine differs in the two conditions, and that urine of patients with early and late pregnancy toxemia, when injected into experimental animals, produces different alterations in the thyroid, adrenals, kidney and liver.

Role of Hormones.—A number of observers have attempted to explain nausea and vomiting of early pregnancy on a hormonal basis. Hirst[4] proposed that a deficiency of *corpus luteum hormone* is a causative factor. More recently, Finch[5] suggested that women with hyperemesis gravidarum are allergic to some corpus luteum principle distinct from progesterone. In support of this assumption he points out that symptoms usually appear shortly after the corpus luteum of pregnancy forms, and tend to subside spontaneously about the fourth month when it begins to regress.

Legrand[6] has advanced the theory that the *gonadotropes* are absorbed by the serum proteins in normal pregnancy but not in hyperemesis, and it is the unabsorbed hormone which consequently accumulates in the blood and gives rise to nausea and vomiting. Anselmino[7] attributes hyperemesis to an excess of the so-called "carbohydrate" and "fat-metabolism" principles of the anterior hypophysis (see Chap. XIII). Kemp[8] believes that the malady is due to *adrenal cortical insufficiency*, resulting from the gland's failure to hypertrophy with sufficient rapidity to meet the increasing demands of pregnancy. This he bases on the observations that the maternal adrenal cortex normally hypertrophies during gestation; nausea and vomiting constitute the earliest symptoms of adrenal cortical insufficiency in the adrenalectomized animal; anorexia and morning sickness are the earliest manifestations of Addison's disease; and the postmortem findings in early toxemia of pregnancy, Addison's disease, and the adrenalectomized animal, are identical.

Parathyroid deficiency has also been considered as a possible etiologic factor.[9] A number of observers have reported low serum calcium values in early pregnancy toxemia, but the findings have been too inconstant to warrant any conclusions.

Quantitative determinations of the gonadotropin, estrogen and pregnanediol content of the body fluids have been of little help in the solution of this problem. Studies of the serum gonadotropin have yielded high,[10, 11] normal,[12] and low values. The results of urine tests have been equally conflicting.[13, 14, 15] Values for estrogen and pregnanediol have been recorded in only a limited number of cases. Rakoff[2] found the estrogen content of the blood normal. In the urine, both low[16] and normal[17] levels have been observed. According to Browne and associates,[18] the pregnanediol level of the urine is within normal limits.

Treatment.—The therapeutic agents advocated for this condition are too numerous to list here. Among those which have found favor in recent years are adrenal cortical extract, parathyroid hormone, estrogen, progesterone, thyroid substance, and the gonadotropic hormones. Dominance of the psychic factor in hyperemesis, and the fact that the symptoms usually subside spontaneously after a varying period of time, makes it difficult to evaluate any form of treatment. In the author's experience, reassurance, psychotherapy, and sedation, supplemented by restorative therapy, particularly glucose, sodium chloride, water and the essential vitamins, have given far better results than may be claimed for any of the endocrine products.

LATE TOXEMIAS OF PREGNANCY

Definition.—The term "late toxemia of pregnancy" describes a symptom-complex encountered during the third trimester of gestation. The more severe forms of the malady are known as *preeclampsia* and *eclampsia*. The former is characterized by albuminuria, hypertension, oliguria, edema, precordial pain, headache, visual disturbances and various nervous manifestations. In the latter, this symptomatology is very much exaggerated and convulsions appear. This form of the disease may be fatal.

ETIOLOGY

The etiology is obscure. During the last two decades many observers have attempted to relate the malady to some endocrine disorder. Disturbances of the hypophysis, parathyroids, adrenals, thyroid, and placenta have been considered as possible causative factors. Despite the considerable literature that has accumulated, there is no valid evidence directly linking the incretory glands with the late toxemias of pregnancy. It should be emphasized that any attempt to implicate a particular gland must prove that (1) its secretory products are either deficient, excessive or perverted; (2) that the altered function is due to some fault inherent in the gland and not merely secondary to some condition prevailing elsewhere in the organism, and (3) that a similar glandular disturbance, if experimentally induced, will give rise to typical toxemic manifestations. In no case have all these prerequisites been fulfilled.

Role of the Posterior Hypophysis.—Hofbauer,[1] in 1918, first proposed that an excess of the *vasopressor and antidiuretic principle* of the posterior hypophysis is an important link in the chain of effects leading to preeclampsia and eclampsia. Proof of this hypothesis is still lacking. Cushing[2] called attention to massive basophil cell infiltration in the posterior hypophysis in fatal cases of eclampsia and suggested a causal relationship. Other competent observers[3-4] could find no constant relationship between the degree of basophil cell infiltration and the presence or absence of hypertension. Fauvet[5] described liver and kidney lesions, similar to those seen in women dying of eclampsia, in guinea pigs subjected to protracted treatment with posterior lobe extract. Scheps[6] was unable to duplicate these effects, though he used larger doses over a more protracted period of time. Byrom[7] observed morbid effects, including eclamptic-like manifestations in the rat following repeated injections of vasopressin. Though his findings lend some support to the theory that the lesions of preeclampsia and eclampsia are due to vasospasm, he admits that they do not necessarily prove that the vasospasm is attributable to a simple oversecretion of vasopressin. Sullivan and Heffernan[8] have recently reported the appearance of postpartum convulsions in an apparently non-toxic parturient patient following the intravenous administration of 3 minims of posterior pituitary extract.

Attempts to demonstrate the presence of a pituitrin-like substance in the body fluids of eclamptic women have yielded conflicting results. Anselmino and his associates[9] obtained from the blood of eclamptic women a substance possessing both vasopressor and antidiuretic properties. Its concentration varied in direct proportion to the severity of the symptoms. Page[10] and Dexter and Weiss[11] were unable to corroborate their report. Teel and Reid[12] found that concentrates of urine, collected from preeclamptic women during the phase of acute water retention, exerted a marked antidiuretic effect in rats. The urine of normal pregnant women possessed little or no antidiuretic activity, but when such women were first dehydrated by withholding water, their urine acquired antidiuretic activity comparable to that of preeclamptics. These observers concluded that this pituitrin-like substance, acting in excessive amounts on the kidney, or perhaps inadequately opposed by an antagonist, offers an immediate mechanism for the water retention of preeclampsia and eclampsia. It should be emphasized that, even if it is granted that late pregnancy toxemia is associated with an excess of vasopressor and antidiuretic substances in the blood and urine, we are not justified in concluding that posterior pituitary hyperactivity is the primary cause, for there is as yet no conclusive proof that these blood-borne substances are derived from this gland.[13]

In a recent communication, Hofbauer[14] reiterated his theory with additional details based on evidence now available. He calls attention to the consistent occurrence in the normal placenta of remarkable quantities of acetylcholine. This, he believes, acts as a potent vasodilator through its restraining influence on the tone of the vascular musculature, and offsets the effect of vasopressin, and of the estrogenic and gonadotropic hormones as well as certain split proteins, which increase the vascular reactivity to vasopressin. He suggests that a disturbance of the delicate balance between blood pressure activating and restraining principles, peculiar to normal gestation, constitutes the real determinant in the pathogenesis of toxemia, but he makes no attempt to identify the factor or factors capable of upsetting this balance.

Role of the Thyroid Gland.—In view of the thyroid's role in the regulation of water metabolism (see Chap. XVI), a *deficiency* of its specific hormone may conceivably be a contributory cause of the water retention which is so prominent a feature of late pregnancy toxemia. Support for this supposition is provided by reports[15, 16, 17] that a low basal metabolic rate is often encountered during early pregnancy in women who subsequently develop toxemic symptoms. Hughes[18] observed that preeclampsia tends to develop when the basal rate is abnormally low in the first trimester and fails to rise during the course of pregnancy, or drops to a low value in early pregnancy and remains so thereafter. These findings are significant in view of the evidence that the basal metabolic rate normally tends to be low during early pregnancy but gradually increases as gestation advances. Among a group of more than 500 women receiving routine prenatal care, preeclampsia and eclampsia developed in 5.2 per cent of the cases. In a second group of approximately the same size, where routine measures were supplemented by thyroid therapy in cases with a low basal metabolic rate, only 2.5 per cent developed toxemia.

How hypothyroidism leads to toxemic symptoms is not clear. According to one theory[17, 19] it causes hypercholesteremia, which induces vascular changes in the placenta with consequent degeneration and formation of toxins. These presumably cause the toxemic manifestations.

Role of the Adrenal Cortex.—Both *over-* and *underfunction* of the adrenal cortex has been blamed for late pregnancy toxemia. According to Hofbauer,[20] hyperactivity of both the posterior hypophysis and adrenal cortex may be at fault. Fauvet[21] blames adrenal cortical insufficiency on the basis of his observation that the adrenal cortex of the toxemic patient markedly diminishes in size, instead of undergoing hypertrophy as in the normal pregnant woman. The fact that the clinical picture of late pregnancy toxemia is in many respects opposite to that which characterizes adrenal cortical insufficiency (see Chap. XXXV), argues against this possibility.

The Parathyroids.—That parathyroid *deficiency* may be a cause is suggested by the observation that eclampsia is not infrequently associated with low serum calcium levels and that the convulsions resemble those of maternal tetany due to hypocalcemia. Apparently supporting this possibility is Lopez'[22] report that parathyroid hormone is effective therapy in some cases.

Role of the Placenta.—The fact that preeclamptic and eclamptic manifestations occur only during pregnancy and often disappear dramatically soon after delivery or fetal death, suggests that the cause may be some factor emanating from the products of conception. The observation that eclamptic manifestations may appear in molar pregnancy, would seem to eliminate the fetus as the source of this hypothetical factor. Recent attempts to implicate the placenta in the etiology have been inspired by evidence that this organ is the source of most of the gonadotropic, estrogenic and progestational hormones present during gestation, and that the balance of these hormones is disturbed in the toxemic patient. On the basis of extensive quantitative hormone determinations carried out since 1932, Smith and Smith[23, 24, 25] have evolved the following hypothesis: In normal pregnancy, during the third and fourth month, the gonadotropin level falls, coincident with a sharp rise in estrogen, and progestin's excretion product, pregnanediol. The rise in estrogen and progestin production is due to the fact that the placenta takes over the task of elaborating these hormones at this time. The fall in gonadotropin is taken to signify that this hormone is being utilized by the placenta for the production of estrogen and progestin. In toxemic pregnancy, the gonadotropin level is high while that of estrogen and progestin is subnormal. This signifies abnormal utilization of gonadotropin for the production of estrogen and progestin, with consequent deficiency of the latter. The deficiency of progestin, which normally protects estrogen against destruction, permits its rapid destruction. Toxic concentration of nonestrogenic breakdown products resulting from the disturbance in estrogen metabolism, they believe, is responsible for the vascular phenomena of toxemia. These investigators make no attempt to identify the cause of abnormal utilization of gonadotropin by the placenta.

Though several other investigators have likewise demonstrated excessive amounts of gonadotropin in the body fluids of patients with late pregnancy toxemia,[26, 27, 28] a few have found the values normal[29] or low.[30] In a critical study, Taylor and Scadron[31] found that the general average and range for gonadotropin in the blood and urine of toxemic patients were not significantly different from those in normal controls, though the values were a little high in some severe cases presenting all the manifestations of preeclamptic toxemia. Equally divergent are the results of estrogen[32, 33, 34] and pregnanediol[35, 36] determinations.

While the available evidence suggests that a rise in gonadotropin and fall in estrogen and pregnanediol often accompany late pregnancy toxemia, the significance of these findings is not clear. It should be borne in mind that the level of a particular hormone in the body fluids depends on the rate of its production, utilization, inactivation or destruction, and probably also on other as yet undetermined variables. It is obviously difficult to decide which of these is operating abnormally in a given case. Thus, while Smith and Smith consider the low pregnanediol values evidence of progestin deficiency secondary to decreased utilization of gonadotropin, Browne and his associates suggest that it may signify retention of the sterols due to failure of their conjugation with glucuronic acid. For the present, we can only speculate as to whether the altered hormonal conditions are directly or indirectly responsible for the toxemic symptoms, or whether both are independent manifestations of some renal, hepatic, or placental disturbance.

TREATMENT

There is as yet no convincing evidence that organotherapy favorably affects this malady. Estrogen, progesterone, or a combination of both, are advocated by some workers.[28, 37] The results thus far reported are inconstant and inconclusive. According to Brandstrup,[38] estrogen therapy may benefit some and aggravate the symptomatology in others. Taylor[39] could see no improvement after massive doses of estradiol benzoate and progesterone.

Parathyroid hormone has also been recommended for the control of preeclamptic toxemia.[40] As a prophylactic measure, some observers advocate the use of thyroid substance and iodine.[41] Hofbauer[42] stresses the importance of preserving liver function. It should be emphasized that all these measures are empiric and will remain so until the cause of this malady is determined.

ENDOCRINE ASPECTS OF DYSTOCIA

Definition.—The term *dystocia* describes prolonged, difficult, and painful labor. True primary dystocia is relatively rare, occurring in less than 2 per cent of the cases. Most competent observers believe the majority of cases so diagnosed are in reality the result of hasty and injudicious obstetrical intervention.[1]

ETIOLOGY

Fetal and Maternal Causes.—The immediate cause may be some maternal or fetal abnormality which prevents or materially slows down the passage of the fetus through the birth canal. So-called fetal dystocia may result from abnormal size, position or shape of the fetus. The maternal causes include an abnormally small pelvic outlet, inability of the uterus to contract with sufficient force to expel the fetus, and resistance of the soft parts.

Effects of Endocrine Disturbances.—In the light of our present knowledge of the role of the endocrine glands in somatic growth, sexual development, and reproductive function, many cases of dystocia would seem to be at least partly due to abnormal function of one or more members of the endocrine system.

Over-Sized Fetus.—It has been suggested that, in some cases, an over-sized fetus may be the result of maternal hypothyroidism.[2] According to this view, fetal overweight is not due to maternal dietary excesses and cannot be controlled by food restriction, but is attributable to fetal hypothyroidism secondary to deficiency of the maternal thyroid. It has also been suggested that hypofunction of the maternal thyroid may lead to dystocia by postponing the onset of labor so that the fetus is oversized by the time parturition begins.

Abnormal Pelvis.—Maternal abnormalities, such as contracted or abnormal pelvis, and undue rigidity of the soft parts, which make for dystocia, may at times be traceable to endocrine disorders arising during the juvenile or puberal era. Since the incretory glands, particularly the anterior pituitary, thyroid, and parathyroids, play an important part in skeletal growth, it is conceivable that a disturbance in their function during the formative period of development may adversely affect the skeleton as a whole and the pelvic bones in particular. It is noteworthy that abnormalities of pelvic development are a characteristic of pituitary and thyroid dwarfism, while a masculine type of pelvis is common in the heterosexual type of woman with adrenal cortical hyperfunction. Weysser[3] elicited a history of delayed menarche in a large percentage of a group of women with dystocia due to a narrow pelvis. Whether the undersized pelvis is due to a deficiency of the ovarian sex hormones arising at the time when the pelvis undergoes its final growth spurt, or both the delayed menarche and narrow pelvis are independent manifestations of some deficiency in the anterior pituitary or other glands on which somatic and sexual maturity depend, is not certain.

Undue rigidity of the sacro-iliac joints may be attributable, in some cases, to disordered endocrine function. It has been shown experimentally that separation of the pelvic ligaments, which precedes and facilitates parturition in the guinea pig, depends on a hormonal substance secreted by the corpus luteum (see Chap. III). In the pregnant woman, the pelvic ligaments do not actually separate but become considerably loosened with advancing gestation.[4, 5] The demonstration of relaxin in the blood during pregnancy[6] suggests that similar hormonal stimuli are responsible for this alteration. Whether the immobility of the pelvic ligaments, which makes for difficult labor in some women, particularly elderly primiparae, is attributable to hormonal deficiency, or refractoriness of the tissues, we cannot say.

Resistance of the Soft Parts.—Resistance of the soft parts, due to hypoplasia of the cervix and vagina, may possibly be referable to some endocrine disturbance originating early in life. As Sackett[7] points out, cervical dystocia, in the absence of trauma or disease affecting the cervix, occurs in elderly primigravidae with a menstrual and marital history, general habitus, and local findings suggestive of constitutional deficiency and genital underdevelopment. Of interest in this connection is DeLee's[8] description of *dystrophia dystocia*, a syndrome usually encountered in elderly primiparae with a history of menstrual irregularities and dysmenorrhea. Such women are as a rule below average height, squatty and obese, have a coarse skin, show a tendency to hirsutism, and are phlegmatic. Their bones are thick and their fingers spade-like. The external genitalia may be normally developed, but the vagina is hypoplastic and its walls inelastic and of rubbery consistency. The bones of the pelvis are thick, the symphysis deep, and there is a slight narrowing of the pubic arch, though the measurements suggest an ample pelvis. The wide trochanteric diameter is considered a distinguishing feature. These individuals do not conceive readily and pregnancy is attended by an exaggeration of all the manifestations which would normally accompany it. Labor as a rule is prolonged, painful and exhausting. The membranes often rupture early and harrowing pains are associated with weak, ineffectual contractions. Dilatation of the cervix proceeds very slowly and may be incomplete, even after four days of labor. The dystocia in such cases is apparently due to a resistant cervix and narrow pelvic outlet. The primary cause of "dystrophia dystocia" is not clear. The retarded accessory genitalia, menstrual disturbances, lowered fertility, skeletal changes, adiposity and hirsutism, suggest a disturbance in the anterior hypophysis, and possibly also the adrenal cortex and other glands.

Uterine Inertia.—Uterine inertia, a term applied to slow and prolonged labor ascribable to ineffectual uterine contractions, is usually encountered in primiparae and elderly multiparae. In true primary inertia, the contractions are weak from the start and, as labor proceeds, tend to become progressively weaker, irregular and infrequent, eventually ceasing altogether. It has been suggested that weak uterine contractions may be due to some condition residing within the uterus. Paralysis of the nerve centers controlling uterine contractions, abnormal shape and position of the organ, or weakening and stretching of the musculature caused by oft repeated gestations, have been suggested as possible causes. In the absence of local defects, primary inertia may conceivably be due to some disturbance in the hormonal stimuli responsible for the initiation and maintenance of parturition. On the basis of our present understanding of this phenomenon (see Chap. IX), the fault may lie in a deficiency of estrogen, a relative or absolute excess of progestin, or a deficiency of some oxytocic factor of placental or posterior pituitary origin. In support of the last possibility, it has been pointed out that uterine inertia is not infrequently associated with low blood pressure, and that *posterior lobe* extracts may cause a resumption of uterine contractions, provided the uterine muscle is not already exhausted. That a *deficiency of estrogen* may be at least a contributory cause of uterine inertia is suggested by experiments demonstrating that this hormone increases the vascularity and oxygen consumption of the uterus, causes hypertrophy of the uterine musculature, coordinates and increases the power of spontaneous uterine contractions, and heightens myometrial reactivity to oxytocic agents (see Chap. VI). The observation[9] that the estrogen content of the body fluids normally increases rapidly and steadily with the approach of term is suggestive, but there is as yet no proof that uterine inertia is associated with subnormal estrogen values. On the contrary, there are reports[10, 11] that the estrogen content of the blood does not differ significantly from that of normal labor. Reports[12, 13] of the successful termination of labor, following large doses of estrogen, in cases of uterine inertia are unconvincing because in most cases other measures, to which the improvement might be ascribed, were used concurrently. Moreover, the possibility that labor might have set in when it did without treatment was not satisfactorily excluded.

The supposition that a relative or absolute *excess of progestin* may

30

explain some of the cases is based on evidence that this hormone exerts a quiescent effect on the uterine musculature (see Chap. VI). This possibility must remain purely conjectural, for there is as yet no evidence that uterine inertia is associated with an abnormally high concentration of progestin. The observation of Rosenkranz[14] that prolonged pregnancy is associated with a normal amount of progestin and half the normal amount of estrogen in the placenta is not directly in point, but it suggests that uterine inertia may be associated with a relative rather than an absolute excess of the progestational hormone.

It has been suggested that some cases of uterine inertia may be due to a *deficiency* of *serum calcium,* which some observers consider essential for effectual uterine contractions. Abnormal function of the parathyroid and other glands indirectly concerned in calcium metabolism may be at fault in such cases.

DIAGNOSIS

It is of the utmost importance to recognize, early in gestation, the type of labor to be expected. Aside from the presence of a contracted pelvis or some other mechanical obstruction in the generative tract, information relating to a tendency to large babies, or former difficult or prolonged labors may be of value in the management of the impending labor. The constitutional pattern of the patient and the presence of endocrinopathic stigmata may serve as important clues. The time of onset of puberty and the menarche, the subsequent menstrual history, and developmental status of the pelvis and accessory genitalia should be carefully noted with the view of recognizing "dystrophia dystocia." A basal metabolism test may be of value in establishing the status of thyroid function, and determination of the serum calcium may serve as a guide to therapy. Quantitative estimations of the sex hormone content of the blood and urine are of little value in the diagnosis, for there is no proof that the concentration of estrogen, pregnanediol or gonadotropin can serve as a reliable clue to the type of uterine activity which may be expected at the time of parturition.[15] As a *test of labor* in uterine inertia, Weisman[16] employs 1 mg. of estradiol dipropionate intramuscularly at hourly intervals for 6 doses. If there is no response after ten hours, he concludes that spontaneous labor is unlikely. Convincing proof of the reliability of this method is still lacking.

TREATMENT

General Medical Measures.—Where the pelvis is small or the history reveals a tendency to large babies, a restricted diet and, if the basal metabolic rate is low, small doses of thyroid substance, may be prescribed. In the anemic patient or one who has been weakened by the strain of vomiting, rest, ample nourishment, and other hygienic measures calculated to improve the general health, are important. If the serum calcium is low, calcium salts, vitamin D, or small doses of parathormone may be tried.

As term approaches, the patient, particularly if of nervous temperament, should be reassured and kept calm in order to avoid the inhibitory effect of fear on the uterine contractions. With the onset of labor, the accoucheur should adopt a policy of watchful waiting. The duration of labor is no reliable criterion of its progress, for the time required for normal labor varies considerably. The decision to intervene depends on the condition of the mother and fetus, and the accoucheur's judgment as to the probable outcome. To conserve the patient's strength, she should be reassured and warned against undue efforts at expulsion. Nourishing liquid foods at frequent intervals or, if not retained, glucose by the intravenous route may be necessary to fortify her and insure effectual uterine contractions. Analgesia is indicated where the pains are ineffectual and the patient exhausted. A needed rest will often be followed by resumption of uterine contractions. In primary uterine inertia, sedatives should be used with caution lest they further depress an already weakly contracting uterus and stop labor pains altogether. Some observers[17] believe the intravenous administration of calcium gluconate is worth a trial.

Organotherapy.—*Posterior Hypophyseal Extracts.*—Posterior lobe extracts have been used to induce labor or stimulate contractions in uterine inertia. They are *contraindicated* for weak contractions in the presence of disproportion, because of the danger of a retraction ring. In primary uterine inertia of the nonobstructive type, the oxytocics may be used judiciously after conservative measures have failed. They should be administered only after the uterus has been given a chance to rest by means of sedatives, and only if dilatation is far advanced. One minim at 20 to 30 minute intervals for several doses[18] may induce regular, rhythmic and effectual contractions. The physician should be prepared to administer an anesthetic at the first sign of uterine tetany, or if any ill effects on the mother or child become apparent.

Estrogenic Substances.—The estrogens are advocated by some observers as a stimulant for weak uterine contractions. Their efficacy is difficult to determine from the available evidence because in most of the cases other agents, such as pituitrin and quinine, were administered simultaneously or soon after estrogen treatment. Nor has any systematic attempt been made to determine, by use of controls, in what proportion of the "successful" cases the increase in uterine motility was spontaneous.

Jeffcoate[12, 19] has reported a favorable response following the injection of 2 mg. of estradiol benzoate at hourly intervals for 10 doses or at eight hour intervals for seven or eight days. Stilbestrol by mouth in doses of 2 mg. three times a day, or 1 mg. every four hours for seven or eight days also proved effective in a large proportion of his cases. In fourteen women with weak uterine contractions, Kepp[20] observed stronger uterine movements and increased reactivity to pituitrin and quinine after the injection of estrogenic substance in doses ranging from 30,000 to 250,000 units. Lubin and Waltman[21] administered estrogen without any other form of therapy to thirty-six women and concluded that the onset of labor could fairly be attributed to the hormone in eight or possibly twelve cases. Schurger[22] found that while medical induction of labor was effective in only 50 per cent of his cases, the addition of estrogen to the treatment increased the proportion of successful results to 80 per cent. Abarbanel[23] obtained a satisfactory response in two out of three cases of uterine inertia with a total dose of 100 to 150 mg. of stilbestrol by mouth, followed by a potent oxytocic, but not with stilbestrol alone. No untoward effects were noted.

On the whole, the use of estrogen in uterine inertia is worth a trial, for it has a rational basis and, so far as can be judged from the available clinical reports, is harmless. Its value as a direct stimulant of uterine contractions is questionable, but the evidence seems to justify the conclusion that it may prove of value as a priming agent, preparatory to the use of oxytocics.

MATERNAL TETANY

Definition.—Maternal tetany describes a symptom-complex characterized by abnormal excitability of the nervous system, painful muscular spasms, and convulsions, which may appear during pregnancy, the puerperium, or lactation. Klaften[1] found only ten cases in a series of 28,302 births. The malady is most apt to arise during the last few months of gestation. Of sixty-one cases collected by Frankl-Hochwart,[2] twenty-three were affected in the course of gestation, ten following delivery, and twenty-eight during lactation. Maternal tetany is seldom encountered during the first pregnancy, but once it appears, the affected individual becomes suceptible to attacks during subsequent gestations.

ETIOLOGY

Parathyroid Insufficiency.—Maternal tetany is generally conceded to be due to parathyroid insufficiency. A situation analogous to that in human maternal tetany has been observed in partially parathyroidectomized animals, which tend to remain symptomless until the advent of pregnancy or lactation, when manifest tetany develops. The tetanic manifestations are generally attributed to the profound strain on the calcium regulating mechanism during pregnancy and lactation. This is strikingly shown in Kozelka and Hart's[3] observation that the amount of viosterol required to maintain the serum calcium and phosphorus at a normal level, rises from 13 rat units daily in the nonpregnant animal to over 26,000 rat units in the pregnant animal at term, and 60,000 units during lactation. When this added burden is placed on a normal parathyroid gland, it responds with heightened activity, as suggested by Hoffmann's[4] report that the blood of normal pregnant women contains demonstrable quantities of parathyroid hormone. The concentration of this hormone increases slightly up to the eighth month, rises rapidly thereafter to a peak at term, and disappears soon after parturition. Despite the increased production of this calcium-mobilizing hormone, the serum calcium normally falls during pregnancy and lactation,[5] probably because calcium is utilized more rapidly than it can be mobilized. Where the parathyroid gland is for some reason incapable of satisfying the extraordinary demands placed on it, sub-tetanic or tetanic manifestations appear.[6, 7]

Mechanism.—While it is generally agreed that tetany is due to parathyroid insufficiency, the mechanism involved is not clear. It was earlier believed that the symptoms are caused by toxic substances, particularly methyl guanidin, which accumulate in the blood because the organism is unable to metabolize these derivatives of protein metabolism in the absence of the parathyroid hormone. This so-called toxic theory was based on the finding of excessive amounts of guanidin in the blood and urine of parathyroprivic animals, and women with manifest tetany, and the observation that tetanic symptoms can be elicited in animals by administering this substance. It lost favor, however, when it became apparent that the symptoms induced by administering guanidin differed from those of tetany, and the methods used to detect this substance in the blood and urine were unreliable. The toxic theory was finally abandoned when MacCallum and Voegtlin[8] demonstrated that parathyroidectomy is followed almost immediately by a drop in the concentration of serum calcium. This observation was the starting point for the many significant studies which form the basis of our present concept of parathyroid physiology. It is now well established that parathyroid ablation leads to hypocalcemia and manifest tetany, which can be prevented or corrected by administering parathyroid hormone or by means of parathyroid transplants. There is still some uncertainty as to whether the hypocalcemia is the immediate cause of the tetanic manifestations, or both are secondary to some other metabolic disturbance, possibly the retention of inorganic phosphorus.

Causes.—Parathyroid deficiency may result from inflammatory or degenerative lesions, vascular faults, primary or metastatic neoplasms of the gland, or atrophy due to pressure exerted by large thyroid neoplasms. Partial extirpation of parathyroid tissue, incident to thyroidectomy, may account for some cases. Exposure to cold or dampness, ergot or chloroform poisoning, infectious diseases, and traumatic bleeding during labor have been mentioned as contributing causes. Tetanic symptoms have been known to follow uterine contractions induced by suckling, or by inserting a finger into the cervical canal.[9]

A considerable proportion of patients with maternal tetany present no apparent anatomic alterations of the parathyroids. The symptomatology here may perhaps best be explained on a *functional* basis. Conceivably, the parathyroid hypofunction may be secondary to disturbances in other members of the endocrine system, notably the adenohypophysis. Of interest in this connection is the observation of Anselmino and associates[10] that anterior pituitary gland tissue yields a "parathyrotropic" principle capable of inducing parathyroid hypertrophy and hyperplasia of the chief cells, and thus indirectly affecting the serum calcium. Also significant is Houssay and Sammartino's[11] observation that atrophic changes of the parathyroids follow hypophyseal ablation in the dog. On the other hand, more recent studies (see Chap. XIII) have tended to cast doubt on the existence of this principle.

CLINICAL MANIFESTATIONS

Tetany encountered during pregnancy, the puerperium, or lactation, like that arising in the nonpregnant woman, may be acute, latent, or chronic.

Acute or Manifest Tetany.—Manifest tetany is clinically characterized by painful and often powerful muscular spasms, particularly of the extremities. In some instances, the face, trunk, tongue, esophagus, larynx, bronchi, diaphragm, and even the myocardium are affected. The tetanic contractions sometimes appear suddenly and without warning, but more often are preceded by restlessness, nervous irritability, paresthesias, and twitchings of the extremities. The most characteristic signs of manifest tetany are carpopedal contractures and the so-called "obstetrical" position of the hands. In the severe case, the entire skeletal musculature may be affected. Perhaps the gravest manifestation is cardiospasm, which may be fatal. Strabismus, nystagmus, and inequality of the pupils have been reported. In some instances, the muscular contractions may be so severe and painful as to render the patient unconscious. Though the convulsions as a rule are bilateral, they may be limited to one side of the body, or one group of muscles.

The serum calcium, in the acute form of the disease, is usually below 7 mg. per cent and may drop to 4 mg. per cent.

Latent Tetany.—The latent form of the disease is unattended by symptoms. Affected individuals nevertheless show a marked predisposition to manifest tetany, responding with typical manifestations of nervous hyperirritability to mechanical or electrical excitation of the peripheral nerve of the extremities and face (see Diagnosis).

Chronic Tetany.—Under certain circumstances, manifest or latent tetany may persist and become chronic. Chronic tetany is particularly apt to occur in individuals whose parathyroids have been injured or partially destroyed by surgery or disease. In some instances inadequate therapy, or a diet rich in phosphorus and poor in calcium may be the underlying cause. Though unattended by severe manifestations which threaten life, the disease is characterized by troublesome trophic changes. The more conspicuous findings include loss of hair, brittleness, loosening and deformities of the nails, decalcification of the dentine and absorption of the enamel, with attendant pitting and horizontal ridge formation of the teeth, and cataract formations.

DIAGNOSIS

Manifest Tetany.—Manifest tetany can usually be recognized with little difficulty. The typical carpopedal contractures and convulsions, heightened excitability of the neuromuscular system, low serum calcium, high inorganic phosphorus, and immediate alleviation of the threatening symptoms by calcium and parathormone therapy clearly point to this condition.

Latent Tetany.—Latent tetany may be recognized by Chvostek's[12] sign, Trousseau's[13] phenomenon, Erb's[14] sign, and by quantitative estimations of the serum calcium and inorganic phosphorus. *Chvostek's sign* sometimes termed the facial phenomenon, is obtained by tapping the superficial portions of the facial nerves with fingers or percussion hammer. In latent tetany, this manipulation causes marked contraction of the facial muscles innervated by these nerves. *Trousseau's phenomenon* is elicited by compressing the nerves and blood vessels of the upper arm by means of a tourniquet, or sleeve of a sphygmomanometer, which suppresses the circulation temporarily. If latent tetany is present, this procedure will produce a peculiar contracture of the hand and fingers, commonly known as the "obstetrical" hand. *Erb's sign* is evoked by stimulating the ulnar or other peripheral nerves with the galvanic current. The amount of current required to elicit a neuromuscular response in latent tetany is less than in the normal individual.

The *serum calcium* in latent tetany is subnormal, but seldom falls below 7 mg. per cent.

The patient's response to changes in the calcium and phosphorus intake may also serve as a reliable criterion of latent tetany. When affected individuals are maintained on diets containing relatively more phosphorus than calcium, phosphates are retained in the body fluids, the level of the serum calcium falls, the amount of calcium and phosphorus excreted in the urine and feces is markedly diminished, and symptoms of manifest tetany appear. This test should be carried out in a hospital and under constant supervision, and calcium and parathormone medication should be available for immediate intravenous use in the event that signs of impending manifest tetany appear.

Chronic Tetany.—Chronic tetany may be suspected where there is a history of thyroidectomy or recurrent attacks of manifest tetany. With the trophic modifications, these criteria suffice for the diagnosis. Slit lamp examination of the eye is important in the suspected case, for it may reveal incipient cataract formation long before it can be demonstrated by any other method.

Differential Diagnosis.—Parathyroprivic tetany is to be distinguished from tetany unrelated to parathyroid involvement, and from hysteria, epilepsy, tetanus, strychnine poisoning, uremia, and other conditions associated with muscular spasms and convulsions.

In *hysteria*, there may sometimes occur muscular contractures which closely resemble those seen in parathyroprivic tetany. Moreover, Trousseau's phenomenon and, in some cases, Chvostek's sign may be elicited, though both these reactions are mild as compared with those obtained in tetany. Consequently, the quantitative estimation of calcium and inorganic phosphorus is necessarily the only reliable aid in the differential diagnosis.

In *tetanus*, the convulsions affect the entire body, whereas general involvement is rare in tetany. Contractures of the hands, so conspicuous in tetany, are absent in tetanus. In the latter malady, the masseter muscles are involved early and the reflexes are markedly increased. Furthermore, Chvostek's, Trousseau's, and Erb's signs are absent. A history of skin injury, a positive blood culture, and normal serum calcium definitely confirm the diagnosis of tetanus.

Epilepsy may offer difficulty in the differential diagnosis, for it is sometimes associated with tetany. The presence of tongue scars, and urinary or fecal incontinence during the attack speak for epilepsy. A normal serum calcium and the inefficacy of calcium or parathormone therapy in controlling the attack establish the diagnosis.

Strychnine poisoning may cause a muscular spasm which begins with a clonic contraction that soon becomes tonic. In contrast to tetany, the muscles relax between paroxysms. A history of strychnine medication in overdose, and a normal blood chemistry are sufficient to confirm the diagnosis.

Uremic poisoning may be confused with tetany only when the muscular contractions and convulsions are associated with a secondary hypocalcemia caused by phosphate retention. A history of renal disease, the presence of hypertension, arteriosclerosis, and retinal hemorrhages point to renal involvement. Studies of the chemistry of the blood and urine will dispel any doubt.

Convulsions of *eclampsia* may simulate those seen in maternal tetany. Negative facial and electrical phenomena, a normal blood calcium, and the inefficacy of calcium therapy readily distinguish these conditions.

Course and Prognosis

In severe cases of manifest maternal tetany, the life of both mother and fetus may be threatened. Not infrequently, the child is born in a macerated condition or, if born alive, may develop acute tetany a few days after birth and die. In such cases the termination of pregnancy does not check the disease in the mother. Nor does severe tetany arising during lactation subside after weaning. In the mild case, on the other hand, the tetanic manifestations may cease following the termination of pregnancy. Mild *lactation tetany* may either subside spontaneously despite continued suckling, or persist until the child is removed from the breast.

The initial attack of manifest tetany often predisposes the individual to recurrent attacks, particularly in the event of a subsequent pregnancy. In the untreated case of parathyroid hypofunction, attacks of manifest tetany may appear if the weakened gland is subjected to the undue stress of pregnancy, lactation, or faulty diet.

Treatment

Diet.—A history of latent or manifest tetany following thyroidectomy calls for special pre- and postnatal care. It is of prime importance to maintain an adequate calcium balance. This may be accomplished by prescribing a diet rich in calcium and poor in phosphorus. Foods rich in phosphorus, such as meats, milk, cheese, and the yolk of eggs, should be restricted, and those ample in calcium substituted. Milk, though an excellent source of calcium, is also rich in phosphorus and should therefore be used in limited amounts. The observation that maternal tetany is most likely to occur during the first four months of the year suggests that a lack of green vegetables and sunlight are predisposing causes. It is therefore well to expose the patient to as much direct sunlight as possible or, if this is not feasible, to use the ultra-violet lamp and irradiated foods. Vitamin D in doses of 10 to 15 drops daily, either alone or together with 5 gr. of calcium gluconate, may suffice to prevent manifest tetany.

Medical Measures.—Frequent blood calcium determinations should be made throughout gestation to guard against a low concentration of serum calcium, or avoid a state of hypercalcemia, which may follow excessive calcium and vitamin D intake. The patient should be instructed to report to her physician such sub-tetanic manifestations as paresthesias, tingling or twitching of the extremities, undue irritability, and insomnia.

Acute low calcium tetany calls for immediate administration of *calcium,* preferably the gluconate salt. In the severe cases, 20 cc. of a 10 per cent solution should be administered by the intravenous route, care being taken that it is warm and injected very slowly. While this may control the tetanic manifestations, it gives only temporary relief and must therefore be repeated at intervals of three or four hours. 10 to 20 cc. of a 20 per cent solution of calcium gluconate given intramuscularly, and 10 to 15 gm. of calcium lactate or gluconate by mouth may supplement the intravenous injections. Calcium therapy should be pushed until the acute manifestations have subsided and the blood calcium is restored to normal.

Parathormone is effective for maintaining the serum calcium at normal levels. The dose depends on the severity of the symptoms and degree of the hypocalcemia. In the severe case, 100 I.U. of parathormone may be given intramuscularly in a single, or preferably in divided doses. Care should be taken to determine the serum calcium level every few days to avoid overdosage. The serum calcium should be maintained at 8 to 9 mg. per cent.

Viosterol, in doses of 30 to 60 drops daily, is also effective in raising the blood calcium level. It is superior to parathormone because it has a more prolonged effect and is orally active. As with parathormone, its use is attended by the danger of hypercalcemia. Parathormone decreases the blood phosphorus and produces a negative calcium and phosphorus balance, while vitamin D increases the concentration of serum phosphorus and promotes a positive calcium and phosphorus balance. The latter should therefore be given with due caution, the dose not exceeding 10 to 15 drops three times a day.

Dihydrotachysterol, known as A. T. 10, is an antitetanic substance obtained by irradiating ergosterin. It possesses an active calcium-mobilizing principle capable of raising the serum calcium concentration, and has proved effective for the control of manifest tetany.[15, 16] According to Albright and associates,[16] both A. T. 10 and vitamin D have the same fundamental actions, increasing calcium absorption from the gut, and phosphorus excretion in the urine. The ratio of the latter action to the former, however, is apparently greater in the case of A. T. 10, a fact which may explain why this substance is not antirachitic. These observers found that the action of vitamin D is slower, but more prolonged than that of A. T. 10. They state that the parathyroid hormone and A. T. 10 are alike in that both cause a marked increase in phosphorus excretion, but differ in that parathormone has no primary action on calcium absorption from the bowel. A. T. 10 is indicated where the blood calcium level must be maintained for prolonged periods of time. The dose is 2 to 3 cc. once weekly. If used indiscriminately and without frequent blood calcium determinations, it may lead to hypercalcemia. Overdosage may be recognized by such symptoms as anorexia, nausea, vomiting, marked fatigue, and somnolence. Marked overdosage may cause collapse, urinary suppression, and coma. If the blood calcium level exceeds 20 mg., death may ensue.

In order to quiet the hyperirritable nervous system and control the painful muscular spasms and convulsions, deep *sedation or narcosis* may be indicated in the severe attack, especially in the presence of respiratory or cardiac embarrassment. Inhalations of ether or chloroform, or the rectal administration of chloral hydrate (0.5 to 1 gr.), sodium phenobarbital (2 cc. of a 10 per cent solution), or urethane (0.5 to 1 gr.) may be used for this purpose.

The *magnesium salts*, preferably as the gluconate, chloride or the carbonate, in doses of 2 to 5 gms. daily, have been used as an adjuvant to calcium treatment, because of their quiescent effect on the hyperirritable nervous system and their ability to accelerate excretion of phosphorus by the bowel.

While some observers advocate *therapeutic abortion* in the severe case, others report recurrences of the attack soon after emptying the uterus. Considering the high incidence of acute tetany during the puerperium and lactation, it is obvious that therapeutic abortion can contribute little toward combating manifest tetany.

BIBLIOGRAPHY

HYPEREMESIS GRAVIDARUM

1. Ewing, J.: Am. J. Obst. & Gynec. *51*:145, 1905; Am. J. Med. Sc. *139*:828, 1910.
2. Rakoff, A. E.: Am. J. Obst. & Gynec. *38*:371, 1939.
3. Hughes, E. C.: Am. J. Obst. & Gynec. *40*:48, 1940.
4. Hirst, J. C.: J.A.M.A. *76*:772, 1921.
5. Finch, J. W.: J.A.M.A. *111*:1368, 1938; ibid. *119*:400, 1942.
6. Legrand, G.: Bruxelles méd. *19*:84, 1938.
7. Anselmino, K. J.: Arch. f. Gynäk. *161*:273, 1936; Ztschr. f. artzl. Fortbild. *35*:217, 1938.
8. Kemp, W. N.: Endocrinol. *16*:434, 1932.
9. Sussman, W.: Am. J. Obst. & Gynec. *33*:761, 1937.
10. Anselmino, K. J., and Hoffmann, F.: Ztschr. f. Geburtsh. u. Gynäk. *114*:52, 1936.
11. Schoeneck, F. J.: Am. J. Obst. & Gynec. *43*:308, 1942.
12. Bourg, R., and Legrand, G.: Bruxelles méd. *16*:843, 1936.
13. Smith, G. V., and Smith, O. W.: Am. J. Obst. & Gynec. *38*:618, 1939.
14. Schoeneck, F. J.: Am. J. Obst. & Gynec. *32*:104, 1936.
15. Anker, H., and Laland, P.: Norsk. mag. f. laegevidensk. *95*:1217, 1934.
16. Smith, G. V., and Smith, O. W.: Am. J. Obst. & Gynec. *39*:405, 1940.
17. Browne, J. S. L., Henry, J. S., and Venning, E. H.: J. Clin Investigation *17*:503, 1938.

LATE TOXEMIAS OF PREGNANCY

1. Hofbauer, J.: Zentralbl. f. Gynäk. *42*:745, 1918.
2. Cushing, H.: Am. J. Path. *10*:145, 1934; Proc. Soc. Exper. Biol. & Med. *30*:1424, 1933.
3. Spark C.: Arch. Path. *19*:473, 1935.
4. Rasmussen, A. T.: Endocrinol. *20*:673, 1936.
5. Fauvet, E.: Arch. f. Gynäk. *155*:100, 1933.
6. Scheps, M.: Klin. Wchnschr. *13*:1151, 1934.
7. Byrom, F. B., and Wilson, C.: Quart. J. Med. *3*:361, 1934.
8. Sullivan, C. L., and Heffernan, R. J.: Am. J. Obst. & Gynec. *44*:675, 1942.
9. Anselmino, K. J., Hoffmann, F., and Kennedy, W. P.: Edin. Med. J. *39*:376, 1932.
10. Page, E. W.: J. Clin. Investigation *17*:207, 1938.

11. Dexter, L., and Weiss, S., and others: Preeclampsia and Eclamptic Toxemia of Pregnancy. Boston, Little, Brown & Co., 1941.
12. Teel, H. M., and Reid, D. E.: Am. J. Obst. & Gynec. *34*:12, 1937.
13. Ham, G. C., and Landis, E. M.: J. Clin. Investigation *21*:455, 1942.
14. Hofbauer, J.: West. J. Surg. *49*:615, 1941.
15. Bloss, J. R.: South. M. J. *30*:637, 1937.
16. Vorzimer, J. J., Fishberg, A. M., Langrock, E. G., and Rappaport, E. M.: Am. J. Obst. & Gynec. *33*:801, 1937.
17. Colvin, E. D., and Bartholomew, R. A.: Am. J. Obst. & Gynec. *37*:584, 1939.
18. Hughes, E. C.: New York State Med. J. *34*:873, 1934; Am. J. Obst. & Gynec. *40*:48, 1940.
19. Patterson, W. B., Nicodemus, R. E., and Hunt, H. F.: Pennsylvania M. J. *41*:983, 1938; Am. J. Clin. Path. *8*:120, 1938.
20. Hofbauer, J.: Am. J. Obst. & Gynec. *26*:311, 1933.
21. Fauvet, E.: Klin. Wchnschr. *15*:1356, 1936.
22. Lopez, R. E.: Surg., Gynec. & Obst. *49*:689, 1929.
23. Smith, G. V., and Smith, O. W.: Am. J. Obst. & Gynec. *38*:618, 1939.
24. Smith, G. V., and Smith, O. W.: Surg., Gynec. & Obst. *39*:405, 1940.
25. Smith, G. V., Smith, O. W., and Schiller, S.: J. Clin. Endocrinol. *1*:461, 470, 1941.
26. Anselmino, K. J., and Hoffmann, F.: Ztschr. f. Geburtsh. u. Gynäk. *114*:61, 1936.
27. Rakoff, A. E.: Am. J. Obst. & Gynec. *38*:371, 1939.
28. White, E. P., Titus, R. S., Joslin, E. P., and Hunt, H.: Am. J. Obst. & Gynec. *198*:482, 1939.
29. Browne, J. S. L., Henry, J. S., and Venning, H.: J. Clin. Investigation *17*:503, 1938.
30. Young, J.: Brit. Med. J. *1*:953, 1937.
31. Taylor, H. C., Jr., and Scadron, E. N.: Am. J. Obst. & Gynec. *37*:963, 1939.
32. Heim, K.: Klin. Wchnschr. *13*:1614, 1934.
33. Bickenbach, W., and Fromme, H.: Klin. Wchnschr. *14*:496, 1935.
34. Savage, J. E., Wylie, H. B., and Douglass, L. H.: Am. J. Obst. & Gynec. *36*:39, 1938.
35. Cope, C. L.: Lancet *2*:158, 1940.
36. Hain, A. M.: J. Endocrinol. *2*:104, 1942.
37. Smith, G. V., and Smith, O. W.: J. Clin. Endocrinol. *1*:477, 1942.
38. Brandstrup, E.: Acta obst. & gynec. Scandinav. *19*:376, 1939.
39. Taylor, H. C., Jr.: J.A.M.A. *120*:595, 1942.
40. Brougher, J. C.: Am. J. Obst. & Gynec. *43*:710, 1942.
41. Colvin, E. D., Bartholomew, R. A., and Grimes, W. H.: Am. J. Obst. & Gynec. *43*:183, 1942.
42. Hofbauer, J.: Cincinnati J. Med. *23*:107, 1942.

ENDOCRINE ASPECTS OF DYSTOCIA

1. Schumann, E. A.: Med. Rec. *143*:285, 1937.
2. Arnold, L. E.: Am. J. Obst. & Gynec. *39*:99, 1940.
3. Weysser, C.: Zentralbl. f. Gynäk. *60*:728, 1936.
4. Abramson, D., Roberts, S. M., and Wilson, P. D.: Surg., Gynec. & Obst. *58*:595, 1934.
5. Vorzimer, J. J., Fishberg, A. M., Langrock, E. G., and Rappaport, E. M.: Am. J. Obst. & Gynec. *33*:801, 1937.
6. Abramson, D., Hurwitt, E., and Lesnick, G.: Surg., Gynec. & Obst. *65*:335, 1937.
7. Sackett, N. B.: Am. J. Obst. & Gynec. *42*:248, 1941.
8. De Lee, J. B.: Principles and Practice of Obstetrics, 6th ed. Philadelphia, W. B. Saunders Co., 1933.
9. Goldberger, M. A., and Frank, R. T.: Am. J. Obst. & Gynec. *43*:865, 1942.
10. Møller-Christensen, E., and Pedersen-Bjergaard, K.: Acta obst. & gynec. Scandinav. *16*:142, 1936.
11. Tsutsulopulos, G.: Arch. f. Gynäk. *167*:403, 1938.
12. Jeffcoate, T. N. A.: Lancet *1*:1045, 1940.
13. Friedrich, H.: Zentralbl. f. Gynäk. *65*:613, 1941.
14. Rosenkranz, K. D.: Arch. f. Gynäk. *168*:51, 1939.
15. Hain, A. M.: J. Endocrinol. *2*:104, 1942.
16. Weisman, A. I.: Med. Rec. *153*:52, 1941.

17. Danforth, W. C.: Proc. Am. Cong. Obst. & Gynec. 1:81, 1941.
18. Greenhill, J. P.: J.A.M.A. 119:991, 1942.
19. Jeffcoate, T. N. A.: J. Obst. & Gynec. Brit. Emp. 45:893, 1938.
20. Kepp, R. K.: Geburtsh. u. Frauenh. 1:629, 1939.
21. Lubin, S., and Waltman, R.: Surg., Gynec. & Obst. 69:155, 1939.
22. Schurger, S.: Zentralbl. f. Gynäk. 63:207, 1939.
23. Abarbanel, A. R.: Surg., Gynec. & Obst. 73:257, 1941.

MATERNAL TETANY

1. Klaften, E.: Zentralbl. f. Gynäk. 57:2178, 1933.
2. Frankl-Hochwart, L.: Die Tetanie. Wien, 1907.
3. Kozelka, F. L., Hart, E. B., and Bohstedt, G.: J. Biol. Chem. 100:715, 1933.
4. Hoffmann, F.: Arch. f. Gynäk. 153:181, 1933.
5. Thomson, D. L., and Collip, J. B.: Physiol. Rev. 12:309, 1932.
6. Adler, M.: Arch. f. Gynäk. 143:236, 1931.
7. McIsaac, P.: Brit. J. Exper. Biol. 5:233, 1928.
8. MacCallum, W. G., and Voegtlin, C.: J. Exper. Med. 11:118, 1909.
9. Voelker, H.: Monatschr. f. Geburtsh. 19:14, 1904.
10. Anselmino, K. J., Hoffmann, F., and Herold, L.: Klin. Wchnschr. 12:1944, 1933; ibid. 13:44, 45, 1934.
11. Houssay, B. A., and Sammartino, R.: Compt. rend. Soc. de biol. 114:729, 1933.
12. Chvostek, F.: Wien. med. Presse 17:1201, 1225, 1253, 1313, 1876.
13. Trousseau, A.: Gaz. d. hôp. Paris 37:109, 1864.
14. Erb, W.: Arch. f. Psychiat. 4:271, 1874.
15. MacBryde, C. M.: J.A.M.A. 111:304, 1938.
16. Albright, F., Bloomberg, E., Drake, T., and Sulkowitsch, H.: J. Clin. Investigation 17: 317, 1938.

CHAPTER XXXII

ABNORMALITIES OF THE BREAST

With the recognition that mammary growth and function is under hormonal control (see Chap. X), the interpretation of certain breast aberrations, previously considered inflammatory or neoplastic, has been revised, and the therapeutic approach thereto radically modified. It is now generally believed that endocrine factors play a significant role in the etiology of mammary hypoplasia, hypertrophy, and hyperplasia, as well as in disturbances of mammary function, namely hypogalactia and galactorrhea. What part they play and what benefit may be expected from organotherapy and other forms of treatment, is the subject of the present chapter. Brief mention will also be made of "mastitis neonatorum" and precocious mammary development, conditions now generally conceded to be hormonally induced.

PRE-ADOLESCENT ABNORMALITIES OF THE BREAST

Mastitis Neonatorum.—In the newborn, regardless of sex, the infantile mammae not infrequently become swollen and reddened, and secrete a milk-like substance known as "witches' milk." These manifestations usually appear on the second or third day of life and may persist for five or six days, after which the breasts return to their infantile proportions. This relatively common phenomenon varies in intensity, and is often so slight as to pass unnoticed. Formerly considered of infectious origin, it is now generally attributed to the action of estrogenic substances derived from the maternal circulation during fetal life. Whether the mammary secretion formed under these conditions is true milk is still controversial.[1, 2]

Treatment.—Fortunately this condition is self-limited and requires no treatment. Since the swollen, hyperemic breast is a favorable site for infection, it is important to maintain absolute cleanliness and avoid mechanical or other meddlesome manipulation.

Precocious Mammary Development.—Mammary development equivalent to that normally attained at puberty, is usually considered precocious when it is achieved prior to the eighth or ninth year of life. No pathologic alterations are demonstrable in the breast, the sole deviation from normal being the age at which it develops. As a rule, the mammary modifications are accompanied by other manifestations of sexual precocity, and are therefore more appropriately discussed in connection with precocious puberty (see Chap. XXXV).

ABNORMALITIES IN MAMMARY GROWTH

Disturbances in mammary growth may take the form of (1) hypoplasia, in which the size of the breast is below the lower limits of normal for the mature woman; (2) hypertrophy, where the organ attains proportions far exceeding the upper limits of normal; and (3) hyperplasia, a condition characterized by excessive proliferation of one or more of the various constituents of the breast.

MAMMARY HYPOPLASIA

Underdevelopment of the breast may be an expression of general or genital infantilism. Barring developmental anomalies, the hypoplasia may be attributable to a deficiency or absence of the ovarian sex hormones, estrogen and progestin, on which growth of the duct and lobule-alveolar systems depend. The hormonal deficiency may be due to some abnormality inherent in the ovaries per se, or a disturbance in the anterior

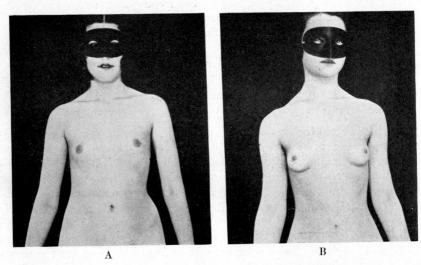

A   B

Fig. 94.—Mammary hypoplasia. A, Marked mammary hypoplasia in a twenty-two-year-old female, associated with primary amenorrhea and negative estrogen and gonadotropin tests. B, Moderate mammary hypoplasia in a twenty-year-old female with secondary amenorrhea and a subthreshold estrogen cycle.

hypophysis or elsewhere in the organism. The severity of the condition varies according to the degree of ovarian hypofunction and the time of its onset. If the ovarian deficiency is marked, involving the follicular and luteal hormones, both the duct and lobule-alveolar systems will be retarded. Where the deficiency is mild, so that follicles mature but fail to rupture and form corpora lutea, some degree of duct growth may be achieved. In such cases, the breast has the peculiar pointed shape which characterizes the gland in which only the duct system has developed.

Prognosis.—Where the ovarian deficiency is irreparable, the outlook is obviously poor. On the other hand, if it is due to some general depressive state which is amenable to treatment, normal ovarian function and with it normal mammary development may eventually be achieved.

Treatment.—The natural and synthetic *estrogens*,[3, 4, 5, 6] administered subcutaneously or orally, or applied directly to the breast in the form of an ointment, may stimulate mammary growth. The dosage found effective by MacBryde[5] is 35 mg. of estradiol benzoate injected subcutaneously once weekly, or the local application of 2.5 mg. of estradiol benzoate in an ointment daily. Breasts so treated retain the pointed shape of the young breast in which only the duct system is developed. Since lobule-alveolar growth depends on the luteal hormone, combined treatment with *estrogen and progesterone* would seem to be rational therapy. According to Werner,[3] estrogen plus progesterone is more effective than estrogen alone in promoting mammary growth. MacBryde[5] found progesterone without effect when given alone, but alternate daily injections of 1 I.U. of proges-

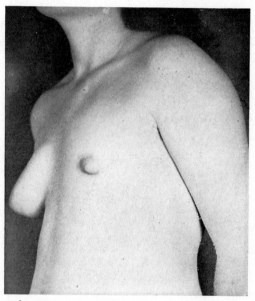

Fig. 95.—Unilateral mammary hypoplasia. Girl aged sixteen. The unequal response of the breasts to a presumably identical hormonal environment emphasizes the importance of local tissue reactivity.

terone and 20,000 to 50,000 I.U. of estrogen caused more rapid and more firm breast growth than that obtained with estrogen. Regression following cessation of treatment was less rapid after the combined treatment than when estrogen alone was used. Where the hypoplasia is unilateral (see Fig. 95), the fault apparently lies in the reactivity of the affected breast, the adequacy of the hormonal stimuli being attested by the normal growth of the other breast. In such cases, watchful waiting until menstruation is established is advisable. If the hypoplasia persists thereafter, local application of estrogen may be tried, but a response is unlikely.[7]

Estrogen may benefit hypoplasia due to ovarian hypofunction, but it cannot correct the underlying ovarian deficiency. The effect is temporary and breasts tend to return to their original hypoplastic proportions soon after treatment is stopped. Long continued treatment with estrogen would seem to be undesirable in view of experimental evidence that its chronic administration may lead to cystic mastitis and, in susceptible breasts, to carcinoma.[8, 9]

Gonadotropic extracts, though capable of stimulating gonadal function and indirectly promoting mammary growth in the lower mammal, are of doubtful value in man. As emphasized elsewhere (see Chap. XII), their ability to stimulate the hypofunctioning human ovary has not been convincingly established.

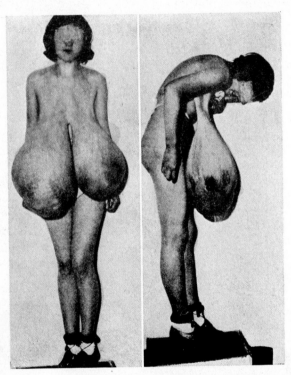

Fig. 96.—Massive puberty hypertrophy of the breasts in a fourteen-year-old girl. (Goodman, B. A.: J.A.M.A. Vol. 103.)

In evaluating the efficacy of organotherapy or any other form of treatment, it must be borne in mind that the *rate of mammary growth* and the *age* at which it is completed shows wide individual variations, being dependent to a large extent on the constitutional make-up of the individual. As Pryor and Carter[10] have pointed out, puberal girls are of two main types, broad-built or "lateral," and slender or "linear." The former begins to mature earlier and more quickly achieves full development of her secondary sex characters (see Fig. 52). Consequently, individuals who are of the same chronological age but of different constitutional type will not show the same degree of mammary development unless both have passed the age at which their respective types normally reach their developmental peak. Unless these individual differences in rate of sexual maturation are recognized, error in evaluating the response to therapy is likely. For example, Kramer and Jacobson[11] diagnosed one of their patients, a "linear" type of individual, as sexually retarded because her development fell short of that achieved by a "lateral" type of girl of the same chronological age. Observing considerable development of the sex characters twenty months after anterior pituitary and thyroid treatment was instituted, they attributed the beneficial effects to the hormonal therapy used. The possibility that the progress noted would have occurred without treatment and was merely equivalent to that which Pryor and Carter[10] have shown occurs spontaneously in the "linear" type of girl at this later age, was not excluded.

Medical and general hygienic measures are probably the most effective therapy for mammary hypoplasia, since they may improve the general physical condition of the individual and thus indirectly fortify a feeble pituitary or gonadal impulse.

MAMMARY HYPERTROPHY

In some women the breasts may achieve enormous proportions. For example, in a fourteen-year-old girl described by Goodman,[12] the beasts attained a weight of 26 and 16 pounds respectively within a period of twenty months (see Fig. 96). Two types of mammary hypertrophy have been described. *Pseudohypertrophy,* the more common form, is due to a marked increase in adipose tissue and is usually unaccompanied by any disturbing symptoms. *True hypertrophy,* on the other hand, is very rare. Here the enlargement is due to a marked increase in all its constituents, particularly the glandular elements. The nipples as a rule are not involved in the general hypertrophy. These two forms are distinguishable only by histologic examination. According to some observers, the breast in true hypertrophy is normal in all respects except for its mammoth size. Others describe areas showing abnormal changes.

Symptomatology.—The condition usually has its inception shortly before or after the menarche, and is therefore often referred to as virginal, puberal, or nongravid hypertrophy. The period of progressive enlargement may vary from several months to over two years. Growth then ceases, though a new spurt of growth may occur in the event of pregnancy. The hypertrophy is usually, though not invariably bilateral, and is often diffuse and somewhat asymmetrical. Because of the rapidity with which the breasts enlarge, the skin overlying the mammae becomes stretched, the nipples flattened, and areolae enlarged. Tortuosity of the superficial veins, chronic edema, and a tendency to ulceration of the skin may be associated findings. The enormous hypertrophy and great weight of the glands give rise to a dragging sensation in the chest, and a feeling of tenseness without pain. The discomfort is usually constant and is not exaggerated at the menstrual flow. No secretion appears except during pregnancy and lactation, though in some cases the enormous size of the breast may interfere with its secretory function. Individuals so afflicted are seldom obese, and as a rule display no endocrinopathic stigmata.

31

Etiology.—The etiology of mammary hypertrophy is obscure. The fact that it is sometimes encountered in several members of the same family suggests that heredity may be a factor. Since its inception often coincides with puberty, mammary hypertrophy has been interpreted as an exaggeration of normal pubescent mammary growth, in which the ovarian sex hormones are etiologic factors. Whether the primary cause lies in excessive hormonal stimulation, or abnormal reactivity of the mammary tissue to normal hormonal stimuli, is not certain. The latter possibility seems likely in view of the fact that all normal puberal girls experience a spurt of ovarian activity, but very few respond with mammary hypertrophy. Of interest in this connection is Gaines'[13] observation

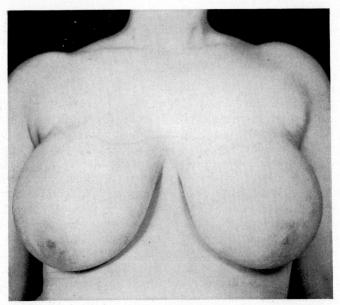

Fig. 97.—Moderate mammary hypertrophy in a sixteen-year-old girl.

that the estrogen content of the body fluids, in a fourteen-year-old girl with massive mammary hypertrophy, was within normal limits. This has also been the author's experience.

Treatment.—The moderate forms may be benefited by an uplift support. In the extreme case, surgery may be unavoidable. For cosmetic reasons, some prefer to retain part of the gland while others favor complete removal lest the retained tissue subsequently become reactivated. Removal of one breast at a time is desirable to minimize shock.

MAMMARY HYPERPLASIA (CHRONIC MASTITIS)

Hyperplasia of the various constituents of the breast is, next to carcinoma, the most common lesion of the female breast. It has acquired a place of importance because some of its forms suggest malignancy and, in the opinion of some investigators, it is a precancerous condition. The protean nature of its histologic pattern and clinical manifestations makes classification exceedingly difficult.

Anatomical Characteristics.—Generally speaking, mammary hyperplasia is characterized by formation of an excessive amount of connective tissue and epithelial elements lining the ducts and acini, with a tendency to cyst formation. In some instances the connective tissue may predominate, while in others cyst formation is the most conspicuous finding. In the majority of cases the two processes are more or less balanced, innumerable tiny cysts appearing embedded in a dense, fibrous tissue.

Types of Hyperplasia.—Though many varieties of mammary hyperplasia have been described, most observers speak of the *cystic* and *non-*

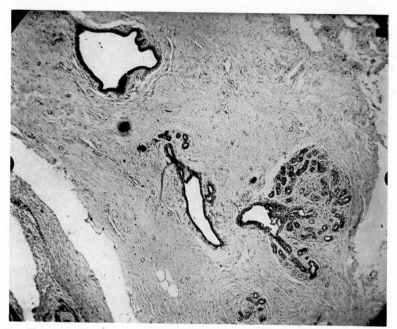

Fig. 98.—Chronic cystic mastitis. Microphotograph of tissue obtained from a twenty-eight-year-old primipara

cystic forms. The latter, as described by Cheatle and Cutler,[14] is "a condition in which a certain type of desquamation of epithelial cells in the terminal ducts and their acini is accompanied by hyperplasia of the pericanalicular and periacinous connective tissue and often by new formation of ducts and acini, but without cysts or papillomatous formation." Cystic hyperplasia, like the noncystic form, begins with a desquamative hyperplasia of the lining epithelium in the terminal tubules, but eventuates in the formation of a varying number of cysts which may involve the acini, milk ducts, and all lobes and lobules. The cysts vary in size, some attaining the proportions of an orange. They may contain a colorless, brown, or bluish-green fluid. Two types of cyst have been described. In one, the epithelium is smooth and of normal thickness, but atrophies and eventually disappears as the cyst enlarges, thus leaving a fibrous wall. In the second, the epithelium undergoes active proliferation and as a result the cells pile up into folds or papillomas, which in extreme cases may entirely fill the lumina of the ducts and acini.

According to Taylor[15] there are at least *two separate entities* which have been termed *chronic mastitis*. The first is characterized by diffuse nodularity and premenstrual pain. The basic lesion is fibrosis or adenofibrosis involving the interstitial, fat, and periacinar tissue, while the ducts are but slightly affected. Taylor considers the condition analogous to adenomyosis of the uterus. The second type is characterized by a discharge from the nipple and is often associated with palpable dilatation of the ducts near the areola. The histologic alterations are edema of the lobules, dilatation of the ducts, periductal inflammation and possibly some hyperplasia of the lining of the ducts. For this form he suggests the terms nonpuerperal lactation, periductal inflammation, or duct hyperplasia. Geschickter[16] distinguishes three forms: (1) premenstrual swelling or *mastodynia*, in which lobule formation is partially suppressed; (2) *adenosis*, characterized by atypical proliferation, within or beyond the ends of the tubules, which replaces normal lobule formation; and (3) *cystic disease*, where the normal lobules have undergone involution and some are replaced by cysts developing in the end buds of the terminal tubules.

Clinical Characteristics.—Mammary hyperplasia may occur at any time from puberty to the menopause. Its most prominent manifestations are nodule formation, pain and sometimes discharge from the nipple.

Mastitis Adolescentium.—The pubescent form of the disease (*mastitis adolescentium*) occurs in boys as well as girls, but is more common in the latter. It tends to appear shortly before the menarche, usually after the eleventh year. One or both breasts may be involved, either simultaneously or in succession. The affected mammary tissue becomes firm and tender and, where a large area is involved, the growth may assume a disc-like or spherical formation, usually situated directly behind the nipple. Occasionally a few drops of an opaque fluid can be expressed, but as a rule there is no discharge unless the nipple has been irritated.

Adult Mastitis.—In the adult, mammary hyperplasia tends to occur in the middle-aged, childless woman, and often affects individuals with pendulous breasts. The lesion may be diffuse, or nodular and shotlike, and may involve one lobe or the whole of one or both breasts. When localized, the nodularity is usually confined to the upper outer quadrant. Unlike true tumors, the margins of such nodular areas are ill defined and cannot be outlined with the breast pressed flat against the chest. If the gland is raised and examined between the fingers, a roughly circumscribed area may be palpated, provided that the breast does not contain too much adipose tissue. The larger cysts as a rule are well defined, fluctuant and movable, and do not distort the nipple.

Tenderness or pain, limited to the breast or transmitted to the axilla, shoulder, arm and lateral thoracic wall, is not uncommon. The pain may be aggravated by movement, exercise, or trauma. Not infrequently, especially in the early stages, it tends to be exaggerated at the premenstruum.

When the condition is fully established, the pain is more constant and sometimes severe. A serous or bloody nipple discharge is not uncommon. In the presence of cysts, a yellow or green fluid can sometimes be expressed.

Etiology.—The pathogenesis of mammary hyperplasia is obscure. Reclus[17] and Schimmelbusch[18] believed it to be neoplastic; Konig[19] considered it of inflammatory origin because of the associated lymphocytic infiltration; while Warren[20] interpreted it as an exaggeration of the normal processes in the involutionary cycle of the breast.

The immediate cause of premenstrual mammary swelling and pain has been the subject of much speculation. It was earlier attributed to venous congestion, but Rosenburg's[21] description of periodic lobule formation during the premenstruum suggested that the swelling and tenderness may be related somehow to this phenomenon. Distention of the ducts and acini by desquamated epithelial cells has been offered by Cheatle and Cutler[14] as a possible explanation. Whitehouse[22] has suggested that excessive epithelialization of the individual acini, hypersecretion of the lobules, or defective absorption and autolysis of the products of secretory activity may be responsible. Intralobular edema, with loosening of the fibers of the mantle tissue about the acini has also been mentioned as a possible cause. An exaggeration of normal premenstrual mammary activity is blamed by Cotte and Pallot,[23] who compared the histologic appearance of the normal and painful breast and found that the latter differed only in degree, presenting no pathologic change but only what appeared to be an exaggeration of a physiologic process. According to Taylor,[15] the histological appearance of the painful breast varies considerably: in some cases, it differs in no way from the normal gland, while in others it shows a striking increase in the density of the connective tissue, disappearance of intralobular fat, and distortion of the lobules by fibrosis of the mantle tissue. In his opinion, the swelling and pain are due to vascular engorgement or an increase in interstitial fluids, while the structural alterations, where present, are the end result of repeated or chronic vascular congestions.

Hormonal Factors.—In seeking to identify the underlying cause of the various forms of mammary hyperplasia, attention has recently been focused on hormonal factors. Recognition of the important part played by the *ovarian sex hormones* in the development of the breast (see Chap. X) is responsible for the belief that a disturbance in the production of estrogen, progestin, or both, may be at fault. That the ovary plays some part in the etiology seems certain in view of the fact that the condition occurs almost exclusively in the female, is usually encountered within the limits of the reproductive period, tends to be exaggerated during the premenstruum, and often regresses following the menopause. There is as yet no agreement as to the nature of the ovarian disturbance which leads to mammary hyperplasia. The observation that the condition tends to regress during pregnancy throws little light on this problem, for the good effect of gestation may be due to the estrogen, progestin, gonadotropin, lactogenic hormone, or any one of numerous other influences known to be operating at this time. The unsettled state of this problem is evident in the number of theories regarding its etiology and the variety of hormones to which relief or cure has been ascribed. An excess of progestin,[22, 23] a deficiency[24, 25] or excess[26, 27] of estrogen, or a normal quantity of estrogen unopposed by an adequate amount of progestin,[28] are among the possibilities that have been considered. Some observers[29] distinguish two types of mammary hyperplasia: that mainly involving the duct system and due to an excess of estrogen, and that in which the lobule-alveolar system is primarily affected and an excess of progestin is at fault.

The view that mammary hyperplasia is due to excessive or protracted *estrogen stimulation unopposed by progestin* rests mainly on the observation that chronic estrogen treatment, in the lower mammal[30, 31] and monkey,[32] induces structural alterations resembling those of human mammary hyperplasia. This evidence is rejected by some observers[33, 34] on the ground that the alterations thus induced in the laboratory animal are not strictly comparable to those which arise spontaneously in the human breast. On the other hand, some support for this theory is provided by Lepper's[35] observation that breast pain was encountered more often among patients with follicular cysts than among those with other types of benign ovarian tumors which contain no estrogen. Preissecker[36] found that estrogen therapy for gonorrheal vaginitis in a group of prepuberal girls, caused asymmetric swelling in three and a painful lump in one case. In a mature woman treated for amenorrhea, an adenoma of the breast developed following estrogen therapy. Of interest also is Scarff and Smith's[37] report of the development of "chronic mastitis" in two stilbestrol workers.

Vascular Factors.—Taylor,[15] who carried out hormonal and endometrial studies in a large series of cases, concluded that an excess or deficiency of the ovarian sex hormones is not a constant finding in "chronic mastitis." On the contrary, the level of these hormones would appear to be within normal limits in most of the cases. He therefore maintains that though an actively functioning ovary is a prerequisite to the development of this disease, it cannot be accounted for by "any simple quantitative abnormality of sex hormone physiology." He advances the theory that premenstrual mammary swelling and pain may be explained on the basis of a vascular reaction with an increase in the fluid content of the mammary tissues. This increase may be due to the ovarian hormones, which have been shown to cause fluid retention,[38] or may be initiated through the nervous system, as suggested by the occurrence of rapid mammary enlargement after psychic stimuli. He considers it likely that "as the result of nervous and perhaps endocrine stimuli the breast becomes the seat of chronic or repeated vascular congestions, producing conditions that lead eventually to a fibrosis or adenofibrosis in which later epithelial changes of all sorts develop." Taylor suggests that hormonal factors may play a more important part in a second type of chronic mastitis, to which he refers as *nonpuerperal secretion.* This is characterized at first by a milky discharge from the nipple and slight hyperplasia of the acini, while later there develops a condition in which dilated ducts become filled with desquamated cells and stagnating secretion. Persistence of this condition, he believes, may lead to periductal inflammation, cysts, and hyperplastic or metaplastic changes in the duct lining. Grossly disturbed menstrual cycles were encountered in many of the cases of this type. It is noteworthy that over 80 per cent of his cases with "nonpuerperal secretion" had had full term pregnancies. He gives as his principal reason for believing that this condition often has an endocrine basis, the fact that hormonal stimuli are the essential causes of milk formation.

Nervous Factors.—According to Atkins,[39] the structural alterations of chronic mastitis may have a hormonal basis, but the associated pain is of nervous origin. Like Taylor, he points out that a general nervous instability is commonly present in these patients. He also calls attention to the fact that the pain in many of the cases is distributed along the course of one or two intercostal nerves, and tends to be intensified by the drag of pendulous breasts, or by cold damp weather. Psychic factors and a lowered pain threshold, he believes, materially contribute to the pain. Sensations which ordinarily pass unnoticed in the normal woman, may be exaggerated in the irritable, sensitive individual, particularly if she harbors phobias of malignancy. The validity of his view is borne out by the fact that placeboes and reassurance are often sufficient to relieve the pain.

Summary.—On the whole, it seems likely that hormonal, vascular, and nervous factors all participate in the etiology, the relative importance of each varying in different individuals. In view of the wide variety of associated hormonal and clinical findings,[15] it would seem that the most important part is played by conditions inherent in the mammary tissue, which are probably genetically controlled and determine the reactivity of the breast to the various stimuli to which it is exposed. Variations in reactivity to identical hormonal stimuli have been observed in the mammae of experimental animals. The fact that the abnormal breast changes in chronic mastitis may involve only one breast or a part of one breast further emphasizes the importance of local tissue reactivity in the etiology. It is possible, as Taylor[15] suggests, that a hypersensitive vascular system may respond excessively to otherwise normal hormonal or nervous stimuli, leading secondarily to abnormal changes in the connective tissue and epithelial elements. On the other hand, it is also conceivable that abnormal stromal and glandular modifications may be due primarily to excessive reactivity of these tissues to hormonal stimuli, which might fail to elicit a similar reaction in the less receptive breast. The confusion surrounding the etiology of "chronic mastitis" may perhaps best be resolved by conceiving of it as the result of the interplay between hormonal, nervous, and possibly other stimuli, on one hand, and genetically controlled conditions within the receptor organ, on the other.

Prognosis.—The pubescent form of mammary hyperplasia is usually transient and self-limited, regressing spontaneously before or with the completion of the puberal epoch. Spontaneous regression is likewise common in the mature woman. Not infrequently, the condition may disappear during pregnancy, lactation, or following the menopause.

Mammary Hyperplasia and Cancer.—Whether mammary hyperplasia is a precancerous condition is controversial. Some believe this is true only of the cystic form of the disease. Others maintain that both the noncystic and cystic forms are precancerous, each representing a different stage of the same pathologic process. A third view considers neither form precancerous. A recent survey of follow-up studies in cases diagnosed as cystic disease led Patey[40] to conclude that "if clinically diagnosable cystic disease is a precancerous condition, in actual practice the danger of carcinoma is very slight." On the other hand, Warren,[41] who studied the relation of cancer to operations for benign noninfectious mammary lesions in 1,206 women, found the cancer rate for women with preexisting breast lesions 4.5 times that for all women. This predominance was especially marked between thirty and forty-nine years of age, when it was 11.7 times as great. Actively proliferating lesions, intraductal papillomas, and cysts with papillary epithelium were followed by cancer more often than the adenofibromas or large cysts with atrophic epithelium.

Diagnosis.—The *history* is of much significance in the diagnosis. The age of the patient, menstrual history, previous occurrence of pregnancy and lactation, and length of time the lump has persisted, are important clues. Also significant is a history of trauma or chronic irritation preceding its appearance, and the presence of pain or discharge from the nipple.

In the *physical examination,* cognizance should be taken of mobility or fixation, fluctuation, size, consistency, location, definition of the tumor, nipple retraction, and the condition of the axillary lymph nodes. While no single bit of evidence is conclusive, the findings in their aggregate may prove valuable.

In benign cystic hyperplasia, the lesion is often multiple, and not infrequently both breasts are involved. There is no fixation or nipple retraction, and the larger cysts may be recognized by transillumination or roentgenograms. Pain, if present, usually precedes the appearance of the lump and, in bilateral involvement, may affect both breasts. Not infrequently, it is exaggerated at the premenstruum and subsides following the flow. Bleeding from the nipple, though suspicious of malignancy, is not as significant as was earlier believed. According to Wainwright,[42] this manifestation is not per se presumptive evidence of malignancy, for statistically it is encountered with equal frequency in benign and malignant lesions.

The *differential diagnosis* between benign cystic hyperplasia and mammary cancer is often difficult, particularly in its early stages. The singularity of the lesion, its fixation to the underlying structures, nipple retraction and, in the later stages, the presence of palpable lymph nodes, point to malignancy. In the older woman, the presence of a lump certainly calls for biopsy. Mammary cancer, if deep seated, may have an elastic consistency resembling that of cyst formation. In such cases, transillumination and roentgenograms may serve as important adjuncts in the diagnosis. If the lesion is solid, biopsy is the only means of distinguishing between benign fibroadenoma and carcinoma.

Treatment.—*General Medical Measures.*—Treatment of mammary hyperplasia is not justified unless malignancy has been excluded. While surgery has been widely practiced for this condition, it is now generally agreed that a policy of watchful waiting and conservative measures should be tried, particularly in young girls or women of childbearing age. Since the etiology of mammary hyperplasia is obscure, treatment is necessarily empirical. The patient should be reassured as to the benign nature of the lesion. This is particularly important in the nervous or cancer-conscious individual. Where feasible, pregnancy and lactation may be advised because these physiologic states are often followed by regression of the lesion. Depressive states, ovarian disturbances, or other endocrine or metabolic faults should be corrected where possible. In the thin individual, a gain in weight may often be beneficial.[7] The author has frequently noted regression of mammary hyperplasia following improvement of the general health.

Organotherapy.—Many endocrine products have been advocated, the one selected varying according to the concept of the etiology favored by the particular observer. Estrogen, progestin, androgen, chorionic gonadotropin, and the anterior pituitary lactogenic hormone have all been used, either singly or in combination. The results of such therapy have varied widely, some reporting cures, others no benefit, or even aggravation of the symptoms.

The *estrogens* have probably been most widely employed for this condition. Some workers[7, 43] resort to their use on the assumption that chronic mastitis is due to a deficiency of estrogen. Those who believe an excess of progestin is responsible for the condition, employ estrogen with the hope that it will either directly neutralize progestin's effect on the mammae, or indirectly lower the progestin level by suppressing production of the luteinizing principle of the anterior hypophysis.[22, 23] According to Lewis and Geschickter,[44] estrogen may improve the condition by carrying the cystic breast modifications to the point of involution and fibrosis. They report good results in *mastodynia* and *adenosis* with 10,000 I.U. of estrogen administered intramuscularly twice weekly until a total of 60,000 I.U. have been given. There are some investigators who maintain that the estrogens may actually aggravate the condition. In view of experimental evidence that the estrogens may induce abnormal mammary alterations and, in the susceptible case, lead to malignant change, *they should be used with caution,* particularly during the cancer age or in women with a family history of mammary cancer (see Chap. II).

A few observers[28] have reported improvement following *progestin therapy* in cases where the hyperplasia chiefly involves the ducts and the condition is presumably due to an absolute or relative excess of estrogen. In the author's experience, this form of treatment has proved of no value in either the cystic or noncystic form of the disease.

Androgenic substances are employed[45, 46, 47] with the aim of inhibiting the anterior pituitary gland and thus indirectly lowering the level of estrogen in the body, or of directly neutralizing the effect of estrogen on the breast. Geist[46] obtained relief of premenstrual mammary pain with 250 mgm. of testosterone propionate during the latter half of the cycle. In the author's experience, such therapy has proved disappointing. Geschickter[16] also failed to see improvement following androgen administration. According to Atkins,[39] the androgens alleviate the symptoms in most cases, but the effect is temporary and may lead to undesirable concomitant effects such as regressive changes of the genital organs, amenorrhea, hypertrophy of the clitoris, deepening of the voice, and hirsutism.

The *chorionic gonadotropes* have been used by a few observers,[48, 49] but their value is questionable, particularly in view of evidence that they may induce cystic changes in the mammae of rodents.[50]

The anterior pituitary *lactogenic principle*, in combination with estrogenic substance, has been employed by Lewis and Geschickter[44] with the aim of simulating conditions prevailing during lactation. They report improvement following the administration of a total of 30,000 I.U. of estrogen followed by 1440 bird units of prolactin in divided doses. Confirmatory reports are still lacking.

In *evaluating the efficacy of organotherapy*, it must be borne in mind that many cases show spontaneous regression, and that the size of the lesion may vary from time to time in the same individual. It is possible that many of the beneficial results ascribed to organotherapy were actually due to spontaneous regression, or correction of some associated disturbance which may have been indirectly responsible for the abnormal mammary modifications. Of interest in this connection is Taylor's[15] recent study comparing the response to organotherapy, and inactive substances or irrelevant methods of treatment. In the control group, three-quarters reported improvement or cure following their supposed treatment. In the group receiving estrogen, progestin, androgen, luteinizing hormone, or lactogenic hormone, permanent results exceeding the anticipated rate of spontaneous improvement were not noted.

X-ray Therapy.—Taylor[15] recommends x-ray radiation of the *ovaries* with the view of depressing their function and thus lowering the estrogen level of the body fluids. Such therapy is definitely contraindicated in young girls or women of childbearing age because of the danger of irreparable damage to the ovarian parenchyma. X-ray radiation of the *breasts* has also been advocated for the treatment of mammary hyperplasia.[51] Here again there is danger of injuring the secretory elements of the mammae,[52] and it should therefore be avoided in the young woman.

In the author's experience, the best results were obtained by applying a tight uplift support, curtailment of the fluid intake, purgation, and use of all measures calculated to correct any existing depressive state, or endocrine and metabolic disturbance. In some instances, use of small doses of thyroid extract, $\frac{1}{2}$ to 1 gr. t.i.d., has proved efficacious. It is possible that the thyroid hormone acts by promoting water elimination and thus preventing an undue shift of fluids to the breast. Assuming that hyperestrinism is responsible for some cases of mammary hyperplasia, thyroid substance may possibly improve the condition through its supposed ability to promote estrogen excretion. Of interest in this connection is Cramer and Hornung's[53] observation that anterior pituitary thyrotropic extract prevented the abnormal mammary modifications, eventuating in carcinoma, which would otherwise follow protracted estrogen administration in the rodent.

ABNORMALITIES IN MAMMARY FUNCTION
DEFICIENT MILK SECRETION (HYPOGALACTIA)

Definition.—Deficient milk secretion is described as *primary* when it is apparent from the outset, and *secondary* when lactation is established at the usual time but then ceases prematurely. Hypogalactia should not be confused with so-called "schwergiebigkeit," where milk is produced but is expressed with difficulty because of some mechanical impediment or other cause.

Etiology.—*Mammary and Hormonal Factors.*—Barring faulty suckling, due to some imperfection in the nipple, or to some oral defect or feebleness of the nursling, the cause of deficient milk secretion may reside in the mammae, or in the hormonal stimuli on which lactation depends. It should be emphasized that the quantity of milk produced depends on the amount of functioning glandular tissue present and not on the size of the breasts. Hypogalactia may be encountered in women whose breasts are large but are composed mostly of fat and connective tissue and contain but little glandular tissue. Where hypogalactia occurs despite an adequate amount of glandular tissue, deficiency of the anterior pituitary lactogenic hormone may be at fault. Of interest is Hoffmann's[54] observation that the lactogenic hormone content of the urine in seven out of eight cases of hypogalactia was significantly lower than in normally lactating women. Meites and Turner[55] likewise found the level of lactogenic hormone in the urine in three cases of hypogalactia below that of mothers producing a normal amount of milk. They suggest that their test for the quantitative determination of lactogenic hormone in the urine may serve as an aid in distinguishing hypogalactia of hormonal origin from that due to other causes.

A deficiency of lactogenic hormone may conceivably result from pituitary exhaustion caused by the extraordinary demands placed on this gland during gestation. Where such a deficiency exists, it is likely to be associated with a deficiency of the adrenocorticotropic factor, which has been shown to augment the effect of the lactogenic principle through its action on important metabolic processes (see Chap. X). In some cases, a deficiency in the quantity or quality of the milk may conceivably be due to a disturbance of the thyroid or adrenal cortex.

Inadequate Nutrition.—Inadequate nutrition may account for the lactational deficiency in some cases.[94] This may be expected to lower the supply of essential food elements that enter into the composition of milk, and may at the same time create a deficiency of the basic materials from which are formed the hormones that support lactation. The importance of the nutritional factor is evident in the high incidence of hypogalactia in Germany during the hunger blockade of the first World War.

Physical and Nervous Stress.—Undue physical or nervous stress may adversely affect milk production. Psychic shock has been known to interfere with lactation, but the mechanism involved is not clear. The impulse may conceivably be carried by way of the hypothalamus to the anterior lobe, suppressing its lactogenic hormone production. On the other hand, it may act by inhibiting release of the hypothetical posterior lobe hormone which, according to Turner,[56] plays an essential role in the removal of milk by stimulating contraction of the smooth musculature of the milk ducts. The observation that adrenalin relaxes this musculature and prevents withdrawal of milk[57] suggests that increased discharge of this hormone may contribute to the transient drop in the output of milk which may follow psychic shock.

Diagnosis.—Before instituting any form of therapy, inadequacy of the glandular tissue and faulty suckling should first be excluded. In addition, one must be certain that he is dealing with true hypogalactia and not merely with a late onset of lactation. As Jaschke[58] has pointed out, a positive diagnosis of hypogalactia is rarely possible the first week postpartum, because of wide individual variations in the time at which milk secretion becomes established. The amount of milk secreted at different times also varies and therefore the quantity of milk withdrawn by the infant at one feeding, or even during the course of an entire day, may often be misleading. These factors must be taken into account, not only in deciding whether an actual deficiency exists, but also when estimating the response to therapy.

Treatment.—The measures advocated for combating hypogalactia have been as varied as the theories advanced to explain its cause.

General Medical Measures.—Milk deficiency due to inadequate mammary secretory tissue is rarely benefited by organotherapy or any other form of treatment. In the presence of ample glandular tissue, on the other hand, much may be accomplished by both general and specific therapy. General medical measures calculated to improve the nutritional status of the nursing mother are of prime importance. A healthy regimen, well balanced diet rich in fat, protein, minerals and essential vitamins, an ample fluid intake, avoidance of dehydrating aperients, and curtailment of mental and physical exertion, may suffice to insure an ample supply of milk in the majority of cases.

Organotherapy.—The value of *lactogenic hormone therapy* cannot be decided from the limited evidence at hand. Kurzrok and his associates[59] found that a total of 75 to 400 bird units of prolactin was followed by a daily increase of as much as 100 grams of milk output in women in whom lactation was not established by the sixth day postpartum. Ross[60] found that a minimum of 1000 units is required to produce an appreciable rise in milk production. Kenny and King[61] observed a rise in milk output in two-thirds of a group of forty-three women, following a total of 900 Riddle units in the course of five days. A favorable response has also been reported by Hoffmann.[54] On the other hand, Preissecker[62] could see improvement in only three of eleven cases and concluded that the relative impotency of the available extracts may be at fault. Since larger doses, administered parenterally, cause unpleasant local and systemic effects, this observer recommends the local application of the hormone in an ointment base,[63] or the use of rectal suppositories containing prolactin.[64] He found a minimum of 300 to 400 mgm. daily per rectum necessary for an effect, as compared with about 100 mgm. daily by the injection route.

The *efficacy* of lactogenic hormone therapy is difficult to estimate because of the occurrence of spontaneous variations in the level of milk production. Significant in this connection is the observation of Stewart and Pratt[65] that the milk output after prolactin therapy did not significantly exceed that which followed injections of saline solution.

Anti-thyroidal therapy, in the form of dijodotyrosine, has been employed on the assumption that overactivity of the thyroid may, by virtue of its diuretic effect, prevent access of an ample amount of fluid to the mammae.[66] Though this would seem to be rational therapy where there is an associated hyperthyroidism, the available data is insufficient to permit an estimate as to its efficacy.

GALACTORRHEA

Definition.—This term describes milk secretion which occurs spontaneously outside the limits of the postpartum lactation period. Galactorrhea has been encountered in association with neoplastic disease of the pituitary[67] or adjacent midbrain structures,[68] or as a sequel of basal meningitis, syringomyelia, craniopharyngeal epidemic encephalitis, tabes, tuberculosis, or typhus. It may appear after castration and, in rare instances, may follow psychic shock or severe nervous upsets.[69] Chiari[70] and Frommel[71] have described a syndrome in which milk secretion persists despite weaning and is associated with progressive utero-ovarian atrophy.

Etiology.—In view of recent experimental evidence establishing the *anterior hypophysis* as the source of the lactogenic hormone, galactorrhea associated with lesions of this gland or its environs is undoubtedly attributable to increased activity of the cells which secrete this principle. The appearance of this symptom following psychic shock may possibly be due to transmission of the nervous impulse to the adenohypophysis by way of the hypothalamus. A somewhat different explanation would seem to apply to the galactorrhea in the syndrome described by Chiari and Frommel. It is noteworthy that the malady tends to develop in individuals who are poorly nourished, and complain of abdominal pain, backache, hysterical manifestations and mental depression. Also significant is Frommel's observation that, though resistant to treatment after it is once established, the condition may be prevented by weaning the child and improving the nutritional status of the mother before genital regression proceeds too far. This would suggest that in the poorly nourished woman, lactation drains the organism of its nutritional stores and at the same time diverts much of the anterior pituitary's energies to the use of the mammae. As a result, the gonads are deprived of the minimum of nutritive and hormonal material necessary to maintain them at the level of activity normally seen during lactation. The progressive atrophy which ensues may also be due in part to an inhibitory effect of the lactogenic hormone (see Chap. X). When weaning once more releases the hormonal resources of the adenohypophysis for the use of the gonads, they are no longer capable of responding. In the absence of effective competition from the ovaries, the still responsive mammae retain the dominant position acquired during lactation, continue to utilize the pituitary's hormonal store, and milk secretion persists.

Treatment.—Galactorrhea due to a lesion of the pituitary or its environs, calls for eradication of the underlying cause by deep x-ray radiation or, where feasible, by surgical removal of the lesion.

X-ray Therapy.—Where spontaneous milk secretion follows castration, some advocate the use of depressive doses of x-ray directed to the *pituitary gland*. The evidence is too limited to permit a fair evaluation of the efficacy of such treatment. X-ray radiation of the *breast* has also been recommended for the suppression of milk secretion. Though it would appear justifiable in the castrate, the danger of injuring the secreting structures[52] makes its use undesirable in cases where the necessity of nursing may arise.

Organotherapy.—Estrogen therapy may be effective in some cases. Whether it acts by inhibiting the lactogenic activity of the adenohypophysis, or by producing some alteration in the mammary epithelium, which prevents its response to the secretion-promoting effect of the lactogenic principle, is not certain. Winter[72] has described a case of galactorrhea associated with amenorrhea and increased gonadotropin excretion, in which the injection of a total of 200,000 mouse units of estrogenic hormone was followed by cessation of milk secretion and a drop in the gonadotropin level of the urine. In a case of acromegaly associated with galactorrhea, Stephens[73] observed suppression of milk secretion during treatment with a total of 190,000 rat units of estradiol monobenzoate over a period of 23 weeks.

General Medical Measures.—Prophylaxis is far more effective than active treatment for the control of milk secretion which persists despite weaning and is associated with utero-ovarian atrophy. As already stated, if the regressive changes in the genitalia are recognized early, the syndrome may be prevented by weaning the child immediately and improving the nutritional status of the mother. Where the condition is already established, the prognosis is much less favorable. General medical treatment aimed at improving the general health may be tried with the hope of reviving gonadal function. At the same time, use of a tight breast binder, restriction of the fluid intake, and the administration of saline cathartics may help to check the secretory activity of the mammae and thus minimize their importance as a competitor for the hormonal products of the anterior hypophysis. The use of estrogen or androgen to check mammary secretion in such cases would seem to be contraindicated because of the possibility of aggravating the regressive changes in the gonads.

POSTPARTUM BREAST ENGORGEMENT AND UNDESIRED LACTATION

General Medical Measures.—Until recently, the routine treatment for the relief of painful breast engorgement and the suppression of undesired lactation consisted of the application of a tight breast binder, curtailment of the fluid intake, administration of saline cathartics, continuous ice-caps, and sedatives. Since this form of treatment requires considerable nursing care, observers have been quick to follow the suggestion that estrogen or androgen may accomplish the same purpose with a minimum of effort.

Estrogen and Androgen Therapy.—Though there is still no agreement as to how estrogen and androgen act, a number of observers have reported rapid relief of painful breast engorgement and gradual cessation of secretory activity following their use. Abarbanel[74, 75, 76] has presented evidence indicating that these hormones may be credited with the relief of painful engorgement which follows their administration. The gradual cessation of secretory activity, on the other hand, is apparently due largely if not entirely to failure to apply the suckling stimulus, for if suckling occurs regularly, even large doses of estrogenic or androgenic substance cannot prevent the initiation of lactation or suppress it after it is established. Abarbanel suggests that breast engorgement and the initiation of milk secretion are distinct physiologic entities, the former being due to lymphatic and vascular stasis and not to distention of the ducts by milk. The relief obtained with estrogen or androgen, he believes, is probably due to their effect on the shifting tides of extracellular fluid.

Observers differ as to the effective *dose* and the best time for beginning treatment. Most begin shortly after delivery and continue for two to six days. Some prefer to wait until the third or fourth postpartum day.[77] Estimates as to the effective dose of natural estrogen by the parenteral route vary from less than 1000[78] to more than 250,000 rat units daily.[79, 80, 81] Stilbestrol has been reported to be effective in doses of 1.0 to 5.0 mg. daily by mouth for two to four days.[82, 83, 84] A favorable response has been reported following the administration of 30 to 150 mg. of testosterone propionate by injection,[85, 86, 87] or about 200 mg. of methyl testosterone by mouth.[88, 89]

Opinions differ as to whether estrogen or androgen therapy is preferable. Some observers[87] object to the estrogens on the ground that they are often followed by considerable after-pains and increased blood flow. On the other hand, Rutherford,[90] who compared the effect of estrogenic and androgenic substances on the genital tract of postpartum women, found that estrogen delayed involution but hastened repair of the endometrium, while androgen had no effect on involution but markedly retarded the process of repair. He suggests that hastening of repair may account for the lowered incidence of postpartum morbidity noted by some observers[91] in women receiving estrogen therapy. He warns, however, that estrogen's stimulative effect on epithelial activity may be dangerous where trophoblastic tissue is present. On the other hand, he points out that androgen's retarding effect on endometrial repair may lessen the resistance to infection and increase the possibility of bleeding.

Thyroid Therapy.—Thyroid therapy for the control of breast engorgement has been employed to a limited extent.[92, 93] The relief noted following its use may be attributable to its diuretic effect.

BIBLIOGRAPHY

1. Grynfeltt, E.: Arch. d'anat. micr. *33*:177, 1937.
2. Davies, W. L., and Moncrieff, A.: Biochem. J. *2*:1238, 1938.
3. Werner, A. A.: Endocrinol. *19*:144, 1935.
4. Bishop, P. M. F., Boycott, M., and Zuckerman, S.: Lancet *1*:5, 1939.
5. MacBryde, C. M.: J.A.M.A. *112*:1045, 1939.

6. MacBryde, C. M., Freedman, H., Loeffel, E., and Castrodale, D.: J.A.M.A. *115*:440, 1940.

7. Adair, F. A.: West. J. Surg. *48*:645, 1940.

8. Allen, E.: Arch. Path. *21*:265, 1936.

9. Lacassagne, A.: Compt. rend. Acad. d. sci. *195*:630, 1932.

10. Pryor, H. B., and Carter, H. D.: California & West. Med. *48*:645, 1940.

11. Jacobson, A. W., and Kramer, A. J.: J.A.M.A. *109*:101, 1937.

12. Goodman, B. A.: J.A.M.A. *103*:335, 1934.

13. Gaines, J. A.: Am. J. Obst. & Gynec. *34*:130, 1937.

14. Cheatle, G. L., and Cutler, M.: Tumours of the Breast, London, Edw. Arnold & Co., 1931.

15. Taylor, H. C., Jr.: Surg., Gynec. & Obst. *62*:129, 562, 1936; ibid. *74*:326, 1942.

16. Geschickter, C. F.: South. Surg. *10*:457, 1941.

17. Reclus, P.: Rev. de chir., Paris *3*:761, 1883.

18. Schimmelbusch, C.: Arch. f. klin. Chir. *44*:117, 1892.

19. König, F.: Zentralbl. f. Chir. *20*:49, 1893.

20. Warren, J. C.: Am. J. Med. Sci. *133*:521, 1907.

21. Rosenburg, A.: Frankfurt. Ztschr. f. Path. *27*:466, 1922.

22. Whitehouse, B.: Surg., Gynec. & Obst. *58*:278, 1934.

23. Cotte, G., and Pallot, G.: Gynéc. et Obst. *33*:113, 1936.

24. Cotte, G., Pallot, G., and Berard, M.: Lyon Chir. *31*:453, 1934.

25. Cutler, M.: J.A.M.A. 96:1201, 1931.

26. Burrows, H.: Brit. J. Surg. *33*:191, 1935.

27. Herold, L., and Effkemann, G.: Arch. f. Gynäk. *163*:85, 94, 1937.

28. Bucher, N. L. R., and Geschickter, C. F.: J. Clin. Endocrinol. *1*:58, 1941.

29. Mazer, C.: Med. Rec. *140*:417, 471, 1934.

30. Heimann, J., and Krehbiel, O. F.: Am. J. Cancer *27*:450, 1936.

31. Astwood, E. B., and Geschickter, C. F.: Arch. Surg. *36*:672, 1938.

32. Geschickter, C. F.: Surgery *3*:916, 1938.

33. MacDonald, I. G.: Surg., Gynec. & Obst. *63*:451, 1939.

34. Taylor, H. C., Jr., and Waltman, C. A.: Arch. Surg. *40*:733, 1940.

35. Lepper, E. H., Pratt, C. L. G., Pratt, F. B., and Vaux, D. M.: Lancet *1*:249, 1938.

36. Preissecker, E.: Zentralbl. f. Gynäk. *63*:451, 1939.

37. Scarff, R. W., and Smith, C. P.: Brit. J. Surg. *29*:393, 1942.

38. Thorn, G. W.: Endocrinol. *22*:155, 1938

39. Atkins, H. J. B.: Lancet *1*:707, 1938; ibid. *2*:411, 1940.

40. Patey, D. H.: Internat. Abst. Surg in Surg., Gynec. & Obst. *68*:575, 1939.

41. Warren, S.: Surg., Gynec. & Obst. *71*:257, 1940.

42. Wainwright, J. M.: Am. J. Cancer *19*:339, 1933.

43. Wanke, R.: Deutsche Ztschr. f. Chir. *250*:234, 1938.

44. Lewis, D., and Geschickter, C. F.: J.A.M.A. *109*:1894, 1937.

45. Nathanson, I. T., Meigs, J. V., and Parsons, L.: New England J. Med. *226*:323, 1942.

46. Geist, S. H.: J. Clin. Endocrinol. *1*:154, 1941.

47. Desmarest and Capitain: Presse Méd. *45*:777, 1937.

48. Campbell, A. D.: Canad. M. A. J. *27*:347, 1932.

49. Goodman, B. A.: Arch. Surg. *38*:917, 1939.

50. Howard, N. J.: Proc. Soc. Exper. Biol. & Med. *34*:732, 1936.

51. Weber, H.: Arch. f. klin. Chir. *187*:715, 1937.

52. Turner, C. W., and Gomez, E. T.: Am. J. Roentgenol. *36*:79, 1936.

53. Cramer, W., and Horning, E. S.: Lancet *1*:72, 1938.

54. Hoffmann, F.: Zentralbl. f. Gynäk. *61*:35, 1937.

55. Meites, J., and Turner, C. W.: J. Clin. Endocrinol. *1*:918, 1941.

56. Turner, C. W., and Cooper, W. D.: Endocrinol. *29*:320, 1941.

57. Ely, F., and Petersen, W. E.: Proc. Am. Soc. Animal Prod., 1939, p. 80; J. Dairy Sci. *23*:536, 1940; ibid. *24*:211, 1941.

58. Jaschke, R. T.: Die Weibliche Brust, in Halban & Seitz' Biologie und Pathologie des Weibes, 1926, vol. 5, part 2, p. 1338.

59. Kurzrok, R., Bates, R. W., Riddle, O., and Miller, E. G., Jr.: Endocrinol. *18*:18, 1934.

60. Ross, J. R.: Endocrinol. *22*:429, 1938.
61. Kenny, M., and King, E.: Lancet *2*:829, 1939.
62. Preissecker, E.: Ergebn. d. inn. Med. u. Kinderh. *54*:702, 1938.
63. Preissecker, E.: Zentralbl. f. Gynäk. *63*:2539, 1939.
64. Preissecker, E.: Wien. klin. Wchnschr. *54*:53, 1941.
65. Stewart, H. L., Jr., and Pratt, J. P.: Endocrinol. *25*:347, 1939.
66. Küstner, H.: Deutsche med. Wchnschr. *62*:304, 1936.
67. Berblinger, W.: Schweiz. med. Wchnschr. *71*:1233, 1941.
68. Salus, F.: Deutsche. arch. f. klin. Med. *177*:614, 1935.
69. Reeb, M.: Gynéc. et Obst. *36*:19, 1937.
70. Chiari, J., Braun, C., and Spaeth, J.: Klin. d. Geburtsh. u. Gynäk., Erlangen, F. Enke, 1855, p. 371.
71. Frommel, R.: Ztschr. f. Geburtsh. u. Gynäk. *7*:305, 1882.
72. Winter, E. W.: Med. Klin. *30*:990, 1934.
73. Stephens, D. J.: Endocrinol. *25*:638, 1939.
74. Abarbanel, A. R., and Goodfriend, M. J.: Am. J. Obst. & Gynec. *40*:1037, 1940.
75. Abarbanel, A. R., and Klein, M. D.: New York State J. Med. *41*:383, 1941.
76. Abarbanel, A. R.: Am. J. Obst. & Gynec. *42*:110, 1941.
77. Duffy, P. V., and Corsaro, J.: J.A.M.A. *116*:33, 1941.
78. Sawizki, W.: Zentralbl. f. Gynäk. *59*:2784, 1935.
79. Hoffmann, F.: Zentralbl. f. Gynäk. *60*:2882, 1937.
80. Ramos, A. P., and Colombo, E. O.: Deutsche med. Wchnschr. *64*:782, 1938.
81. Adrian, J.: Bull. Soc. d'obst. et de gynéc. *27*:331, 1938.
82. Barnes, J.: Brit. Med. J. *1*:601, 1942.
83. Mendel, E. B., Goldman, A. M., and Caire, A.: Am. J. Obst. & Gynec. *42*:528, 1941.
84. Davis, M. E., and Boynton, M. W.: J. Clin. Endocrinol. *1*:339, 1941.
85. Kurzrok, R., and O'Connell, C. P.: Endocrinol. *23*:476, 1938.
86. Birnberg, C. H., Kurzrok, L., and Klor, S. J.: Am. J. Obst. & Gynec. *39*:107, 1940.
87. Siegler, S. L., and Silverstein, L. M.: Am. J. Obst. & Gynec. *39*:109, 1940.
88. Lass, P. M.: Am. J. Obst. & Gynec. *43*:86, 1942.
89. Duckman, S., and Turino, T. R.: Am. J. Obst. & Gynec. *44*:112, 1942.
90. Rutherford, R. N.: Am. J. Obst. & Gynec. *42*:110, 1941.
91. Connally, H. F., Dann, D. I., Reese, J. M., and Douglass, L. H.: Am. J. Obst. & Gynec. *40*:445, 1940.
92. Kraul, L.: Zentralbl. f. Gynäk. *52*:873, 1928.
93. Wachtel, M.: Zentralbl. f. Gynäk. *53*:987, 1929.
94. Ebbs, J. H.: Am. J. Dis. Child. *17*:212, 1942.

32

CHAPTER XXXIII

OBESITY

The importance of obesity as a symptom or contributory cause of serious systemic disorders is well recognized. While the average layman considers excess weight undesirable for esthetic reasons, the internist sees it as a predisposing factor in heart disease and metabolic disturbances, particularly diabetes mellitus. The endocrinologist regards it as possibly presaging some serious endocrinopathy, while the gynecologist views it as a condition which, in some as yet unknown manner, often hinders gonadal function and fertility. It is not surprising that its etiology and treatment have been the subject of extensive investigation.

Definition and Classification.—The term *obesity* describes a condition of overweight due to the accumulation of an excess of fat in the body tissues. Numerous classifications have been proposed, the simplest being the division into *exogenous* obesity, attributable to overeating and insufficient exercise, and the *endogenous* form due to some inherent abnormality. This is rejected by those who question the existence of "exogenous" obesity.[1] Until more is known of the etiology, it will not be possible to arrive at a classification acceptable to all.

ETIOLOGY

Endogenous versus Exogenous Obesity.—It is generally conceded that both internal and external factors may play a part in producing a state of overweight. Observers differ as to the relative importance of each. Some[1] accord internal influences the dominant role, while others believe practically every case is of exogenous origin.

Exogenous Factors.—The exogenous view is based on the reports of Newburgh[2] and others that all types of obesity respond to restriction of the food and fluid intake with a weight loss proportional to the energy deficiency of the diet, and where this does not occur, the explanation may be found in a definitely calculable and temporary water retention. These findings refute the argument, offered in support of the endogenous view, that some individuals gain weight out of proportion to the amount of food ingested, and fail to lose despite a reduced intake. This erroneous impression probably arises partly from failure to take into account the factor of water retention, and partly from an unjustified faith in the patient's veracity regarding the amount of food consumed. In the author's experience, the obese individual, particularly the less intelligent type, is prone to understatement concerning his daily food intake. Of interest in this connection is Hunter's[3] observation that dietary treatment failed in 85 per cent of his obese patients, not because the laws of energy conservation did not apply, but because dietetic rules were broken.

Endogenous Factors.—Though the available evidence indicates that dietary restriction is effective in all types of obesity, and no individual can escape the laws of energy conservation, it does not necessarily follow that practically all cases of obesity are of exogenous origin, and that endogenous factors play at best only a minor role. That an inherent abnormality is responsible for many cases is suggested by the fact that a disposition to adiposity is often inherited, and that a rapid accumulation of fat is a

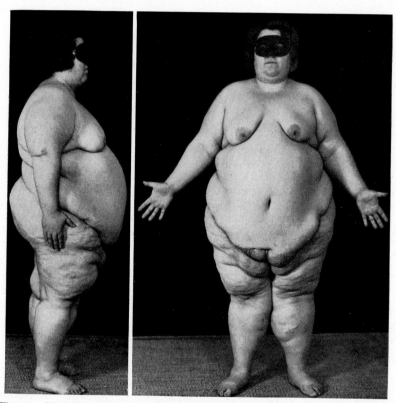

Fig. 99.—Marked generalized obesity. Patient aged twenty-eight, weight 348 pounds. Amenorrhea for fourteen years and primary sterility. Small genitalia; polypoid ("carcinoid") hyperplasia of the endometrium; negative estrogen tests. X-ray of sella turcica negative. After loss of 100 pounds in eighteen months with dietotherapy, regular menses established; pregnancy followed; delivery by cesarean section.

constant finding in certain syndromes with an undoubted endocrinopathic or neurologic basis. The possibility that the weight level is at least partly controlled by some intrinsic mechanism is also suggested by the observation that some individuals maintain a normal weight over a long period of time without conscious effort, while others either gain weight readily and lose with difficulty, or do not gain even on forced feeding. The nature of this hypothetical mechanism, and its mode of operation have been the subject of considerable investigation.

In seeking a solution, studies have been carried out to determine, (1) whether the obese show any deviations from normal which would tend to create a positive energy balance eventuating in adiposity, and (2) what endogenous factors, endocrine or otherwise, may conceivably be blamed for these aberrations. Particular attention has been directed to the appetite, which determines the energy intake, and to the temperament, basal metabolic rate, and specific dynamic action, which influence the total energy expenditure. In addition, the status of fat, sugar and water metabolism in the obese has been studied to determine whether their body tissues possess an unusual capacity for storing fat or retaining water.

CONTROL OF ENERGY INTAKE

The Appetite.—An excessive appetite and abnormal craving for foods of high caloric value are frequently encountered in the obese and undoubtedly play an important part in the etiology. The identity of the factors which control the appetite is obscure. That some intrinsic mechanism regulates the quantity of food consumed is suggested by Harrington's[4] observation that subjects offered unlimited quantities of food show a remarkable constancy in the amount ingested daily. That it also influences the selection of food has not been demonstrated experimentally, but it is significant that normal individuals tend to choose a well balanced diet, while the obese often evince a decided craving for foods of high caloric value, and underweight individuals frequently show unreasonable food dislikes, ingesting foods of high caloric value with difficulty.

Influences on Appetite.—Some observers believe that the appetite and feeling of satiety are controlled by a central nervous influence emanating from the organs of digestion. Others postulate the existence of an appetite controlling center in the brain, which is influenced by the concentration of foodstuffs in the blood. Rony[1] speaks of a "homeostatic body weight regulatory mechanism," which is apparently disturbed in obesity. According to Bauer,[5] the mechanism which regulates the appetite is associated with the intermediary metabolic processes and ultimately with the endocrine system. The situation in obesity, he believes, is analogous to that seen in dogs in which acromegaly is induced by administering anterior pituitary growth extract. Bauer maintains that this hormone produces its effect not through a direct action on the appetite but by intensifying the growth tendency of the tissues, which in turn increases the demand for food. His suggestion is borne out by the recent observation of Evans and associates[6] that growth hormone treated animals, given the same diet as untreated controls, gain significantly more weight. They concluded that the growth hormone causes increased deposition of tissue not as a consequence of increased food intake but through better utilization of food. So also in the obese, an excessive appetite may not be primarily responsible for the obesity, but may itself be the result of a heightened capacity for the absorption of foodstuffs and their deposition as fat.

When considering the causes of excessive appetite, the importance of habit and environment should not be overlooked. It must be emphasized, however, that though some cases may possibly be accounted for on this basis, more than this is required to explain the wide differences in appetite which may exist between individuals who are exposed to identical environmental influences and might therefore be expected to develop similar eating habits. The observation that dietary re-education often corrects an excessive appetite suggests that the abnormal desire for food was originally caused by bad eating habits. On the other hand, it may as reasonably be taken to signify that radical modification of the dietary regimen may permit spontaneous readjustment of a previously disordered appetite-controlling mechanism.

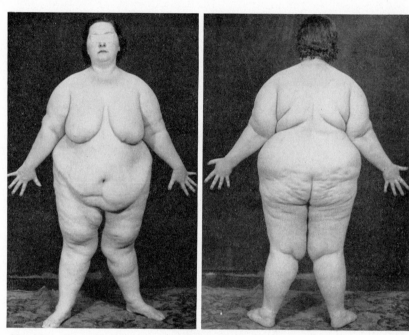

Fig. 100.—Generalized obesity. Patient aged thirty-seven, weight 278 pounds. Eleven children. Menses normal; genitalia normal; estrogen and gonadotropin values within normal limits.

Control of Energy Expenditure

If the energy output is decreased without a corresponding reduction of the food intake, it is obvious that a positive energy balance will result. It follows, therefore, that any factor which appreciably lowers the amount of energy expended is a potential cause of overweight. The total energy expenditure or total metabolism may be defined as the summation of three metabolic processes: (1) the basal metabolic rate, representing the sum of all the oxidative processes of the body when at rest; (2) the accessory oxidative processes due to the specific dynamic action of food; and (3) the accelerated metabolism due to muscular and nervous activity.

The Basal Metabolic Rate.—Studies of the basal metabolic rate in the obese have yielded varying results. Use of the total body weight as a basis for calculation tends to give the obese a low rate, possibly because of the large proportion of relatively inert adipose tissue. Use of the total body surface may also make for error when applied to obese persons. As pointed out by Rony,[1] comparisons of surface area, calculated on the basis of height and weight, with direct measurements of surface area indicate that this calculation is sufficiently exact for normal and most obese persons, but may show an appreciable discrepancy in obese persons with unusual distribution of fat deposits. Most investigators employing these methods have found the rate to be within normal limits in the large majority of obese individuals, being low only where there is an associated hypothyroidism. In the opinion of Strang and Evans,[7] both methods of calculation give misleading results when applied to individuals of abnormal weight. They consider it fallacious to compare an obese person with a normal one of the same weight, and maintain that the probable mass of active tissue rather than the actual weight should be employed, the figure used being the ideal weight of a person of the same age, sex and height. In their own series, and on recalculating the results of other observers, they found that the obese tend to show rates 25 to 30 per cent above normal, except where there is an associated hypothyroidism.

Without attempting to decide the relative merits of the various methods employed, we would seem to be justified in concluding from the evidence at hand that a low basal metabolic rate is of minor importance in the maintenance of a state of overweight. Whether it plays an equally minor role in the production of such a state cannot be decided from the available data, for tests performed after obesity has developed can hardly be employed as a measure of the individual's metabolic status at the inception and during the formative stages of the condition. A normal rate may signify that metabolic activity has been normal from the outset, or may be the end-result of a long series of adjustments, whereby an originally disordered metabolism has achieved a balance.[8] On the other hand, a low rate may conceivably indicate that the rate has always been low or, alternatively, that it has become low as the result of exhaustion of the overburdened metabolic apparatus.

Specific Dynamic Action of Foodstuffs.—A lowered response to the specific dynamic action of foodstuffs is considered by some investigators to be a contributory cause of obesity.[9] In the normal individual, following the ingestion of food, the basal metabolic rate rises for several hours and then returns to normal. The rise is most marked after the ingestion of protein, much less after carbohydrate, and negligible after fat. Attempts to demonstrate that this capacity for increased oxidative response is deficient in the obese have yielded inconstant results. In some obese individuals, it has been found to be diminished or completely absent, but in the large majority of cases, normal or above normal values have been obtained. Strang and McClugage[10] observed that in obese subjects, the rise in the basal metabolic rate after eating is the same as in normal individuals, but reaches its climax an hour later. They offer this as evidence that the physiologic load imposed by the ingestion of food is less in the obese, and suggest that this may account for the fact that obese individuals are slow in reaching a state of satiety.

From the available evidence, it would appear that an appreciable drop in the basal metabolic rate and specific dynamic action occurs in only a small percentage of all cases of obesity. Even where such a drop is demonstrable, it is probably not the sole factor operating. This is suggested by the fact that hypothyroidism, in which the basal metabolism and oxidative response to foods are characteristically depressed, may often be unaccom-

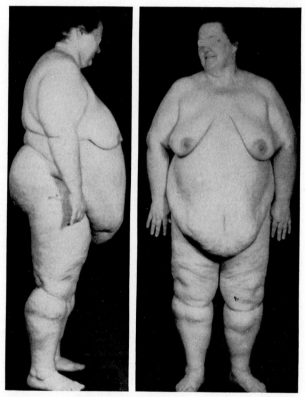

Fig. 101.—Marked generalized obesity. Patient aged forty-seven, weight 293 pounds. Four children. Irregular uterine bleeding for four years. Obesity developed during past seven years. Hyperplastic endometrium. Estrogen and gonadotropin values within normal limits.

panied by adiposity, while Simmonds's disease, in which a similar depression occurs, is characterized by emaciation.

Luxury Consumption Theory.—According to the so-called "luxury consumption" theory sponsored by von Grafe,[11] the normal organism reacts to overnutrition by progressive increases in metabolism, presumably as a protection against an undue gain in weight. Obesity develops when this capacity is diminished or absent. The evidence on which this theory is based is considered by some to be inadequate, because progressive increases in metabolism during overfeeding were established in subjects who were in a state of undernutrition at the beginning of the experiment. Though convincing proof of this hypothesis is still lacking, it is not unreasonable to suppose that a normal organism, which is admittedly equipped to decrease its consumption in undernutrition, should also be capable of increasing it in overnutrition, the purpose in the one case being to conserve energy, in the other to prevent excessive weight.

Accelerated Metabolism Due to Muscular and Nervous Activity.— In addition to the basal metabolism and specific dynamic action of foodstuffs, muscular and nervous activity materially contribute to the total energy expenditure. The latter cause a much more marked increase in metabolism than the ingestion of food. Though their effect is difficult to measure, they undoubtedly account for a large proportion of the total energy expenditure. Since the muscular and nervous activity of the individual depends to a large extent on his temperament, it can readily be seen that wide differences in total energy expenditure will exist between an individual who is physically active and emotionally responsive, and one who is sluggish, emotionless and phlegmatic. Such differences may help to explain why one individual is obese while another is of normal weight, though both ingest equal quantities of food and their basal metabolic rate and specific dynamic reaction to foodstuffs are within normal limits.

Though excessive accumulation of adipose tissue may be partly explained by an inability to properly oxidize the elements which contribute to the formation of fatty tissue, an unusual capacity for absorbing and storing these fat-forming elements probably plays an even more important role. Since adipose tissue is derived mainly from fat and carbohydrate, evidence that the obese show increased tolerance for either or both would appear significant from the etiologic standpoint.

Sugar and Fat Metabolism.—There is evidence[12] that when obesity first develops, the *sugar* tolerance may be increased but is more often normal. Later it diminishes steadily, often eventuating in spontaneous hyperglycemia and glycosuria. The extent to which the sugar tolerance falls is apparently dependent on the duration rather than the degree of adiposity. That it is not due to loss of the ability to oxidize sugar and deposit it as glycogen in the liver, is indicated by the observation that obese persons who show spontaneous glycosuria when on an unrestricted diet, have a normal dextrose tolerance curve after a low caloric diet restores their weight to normal.[13] The interpretation of these findings is not altogether clear. Though the developing adiposity and decreasing sugar tolerance are probably causally related, it is not certain how this effect is produced or whether it involves any alteration in the pancreas. So far as it goes, the evidence suggests that a heightened tolerance for sugar may be a contributory cause of the adiposity in only a small percentage of the cases. In the majority, any deviation from normal is in the direction of a decrease[14] rather than an increase in the sugar tolerance, and would seem to be the result rather than the cause of the obesity.

Attempts to demonstrate that obese subjects have an increased capacity for digesting and absorbing *fat*, or that their fat stores are less available for mobilization and utilization, have yielded conflicting results. MacKay and Sherrill[15] speak of "locked fat" on the basis of their observation that the ketonuria which develops during fasting is less in obese than in normal persons. Hetenyi[16] observed that the lipoid level of the blood remained unchanged in normal persons on a subnutrition diet but dropped 18 to 43 per cent in obese individuals whose intake was similarly restricted. The oral or parenteral administration of fat was followed by a rise in the blood fat level which was much more marked in normal than obese individuals.

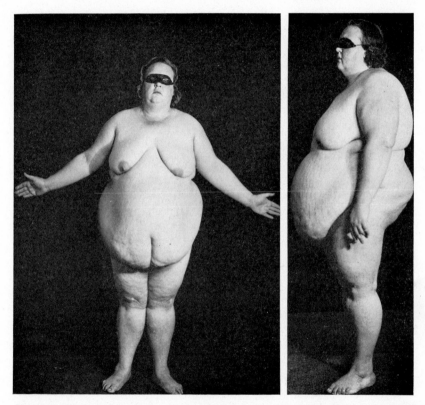

Fig. 102.—Marked abdominal and upper girdle obesity. Married woman aged thirty-two, weight 310 pounds. Genitalia normal; menses regular; mother of five children, each weighing 15 pounds at birth. X-ray of sella turcica negative. Case emphasizes fact that enormous obesity may be compatible with normal gonadal and reproductive function.

He interpreted his findings as evidence that the fat of obese persons cannot be mobilized for heat production, thus supporting von Bergmann's[17] view that the adiposity in some cases is due to a lipomatous tendency of the tissues or, in the words of Wilder,[18] "a condition of abnormally facilitated fat production and impeded fat destruction." Hetenyi's conclusions have been questioned by Block,[19] who found that obese women on a submaintenance diet maintained a positive nitrogen balance throughout. The blood lipoids varied in essentially the same manner as those of normal women on a submaintenance diet. He concluded that the obese women were utilizing their own body fat, which appeared to be as readily available for heat production as that in the normal individual.

Water Metabolism.—The importance of hidden water retention in obesity is now recognized by most competent observers. Von Noorden[20] recognized this when he stressed the value of water and salt restriction in the treatment of obesity. Zondek[21] and Bauer[5] apply the terms *water-salt obesity* and *hydrophilia* to cases in which retention of water plays a prom-

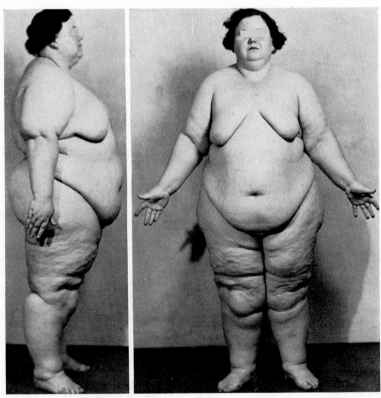

Fig. 103.—Marked generalized obesity. Female aged thirty-six, weight 340 pounds, height 61 inches. Eleven children. Amenorrhea for three years. Vasomotor symptoms. Atrophic changes in endometrium. Estrogen tests negative; gonadotropin test mildly positive. Loss of 140 pounds in two years with dietotherapy, followed by return of normal menses.

inent part. Retention of water is often overlooked as an etiologic factor, probably because water has no caloric value and therefore need not be taken into account when calculating the energy intake and expenditure. Its role in producing corpulency can readily be appreciated when it is recalled that water makes up 60 to 75 per cent of the total body weight, and its retention is a necessary concomitant of fat deposition. As von Grafe[11] has pointed out, "fatty tissues absorb water like a sponge without circulatory disturbances and with no evidence of edema." A few observers have attempted to prove, by means of the Volhard dilution test, that the ability to retain water is increased in the obese. Wohl[22] found that over half of his obese subjects retained more than normal quantities of water. Rowntree[23] has reported similar findings in two instances. In patients who reacted positively to the test, diuretics were effectual in reducing the corpulency after a submaintenance diet had ceased to have this effect. Water not only makes up a large part of the total weight of obese individuals, but is apparently not readily surrendered by the tissues, as suggested by the observation[2] that obese subjects on a restricted diet may fail to lose at first, due to temporary water retention.

Summary.—In summation, it may be stated that obesity may conceivably result from a disturbance in one or more of the many factors which influence energy intake and expenditure, and regulate the storage of fat and water in the body tissues. In the normal individual, the anabolic and catabolic processes are apparently so evenly balanced as to prevent an undue gain or loss of weight. In the obese, on the other hand, this balance would appear to be disturbed.

In seeking to identify the forces which control anabolic and catabolic activity and may, if disturbed, conceivably cause obesity, investigators have stressed heredity and constitution, and endocrine and nervous factors.

HEREDITY AND CONSTITUTION

It is generally agreed that an inherited predisposition to adiposity plays a part in many cases of obesity. Adiposity was a familial trait in 70 per cent of a group observed by von Noorden,[20] 88 per cent of Bauer's[24] series and 75 per cent of Nixon's[25] cases. Danforth[26] observed a strain of mice in which adiposity was transmitted as a dominant mendelian unit, while Gurney[27] has submitted evidence of segregation pointing to the mendelian inheritance of obesity in man. Among a group of obese patients this observer found 43 per cent had a stout mother, 15 per cent a corpulent father; in 24 per cent both parents were obese, a total of 82 per cent with one or two obese parents. In a control group, on the other hand, only 38 per cent had one or two stout parents. Study of the progeny showed that where both parents were obese, 73 per cent of the offspring were corpulent; where only one parent was overweight, 41 per cent of the children were similarly affected. Where neither parent was stout, only 9 per cent of the progeny were obese. The fact that fat accumulates in certain regions of the body, and the sites of predilection tend to be the same in several members of the same family, suggests that what is transmitted is not only a disposition to accumulate but also a tendency to deposit fat in certain areas of the body. While these observations strongly suggest that many cases of obesity are due to an abnormal gene transmitted from parent to child, it is not certain through what agents it impresses its will on the developing organism. It has been proposed that what is inherited is a peculiar ability of certain tissues to store excessive fat. Besides this tendency, there is evidence that the gene for adiposity probably also acts through endocrine and neural channels.

The Endocrine Glands in Obesity

Participation of the endocrine glands in the production of adiposity is suggested by the observation that obesity is a cardinal manifestation of certain endocrinopathies. The peculiar localization of the fat deposits has led observers to distinguish several "endocrine" types of obesity, naming each according to the gland principally involved. It has thus become customary to speak of "pituitary," "thyroid," "gonadal," "interrenal," and "pineal" obesity. Whether each of these is to be explained on a different basis, or all represent variants of a common morbid process, is still uncertain. The available clinical and experimental evidence suggests that some glands contribute more than others to the development of obesity. Because

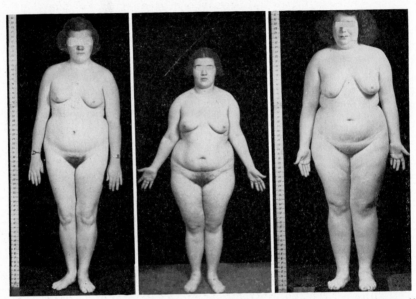

Fig. 104.—Moderate obesity associated with a low basal metabolic rate and other manifestations of hypothyroidism.

of their close functional interrelationship, all are implicated to a varying degree, some exerting a direct, others an indirect effect. By extirpating each gland, or noting the effects of its extracts, it has been found that none is without some influence on the oxidation or synthesis of fat, carbohydrate and protein, and on the water exchange. The actual production of obesity through these experimental procedures has been accomplished only occasionally, and then under circumstances not sufficiently well defined to permit definite conclusions. Though much has yet to be learned, the intricate interrelationships between the various endocrine glands and the metabolic activities of the organism are gradually being clarified.

Role of the Thyroid Gland.—The essential function of the thyroid is to promote cellular oxidation and maintain the general metabolic rate of the organism at its proper level. In addition, this gland influences water metabolism by promoting water elimination (see Chap. XVI). Since both these factors play a part in maintaining the normal weight balance, it might be expected that a deficiency or absence of thyroid function would make for corpulency by curtailing energy expenditure and water elimination. This supposition is not borne out by clinical evidence, for cachexia strumi priva is characterized by emaciation, while true myxedema is only occasionally associated with true adiposity, the corpulency being more accurately described as a "pseudo-obesity," since it is due chiefly to fluid retention in the subcutaneous tissue and skin.

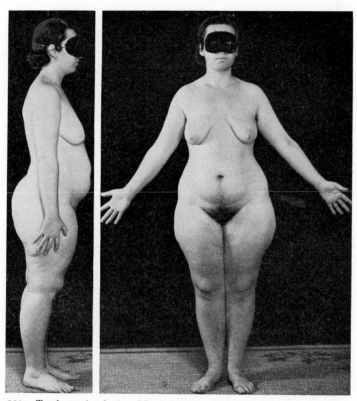

Fig. 105.—Trochanteric obesity. Married woman aged thirty; weight 160 pounds. Amenorrhea for three years associated with sterility. Hypoplastic genitalia; proliferative type of endometrium and subthreshold estrogen cycle. Note lower body obesity, particularly about the trochanteric region.

The absence of adiposity in severe *hypothyroidism*, despite a low basal metabolic rate and specific dynamic action, may possibly be explained by assuming that depression of thyroid function, if sufficiently marked, may directly or indirectly depress the anabolic as well as the catabolic activities of the organism, preventing a positive energy balance. A somewhat analogous situation apparently exists in Simmonds's disease, where severe anterior pituitary deficiency is associated with a marked depression of all vital processes, and emaciation develops despite a low basal metabolic rate and specific dynamic action. Whether the true adiposity sometimes associated with mild thyroid hypofunction is causally related to it, or is traceable to some abnormality outside the thyroid's sphere, is not clear. Participation of other factors seems likely in view of the fact that hypothyroidism rarely exists as such, being associated usually with disturbances of other members of the endocrine chain. On the other hand, the favorable response to thyroid therapy in obesity associated with a low basal metabolic rate suggests that the thyroid deficiency is at least partly responsible

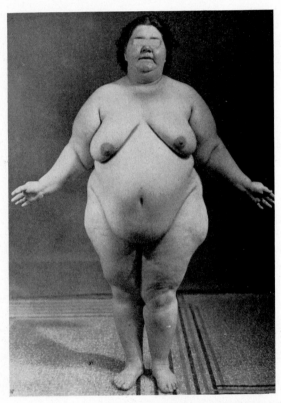

Fig. 106.—Trochanteric and upper body obesity. Patient aged thirty-two, weight 268 pounds. Five children. Oligomenorrhea. Obesity acquired gradually since birth of first child.

for the excess weight. To explain why mild thyroid deficiency may be associated with adiposity, while the weight is normal or subnormal in marked hypothyroidism, it may be suggested that the first effect of thyroid deficiency is a lowering of the metabolic level of the organism and a corresponding drop in the total energy expenditure. This creates a positive energy balance and leads to obesity. As the thyroid deficiency becomes more marked, however, the general depression of cellular activity may involve other incretory glands and tissues on which the anabolic activities of the organism depend. In this event, a positive energy balance is precluded, no obesity develops and if the depression is sufficiently profound, emaciation may result.

Role of the Gonads.—That *hypogonadism* may be an etiologic factor is suggested by the observation that obesity may develop for the first time following the natural or artificial menopause, or coincident with the onset of menstrual disorders, particularly amenorrhea. Whether the adiposity is due to loss of some ovarian metabolic principle, or is attributable to secondary alterations in other glands more directly implicated in maintaining the normal weight level is not certain.

Influence on Metabolism.—Attempts to prove that the gonads exert a direct influence on general metabolism have yielded conflicting results. Some observers[28, 29] have noted a cyclic rise in the basal metabolic rate during the premenstruum, while others[30] could observe no significant change. According to some workers,[31] the basal metabolic rate falls following castration, but this is apparently not a constant finding for many cases show no appreciable alteration. In experimental animals receiving estrogen, some have noted a rise, others a fall or no change whatsoever in the basal metabolic rate. According to Anselmino,[32] follicular fluid yields a metabolism-stimulating substance distinct from estrogen, which is ineffective in the absence of the thyroid, but Guggisberg[30] could not confirm his observation. Nor could he detect any appreciable change in the basal metabolic rate of castrated rats or women with ovarian deficiency, following the administration of large doses of estrogen. Negative results in the human being have also been reported by Stokes.[33]

Evidence relating to the gonad's influence on the specific dynamic action is limited. That its effect is stimulative is implied in Rolly's[34] observation that the oxidative response to foods decreases following castration. Attempts to demonstrate that the gonads influence *carbohydrate metabolism* have yielded varying results.[35] Though some observers report an increase in the sugar tolerance during the menstrual flow, the concensus of opinion is that cyclic changes in carbohydrate metabolism are not demonstrable in the course of the menstrual cycle. According to some workers,[36] estrogen lowers the blood sugar, increases insulin hypoglycemia and decreases the sensitivity to the hyperglycemic action of adrenalin. Barnes and associates[37] believe it acts indirectly by inhibiting the secretion of the anterior pituitary diabetogenic hormone. Of interest in this connection is Ogilvie's[12] observation that the fall in the sugar tolerance of the obese is particularly marked in patients with a history of ovarian deficiency. The effect of estrogen on the glycogen content of the liver is not clear. According to Raab[38] estrogen treated animals show an increase in hepatic glycogen due to increased gluconeogenesis, but Gulick and his associates[39] found that the glycogen store of the liver increased following castration and could be reduced by administering estrogen.

The ovary's role in *fat metabolism* is likewise uncertain. Lipemia has been reported following injections of the estrogens, but according to Neumann and Hermann,[40] the lipoid substances are increased in the blood of climacteric women.

An association between ovarian function and *water metabolism* is suggested by the observation that many women show a temporary gain of 1 to 4 pounds during the premenstruum.[41, 42] The author has often observed obese patients on a restricted diet who failed to lose or even gained weight during this phase of the cycle. Significant in this connection is Thorn's[43, 44] observation that dogs given estradiol or progesterone while on a constant food, fluid and mineral intake, gained weight due to temporary sodium chloride and water retention. Also noteworthy is the observation that normally menstruating monkeys show a cyclic increase in weight, trace-

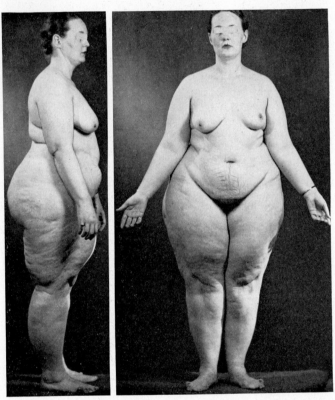

Fig. 107.—Lower body obesity. Single girl aged twenty-nine, weight 300 pounds, height 65 inches. Normal menses; pelvic findings normal. Sex hormone values within normal limits. Limited response to dietotherapy and thyroid extract.

able to sex skin swelling resulting from water retention,[45] and that monkeys subjected to protracted estrogen stimulation may develop edema in nonsexual areas of the body. It would thus appear that the estrogens promote water retention, though it is not clear whether they act directly on the tissues or through the mediation of some other gland.

Secondary Effects—Granting that the ovarian hormones exert some influence over the metabolic activities of the organism, the fact that adiposity does not invariably follow partial or complete suppression of gonadal function suggests that where it does develop, it is due to more than mere loss of the ovarian hormones. Gurney's[27] observation that adiposity develops after castration only in individuals whose family history points to an inherited predisposition to adiposity implies that some hereditary factor is implicated. It would thus appear that castration may be considered a cause of obesity only in the sense that it acts as a precipitating factor which causes a latent genetical tendency to adiposity to become

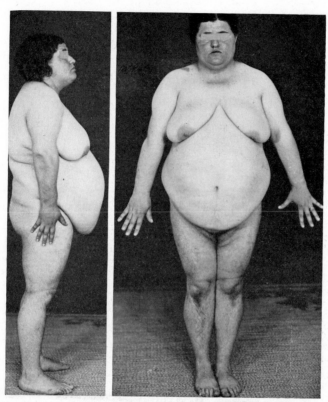

Fig. 108.—Upper girdle obesity. Nullipara aged twenty-eight. Amenorrhea for five years associated with primary sterility. External and internal genitalia hypoplastic. Negative estrogen tests; increased gonadotropin excretion; above normal androgen values. Atrophic changes in endometrium. X-ray of sella turcica negative. The moon-face, short neck, buffalo type of obesity, hirsutism, and decreased sugar tolerance suggest adrenal cortical involvement.

phenotypically manifest. That the *hypophysis* is a link in the chain of effects leading from ovarian withdrawal to adiposity is suggested by Schultze's[46] observation that the adenohypophysis of rats which develop adiposity following castration contains more enlarged basophiles than that of castrate animals which maintain a normal weight. It may be recalled in this connection that adiposity is a cardinal manifestation of *pituitary basophilism* (see Chap. XXXV).

Role of the Adrenal Glands.—That disturbances of suprarenal func-

33

tion may be a contributory cause is suggested by the association of adiposity with *adrenal cortical tumors* (see Chap. XXXV). Whether this manifestation is directly traceable to the abnormal state of the adrenals or is produced through the mediation of the adenohypophysis, is not clear. This uncertainty arises from the fact that the adiposity incident to adrenal cortical disease is indistinguishable from that of pituitary basophilism. While there is evidence that partial or complete suppression of adrenal

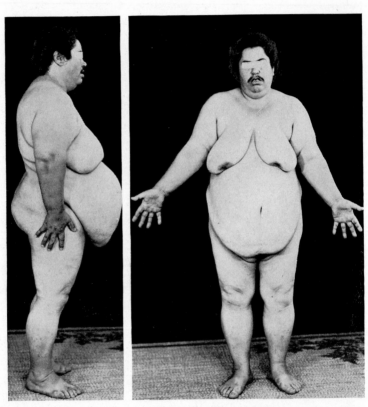

Fig. 109.—Obesity and hirsutism in an Italian woman aged forty-seven, mother of six children. Weight 252 pounds. Normal menses; pregravid endometrium; sex hormone values within normal limits. In view of normal menstrual and reproductive function, the hirsutism and adiposity are probably better explained on racial than on endocrinopathic basis.

cortical function may lead to emaciation, and that adrenal cortical extracts influence *fat and carbohydrate metabolism* (see Chap. XVII), there is no convincing proof that the administration of any of the available adrenal extracts will produce obesity. Of interest is Bomskov and Schneider's[47] observation in rats subjected to bilateral adrenalectomy. Some of the animals showed evidence of marked thyroid activity associated with a rapid loss of fat, eventuating in emaciation and death. Others showed a marked gain in weight associated with compensatory hypertrophy of the accessory adrenals, which attained a size greatly exceeding that of the glands removed.

Role of the Pancreas.—*Obesity and Diabetes Mellitus.*—The frequent association of obesity and diabetes mellitus suggests that pancreatic deficiency may be related in some way to excessive fat accumulation. Falta[48] suggested that both conditions may result from a state of *hyperinsulinism.* According to his theory, hyperinsulinism produces obesity by increasing the appetite, but sooner or later the pancreas becomes exhausted and diabetes results. Reports of the successful use of insulin for increasing the weight of the undernourished are significant in this connection. MacKay[49] recently induced obesity in rats by injecting protamine insulin over considerable periods. Of interest also is Ogilvie's[12] observation that the sugar tolerance was increased in one-third of his obese patients when adiposity first began to develop. Falta's theory has been questioned, however, on the ground that hyperinsulinism due to tumors of the islets is associated with emaciation and that such patients fail to gain weight even when large quantities of carbohydrates are administered to combat the associated hypoglycemia.

A view, advanced by von Noorden,[50] proposes that the diabetes is the cause of the associated adiposity. According to this theory, the fixing of sugar and glycogen is disturbed in diabetes, but the formation of fat from carbohydrates continues, the adipose tissue taking up the excessively formed carbohydrate and fat. This seems doubtful in view of Ogilvie's[12] report that the onset of obesity was associated with a normal or high, but in no case with a low sugar tolerance. His observation that the sugar tolerance gradually falls as obesity develops, and where the condition persists, often culminates in diabetes, seems rather to support the view that so-called "pancreatogenic" obesity is actually an exogenous form in which overeating and digestive stress have brought on both the obesity and the diabetes. According to this interpretation, a vicious cycle is set up in which overeating leads to hypertrophy of the islets. This results in hypoglycemia, which is in turn responsible for hunger contractions and increased food consumption.

The Anterior Hypophysis and the Pancreas.—A theory, recently evolved by Young,[51] is based on the newer knowledge of the role of the anterior pituitary gland in carbohydrate metabolism (see Chap. XIII). He attributes the adiposity and diabetes to anterior pituitary *hyperactivity,* involving particularly its growth, pancreatropic and diabetogenic factors. The pancreatropic hormone stimulates the islets and insulin production, and is at least partly responsible for the nitrogen retention necessary for increased body growth. The diabetogenic factor causes hyperglycemia either by suppressing carbohydrate oxidation or causing increased sugar formation from fatty acids. This effect is masked so long as the pancreas is capable of responding to the pancreatropic factor with hypertrophy and increased insulin production. With time, it becomes exhausted, the blood sugar level rises, and eventually irreparable damage to the islet tissue and persistent diabetes result. Young suggests that the prediabetic increase of height in children and of weight in the adult may be regarded as a reactive or protective mechanism for the storage of the carbohydrate, of which the oxidation is suppressed, and of the nitrogen retained under the influence of the anterior pituitary hormones.

Young makes no attempt to explain why the adult responds with adiposity instead of acromegaly to a situation which, in the prepuberal individual, leads to an increase in height. The answer may lie in age differences in the reactivity of the various incretory glands, and other organs and tissues through which the anterior pituitary influences metabolism.

Role of the Pineal and Thymus Glands.—Tumors of the pineal body are sometimes associated with adiposity, similar in distribution to that associated with lesions of the hypophysis or hypothalamus (see below). It is not certain whether this manifestation is due to a disturbance of pineal function, or to alterations in the neighboring pituitary and hypothalamus, caused by the pressure of the tumor. The latter possibility seems more likely in view of the fact that the pineal body has not been conclusively shown to possess endocrine function, whereas the hypophysis and hypothalamus are known to play a dominant role in regulating important metabolic processes of the organism (see below).

Obesity may sometimes accompany hypertrophy of the *thymus* in children, but since it is not a constant finding, the association is probably coincidental. The observation that structural alterations in the adrenals, gonads, and pituitary are not infrequent findings in cases with thymus hypertrophy suggests that the cause of the obesity may be found in these glands. Leschke[52] attributes the adiposity to a disturbance of the sympathetic regulation of metabolism, on the ground that irritability of the parasympathetic nervous system and salt and water retention are characteristic findings in this disease.

Role of the Hypophysis.—The available evidence suggests that the hypophysis plays an important part in the etiology. It is significant that adiposity is a cardinal manifestation of Fröhlich's syndrome and Cushing's disease (see Chap XXXV), conditions in which a lesion of the pituitary is believed to be an important etiologic factor. Experimental attempts to establish a causal relationship between this gland and adiposity have been hampered by technical difficulties involved in removing it without disturbing important adjacent nerve centers, and by the fact that its various hormonal principles have thus far resisted complete separation and purification. Despite these handicaps, recent investigations have yielded a number of significant observations which shed some light on this subject (see Chap. XIII).

In the earlier hypophysectomy experiments, adiposity developed following operation and it was therefore inferred that lack of the hypophyseal hormones is a causative factor in obesity With the adoption of more refined techniques,[53] it was found that adiposity followed hypophysectomy only if adjacent nerve centers were also damaged. When the hypophysis alone was completely destroyed, loss of weight occurred. These experiments, coupled with the clinical observation that marked hypophyseal deficiency, as in Simmonds's disease, is associated with cachexia, strongly indicate that complete suppression of hypophyseal function is not a cause of adiposity. A few observers[54, 55] have reported the development of adiposity following protracted administration of anterior pituitary extracts, but these observations are inconclusive because of the limited number of animals observed, and failure to determine the precise nature of the hormonal constituents of the crude extracts used. There is, however, ample evidence that the pituitary plays an important part in the *regulation of*

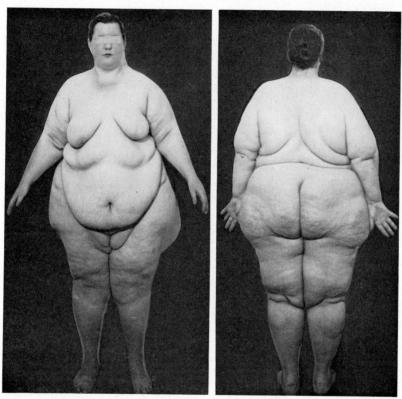

Fig. 110.—Marked generalized obesity. Single girl aged twenty-three, weight 420 pounds. Fatigue, dyspnea, and ankle edema. Irregular uterine bleeding associated with endometrial hyperplasia. Estrogen values slightly elevated. X-ray of sella turcica negative; eye-grounds normal. Note huge fat deposits in roll formation, particularly on the abdomen and trochanteric region. Loss of 102 pounds within ten months as result of dietotherapy combined with small doses of thyroid.

the metabolic activities of the organism (see Chap. XIII). Acting directly on the periphery and indirectly through other glands, particularly the thyroid, adrenal cortex and pancreas, it apparently influences both anabolic and catabolic activity. It has been shown to exert a profound influence over the basal metabolic rate and specific dynamic action, and also over the metabolism of fat, sugar, protein, minerals, and water. Though the evidence is still far from complete, it would appear that, under normal conditions, the anterior pituitary plays a major role in main-

taining the weight level, so that disturbances in its function may make
for adiposity or wasting, depending on the nature of the disorder. The fact
that its complete destruction is followed by emaciation may possibly be
explained by assuming that withdrawal of those principles which promote
anabolic activity more than offsets the loss of those which stimulate catabolic activity. On the other hand, lesions of this gland, such as are encountered in Cushing's disease and Fröhlich's syndrome, of which adiposity
is a cardinal manifestation, may conceivably produce this manifestation
by either increasing the production of those pituitary factors which favor
anabolism, or suppressing those which promote catabolism. The differences
in fat distribution in Fröhlich's and Cushing's disease suggest that the

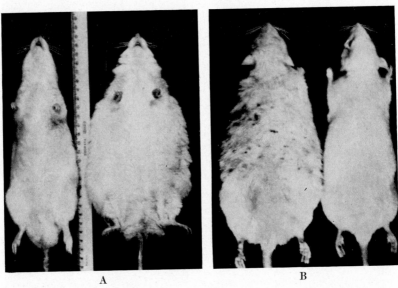

A   B

Fig. 111.—Hypothalamic lesions and adiposity in the rat. A, Left, control rat; right,
animal photographed at autopsy eight months after lesion was placed in hypothalamus by
Horsley-Clarke technique. B, Right, control rat; left, animal photographed at autopsy four
and a half months after operation. (A. W. Hetherington and S. W. Ranson: Anat Rec.
Vol. 78.)

disturbance assumes a different form in each case. Of interest is Thompson
and Cushing's[55] observation that adiposity resembling that of Cushing's
disease appeared in a group of rats and dogs following protracted treatment with anterior pituitary extract. This would suggest that this type
of adiposity is due to an excess of some pituitary hormone or hormones.
Unfortunately, the identity of the principles involved was not established.
A precise definition of the pituitary's role in obesity must await complete
chemical separation of its hormones, for only then will it be possible to
note their effect on fat deposition in different regions of the body, when
given singly and in various combinations.

   Neural Factors in Obesity: Role of the Hypothalamus.—The rapid
accumulation of fat in diseases of the brain or meninges suggests that the

nervous system also plays a part in the etiology of obesity. The association of lesions at the base of the diencephalon with abnormal obesity has been observed in both man and animals, but there has been considerable controversy as to whether a neural or glandular structure is primarily at fault. Of particular interest are the recent studies of Hetherington and Ranson,[57-64] demonstrating that adiposity follows experimentally induced degenerative lesions of the hypothalamus in the rat, dog, and monkey. The center whose destruction is responsible for this effect has not yet been precisely defined, though these observers are making steady progress in this direction. The hypophysis is apparently not involved, except perhaps secondarily, for marked adiposity may develop in the absence of any specific morphologic change in this gland or any disturbance in growth and sexual function. The adiposity is apparently not dependent on damage to the median eminence or hypophyseal stalk for it may develop in the absence of diabetes insipidus, and does not follow destruction of the infundibulum. Hetherington and Ranson concede, however, that their findings do not exclude the possibility that there may exist a hypophyseal adiposity as an entity apart from hypothalamic obesity. Nor do they exclude the possibility that the hypophysis participates in some secondary way in the altered physiological state attending the body's augmented fat supply. This much they hold to be certain, namely, that direct innervation of the hypophysis from the hypothalamus via the stalk is not necessary for the processes concerned in fat metabolism to proceed in an apparently normal fashion. That the hypophysis does participate, at least secondarily, is indicated by the observations of Heinbecker and White[65] in dogs subjected to various operations on the hypophysis and hypothalamus. On the basis of their findings, they reached the following conclusions: (1) Obesity in the dog results from partial destruction or retrograde degeneration of the paraventricular hypothalamic nuclei, particularly of their caudal portions. (2) Marked obesity results when destruction or denervation of the neurohypophysis and partial destruction or retrograde degeneration of the caudal paraventricular nuclei coexist. (3) Removal of the pars distalis in itself does not result in significant obesity. (4) The presence of the pars distalis in animals with partial destruction or degeneration of the supraoptic and paraventricular nuclei is favorable to the development of marked adiposity. (5) The results suggest that a lessening or lack of secretion of the neurohypophysis may aid in fat storage in the presence of a diminution in the number of cells of the caudal portion of the paraventricular nuclei.

Summary.—Though the available evidence leaves many questions unanswered, it clearly indicates that the metabolic processes are controlled to a large extent by the endocrine system, of which every member plays a part. Under normal conditions, these are apparently so adjusted as to maintain a normal weight level, but disease or functional disturbances in any one or more may upset the delicate metabolic equilibrium, with a resulting gain or loss of weight. Whether the weight level will rise or fall depends on the gland primarily involved, how its function is affected, and what reaction the disturbance evokes in other members of the endocrine chain. This may help explain why under- or overweight is frequently associated with gonadal and reproductive disorders, and why, as the author and others have repeatedly demonstrated, measures calculated to restore the weight to normal often simultaneously correct the associated gonadal disturbance. Since the endocrine system, and particularly the adenohypophysis, is intimately concerned with both metabolic and gonadal activity, incretory disturbances sufficiently marked to affect the metabolic equilibrium may also lead to gonadal disorders. Correction of the latter, following weight reduction in the obese, may conceivably be due to the fact that the endocrine glands are relieved of an excessive burden and are thus rendered more efficient for their task of maintaining gonadal function. This sequence of events may be expected to occur where the incretory disturbance is functional and therefore reversible, but not in cases where some irreversible organic alteration in one or more members of the endocrine system is at fault. In the functional case, the disturbance is apparently such that it may be aggravated if left unrestrained through failure to restrict the supply of material, liquid and solid, available to the deranged metabolic machinery. On the other hand, if the exogenous supply of such material is controlled through dietotherapy, the disordered metabolic machinery is enabled to achieve spontaneous adjustment, or at least is prevented from attaining full expression of its perverted tendency. The endocrine glands, which apparently provide the motive power required for its operation, are thereby permitted to divert their energies to other functions, among them the maintenance of gonadal activity. Here again, the principle enunciated by Allen[56] would seem to apply, namely that "interrelations of endocrine glands seem best interpreted by inclusion of a concept of balance through competitive utilization of certain limited vital necessities by successively dominant organs and tissues."

Though there is still much to learn, it seems likely from the information now available, that the coordinated activity of both the endocrine and neurovegetative systems is essential for the maintenance of the weight equilibrium. While a disturbance in either one may be the primary cause of obesity, secondary alterations in the function of the other probably contribute to this result.

COMPLICATIONS AND SEQUELAE

Adiposity, particularly when marked, may have an unfavorable effect on the organism. Fatty infiltration of the heart muscle and other vital organs may interfere with their function or eventuate in serious damage. Myocardial insufficiency, cardiac arrhythmias, renal disease, hypertension, arteriosclerosis, and coronary disease may complicate the obese state. Poor ventilation secondary to cardiac insufficiency, and mechanical impediments offered by the fat pads, may embarrass respiratory movements and make for troublesome pulmonary affections. The undue burden of overweight on the digestive and metabolic processes predisposes the obese to diabetes, gout, obstinate constipation, liver affections, gall bladder disease, and calculi formation.

Disturbances in gonadal and reproductive function are frequently associated with obesity. Amenorrhea and sterility in the female, and loss of libido, impotence and azoospermia in the male are frequent manifestations, particularly in the obesities of endocrinopathic origin (see Chap. XXXV). Obese women are more prone to toxemia of pregnancy, show a higher maternal and fetal mortality, and more postpartum complications.[66, 67]

Skin diseases, varicose veins, hernias, neuralgias, and psychic disturbances are common sequelae of obesity.

PROGNOSIS

In obesity unassociated with any demonstrable lesion in the endocrine glands or neurovegetative system, the outlook as a rule is good. Such individuals, if cooperative, respond readily to simple dietetic measures without endocrine therapy. Where the obesity has some organic basis, the prognosis necessarily depends on the underlying cause and its amenability to treatment. Where it is traceable to some adrenal cortical, pituitary, or midbrain lesion which can be controlled by x-ray radiation or eradicated by surgery, the prognosis is favorable. Obesity associated with hypothyroidism usually responds to thyroid therapy. Where the primary cause is obscure or resists therapy, as in *lipodystrophia progressiva, Dercum's disease,* and certain forms of *cerebral obesity,* the prognosis is poor.

Obesity, of whatever origin, is a menace to health and tends to shorten the life span. Obese individuals are peculiarly susceptible to infection and are poor surgical risks. In the presence of complications, such as diabetes or heart disease, the prognosis should be guarded.

DIAGNOSIS

In the absence of ascites or edema, the existence of an obese state can be established readily by an inspection in the nude. Comparison with standard height-weight tables is of some value but may sometimes be misleading, as recently pointed out by Behnke and his associates.[68, 69] These observers suggest that the decision should also rest upon the specific gravity (body weight divided by volume) of the individual, which is lower where fat tissue is excessive, than in the normal healthy individual.

History and Physical Examination.—The underlying cause of an obese state is less readily determined. A careful history, painstaking physical examination in the nude, and laboratory tests are essential. Significant in the diagnosis is a familial tendency to obesity or endocrinopathic disease, and a history of epidemic paratitis, lues, encephalitis lethargica or other diseases likely to cause endocrine or cerebral damage. Also important in the history are operations or x-ray radiation of the endocrines, and brain injuries. A valuable clue may be obtained from the events which immediately preceded or coincided with the onset of the adiposity, and the rapidity of its development. In the physical examination, particular attention should be directed to the type of fat distribution, and a careful search should be made for the presence of endocrinopathic stigmata. Tests of the basal metabolic rate, blood cholesterol, sugar tolerance, and specific dynamic action may yield significant information. In addition, roentgenologic studies of the skeletal system and sella turcica, and ophthalmologic examinations may be indicated, particularly where pituitary or midbrain pathology is suspected.

The diagnosis of Fröhlich's syndrome, Cushing's disease, and adrenogenitalism, of which adiposity is a cardinal manifestation, is considered in detail elsewhere. Lipodystrophia progressiva and Dercum's disease, whose etiology is still obscure, are also discussed with the endocrinopathies (see Chap. XXXV).

Thyrogenic Obesity.—Thyrogenic obesity is comparatively rare and usually of moderate degree. The fat deposits show a predilection for the face, nucha, supra and infra-clavicular region, and abdomen. In contrast to the Fröhlich's type of obesity, the forearms, wrists, dorsum of the hands, fingers, legs, and feet are involved. A history of disease or operation of the thyroid gland is important in the diagnosis. Recognition of this type of obesity is easy where it is associated with myxedema, a dry, thick skin, loss of hair, short, broad hands and feet, mental and physical sluggishness, hypothermia, slow pulse, and other manifestations of thyroid insufficiency. These, together with a low basal metabolic rate, high serum cholesterol, decreased urinary excretion and creatinuria, clinch the diagnosis. Since the basal metabolism test is not feasible in children, the serum cholesterol estimation is a valuable aid. An important therapeutic test of thyrogenic obesity is its striking response to thyroid therapy.

Hypogonadal Obesity.—Where the adiposity develops abruptly after the natural or artificial menopause, or coincident with cessation of menstrual function during the reproductive period, secondary changes in the anterior pituitary and other glands, precipitated by the withdrawal of the ovarian secretions, may possibly be at least contributory factors. So-called "hypogonadal" obesity often but not invariably shows a predilection for the breasts, abdomen, mons, proximal portions of the thighs, and especially the trochanteric regions.

Neurogenic Obesity.—A nervous origin may be suspected where the adiposity develops abruptly following disease of the midbrain or head injury. The presence of cranial manifestations, together with evidence obtained by roentgenological and ophthalmologic studies, are important in the diagnosis. In the physical examination, the clinician should be on the lookout for manifestations of the *Laurence-Moon-Biedl syndrome*, which is believed to have a neural basis. Considered by some a cerebral form of Fröhlich's syndrome, it is characterized by manifestations of dystrophia adiposa genitalis (see Chap. XXXV) plus retinitis pigmentosa, retarded mental development, atresia ani, cortical cataracts, poly- and syndactylia, skull deformities, strabismus, congenital nystagmus, and tremors.

The obesity encountered in *postencephalitis lethargica* is characterized by a sudden gain in weight, associated with progressive paresis. The fat deposits may be unilateral or bilateral.

TREATMENT

It is far simpler to prevent than to treat obesity after it has developed. Prophylaxis is particularly indicated for individuals with a familial his-

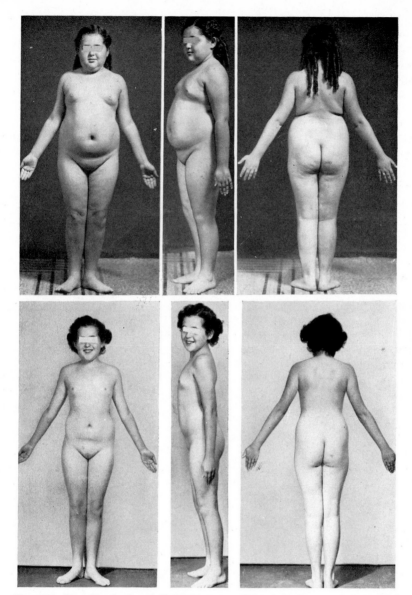

Fig. 112.—Juvenile obesity of Fröhlich's type. (Upper) Patient aged nine, weight 125 pounds, height 53½ inches. (Lower) Same patient one year later following dietotherapy plus small doses of thyroid. Progress in school studies much improved. Case constitutes example of childhood adiposity often erroneously diagnosed as Fröhlich's syndrome and treated with pituitary products.

tory of adiposity. Such persons should be carefully watched, especially at puberty, following childbirth, and after the menopause. Attention to weight is also important during convalescence from infectious diseases, or follow- ing surgical operations, for at such times patients often develop ravenous appetites and may become obese. The physician should warn his patients of the dangers inherent in obesity and encourage a habit of frequent weight check-ups. Any sudden or progressive gain in weight should be reported to the physician, so that appropriate measures may be instituted before the condition progresses too far.

Active Treatment.—Active treatment is indicated in individuals who are 20 per cent or more above normal weight. The aim is not only to effect a material loss of weight, but where possible, to eradicate the underlying cause. Close cooperation between patient and physician is of paramount importance. The aim of the treatment is to create a negative energy balance by increasing the energy expenditure and decreasing the energy intake. The methods employed for this purpose will vary according to

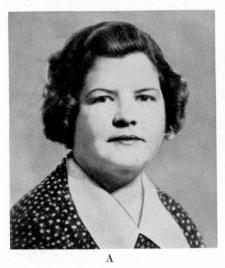 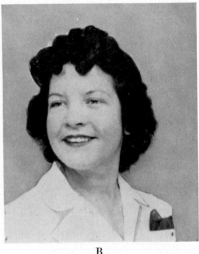

A   B

Fig. 113.—Female aged twenty-four, weight 190 pounds; height 62 inches. Amenorrhea and primary sterility. A, Before treatment. B, After dietotherapy and thyroid substance over a period of eight months. Weight now 126 pounds; menses regular.

the particular individual. To avoid untoward effects, the physician should be guided in his selection by the type and degree of adiposity, and the age and physical status of the patient.

Dietotherapy.—Regardless of the underlying cause of the adiposity, restriction of the caloric intake constitutes the most effective and often the only certain means of removing excess fat. This is not surprising for, no matter what is responsible for the abnormal operation of the mechanism controlling the weight equilibrium, it cannot express its perverted tendency without the materials essential for fat formation.

The diet should be low in calories but adequate in all other respects. It should be rich in *minerals* and *vitamins*, and include the three basic foodstuffs, protein, carbohydrate, and fat. The proportion of these elements should be such as to maintain the nitrogenous equilibrium and keep the relationship of fat to carbohydrate in accordance with the anti-ketogenic ratio. The diet should be attractive, varied, bulky, and have satiety value. *Fat* and *carbohydrate*, the main sources of adipose tissue, should be curtailed. Fat should be cut to a minimum, since it is the most concentrated of foods, and greatest calorie producer. *Protein*, on the other hand, is a desirable constituent of the anti-fat diet and should be prescribed in ample amounts. Besides promoting dehydration, it increases the energy expenditure by raising the specific dynamic action, and possesses greater satiety value than carbohydrate or fat. One to 2.5 grams of protein per kilogram of body weight may be prescribed unless a contraindication exists. The total number of *calories* may be made up with carbohydrates, preferably in the form of vegetables and fruits of low caloric value. The number of calories prescribed will depend on the degree of adiposity and rapidity with which weight loss is to be effected. Too severe a reduction in the caloric intake is not advisable, especially at the outset, for this may make the patient weak and irritable, and discourage her from continuing treatment. Caution is also necessary when prescribing a restricted diet for growing, obese children, who are otherwise healthy and active, for if too stringent, it may interfere with normal growth processes. A maximum loss of two pounds per week is a reasonably safe goal. In the average case, from 800 to 1200 calories may be prescribed. The rules to be followed in determining the number of calories in a specific instance, and a detailed description of anti-fat diets which fulfil all the requirements mentioned previously, may be found in any of the standard works on dietetics.

Since water retention is often a contributory factor in obesity, the *fluid intake* should be restricted to from 1,000 to 1,500 cc. daily. Alcoholic beverages should be avoided because of their high caloric value. *Salt* favors water retention, and should therefore be restricted or replaced by salt substitutes.

Water Elimination.—Turkish or cabinet *baths* are useful adjuncts in the treatment. Besides causing a temporary loss of water by way of the skin, the external application of heat may heighten the oxidative processes and thus increase the energy expenditure. Sweat baths should be taken under medical supervision, especially if the patient is old. They are contraindicated in obesity complicated by cardiovascular disease, because of the danger of cardiac failure or vascular accident.

Diuretics, such as ammonium chloride, neptal, salyrgan, and saline cathartics may be of value, particularly in obesity associated with water retention. These drugs should not be used over protracted periods of time, and only on the recommendation of a physician.

Organotherapy.—*Thyroid Substance.*—With the possible exception of thyroid substance, there is no convincing evidence that the available endocrine products are of value in the treatment of obesity. It is generally conceded that thyroid substance gives striking results in obesity associated with hypothyroidism. Whether it is also of value in other types of adiposity is controversial. Some observers contend that thyroid substance may injure the cardiovascular system and produce symptoms of thyrotoxicosis. Others advocate its use in any form of obesity so long as the basal metabolic rate is not elevated and it is well tolerated. In the author's

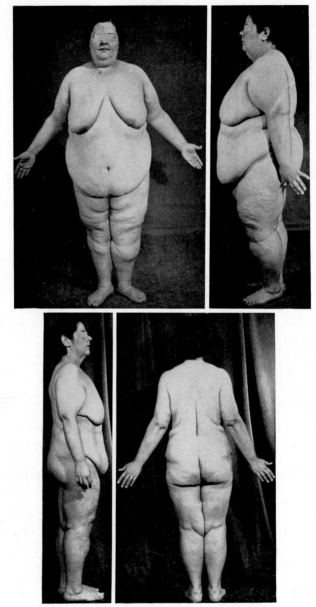

Fig. 114.—Marked generalized obesity. (Upper) Patient aged thirty-two, weight 300 pounds, height 61 inches. Painful fat deposits. Amenorrhea, proliferative type of endometrium, and subthreshold estrogen cycle. X-ray of sella turcica negative. B.M.R. —15. (Lower) Same patient two years later after loss of 125 pounds with dietotherapy and small doses of thyroid. Menses now regular; pregravid endometrium.

experience, thyroid substance may be used with good effect, even when the basal metabolic rate is normal, provided that it is administered in small doses, under careful medical supervision. Whether the weight loss which follows its use is due to its diuretic action,[70] to its pharmacodynamic effect on the oxidative processes, or its favorable effect on other endocrine glands more directly concerned in the etiology, is not clear. The dose is ½ to 1 grain of desiccated extract three times a day. This may be increased to two or more grains t.i.d. in cases of obesity associated with hypothyroidism. To avoid untoward effects, the pulse and basal metabolic rate should be checked at frequent intervals.

Anterior Hypophyseal Extracts.—Anterior pituitary preparations are advocated by some clinicians, particularly for the so-called "pituitary" obesities, on the assumption that the cause is anterior pituitary hypofunction. In the light of our present concept of the pituitary's role in general metabolism and its probable contribution to the causation of obesity, this explanation is obviously inadequate and therapy based upon it hardly rational. Any attempt to treat obesity with extracts of the anterior lobe must remain purely empirical until the precise nature of the pituitary's contribution to this condition is defined. In the author's experience, hypophyseal substance has proved of no avail. Claims that such therapy can influence adiposity are unconvincing because of the concomitant use of thyroid substance and an anti-fat diet. The author, like Rony[1] and others, has found human chorionic gonadotropin equally ineffective. Use of thyrotropic hormone and Collip's metabolic principle (see Chap. XIII) would seem rational, but these substances are still in the experimental stage and a decision as to their efficacy must await clinical trial. The author has employed thyrotropic extract in obesity associated with thyroid hypofunction, but the cases have been too few to permit any conclusions.

Ovarian Extracts.—Ovarian extracts, used by some for the treatment of obesity, are of questionable value. As previously noted, Guggisberg[30] was unable to increase the basal metabolic rate even with huge doses of estrogenic hormone. Convincing clinical evidence that ovarian extracts are effective in causing weight loss is still lacking.

Dinitrophenol.—This powerful metabolic stimulant is mentioned only to warn against its use. Since its introduction in 1933, there have accumulated many reports indicating its toxic nature. Skin eruptions, cataracts, hyperpyrexia, and granulocytopenia have been observed following its use. Since there is no reliable criterion by which the patient's reaction to this may be judged, and no suitable antidote is available, its use is contraindicated in any event.

Benzedrine Sulfate.—Amphetamine (benzedrine) sulfate is employed in the treatment of obesity because of its ability to cause anorexia.[71, 72, 73] Some observers[74] claim that it also has a calorigenic effect but others[75] find its effect on the basal metabolic rate inconstant. The loss of weight seen following its use is apparently due to the loss of appetite and restlessness which occurs under its influence. While this drug may facilitate adherence to a restricted diet, the occurrence of disagreeable side effects and the absence of proof that its protracted administration is harmless, make its use undesirable. Other more conservative means of gaining the patient's cooperation are preferable, though they may entail more effort on the part of the physician and patient. Significant in this connection is Bruch's[72] observation that children receiving 10 mg. of benzedrine sulfate daily did not lose significantly more weight than those given tablets resembling the drug. The best results occurred in a control group who showed good cooperation. In general, the loss of weight seemed to be proportional to the enthusiasm and cooperation of the patient.

BIBLIOGRAPHY

1. Rony, H. R.: Obesity and Leanness. Philadelphia, Lea & Febiger, 1940.
2. Newburgh, L. H.: Ann. Int. Med. *3*:815, 1930.
3. Hunter, D.: Proc. Roy. Soc. London, s.B. *29*:426, 1936.
4. Harrington, M. H.: J. Am. Dietetic Assoc. *6*:101, 1930.
5. Bauer, J.: Med. Klin. *29*:1297, 1933.
6. Marx, W., Simpson, M. E., Reinhardt, W. O., and Evans, H. M.: Am. J. Physiol. *135*: 614, 1942.
7. Strang, J. M., and Evans, F. A.: J. Clin. Investigation *6*:277, 1928.
8. Epstein, A. A.: Bull. New York Acad. Med. *10*:389, 1934.
9. Wang, C. C., and Strouse, S.: Arch. Int. Med. *34*:573, 1924.
10. Strang, J. M., and McClugage, H. B.: Am. J. Med. Sc. *182*:49, 1931.
11. von Grafe, E.: Metabolic Diseases and Their Treatment. Philadelphia, Lea & Febiger, 1933.
12. Ogilvie, R. F.: Quart. J. Med. *4*:345, 1933; Lancet *2*:885, 1935.
13. Newburgh, L. H., and Conn, J. W.: J.A.M.A. *112*:7, 1939.
14. Embleton, D.: Brit. Med. J. *2*:739, 1938.
15. MacKay, E. M., and Sherrill, J. W.: Endocrinol. *21*:677, 1937.
16. Hetenyi, G.: Deutsche Arch. f. klin. Med. *179*:134, 1936.
17. von Bergmann, G., and Goldner, M.: Functional Pathologie. Berlin, Springer, 1932.
18. Wilder, R. M., and Wilbur, D. L.: Arch. Int. Med. *61*:297, 1938.
19. Block, M.: Proc. Soc. Exper. Biol. & Med. *49*:496, 1942.
20. von Noorden, C.: Med. Klin. *5*:1, 1909.
21. Zondek, H.: Diseases of the Endocrine Glands. Baltimore, Wm. Wood & Co., 1936.
22. Wohl, M.: Am. Therap. Soc. *31*:211, 1932.
23. Rowntree, L. G., and Brunsting, L. A.: Endocrinol. *17*:377, 1933.
24. Bauer, J.: Verhandl. d. gesellsch. f. Verdauungs. u. Stoffwechselkr. *9*:116, 1929.
25. Nixon, N. K.: J. Pediat. *4*:295, 1934.
26. Danforth, C. H.: J. Heredity *18*:153, 1927.
27. Gurney, R.: Arch. Int. Med. *57*:557, 1936.
28. Wakeham, G.: J. Biol. Chem. *56*:555, 1923.
29. Lanz, W.: Ztschr. f. Geburtsh. u. Gynäk. *89*:133, 1925.
30. Guggisberg, H.: Helvet. med. Acta *1*:271, 1935.
31. Loewy, A., and Richter, P. F.: Zentralbl. f. Physiol. *16*:449, 1902.
32. Anselmino, K. J., and Hoffmann, F.: Arch. f. Gynäk. *162*:176, 1936.
33. Stokes, E. H.: Med. J. Australia *1*:804, 1934.
34. Rolly: Deutsche med. Wchnschr. *47*:887, 917, 1921.
35. Cramer, H. I.: Canad. M. A. J. *47*:51, 1942.
36. Elek, L.: Ztschr. f. exper. Med. *85*:227, 1932.
37. Barnes, B. O., Regan, J. F., and Nelson, W. O.: J.A.M.A. *101*:926, 1933.
38. Raab, W.: Arch. f. Gynäk. *144*:284, 1931.
39. Gulick, M., Samuels, L. T., and Deuel, H. J., Jr.: J. Biol. Chem. *105*:29, 1934.
40. Neumann, R., and Hermann, W.: Arch. f. Hyg. *45*:1, 1902.
41. Thomas, W. A., and Sweeney, J. S.: J.A.M.A. *103*:234, 1934.
42. Atkinson, A. J., and Ivy, A. C.: J.A.M.A. *106*:515, 1936.
43. Thorn, G. W., and Harrop, G. A.: Science *86*:40, 1937.
44. Thorn, G. W., Nelson, K. R., and Thorn, D. W.: Endocrinol. *22*:155, 1938.
45. Krohn, P. L., and Zuckerman, S.: J. Physiol. *88*:369, 1937.

46. Schultze, K. W.: Arch. f. Gynäk. *158*:555, 1934.
47. Bomskov, C., and Schneider, E.: Klin. Wchnschr. *18*:12, 1939.
48. Falta, W.: Endocrine Diseases. London, Churchill, 1923.
49. MacKay, E., personal communication to D. P. Barr, in Internat. Clin. *3*:134, 1941.
50. von Noorden, C.: Die Fettsucht, Nothnagel's spez. Path. u. Therap. *8*:4, 1900.
51. Young, F. G.: Brit. Med. J. *2*:897, 1941.
52. Leschke, E.: Stoffwechsel Krankheiten. Leipzig, T. Steinkopff, 1930.
53. Smith, P. E.: Am. J. Anat. *45*:205, 1930.
54. Evans, H. M., Meyer, K., Simpson, M. E., and Reichert, F. L.: Proc. Soc. Exper. Biol. & Med. *29*:857, 1932.
55. Thompson, K. W., and Cushing, H.: Proc. Roy. Soc. London, s.B. *115*:88, 1934.
56. Allen, E.: J.A.M.A. *116*:405, 1941.
57. Hetherington, A. W.: Anat. Rec. *76*(Suppl.):30, 1940.
58. Hetherington, A. W.: Endocrinol. *26*:264, 1940.
59. Hetherington, A. W., and Ranson, S. W.: Proc. Soc. Exper. Biol. & Med. *41*:465, 1939.
60. Hetherington, A. W., and Ranson, S. W.: Anat. Rec. *78*:149, 1940.
61. Hetherington, A. W., and Ranson, S. W.: Proc. Soc. Exper. Biol. & Med. *49*:321, 1942.
62. Hetherington, A. W., and Ranson, S. W.: J. Comp. Neurol. *76*:475, 1942.
63. Hetherington, A. W., and Ranson, S. W.: Am. J. Physiol. *136*:609, 1942.
64. Hetherington, A. W., and Ranson, S. W.: Endocrinol. *31*:30, 1942.
65. Heinbecker, P., and White, H. L.: Proc. Soc. Exper. Biol. & Med. *49*:324, 1942.
66. Matthews, H. B., and der Brucke, M. G.: J.A.M.A. *110*:554, 1938.
67. Koller, T., and Zoller, C. M.: Schweiz. med. Wchnschr. *71*:1296, 1941.
68. Behnke, A. R., Feen, B. G., and Welham, W. C.: J.A.M.A. *118*:495, 1942.
69. Welham, W. C., and Behnke, A. R.: J.A.M.A. *118*:498, 1942.
70. Handelsmann, M. B., and Gordon, M. B.: J. Clin. Endocrinol. *1*:612, 1941.
71. Ersner, J. S.: Endocrinol. *27*:776, 1940.
72. Bruch, H., and Waters, I.: J. Pediat. *20*:54, 1942.
73. Chrisman, R. B., Jr.: South. Med. & Surg. *104*:200, 1942.
74. Dill, D. B., Johnson, R. E., and Daly, C.: Am. J. Med. Sc. *198*:702, 1939.
75. Altschule, M. P., and Iglauer, A.: J. Clin. Investigation *19*:497, 1940.

34

CHAPTER XXXIV

CONSTITUTIONAL TYPES

Definition.—Constitution, as defined by Pende,[1] is the "morphological, physiological, and psychological resultant of the properties of all the cellular and humoral elements of the body; this resultant is determined by the laws of heredity and by the influence of environment." While no two women are identical in their physical and mental makeup, certain general types are readily definable. Many classifications are found in the world

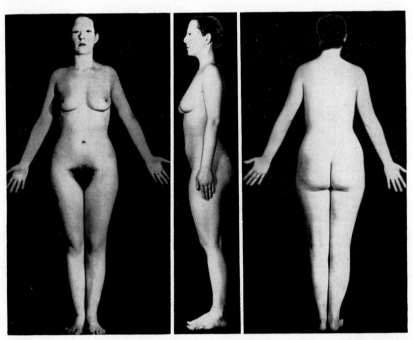

Fig. 115.—Normal type. Single woman aged twenty-five. Anthropometric measurements normal (upper measurement equals lower and span equals height). Normal development of primary and secondary sex characters. Menses regular. Note feminine body contours and normal fat and hair distribution.

literature, some based on morphological,[2, 3] others on functional characteristics.[4] In the present writing, Tandler's[5] division into the normal, hypotonic, and hypertonic types will be followed.

DESCRIPTION OF TYPES

Normal Type.—The so-called "normal" woman, as described by Gellhorn,[6] is of moderate height and weight, and endowed with a physical and mental makeup conducive to good health and a fruitful life. Her skeletal frame is well proportioned, the upper measurement (scalp to pubic bone) equalling the lower one (pubic bone to soles), and the span being equivalent to the height. The subcutaneous adipose tissue is ample without being excessive, and its even distribution makes for soft, graceful body contours. The soft, clear, and elastic skin is devoid of hair, except in the pubic and axillary regions. The face is small with delicate features, the neck well rounded, and the clavicles, scapulae and ribs well padded with subcutaneous fat. The costal angle is greater than 90 degrees, and the scapulae lie flat against the thorax. The musculature and connective tissue of the abdomen and pelvic floor are of good tone, furnishing adequate support for the abdominal viscera and pelvic organs. Also characteristic are the wide pelvis with ample outlet, broad hips, prominent and firm buttocks, and tapering thighs in close approximation.

The primary and secondary sex characters are well developed. The firm, well rounded breasts contain ample glandular tissue. Both the external and internal genitalia are fully matured, and menstruation is regular and painless. Conception occurs readily, pregnancy is usually uneventful, and labor offers little difficulty. Because of her normal physical and mental makeup, she adapts herself readily to changing environmental conditions, and passes through the climacteric with a minimum of discomfort.

Hypotonic Types.—To this group belong the tall and thin or "linear" asthenic, the short and broad or "lateral" hypotonic, and the infantile individual.

Linear Asthenic.—The linear asthenic may be of normal height, but is more often tall. Her angular body contours sharply contrast with the soft graceful curves of the normal woman. Her skeletal frame is frail, while her musculature, and subcutaneous tissue and fat are inadequate and of an inferior quality. Frequently there is a high dorsal kyphosis and low lumbar lordosis, with resultant poor posture. A long, narrow, sharp featured "hatchet-face" is characteristic. The neck is long and thin, and the larynx very prominent. The deficiency in subcutaneous fat makes the clavicles, ribs and vertebrae conspicuous. The thorax is long, narrow, and flat, the scapulae project outwards, and the ribs are acutely angulated. The upper and lower extremities are long and thin, and the thighs widely spaced. Because of the inadequate musculature, connective tissue, and intra-abdominal fat, general visceroptosis is a frequent finding. The internal and external genitalia are often poorly developed and the inferior quality of the pelvic connective tissue makes for uterine displacements, prolapse, and vaginal relaxation.

Thanks to the protection and special care often afforded them, asthenics may outlive normally constituted individuals who are subjected to the rigors and stresses of life. The demands incident to the reproductive period are, however, often too much for the asthenic woman. This probably explains why these individuals make up a large percentage of gynecologic patients.

Lateral Hypotonic (Pyknic).—The "lateral" hypotonic or "pyknic" type is characterized by a rather marked lateral development of the thorax and abdomen, and frequently by adiposity. The skeleton is delicate and deficient in calcium. Such individuals as a rule are short in stature, and their body proportions are not unlike those of the child. The head is short and broad, and the features distinctly puerile. The body is usually very well padded, the adiposity showing a predilection for the lower chin, neck, breasts, abdomen and hips. The cardiovascular system is often poorly developed, while the veins and lymphatics are rather prominent.

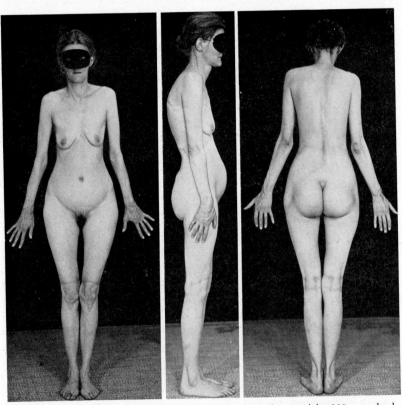

Fig. 116.—Asthenic type. Married woman aged thirty-four, weight 105 pounds, height 66 inches. Asthenic constitution associated with amenorrhea, sterility, frigidity, and nervous and psychic manifestations.

The primary and secondary sex characters may be normal, but more often are hypoplastic.

Infantile Type.—The infantile type of woman presents the physical and psychic pattern of the prepuberal girl. The rounded chin, full cheeks, high, narrow, hard palate, receding lower jaw, and widely spaced teeth suggest the features of the child. Her thorax is narrow and barrel-shaped, and her ribs, like those of the young girl, run at right angles to the spine. The pelvis is small, its outlet narrow and funnel-shaped. The bones of the lower girdle, like the rest of the skeleton, are light and delicate.

The *endocrine glands,* particularly the hypophysis and ovary, are apparenty implicated in the general arrest of somatic development, as indicated by the retardation of the primary and secondary sex characters. The vulva and vagina are ill-developed, the uterus small and acutely anteflexed, and the cervix narrow, elongated, and nipple-shaped. The ovaries are likewise small, with a thick, smooth capsule, indicating that ovulation has never occurred. In some instances, they may be enlarged to oyster size and contain numerous cystic follicles of varying size, but no corpora lutea. In the severe case, primary amenorrhea and permanent sterility are

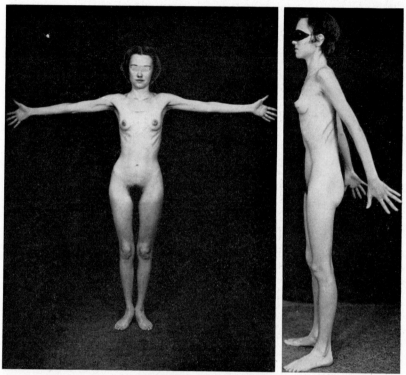

Fig. 117.—Infantile type. Single woman aged twenty-three, weight 71 pounds, height 57 inches. Petite, delicate, and small boned. No disproportion between upper and lower measurements. Small breasts; internal and external genitalia small. Oligomenorrhea with subthreshold estrogen cycle.

the rule. The mild case, on the other hand, may present some degree of genital development. In this event the menarche may be late and the periods scanty and infrequent. Should conception occur, the hypoplastic uterus is likely to be inadequate to accommodate the growing fetus and abortion is therefore frequent. Should pregnancy continue uninterrupted to term, the narrow pelvis and poorly developed supports may make labor difficult and result in serious obstetrical trauma. Under these circumstances, vaginal delivery may be difficult or impossible.

Occasionally individuals are encountered who give the general impression of infantilism, but whose behavior and functional status are those of the normal woman. Though their body build is small and delicate, they possess well developed primary and secondary sex characters, and menstrual function is normal. Such individuals conceive readily and as a rule encounter comparatively little difficulty during labor and the puerperium. Often the entire body undergoes a marked degree of development during gestation. This type has been described as a miniature edition of the normal adult woman.

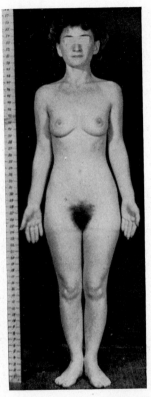

Fig. 118.—Infantile type with fair degree of sexual development. Single girl, aged thirty; weight 74 pounds, height 57 inches. Oligomenorrhea and psychoneurotic manifestations.

Hypertonic Types.—To this group belong the tall or linear sthenic, the broad or lateral sthenic, and the heterosexual or masculine type.

Linear Sthenic.—The tall or linear sthenic may be described as a large, robust, powerful woman, who is sometimes classified as a physiologic giant because of her great stature and proportionate body build. She is endowed with a well formed, strong skeletal frame, powerful musculature, long strong limbs, and normal viscera. Her primary and secondary sex characters are well developed, she menstruates normally, conceives readily, and her large, roomy pelvis makes labor easy and safe. She enjoys good health and has a cheerful disposition.

Lateral Sthenic.—The broad or lateral sthenic type of woman is a short, broad-boned, stocky, closely knit individual, with a strong, thick skeletal frame, powerful musculature, and a large massive trunk. Her features are strong and angular, her complexion ruddy. Her primary and secondary sex characters are well developed and her menstrual and reproductive potentialities are normal.

Heterosexual Type.—The heterosexual or masculine type is usually above the average in height and weight. Her skeleton is massive and her

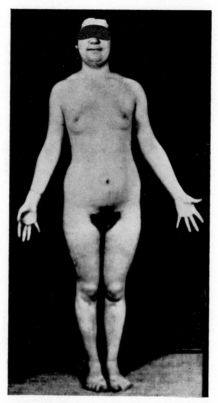

Fig. 119.—Heterosexual constitutional type. Female aged twenty-five years; weight 150 pounds. Late puberty, amenorrhea alternating with menorrhagia; hypoplastic genitalia; small breasts; tendency to masculine contours; facial hirsutism. Atrophic changes of endometrium. Subthreshold estrogen cycle. Sella negative.

musculature unusually well developed for a woman. Her features are coarse and her skin thick and often pigmented. She has broad shoulders and a large voluminous thorax. Her body hair is distinctly of the male type and distribution, the hirsutism showing a predilection for the upper lip, chin, chest, abdomen and extremities. Her pelvis is large, of the masculine type with narrow, funnel-shaped outlet, and thick, massive bones compose the pelvic girdle. The developmental and functional status of her secondary sex characters varies according to the degree of genital development she has achieved. If her development has been arrested during early life, her primary and secondary sex characters will be ill developed, often precluding menstrual and reproductive function. In some instances, however, complete sexual development is attained, in which case the uterus is unduly large and the clitoris oversized. Normal marital relations and conception are then possible, and pregnancy may proceed to a successful conclusion. The large majority of heterosexual women suffer severe mental distress because of their physical incompleteness. Some rebel against their

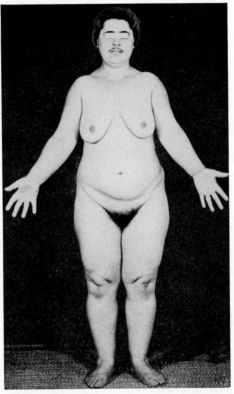

Fig. 120.—Heterosexual type with fair degree of sexual development. Amenorrhea and primary sterility; hypoplastic genitalia; androgen values above normal.

femininity, and find menstruation, coitus, and the thought of childbirth obnoxious. Though frigidity is the rule, some are oversexed.

SIGNIFICANCE OF CONSTITUTION IN GYNECOLOGY

Genital Disorders.—Due appreciation of constitution may aid in the diagnosis, prognosis, and treatment of menstrual disturbances, dysmenorrhea, dyspareunia, sterility, lower abdominal pain, and backache. As Bauer[7] points out, disorders of constitutional origin are often labelled as endocrine cases and treated accordingly. This error may arise either because the individual exhibits endocrinopathic stigmata actually unrelated to the constitutional anomaly; because the endocrines act, in the particular case, as the agents through which the genetically determined abnormality is phenotypically expressed, or because the clinician is a faddist who prescribes hormonal preparations indiscriminately.

Surgery.—It is especially important to consider the constitutional makeup of the individual when contemplating surgery in the asthenic woman. Because of the general visceroptosis and low pain threshold which characterizes such individuals, they often complain of lower abdominal discomfort or pain, frequently erroneously diagnosed as chronic appendicitis and treated surgically. Dysmenorrhea and backache, common complaints in such women, are too often treated by surgical means on the assumption that the symptoms are due to uterine displacement. Suspension operations are apt to be unsuccessful because of the inferior quality of the pelvic connective tissue and uterine ligaments. Temporary relief is sometimes obtained, but this is probably due to the prolonged rest in bed necessitated by the operation. Sooner or later, as the good effects of hospitalization wear off, the symptoms recur.

Course of Climacteric.—An appreciation of the individual's constitutional makeup may enable the observer to predict to some extent the course of her climacteric. As a rule, the woman of normal constitution may be expected to pass through this transitional period with little or no physical or psychic upheaval. The constitutionally inferior woman, on the other hand, will probably suffer severely. This is especially true of the asthenic woman who experiences her usual complaints in exaggerated form during the climacteric. Heterosexual women either improve or become worse. For some, the menopause resolves the disharmonies of their torn personality;[8] in others, the masculine traits become intensified. The infantile type of woman may pass through the climacteric with very little discomfort for, having never actually matured, she undergoes no appreciable "change of life."

TREATMENT OF CONSTITUTIONAL INFERIORITY

Since, by definition, constitution is the resultant of hereditary and environmental factors, the ideal therapy would be to correct or improve both of these. An attempt at selective breeding in the human is unfortunately far from practicable at the present time. We are therefore necessarily limited to the prevention or correction of all unfavorable environmental influences. It should be emphasized that prophylaxis is far more effective than treatment of an established abnormality. Preventive measures should be utilized early in life, before epiphyseal union takes place. Children of constitutionally inferior women should be closely watched, and the physician should be on the lookout for any abnormal deviation in growth and development. A healthy regimen, including an abundance of fresh air and sunlight, a well-balanced diet rich in the essential vitamins, proper exercise, and corrective supports, where indicated, can do much to minimize or forestall many of the physical and nervous manifestations which may appear later in life.

Asthenic Types.—Adult women of the hypotonic or asthenic constitutional type should be spared unnecessary physical and mental strain. They should be cautioned against too frequent gestations and prolonged lactation. Such individuals require special prenatal care, and all available means should be employed to minimize the burdens of labor and avoid obstetrical trauma.[9] The physician should guard against such complications as uterine inertia, puerperal infections, and postpartum hemorrhage. Following delivery, such women require a longer period of rest in bed than the normal woman, and should be spared the burden of lactation.

Surgical procedures, unless urgent, should be avoided, for unless definite pelvic pathology is present, abdominal or pelvic operations merely agravate the symptomatology. Asthenics are often greatly benefited by a gain in weight. This may be achieved by prescribing plenty of rest and a high caloric diet, rich in carbohydrate and fat. Backache, visceroptosis, and pelvic relaxation are best treated by use of proper supports and pessaries. Proper elimination is important and should be aided, where necessary, by mild laxatives, proper exercise, and abdominal massage.

Infantile Type.—The infantile type of woman may or may not benefit by marriage and pregnancy. In the mild case, where conception is possible, the pelvic organs may attain almost normal proportions during gestation. Although infantile women often abort, they may, after oft-repeated abortions, finally carry to full term. Here again, prenatal care is important, and expert management of labor imperative. Congenital retroflexion is now considered to be almost always associated with the other stigmata of infantilism, and does not justify indiscriminate operations. The pelvic complaints of these patients are seldom caused by uterine displacement, but are due rather to their inferior constitutional makeup and low pain threshold.

Heterosexual Type.—The heterosexual type rarely benefits from any form of treatment. Should conception occur and the outcome of pregnancy be successful, happy marital relations may follow and the mental conflicts may come to an end.

Organotherapy.—Organotherapy is of little value in constitutionally inferior women. Notwithstanding this fact, many of these unfortunates are subjected to prolonged and useless endocrine treatment, because of failure to interpret their symptoms in the light of their constitutional background.

BIBLIOGRAPHY

1. Pende, N.: Constitutional Inadequacies, Trans. by Sante Naccarati, Philadelphia, Lea & Febiger, 1928.
2. Sheldon, W. H., Stevens, S. S., and Tucker, W. B.: The Varieties of Human Physique, New York and London, Harper & Brothers, 1940.
3. Pearl, R.: Human Biol. *8:*92, 1936.
4. Bayer, L. M.: Endocrinol. *24:*260, 1939.
5. Tandler, J.: Wien. klin. Wchnschr. *43:*626, 1930.
6. Gellhorn, G.: Am. J. Obst. & Gynec. *24:*481, 1932.
7. Bauer, J.: Wien. klin. Wchnschr. *49:*504, 1936.
8. Mayer, A.: Die Bedeutung der Konstitution fur die Frauenheilkunde, In: Veit-Stoeckel's Handb. d. Gynäk. *3:*279, München, J. T. Bergmann, 1928.
9. Saltykow, S.: Virchows Arch. f. d. ges. Physiol. *272:*442, 1929.

CHAPTER XXXV

ENDOCRINOPATHIES

HYPOPHYSEAL INFANTILISM

Definition.—Hypophyseal infantilism (pituitary dwarfism, nanosomia pituitaria, ateleiosis) describes a condition in which somatic growth and sexual development are arrested some time before puberty, with subsequent retention of the body build and sexual status of the child. The somatic and sexual retardation is presumably caused by a deficiency of the anterior hypophyseal hormones.

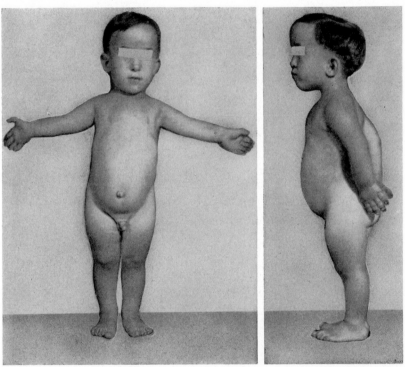

Fig. 121.—Pituitary dwarf. Boy aged seven, weight 28 pounds, height 31½ inches, span 26 inches. Upper measurement 20 inches, lower measurement 11½ inches. Note large head, pot belly, baby hands. Mentally very alert. Testicles descended. After growth hormone, small doses of thyroid, and general medical measures for one and one-half years, weight 29 pounds, height 32 inches.

Incidence.—The condition may develop at any time during childhood. In rare instances it may be congenital, so that the retardation of growth is already apparent at birth. It affects both sexes with equal frequency.

The severe forms of pituitary infantilism are rare; the milder types are not uncommon but often go unrecognized.

Clinical Characteristics.—The degree of undergrowth and genital infantilism depends on the extent of the anterior pituitary deficiency, and the age at which it develops. It is obvious that the retardation will be most marked where the condition arises at birth or during infancy.

The classical case is characterized by a *well proportioned, diminutive body*. The upper measurement exceeds the lower, thus corresponding to

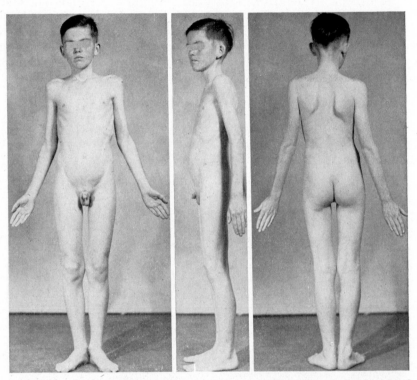

Fig. 122.—Pituitary infantilism. Male aged fifteen, weight 65 pounds, height 56 inches. Small genitalia, testes descended but tiny. Pubic and axillary hair absent. X-ray of long bones shows some retardation of epiphyseal lines. X-ray of skull negative. Unsatisfactory response to organotherapy.

the normal values for childhood. The head is spherical, and large in proportion to the rest of the body. The small, rounded face, recessive chin, high, narrow palatal arch, crowded teeth, and poorly delineated features, all characteristic of the child, are retained throughout life. The hands and feet are small, the thorax narrow and flat, and the abdomen slightly protuberant. The skin is smooth, soft, and delicate, its texture being not unlike that of the infant or young child. With advancing years, and occasionally at a relatively early age, it may become dry, wrinkled, and pigmented, giving the affected individual a wizened, oldish look. This premature aging may be associated with cachexia, the resultant picture being that of Simmonds' disease superimposed on pituitary infantilism.

The pituitary dwarf has a light and delicate *skeleton*, with small, thin, fragile, long bones, and short but pointed phalanges. In the severe case, the calvarium is very thin, and the convolutional markings pronounced. The facial bones are small, and the accessory sinuses markedly hypoplastic or absent. The sella turcica, unless it be the seat of a neoplasm, is small and partially or completely bridged. The ossification centers appear late,

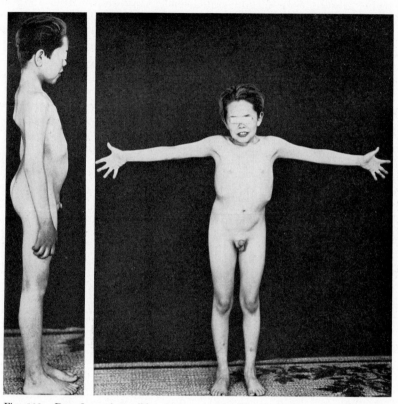

Fig. 123.—Dwarfism of possible pituitary origin. Boy aged fifteen, weight 49 pounds, height 47 inches. Note stunted body growth, pigeon chest, and lumbar lordosis. Small genitalia. Mentally alert.

and the epiphyseal lines remain open much longer than normal, in some cases well into advanced adult life. The bone nuclei may be normal or slightly retarded.

The *primary and secondary sex characters*, in the severe case, retain their infantile or juvenile status in adult life. In the female, menstruation may never appear, and procreation is precluded. The breasts remain infantile or may develop slightly. Pubic and axillary hair is sparse or absent, depending on the severity of the glandular deficiency. In the male, the penis and scrotum are often of infantile proportions, and unilateral or bilateral cryptorchidism is common. The prostate may be markedly hypoplastic or rudimentary. Libido sexualis and spermatogenic function are absent.

Etiology and Pathology.—Pituitary infantilism is presumed to be primarily due to a deficiency or absence of the anterior pituitary growth promoting and gonadotropic hormones, arising some time during childhood. Other incretory products of the adenohypophysis, particularly the thyrotropic and adrenocorticotropic factors, are probably also deficient to a varying degree. The pituitary deficiency may result from congenital absence of its incretory elements, or from acquired lesions which destroy or inactivate them. Atrophy of the adenohypophysis resulting from emboli or infarction, and destruction of the gland by inflammatory processes or destructive neoplasms situated in or near the hypophysis, have been recorded at autopsy in some of the cases. In others, the anterior lobe pre-

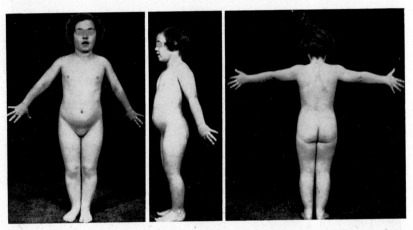

Fig. 124.—Stunting of growth associated with coarse hair, facial myxedema and mental sluggishness, suggesting a hypothyroid origin. Patient aged eleven, height 42 inches. After one and one-half years of thyroid therapy and general hygienic measures, height 46½ inches. Pituitary extract for six months without apparent effect.

sented no demonstrable pathology, suggesting that the deficiency is of a functional nature, resulting from inactivity or stagnation of the gland. Such a condition may conceivably be caused by constitutional depressive states, chronic infections, or deficiency diseases.

Diagnosis.—Though stunting of growth and genital infantilism are readily recognized by comparing the height of the patient with standard tables, and by physical examination in the nude, the underlying cause is often difficult to ascertain.

The responsibility of the hypophysis can readily be established where suppression of its function is due to a destructive tumor, large enough to produce intracranial pressure symptoms or distort the sella. In such cases roentgenography of the skull may provide valuable information. In the absence of demonstrable cranial pathology, the diagnosis is difficult and can only be made by excluding other causes of arrested skeletal growth. A careful history and thorough physical examination, combined with routine laboratory and roentgenologic studies, may help to eliminate such causes of retarded skeletal growth as chronic infectious diseases, nutritional and deficiency diseases, intestinal parasites, celiac disease, as well as rickets, achondroplasia, and other bone diseases.

Differential Diagnosis.—Pituitary infantilism is readily distinguished from *infantile hypothyroidism*, for though victims of both types of dwarfism are well proportioned, the hypothyroid dwarf presents such distinctive features as mental retardation, a slow, clumsy gait, thick, dry or puffy skin, enlarged protruding tongue, short thick neck, prominent molar and alae nasi bones, and delayed or defective dentition.

The *achondroplastic dwarf* is easily recognized by the large head, relatively long trunk, extremely short arms and legs, wobbly gait and grotesque

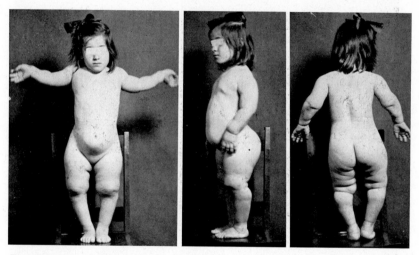

Fig. 125.—Achondroplastic dwarf. Girl aged ten, weight 50 pounds, height 38 inches.

appearance. The normal sexual development of such individuals is also an important distinguishing feature.

The absence of adiposity distinguishes the pituitary dwarf from the *juvenile form of Fröhlich's syndrome* associated with skeletal undergrowth. Hypophyseal infantilism of organic origin may be differentiated from the functional type, secondary to some constitutional depressive state, by testing the patient's response to ideal dietetic and nonendocrine treatment calculated to stimulate somatic growth. If, at the end of one year, the growth deficiency persists, it may be inferred that an inherent defect in the pituitary is the primary cause.

According to Albright and his associates,[20] pituitary dwarfism ("panhypopituitarism") is to be distinguished from a syndrome described by them as having the following characteristics: infantile sexual organs, complete absence of breast development, small to moderate amounts of axillary and pubic hair (contrasting with complete absence in panhypopituitarism), and short stature (in contrast to dwarfing in panhypopituitarism). It is frequently associated with congenital anomalies such as webbing of the neck and coarctation of the aorta. Osteoporosis and precocious senility are also often encountered. The bone age is less markedly retarded than in pituitary dwarfism, and such individuals are stronger and better nourished. Their urine contains more than normal amounts of follicle stimulating hormone, contrasting with the negative findings in the pituitary dwarf. Determinations of 17-ketosteroid excretion show a decrease but not the marked drop characteristic of panhypopituitarism. In the insulin tol-

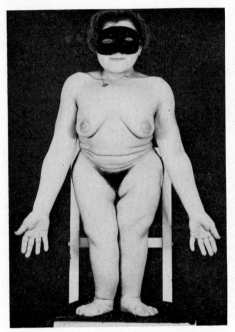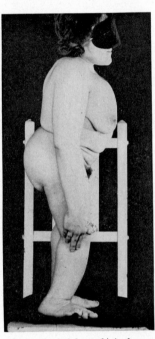

Fig. 126.—Achondroplastic dwarf. Female aged twenty-seven, height 38½ inches, weight 70 pounds. History of numerous pathologic fractures during childhood. Note marked telescoping of body, marked lordosis and dorsal kyphosis, barrel-shaped chest, short legs and long arms.

erance test, such individuals exhibit normal hypoglycemia responsiveness in contrast to the unresponsiveness of the pituitary dwarf.

Course and Prognosis.—The pituitary dwarf may live to a ripe old age. Priesel's[1] dwarf was 91 years old at the time of his death. The chances of achieving further growth and sexual development largely depend on the cause of the pituitary deficiency, its severity and amenability to treatment, and the age of the patient when treatment is instituted. The earlier specific treatment is begun, the more favorable the prognosis. It is obvious that once the dwarf reaches adult years, very little can be expected.

Treatment.—*Anterior Lobe Extracts.*—Since the growth deficiency is primarily due to a lack or deficiency of anterior pituitary growth hormone, replacement therapy with a potent growth-promoting extract of anterior lobe tissue would seem to be rational therapy. Unfortunately, the potency of the available preparations is relatively low. This probably accounts for the varied and inconsistent results reported thus far.[2, 3, 4] In the post-puberal case, most competent observers agree that very little may be expected from this or any other known form of treatment. In the pre-puberal pituitary dwarf, some growth may be induced if treatment is instituted early and continued throughout the growth period, but complete physiologic rehabilitation is not possible. The *dose* is 2 to 5 cc. (20 to 50 growth units) for 5 days of each week.[5] Some observers prefer crude pituitary extract to the purified growth principle. A few[6] report good results with *anterior lobe implants,* but these observations are unconvincing because they were not adequately controlled. *Desiccated thyroid,* in doses of $\frac{1}{4}$ to 1 grain three times daily, if well tolerated, is a useful adjuvant in the treatment, especially where there is an associated thyroid deficiency. These measures should always be supplemented by a well balanced, high caloric *diet,* rich in vitamins, calcium, and other essential minerals, without which no growth-promoting stimulus can exert its maximum effect.[7]

Where stunting of growth is associated with *genital retardation,* the available *gonadotropes* of hypophyseal, equine and human chorionic origin may be tried. The *dose* ranges from 100 to 500 international units every two to three days for one or two months, with intervening rest periods of two to four weeks. Thus far, the most consistent results have apparently followed human chorionic gonadotropin in the male. Even here, however, the effect is limited to the interstitial cells, which are stimulated to secrete male sex hormone.

Sex Hormone Therapy.—The use of gonadal sex hormones to stimulate growth in individuals with retarded growth and sexual development is finding increasing favor in recent years. For some time, it has generally been assumed that these substances have a retarding effect on longitudinal growth, due to their ability to cause closure of the epiphyses, and their inhibitory effect on anterior pituitary function. This belief is based on the observation that individuals who achieve sexual maturity at an early age tend to be short, while those who mature late or not at all, are usually tall. Experimental evidence that protracted treatment with sex hormones inhibits the anterior pituitary gland, with consequent stunting of growth,[8, 9] and also causes premature closure of the epiphyses,[10, 11] has also seemed to substantiate this view. More recent experimental and clinical investigations suggest that these substances may either stimulate or retard body growth, depending on the dosage and length of treatment.[11–16] Stimulation of body growth has thus far been noted almost exclusively in hypogonadal males, of puberal or prepuberal age, during treatment with male sex hormone (*testosterone propionate*) in *doses* ranging from 5 to 125 mg. weekly. These observations suggest that the body growth also observed[17, 18] following human chorionic gonadotropin therapy in males was due to the male sex hormone secreted under its influence. In the female, only a few instances have been reported[13] in which *estrogenic hormone*

35

seemed to stimulate growth, while no instance of accelerated growth during chorionic gonadotropin therapy has come to the author's attention.

That the gonadal sex hormones should have a stimulative effect on body growth is not entirely unexpected in view of the clinical observation that hormone-secreting gonadal tumors, arising before puberty, are associated with general body growth as well as sexual precocity (see p. 595). But while these individuals exceed for a time the size of normal individuals of the same chronological age, their epiphyses unite and longitudinal growth ceases earlier than in persons maturing at the normal time. For this reason, the sexually precocious individual tends to be under average height on reaching adult years.

Though the growth retardation which occurs when large doses of sex hormone are administered over a protracted period would appear to be due partly to acceleration of epiphyseal closure and partly to inhibition of anterior pituitary function, the explanation of the growth stimulation apparently produced with smaller doses over a short period of time, is not clear. From the available clinical and experimental evidence, it would appear that the attainment of normal statural growth depends on the interaction of the gonadal sex hormones and extragonadal growth stimuli, particularly those of anterior pituitary origin. The amount of each that is available, the time when it begins to act, and the length of time that it is permitted to act, are apparently important factors in determining whether or not growth will be normal. If proper quantitative and temporal relationships are preserved, longitudinal growth will be neither deficient nor excessive; but if the delicate balance is disturbed, statural deviations are likely to result.

In the absence of precise information concerning the quantity and time relations involved, caution should be exercised when contemplating sex hormone therapy for the purpose of stimulating body growth. The danger of depressing the already hypo-active gonad, and the unfavorable psychologic effect of premature development of the accessory genitalia and secondary sex characters, should always be borne in mind. If used at all, repeated x-ray examination of the epiphyses is important to avoid premature closure. Though most observers employing this form of treatment could observe no evidence of premature epiphyseal union with the doses used, there is always the possibility that, due to individual variations, a dose which is safe in one case may accelerate epiphyseal union in another.

HYPOPHYSEAL GIANTISM

Definition.—Hypophyseal giantism is characterized by an abnormally tall stature, and marked overgrowth of the long bones, musculature and viscera. It is far more common in the male, and may have its inception during fetal life or childhood, but is particularly apt to arise at the puberal epoch. The manifestations of the disease are ascribed to an excess of the anterior pituitary growth hormone, acting before epiphyseal closure. Hyperplasia or adenoma of the acidophil cells of the adenohypophysis is generally conceded to be the primary cause.

Symptomatology.—Excessive tallness and prodigious muscular prowess may be the only manifestations in the prepuberal giant. If the age of puberty has been reached, abnormal sexual modifications may be added to the picture. The nature of the somatic, sexual and metabolic alterations depends largely on the stage of the disease.

The early, *formative or hyperactive stage* is characterized by rapid and pronounced increase in skeletal growth, marked muscular development

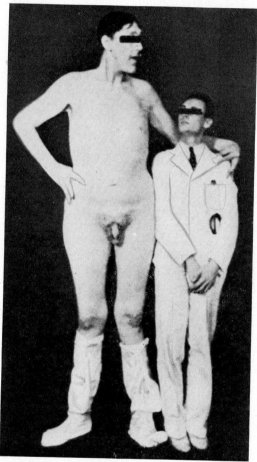

Fig. 127.—The Minneapolis giant, 2134 mm. (7 ft. 0 in.) beside Dr. J. S. M., 1763 mm. (5 ft. 9½ in. net). (Gray, H.: Ann. Int. Med. Vol. 10.)

and general splanchnomegaly. Genital development and function may be normal in some cases, while others may show varying degrees of genital hypoplasia. Not infrequently, the hyperactive phase in the male is associated with hypertrichosis, enlargement of the penis, and heightened libido sexualis. These manifestations are often accompanied by elevation of the basal metabolic rate and specific dynamic action, hyperglycemia, glycosuria and a low sugar tolerance.

Excessive skeletal growth is the most conspicuous sign. The height may vary from six feet six inches to well over eight feet. The long bones are particularly affected. The arms, hands and fingers, legs, feet and toes are considerably lengthened. As a result, the lower measurement exceeds the upper one, and the span is greater than the height. Roentgenograms of the long bones show overgrowths of tuberosities and exostoses at the muscle insertions. There is no tufting of the terminal phalanges, unless the disease is complicated by acromegaly.

In the *retrogressive and terminal stages* of the disease, the manifestations of the active period are reversed. The giant loses height because of the thoracic kyphosis and bowing of the shoulders. In addition there is progressive and profound muscular weakness, asthenia, loss of body hair, and involutionary changes in the sex organs. These changes may be accompanied by depression of the basal metabolic rate and specific dynamic action, hypoglycemia and increased sugar tolerance, hypotension, hypothermia, and bradycardia.

Associated Symptoms.—Distention of the sella turcica by the expanding pituitary neoplasm may give rise to neighborhood pressure symptoms, which vary according to the extent of midbrain involvement. Excruciating headaches, projectile vomiting, bilateral hemianopsia, optic atrophy, oculomotor palsies, disturbances of taste and smell, and nervous hyperirritability are not uncommon. Incoordination, loss of memory, and other manifestations of mental deterioration may be encountered during the terminal phases.

Etiology and Pathology.—The first inkling of a possible association between the hypophysis and giantism came in 1872, when Langer[1] distinguished between physiologic and pathologic giants, and pointed out that the sella turcica is often enlarged in the latter. A connection between giantism and acromegaly was suggested by Sternberg,[2] who found that 40 per cent of giants present acromegalic manifestations, while 20 per cent of acromegalics are giants. Brisseaud and Meige[3] were the first to recognize a causal relationship between pituitary disease and giantism. They proposed that the hypophyseal disorder which causes acromegaly in the adult, may lead to giantism before the advent of epiphyseal closure.

In the vast majority of cases, hyperplasia or adenoma of the acidophil cells of the anterior hypophysis has been demonstrated at autopsy. Experimental evidence linking the malady to a disturbance of hypophyseal function was provided by Evans and Long,[4] who induced giantism in rats by protracted treatment with extract of beef anterior pituitaries. On the basis of this evidence, pituitary giantism is now generally conceded to be due to production of excessive amounts of growth hormone by the acidophilic cells of the anterior hypophysis.

The contrasting symptomatology of the early and late stages of the disease suggests that the adenohypophysis, and particularly the acidophilic cells, are hyperactive during the formative and inactive during the later or terminal stages, when the gland is exhausted or has degenerated.

Individual variations in the degree of sexual development attained by the pituitary giant can perhaps be explained by assuming that the source of the gonadotropes, which is generally believed to be the basophils, may function normally or be disturbed to a varying extent. The level of gonadotropic hormone production will vary, depending on whether the activity of the basophils remains unaffected, increases, or diminishes. Where excessive activity of the acidophils is associated with normal function of the basophils, full sexual development may be attained and reproductive function may be normal at least during the earlier stages. On the other hand, if the tumor causes pressure atrophy of the basophils before the advent of puberty, it may lead to varying degrees of sexual retardation. Where giantism is associated with hypertrophy of the penis, hypertrichosis, and increased libido, hyperactivity of the basophils, or adrenal cortical hyperfunction with consequent excessive androgen production may be at fault. The latter possibility is suggested by the observation that the adrenal cortex is often hyperplastic, due possibly to increased production of adrenocorticotropic hormone by the anterior pituitary.

Diagnosis.—The abnormally tall stature and associated symptomatology usually suffice for the diagnosis. In the atypical case, roentgenograms of the skull and long bones will dispel any doubt. Difficulties in diagnosis may arise in the prepuberal individual. Pathologic overgrowth in children may be suspected where the height is excessive for the age and race, or skeletal growth shows an abrupt and rapid spurt. During the juvenile period, particularly between the twelfth and fifteenth year, it may be very difficult to decide whether the excessive height is pathological, or merely an expression of a physiologic growth spurt which will equalize itself when the normal age for epiphyseal union is attained. The nature of the osseous overgrowth, the size of the sella turcica, and the presence of other endocrinopathic stigmata are far more significant in the diagnosis than mere tallness.

Differential Diagnosis.—The accelerated statural growth incident to *macrogenitosomia praecox* of adrenal cortical, pineal, or gonadal origin, may be differentiated from juvenile pituitary giantism by the associated sexual precocity, the advanced state of ossification and the presence of pathology in the affected glands.

The *physiologic giant* is distinguishable from the pituitary giant by the normal body proportions, absence of endocrinopathic stigmata, normal sella turcica, and occurrence of epiphyseal union at the normal age.

Eunuchoid tallness may be differentiated from pituitary giantism by the normal size of the sella and associated genital hypoplasia. Though such individuals may be very tall, they do not attain the extreme height of the pituitary giant. In distinguishing between eunuchoidism and pituitary giantism associated with genital hypoplasia, the sex hormone content of the blood and urine may be of some value. The presence of gonadotropin, and absence of estrogen in the female or androgen in the male, suggests eunuchoidism. In the pituitary giant, where the genital retardation is secondary to a deficiency of the pituitary gonadotropes, the latter may be expected to be absent from the blood and urine either because none are produced, or the small amounts secreted are utilized by the responsive gonads.

Prognosis.—The prognosis of pituitary giantism is grave. Death may result from the intracranial neoplasm or from intercurrent infection, to which such individuals are highly susceptible. In the presence of a malignant tumor, the life span will obviously be materially shortened. Where the cause is hyperplasia or a benign tumor, the outlook is more hopeful. Early recognition of the disease, and prompt institution of treatment may check the progress of the lesion and prevent further skeletal growth, at the same time preventing or at least postponing exhaustion or destruction of the gland.

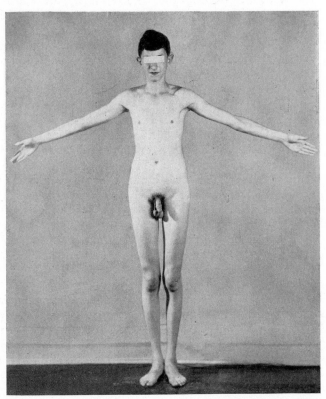

Fig. 128.—Physiologic giant. Boy aged fourteen; height 72 inches. Roentgenograms of skull and long bones show no abnormalities.

Treatment.—The treatment is identical with that of acromegaly (see p. 555). Here, as in acromegaly, sex hormone therapy has been tried with the hope of inhibiting the overactive pituitary,[5, 6, 8] but convincing proof of its efficacy is still lacking.

ACROMEGALY

Definition.—The term "acromegaly," introduced by Marie[1] in 1886, describes a syndrome whose cardinal features are marked enlargement of the acral parts of the body, and hypertrophic alterations of the osseous system and soft parts. It is generally attributed to hyperplasia or adenoma of the acidophilic cells of the anterior pituitary gland.

Incidence.—In a survey of the world literature between 1886 and 1938, Atkinson[2] could find only 1606 cases. The disease affects the male and female with equal frequency. It develops as a rule at some time after epiphyseal union, but is most often encountered during the third decade of life.

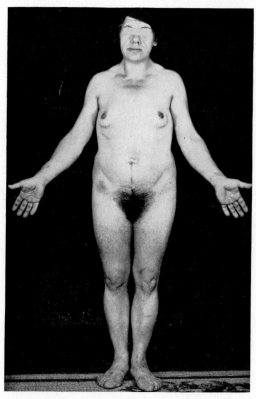

Fig. 129.—Acromegaly. Single woman aged forty, six years after onset of disease. Amenorrhea alternating with menorrhagia. Note large feet and hands with spadelike fingers, and heterosexual distribution of pubic hair.

SYMPTOMATOLOGY

The manifestations of acromegaly may be referable to disturbed pituitary function, or result from pressure of the pituitary adenoma on adjacent areas in the midbrain.

Skeletal Alterations.—Most conspicuous and constant signs of the disease are the pronounced hypertrophic changes of the facial skull, vertebrae, and long bones. The cranial vault is irregularly thickened and the accessory sinuses enormously enlarged. A narrow and recessive forehead, with a prominent and elongated external occipital protuberance are characteristic. The zygomatic process and lower jaw are particularly enlarged and protruding, resulting in a typical prognathism. Enlargement of the mandible is responsible for the wide separation of the teeth seen in such individuals.

Marked broadening of the epiphyses of the long bones, and tufting of the terminal phalanges, especially of the hands and feet, are probably the most prominent skeletal alterations. The clavicles are large and thick, the sternum protuberant. The vertebrae undergo marked hypertrophy and become ankylosed in the later stages of the disease. The resulting high dorsal kyphosis, lumbar lordosis, prominent sternum, and bowed shoulders are responsible for the apelike stature of the classical acromegalic. Fortunately, such extreme skeletal changes are not the rule, for many patients may go on for years with only minor alterations of the facial skull, or other parts of the osseous system.

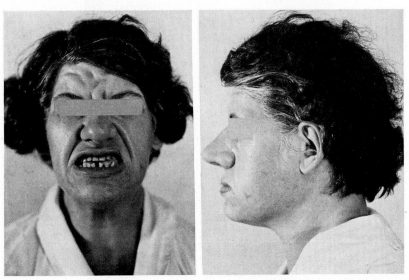

Fig. 130.—Close-up of patient in figure 129. Note coarse features, thickened skin, large thick nose with bulbous tip and deep nasolabial folds, widely spaced teeth and prognathous jaw.

Alterations of the Soft Parts.—The ears, lips, finger tips, and particularly the nose are enormously enlarged and thickened. The tongue is often huge and, in the extreme case, forces the mouth open, interfering with mastication and speech. Hypertrophy of the soft palate, uvula, larynx, and vocal cords gives the voice a deep, discordant pitch. The neck of the acromegalic is short, thick, and sunken between the shoulders. The skin is thick and moist, and usually dark-complexioned. Pigmentation, fibromata, and lipomata are common. These alterations, together with the hypertrophy of the subcutaneous tissue, produce deep furrows which are most pronounced on the forehead and nasolabial folds, and are responsible for the ugly, distorted, bulldog-like features of the classical acromegalic. In the later stages of the disease, the skin undergoes atrophic changes, becoming dry and wrinkled.

General splanchnomegaly is a common finding and may cause much distress. The heart,[3] stomach, liver, spleen, kidneys, colon, and other viscera may be enormously enlarged

Sexual Manifestations.—In the early stages, before enlargement of the sella is apparent, gonadal and reproductive function may be normal.[4] In the male acromegalic, the formative or hyperactive phase may be associated with a marked increase in libido sexualis and enlargement of the genital organs, but diminution or loss of sexual function marks the later stages. In the female, the terminal or retrogressive stages of the malady are as a rule accompanied by oligomenorrhea or amenorrhea, sterility, and regressive alterations of the genital organs. Mammary enlargement and secretion, in the absence of pregnancy, have been observed in some instances. Hirsutism may be an early manifestation in both sexes, but in the terminal stage hypotrichosis is a common finding.

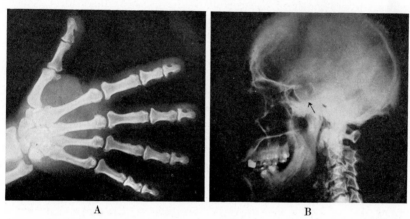

Fig. 131.—X-ray of skull and right hand of patient in Fig. 129. A, Note tufting of phalanges; B, note markedly enlarged sella turcica and hypertrophy of the mandible.

Neighborhood Symptoms.—The presence of a small or slowly proliferating *adenoma* may be compatible with normal mental and physical vigor for many years. On the other hand, a large, rapidly growing tumor may be accompanied by a long train of troublesome symptoms, which vary according to the cranial structures involved. The *formative stage* may be attended by excruciating headaches, projectile vomiting, hyperirritability, paresthesias, perversion of taste or smell, emotional and mental disorders, insomnia, and convulsions. Bitemporal hemianopsia, optic atrophy, oculomotor palsy, and other signs of intracranial pressure may also be encountered, while polyphagia and polydipsia are not uncommon. The *terminal stages* may be accompanied by asthenia, loss of memory, mental deterioration, somnolence, apathy, stupor, and occasionally by dementia.

Disturbances in Metabolism.—A rise in the basal metabolic rate and specific dynamic action is common, particularly in the early stages. Later, the values for both may be materially lowered. Hyperglycemia and glycosuria are common in the formative stage, but during the later stages there may be hypoglycemia and increased sugar tolerance. Among 153 cases reviewed by Coggeshall and Root,[5] 17 per cent developed diabetes mellitus an average of 9.5 years after the onset of the acromegaly; glycosuria occurred in 36 per cent.

Alterations in the Endocrine Glands.—*Thyroid enlargement* is a common finding. It was observed in 50 per cent of a group of 166 cases reviewed by Davis.[6] Of the 1606 cases collected by Atkinson,[2] the status of the thyroid was recorded at autopsy in 167. It was found to be enlarged in 96, cystic, fibrous, or adenomatous in 32, atrophic in 14, and normal in 25. The *thymus* was mentioned in 116 of the autopsied cases: it was present in 62, absent in 45, and replaced by fat in 9. *Hyperplasia or adenomas of the parathyroids* were fairly common. In some instances, the *pancreas* was enlarged. The size of the *adrenals* was significantly increased, due chiefly to hypertrophy of the cortex. While these findings are significant, it should be emphasized that in many instances they represent the status of the endocrine glands in the terminal stages of the disease.

ETIOLOGY AND PATHOLOGY

Hyperpituitarism.—Marie,[1] in 1886, found a pituitary tumor in his acromegalic patient, but it was not until the following year that Minkowski[7] suggested that the disease may be due to *hyperpituitarism*. Benda[8] was the first to emphasize the role of the acidophilic cells as the source of the stimulus responsible for the characteristic manifestations. This hypothesis has been substantiated by both histologic and physiologic studies. *Hyperplasia or adenoma of the acidophils* has been demonstrated at autopsy in the large majority of the cases. An increase in the number of acidophils was observed in all of 62 cases reviewed by Bailey and Cushing[9] in 1928. Atkinson's[2] survey of the literature to 1938 revealed that the pituitary had been described at autopsy in 287 cases, of which 124 presented adenomata. In a few instances no pituitary lesion could be demonstrated, but in some of these hyperplastic pituitary tissue was present in the cranio-pharyngeal canal, or at the site of the pharyngeal pituitary.

Experimental Evidence.—Direct evidence that acromegaly is due to hyperactivity of the anterior hypophysis was provided by Putnam and his associates[10] in 1929. These observers induced acromegalic manifestations in certain breeds of dogs by protracted treatment with an anterior pituitary extract containing the growth principle. This was subsequently confirmed by Evans and his coworkers.[11] Putnam and Wilcox[12] found that the acidophilic granules present in adenomas removed from acromegalic patients contained a specific reducing substance, which was also present in Evans' anterior pituitary growth-promoting extract. This would seem to substantiate the hypothesis that the acidophils are the source of the growth stimulus responsible for the skeletal changes in acromegaly. On the other hand, this assumption is apparently contradicted by the observation that typical acromegalic manifestations may sometimes occur without demonstrable hyperplasia or adenoma of the acidophils, or be absent despite the presence of such pathology.[13] Though such exceptional cases are of interest, they do not necessarily detract from the validity of the view that hyperactivity of the acidophils is the primary cause. It is possible that acromegalic manifestations associated with a normal pituitary are due to aberrant herds of acidophilic cells which have wandered from the anterior lobe to such extrasellar locations as the sphenoidal and pharyngeal vault. To account for rare instances in which an acidophilic adenoma has been found without acromegaly, it has been suggested that mere morphologic hyperplasia of secreting tissue does not necessarily imply a corresponding increase in secretory function.

Though acromegaly usually develops after epiphyseal union is complete, the syndrome may occasionally appear *in children or young adults*,[14] and has been experimentally induced in certain species prior to closure of the epiphyses. It would thus appear that epiphyseal closure is not an essential prerequisite for the production of acromegalic manifestations.

Sexual Alterations.—It is not certain whether the regressive sexual alterations of the later stages of the malady are due to exhaustion of the hypophysis following a period of hyperactivity, or compression of the basophil cells by the growing pituitary adenoma. The latter possibility finds support in the observation that after enucleation of the acidophilic adenoma, the atrophic genitalia may return to normal, with restoration of the menstrual rhythm.

Hirsutism.—The hirsutism often seen in both the male and female acromegalic is probably attributable to adrenal cortical hyperactivity, resulting from increased adrenocorticotropic hormone production by the hyperactive adenohypophysis.

Basal Metabolic Rate.—The *high basal metabolic rate* in acromegaly would appear at first sight to be an expression of hyperthyroidism secondary to heightened thyrotropic hormone secretion by the anterior lobe. The observation that the rate may remain high despite thyroidectomy[15] indicates that the increased metabolism is at least partly due to an excess of some pituitary principle or principles which stimulate oxygen consumption without the intervention of the thyroid gland (see Chap. XIII).

Diabetes Mellitus in Acromegaly.—Recent studies of the role of the anterior pituitary gland in carbohydrate metabolism (see Chap. XIII) suggest a possible explanation for the diabetes mellitus of the acromegalic. There is evidence that the anterior lobe secretes a diabetogenic and possibly also a pancreatropic principle. The former causes hyperglycemia and glycosuria, while the latter apparently stimulates the pancreas to elaborate insulin. According to Young,[16] the growth, diabetogenic and pancreatropic factors are closely associated chemically, though they are not identical. If this is true, it might be expected that an excess of the growth principle would be associated with increased production of the diabetogenic and pancreatropic principles. Young believes that the diabetogenic effect is masked so long as the pancreas continues to respond to the pancreatropic factor with adequate insulin production. Should the strain of prolonged stimulation lead to exhaustion of this gland, diabetes will result.

That the *thyroid gland* contributes to the glycosuria of the acromegalic is suggested by Lammli's[17] observation that glycosuria persisted following surgical removal of the pituitary tumor, but disappeared after thyroidectomy performed subsequently. Of interest in this connection is the case reported by Hart and Greene,[18] in which operation on the pituitary checked the acromegaly and even caused some regression, but did not affect the glycosuria. In view of the important part played by the adrenal cortex in carbohydrate metabolism (see Chap. XVII), and the fact that this gland is often enlarged in acromegaly, it seems likely that it also contributes to the glycosuria.

On the whole, the available evidence suggests that the development of diabetes mellitus in the acromegalic depends on whether the excess of growth hormone is associated with increased production of the diabetogenic, pancreatropic, thyrotropic, and adrenocorticotropic principles, on the reactivity of the thyroid and adrenal cortex, and the ability of the pancreas to withstand the strain of protracted stimulation. Individual variations in one or more of these factors may account for the fact that only some acromegalics become diabetic.

The diabetes of acromegalics is said by some observers[19] to be resistant to insulin, but others[5] maintain that their response to this drug is essentially the same as that of the nonacromegalic diabetic.

Precipitating Causes.—The precipitating causes of the pituitary pathology primarily responsible for this syndrome are obscure. In the large majority of the cases, there was no specific event in the history to which the onset of the malady could be attributed. In some instances, there was a family history of acromegaly, but most observers attach little significance to this. Occasionally the onset of the disease coincides with *acute illness* or *head injury*. It has been suggested that *ovarian ablation* or *pregnancy* may be possible predisposing causes, since the hypophysis enlarges under these conditions, and the number of acidophils, supposed source of the growth hormone, is appreciably increased. Such pituitary modifications may account for the transient acromegalic manifestations which sometimes appear in the pregnant woman, but disappear soon after delivery. This tendency, if exaggerated for some reason, may conceivably lead to acromegaly.

DIAGNOSIS AND DIFFERENTIAL DIAGNOSIS

In the classical case, the diagnosis is simple and can be made by mere inspection. In the early stages of the disease, before the physical signs become pronounced, roentgenograms of the facial skull, sella turcica, and long bones, and ophthalmologic examination will dispel any doubt. In determining whether a tumor is present, x-ray of the sella is of value only where marked enlargement of the hypophysis has caused it to encroach on its bony envelope. Failure to demonstrate such encroachment does not necessarily exclude the presence of a tumor.[26]

Though acromegaly, in its fully developed form, can hardly be confused with any other condition, difficulties may arise in the fugitive forms of the disease. *Paget's disease* differs from acromegaly in that it occurs in old individuals, and affects the cranial rather than the facial skull. In addition there is curving and enlargement of the shafts of the long bones, asymmetrical osseous enlargements, and characteristic cotton batting appearance of the skull.

Pulmonary osteo-arthropathy may be distinguished from acromegaly by the characteristic drum-stick fingers, curved finger nails, deformities of the hands and feet, normal facial skull, and presence of pulmonary pathology.

Giantism is easily differentiated from acromegaly by the tapering phalanges, and the absence of tufting and enlargement of the acra.

COURSE AND PROGNOSIS

The disease as a rule runs a chronic progressive course, and may extend over several decades, even without effective treatment. It is often compatible with great physical and intellectual vigor and skill, particularly in the early stages. If a tumor is present, the prognosis depends on its nature and size, the direction of its growth, the extent of the damage to the midbrain, and the nature of the secondary changes induced in other organs of the body. Where the adenoma is malignant, or involves vital neighboring structures, the outlook is poor unless the growth can be removed or inactivated. While enucleation may relieve many of the intracranial pressure symptoms, it obviously cannot reverse the acromegalic skeletal alterations.

Where the diagnosis is made early and appropriate therapy instituted, the disease may be checked, but once it is fully established, the prognosis is unfavorable. Fortunately, many of the cases are self-limited. Such patients may live in comparative comfort to a ripe old age, and die of other causes.

TREATMENT

Intensive *x-ray radiation* of the hypophysis is indicated in the early or formative phases of the disease.[20, 21] Three portals are used, one on each temple and one in the midfrontal region. Through each portal, a total of 800[22] to 900 r[23] may be given in divided doses of 200 or 300 r daily or every other day. Davidoff[22] employs the following factors: 200 KV, 8 milliamp., 1 mm. Al., 0.5 mm. Cu, 50 cm. (distance from skin), 20 r per min.

While observers are not agreed as to the efficacy of x-ray therapy in arresting the hypophyseal adenoma, it is nevertheless worth a trial before resorting to hypophyseal surgery, for the acidophil cell adenomas are most sensitive to the x-rays. Such therapy is obviously contraindicated in the retrogressive stages of the disease when the hypophysis is either exhausted or destroyed.

In the presence of intracranial symptoms or where the adenoma invades important neighborhood structures, *decompression or enucleation* may become urgent to save sight or life.

A few observers have employed *estrogen or androgen* with the aim of inhibiting the hyperactive pituitary. Goldberg and Lisser[21] observed two patients who seemed to benefit from such treatment. Schrire and Sharpey-Schafer[24] noted a drop in the urinary level of creatine and creatinine following sex hormone therapy and interpreted this as evidence of inhibition of the growth-promoting activity of the anterior hypophysis. Some of their patients complained of greater frequency and intensity of headaches during the course of treatment. In general, the available clinical reports fail to provide convincing proof of the efficacy of such therapy. To achieve inhibition of pituitary function, large doses must be given continuously over a protracted period of time. An obvious disadvantage of such treatment is that it may simultaneously suppress the gonadotropic activity of the gland. In addition, it may encourage dangerous delay in instituting other forms of therapy.

In the presence of an enlarged thyroid and persistently high basal metabolic rate, some workers recommend *thyroidectomy*. Though the ensuing drop in the metabolic rate is less marked and less consistent than in primary hyperthyroidism, operation is deemed advisable to prevent diabetes and heart failure.[25] According to Davis,[6] thyroidectomy in the presence of acromegaly has a high surgical risk.

In the terminal phases of the disease, *substitutive organotherapy* is indicated for the secondary pluriglandular insufficiency which characterizes the malady at this time.

DYSTROPHIA ADIPOSOGENITALIS (FRÖHLICH'S SYNDROME)

Definition.—Babinski,[1] in 1900, first described a clinical syndrome whose salient features, adiposity and genital hypoplasia, prompted Bartel's[2] subsequent use of the term "dystrophia adiposogenitalis." Though a pituitary neoplasm was known to be present in the case reported by Babinski, it was not until the following year that the importance of the hypophysis in the etiology was emphasized by Fröhlich.[3] The term "Fröhlich's syndrome" has since been generally applied to this disease. Most observers, however, prefer to reserve this designation for the rare cases in which a tumor is present, and describe the much more common cases without demonstrable pathology as adiposogenital dystrophy.

CLINICAL CHARACTERISTICS

The essential manifestations of the disease are a feminine type of adiposity and genital hypoplasia. In addition, there may be skeletal under- or overgrowth, and metabolic disturbances. Some observers classify cases with skeletal overgrowth as a separate clinical entity which they describe as the *Neurath-Cushing type* of adiposogenital dystrophy.[4] In the presence of a neoplasm, intracranial pressure symptoms may appear. The clinical picture varies, and depends largely on the age and degree of sexual development achieved at the onset of the malady.

Adiposity.—Adiposity is a constant manifestation of the syndrome. It appears early, is often acquired rapidly, and shows a predilection for the breasts, abdomen, mons veneris, hips, buttocks, and proximal parts of the upper and lower extremities. The face, neck, and distal portions of the arms and legs are usually exempt, and appear thin in contrast to the large torso. In some instances, particularly in the adult female, the fat deposits are enormous and involve the entire body, though more pronounced at the sites of predilection. The lipomatous masses of the abdominal wall often form large apron-like folds, which cover the genitalia and upper thighs. The breasts may likewise be the site of enormous fat deposits, becoming huge and pendulous.

Genital Hypoplasia.—The degree of genital hypoplasia will obviously depend on the developmental status of the sex organs at the inception of the disease. The infantile and juvenile forms of the malady are characterized by the most pronounced sexual retardation. The primary and

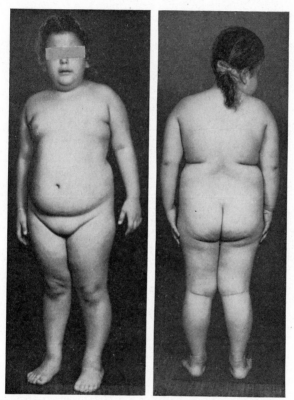

Fig. 132.—Fröhlich's type of obesity in a five-year-old girl. Weight 92 pounds, height 40 inches.

accessory genital organs remain immature or, where the disease begins in late childhood, may attain at best only a slight degree of development. In such individuals, the normal age of puberty is reached and passed without the appearance of secondary sex characters. In the *female*, menstruation may never appear and reproductive function is precluded. When the disease arises during adolescence, the gonads and accessory genitalia may mature to some extent. The secondary sex characters may be only partially developed and retain their pubescent form in adult life. A late menarche and hypomenorrhea or oligomenorrhea are common in the

milder cases. In the more severe forms, menstrual function may fail to
appear or, though already initiated, may cease as the disease progresses.
In the adult form of the disease, the normally developed primary and
secondary sex characters undergo retrogressive changes. Menstruation
becomes scanty, infrequent and finally ceases. The libido is diminished and
sterility is the rule.

In the *male*, as in the female, the preadolescent form is characterized
by the most marked degree of genital hypoplasia. The penis, scrotum, and
prostate are markedly hypoplastic, the testes minute and often undescended. When the normal age for adolescence is reached, the secondary
sex characters fail to appear. The facial hair is absent or barely per-

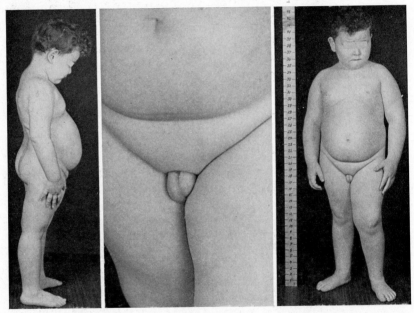

Fig. 133.—Fröhlich's type of adiposity in a four-year-old boy. Weight 80 pounds; height 44
inches. Penis infantile though testicles are fully descended.

ceptible. The pubic hair may likewise be absent or sparse, assuming the
female distribution. Libido and ejaculation are absent, and the voice retains
its high pitch. In the adolescent form, the primary and secondary sex
characters may show a fair degree of development, but undergo regressive
changes as the disease becomes established. When the malady arises during adult life, the fully developed primary and secondary sex characters
undergo retrogressive alterations. Libido sexualis, potentia and spermatogenic function may be markedly diminished and, in the severe case, absent.

Somatic Alterations.—In the juvenile form, skeletal growth may
sometimes be retarded, but is more often normal for the age or excessive. Where excessive, the lower measurement may exceed the upper one,
the clinical picture simulating the mild form of obese eunuchoidism. In

the adult form of the disease, skeletal growth shows no significant deviations from the normal.

In both sexes, the skin is soft, smooth and has a delicate texture. The face is small and doll-like, and the complexion is of the so-called "peaches and cream" variety. These characteristics, together with the absence of body hair, soft body contours, tendency to lay on mammary and abdominal fat, broad pelvis, genu valgum, small hands and feet, tapering fingers, and high pitched voice give such males a distinctly feminine appearance.

Metabolic Disturbances.—Metabolic disturbances are common. The sugar tolerance, as a rule, is increased and the blood sugar lowered. Affected

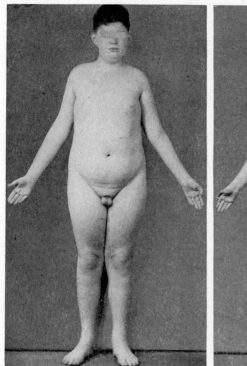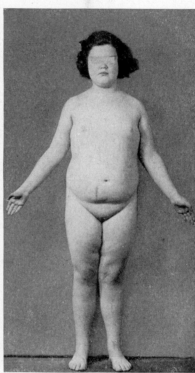

Fig. 134.—Fröhlich's type of adiposity and sexual retardation occurring in a brother and sister, aged fourteen and nine, respectively.

individuals often evince a decided craving for sweets, a factor which may play a significant role in producing the enormous obesity. The basal metabolic rate is within normal limits in the majority of cases, though low rates are encountered in cases associated with hypothyroidism. It should be emphasized that basal metabolic estimations in children are unreliable and that calculations on the basis of total body weight may give misleading results (see Chap. XXXIII).

Nervous and Psychic Manifestations.—Nervous manifestations are absent as a rule, unless the disease is due to an expanding cranial neoplasm. Under such circumstances, headaches, projectile vomiting, vertigo, bitemporal hemianopsia, optic atrophy, oculomotor palsies, epilepsy, and other manifestations of intracranial pressure may ensue.

In harmony with their feminine physical appearance, males have a distinctly effeminate demeanor, and prefer artistic and cultural pursuits to activities entailing physical exertion. In the female, the marked adiposity constitutes a distinct social and physical handicap, and often makes for introspection and psychic disturbances. As a rule, the disease does

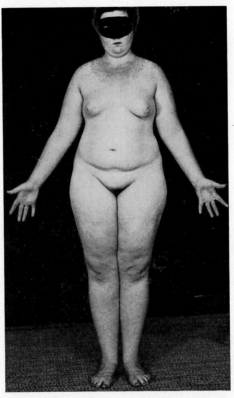

Fig. 135.—Adolescent hypogonadism with Fröhlich's type of adiposity. Girl aged sixteen, weight 175 pounds. Primary amenorrhea; hypoplastic genitalia, axillary hair absent, pubic hair scanty; subthreshold estrogen cycle.

not affect the mentality, and most cases possess average or even above average intelligence.

ETIOLOGY AND PATHOLOGY

Role of the Hypophysis and Hypothalamus.—The cause of adiposogenital dystrophy is not clear. The existing confusion is largely due to the varied pathologic findings recorded at autopsy. Neoplasms, cysts, hemorrhage, and other lesions have been found confined to the hypophysis or midbrain. In some cases no pathology could be demonstrated in either structure. Fröhlich and other early observers believed the disease to be of hypophyseal origin. Marburg[5] was the first to attribute it to hypopituitarism. Erdheim[6] maintained that both the pituitary and hypothalamic region are implicated, and interpreted the syndrome as pituitary nanosomia plus obesity due to disturbance of a trophic center in the midbrain. A purely midbrain origin was favored by some observers,[7, 8, 9] on the basis of the observation that the syndrome may occur with a lesion of the midbrain and an apparently normal hypophysis, and that damage to the tuber cinereum in experimental animals results in obesity and genital atrophy. Biedl[10] attempted to reconcile the varied pathologic findings by distinguishing between a hypophyseal and cerebral form of adiposogenital dystrophy, according to the site of the primary lesion.

Experimental studies during the past decade have shed some light on this problem. In view of evidence establishing the anterior pituitary as the primary gonad-stimulating gland, it would seem reasonable to assume that a deficiency of its gonadotropic hormones is responsible for the genital retardation in dystrophia adiposogenitalis. Recent experiments demonstrating that removal of the hypophysis without injury to adjacent centers in the midbrain does not cause obesity, have cast doubt on the view that the adiposity of Fröhlich's syndrome is an expression of hypopituitarism. The studies of Hetherington and Ranson,[11] and of Heinbecker and White[12] strongly suggest that the cause of the adiposity probably resides in the hypothalamus, while the hypophysis plays at best only a contributory role (see Chap. XXXIII). Though the available evidence permits no final conclusion, it seems likely that both the hypophysis and hypothalamus are implicated in the production of adiposogenital dystrophy, the former being chiefly responsible for the genital atrophy, the latter for the adiposity.

Observers have long been at a loss to explain why identical clinical manifestations may result from lesions confined to the hypophysis or hypothalamus exclusively. This is becoming more understandable with the accumulation of histologic and experimental evidence pointing to a close anatomic and functional relationship between these structures (see Chap. XV). It is conceivable that, by reason of their neural and vascular connections, a lesion in one may be reflected in the other, disturbing its function without causing any demonstrable morphologic modifications.

Associated Skeletal Findings.—The associated skeletal findings in dystrophia adiposogenitalis have puzzled observers, who find it difficult to account for the fact that growth is retarded in some cases and accelerated in others. *Skeletal retardation* may perhaps best be explained by assuming that the disturbance of anterior pituitary function involves suppression of its growth as well as its gonadotropic function. *Skeletal overgrowth,* on the other hand, is less easily explained. One possibility is that the gonadotropic hormone deficiency is associated with overproduction of the growth factor. On the other hand, the anterior lobe may be producing normal amounts of growth hormone but the deficiency of its sex principles and consequent absence of gonadal function results in delayed epiphyseal closure, permitting growth of the long bones beyond the time when it would normally cease.

DIAGNOSIS

Prepuberal Cases.—In the classical case, where the individual has already passed the puberal age, the characteristic distribution of the fat deposits, and genital hypoplasia strongly suggest adiposogenital dystrophy. Difficulties often arise in the prepuberal case.[13, 14] The fat boy or girl may closely resemble the true Fröhlich's type, for in both there is adiposity and the genitalia are undeveloped. Except in the presence of marked skeletal anomalies, metabolic disturbances, or a demonstrable lesion in the hypophysis or its environs, the diagnosis is necessarily tentative, and

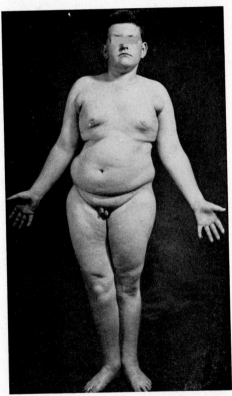

Fig. 136.—Adiposogenital dystrophy. Boy aged sixteen, weight 185 pounds. Note typical fat padding and tiny genitalia, absence of facial and pubic hair.

can only be established after the puberal age is passed. It must be emphasized that in many obese boys and girls, positively classified as cases of Fröhlich's syndrome, normal development of the primary and secondary sex characters, and disappearance of the adiposity occurs spontaneously when the age of puberty is reached.[15, 20] Such cases probably account for many of the cures attributed to organotherapy (see below). The adiposity and small genitalia in these individuals may conceivably be due to a purely functional, and therefore reversible disturbance in the anterior pituitary and hypothalamus, which develops in the course of the endocrine and metabolic upheaval that marks the transition from child-hood to adulthood, but rights itself with the completion of this epoch.

Adult Cases.—The diagnosis is comparatively simple when typical adiposity and sexual retardation is encountered in an individual already past the puberal age. Uncertainty may arise where skeletal development is excessive and the body proportions altered. Such cases may be clinically indistinguishable from the obese form of eunuchoidism. Unless a demonstrable intracranial lesion is present or there is a history of gonadal damage, it may be difficult to decide whether the pituitary or gonads are primarily at fault. The gonadotropin tests of the blood and urine may be of value in the differential diagnosis. The value of 17-ketosteroid determinations is not established.

In the absence of a demonstrable intracranial lesion, recognition of adiposogenital dystrophy arising during adult life may be difficult, especially in the female. In the male, the rapid development of a feminine type of adiposity, together with loss of libido and potentia, constitute significant presumptive evidence.

COURSE AND PROGNOSIS

The degree of genital development achieved by the individual will depend on the time of onset of the disease. In the presence of a lesion of the hypophysis or its environs, the outlook is obviously grave unless the neoplasm can be eradiated by surgery or arrested by deep x-ray radiation.

TREATMENT

The object of the treatment is to eliminate the primary cause where possible, prevent or correct the genital hypoplasia, reduce the abnormal adiposity, stimulate skeletal growth where necessary, and relieve the patient of troublesome symptoms.

Surgery.—The presence of a hypophyseal or cerebral neoplasm, particularly when associated with intracranial pressure symptoms, obviously calls for surgery. Deep x-ray therapy, according to some observers, is of doubtful value, since the tumors associated with adiposogenital dystrophy are often resistant to the rays.

Organotherapy.—Organotherapy has been employed not only to stimulate sexual development, but also as an aid in promoting skeletal growth. The empirical use of *thyroid* (gr. ½ to 1½ daily, or more if well tolerated) is always indicated. Where skeletal retardation is an associated finding, a potent anterior hypophyseal growth-promoting preparation may be tried (see Chap. XIII).

The available *gonadotropins* of hypophyseal, chorionic and equine origin have been recommended as a prophylactic measure in obese children where sexual retardation is suspected, and as active treatment to combat genital hypoplasia in individuals past the puberal age. The *dose* commonly employed varies from 100 to 200 international units every other day for one to two months, with intervening rest periods of two to four weeks.

The efficacy of gonadotropic hormone therapy in the juvenile case is difficult to evaluate. Striking improvement has thus far been noted only in cases free from intracranial neoplasms. As already pointed out, such individuals often achieve normal sexual development at puberty without treatment or following weight reduction by dietary means.[16, 17] The possibility of spontaneous correction, coupled with the fact that thyroid substance and dietotherapy were employed concurrently in many of the cases, makes it difficult to decide what benefit was actually derived from the gonadotropic hormones.

As may be expected, the results claimed for gonadotropic hormone therapy have been much less spectacular in the postpuberal than in the prepuberal cases. Convincing proof that any of the available gonadotropes can stimulate spermatogenesis in the hypofunctioning male gonad is still lacking. For the stimulation of male sex hormone production by the interstitial cells of the testis, human chorionic gonadotropin would appear more effective than the hypophyseal or equine hormones. In the female, gonadotropic hormone therapy has proved of doubtful value. None of the available preparations, whether given singly or in combination, has been conclusively shown to be effective in restoring normal cyclic activity in the hypofunctioning ovary (see Chap. XII).

Where the gonadotropes fail to evoke a response, some workers advocate the use of the *gonadal sex hormones* to stimulate development of the accessory genitalia and secondary sex characters. Since such therapy cannot stimulate and may even depress anterior pituitary and indirectly gonadal function, it should be avoided in the prepuberal case. Its use is justified in the postpuberal case where hope of spontaneous correction no longer exists and the favorable psychologic effect of the genital development achieved thereby justifies the trouble and expense involved. It should be emphasized, however, that the effects of the sex hormones regress rapidly unless treatment is continued. Moreover, the response to these substances diminishes after a time, so that increasingly large doses become necessary to elicit any reaction.[18]

X-ray Therapy.—Low dosage x-ray radiation directed to the hypophyseal region (for dosage see Chap. XXV) is employed by some workers[19] with the hope of stimulating stagnant hypophyseal function. In the absence of satisfactory proof that such treatment has a stimulative effect, and in view of the possibility that it may harm the pituitary or adjacent structures, it should be undertaken with caution and only after conservative measures have failed.

SIMMONDS' DISEASE (HYPOPHYSEAL CACHEXIA)

Definition.—The term "Simmonds' disease" describes a symptom-complex characterized by a progressive and profound emaciation, and regression of the primary and secondary sex characters.[1] Some investigators reserve this term for those cases in which pituitary pathology was demonstrated at autopsy. Where typical manifestations arise in the absence of demonstrable organic disease, they apply the terms "pituitary emaciation," "von Bergmann's magersucht,"[2] or "functional Simmonds' disease."[3]

Incidence.—Proved cases of Simmonds' disease are rare. In a survey

of the world literature to 1940, Lisser and Escamilla[4] found only 101 verified cases among a total of 595 patients with symptoms suggestive of Simmonds' disease. The syndrome is most apt to develop during middle life
and is only occasionally encountered in the young or aged. It is far more
common in women than in men; of the 101 verified cases, 65 were female.

CLINICAL CHARACTERISTICS

Somatic Alterations.—The malady is marked by a severe and progressive emaciation with terminal cachexia, loss of axillary and pubic hair,

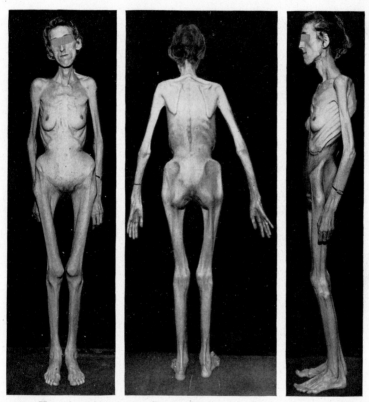

Fig. 137.—Hypophyseal cachexia (Simmonds' disease). Single woman aged twenty-nine
in terminal stages of disease. Weight 49 pounds, after loss of 82 pounds in three years.
Amenorrhea associated with atrophic genitalia and negative estrogen tests. Anorexia: hypotension, hypothermia, hypoglycemia and low basal metabolic rate (—40). Note extreme
emaciation and loss of pubic hair.

genital atrophy, and profound depression of all endocrine and metabolic
functions. The extreme emaciation, which is the most prominent manifestation of the disease, is due to complete loss of subcutaneous and visceral
fat, and general atrophy of musculature and viscera (microsplanchnia).
Losses up to 65 per cent of the original body weight have been recorded,
and in the terminal phases the patient is literally skin and bone. The pronounced loss of weight is accompanied by profound asthenia, particularly

in the later stages. Early graying, loss of teeth with atrophy of the jaw, a dry, sallow, wrinkled skin, and loss of pubic and axillary hair combine to give the sufferer a prematurely senile appearance. Amenorrhea, loss of libido, and marked retrogressive alterations of the reproductive organs and secondary sex characters are constant findings, particularly in the advanced case.

Metabolic Disturbances.—All metabolic activities are profoundly depressed. The basal metabolic rate is markedly lowered. Readings of minus 30 to minus 49 have been recorded. These values are lower than those

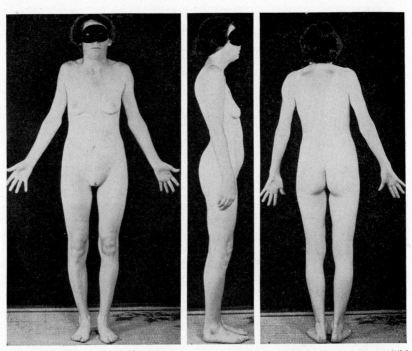

Fig. 138.—Early Simmonds' disease. Patient aged thirty-five; mother of three children born within period of three years. In course of four months following last childbirth, weight dropped from 150 to 105 pounds, associated with loss of pubic and axillary hair, regression of breasts and of internal and external genitalia. Asthenia, hypothermia, hypoglycemia, hypotension. B.M.R. —30. Atrophic changes of endometrium; negative estrogen and gonadotropin tests.

recorded following thyroidectomy. This is not surprising in view of recent evidence (see Chap. XIII) that the anterior hypophysis secretes, in addition to its thyrotropic factor, a principle capable of increasing the basal metabolic rate without the intervention of the thyroid gland. The specific dynamic action is likewise materially reduced or absent. Carbohydrate metabolism is disturbed, and hypoglycemia is often encountered. Spontaneous drops in the blood sugar may explain the attacks of severe abdominal cramps, fainting spells, cold sweats, and epileptiform seizures, all suggestive of hypoglycemic shock. Disturbances of the water, salt, and calcium metabolism are not uncommon. Hypotension is a frequent finding, and in the severe case the systolic pressure may fall to 60 mg. Hg or lower. The arterial tension in the Simmonds' patient has a peculiar tendency to fall on the slightest exertion. The pulse is weak and slow, and in the advanced stages bradycardia is a frequent finding. The blood picture is that of a severe secondary anemia, and the eosinophiles and lymphocytes are often increased. Hypochlorhydria and achylia have been reported in many of the cases. Considered in conjunction with the cachexia, the picture suggests gastric malignancy.

Subjective Symptoms.—The most striking subjective symptoms are anorexia, aversion for water, profound asthenia, hypothermia, vertigo, headaches, nausea and vomiting, obstinate constipation, epigastric distention, and attacks of severe abdominal cramps. Profound depression, apathy, delusions, and mental deterioration are not uncommon in the advanced stages.

ETIOLOGY AND PATHOLOGY

Role of the Anterior Hypophysis.—Simmonds' disease may arise from any one of many causes which profoundly depress, render inactive or completely destroy the secretory elements of the anterior hypophysis. Embolism, thrombosis, hemorrhage, simple atrophy or fibrosis, cyst or abscess formation, primary or metastatic neoplasms of the pituitary or its environs, lues, tuberculosis, trauma, and intensive hypophyseal radiation have been recorded. The importance of embolism as an etiologic factor is borne out by its presence in twenty-five of forty cases reviewed by May and Robert.[5] The syndrome not infrequently follows oft *repeated gestations,* or *pregnancy complicated by toxemia or dystocia.*[6] According to Sheehan,[7] the commonest cause is necrosis of the anterior lobe following difficult puerperium with hemorrhage. According to this observer, the pituitary undergoes rapid involution at the time of the puerperium. If the sudden reduction in the blood flow which occurs at this time is complicated by circulatory collapse due to hemorrhage, the blood flow may be reduced to almost nothing. This may result in thrombosis in the sinuses of the gland with consequent infarction and necrosis. Effkemann and Müller-Jager,[8] on the other hand, deny that the endocrine disturbance is related to the difficult puerperium. They believe that women with a latent predisposition to endocrine disorders are also predisposed to difficult labor with hemorrhage.

The well established role of the anterior hypophysis in gonadal function and general metabolic activity, is responsible for the view that the clinical manifestations of Simmonds' disease are due to marked deficiency or absence of most or all the anterior pituitary hormones. In view of this gland's trophic effect on other members of the endocrine system, the pluriglandular insufficiency which marks this malady is considered to be secondary to the hypophyseal deficiency. The experimental observation that animals subjected to partial or total hypophysectomy show emaciation and genital atrophy, which can be corrected by administering anterior pituitary extracts or implants,[9] would seem to substantiate this interpretation.

Role of the Hypothalamus.—The appearance of the syndrome in patients with extrasellar lesions and an intact hypophysis,[10] and occasional instances of partial or complete pituitary atrophy without symptoms of Simmonds' disease,[11] have led some investigators[12, 13] to attribute the malady to a break in the connections between the pituitary and vegetative centers in the midbrain (see Chap. XV). According to this view, the primary cause of the emaciation is a disturbance in the diencephalic centers concerned with the regulation of metabolism. Protagonists of this theory attribute the cachexia which follows experimental hypophysectomy to incidental injury to the midbrain.

The close anatomic and functional relationship between the hypophysis and *hypothalamus* probably accounts for the fact that identical clinical manifestations may result from lesions confined to either one exclusively. Since the hypophysis is the primary gonad-governing gland, it is very likely that a disturbance in its function is the immediate cause of the genital atrophy. Whether the emaciation is of purely hypothalamic origin or is due to a deficiency of the anterior pituitary hormones concerned with growth and metabolism cannot be decided definitely from the evidence at hand.

Diagnosis and Differential Diagnosis

In the presence of a discernible intrasellar tumor, the differential diagnosis between Simmonds' disease and other conditions attended by marked emaciation offers no difficulty. Where no pituitary lesion is demonstrable, the diagnosis of hypophyseal insufficiency is necessarily one of exclusion. Emaciation or cachexia incident to progressive muscular dystrophy (see Fig. 140), advanced tuberculosis, malignancy, diabetes, blood dyscrasias, or other constitutional depressive states can be excluded by the history, physical findings, laboratory studies, and x-ray examinations.

Anorexia nervosa is very often confused with Simmonds' disease and as yet no reliable means of distinguishing the two has been found. A history of infection or pregnancy just preceding the appearance of symptoms points to Simmonds' disease.[4] Significant in the differential diagnosis is the fact that anorexia nervosa occurs as a rule in young women with a psychoneurotic background. In contrast to the dull, apathetic Simmonds' patient, the individual with anorexia nervosa is active, restless, and conscious of a sense of well-being, despite the extreme emaciation.[14] There is usually no loss of teeth, or of pubic and axillary hair. Nor do the primary and secondary sex characters, particularly the breasts, undergo the marked degrees of atrophy seen in the Simmonds' patient. Psychiatric examination may be of value in the differential diagnosis. Probably the most decisive evidence pointing to anorexia nervosa is the favorable response to psychotherapy.

Simmonds' disease may often be confused with *multiple glandular sclerosis,* which may be accompanied by an almost identical symptomatology. According to Falta,[15] the presence of myxedema in the latter may be the only distinguishing feature, but the recent studies of Means and his associates[16] indicate that this manifestation may also be encountered in Simmonds' disease. In the opinion of Falta,[15] multiple glandular sclerosis is a distinct clinical entity due to a simultaneous fibrosis involving several of the ductless glands. Lisser and Escamilla[4] question his theory and believe that cases described as multiple glandular sclerosis or pluriglandular insufficiency were actually examples of Simmonds' disease.

Addison's disease associated with pigmentation of the skin and mucous membranes is easily distinguished from Simmonds' disease. In the absence of pigmentation, a history of remissions and acute crises, and a favorable

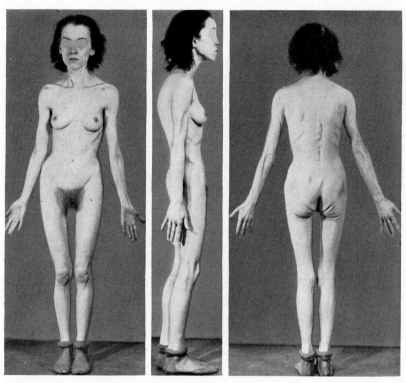

Fig. 139.—Anorexia nervosa. Single girl aged twenty-four, weight 70 pounds. Amenorrhea for one year associated with loss of 25 pounds. Nervous and psychic instability, anorexia, headaches, weakness, hypoglycemia and low basal metabolic rate. Atrophic type of endometrium; negative estrogen tests. Favorable response to psychotherapy and dietary measures.

response to adrenal cortical extract and salt therapy are significant. Also significant is the fact that the Addisonian patient does not show the extreme wasting or the profound regressive changes in the generative organs and secondary sex characters which mark Simmonds' disease. In Addison's disease, the gastrointestinal symptoms are more intense, the hypotension more pronounced, and the depression of the basal metabolic rate less marked than in Simmonds' disease. Quantitative determinations of the 17-ketosteroids in the urine (see Chap. XXXIX) are of limited value in the differential diagnosis. In the female, both Addison's and Simmonds' disease are associated with a marked decrease[17] or disappearance[18] of these substances. In the male, the drop is less marked in Addison's disease because of the presence of small quantities derived from the testes.[17, 18] Whether the adrenocorticotropic hormone content of the body fluids, and the response to therapy with this hormone differs in the two conditions has not yet been investigated.

Simmonds' disease associated with *myxedema* is often erroneously diagnosed as *primary hypothyroidism* and treated as such. The observation that thyroid therapy may prove harmful and even fatal in these individuals emphasizes the importance of distinguishing between myxedema due to primary hypothyroidism and that resulting from hypothy-

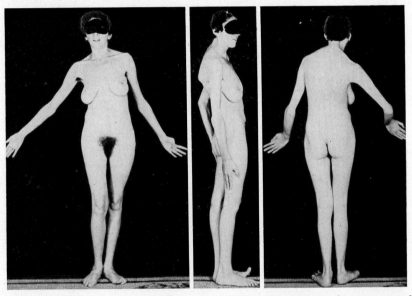

Fig. 140.—Progressive muscular dystrophy. Single girl aged twenty-six, two years after onset of disease precipitated by psychic shock. Gradual, progressive emaciation with atrophy of muscles; inability to walk, loss of speech, and marked difficulty in swallowing. Amenorrhea. Note well preserved breasts and pubic hair, contrasting with Simmonds' disease. Fatal outcome.

roidism secondary to pituitary deficiency. According to Means and associates,[16] the presence of other symptoms of pituitary hypofunction, particularly adrenal cortical and gonadal insufficiency, is significant in the differential diagnosis. They recommend the use of the insulin tolerance test to establish a deficiency of the anterior pituitary diabetogenic factor. In addition, the gonadotropin content of the body fluids may provide a further clue to the status of pituitary function. A history of untoward effects following previous thyroid therapy is significant. A therapeutic test with thyrotropic hormone might also prove of value in determining whether the thyroid depression is due to some inherent defect or to a deficiency of this pituitary factor. Adrenal cortical extract and salt solution should be at hand in the event that symptoms of adrenal cortical insufficiency develop.

COURSE AND PROGNOSIS

The onset and course of Simmonds' disease may vary considerably. Cachexia develops gradually or rapidly. In the acute case, death may occur within a few months, but as a rule the disease is chronic and the individual may survive for many years. In one case reported by Reiche,[19] the patient lived forty-four years after the appearance of the first symptoms. The author's case (see Fig. 137) lived five years after the onset of the malady. The outlook obviously depends on the nature of the underlying cause. Where the secretory elements of the adenohypophysis are destroyed or markedly atrophic, the prognosis is poor. If the pituitary depression is due to lues, and specific therapy is instituted before irreparable damage is incurred by the hypophysis, the prognosis is much brighter. In the functional case, spontaneous remissions are common, and such individuals usually respond to therapy calculated to eradicate the condition responsible for the hypophyseal depression.

TREATMENT

Organotherapy.—If anterior pituitary insufficiency may properly be regarded as the primary cause of this malady, replacement with anterior pituitary extracts would seem to be rational therapy. In addition, other endocrine products would seem to be indicated to combat the concomitant pluriglandular insufficiency. Observers differ as to the efficacy of organotherapy for the control of the disease. Many could see no improvement with any of the available endocrine products,[20] while a few report improvement or cure with a variety of hormone preparations.[2, 5] In true Simmonds' disease, due to marked atrophy or destruction of the adenohypophysis, no endocrine preparation, regardless of its potency, can be expected to effect a cure, for the underlying deficiency persists and its manifestations are bound to recur when treatment is stopped. It is likely that the cures attributed to organotherapy occurred in cases where the pituitary deficiency was of purely functional origin and therefore capable of spontaneous correction, or in patients with anorexia nervosa who benefited from the psychotherapeutic effect of the treatment.

The good effects ascribed by some workers to oral therapy with *anterior lobe substance* may well be questioned in view of evidence that the hypophysectomized animal is not benefited when fed large quantities of gland substance.[21] Anterior lobe *implants* are advocated by a few observers.[22, 23, 28] While repeated implants constitute effective replacement therapy in the hypophysectomized animal, there is no satisfactory proof that it is of value in the human. No one has thus far convincingly demonstrated that such transplants remain functionally active for any length of time. On the contrary, there is ample evidence that they rapidly undergo retrogression and become inactive. Unless an implant remains functional, its contribution to the hormonal store of the host cannot exceed its hormonal content at the moment of implantation. Of interest is Kylin's[2] report that improvement or cure occurred in eighteen out of twenty-three cases receiving hypophyseal implants. Since his patients were all adolescent girls or young women, it is possible that they were actually cases of anorexia nervosa which responded favorably to the psychotherapeutic effect of the implants.

Crude *extracts* containing several or all the known active principles of the adenohypophysis would seem to be the therapy of choice. Here again, reported results have been either brilliant or disappointing.[24] Failures with anterior pituitary extracts may be due to the relative impotency of the available preparations, inadequate dosage, and institution of therapy late in the disease, when the responding endocrine glands are too depressed to be capable of reactivation. Those who believe the midbrain is implicated to some extent in the etiology, argue that anterior pituitary hormone therapy is at best only a partial attack upon the disease. Despite the prevailing pessimism, crude anterior pituitary extracts are worth a trial.

Though the concomitant pluriglandular insufficiency would seem to call for substitutive organotherapy in the form of thyroid substance, adrenal cortical extract, and other glandular products,[25, 26, 27] caution must be exercised in employing these substances. *Adrenal cortical extract,* if well tolerated, is worth a trial, particularly where the electrolytes of the blood point to adrenal cortical insufficiency (see p. 588). *Thyroid substance* or any other metabolic stimulant is contraindicated in Simmonds' disease, for there is reason to believe that the low rate of oxidation in the emaciated or cachectic patient is a conservative mechanism designed to prevent further weight loss. Some employ thyroid therapy where there is an associated myxedema, due to secondary hypothyroidism. Adrenal cortical extract and salt solution should be available for immediate use, for recent studies indicate that thyroid substance may aggravate the secondary adrenal cortical insufficiency usually present in such individuals and precipitate a crisis. Insulin has been recommended as an adjuvant in combating the anorexia and thus favorably influencing the nutritional status. In view of the frequent tendency to hypoglycemia in the Simmonds' patient, it should be used with extreme caution and only when combined with adequate amounts of glucose. A favorable response has been reported following corticotropic hormone therapy.[25]

The *gonadotropes* and *gonadal sex hormones* have no place in the therapeutic armamentarium, for the gravity of the disease overshadows the importance of reestablishing gonadal function. Even were such therapy effective, the occurrence of periodic uterine bleeding in the female patient would tend to aggravate the general depression by further sapping the patient's limited resources. The gonadal sex hormones are contraindicated because of their possible inhibitory effect on anterior pituitary function.

General Medical Measures.—General medical measures calculated to improve the nutritional status and relieve the sufferer of troublesome symptoms, are of prime importance in the treatment. Frequent small feedings are preferable to large meals. The diet should be of high caloric value, well balanced, not bulky, and ample in vitamins and minerals. In the severe case, highly concentrated fluid foods, or feeding by tube may be indicated. Fresh air, ample sunlight and good nursing may do much for the functional case, and may comfort and prolong the life of the true Simmonds' patient. Utmost care should be exercised to avoid exposure to infection, because of the lowered resistance.

CUSHING'S SYNDROME (PITUITARY BASOPHILISM)

Definition.—Cushing,[1] in 1932, called attention to a clinico-pathological entity, which he designated "pituitary basophilism" on the assumption that the primary cause is hyperplasia or adenoma of the basophil cells of the adenohypophysis. Since his original communication, the cardinal features of this syndrome have been encountered with other types of pituitary

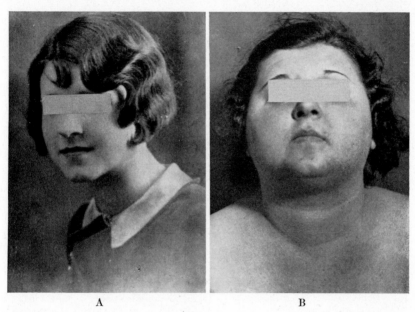

A   B

Fig. 141.—Cushing's Syndrome. A, Patient aged twenty-three, prior to onset of disease. B, Same patient four years later, showing typical manifestations of Cushing's disease, which first appeared following an ovarian operation about three years ago.

tumor, lesions of the adrenal cortex, thymus, or parathyroids, or in the absence of any demonstrable lesion. Because of the existing uncertainty as to the etiology, the term "Cushing's syndrome" will be used here to designate all cases presenting this symptom-complex, while "pituitary basophilism" will be applied only where the presence of basophil cell hyperplasia or adenoma is definitely established.

Incidence.—Pituitary basophilism is comparatively rare. Eisenhardt and Thompson,[2] who reviewed the world literature to 1939, could find only forty-eight cases in which a basophil adenoma was found at autopsy. While the malady may develop at any age, its incidence is highest during the third decade of life. According to some workers, the disease is much more common in the female. Others believe it occurs with equal frequency in both sexes, but that women appear to be affected more often because the manifestations of the malady are more pronounced and therefore more readily recognized.

SYMPTOMATOLOGY

The cardinal manifestations of Cushing's syndrome are a buffalo type of obesity, osteoporosis, hirsutism, purplish-red striae and a plethoric appearance of the skin, hypertension, glycosuria, and depression of gonadal function.

Obesity.—The obesity is rapidly acquired and often painful. It shows a predilection for the face, neck, trunk, and abdomen, but spares the

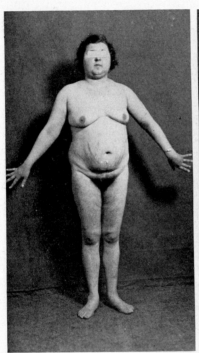
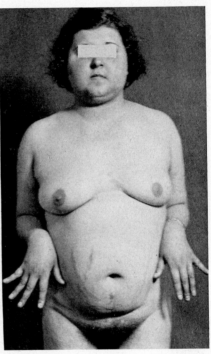

Fig. 142.—Same patient as in Fig. 141. Note buffalo type of obesity, facial hirsutism and purplish striae on lower abdomen. Blood pressure 160/90. Very low sugar tolerance; B.M.R. —12. Sella turcica negative. Exploratory operation revealed adrenal cortical hyperplasia, without tumor formation. Partial regression of facial hirsutism followed x-ray radiation of pituitary and adrenal regions.

hips and extremities. The facial adiposity may materially alter the normal features and is responsible for the "moon face" and "pig-eyed" expression of the classical case.

Skin and Hair Changes.—The skin as a rule is dry and pitted, and of a dusky, plethoric, or cyanotic hue. Transitory mottling, petechial hemorrhages, and purpuric spots are common. Purplish-red striae of the lower abdomen, hips, thighs, axillae, or mammae are a constant manifestation

Hirsutism of the face, with mustache and beard formation, and masculine distribution of the pubic hair are conspicuous in the female and preadolescent male. In the adult male, hirsutism is absent, and some cases may show an actual loss of head and body hair.

Bone Changes.—Osteoporosis and decalcification, particularly of the spine, have been reported in the majority of the cases. Ankylosis of the vertebrae, rounding of the shoulders, shortened stature, kyphosis, spontaneous fractures, and lumbar pain are some of the manifestations which may be attributed to the bone changes.

Hypertension.—Hypertension, usually of the fluctuant type, is also a common finding. A substantial rise in blood pressure was observed in 85.5 per cent of a group of cases observed by Jonas.[3] Of sixty-seven cases reviewed by Eisenhardt and Thompson,[2] the blood pressure was high in

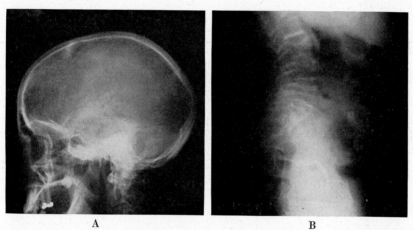

A   B

Fig. 143.—Bone changes in Cushing's syndrome. A, Roentgenogram of skull taken shortly before death in a patient with Cushing's disease. Note marked demineralization of vault. B, Roentgenogram of spine from same patient. Note decompression fractures due to demineralization.

forty-six, or 68.6 per cent. This may partly explain the cardiovascular embarrassment and apoplexy encountered in some young adults with this malady.

Sexual Disturbances.—In women, the early stages of the disease may be compatible with normal menstrual and reproductive function, but as it progresses, amenorrhea, sterility, and regressive changes of the ovaries are common. In the male, the later stages of the malady are often accompanied by marked diminution of libido sexualis and potentia, and partial or complete suppression of spermatogenesis.

Metabolic Disturbances.—Hyperglycemia, glycosuria, and a lowered sugar tolerance have been observed in a large percentage of the cases. The basal metabolic rate and specific dynamic action show individual variations, in some instances being normal, in others high or low.

Associated Symptoms.—Headache, which is often severe and of the

37

pituitary type, may be an associated complaint. Since the adenoma is minute in most cases, signs of intracranial pressure are only rarely encountered. Severe backache and pain in the extremities may result from the skeletal changes. Fatigability, asthenia, dyspnea, and other symptoms of cardiac decompensation are relatively common in the terminal stages. Aching pains in the eyes, insomnia, and mental changes have been recorded.

PATHOLOGY

Of Cushing's[1] original twelve cases, eight came to autopsy, and in six a *pituitary adenoma* was found. Three of the adenomas were composed of basophil cells. In 1935, Jonas[3] collected a group of thirty-five cases, of which twenty-one presented a *basophil adenoma* or significant increase in the number of basophil cells. Eisenhardt and Thompson,[2] in 1939, reviewed the findings in sixty-seven cases in which a pituitary lesion had been found at autopsy. An adenoma was present in fifty-eight, of which forty-eight were of the basophilic type. The basophil adenomas found associated with Cushing's syndrome were of minute size, their presence being established in many instances only by serial section of the gland. In only a few instances was the tumor discernible macroscopically, or large enough to distend the sella or give rise to intracranial pressure symptoms.

While a basophil adenoma is unquestionably a frequent finding, the cardinal manifestations of the disease have been encountered in many cases in which autopsy revealed other types of pituitary tumor, or lesions of other glands. Thus, in the sixty-seven cases reviewed by Eisenhardt and Thompson, a chromophobic adenoma was present in three, an acidophilic adenoma in one, a mixed type in two, and an atypical adenoma in one. Two cases with a fibro-adenoma of the pituitary, and two with a malignant tumor of this gland were also encountered in this series.

Hyperplasia or adenomas of the adrenal cortex, either with or without pituitary pathology, have been observed in a large percentage of the cases. In Eisenhardt and Thompson's series, nine cases revealed an adenoma and thirty-six hyperplasia of the adrenal cortex. Cushing's syndrome has also been found associated with an oat-cell *carcinoma of the thymus*, and with *hyperplasia or adenoma of the parathyroids*. It is significant that Eisenhardt and Thompson were able to find nine cases with the typical features of the syndrome, in which no adenoma or other tumor of any of the endocrine glands was demonstrable at autopsy.

ETIOLOGY

Role of the Adrenal Cortex and Hypophysis.—The presence of hyperplasia or adenoma of the adrenal cortex in many of the cases led earlier observers to blame adrenal cortical pathology for the symptom-complex now known as Cushing's syndrome. In 1924, Raab[4] found a basophilic adenoma at autopsy in a case presenting the cardinal manifestations of this disease, and a similar observation was subsequently made in two additional cases, but no significance was attached to these findings until 1932, when Cushing[1] emphasized the importance of the basophil cell adenoma in the etiology. He proposed that the adrenal cortical alterations so frequently encountered in this disease, are secondary manifestations of the pituitary disturbance, being due to overproduction of the hypophyseal adrenocorticotropic principle. The demonstration of a substance possessing adrenocorticotropic properties in the body fluids of some patients with this malady,[5, 6] and reports of improvement following depressive doses of x-ray directed to the pituitary,[7] seem to lend support to this view. On the other hand, doubt is cast on it by the occurrence of the syndrome without basophil hyperplasia or tumor,[8] and its absence in many cases despite the presence of such pathology.[9, 10]

In 1935, Crooke[11] called attention to a peculiar *hyaline change in the cytoplasm of the basophils*, which he found in twelve cases with Cushing's syndrome. In six, this change was associated with a basophil-cell adenoma,

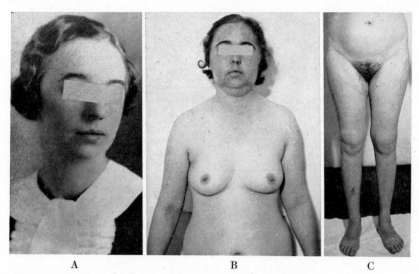

A   B   C

Fig. 144.—Cushing's syndrome. A, Patient at nineteen years of age, prior to onset of disease. B and C, Same patient three years later. Note buffalo type of obesity; hirsutism, particularly of the face; purplish striae on abdomen and thighs.

in three with a thymic neoplasm, and in three with adrenal cortical pathology. He also observed this alteration in a few cases of Cushing's disease, in which no pathology was demonstrable in any of the endocrine glands. He concluded that it represents the single common denominator of the syndrome, and is of fundamental significance in its causation, indicating increased activity of the basophils. Crooke's findings have been confirmed by Rasmussen.[12] His interpretation has been questioned by Severinghaus and Thompson,[13] who believe this hyaline change signifies degeneration following a period of hyperactivity. Bauer[14] deems it of no etiologic significance, and holds that it merely represents a reaction of the hypophysis to heightened activity of the adrenal cortex.

In the recent literature, there has again been a growing tendency to stress adrenal cortical hyperactivity as the primary cause of this syndrome.

On the basis of recent advances in adrenal cortical physiology (see Chap. XVII), Haymaker and Anderson[15] have suggested that Cushing's syndrome be classed, together with adrenogenitalism (see p. 581), under the common head of *adrenal cortical syndrome*. Both entities, they believe, are of adrenal cortical origin, but in adrenogenitalism there is an overproduction of an adrenal cortical masculinizing hormone, while in Cushing's disease there is an excess of the adrenal cortical hormones concerned with metabolism. According to this view, an excess of both the androgenic and metabolic principles of the adrenal cortex is responsible for a mixed type of syndrome, in which manifestations of Cushing's disease and adrenogenitalism appear.

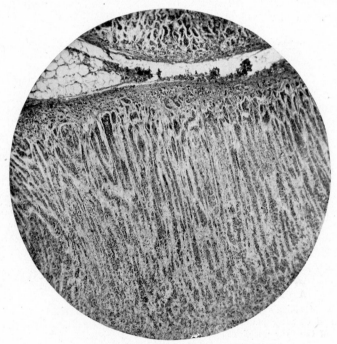

Fig. 145.—Adrenal Cortical Hyperplasia. Gland obtained at autopsy from a patient with Cushing's syndrome.

It is thus apparent that one school of thought accords the hypophysis the primary role, while another favors the adrenal cortex as the dominant factor. In view of the varied pathologic findings recorded in this disease, it seems likely that both glands are implicated, and that either may be the site of the primary lesion, the other being secondarily affected because of their close functional interrelationship (see Chap. XIII). Where no pathology is demonstrable in any of the ductless glands, the cause may conceivably be a functional disturbance in both the anterior pituitary and adrenal cortex. Rare instances in which a neoplasm was found in the thymus, parathyroid, or ovary, are difficult to explain unless it is assumed that such lesions lead secondarily to a disturbance of anterior pituitary and adrenal cortical function. Whatever the primary site of the lesion, it may be expected that repercussions will occur in other endocrine glands. The resulting pluriglandular involvement probably accounts for the varied symptoms, some referable to the pituitary, others to the adrenals, gonads, parathyroids, and pancreas.

Causes of Specific Symptoms.—The lack of accord as to the primary cause of the syndrome is evident in the variety of explanations offered to account for the individual manifestations of the disease. Cushing attributed the characteristic *adiposity* to a disturbance of the hypophyseal-hypothalamic connections. This suggestion has been challenged on the ground that the nature and distribution of the fat deposits in no way resemble those which accompany lesions of the tuber-hypophyseal region.[14] An excess of the parathyrotropic factor of the anterior pituitary gland was blamed by Cushing for the *osteoporotic changes*. Aside from the fact that the existence of this principle is still doubtful (see Chap. XIII), participation of the parathyroids has been questioned on the ground that the *skeletal changes* seen in Cushing's disease are unlike those of osteitis fibrosa, a disease attributed to hyperparathyroidism. It may also be pointed out that, except for the few cases with a parathyroid adenoma, the vast majority thus far encountered presented no histologic evidence indicative of parathyroid hyperactivity. Cushing[16] believed that the *hypertension* characteristic of this malady is due to increased production of the posterior pituitary pressor principle, resulting from invasion of the posterior lobe by basophil cells from the adenohypophysis. Attempts to prove this have yielded conflicting results. The possibility that the anterior lobe may be responsible for this manifestation has likewise been considered, but the evidence on this point has been equally inconclusive.[17, 18] According to Haymaker and Anderson,[15] the rise in *blood pressure*, like the other manifestations of the disease, is due to adrenal cortical hyperactivity, the situation being the reverse of that in Addison's disease, which is associated with hypotension.

The cause of the *gonadal depression* in Cushing's disease is not clear. If it is true that the basophils are the source of the gonadotropic principles, as is generally believed, then hypergonadism should characterize pituitary basophilism. It has been suggested[19] that the gonadotropes produced by the presumably hyperactive basophils cause excessive luteinization of the ovary, which is ultimately transformed into fibrous tissue. This sequence of events is reflected in the transition from normal menses during the early phases of the disease, to menstrual irregularities and complete cessation of menstrual function in its later stages. Another explanation, offered by Severinghaus and Thompson,[13] is that the protracted elaboration of excessive amounts of gonadotropic hormone leads to the formation of antigonadotropic substances which inhibit the gonadal response to the hypophyseal gonadotropes. As yet, there is no convincing proof that gonadotropic hormone production is consistently increased in this disease. On the contrary, some workers report low gonadotropin titers in many of the cases.[20, 21, 22] Though a few cases with evidence of gonadal stimulation,[23] or a history of an early menarche preceding the onset of the disease, have been encountered, in the vast majority, hypoplasia of the gonads has been observed. As emphasized by Goecke,[21] the gonadal depression which marks this syndrome points to a deficiency rather than an excess of gonadotropic hormone. If this is true, how may it be reconciled with the presence of basophil cell hyperplasia or adenoma? It may signify that the basophils are not the source of the gonadotropes, or that they are not hyperactive, except possibly during the earliest stages of the disease. On the other hand, it may mean that these cells normally secrete gonadotropic hormones, but under pathologic conditions produce substances which are closely related chemically to the gonadotropes but lack gonadotropic activity or possess a limited activity which enables them to induce the thecal luteinization without follicular maturation or corpus luteum formation, described in some of the cases.[24] It is also conceivable that the basophils secrete both the gonadotropic and adrenocorticotropic factors, and that the stimulative effect of the former is offset by the inhibitory action of androgens produced by the adrenal cortex under the influence of the latter.

DIAGNOSIS AND DIFFERENTIAL DIAGNOSIS

Cushing's syndrome is readily recognized, particularly in the classical case, but its primary cause is very difficult and often impossible to determine from the clinical manifestations alone. The diagnosis is therefore necessarily one of exclusion.

Since the clinical manifestations of pituitary basophilism and adrenal cortical tumors may be identical, and the pituitary lesion is usually too small to be detected by the x-rays, the site of the primary lesion must often remain uncertain until autopsy, unless an adrenal neoplasm can be demonstrated by aerogram or by surgical inspection of the adrenals. It should be emphasized that even where roentgenograms reveal definite alterations in the adrenals, the presence of a pituitary lesion is not thereby excluded, for simultaneous involvement of both glands is not uncommon.

Crooke and Callow,[25] in 1939, suggested that the presence of excessive amounts of neutral *17-ketosteroids in the urine* may serve as a useful clue in distinguishing between cases of adrenal cortical and pituitary origin. Of four cases of Cushing's syndrome investigated by them, the excretion of these substances was increased in two with adrenal cortical tumors. Broster[26] made a similar observation in two patients. In none of the cases studied was the status of the hypophysis determined. For this reason, their findings only justify the conclusion that the level of neutral 17-ketosteroids may be used as a clue to the condition of the adrenal cortex, but cannot be made the basis for any decision as to the functional status of the anterior pituitary gland. More recent investigations of 17-ketosteroid excretion indicate that the values in adrenal cortical carcinoma are significantly elevated, whereas in adrenal cortical hyperplasia or benign adenoma the increases noted are too slight and the values too variable to constitute a reliable aid in the differential diagnosis between Cushing's disease of adrenal cortical and pituitary origin (see Chap. XL).

The observation that the adrenocorticotropic hormone content of the body fluids is increased in some cases of Cushing's disease,[5, 6] raised the hope that this might serve as a clue in the differential diagnosis between primary adrenal cortical hyperactivity and that secondary to hyperactivity of the anterior hypophysis. The number of cases studied thus far[27, 29] is still too limited to permit any conclusions.

COURSE AND PROGNOSIS

The duration of the disease varies considerably, the average being five years. Some cases develop rapidly and run a short, fatal course. In others, the malady may reach its peak within a short time and remain more or less quiescent for many years. Chronic cases have been known to live twenty years or more after the onset of the disorder. No case of spontaneous cure has been recorded.

The outlook, so far as life is concerned, is usually grave and depends on the nature of the underlying cause, its amenability to treatment, and the general state of the patient's health. Such individuals are highly susceptible to pyogenic infections. The disease is usually terminated by pneumonia, uremia, cerebral hemorrhage, apoplexy, or heart failure.

TREATMENT

In the presence of a pituitary tumor, deep *x-ray radiation* of the hypophyseal region is the therapy of choice. Partial or complete remission of some of the manifestations has been reported following such treatment.[7] *Cranial surgery* is not practicable because of the minute size of the adenoma, and there is no record of any case in which this was attempted with a successful outcome.[28] Since adrenal cortical hyperplasia is often an associated finding, some workers advocate x-ray radiation of both the adrenals and the hypophysis. In the presence of adrenal cortical tumor, surgery is obviously indicated. Surgical procedures may be fraught with danger because of the low resistance to infection, and adequate pre- and postoperative treatment (see p. 587) is therefore of the utmost importance.

Sex hormone therapy has been employed by a few observers with the hope of inhibiting the presumably hyperactive basophil cells. The number of cases so treated is too few and the results too conflicting to permit any conclusions as to the efficacy of such treatment. Rakoff and his associates[29] report good results with stillbestrol, while Gill[30] could see no effect after estrogen therapy. Albright and his coworkers[31] found that testosterone propionate caused nitrogen and phosphorus retention, reduced the urinary calcium output, and resulted in a gain in weight and strength. The administration of estrogenic substance reversed these effects. Bennhold[32] reports a favorable response to progesterone supplemented by thyroid substance.

THE ADRENOGENITAL SYNDROME

Definition.—The so-called "adrenogenital syndrome" is characterized by profound sexual and somatic alterations, usually in the male direction, occurring in the presence of adrenal cortical tumor or hyperplasia. The disease may have its inception before birth or at any time during postnatal life, but is most often encountered in the adolescent or young adult. It affects the female much more often than the male.

CLINICAL CHARACTERISTICS

The clinical manifestations vary according to the age of the patient and degree of genital development achieved at the inception of the disease. It is customary to speak of the congenital, juvenile, adult, and climacteric forms.

Congenital Form.—*Feminine pseudohermaphrodism,* associated with hyperplasia or tumor of the adrenal cortex, is classified by many observers as *interrenal pseudohermaphrodism* on the assumption that the adrenal pathology and sexual anomaly are causally related. If this assumption is

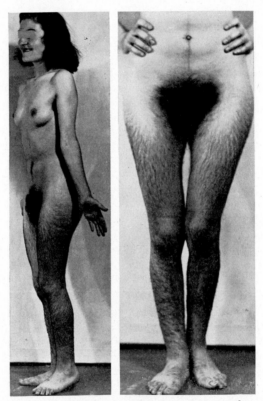

Fig. 146.—Hirsutism associated with amenorrhea, low estrogen and normal androgen values. Note marked hirsutism of lower extremities. Suggests possible adrenal cortical involvement.

correct, such cases must be taken to represent the most complete form of the adrenogenital syndrome. The external genitalia are modified in the male direction, while the ovaries, uterus, and tubes remain more or less normal. The vagina is incompletely separated from the urogenital sinus, and opens into the urethra. The most striking manifestation is a marked hypertrophy of the clitoris, which may assume penile proportions with a definite glans or prepuce. Some cases have a distinct scrotum.

Juvenile Form.—In the *young boy,* adrenogenitalism is characterized as a rule by marked muscular development and strength (Infant Hercules), though occasionally such individuals are obese. Somatic growth is accelerated at first, but premature ossification and epiphyseal closure is responsible for their relatively short stature on reaching adult life. Hirsutism is a cardinal manifestation. A profuse growth of dark, coarse hair first becomes apparent on the genital and anal regions, followed by the appearance of a luxuriant hair growth on the face, body and extremities. The penis, even in very young boys, is considerably enlarged and may attain adult proportions. The testicles as a rule remain small and infantile, though occasionally spermatogenesis and other manifestations of precocious sexual activity are encountered.

In the *young girl*, the most prominent features are hirsutism and hypertrophy of the external genitalia. The hair growth is of the male type and distribution, appearing in profusion on the genital region as well as the face, torso, and extremities. Especially striking is the enlargement of the clitoris, which may attain penile proportions, and at times even presents a definite glans and prepuce. The labia may be markedly enlarged and in some cases resemble a scrotum. The ovaries, tubes and uterus remain unaltered, retaining their infantile or juvenile status. With rare exceptions, menstruation and other signs of true sexual precocity, such as mammary enlargement, are absent.

The skin is usually dry, coarse and of a dusky red hue. In the obese case, the fat deposits show a predilection for the face, neck and trunk, but spare the girdle and extremities. In the muscular form of juvenile adrenogenitalism, the individual is endowed with a powerful musculature which is particularly pronounced in the extremities. Such girls are of short stature, stocky, broad-shouldered and deep-chested. Because of the sparsity of subcutaneous fat, they lack the soft body curves which characterize the normally developing female. As a rule, the mammae remain undeveloped and resemble those of the adolescent male. The psyche and demeanor are usually in the male direction.

Adult Form.—The adult form of the syndrome occurs almost exclusively in the female. The few instances thus far encountered in the male have shown very little or no exaggeration of masculine traits. Indeed, gynecomastia and other evidence of feminization have been recorded in some of the cases.[1]

In the *adult female*, the adrenogenital syndrome is characterized by retrogression of the female sex characters and the appearance of sex characters of the male type. The *cardinal manifestations* are hirsutism of the male type and distribution, deepening of the voice, enlargement of the clitoris, and a buffalo type of obesity. The ovaries, tubes and uterus undergo marked retrogressive changes. Disturbance of the menstrual rhythm is often an early manifestation. The periods become scanty, infrequent, and eventually cease. The mammary parenchyma may undergo involution or be replaced by large accumulations of fat. Libido sexualis may be diminished or absent, and sterility is the rule. The presence of osteoporosis, striae distensae, hypertension, and glycosuria makes this form of adrenogenitalism practically indistinguishable from pituitary basophilism.

Climacteric Form.—In the climacteric woman, the malady does not present the striking somatic and genital alterations seen in the juvenile form. Hirsutism and occasionally baldness have been reported. Since regressive changes in the sex sphere normally accompany the climacteric, the defeminizing effects of the adrenal cortical lesion are not conspicuous.

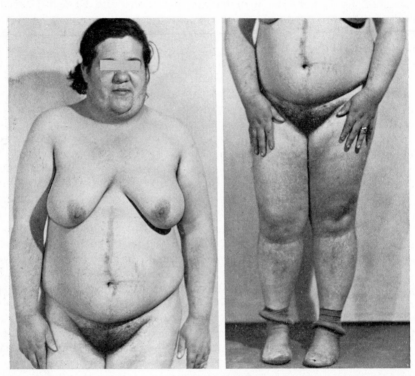

Fig. 147.—Obesity associated with hirsutism. Patient aged thirty, weight 180 pounds. Note facial and body hirsutism, and abdominal striae. Amenorrhea, negative estrogen and above normal androgen findings. X-ray of sella turcica and adrenals negative. Low sugar tolerance; mild hypertension. Symptomatology suggestive of adrenal cortical involvement.

ETIOLOGY AND PATHOLOGY

The adrenogenital syndrome is associated as a rule with diffuse *hyperplasia,* or with benign or malignant *neoplasms of the adrenal cortex.* Though it is generally agreed that the sexual alterations are due to the associated adrenal pathology, there is considerable uncertainty regarding the identity and source of the hormonal factors concerned.

Adrenal Cortical Causative Factors.—Earlier observers attributed the syndrome to *hyperfunction of the adrenal cortex,* with consequent overproduction of its specific life-sustaining hormone. This assumption has been questioned on the ground that tumors of the interrenal system may exist without virilism, and that the syndrome cannot be reproduced in experimental animals by administering large quantities of potent life-sustaining cortical hormone.

Another theory ascribes the syndrome to a *masculinizing substance,* produced by adrenal cortical cells distinct from true interrenal tissue. According to Krabbe,[2] this substance is secreted by reactivated fetal testicular cells incorporated within the substance of the developing adrenals during embryonic life. Since the adrenal cortex arises in the genital ridge, from which the gonads are also derived, Krabbe reasons that the medullary or male constituent of the embryonic gonad, which normally remains rudimentary in the female, may, as the result of a developmental anomaly, become part of the adrenal gland. Under pathologic conditions, these fetal "testicular" cells develop into tumors which physiologically manifest their testicular origin, causing virilism.

Grollman[3] has advanced the theory that the adrenal contains a third type of tissue, distinct from the cortical and medullary components of the gland. This so-called *androgenic tissue,* he believes, is normally present before birth, disappearing in the course of the first few years of postnatal life. At times, it may persist in the adult as small aggregations of dormant cells which, under pathologic conditions, undergo hyperplasia or become the site of neoplasms, and exert a masculinizing influence. While recognizing that the exact embryologic origin of this tissue is obscure, Grollman suggests that it may have a common origin with the "testicular" cells which Krabbe considers the source of the virilizing stimulus.

Broster and Vines,[4] in 1933, observed that, in cases where adrenal cortical hyperplasia or tumor was associated with virilism, certain cells in the adrenal cortex stained positively with Poinceau fuchsin. A negative or weakly positive reaction was obtained in adrenal cortical hyperplasia or tumor unassociated with masculinization, although the lesions in both cases were histologically indistinguishable. They concluded that the presence of a *fuchsinophile material* in the adrenal cortex is associated with virilism. Attempts to corroborate their claim as to the specificity of this stain have yielded conflicting results.[5-8] It is noteworthy that Broster[9] recently obtained a positive reaction with tissue removed from the hyperplastic adrenal cortex of a male showing evidence of demasculinization.

Androgenicity of Body Fluids.—In 1937, Broster and Vines,[10] in collaboration with Marrian and Butler,[11] detected excessive androgenic activity in the urine of patients with adrenal virilism. In addition, they isolated a crystalline compound, pregnane-3 (alpha) 17,20-triol, which they believed to be specific to adrenal virilism, since they could not find it in the urine of normal men and women. Their observation that the concentration of these substances diminished following unilateral adrenalectomy, clearly established their adrenal cortical origin. In a more recent study, Wolfe and his associates[12] found that the urine of a girl, with adrenal tumor and virilism, possessed excessive androgenic activity and contained a normal amount of androsterone, ten times the normal amount of 3-alpha-hydroaetiocholanone-17, and about 100 times the normal amount of dehydroisoandrosterone. They also isolated $\triangle^{3, 5}$-androstadienone-17, a steroid found in the urine of males with adrenal tumor but not in that of normal males or females, and a new steroid, characterized as 3-alpha-hydroxy-androstenone-17. These and other similar studies[13] have clearly established an association between adrenal cortical hyperactivity and increased androgenicity of the body fluids (see Chap. XL). It has also been shown that adrenal cortical tissue yields adrenosterone[14] and other crystalline compounds which possess varying degrees of androgenic activity.

There would therefore seem to be no doubt that the masculinization associated with adrenal cortical disease is due to androgenic substances derived from the adrenal cortex. The evidence suggests that these substances are physiologically and chemically distinct from the specific adrenal cortical life-sustaining principle, but fails to indicate whether they are secreted by distinct androgenic cells, or are merely products of perverted function of the true interrenal cells which, under normal conditions, secrete the life-sustaining principle. The latter possibility seems more likely in view of the fact that the cells in adrenal cortical hyperplasia or tumor associated with virilism are histologically indistinguishable from those in adrenal cortical hyperplasia or neoplasms unassociated with such manifestations. The mere fact that the cortical cells in adrenal virilism contain a peculiar fuchsinophile material, which is lacking in cases free from virilism, does not justify the conclusion that the two types of cells are anatomically and functionally distinct. In view of the close chemical relationship existing between cortical compounds with life-sustaining properties, and the androgens obtained from adrenal cortical tissue and urine of patients with adrenal virilism, it is conceivable that, under pathologic conditions, the metabolism of the true interrenal cells may be so disturbed that the specific life-sustaining principle is converted into a closely related chemical compound with androgenic activity. The fuchsinophile material present in adrenal virilism may be identical with this perverted secretion, or represent an intermediary product in the process leading to androgen formation. Significant in this connection is the observation of Lawrence[15] that administration of desoxycorticosterone acetate, for the control of adrenal cortical insufficiency in an adult male, caused gynecomastia associated with intense libido and erections.

DIAGNOSIS AND DIFFERENTIAL DIAGNOSIS

Since masculinization may arise from any one of several causes, the diagnosis of adrenal virilism is possible only in the presence of a discernible adrenal tumor. This may be established by Cahill's[7] method of x-ray visualization of the adrenals. Where the neoplasm is small, or the syndrome is due to adrenal cortical hyperplasia, the diagnosis is only possible after exploration and inspection of both adrenals. This formidable procedure should not be undertaken unless pituitary basophilism and other causes have been excluded.

Pseudohermaphrodism of adrenal origin may be diagnosed by inspecting the external genitalia and establishing the presence of a tumor in the region of the adrenal glands.

Macrogenitosomia praecox of cerebral or pineal origin may be distinguished from the juvenile form of adrenogenitalism in the male by the associated intracranial symptomatology. Where the neoplasm is appreciably enlarged, roentgenograms of the skull may be of value. An embryonal testicular neoplasm may be suspected where there is a palpable testicular mass and increased amounts of gonadotropin in the blood and urine (see Chap. XL).

The differential diagnosis between pseudosexual precocity of adrenal origin in the female, and isosexual precocity incident to *granulosa cell tumors of the ovary* (see p. 595) offers no difficulty. Precocious development of the primary and secondary sex characters, and the occurrence of menstruation in the prepuberal girl points to granulosa cell tumor. In addition, there may be a palpable tumor in the region of the adnexa, hyperplasia of the endometrium, and an increase in the estrogen content of the blood and urine. There is no enlargement of the clitoris and no hirsutism.

The adult form of adrenogenitalism in the female may be confused with *pituitary basophilism*, or masculinization due to *arrhenoblastoma of the ovary* (see p. 600) or *oat-cell carcinoma of the thymus*. The differential diagnosis between adrenogenitalism and pituitary basophilism is considered elsewhere (see p. 580). Arrhenoblastoma may be suspected where there is a palpable ovarian mass, but if the pelvic findings are negative, laparotomy and inspection of the ovaries may be necessary to establish the diagnosis. This should not be undertaken unless all extra-ovarian causes have been excluded. The presence of androgenic substances in the urine is of little help in the differential diagnosis, since a moderate rise occurs in both arrhenoblastoma and adrenal virilism.[16] This is apparently also true as regards increased excretion of pregnanediol.[17] On the other hand, a marked rise in the androgen level, or a considerable elevation of the estrogen level,[18, 19, 20] points to adrenal cortical carcinoma. According to Kantner and Klawans,[21] decreased serum sodium, increased serum potassium, and increased retention of nitrogen occurs in adrenal cortical hyperactivity but not in arrhenoblastoma, and may therefore prove a useful aid in the differential diagnosis.

PROGNOSIS

The prognosis depends on the time of onset and nature of the adrenal pathology. It is obvious that very little can be done for the congenital form of the disease, inasmuch as the structural changes in pseudohermaphrodism are irreversible. In cases associated with malignant neoplasms, the outlook is obviously grave unless the growth is removed before metastases occur.

TREATMENT

Surgery.—The presence of an adrenal cortical neoplasm, whether benign or malignant, obviously calls for surgery. If the lesion is unilateral, partial or total extirpation of the involved gland should not be undertaken unless it is certain that a normal adrenal is present on the opposite side. If the tumor is encapsulated, its removal before metastases have occurred may be followed by loss of masculine traits and reappearance of female sex characters. In the presence of diffuse bilateral hyperplasia, some observers recommend resection of one or both adrenals. This procedure is of only temporary value, for recurrences are common.

Though a high incidence of mortality was reported by earlier observers following adrenal surgery, the death rate has recently been materially reduced, thanks to improvements in surgical technique, and the realization that many of the earlier fatalities were due to acute adrenal insufficiency. To guard against this accident, the patient should receive adequate amounts of life-sustaining cortical hormone as well as salt, before and after operation. In addition, the postoperative diet should be high in salt and low in potassium content.

X-ray Therapy.—Deep x-ray radiation of the hypophyseal region is advocated by some with the view of suppressing its corticotropic hormone production, thus preventing compensatory hypertrophy of retained cortical tissue. X-ray radiation of both the hypophyseal and adrenal regions has also been recommended, but most conservative observers consider such therapy of little value.

CHRONIC ADRENAL INSUFFICIENCY (ADDISON'S DISEASE)

Definition.—Addison's disease is a progressive and fatal malady due to atrophy or destruction of the adrenal cortex. It is comparatively rare and affects men more often than women. Its incidence is highest between the twenty-fifth and forty-fifth year.

CLINICAL CHARACTERISTICS

The disease is characterized by profound asthenia, pigmentation of the skin and mucous membranes, hypotension, gastro-intestinal symptoms, and loss of weight.

Skin Changes.—The peculiar *pigmentation* of the skin and mucous membranes is the most conspicuous sign, and may either precede or follow its other manifestations. It may vary in intensity from time to time, and between one individual and another. In some cases, the skin assumes a light tan shade, while others show dark brown bronzing, approaching that of the Negro. The pigmentation is confined as a rule to portions of the body exposed to light or pressure of clothing. The sites of predilection are the face, neck, upper chest, forearm, back of the hands, and the skin surrounding the nipples and genitalia. The mucous membrane, particularly that of the lips, gums, hard palate, tongue, inside of the cheek and vagina, is also involved.

Asthenia.—Profound asthenia, involving both voluntary and involuntary muscle, is probably the most constant manifestation. In the advanced stages of the disease, the asthenia may be so profound as to totally incapacitate the sufferer. The slightest movement and even speech is an effort. Adynamia of the heart muscle is evident in the weak cardiac action and small, feeble, easily compressible pulse. Occasionally this may lead to a fatal syncope.

Blood Pressure.—Hypotension is a frequent finding. Whether it is the result of the decreased blood volume, myocardial asthenia, or associated electrolytic disturbance, is not certain.

Gastro-intestinal Symptoms.—A troublesome gastro-intestinal symptomatology almost always accompanies Addison's disease. Anorexia, nausea, vomiting, diarrhea alternating with constipation, dyspepsia, gaseous distention, and hiccoughs contribute to the inanition, wasting, and dehydration of the Addisonian patient. During a crisis, the vomiting may become incessant and uncontrollable. Attacks of intense abdominal pain, simulating that of a surgical abdomen, are not uncommon.

Nervous and Psychic Disorders.—Nervous and psychic disorders are late manifestations. Headaches, drowsiness, vertigo, hyperirritability, insomnia, mental apathy, epigastric and lumbar pain, rheumatoid pains in the extremities, and disturbances of vision, hearing, and speech have been recorded.

During a crisis, or in the terminal stages of the disease, these symptoms are greatly accentuated. The acute mental confusion, chronic convulsions, and coma frequently seen under such conditions, are not unlike those of insulin poisoning, and have been attributed by some observers to the associated hypoglycemia.

Genital Alterations.—Disturbances of sexual and reproductive function are common, particularly in the advanced stages. Progressive atrophy of the genital organs is accompanied by gradual loss of libido and impotence in the male, and by prolonged periods of amenorrhea and sterility in the female.

Temperature.—The temperature may be normal or low, but a rise may occur during a crisis, or in the terminal stages. The hyperpyrexia sometimes encountered may be due to an associated generalized tuberculosis, or to the same factor, as yet unindentified, which causes the temperature to rise in the partially adrenalectomized experimental animal.

Basal Metabolic Rate.—The basal metabolic rate is usually within normal limits, but at times is low or, in the presence of fever, elevated.

Blood.—The blood exhibits no striking alterations except during a crisis, when there is hemo-concentration with a decrease in the plasma volume, a material reduction of serum sodium, chloride and bicarbonate concentration, and a rise in the serum potassium. The excretion of sodium and chloride increases while that of potassium falls. The blood sugar as a rule is low, and the non-protein nitrogen, urea and creatine values are elevated. Elimination of phenolsulphonphthalein is reduced and urea clearance decreased.

ETIOLOGY AND PATHOLOGY

Addison's disease is generally conceded to be due to *chronic adrenal cortical insufficiency* resulting from atrophy or lesions which gradually destroy both suprarenal glands. *Bilateral caseous or fibrocaseous tuberculosis,* usually secondary to pulmonary involvement, is by far the most frequent lesion. The next most common cause is simple atrophy. Syphilis, amyloid disease, destructive neoplasms, hemorrhages or infarction are occasional causes. In 566 cases reviewed by Guttman,[1] bilateral suprarenal tuberculosis was found in 68.3 per cent, primary atrophy in 19.4 per cent, amyloid disease in 1.7 per cent, and neoplasms in 1.2 per cent. The remaining 9.4 per cent were due to fatty degeneration, pressure atrophy, venous thrombosis, arterial emboli, and syphilis.

DIAGNOSIS

In the typical case, the characteristic pigmentation of the skin and particularly of the mucous membranes, together with the profound asthenia, loss of weight, and hypotension, suffice to establish the diagnosis. In the absence of pigmentation, recognition of the malady may be exceedingly difficult.

Diagnostic Procedures.—In the atypical case, *Harrop's salt-deprivation test*[2] may be an aid in the diagnosis. A salt-poor diet is instituted for five to six days. The test is positive if it precipitates a crisis and brings about alterations in the blood chemistry like those seen in the adrenalectomized animal. This procedure may prove harmful and the crisis thus precipitated may end in death.[3, 4] A more rapid technique, requiring fifty-two hours, has been developed by Cutler and his associates.[5] It is based on the observation[6] that the administration of potassium to the Addisonian patient may provoke an increased excretion of sodium and chloride and precipitate a crisis. A low sodium chloride and high potassium diet is instituted and the amount of sodium and chloride in the urine is then measured. The test is positive if the urinary chloride output on the morning of the third day exceeds 225 mg. per cent. This procedure is also fraught with danger and, if used, the patient should be hospitalized and kept under constant observation. An adequate supply of potent adrenal cortical extract and sterile salt solution for intravenous use should be kept close at hand and administered immediately when a crisis threatens.

Robinson and his associates[7] have recently devised two closely related procedures which may help in the diagnosis of Addison's disease without endangering the life of the patient. One is based on the fact that normal, prompt diuresis does not follow the ingestion of large amounts of water in the Addisonian patient. On the day preceding the test the patient eats his usual three meals but omits extra salt; after 6 P.M. he neither eats nor drinks. At 10:30 he voids and discards the urine. All urine voided between 10:30 P.M. and 7.30 A.M. is collected, measured, and saved. At 8:30 A.M. the patient voids again if possible and discards the urine. In the course of the next 45 minutes, he receives water (9 cc. per pound of body weight). He is then asked to void at 9:30, 10:30, and 11:30 A.M. and at 12.30 P.M. Each of the specimens is measured. Addison's disease is excluded if the volume of urine voided during the night is less than the volume of the largest single hourly specimen voided between 8:30 A.M. and 12:30 P.M. If it is more, then the patient may or may not have Addison's disease. In the latter event, the second procedure is carried out. This involves analysis of the concentration of urea and chloride in the urine voided during the night and in specimens of blood drawn under oil at 11:30 A.M. or 12:30 P.M. From the values obtained a ratio is calculated as follows:

$$A = \frac{\text{Urea in urine (mg./100 cc.)}}{\text{Urea in plasma (mg./100 cc.)}} \times \frac{\text{Chloride in plasma (mg./100 cc.)}}{\text{Chloride in urine (mg./100 cc.)}} \times \frac{\text{Volume of day urine (cc.)}}{\text{Volume of night urine (cc.)}}$$

On the basis of their studies of ninety patients including forty with Addison's disease, they concluded that Addison's disease may be suspected when A equals twenty-five or less.

The observation that patients with Addison's disease tend to excrete subnormal amounts of neutral 17-ketosteroids (see Chap. XL) suggests that quantitative determination of these substances in the urine may serve as a useful adjunct in the diagnosis.

Diagnosis through Therapy.—The response to specific therapy is preferred by some observers as a clue to the diagnosis. Gordon and his associates[8] consider a rise in blood pressure and favorable symptomatic response following cortical hormone therapy as evidence that Addison's disease is present. A more reliable method is that of Thorn and associates[9] who determine the presence of Addison's disease by the effect of cortin on the sodium, potassium, chloride, inorganic phosphorus, and total nitrogen balance as determined by chemical analysis of the urine.

The roentgen rays may sometimes prove of diagnostic value, particularly where there is calcification of the adrenals. Rowntree and Boll[10] found positive signs of adrenal calcification in 31.5 per cent of their cases, especially those due to adrenal tuberculosis.

COURSE AND PROGNOSIS

The disease, particularly when due to tuberculosis, has an insidious onset and runs a slow chronic course. It is characterized by periodic exacerbations and remissions. The patient constantly loses ground, until a crisis finally proves fatal. During a remission, the strength increases, but sooner or later another crisis depresses the patient's health even more than before. Many remissions and crises may occur before the terminal fatal stage is reached.

The *duration* of the disease varies considerably, depending to a large extent on the nature of the underlying cause. In Guttman's 566 cases, the average duration was thirteen months in those due to tuberculosis, and thirty-four months where adrenal atrophy was the cause. Instances have been reported in which its course extended over nearly two decades. In the absence of pigmentation, it is generally conceded to run a more rapid course.

The *outlook* in a particular instance depends on the degree of adrenal cortical insufficiency, availability of potent cortical extracts, and the presence of complications capable of precipitating a crisis. In cases due to syphilis, antiluetic treatment may improve the outlook, but in those with active generalized tuberculosis, the prognosis is distinctly unfavorable. Marked bronzing is usually considered a favorable sign. Rowntree and Boll[10] stress progressive wasting as an important prognostic sign suggesting a grave outlook. Other unfavorable signs are extreme loss of weight, a systolic blood pressure of less than 70 mm. Hg, a concentration of urea exceeding 60 mg. per 100 cc. of blood and a poor response to treatment. It must be emphasized that, even under the most favorable conditions, a crisis with sudden death is ever a possibility.

38

TREATMENT

The aim is to substitute for the deficient cortical hormone, correct any disturbance in the electrolytic balance, combat acute crises, guard the compensated case against all unfavorable influences which may precipitate a crisis, and, where possible, correct or eradicate the underlying cause. Recent evidence that the symptoms of Addison's disease are in large part due to a disturbance of the electrolytic balance which can be corrected by sodium chloride therapy, and the availability of natural and synthetic cortical hormone, has greatly facilitated the management of chronic adrenal insufficiency, particularly during a crisis.

General Care of the Addisonian Patient.—General medical care is of the utmost importance, for even minor unfavorable influences may throw a compensated case into an acute or even fatal crisis. To guard against this danger, physical and mental stress should be radically curtailed and periods of complete rest in bed prescribed. Care should be taken to avoid exposure to sudden changes in temperature, or to infection, which is the greatest danger to the Addisonian patient.

Affected individuals are very *poor surgical risks*. Even minor surgery has been known to precipitate a crisis or cause sudden death. Should surgery become urgent, large doses of sodium chloride and potent cortical extracts should be administered before and after operation. For this purpose, 40 cc. of potent cortical hormone is given daily for 2 days preceding operation, 20 cc. immediately after, and 10 cc. twice daily, plus sodium chloride intravenously for several days after operation. Local rather than general anesthesia should be used, for the latter is poorly tolerated. Drugs should be avoided where possible, or used with caution.

An easily digestible salt-rich and potassium-poor *diet*, given preferably in small but frequent meals may prevent some of the troublesome gastrointestinal manifestations and help maintain a normal electrolytic balance. Ample quantities of fluid are desirable, if well tolerated. Vitamins C and B_2 have been recommended to enhance the efficacy of the cortical hormone. For relief of constipation, small enemas, mineral oil, or mild laxatives are indicated. Purgatives should be avoided, because of the danger of dehydration which may precipitate a crisis.

Organotherapy.—*Adrenal Cortical Extracts.*—The potent cortical hormones (*eschatin, cortin, interrenin*) are at best merely substitutive therapy, since they obviously cannot stimulate cortical function. The brilliant results obtained with these extracts in the adrenalectomized animal have unfortunately not been duplicated in the Addisonian patient. This is possibly due to the fact that animals subjected to adrenalectomy are otherwise essentially normal, while patients suffering with Addison's disease are often afflicted with grave systemic disease. The varied results reported with the commercial extracts may be at least partly due to differences in potency.

Cortical extracts have proved efficacious as a prophylactic measure and are often life-saving during a crisis. Such therapy is always indicated when the Addisonian patient becomes ill, or is in urgent need of a surgical operation. The dosage obviously depends on the extent of the cortical deficiency. This can be gauged by estimating the serum sodium and chloride, or determining the level of these electrolytic ions in the urine. During a crisis, huge doses ranging from fifty to several hundred cubic centimeters (1 cc. of cortin equals 40 grams of fresh adrenal cortical substance) may be required to combat the menacing manifestations and restore the normal electrolytic balance. After the acute symptoms subside, smaller doses may suffice. The maintenance dose varies from 2 to 10 cc. once or twice weekly. In the chronic case, 2 to 5 cc. parenterally, or glycerinized cortical substance taken orally, may be used. The oral dose is at least three times the hypodermic one.

Desoxycorticosterone.—Desoxycorticosterone, a crystalline compound prepared from adrenal cortical tissue or by synthesis from stigmasterol (see Chap. XLI), has been found effective in restoring the electrolyte balance, hydration and blood pressure in the Addisonian patient. It does not constitute complete replacement therapy, however, for it has no effect on the disturbance in carbohydrate metabolism associated with adrenal cortical insufficiency. To prevent or control hypoglycemia, large doses of whole adrenal cortical extract, or the ingestion of carbohydrate at frequent intervals is recommended. It is to be hoped that other adrenal cortical compounds, namely corticosterone, dehydrocorticosterone, and 17-hydroxy-11-dehydrocorticosterone, which are apparently capable of correcting the disordered carbohydrate metabolism of the adrenalectomized experimental animal,[11] will eventually become available for clinical use in a potent and inexpensive form.

Desoxycorticosterone acetate or propionate may be administered by the subcutaneous or intravenous route. Ferrebee and associates[12] have reported favorable results with 25 mg. daily for four days followed by 10 mg. for the next five days. During this time, the patient is kept on a constant food, fluid and mineral intake. After the ninth day, he is permitted to eat as he likes and is kept on a maintenance dose of 5 mg. daily. According to Thorn,[13] desoxycorticosterone acetate may be administered by *intramuscular injection*, by the *sublingual route* in propylene glycol, or by *subcutaneous implantation* in pellet form. The relative efficacy of the implantation, intramuscular and oral routes is 1:3:5. Thorn estimates the number of pellets to be implanted by determining what quantity, given daily by intramuscular injection, is required for maintenance purposes in the particular individual. In his experience, "one pellet of 125 mg. is required for each 0.5 mg. of hormone in oil necessary for maintenance on the same regimen." Though such pellets may remain effective for twelve to fifteen months and thus insure a constant supply of hormone without the necessity of repeated injections, the implantation method is open to the objection that the supply of hormone cannot be controlled in the event that symptoms of overdosage should appear. This eventuality may be avoided to a certain extent by carefully estimating the amount of pellets to be implanted, but variations in the rate of absorption of the hormone between different individuals and at different times in the same individual may result in overdosage despite this precaution. To meet such a situation, Thorn recommends withdrawal of supplementary sodium chloride therapy, a diet low in sodium chloride, and the administration of potassium citrate solution (10 per cent solution in fruit juices).

Since 1939, when desoxycorticosterone was first made available for clinical use, a number of observers have described *ill effects resulting from overtreatment*. These include edema associated with headache, hypertension, and dyspnea with signs of pulmonary edema (particularly in patients with pre-existing myocardial damage and vascular disease). Abnormal lowering of the blood potassium associated with muscular weakness and paralysis, neuromuscular pains referable to the joints, and hypoglycemia have also been reported. To avoid such untoward effects, it is necessary to regulate the dose carefully and follow the blood pressure and body weight. McGavack[14] suggests that electrolyte therapy be stopped when the blood and urine sodium values approach normal, and that vitamin B be made a standard part of the therapeutic regimen. He also uses cardiac mensuration as an index of treatment, a cardiac-thoracic ratio of 0.32 signifying a crisis. The low potassium diet which has been found to enhance the good effect of sodium chloride therapy in patients receiving adrenal cortical extract, is now recognized to be dangerous in the patient on desoxycorticosterone therapy.

Corticotropic Hormone Therapy.—The anterior pituitary corticotropic principle, used for stimulative purposes, could hardly be expected to be of any value in Addison's disease, where the adrenal cortical insufficiency is due to some inherent defect which renders the gland incapable of responding to stimulation. This hormone would seem to be indicated only in cases of adrenal cortical insufficiency secondary to pituitary hypofunction. To distinguish between the primary and secondary forms, the response to corticotropic hormone therapy might prove of some value.

Sodium Chloride Therapy.—The sodium salts have proved effective in restoring the sodium loss and combating the accompanying dehydration.[15] During a crisis, the intravenous administration of physiologic and hypertonic saline solution combined with glucose is often a life-saving measure. One thousand cubic centimeters of a warm sterile solution, containing 10 grams of sodium citrate and 50 grams of glucose, to which may be added 20 to 50 cc. of active cortical extract, is given intravenously and repeated several times a day. During remissions, 20 to 30 grams of sodium chloride, alone or with sodium bicarbonate, in an enteric-coated capsule or taken with foods, will usually suffice to maintain the normal electrolytic balance of the blood. The compensated case can be carried along with comfort by sodium chloride therapy (about 10 grams daily in addition to that in the diet) either alone or with small doses of cortical extract (2 to 5 cc. daily).

Treatment of the Underlying Cause.—Addison's disease of syphilitic origin may benefit from antiluetic therapy. Caution should be exercised in resorting to antiluetic drugs, for they may precipitate a crisis unless the patient is fortified by cortical extract and sodium chloride. Tuberculosis and other systemic diseases should be treated by the accepted methods.

HORMONE SECRETING TUMORS OF THE OVARY

Ovarian neoplasms possessing endocrine function include the so-called granulosa and theca cell tumors, which exert a feminizing action on the host, and the luteoma and arrhenoblastoma, whose effect is masculinizing.

GRANULOSA CELL TUMOR

This ovarian neoplasm was first described by Rokitansky[1] in 1855. Von Kahlden[2] designated it "graafian follicle adenoma," but Von Werdt[3] later applied the term *granulosa cell tumor*, since generally adopted. The term *granulosa cell carcinoma* is used to distinguish the malignant from the benign form, a distinction based on the clinical course rather than on any appreciable histological differences.

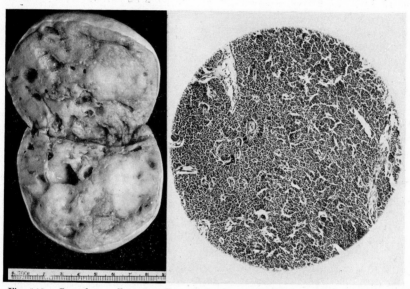

Fig. 148.—Granulosa cell tumor. Gross and microscopic appearance of ovarian neoplasm removed from postmenopausal woman aged fifty, with irregular uterine bleeding, endometrial hyperplasia, and high estrogen titers in the urine.

Granulosa cell tumors are relatively uncommon, and are estimated to comprise from 2 to 10 per cent of all solid ovarian neoplasms. While they may occur at any age, their incidence is highest between the fortieth and fiftieth year.

The size, shape and consistency of these tumors show wide variations. They may appear as tiny nodules, hardly detectable by the naked eye, or be twice the size of an adult's head. In one recorded instance, the neoplasm weighed 34 pounds.[4] Over 90 per cent are unilateral. The tumor may be solid, cystic or both. The solid portions have a granular consistency.

Classification and Histology.—Marked variations in the histology of these neoplasms make classification very difficult. R. Meyer,[5] in 1915, distinguished *four main types:* folliculoid, cylindroid, diffuse, and sarcomatoid. Of these, the *folliculoid* is the most common and best differentiated form. It is characterized by follicle-like or acinar arrangements of granulosa cells, which may be small (micro-folliculoid) and resemble the primordial follicle, or large (macro-folliculoid), suggesting the mature graafian follicle. Theca cells may be present in small numbers or be entirely absent. Cyst formation is common. In the *diffuse* form, the granulosa cells show little or no tendency to follow a folliculoid pattern, but are arranged in large diffuse fields. The *cylindroid* form is characterized by dense columns or strands of granulosa cells, separated by bands of fibrous connective tissue. Cyst formation is rarely encountered and the tumor as a rule presents a solid adenoma-like appearance. In the fourth and least differentiated form, which is described as *sarcomatoid* because it resembles sarcoma, the cells are arranged in trabeculae formation.

Since 1915, two additions have been made to the class of granulosa cell neoplasms. One, a rare growth originally designated *folliculoma lipidique,* was first described by Marion in 1910 and interpreted as a luteinized granulosa cell tumor by Plate.[6] It is grossly characterized by its yellow color. Histologically it resembles the diffuse type of granulosa cell tumor, except for the abundance of lipoid material which crowds the cells and gives it an appearance not unlike that of the mature corpus luteum or adrenal cortex. The second, a *tubular* form of granulosa cell tumor, is composed of single rows of cells, arranged about a central acinus as though it were a duct. The system of tubules strongly suggests Pick's[7] testicular tubular adenoma, the most differentiated form of the masculinizing arrhenoblastoma (see p. 600).

Some observers maintain that the so called theca cell tumor or thecoma should be included among the granulosa cell tumors. The merits of this contention will be discussed later (see Thecoma).

Histogenesis.—According to R. Meyer,[8] the granulosa cell tumor springs from unused granulosa cell rests or pre-granulosa cells present in the medulla near the hilum of the ovary. These so called "granulosaballen," often present in the fetus, may also be found in the young girl, mature woman, and in women past the menopause. He questions the possibility that granulosa cell tumors may also arise from cells of the mature graafian follicle, on the ground that they usually appear after the menopause, when mature follicles no longer develop. He argues, moreover, that since the granulosa cells of the follicle depend on the ovum for their continued integrity and are short lived, it is unlikely that they could be the source of neoplastic growth. Furth and Butterworth,[9] on the other hand, maintain that tumors may arise from the granulosa cells of the mature follicle. This they base on their observation that new growths, histologically and functionally comparable to granulosa cell tumors in women, can be induced in mature mice by irradiating the ovaries. These experimentally induced tumors, they believe, arise directly from the degenerating epithelium of the damaged follicles. Geist and his associates[10] have reported similar findings. Since there is no convincing proof that the neoplasms thus induced are strictly analogous to granulosa cell tumors in the human, the question must remain open.

Another view, favored by Novak[15] and others, traces these tumors, as well as the so-called thecomas, to the ovarian mesenchyme, which is assumed to be the common source of both the theca and granulosa cells. This theory would help to explain why some of the tumors encountered are composed of a mixture of both types of cell.

Clinical Characteristics.—Except for occasional instances where the tumor is large enough to elicit local pressure symptoms, the manifestations are traceable to the estrogens which they apparently secrete.

Childhood.—When such neoplasms develop during childhood, they may be associated with marked acceleration of skeletal growth, enlargement of the external genitalia and uterus, development of the breasts, premature appearance of pubic and axillary hair, typical feminine body contours, and more or less periodic uterine bleeding from an estrogen-prepared endometrium. The mental age is normal.

Maturity.—When encountered in the sexually mature woman, granulosa cell neoplasms are as a rule accompanied by excessive uterine bleeding alternating with amenorrhea. A proliferative type of mucosa and hypertrophy of the uterine musculature are associated findings. Ovulation is usually absent and sterility is the rule so long as the tumor persists. Occasionally there may be mammary enlargement and secretion. While the occurrence of excessive uterine bleeding in women bearing these estrogen producing tumors can readily be understood, it is difficult to account for occasional instances in which the growth is associated with protracted amenorrhea. Conceivably, the amount of estrogen produced by the tumor may be below that required to bring the mucosa to the threshold for bleeding, or the supply of hormone may be maintained at a level which does not permit withdrawal bleeding. On the other hand, the amenorrhea may be due to some fault inherent in the endometrium which precludes estrogen-priva bleeding.

Postmenopause.—Where the neoplasm develops after the menopause the cardinal symptom is uterine bleeding. This is usually irregular, but at times shows some semblance of cyclicity. Endometrial proliferation and myometrial hypertrophy are related findings. The secondary sex characters usually remain unaffected, but occasionally the atrophic mammae show considerable development and secretory activity.

Symptoms of Virilism.—In rare cases, hirsutism and other manifestations of virilism have been recorded in association with what was histologically diagnosed as granulosa cell tumor.[11] Such cases may possibly be explained by assuming that the neoplasm was actually a gynandroblastoma, which is a combination of granulosa cell tumor and arrhenoblastoma, or that it contained adenomatous elements of the adrenal cortex, as Traut and Butterworth[12] have suggested.

Course and Prognosis.—There is considerable controversy as to the degree of malignancy of granulosa cell tumors. Some observers contend that the neoplasm is benign in the vast majority of the cases and recur-

rences rarely follow its removal. Others point out that insufficient time
has elapsed since operation in many of the reported cases. In a follow-up
study of thirty-six cases, Novak and Brawner[13] found the clinical malignancy to be 28.1 per cent. Dockerty and McCarty,[4] on the other hand, in a
study of thirty cases, found there was no recurrence in at least twenty-five.

Removal of the tumor is as a rule followed by regression of the estrogen
induced symptomatology. In the prepuberal case, uterine bleeding ceases
and the precociously developed genitalia and secondary sex characters
regress. Barring a recurrence, puberty occurs at the usual time and the
individual's subsequent function may be entirely normal. Removal of the
neoplasm in the sexually mature woman is usually followed by a return to
normal menstrual periodicity and fertility. In the postmenopausal case,
bleeding ceases, the uterine mucosa reverts to its former atrophic state,
and evidence of mammary stimulation, if present, disappears.

Diagnosis.—In the prepuberal girl, precocious sexual development,
bleeding from a proliferative type of mucosa, and increased estrogen in
the body fluids suggests granulosa cell tumor, particularly when associated
with a palpable ovarian mass. In the postclimacteric woman, recurrent
uterine bleeding from a hyperplastic endometrium, associated with high
estrogen values in the blood and urine is significant presumptive evidence,
even when no ovarian tumor can be palpated. The diagnosis of granulosa
cell tumor in the sexually mature woman is exceedingly difficult, especially
where there is no appreciable adnexal enlargement. Since menstrual irregularities and endometrial hyperplasia may be traceable to a wide variety of conditions (see Chap. XXV), the diagnosis is possible only after
laparotomy.

Treatment.—Removal of the neoplasm is the therapy of choice. Radiation is of doubtful value, for this type of tumor is as a rule resistant
to the x-rays. In the young woman, surgery, with conservation of as much
ovarian tissue as possible, is desirable. In the menopausal and postmenopausal woman, removal of both adnexa together with the uterus, followed
by deep x-ray radiation of the pelvis, is indicated.

Repeated determinations of the estrogen content of the blood and urine
should be carried out to make sure there is no recurrence, particularly
after conservative surgery.

THECA CELL TUMOR (THECOMA)

The so-called *thecoma* was first described in 1932 by Löffler and
Priesel.[14] This ovarian neoplasm is rare, only thirty-five cases having thus
far been recorded in the world literature. The large majority of the cases
were postmenopausal women. In no instance was the neoplasm encountered before puberty, the youngest case recorded being eighteen years of
age. In all but one the growth was benign.

The thecoma is rarely bilateral, is nodular and firm in consistency and
resembles an ovarian fibroma. It varies from a few centimeters in diameter
to the size of an adult's head. The cut surface appears to be composed of
islands of yellowish white tissue. Cyst formation and small hemorrhagic
areas are not uncommon.

Histology.—Histologically, the thecoma suggests the diffuse form of granulosa cell tumor. It is made up of a considerable amount of connective tissue and islands of cellular tissue composed of polygonal or large spindle cells, with darkly staining protoplasm and oval shaped or elongated, eccentrically situated nuclei. These cells have an epithelioid appearance and contain fat globules. The adjoining interstitial tissue likewise contains double refractile fat and often hyaline plaques. According to Novak,[15] areas of what are apparently definite granulosa cells are often present.

Histogenesis.—There is considerable controversy as to whether the thecoma is a distinct pathologic entity or simply a variant of the granulosa cell tumor. Geist[16] maintains that the granulosa and theca cell neoplasms are separate entities. He argues that the ovarian parenchyma contains granulosa cell forerunners and theca cell forerunners, from which two distinct types of tumor may develop. In support of this view, he points out that the granulosa and theca cell neoplasms differ in their histological, chemical and clinical characteristics. The thecoma is a hard, fibrous, yellowish growth, whereas the granulosa cell tumor is softer, more cellular, medullary, and whiter. He insists that nowhere in the thecoma are there areas suggesting the pattern of the granulosa cell tumor. Another distinguishing point is the nature and distribution of fat. In the thecoma, the fat is a cholesterol and cholesterol ester, is limited almost entirely to the cellular elements comprising the tumor, and is found only in tiny scattered globules in the connective tissue. The fat in the granulosa cell neoplasm is usually a phospholipid and is confined mainly to the connective tissue. Clinically the tumors differ in that no thecoma has thus far been encountered in children, whereas about 8 per cent of the granulosa cell tumors develop before puberty. In addition, the thecoma is usually benign, while the granulosa cell neoplasm is sometimes malignant.

Geist's interpretation is opposed by Novak,[15] who believes that the thecoma is a subdivision of the larger group of ovarian neoplasms commonly classed as granulosa cell tumors. This observer contends that both granulosa and theca tumors have a common origin from the embryonic ovarian mesenchyme, the corresponding tumors developing most often as frankly granulosal, occasionally as theca cell neoplasms, and sometimes as intergrades or interminglings of the two. He points out that a careful examination of undoubted granulosa cell tumors will often disclose areas identical with those which Geist considers peculiar to the thecoma, and conversely that areas presenting the pattern of the granulosa cell tumor may be found in the thecoma. This view has been adopted by Greenhill and Greenblatt,[17] Dockerty[18] and others, who have also recorded examples of tumors containing neoplastic elements markedly resembling both granulosa and theca cells.

Clinical Characteristics.—The clinical manifestations of the thecoma are practically identical with those of the granulosa cell tumor. This is presumably due to the fact that both secrete estrogenic substances. In *young women*, endometrial hyperplasia and amenorrhea alternating with irregular uterine bleeding, are the cardinal features. *Postmenopausal women* often experience atypical uterine bleeding. In rare instances, the thecoma may be associated with *virilism*. Not infrequently, evidence of hormonal influence may be completely lacking. This was true in 28.3 per cent of a series studied by Traut and Marchetti,[19] and in one case reported by Danforth.[20] The latter suggests that the hormonal influence exerted by a thecoma is inversely proportional to its age and the proportion of theca cells present.

There is very little data relating to the associated hormonal findings. In cases where endometrial hyperplasia and uterine bleeding are associated findings, it seems reasonable to assume that estrogen excretion is fairly continuous and possibly above normal.

Diagnosis.—Since the symptomatology of both the granulosa and theca cell tumor is practically identical, the diagnosis must await histologic and

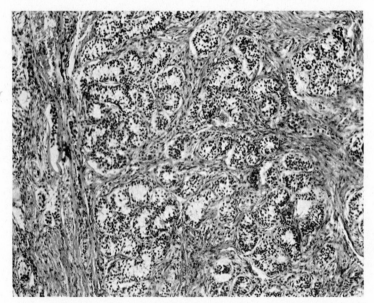

Fig. 149.—Microphotograph of arrhenoblastoma of ovary.

chemical examination of the growth. The age of the patient may serve as a clue since the thecoma usually affects older women.

Prognosis.—The thecoma is as a rule benign. Its extirpation with retention of the uninvolved normal portion of the ovary may be expected to effect a return of normal menstrual periodicity in the young woman, and cessation of bleeding in the postmenopausal individual.

ARRHENOBLASTOMA

The arrhenoblastomata are the chief masculinizing neoplasms of the ovary. R. Meyer,[21] in 1930, first called attention to this type of ovarian neoplasm and designated it arrhenoblastoma because of its masculinizing effect on the host. This type of tumor is rare. In 1941, Krock[22] could find only 70 cases. It is most frequently encountered during the second and third decades of life. The youngest recorded case was sixteen, the oldest sixty years of age.

Histology.—These interesting ovarian neoplasms show a wide variation in their histologic pattern. At one extreme are the highly differentiated tumors (*Pick's*[7] *testicular adenoma*), and at the other the undifferentiated or atypical form, whose histological structure is essentially that of sarcoma. Between these extremes there is a third form which holds an intermediate position.

The typical form of arrhenoblastoma, the so-called *adenoma tubulare testiculare* has no masculinizing effect upon the host and is not malignant. The neoplasm is usually small, firm, well encapsulated and often deeply embedded in the ovary. It is composed of perfectly formed mature seminiferous tubules, resembling those of the normal testicle, supported by a dense connective tissue, which may also harbor rete structures.

The *intermediate group* of neoplasms have only a slight masculinizing effect on the host. They are composed of interstitial cells with characteristic lipoid content and incomplete or imperfectly formed tubules or cell columns arranged in various patterns.

The undifferentiated, *atypical arrhenoblastoma* is associated with the most pronounced masculinizing effects. These neoplasms vary from minute nodules to the size of a human head. They are as a rule firm in consistency, though cystic formations may be encountered. On cut section the tumor assumes a multicentric pattern and is of a gray or yellowish hue. The growth is composed for the most part of spindle cell elements not unlike those of the undifferentiated form of granulosa cell tumor. Its arrhenoblastomatous nature is suggested by the presence of occasional cord-like arrangements of cells or imperfect tubule formation.

Histogenesis.—According to Robert Meyer,[21] these masculinizing neoplasms are derived from certain male directed cells which persist in the ovary from the early stages of gonadogenesis. He believes that the hilum of the embryonic sex gland harbors cells, the so-called "blastema," which normally give rise to the rete ovarii and some medullary cords or tubules which are homologous to the rete testis and tubuli efferentes of the male gonad. Should this bisexual anlage of the gonads persist in an undifferentiated state and later proliferate, neoplasms exerting an influence in the direction of maleness may result.

Pick,[7] in 1905, called attention to an ovarian neoplasm which he named "adenoma tubulare testiculare" because it resembled adenoma of the testis. This neoplasm, in which the testicular apparatus is perfectly developed, he believes is derived from the testicular portion of an ovariotestis. Robert Meyer,[21] on the other hand, holds that these, like the atypical masculinizing neoplasms of the ovary, have a common origin from undifferentiated germ cells not utilized during embryonic development. He questions Pick's assertion that they originate from a true ovariotestis, on the ground that women harboring such neoplasms do not exhibit signs of intersexuality from birth, as would be the case with true ovariotestis. He also points out that hermaphrodites with testicles or ovariotestes have never been known to develop tumors which alter their female characters in the direction of maleness. The fact that Pick's adenoma only rarely causes masculinization, while the atypical neoplasm as a rule does so, may be accounted for by a difference in the degree of development of the anlage and need not imply a different origin.

Clinical Characteristics.—As stated above, the degree of masculinization which the arrhenoblastoma produces in the host is inversely proportional to the maturity of the tubules. The highly differentiated neoplasms, composed of perfectly formed tubules, do not give rise to heterosexual manifestations, while the undifferentiated or atypical tumors are almost invariably associated with varying degrees of masculinization. The latter first defeminize and then masculinize the individual. The sequence of events in the classical case are as follows: menstruation ceases, the head hair falls out, the breasts atrophy, the feminine body contours are lost, and the genital organs, with the exception of the clitoris, regress. At the same time there appears such manifestations of masculinization as hirsutism of the male type and distribution, enlargement of the clitoris, and hypertrophy of the larynx with deepening of the voice. It is significant that removal of the growth is followed by partial or complete disappearance of the heterosexual manifestations.

Diagnosis.—Sexual reversion in a previously normal female, particularly when associated with a palpable ovarian mass, strongly suggests the undifferentiated or atypical type of arrhenoblastoma. Decision as to the nature of the ovarian neoplasm must await microscopic examination. (For differential diagnosis see p. 587.)

Prognosis.—If the tumor is benign, its removal may be expected to be followed by gradual retrogression of the heterosexual symptomatology, return of the feminine characteristics and re-establishment of menstruation. The hirsutism may disappear slowly, but the clitoris, if markedly hypertrophic, may remain so. In a few reported cases the tumor was malignant and terminated fatally.[23, 24]

Treatment.—Extirpation of the affected ovary usually effects a cure. If the opposite ovary is uninvolved, it should be conserved, particularly in the young woman.

GYNANDROBLASTOMA

This term describes an ovarian neoplasm composed of both granulosa cell tumor and arrhenoblastoma elements. Plate[25] believes that both types of tumor arise simultaneously from epithelium of the same degree of maturation. If this be true it explains why both can occur in the same growth. Of interest is a case cited by Geist[26] in which an ovarian neoplasm developed in a postmenopausal woman. This tumor, which R. Meyer diagnosed as an arrhenoblastoma, contained appreciable amounts of estrogenic hormone. This finding and the associated uterine bleeding led Geist to assume that the neoplasm was a combination of an arrhenoblastoma and granulosa cell tumor. The existence of such neoplasms may account for cases of masculinization associated with what appeared to be typical granulosa cell tumors. The thought suggests itself that serial sections of such neoplasms might have disclosed arrhenoblastoma elements, possibly of the undifferentiated type, which, as already noted, may closely resemble certain diffuse forms of granulosa cell tumor.

LUTEAL CELL TUMOR (LUTEOMA)

The so-called *luteoma* is a rare ovarian neoplasm, only twelve cases having thus far been recorded. The youngest case was fifteen and the oldest sixty-five years of age. The neoplasm is as a rule unilateral, of moderate size, more often solid than cystic, and of a bright canary yellow color. Grossly and microscopically the luteoma resembles the adrenal cortex or mature corpus luteum. In the majority of cases the neoplasm is benign.

Histogenesis.—The origin of these lipoid-rich ovarian neoplasms is not clear. Some observers[27] contend that the true luteoma, particularly when

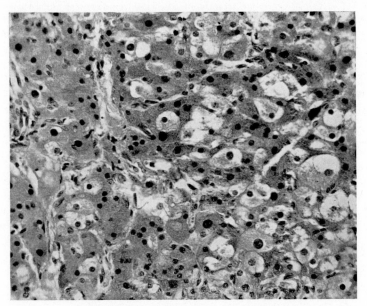

Fig. 150.—Luteoma of the ovary (× 300).

associated with masculinization, is of adrenal cortical origin and represents a metastatic nephroma. This view finds support in the observation that aberrant adrenal tissue or rests have been demonstrated in the broad ligament, along the course of the ovarian hilum and in the ovary itself; that in some cases of supposed luteoma, the clinical manifestations, particularly masculinization, are like those found with adrenal cortical neoplasms; and that the luteoma grossly and microscopically resembles adrenal cortical tissue. On the other hand, some observers maintain that the luteoma is derived from the cells which comprise the corpus luteum and is therefore a true ovarian neoplasm, that is, a "luteal cell blastoma."[28] According to Traut and Butterworth,[12] the luteoma does not arise from completed granulosa luteal cells, but comes into being through luteiniza-

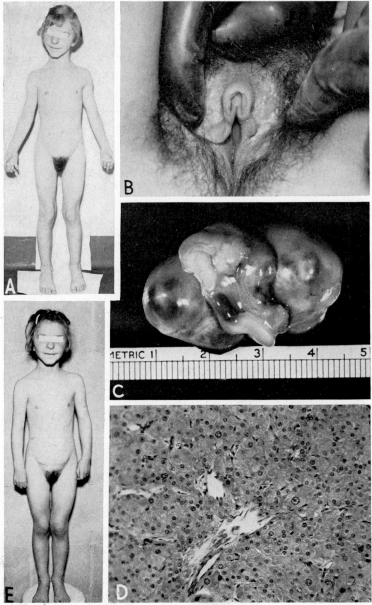

Hormone Findings:	Preoperative	Postoperative
Urine estrogen	32–44 m.u./24 hours.	Less than 13 m.u. in 24 hours.
Gonadotropins	35 m.u./24 hours.	Less than 8 m.u. in 24 hours.
Androgens	40 I.U.	20 I.U.
17-ketosteroids	9.7 mgms. equivalent of androsterone.	4.7 mgms. equivalent of androsterone.

Fig. 151.

tion of either granulosa or theca cell tumors. Novak and Brawner[13] also interpret the luteoma as a granulosa cell tumor which has been transformed by a secondary process of luteinization. As proof, they offer the observation that the luteoma is at first frequently associated with profuse uterine bleeding, probably due to hyperestrinism, and later with amenorrhea, presumably attributable to a persistent luteal effect. Its luteomatous nature is emphasized by the striking progestational effect observed in the endometrium of a forty-eight year old woman with such a tumor, encountered by Henriksen.[29] Schiller[30] also considers it unlikely that the luteoma springs from the corpus luteum. It is possible that both views are correct. Some tumors classified as luteomas may be true ovarian neoplasms, particularly those which exert an estrogenic or luteal effect upon the host. The association of masculinizing effects with some luteomas may perhaps be explained on the basis of the close chemical and biological relationship existing between progesterone and testosterone. Of interest in this connection is Greene's[31] observation that progestin, in large doses, may act as an androgen in that it will maintain the prostate in the castrate male and induce growth of the clitoris in the immature female rat.

Clinical Characteristics.—The luteoma, like the arrhenoblastoma, may both defeminize and masculinize the host. Profuse uterine bleeding, followed by amenorrhea, has been noted in some of the cases. This symptom may be explained on the basis of suppression of ovarian function by androgens produced by the neoplasm, or postponement of endometrial disintegration by reason of the presence of excessive amounts of progestin secreted by the luteoma.

Prognosis.—In the majority of the cases the luteoma is a benign neoplasm and extirpation is followed by disappearance of the masculine manifestations and reappearance of feminine traits.[32]

PRECOCIOUS PUBERTY (MACROGENITOSOMIA PRAECOX)

Definition.—The term *macrogenitosomia praecox* describes a clinicopathological symptom-complex, characterized by precocious genital and somatic development. This syndrome is attributed to a temporal disturbance in the growth and sex-promoting factors. In a review of the world literature to 1938, Bing and associates[1] could find only 565 cases of precocious sexual maturity. The malady is much more common in the female: of 440 cases collected by Reuben and Manning,[2] 338 were girls.

ETIOLOGY

Sexual Precocity of Gonadal Origin.—Precocious puberty in girls may be caused by an estrogen-secreting granulosa cell tumor of the ovary (see p. 595). Up to 1935, Bland and Goldstein[3] could find, among 250 patients bearing such neoplasms, only seven who were under ten years of

---

Fig. 151.—Heterosexual precocity in a six-year-old girl, due to an ovarian neoplasm, probably of adrenal cortical derivation. A, Note profuse growth of pubic hair, and sturdy, boyish figure. Voice deep and husky in tone. B, Clitoris several times larger than that of adult female; labia and vulva slightly hypertrophied. C and D, Gross and microscopic appearance of neoplasm. E, Same patient six months after removal of growth. Note partial loss of pubic hair. (Courtesy of Drs. D. M. Davis and A. E. Rakoff.)

age. The precocity, which is isosexual in nature, is characterized by uterine bleeding, enlargement of the breasts, uterus and accessory genitalia, growth of axillary and pubic hair, and acceleration of skeletal and somatic growth. Fat deposition, particularly in the region of the hips, thighs, buttocks and

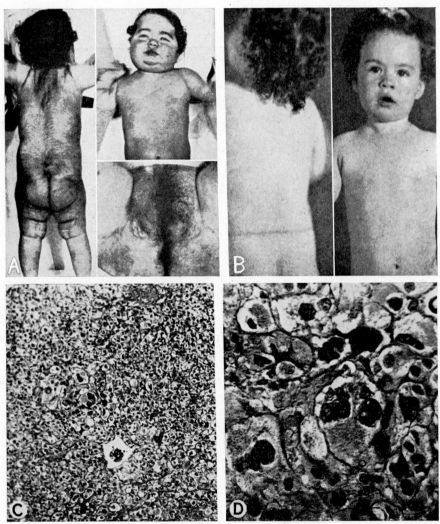

Fig. 152.—Pseudosexual precocity due to adrenal cortical tumor. A, Appearance of infant on admission to hospital at age of sixteen months. B, Appearance of child at two years of age, nine months after operation for removal of adrenal tumor. C and D, Photographs of tumor sections, magnified 100 and 460 times, respectively. (F. C. Neff, et al., in J. Clin. Endocrinol. *2:*125, 1942.)

calves, is responsible for the mature feminine body contours of such sexually precocious children. Mental and psychic precocity may or may not accompany the somatic and genital modifications.

Sexual Precocity of Adrenal Cortical Origin.—Hyperplasia, or benign or malignant neoplasms of the adrenal cortex may sometimes be associated with sexual and somatic precocity. In boys, the precocity is almost invariably isosexual, while in girls it is as a rule heterosexual. In the latter, the malady is characterized by hirsutism of the male type. The clitoris and labia are markedly hypertrophied, but the internal genitalia remain immature and menstruation is precluded. For this reason, the condition is more accurately described as "pseudoprecocity." In boys, there is hirsutism and marked enlargement of the penis. The testes as a rule remain undeveloped and without spermatogenic function. The sexual modifications may be associated with marked muscular development, or with adiposity which shows a predilection for the face and trunk, but spares the extremities (see p. 582).

Sexual Precocity of Hypophyseal Origin.—Since genital development and function is primarily dependent on the anterior hypophysis, it might be supposed that a disturbance in this gland, arising during childhood, would be a relatively frequent cause of isosexual precocity, involving stimulation of the gonads and development of secondary sex characters. In reviewing the world literature in 1922, Reuben and Manning[2] were unable to find a single instance of isosexual precocity definitely attributable to anterior hypophyseal pathology. In 1932, Cushing[4] reviewed the findings in a group of 15 cases of the syndrome now generally known by his name (see p. 573). Among these were two females who gave a history of early menarche, occurring at the age of 9 and 10 years, respectively. In only one was the presence of a basophil cell adenoma of the pituitary verified at autopsy. In a third case, where the syndrome developed at the age of six, facial, pubic and axillary hair appeared at the age of eleven, but no menstruation occurred. Menstruation was also absent in a fourth case where typical adiposity and other features of the syndrome first appeared at the age of ten. The significance of these findings and other similar cases reported since 1932,[21] is not altogether clear. It is noteworthy that in the cases with a history of early menarche, the adiposity and other characteristic manifestations of the disease did not appear until a few years later, their development coinciding with menstrual irregularity and amenorrhea. Whether the early menarche is to be interpreted as a manifestation of the basophil cell adenoma in the earlier stages of its development, or was purely coincidental, occurring before abnormal changes began to develop in the anterior hypophysis, cannot be decided from the limited evidence. Further evidence is desirable before we are justified in considering hyperactivity of the anterior hypophyseal basophils a cause of true, isosexual precocity.

Sexual Precocity of Pineal Origin.—Of the 177 cases with a pineal neoplasm, collected by Bing[1] in 1938, fifty-six were under fifteen years of age. Of these, twenty-one showed sexual precocity. Precocity associated with verified pineal neoplasms is of the isosexual type and almost invariably occurs in the male. The precocity in such cases is often associated with intracranial pressure symptoms, due to mechanical obstruction of the ventricular system, or pressure on adjacent nerve centers in the midbrain.

39

There has been considerable controversy as to whether the pineal tumor is responsible for the associated sexual precocity. According to one view the pineal body produces a maturity-inhibiting substance, which is deficient when the gland is the seat of a destructive neoplasm.[6] As a result, the maturity-promoting factors elaborated elsewhere in the organism gain the ascendancy and cause premature sex ripening. This interpretation is based on the observation that pineal involution occurs with the onset of puberty, while pinealectomy is followed by acceleration of sexual and somatic development.[7, 8] Engel's[9] experiments demonstrating the presence of a so-called "antigonadotropic" substance in pineal extract would seem to favor this view. Damaging evidence against it has been provided by more recent controlled experiments[10] demonstrating that the rate of sexual or somatic development is unaffected by pineal ablation (see Chap. XXI). Another theory attributes the sexual precocity to hyperpinealism.[11] It assumes that the pineal elaborates a sex-stimulating principle which is secreted in excessive amounts by the pineal neoplasm. This view finds support in Rowntree's[12] as yet uncorroborated report that sexual development is accelerated in rodents, whose parents have received pineal extract.

Neither the apinealism nor the hyperpinealism theory can account for the clinical observation that sexual precocity associated with pineal tumor occurs almost exclusively in boys, or explain why such neoplasms may often occur without sexual precocity.

Hypothalamic Involvement.—On the basis of recent findings, it has been suggested that the precocity associated with neoplasms of the pineal body or its environs, is due to concomitant hypothalamic involvement rather than a deficiency or excess of some pineal hormone.[13, 14] This view assumes that the hypothalamus harbors a nervous center for the regulation of sexual function which, if disturbed, may cause sexual precocity, possibily through the mediation of the hypophysis, adrenals or gonads. It is noteworthy that in all the twenty-one cases of pineal tumor associated with sexual precocity, which Bing and associates[1] collected, the neoplasm invaded other regions of the brain, particularly the diencephalon. In fifteen of the twenty-one cases, the precocity was associated with polydypsia, polyphagia, polyuria, somnolonce, obesity, and other manifestations referable to a disturbance of the vegetative nerve centers in the midbrain. These findings, coupled with the observation that anatomical disturbances in and about the diencephalon, but not involving the pineal, are often accompanied by sexual precocity (see below), suggest that the cause of the syndrome is to be sought in the hypothalamus.

Cerebral Causes of Sexual Precocity.—Precocious puberty may sometimes follow encephalitis, grippe, infectious diseases, internal hydrocephalus, astrocytoma of the third ventricle, non-neoplastic lesions in the neighborhood of the hypothalamus, and other conditions which may directly or indirectly affect the vegetative nerve centers of the midbrain. It has been suggested that the sexual precocity may be due to a disturbance of a hypothetical sex center situated in the hypothalamus, or of the hypothalamico-hypophyseal connections (see Chap. XV).

Sexual precocity has also been observed in association with, or as a sequel of chlorosis, extirpation of the spleen, chondrodystrophia, osteo-dystrophia fibrosa, and osteogenesis imperfecta. Albright[15] and others[16, 17] have described a syndrome characterized by multiple bone cysts, pig-mentation and isosexual precocity. The relationship of these alterations to the precocity is obscure.

Constitutional Precocity.—Sexual and somatic precocity without a demonstrable organic basis is usually considered of constitutional origin and attributed to some peculiarity in the chromosomal constitution. Gold-

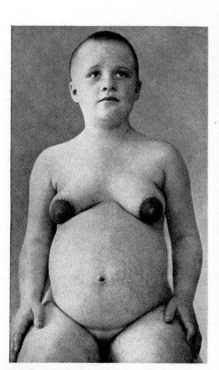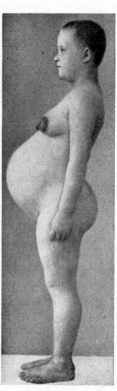

Fig. 153.—Constitutional precocity. Child six and a half years old, in the tenth month of gestation. Subsequently gave birth to a six-pound baby which died in the course of delivery. (Chaschinsky, P. Ch., and Jerschow, S. I.: Zentralbl. f. Gynäk., Vol. 57.)

schmidt suggests that the increased rate of development is due to an excess of the dominant sex gene. Precocity of constitutional origin is invariably of the isosexual type. It is a true precocity, in which conception is possible, even at the chronological age of five or six, and pregnancy may proceed normally and terminate in normal labor.[18] This type of precocity may be encountered in several members of the same family.[19]

DIAGNOSIS

Isosexual or heterosexual precocity can readily be established by physi-cal examination in the nude. It is necessary to distinguish between *pre-cocious* and *early* puberty. The dividing line between the two is necessarily arbitrary and most observers consider sexual ripening precocious when it occurs before the eighth or ninth year. The sex and age of the patient, type of precocity, associated nonsexual manifestations, and location of the lesion, if one is present, are important factors in evaluating a given case.

Isosexual precocity in the female is most likely to be due to granulosa cell tumor of the ovary, which may be suspected where there is a palpable adnexal mass, endometrial hyperplasia and an excess of estrogen in the blood and urine. Heterosexual pseudoprecocity in girls suggests primary adrenal cortical pathology or adrenal cortical hyperactivity secondary to pituitary basophilism (see p. 573).

Where isosexual precocity is encountered in the male, search should be made for testicular, pineal or adrenal cortical pathology. Testicular neoplasms are readily recognized by palpation and should be suspected where the sexual precocity is associated with undescended testes. A pineal tumor, if sufficiently large, may be recognized by roentgenograms of the skull and the presence of intracranial pressure symptoms. Adrenal cortical tumors may sometimes be demonstrated by the Cahill[20] method of perirenal insufflation. The diagnosis of constitutional precocity is necessarily one of exclusion.

PROGNOSIS AND TREATMENT

The outlook in sexual precocity due to a granulosa cell tumor is good, for extirpation of the growth, particularly if it is benign, may be followed by retrogression of the prematurely developed sex characters. Where the precocity is due to a testicular or adrenal neoplasm, the prognosis depends on whether the growth is benign or malignant. If benign, its removal will be followed, in the large majority of cases, by a return to normal. If malignant, the outlook is poor unless the growth is removed before metastases have occurred. In the presence of a pineal tumor, the prognosis is unfavorable, for such neoplasms are not readily accessible and their surgical removal is therefore attended by danger. The extent to which the midbrain is damaged by the tumor will also affect the outcome.

The *treatment* of sexual precocity due to tumors of the gonads, adrenal cortex, or pineal is surgery or x-ray irradiation. Constitutional precocity obviously does not call for any treatment.

LIPODYSTROPHIA PROGRESSIVA

Lipodystrophia progressiva describes a' syndrome characterized by extreme emaciation of the upper half and adiposity of the lower half of the body. This relatively rare disease is encountered more often in women than in men. It may develop during the first decade of life, particularly just before the onset of puberty, or after the puberal epoch, especially between the twentieth and fortieth year.

Symptomatology.—The face, neck, upper extremities, and entire thorax except the breasts, are extremely emaciated. In the classical case, the face loses nearly all its subcutaneous fat and is literally skin and bone. Marañón[1] has likened it to a death's head. The contrasting adiposity of the lower girdle, thighs, and lower extremities gives the body an extraordinary, grotesque appearance. As aptly described by Weber,[2] the lower portion of the body suggests that of a Venus in an ultra-Rubens style, while the upper part has the semblance of a witch.

The peculiar body configuration may be the only manifestation of the disease, or it may be accompanied by polyuria, oliguria, glycosuria, hyperhydrosis, acrocyanosis, and other symptoms of midbrain involvement. Psychic disturbances are sometimes encountered. Disorders of menstruation have been reported in many of the cases. The basal metabolic rate may be normal, elevated, or low. Roentgenograms of the skull as a rule reveal no abnormal change.

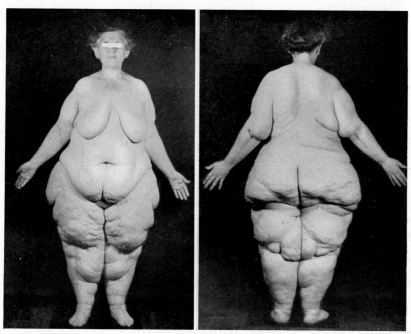

Fig. 154.—Marked lower body obesity. Multipara aged fifty, height 58 inches, weight 300 pounds. Note marked contrast between upper and lower half of body.

Etiology.—The cause of lipodystrophia progressiva is still unknown. It has been attributed, at one time or another, to acute infectious disease, trauma, and tuberculosis. Heredity may play a part, for the disease not infrequently affects several members of the same family. Van Leeuwen[3] encountered it in three out of seven sisters, while Barraquer-Ferré[4] observed it in a grandmother, mother and daughter. The thyroid, pituitary, pineal, and ovary have all been suspected as possible etiologic factors, but the negative autopsy findings and absence of clinical signs of endocrine disturbance would seem to absolve the incretory glands of any responsibility. A central nervous origin is suggested by the peculiar fat distribution, segmental emaciation and presence of symptoms of diencephalic involvement. Many observers[5-8] attribute the malady to a trophoneurotic disturbance, with its primary seat in the diencephalon. Others believe it is a purely local disturbance, like that in lipotrophia circumscripta, where there is retention of lipomatous tissue despite a general emaciation.

Diagnosis.—In the advanced case, the segmental emaciation and adiposity are so characteristic that the diagnosis can readily be made by mere inspection of the patient in the nude.

Prognosis.—The disease runs a chronic course and many years may elapse before it is fully developed. The loss of subcutaneous fat begins in the face and gradually travels downward. The adiposity of the lower part of the body becomes apparent during the later stages of the disease. These alterations are compatible with good health. From the cosmetic standpoint, the prognosis is very poor, for the grotesque body configuration, once established, persists and is not amenable to treatment.

Treatment.—To correct the marked facial emaciation, Hollander[9] has resorted to injections of a mixture of human and mutton fat. This form of treatment, like others that have been tried, is unsatisfactory.

DERCUM'S DISEASE (ADIPOSIS DOLOROSA)

Dercum's[1] disease is a syndrome characterized by painful adiposity, asthenia, and psychic disturbances. The malady is comparatively rare and affects approximately five times as many women as men. It is most often encountered between the forty-fifth and sixtieth year.

Symptomatology.—The *adiposity* is not unlike that of Fröhlich's syndrome. It is sometimes diffuse but more often assumes a symmetrical, nodular formation. The back of the neck, shoulders and arms, particularly the deltoid region, the trunk, abdomen, hips, thighs, and medial aspects of the knees are usually involved. The face and hands are only rarely affected. The fat nodules are of a rather firm consistency and vary in size. They may be symmetrically or irregularly distributed, are separated by deep furrows, and may be covered with a tense, red, and shiny skin. Paresthesia, formication and undue sensitivity of the affected areas to cold, have been reported in some cases. Because of the peculiar condition of the skin, minor injury or vigorous massage may readily provoke bleb formation or ecchymosis.

A striking feature of the disease is the *painful nature of the fat deposits.* The patient may complain of sensations varying from slight tenderness to spontaneous attacks of exquisite pain.

Asthenia and muscular weakness are prominent symptoms. The asthenia varies from mere fatigue on exertion to marked prostration, which may simulate the adynamia of Addison's disease. In can readily be understood how, in severe cases, the painful adiposity and marked asthenia may be incapacitating.

Where the disease develops during the reproductive period, amenorrhea, sterility, and frigidity are associated findings. *Nervous instability,* melancholia, hysteria, impairment of memory, mental confusion, and actual dementia have been encountered.

Etiology.—The etiology is obscure. Dercum[1] originally attributed the syndrome to atrophy or some perversion of thyroid function. Attempts to corroborate his view have thus far been unconvincing. The pituitary has likewise been considered as a possible factor. Though anatomic alterations in this gland have been demonstrated at autopsy in some of the cases, these have been too varied to warrant any conclusion as to its role in the etiology. Winkelman and Eckel,[2] who reviewed 200 cases collected from the world literature, suggested a pluriglandular origin. Marañón[3]

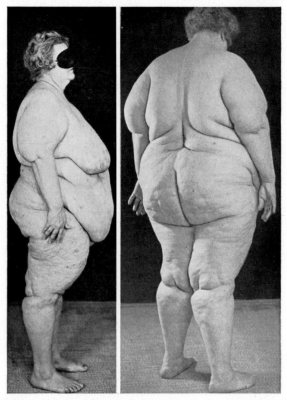

Fig. 155.—Adiposis dolorosa (Dercum's Disease). Patient aged forty-two; weight 327 pounds, after gain of 120 pounds in two years. Amenorrhea, asthenia, nervous and psychic manifestations, and tender fat deposits.

attributed the disease to ovarian insufficiency. He maintained that the adiposity differs in no way from other forms of obesity, while the pain is the result of a temperamental factor. Many observers favor a neuropathic origin, but differ as to whether the abnormality is central,[4] peripheral,[5] or both. Trizzino[6] believes both nervous and endocrine factors are involved in the etiology. Boller[7] recently collected a total of twenty cases in which autopsy findings were recorded. Abnormal changes were observed in the thyroid in sixteen, and in the anterior pituitary in ten cases. The adrenals were altered in five, while ovarian atrophy or sclerosis was noted in eight cases. Neuritis was mentioned in six instances. Boller suggests that the disease is a "polyneuritis" on the basis of his observation that injection of novocaine into the fat deposits relieves the pain.

Diagnosis.—The diagnosis can be readily made from the painful nature of the fat deposits, and the associated asthenia and psychic disturbances.

Course and Prognosis.—The onset of the disease is insidious and it may run a chronic course extending over several decades. The life expectancy is good, but cures are seldom effected by any known form of therapy. In the severe case, the asthenia may be so marked as to incapacitate the individual, and occasionally may even lead to death.

Treatment.—Because of the obscure etiology, the therapy is necessarily empirical. The aim of the treatment is to effect an appreciable reduction in weight (see Chap. XXXIII), allay the pain, and combat the asthenia and psychoneurotic manifestations. The salicylates (gr. xx t.i.d.) or other coal tar derivatives may aid in alleviating the pain. Where the pain is very severe, use of morphine is unavoidable, but should be employed with due caution and no longer than absolutely necessary. In some cases, excision of the most tender fat nodules has been carried out. Several investigators[7] have reported relief with procaine or novocaine injections, using a 2.5 per cent solution in increasing doses beginning with 10 to 60 cc. daily. The troublesome psychoneurotic manifestations may be ameliorated by the use of the bromides (gr. xx t.i.d.) or phenobarbital (gr. ½ to ¾ t.i.d.).

There is no proof that organotherapy in any form has been of any value, either for controlling the adiposity or relieving the pain. Thyroid, pituitary, and ovarian sex hormones have all been tried on the assumption that a deficiency of these hormones is an etiologic factor. On the whole, the treatment of the disease has thus far proved very discouraging.

BIBLIOGRAPHY

Hypophyseal Infantilism

1. Priesel, A.: Beitr. z. path. Anat. u. z. allg. Path. *117*:220, 1919.
2. Shaefer, R. L., and Strickroot, F. L.: Endocrinol. *26*:599, 1940.
3. Greene, J. A., and Johnson, J. A.: J. Clin. Endocrinol. *1*:327, 1941.
4. Shelton, E. K.: Endocrinol. *30*:1000, 1942.
5. Shelton, E. K.: California & West. Med. *45*:20, 1936.
6. Waldorp, C. P., Reforzo Membrives, J., and Luchetti, S. E.: Semana méd. *2*:1277, 1936.
7. Evans, H. M.: J.A.M.A. *117*:287, 1941.
8. Zondek, B.: Am. J. Obst. & Gynec. *33*:979, 1937.
9. Richards, R. K., and Kueter, K.: Endocrinol. *29*:990, 1941.
10. McCullagh, E. P., and McGurl, F. J.: Endocrinol. *26*:377, 1940.
11. Gaarenstroom, J. H., and Levie, L. H.: J. Endocrinol. *1*:420, 1939.
12. Webster, B., and Hoskins, W. H.: Proc. Soc. Exper. Biol. & Med. *45*:72, 1940.
13. Goldzieher, M. A.: J. Clin. Endocrinol. *1*:924, 1941.
14. McCullagh, E. P., and Rossmiller, H. R.: J. Clin. Endocrinol. *1*:507, 1941.
15. Rubinstein, H. S., and Solomon, M. L.: Proc. Soc. Exper. Biol. & Med. *44*:442, 1940.
16. Lurie, L. A., and Hertzman, J.: J. Clin. Endocrinol. *1*:717, 1941.
17. Howard, J. E.: Bull. New York Acad. Med. *17*:519, 1941.
18. Dorff, G. B.: Endocrinol. *27*:403, 1940; Arch. Pediat. *59*:791, 1942.
19. Dorff, G. B.: J. Clin. Endocrinol. *1*:940, 1941.
20. Albright, F., Smith, P. H., and Fraser, R. W.: Am. J. Med. Sc. *204*:628, 1942.

Hypophyseal Giantism

1. Langer, K.: Denkschr. d. Acad. Wissensch., Math. Naturw. Kl. *31*:50, Wien, 1872.
2. Sternberg, M.: Die Acromegalie, Spez. Path. u. Therap., Nothnagel, 7, Wien, 1897. Translated by F. R. B. Atkinson, London, New Sydenham Soc., 1899.
3. Brissaud, E., and Meige, H.: Rev. Scient. Paris, *45*:3, 1895.
4. Evans, H. M., and Long, J. A.: Anat. Rec. *21*:26, 1921.
5. Von Drigalski, W.: Klin. Wchnschr. *16*:628, 1937.
6. Currier, F. P., Frantz, C. H., and Van der Meer, R.: J.A.M.A. *117*:515, 1941.
7. Goldzieher, M. A.: J. Clin. Endocrinol. *1*:924, 1941.
8. Hurxthal, L. M.: J. Clin. Endocrinol. *3*:12, 1943.

Acromegaly

1. Marie, P.: Rev. de Méd. *6*:297, 1886.
2. Atkinson, F. R. B.: Endokrinol. *20*:245, 1938.
3. Courville, C. B., and Mason, V. R.: Arch. Int. Med. *61*:704, 1938.
4. Kloppner, K.: Geburtsh. u. Frauenh. *1*:709, 1939.
5. Coggeshall, C., and Root, H. F.: Endocrinol. *26*:1, 1940.
6. Davis, A. C.: J. Clin. Endocrinol. *1*:445, 1941.
7. Minkowski, O.: Klin. Wchnschr. *24*:371, 1887.
8. Benda, C.: Arch. f. Anat. u. Physiol. Abst. 1900, p. 373.
9. Bailey, P., and Cushing, H.: Am. J. Path. *4*:545, 1928.
10. Putnam, T. J., Benedict, E. B., and Teel, H. M.: Arch. Surg. *18*:1708, 1929.
11. Evans, H. M., and Long, J. A.: Anat. Rec. *21*:62, 1921. Reichert, F. L., Simpson, M. E., Cornish, R. E., and Evans, H. M.: Mem. Univ. California. *11*:409, 1933.
12. Putnam, T. J., and Wilcox, H. B.: Am. J. Path. *9*:649, 1933.
13. Kraus, E. J.: Handb. d. spez. path. Anat. *8*:818, Berlin, Springer, 1926.
14. Schultze, F., and Fischer, B.: Mitt. a. d. Grenzgeb. d. Med. u. Chir. *24*:607, 1911-1912.
15. Cushing, H., and Davidoff, L. M.: Arch. Int. Med. *39*:673, 751, 1927.
16. Young, F. G.: Brit. Med. J. *2*:897, 1941.
17. Lammli, K. A.: Deutsche med. Wchnschr. *63*:1568, 1937.
18. Hart, F. D., and Greene, R.: Proc. Roy. Soc. Med. *35*:17, 1941.
19. Ulrich, H.: Arch. Int. Med. *43*:785, 1929.
20. Weinstein, A.: Ann. Int. Med. *13*:715, 1939.
21. Goldberg, M. B., and Lisser, H.: J. Clin. Endocrinol. *2*:477, 1942.
22. Davidoff, L. M.: Bull. New York Acad. Med. *16*:227, 1940.
23. Vaughan, W. W.: Am. J. Roentgen. *40*:660, 1938.
24. Schrire, I., and Sharpey-Schafer, E. P.: Clin. Sc. *3*:413, 1938.
25. Aub, J. C., and Karnofsky, D.: New England J. Med. *226*:759, 1942.
26. Spark, C., and Biller, S. B.: Arch. Path. *35*:93, 1943.

Dystrophia Adiposogenitalis (Fröhlich's Syndrome)

1. Babinski, J.: Rev. Neurol. *8*:531, 1900.
2. Bartel, M.: Munch. med. Wchnschr. *55*:201, 1908.
3. Fröhlich, A.: Wien. klin. Rundschau *15*:883, 1901.
4. Raybaud, A.: Les syndromes hypophysaires et infundibulotuberiens, Paris, G. Doin et Cie, 1933.
5. Marburg, O.: Deut. Ztschr. f. Nervenh. *36*:14, 1908.
6. Erdheim, J.: Beitr. z. path. Anat. u. z. allg. Path. *112*:302, 1916.
7. Leschke, E.: Deutsche med. Wchnschr. *96*:959, 1920.
8. Camus, L., and Roussy, G.: Compt. rend. Soc. de biol. *115*:483, 1913.
9. Fulton, J. F., and Bailey, P.: J. Nerv. & Ment. Dis. *119*:164, 1929.
10. Biedl, A.: Deutsche med. Wchnschr. *98*:1630, 1922.
11. Hetherington, A. W., and Ranson, S. W.: Anat. Rec. *78*:149, 1941.
12. Heinbecker, P., and White, H. L.: Proc. Soc. Exper. Biol. & Med. *49*:324, 1942.
13. Mittelmann, B.: Endocrinol. *23*:637, 1938.

14. Bauer, J.: Med. Rec. *151*:89, 1940.
15. Bruch, H.: J. Pediat. *19* (Supp.) :365, 1941.
16. Aub, J. C., and Karnofsky, D.: New England J. Med. *226*:759, 1942.
17. Werner, S. C.: J. Clin. Endocrinol. *1*:134, 1941.
18. Pratt, J. P.: J. Clin. Endocrinol. *2*:460, 1942.
19. Roussy, G., Bollack, J., and Pages, R.: Rev. Neurol. *1*:491, 1932.
20. Bronstein, I. P., Halpern, L. J., and Brown, A. W.: J. Pediat. *21*:485, 1942.

Simmonds' Disease (Hypophyseal Cachexia)

1. Simmonds, M.: Deutsche med. Wchnschr. *40*:322, 1914.
2. Von Bergmann, G.: Deutsche med. Wchnschr. *60*:123, 159, 1934.
3. Sheldon, J. H.: Lancet *1*:369, 1937; Proc. Roy. Soc. Med. *32*:738, 1939.
4. Escamilla, R. F., and Lisser, H.: J. Clin. Endocrinol. *2*:65, 1942.
5. May, E., and Robert, P.: Ann. de méd. *38*:317, 1935.
6. Silver, S.: Arch. Int. Med. *51*:175, 1933.
7. Sheehan, H. L.: Quart. J. Med. *8*:277, 1939.
8. Effkemann, G., and Müller-Jager, F.: Arch. f. Gynäk. *168*:867, 1939.
9. Smith, P. E.: Am. J. Anat. *45*:205, 1930.
10. Lang, F. J.: Wien. klin. Wchnschr. *37*:977, 1924.
11. Gunther, L., and Courville, C. B.: J. Nerv. & Ment. Dis. *82*:40, 1935.
12. Urechia, C. I., and Elekes, N.: l'Encéphale *21*:352, 1925.
13. Roussy, G., and Mosinger, M.: Ann. de méd. *33*:193, 1933.
14. Nicolle, G.: Proc. Roy. Soc. Med. *32*:153, 1939.
15. Falta, W.: Die Erkrankungen der Blutdrüsen, Berlin, Springer, 1913.
16. Means, J. H., Hertz, S., and Lerman, J.: Tr. A. Am. Phys. *55*:32, 1940.
17. Callow, N. H., Callow, R. K., and Emmens, C. W.: J. Endocrinol. *2*:88, 1940.
18. Fraser, R., and Smith, P. H.: Quart. J. Med. *10*:297, 1941.
19. Reiche, F.: Med. Klin. Berlin *14*:690, 1918.
20. Regester, R. P., and Cuttle, T. D.: Endocrinol. *21*:558, 1937.
21. Smith, P. E.: Am. J. Physiol. *81*:20, 1927.
22. Kylin, E.: Deutsche Arch. f. klin. Med., *180*:115, 1937.
23. Von Bergmann, G.: München. med. Wchnschr. *82*:5, 1935.
24. Escamilla, R. F., and Lisser, H.: California & West. Med. *48*:343, 1938.
25. Hemphill, R. E., and Reiss, M.: J. Mental Sc. *88*:559, 1942.
26. Prout, T. P., and Thomson, C. S.: J. M. Soc. New Jersey *39*:376, 1942.
27. Williams, R. H., and Whittenberger, J. L.: J. Clin. Endocrinol. *2*:539, 1942.
28. Rochat, R. L.: Helvet. med. Acta *9*:243, 1942.

Cushing's Syndrome (Pituitary Basophilism)

1. Cushing, H.: Bull. Johns Hopkins Hosp. *50*:137, 1932.
2. Eisenhardt, L., and Thompson, K. W.: Yale J. Biol. & Med. *11*:507, 1939.
3. Jonáš, V., Časop. lék. česk. *74*:1313, 1349, 1372, 1413, 1439, 1462, 1935.
4. Raab, W.: Wien. Arch. f. inn. Med. *7*:443, 1924.
5. Jores, A.: Klin. Wchnschr. *14*:1348, 1935; Klinische Endokrinologie, Berlin, Springer, 1939.
6. Jacobi, J., and Tigges, F.: Münch. med. Wchnschr. *86*:1665, 1939.
7. Freyberg, R. H., Barker, P. S., Newburgh, L. H., and Coller, F. A.: Arch. Int. Med. *58*:186, 1936.
8. Ulrich, H. L.: Minnesota Med. *19*:535, 1936.
9. Ecker, A. D.: Endocrinol. *23*:609, 1938.
10. Silver, S.: Bull. New York Acad. Med. *16*:368, 1940.
11. Crooke, A. C.: J. Path. & Bact. *41*:339, 1935.
12. Rasmussen, A. T.: Endocrinol. *20*:673, 1936.
13. Severinghaus, A. E., and Thompson, K. W.: Proc. Soc. Exper. Biol. & Med. *40*:627, 1939.
14. Bauer, J.: Klin. Wchnschr. *14*:361, 1935; Schweiz. med. Wchnschr. *66*:938, 1936.
15. Haymaker, W., and Anderson, E.: Internat. Clin. *4*:244, 1938.
16. Cushing, H.: Proc. Soc. Exper. Biol. & Med. *30*:1424, 1933.

17. Kylin, E.: Deutsche Arch. f. klin. Med. *176*:301, 1934.
18. Scarf, M., and Israel, S. L.: Endocrinol. *20*:180, 1936.
19. Thompson, K. W., and Cushing, H.: Proc. Roy. Soc. Lond., s.B. *115*:88, 1934.
20. Gerard-Lefebre, M.: Bull. Soc. pédiat. de Paris *37*:326, 1939.
21. Goecke, H.: Wien. med. Wchnschr. *31*:571, 1940.
22. MacCallum, W. G., Futcher, T. B., Duff, G. L., and Ellsworth, R.: Bull. Johns Hopkins Hosp. *56*:350, 1935.
23. Bergstrand, H.: Virchows. Arch. f. path. Anat. *293*:413, 1934.
24. Geist, S. H., and Gaines, J. A.: Am. J. Obst. & Gynec. *44*:975, 1942.
25. Crooke, A. C., and Callow, R. K.: Quart. J. Med. *8*:233, 1939.
26. Broster, L. R.: Brit. Med. J. *1*:425, 1940.
27. Paschkis, K. E., Rakoff, A. E., and Cantarow, A.: Endocrinol. *30*:523, 1942.
28. Davidoff, L. M.: Bull. New York Acad. Med. *6*:227, 1940.
29. Rakoff, A. E., Cantarow, A., and Paschkis, K. E.: J. Clin. Endocrinol. *1*:912, 1941.
30. Gill, A. M.: Lancet *1*:72, 1937.
31. Albright, P., Parson, W., and Bloomberg, E.: J. Clin. Endocrinol. *1*:375, 1941.
32. Bennhold, H.: Verhandl. d. deut. Gesellsch. f. inn. Med. Kong. 52, 1940, p. 448.

THE ADRENOGENITAL SYNDROME

1. Levy-Simpson, S., and Joll, C. A.: Endocrinol. *22*:595, 1938.
2. Krabbe, K. H.: New York Med. J. *114*:4, 1921.
3. Grollman, A.: The Adrenals, Williams, Wilkins Co., Baltimore, 1936.
4. Broster, L. R., and Vines, H. W. C.: The Adrenal Cortex, London, H. K. Lewis, 1933.
5. Fujiwara, T. F.: Arch. Path. *27*:1030, 1939.
6. Howard, J. E., and Whitehall, M. R.: Internat. Clin. *4*:50, 1937.
7. Cahill, G. F.: J. Urol. *34*:238, 1935.
8. Mintz, N., and Geist, S. H.: J. Clin. Endocrinol. *1*:316, 1941.
9. Broster, L. R.: Brit. Med. J. *1*:117, 1941.
10. Broster, L. R., and Vines, H. W. C.: Brit. Med. J. *1*:662, 1939.
11. Marrian, G. F., and Butler, G. C.: J. Biol. Chem. *119*:565, 1937; ibid. *124*:237, 1938.
12. Wolfe, J. K., Fieser, L. F., and Friedgood, H. B.: J. Am. Chem. Soc. *63*:582, 1941.
13. Hamblen, E. C., Cuyler, W. K., and Baptist, M.: J Clin. Endocrinol. *1*:763, 1941.
14. Reichstein, T.: Helvet. chim. Acta *19*:223, 1936.
15. Lawrence, R. D.: Brit. Med. J. *1*:12, 1943.
16. Dorfman, R. I., Wilson, H. M., and Peters, J. P.: Endocrinol. *27*:1, 1940.
17. Salmon, U. J., Geist, S. H., Salmon, A. A.: Proc. Soc. Exper. Biol. & Med. *47*:279, 1941.
18. Frank, R. T.: Proc. Soc. Exper. Biol. & Med. *31*:1204, 1934.
19. Silver, S.: Bull. New York Acad. Med. *16*:638, 1940.
20. McGavack, T. H.: Endocrinol. *26*:396, 1940.
21. Kanter, A. E., and Klawans, A. H.: Am. J. Cancer *40*:474, 1940.

CHRONIC ADRENAL CORTICAL INSUFFICIENCY (ADDISON'S DISEASE)

1. Guttman, P. H.: Arch. Path. *10*:742, 895, 1930.
2. Harrop, G. A., Weinstein, A., Soffer, L. J., and Threscher, J. H.: J.A.M.A. *100*:1850, 1933.
3. Lilienfeld, A.: J.A.M.A. *110*:804, 1938.
4. Garvin, C. F., and Reichle, H. S.: Ann. Int. Med. *14*:323, 1940.
5. Cutler, H. H., Power, M. H., and Wilder, R. M.: J.A.M.A. *113*:117, 1938; Proc. Staff Meet. Mayo Clin. *13*:244, 1938.
6. Wilder, R. M., Kendall, E. C., Snell, A. M., Kepler, E. J., Rynearson, E. H., and Adams, M.: Arch. Int. Med. *59*:367, 1937.
7. Robinson, F. J., Power, M. H., and Kepler, E. J.: Proc. Staff Meet. Mayo Clin. *16*:577, 1941.
8. Gordon, E. S., Sevringhaus, E. L., and Stark, M. E.: Endocrinol. *22*:45, 1938.
9. Thorn, G. W., Garbutt, H. R., Hitchcock, F. A., and Hartman, F. A.: Endocrinol. *21*:202, 1937.

10. Rowntree, L. G., and Boll, R. G.: Endocrinol. *17*:263, 1933.
11. Thorn, G. W., Engel, L. L., and Lewis, R. A.: Science *94*:348, 1941.
12. Ferrebee, J. W., Ragan, C., Atchley, D. W., and Loeb, R. F.: J.A.M.A. *113*:1725, 1939.
13. Thorn, G. W., Engel, L. L., and Eisenberg, H.: J. Exper. Med. *68*:161, 1938; Bull. Johns Hopkins Hosp. *64*:339, 1939.
    Thorn, G. W., Howard, R. P., Emerson, K. Jr., and Firor, W. M.: Bull. Johns Hopkins Hosp. *64*:339, 1939.
    Thorn, G. W.: J. Mt. Sinai Hosp. *8*:1177, 1942.
14. McGavack, T. H.: J. Clin. Endocrinol. *1*:68, 1941.
15. Loeb, R. F., Atchley, D. W., and Stahl, J.: J.A.M.A. *104*:2149, 1935.

HORMONE SECRETING TUMORS OF THE OVARY

1. Rokitansky, C.: Wien. Allg. med. Zeitung *34*:35, 1859.
2. Von Kahlden, C.: Zentralb. f. allg. Path. u. path. Anat. *6*:257, 1895.
3. Von Werdt, F.: Beitr. z. path. Anat. u. allg. Path. *59*:453, 1914.
4. Dockerty, M. B., and MacCarty, W. C.: Am. J. Obst. & Gynec. *37*:425, 1939; ibid. *38*:698, 1939.
5. Meyer, R.: Ztschr. f. Geburtsh. u. Gynäk. *77*:506, 1915.
6. Plate, W. P.: Arch. f. Gynäk. *153*:318, 1933.
7. Pick, L.: Arch. f. Gynäk. *76*:191, 1905.
8. Meyer, R.: Arch. f. Gynäk. *145*:2, 1931; Am. J. Obst. & Gynec. *22*:697, 1931; Zentralbl. f. Gynäk. *56*:770, 1932.
9. Furth, J., and Butterworth, J. S.: Am. J. Cancer *28*:66, 1936.
10. Geist, S. H., Gaines, J. A., and Escher, G. C.: Endocrinol. *29*:59, 1939.
11. Bergstrand, H.: Acta obst. & gynec. Scandinav. *13*:336, 1934.
12. Traut, H. F., and Butterworth, J. S.: Am. J. Obst. & Gynec. *34*:987, 1937.
13. Novak, E., and Brawner, J. N.: Am. J. Obst. & Gynec. *28*:637, 1934.
14. Loeffler, E., and Priesel, A.: Beitr. z. path. Anat. u. z. allg. Path. *90*:199, 1932.
15. Novak, E.: Gynecological and Obstetrical Pathology, Philadelphia, W. B. Saunders Co., 1940, chap. 27.
16. Geist, S. H.: Am. J. Obst. & Gynec. *30*:480, 650, 1935.
17. Greenhill, J. P., and Greenblatt, R. B.: Am. J. Obst. & Gynec. *36*:684, 1938.
18. Dockerty, M. B.: Proc. Staff Meet. Mayo Clin. *14*:298, 1939; Am. J. Obst. & Gynec. *39*:431 1940.
19. Traut, H., and Marchetti, A. A.: Surg., Gynec., & Obst. *70*:632, 1940.
20. Danforth, W. C.: Am. J. Obst. & Gynec. *43*:526, 1942.
21. Meyer, R.: Verhandl. d. deutsch. path. Gesellsch. *25*:328, 1930; Am. J. Obst. & Gynec. *22*:697, 1931.
22. Krock, F., and Wolfermann, S. J.: Ann. Surg. *114*:78, 1941.
23. Novak, E., and Long, J. H.: J.A.M.A. *101*:1057, 1933.
24. Taylor, J. M., Wolfermann, S. J., and Krock, F.: Surg., Gynec. & Obst. *56*:1040, 1933.
25. Plate, W. P.: J. Obst. & Gynec. Brit. Emp. *45*:254, 1938.
26. Geist, S. H., and Spielman, F.: J.A.M.A. *104*:2173, 1935.
27. Geist, S. H.: Am. J. Obst. & Gynec. *30*:480, 1935.
28. Saphir, O.: Am. J. Obst. & Gynec. *37*:1008, 1939.
29. Henriksen, E., cited by E. Novak, in Gynecological and Obstetrical Pathology (*supra* 15).
30. Schiller, W.: Pathologie u. Klinik der Granulosazelltumoren, Wien, Maudrich, 1934.
31. Greene, R. R., Burrill, M. W., and Ivy, A. C.: Endocrinol. *24*:351, 1939.
32. Bingel, A.: Deutsche. med. Wchnschr. *50*:330, 1924.

PRECOCIOUS PUBERTY

1. Bing, J., Globus, J., and Simon, H.: J. Mt. Sinai Hosp. *4*:935, 1938.
2. Reuben, M. S., and Manning, G. R.: Arch. Pediat. *39*:769, 1922.
3. Bland, P. B., and Goldstein, L.: Surg., Gynec. & Obst. *61*:250, 1935.
4. Cushing, H.: Bull. J. Hopkins Hosp. *50*:137, 1932.

5. Bronstein, I. P.: J. Pediat. *14*:203, 1939.
6. Marburg, O.: Arb. a.d. neurol. Inst. a.d. Wien. Univ. *17*:217, 1909.
7. Foa, C.: Arch. ital. de biol. *57*:137, 1912.
8. Horrax, G.: Arch. Int. Med. *17*:607, 1916.
9. Engel, P.: Klin. Wchnschr. *13*:266, 1934; Wien. klin. Wchnschr. *48*:1160, 1935; Ztschr. f. d. ges. exper. Med. *95*:44, 1935.
10. Anderson, D. H., and Wolf, A.: J. Physiol. *81*:49, 1934.
11. Askanazy, M., Verhandl. d. deut. path. Gesellsch., 1906, p. 58.
12. Rowntree, L. G., Clark, J. H., Steinberg, A., and Hanson, A. M.: J.A.M.A. *106*:370, 1936; Endocrinol. *20*:348, 1936.
13. Le Marquand, H. S., and Russell, D. S.: Roy. Berkshire Hosp. Rep. 1934-35, pp. 31-61.
14. Roussy, G., and Mosinger, M.: Rev. Neurol. *1*:459, 1938.
15. Albright, F., Butler, A. M., Hampton, A. O., and Smith, P.: New England J. Med. *216*:727, 1937.
16. Summerfeldt, P., and Brown, A.: Am. J. Dis. Child. *57*:90, 1939.
17. Robson, K., and Todd, J. W.: Lancet *1*:377, 1939.
18. Chaschinsky, P. C., and Jerschow, S. I.: Zentralbl. f. Gynäk. *57*:2252, 1933.
19. Rush, H. P., Bilderback, J. B., Slocum, D., and Rogers, A.: Endocrinol. *21*:404, 1937.
20. Cahill, G. F.: J. Urol. *34*:238, 1935.
21. Farber, J. E., Gustina, F. J., and Postoloff, A. V.: Am. J. Dis. Child. *65*:595, 1943.

LIPODYSTROPHIA PROGRESSIVA

1. Marañón, G.: The Climacteric Age, trans. by K. S. Stevens, ed. by C. Culbertson, St. Louis, C. V. Mosby Co., 1929, p. 250.
2. Weber, F. P.: Proc. Roy. Soc. Med. VI Sect. Neurol. 1912–13, p. 127.
3. van Leeuwen, H. C.: Ztschr. f. klin. Med. *123*:534, 1933.
4. Barraquer-Ferré, L.: Presse méd. *43*:1672, 1935.
5. Klein, H.: München. med. Wchnschr. *1*:206, 1921.
6. Curschmann, H., and Kramer, F.: Lehrbuch d. Nervenkrankh., Berlin, J. Springer, 1925.
7. Marburg, O.: Arb. a.d. neurol. Inst. a.d. Wien. Univ. *30*:1, 1927.
8. Pollock, F.: Ztschr. f. Neurol. *127*:415, 1930.
9. Hollander, E.: München. med. Wchnschr. *57*:1794, 1910.

DERCUM'S DISEASE (ADIPOSIS DOLOROSA)

1. Dercum, F. X.: Am. J. Med. Sc. *104*:521, 1892.
2. Winkelman, N. W., and Eckel, J. L.: J.A.M.A. *85*:1935, 1925.
3. Marañón, G.: The Climacteric Age, trans. by K. S. Stevens, ed. by C. Culbertson, St. Louis, C. V. Mosby Co., 1929.
4. Waldorp, C. P.: Endocrinol. *8*:54, 1924.
5. Maddox, K.: M. J. Australia *2*:817, 1931.
6. Trizzino, E.: Sperimental, Arch. di biol. *92*:66, 1938.
7. Boller, R.: Med. Welt *13*:329, 1939.

CHAPTER XXXVI

CRYPTORCHIDISM AND MALE HYPOGONADISM

CRYPTORCHIDISM

Definition.—The term *cryptorchidism* describes a genital anomaly in which one or both testes fail to reach the scrotum and remain instead in the abdominal cavity or inguinal canal. Unilateral nondescent is much more common than the bilateral form. The location of the undescended testes varies. Among ninety-six cases observed by Thiessen and Walters,[1] nineteen were intra-abdominal, three at the internal inguinal ring, forty-two in the inguinal canal, and thirty-seven at the external inguinal ring.

Incidence.—Estimates as to the incidence of cryptorchidism vary considerably, due possibly to differences in the care taken to exclude pseudocryptorchidism. Another factor which may account for the widely differing estimates is the fact that a large number of cases are corrected spontaneously at or shortly after the onset of puberty.[2, 3, 4] The number of cases with undescended testes may thus be expected to be much greater among boys under twelve than among those past this age. In this connection, Smith[2] found undescended testes in nine out of 267 boys under fourteen as compared with four out of 705 males over fourteen. On the basis of observations among recruits in the first[5] and second World War,[6] true cryptorchidism would appear to be relatively rare.

Etiology.—The cause of cryptorchidism may be mechanical or hormonal. Among the mechanical causes may be mentioned an oversized testicle, anomalies of the mesorchium, gubernaculum, or cremaster, a narrow processus vaginalis, short spermatic cord, and rudimentary or obliterated scrotum. Premature obliteration of the inguinal canal, hernia, fat masses constricting the external ring, and fibrosis between the testes and groin may also interfere with testicular descent. Barring these mechanical obstructions, failure of descent may be due to endocrine deficiency, particularly of the anterior hypophysis on which testicular development and function primarily depend.

Cryptorchidism and Sexual Development.—Cryptorchidism is compatible with normal development of the genitalia and secondary sex characters. This is due to the fact that, though the germinal tissue of the undescended testis in the adult may show evidence of degeneration,[7, 8] the interstitial cells, which are the source of the male sex hormone, apparently remain unaffected.[9] Degeneration of the seminiferous tissue in cryptorchidism is generally attributed to the fact that the temperature in the ectopic position is relatively higher than that prevailing in the scrotum. The scrotal sac is believed to function as a thermoregulator, producing a localized environment a few degrees cooler than that of the abdomen.[10] That

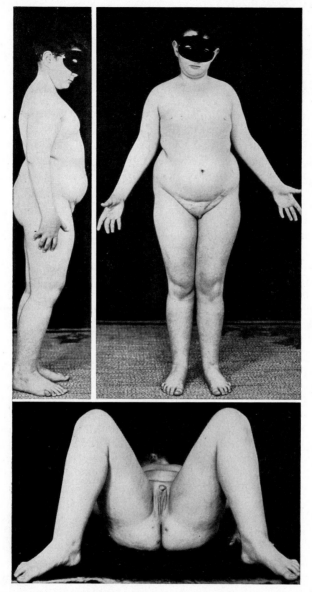

Fig. 156.—Adiposity of Fröhlich's type with marked genital hypoplasia. Boy aged ten, weight 100 pounds. Following tonsillectomy at three and one-half years, gradual gain of weight, headache, fatigability and polyuria. Note feminine body contours, tiny penis resembling enlarged clitoris, and scrotum suggesting labia. Testes hypoplastic and undescended; operative intervention unsuccessful.

this is essential for normal sperm production is suggested by the observation that normally developed rabbit testes, transplanted from the scrotum to the abdomen, undergo degenerative changes similar to those in cryptorchidism, despite the fact that the vascular pedicle and nerves are kept intact. On the other hand, they function normally when transplanted to the ear, where the temperature approaches that of the scrotum.[11]

Diagnosis.—It is of the utmost importance to exclude *pseudocryptorchidism,* in which descent has occurred but the testes are of the migratory type, moving up and down spontaneously or on manipulation. A diagnosis of true cryptorchidism is justified only when it is impossible, on repeated examination, to displace the testis into the scrotum in any position of the body. To encourage descent of a migratory testis, pressure over the external inguinal ring, and local application of heat to relax the muscles concerned in spastic retraction of the testis, may be tried.[6, 12] Hyperextension, and the application of suction to stretch the scrotum and gubernaculum are also recommended.[12]

Various criteria have been recommended for the purpose of distinguishing between cases requiring surgery and those which may be expected to descend spontaneously or in response to organotherapy.[1] Smith[2] believes that surgery should be undertaken only in cases where nondescent is associated with hernia; all others should be given a chance to descend spontaneously at puberty. According to Browne,[13] spontaneous descent will eventually occur in all cases in which the testis can be pushed down over the pubic bone. Where this is not possible, descent is not likely to occur either spontaneously or as the result of hormone therapy, and surgery is indicated. Schonfeld[12] recommends a therapeutic test with gonadotropic hormone to determine whether nondescent is due to some mechanical obstruction correctable only by surgery, or to hormonal deficiency.

Treatment.—The management of cryptorchidism depends on the underlying cause and the age of the patient. Where nondescent is due to mechanical obstruction, surgery is indicated. Some recommend a preoperative course of gonadotropin therapy, which facilitates operation by increasing the size of the testis and the length of the cord. Where no obstruction is demonstrable, opinions differ as to whether gonadotropic hormone therapy should be instituted to accelerate descent, or a policy of watchful waiting should be adopted. Most conservative investigators prefer to wait until puberty because of the large percentage of spontaneous cures which occur at this time.[2, 3, 4]

Organotherapy.—Among those who favor the use of organotherapy, particularly *chorionic gonadotropin,*[14, 15] there is as yet no accord as to the dosage, duration of treatment, or age at which organotherapy should be instituted. Some begin treatment as early as the fourth year, while others wait until the tenth year or later.[27] The *dose* varies from 100 to 500 I.U. two to three times weekly for several months, with intervening periods of rest to avoid anti-hormone formation. Cures have been reported in from 20 to 80 per cent of the cases. Critics of the endocrine treatment of cryptorchidism attribute the cures to self-correction. As proof, they point out that the best results have been observed in boys under 15, while older males have generally proved unresponsive. Some observers[16, 17] warn against gonadotropin therapy on the ground that it may injure the testicular structures or disturb the delicate endocrine balance. The danger of causing the premature appearance of secondary sex characters is another disadvantage of such treatment. The merit of these opposing views must await further evidence as to whether the testes are more likely to suffer from a prolonged stay in their ectopic position, or from premature stimulation by exogenous gonadotropins, while thus abnormally situated. According to Wangensteen,[18] testes which are undescended during prepuberty but later descend spontaneously or are brought down by surgery, may be capable of spermatogenic function. In the opinion of Rieser,[17] glandular therapy has no harmful effect on the normally situated testis but may produce definite degenerative changes in the retained testis. This was also the experience of Eisenstaedt and his associates.[16]

To secure the benefits of chorionic gonadotropin therapy without its disadvantages, Lapin and Klein[27] recommend the following procedure: Treatment is withheld until the fourteenth year, when a maximum dosage of 6000 I.U. is given in small, frequent doses over a six-week period. If it proves ineffective, operation is performed immediately to avoid the degenerative changes which may occur if the artificially stimulated testes remain in their ectopic position.

Testosterone propionate by injection, or *methyl testosterone* by mouth have also been employed for cryptorchidism.[19, 20] Aside from the fact that their ability to accelerate descent is questionable,[18] their protracted use may damage the testicular structures and would therefore appear to be injudicious. The possibility that they may cause premature development of secondary sex characters should also be borne in mind.

General Medical Measures.—The spectacular results claimed for the various endocrine preparations have obscured the value of general medical measures. In the author's experience, hygienic and dietary measures, and thyroid extract where indicated, have proved efficacious in the treatment of non-obstructive cryptorchidism, particularly when associated with adiposity of the Fröhlich's type. In the undernourished cryptorchid patient, a diet rich in carbohydrate, fat, and essential vitamins, is often a valuable adjunct.

MALE HYPOGONADISM

Eunuchism (Agonadism).—A eunuch may be defined as a male devoid of testicular function. Some observers limit the term to castrates and hold that where rudimentary testes are present, the condition is more properly described as *eunuchoidism.*

Clinical Manifestations.—The clinical manifestations vary according to whether loss of the gonads precedes or follows puberty. Castration during the juvenile period precludes subsequent development and function of the accessory genitalia and secondary sex characters. The penis remains infantile, the scrotal sac is ill developed, and the prostate and seminal vesicles remain rudimentary. Libido sexualis and potentia are markedly diminished or absent. The male secondary sex characters do not appear at the normal age. There is no beard formation, and the axillary and pubic hair may be very sparse or show the female type of distribution. The laryngeal cartilages do not chondrify at puberty and the voice remains high

40

pitched. The sexual retardation is associated with profound somatic modifications. The prepuberal eunuch is either excessively tall and slender, or obese. In the latter, there is an excessive accumulation of fat about the lateral aspects of the eyelids, on the mammae, lower abdomen, mons, buttocks, and trochanteric regions.

The postpuberal eunuch differs but little in appearance from the normal adult male, since full somatic and genital development have already been attained. The accessory genitalia as a rule are but little affected, though

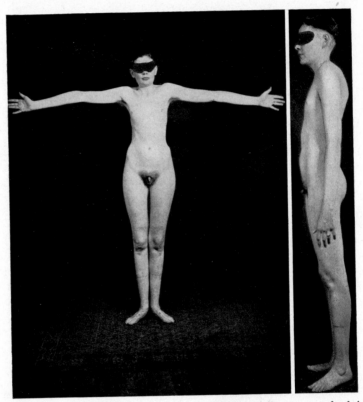

Fig. 157.—Male eunuchoidism. Patient aged thirty, weight 138 pounds, height 73½ inches. Lower measurement exceeds the upper, and the span is greater than the height. Note absence of facial and body hair, and scant pubic hair. Penis tiny (1 inch long); testes hypoplastic but descended; low androgen values in the urine.

there may be some retrogression. Castration in the mature male does not necessarily abolish libido and potentia, though breeding capacity is obviously destroyed. There is usually a slow but progressive accumulation of fat about the mammae, abdomen, mons and trochanteric regions.

Eunuchoidism.—The eunuchoid male may present the same features as the juvenile castrate, the only difference being that some degree of testicular function may be present.

Etiology.—Primary eunuchoidism may be due to a congenital anomaly of the testes, or a deficiency of the gonadotropic hormones of the anterior hypophysis arising during the prepuberal period. Secondary or acquired eunuchoidism may result from trauma, radiation, destructive neoplasms, or inflammatory lesions of the testes during childhood. Nutritional faults, vitamin deficiency, severe systemic disease, or other debilitating states which depress the hypophysis and with it the gonads, account for some of the cases.

Clinical Manifestations.—The *somatic and sexual manifestations* vary with the degree of testicular insufficiency, and the state of sexual maturity attained at the time the deficiency arises. In the severest form of eunuchoidism, the patient may closely resemble the juvenile castrate. The testicles and accessory genitalia are markedly hypoplastic, the secondary sex characters fail to appear, and the individual retains his childhood characters on reaching adult life. The eunuchoid patient is usually tall due to the fact that the epiphyseal lines remain open beyond the normal age for closure. Because of his excessively long extremities, the span of the eunuchoid male is greater than his height and the lower measurement (symphysis to feet) exceeds the upper one (symphysis to top of head). The fingers and toes are markedly elongated and pointed, the wrists and ankles narrow and long. The pelvis is either infantile or of the female type.

The *features* and *body contours* are reminiscent of childhood. The face is elongated, narrow and angular, with prominent cheek bones and a receding chin. The skin is smooth, thin and sallow, the eyes small and deeply sunken, and the nose thin and small. The eyebrows are sparse and there is no mustache or beard formation. In the obese case, the face is rounded and double-chinned, and fat deposits are characteristically present about the lateral aspect of the upper eyelids. The chest is often rounded, hairless, and presents large fat deposits about the mammae.

The eunuchoid individual retains his *infantile accessory genitalia* on reaching adulthood. The penis is very small and, in the obese individual, may be obscured by fat deposits. The scrotal sac is markedly underdeveloped, and cryptorchidism is common. The prostate and seminal vesicles are rudimentary. Libido sexualis and potentia are either absent or markedly diminished. Occasionally, there may be feeble erections and sterile ejaculations. The male secondary sex characters fail to appear at the usual age for the onset of puberty. The axillary and pubic hair is very scant and of a distinct feminine distribution. The laryngeal cartilages do not chondrify, and the voice retains its boyish quality.

In the *mild case*, the penis and other accessory genital organs may attain an appreciable size, and the testes may be normal in size and fully descended into the scrotum. The secondary sex characters appear at puberty, but are less pronounced than in the normal male. Azoospermia, oligospermia, and some depression of libido sexualis and potentia are frequent findings.

Between the severest and mildest forms, there are many gradations.

Treatment of Eunuchism.—In the prepuberal eunuch, the object is to develop the accessory genitalia and secondary sex characters. Since such individuals are devoid of gonadal tissue, testicular transplants, preferably from primate donors, would constitute the ideal form of therapy. Unfortunately, even under the most favorable conditions, transplants do not take or are resorbed within a short time, and are therefore of little value. The availability of potent androgens has made substitution therapy possible. These may be administered by mouth,[21, 22] inunction, or by intramuscular injection.[23] Since treatment must be continued throughout reproductive life, the subcutaneous implantation of *crystalline testosterone* appears ideal therapy since it assures a continuous release of hormone over a fairly long period. This method of administration has thus far been em-

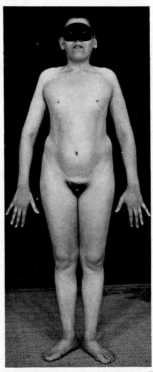

Fig. 158.—Male eunuchoidism. Patient aged thirty-two. Tiny genitalia, absence of facial and body hair, and feminine body contours. High pitched voice and feminine demeanor. No response to gonadotropic extracts. Anterior pituitary implants likewise of no avail.

ployed in only a limited number of cases[24, 25] and a decision as to its practicability is not yet justified. The availability of orally active androgens would seem to make implantation unnecessary.

In the adult castrate, where the genital organs and secondary sex characters have already attained full maturity, substitution with the male sex hormone may prevent regressive changes and maintain the sexual powers.

Dosage.—The dosage and duration of treatment depends upon what is to be accomplished. In the adult eunuch small maintenance doses usually

feld[12] has recently emphasized, normal boys show a great variation in the age at which development of the genitalia and secondary sex characters begins, and the rate at which it proceeds. Since development may begin spontaneously at any age from ten to sixteen and occasionally even later, any improvement observed during this period may not be credited with certainty to organotherapy concurrently employed.

If a trial of gonadotropin therapy indicates that it is unlikely to evoke a response, and the normal age for the attainment of sexual maturity passes without any evidence of improvement, *androgen therapy* is justified to insure at least an outward semblance of maleness. In view of the possible inhibitory effect of the androgens on the testis,[21] this form of treatment should be used only after all attempts to stimulate testicular function have failed.

In the adult eunuchoid male, the *gonadotropins* are worth a trial. Should no improvement follow their use, it may be assumed that the testicular tissue is incapable of responding to these substances. The only recourse left is substitution therapy with the *androgens,* which may effect an appreciable growth of the penis and cause some development of the male sex characters. The dose is approximately the same as that recommended for the prepuberal eunuch. Unfortunately, the effects produced by this means are transient and regression sets in soon after such therapy is stopped. It is therefore necessary to continue the treatment indefinitely. Increasing refractoriness may necessitate the use of larger doses.[26]

It should be emphasized that *general medical measures,* calculated to eradicate or correct associated depressive states, are an important adjunct in the treatment, particularly in the prepuberal case, where there is still some chance of favorably influencing the maturation processes by improving the general condition of the patient. This may sometimes be accomplished by proper hygiene, ample sunlight, a well balanced, vitamin-rich diet, and small doses of thyroid extract, where indicated.

BIBLIOGRAPHY

Thiessen, N. W., and Walters, W.: Proc. Staff Meet. Mayo Clinic *10*:132, 1935.
Smith, R. E.: Lancet *1*:747, 1941.
Johnson, W. W.: J.A.M.A. *113*:25, 1939.
Drake, C. B.: J.A.M.A. *118*:479, 1942.
MacKenzie, cited by Hinman, F., and Benteen, F. H.: J. Urol. *35*:378, 1936.
Hamilton, J. B., and Hubert, G.: Internat. Clin., n.s. *2*:16, 1941.
ce, N. M.: Proc. Staff Meet. Mayo Clinic *10*:726, 1935.
isman, A. I.: Human Fertility *6*:45, 1941.
C. E.: Arch. Surg. *38*:1054, 1939; ibid. *44*:27, 1942.
e, C. R., and Quick, W. J.: Am. J. Physiol. *68*:70, 1924.
, C. R.: Endocrinol. *8*:493, 1924.
ld, W. A.: J.A.M.A. *121*:177, 1943.
D.: Brit. Med. J. *2*:168, 1938.
, W. O., and Heckel, N. J.: J.A.M.A. *117*:1953, 1941.
. H., and Rowntree, L. G.: J. Clin. Endocrinol. *1*:649, 1941.
J. S., Appel, M., and Fraenkel, M.: J.A.M.A. *115*:200, 1940.
outh. Surgeon *11*:90, 1942.
O. H.: Ann. Surg. *102*:875, 1935.

19. Jaffe, I., and Brockway, G.: J. Clin. Endocrinol. *2:*189, 1942.
20. Gordon, M. B., and Fields, E. M.: J. Clin. Endocrinol. *2:*531, 1942.
21. McCullagh, E. P., and Rossmiller, H. R.: J. Clin. Endocrinol. *1:*496, 1941.
22. Kearns, W. M.: J. Clin. Endocrinol. *1:*126, 1941.
23. Tager, B. N., and Shelton, E. K.: J. Clin. Endocrinol. *1:*131, 1941.
24. Biskind, G. R., Escamilla, R. F., and Lisser, H.: J. Clin. Endocrinol. *1:*38, 1941.
25. Eidelsberg, J., and Ornstein, E. A.: J.A.M.A. *117:*1068, 1941.
26. Pratt, J. P.: J. Clin. Endocrinol. *2:*460, 1942.
27. Lapin, J. H., and Klein, W.: J. Pediat. *22:*175, 1943.

CHAPTER XXXVII

SEX DETERMINATION AND DIFFERENTIATION
OF SEX CHARACTERS

INTRODUCTION

A fascinating though complex phase of sexuality is the question of what determines maleness and femaleness. An appreciation of the various aspects of this problem is indispensable for a proper understanding and evaluation of normal and abnormal sexual phenomena, such as pseudo- and true hermaphrodism (see Chap. XXXVIII).

It is necessary to distinguish between *sex determination* and *sex differentiation*. Lillie[1] defines sex determination as the establishment in the fertilized ovum, of internal conditions leading to the development of one or the other set of sex characters in the embryo and adult. Sex differentiation, on the other hand, refers to the process of development by which originally indifferent sex character rudiments acquire the specific characteristics peculiar to one or the other sex.

Biedl[2] divides the so-called sex characters into three groups: (1) the *primary sex organs*, or gamete-producing tissues; (2) the *secondary sex organs*, which include the internal and external genitalia and breasts; and (3) the *secondary sexual characteristics*, which are those somatic characters that normally distinguish the male from the female, and are dependent for their development on the sex hormones, but apparently play no essential role in sex function. In man, the contrasting features of the mature male and female are as follows:

Female	Male
Primary Sex Organs	
Ovary (containing ova)	Testis (containing sperm)
Secondary Sex Organs	
Uterus	
Fallopian tubes	Prostate
Vagina	Vas deferens
Hymen	Epididymis
Vulva	Scrotum
Clitoris	Penis
Breasts—full and well developed	Breasts—rudimentary
Secondary Sexual Characteristics	
Hair on head, pubes and axillae; absent or scanty elsewhere, depending on race	Hair on head, axillae and genital region; also on face, trunk, arms and legs
Skin fine and delicate	Skin coarse
Larynx small, voice high pitched	Larynx large, voice deep
Thorax relatively short	Thorax relatively long
Abdominal cavity large	Abdominal cavity short
Bones relatively light and small	Bones heavy and large
Muscles relatively weak	Muscles powerful
Pelvis shallow and wide	Pelvis deep and funnel-shaped
Psychically submissive	Psychically dominant

PREVAILING THEORIES ON THE CONTROL OF SEX

The causes of maleness and femaleness have been the subject of much controversy, engaging the attention of the geneticist, biologist and endocrinologist. Despite the wealth of data relating to the sex-controlling mechanism, its nature and operation is not yet completely understood. The theories currently favored are based largely on observations in species whose sexual and somatic constitution differs considerably from that of man. Hence, their application to the latter must be made tentatively and with due reservations.

Sex in mammals and man is generally attributed to the interaction of genetic and hormonal factors. It is believed that genetic factors determine the sex of the individual, while the execution of the predetermined plan is effected through hormones or hormone-like agents. There is, how-

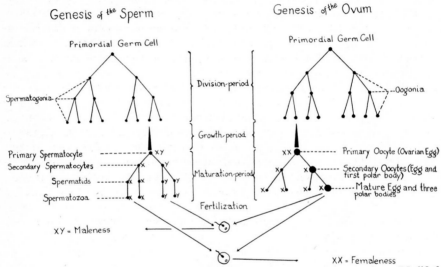

Fig. 161.—Diagram illustrating the chromosomal theory of sex determination. (Modified after Boveri and Wilson.)

ever, considerable uncertainty as to the relationship between the two types of control, the point at which the influence of each begins and ends, and the exact manner in which each exerts its effect.

Genetical Sex Determination.—The nucleus of every germ cell harbors *chromosomes*, rod-shaped structures which carry the ultramicroscopical genes, determiners of hereditary characteristics. The number of chromosomes shows species variations. In man, before maturation division begins, there are forty-eight, including twenty-three pairs of autosomes (body chromosomes) and one pair of sex chromosomes. While the autosomes of the male and female germ cells are structurally identical, the sex chromosomes differ. In the female, the two members of the pair are alike and are designated XX; but in the male, they are dissimilar and are accordingly named XY. The number of chromosomes is halved through reduction division in the process by which the male and female germ cells become ripe for fertilization (see Fig. 161). As a result, the female germ cell is transformed into an ovum containing twenty-three autosomes and an X chromosome. In the male, the maturation process culminates in the formation of two types of spermatozoa, one containing twenty-three autosomes and an X chromosome, the other twenty-three autosomes and a Y chromosome. It is generally conceded that the XX combination is associated with femaleness, the XY combination with maleness. Fertilization results in a male or female offspring depending on whether the X-containing ovum is impregnated by an X- or Y-containing sperm. Thus, at the time of fertilization, there is created in the ovum a condition which will direct the development of the embryo in the male or female direction. The creation of this bias in favor of one or the other sex is called *genetical sex determination,* the favored sex being described as the genetical sex.[3]

Potential Bisexuality of the Fertilized Ovum.—All observers agree that the fertilized ovum contains both male and female determining factors. It develops into one or the other sex because one of the two factors is normally dominant, and not because the egg embodies the genes of that sex exclusively. Evidence of this primordial or potential bisexuality is provided by the presence of homologous organs and tissues in both sexes. The early embryo, regardless of its genetical sex, possesses the rudiments of all the organs and tissues which, in their developed form, characterize the male and female respectively. The embryonic gonad consists of a cortex, forerunner of the ovary, and a medulla, forerunner of the testis. Also present in the embryo are wolffian and müllerian ducts, primordia of the male and female genitalia respectively. The primordia of the external genitalia are identical in early embryos of both sexes and are capable of differentiating in either the male or female direction.

Difference between Male-Determined and Female-Determined Zygote.—While it is generally believed that every zygote, no matter what its genetical sex, contains both male and female determiners, there is some uncertainty as to their number and location or how one type gains the ascendancy over the other. The observation that in some species sex is correlated with the presence of an XX or an XY combination of chromosomes, suggested at first that the difference between a male-determined and a female-determined ovum is quantitative. Studies in other species, however, indicate that two eggs may be of opposite sex although there is no visible chromosome difference between them, suggesting that the essential difference between the two is something not detectable by cytological investigation alone.

The Sex-Determining Genes.—In seeking to define the nature of the sex-determining genes and determine how they differ in the two sexes, several possibilities have been considered. According to Goldschmidt,[4] there is but a single pair of sex genes, which differ quantitatively in the two sexes. In the human being the female factor F is in the X chromosome, the male factor M in the autosomes. In the male, two M genes are pitted against only one F gene in the one X chromosome, but in the female the M genes compete with two F genes in the two X chromosomes. He assumes that F is quantitatively superior to M.

A qualitative difference has been postulated by Bridges[5] to explain why one ovum develops in the male, another in the female direction. This observer proposes that there are a number of sex genes which are distributed to all the chromosomes and are balanced against each other in such a way that the effect of one or the other normally predominates. Their joint action produces each character or feature of the adult.

Another explanation offered by Lebedeff[6] is that there are two factors M and F, which are equally potent, but that there is a special mechanism which decides which of these will function in the zygote. This mechanism consists of a set of suppressors which, though themselves neutral, determine the balance between the M and F factors by inhibiting the male gene.

Leaving open the question of the number of sex genes, and how one or the other type becomes dominant, it may be assumed that both male and female determining factors are invariably present and that the embryo possesses primordia of both male and female sex characters. Some of these, such as for example the wolffian and müllerian ducts, may either develop or regress, while others, notably the external genitalia, may develop in either of two directions. At a certain stage in the evolution of the individual, each sex character primordium must "choose," so to speak, between the two alternatives. While most authorities agree that the selection is genetically determined, the exact manner in which the dominant genes impress their "will" on the developing sex organs and tissues, and the identity of the agents through which they act are still uncertain. Some observers stress hormonal and, to a lesser extent, metabolic factors.

Metabolic Factors in Sex Differentiation.—A theory, sponsored by Riddle,[7] proposes that the sex genes produce maleness or femaleness through their effect on *cellular metabolism.* Differing quantitatively and qualitatively in the two sexes, they exercise their influence on developing sexuality by establishing a higher or lower rate of oxidation. A high rate results in maleness, a low one in femaleness. Thus, the primary and decisive element in normal sex determination and differentiation is an initial and sustained difference in the intensity and rate of oxidation.

Although variations in the metabolic rate, experimentally induced by temperature changes or other means, appear to play a role in sex differentiation in certain lower forms, evidence that this may influence sex differentiation in man is still fragmentary and unconvincing. Thus far, it consists mainly of observations that the basal metabolic rate is characteristically higher in the male than in the female, and then only in the average and within homogeneous racial groups. In the opinion of Witschi,[8] the role of the metabolic rate in sex differentiation has been definitely ruled out, at least so far as the higher vertebrates are concerned.

Hormonal Factors in Sex Differentiation.—It has been suggested that the particular set of genes assembled in the fertilized egg directs sex development into one channel or another by producing the appropriate type of endocrine or "inductor" (Witschi) system, which supplies the stimuli necessary for the realization of the kind of sexuality foreshadowed in the fertilized ovum.[3]

That sex differentiation in mammals is influenced to a certain extent by hormones or hormone-like substances was first suggested by the occurrence of the free martin among heterosexual cattle twins. As distinguished from its normal male co-twin, the free martin presents sterile male gonads, more or less completely male internal genitalia, and external sex characters which are mainly of the female type. Tandler and Keller,[9] and Lillie[10] first suggested that the free martin is a genetical female, whose sex has been modified in the male direction by factors operating during embryonic life. The hormonal nature of the modifiers and their origin in the male twin seemed likely in view of the fact that anastomosis of the two chorionic circulations in such pairs permits the blood streams of the two partners to mingle. This observation suggested at once that genetical determination is not irrevocable, and that the actual control of sex differentiation passes from the genes to extra-cellular agents, which are hormones in the sense that they act on tissues removed from their site of origin.

To demonstrate these inferences experimentally, three types of procedure have been carried out: (1) parabiosis of amphibian embryos; (2) grafting of adult gonads into embryos of the opposite sex, or embryo gonads into adult hosts of the opposite sex; and (3) introduction of the sex hormones of the mature ovary and testis into the water in which amphibian larvae live, and into hens' eggs, new-born animals, pregnant animals near term, or females just before coitus. In the course of these investigations, the following questions have been raised but only partially answered: Where are the substances which control embryonic sex differentiation produced? How early do they become effective? How do they produce their effect? Are they similar to or identical with the substances elaborated by the adult gonad after differentiation is complete? Do they entirely replace or merely supplement intra-cellular forces in the control of somatic sex differentiation?

Site of Origin of Embryonic Sex-Differentiating Substances.—The studies of Witschi,[8] Burns[11] and others, carried out with parabiotic amphibian embryos of opposite sex, indicate that the substances concerned in embryonic sex differentiation originate in the gonad primordium. The *cortex* apparently produces the female differentiating substance; the *medulla* the male differentiating substance, thus acting as female and male "inductors" or "organizers" respectively. Each inductor apparently acts positively by stimulating specific differentiation. For example, the medulla stimulates development of the wolffian ducts. At the same time, each inductor acts negatively, antagonizing or inhibiting the other inductor. Witschi[8] believes the stimulating and inhibitory effects are produced by two distinct substances. Which of the two inductors will predominate is apparently controlled by the genes, which find their first visible expression with the appearance of these separate inductive areas in the early undifferentiated gonad.

Though the findings in amphibians strongly suggest the existence of hormone-like sex-differentiating substances, which originate in the gonad primordium, studies in other species have yielded less clear-cut results. Parabiotic experiments, similar to those carried out with amphibian embryos, are not feasible in mammals. Grafting experiments have been unsatisfactory, because the delay before the graft "takes" may bring the heterosexual hormones to bear too late to influence the differentiation of the embryonic gonad. Moreover, unfavorable vascular conditions in the graft may prevent it from either sending forth, or being exposed to, an adequate amount of heterosexual substances. In the absence of evidence to the contrary, however, it seems reasonable to assume that in mammals, as in amphibians, the sex-differentiating substances present in the embryo originate in the primordial gonad, the masculinizing substances in the medulla, the feminizing ones in the cortex.

Time of Transfer from Genic to Inductor Control.—The moment when control of sex differentiation passes from the genes to the inductors has not been exactly defined. Observations in chicks, bearing grafts, and in the free martin suggest that the inductor substances first become effective after the sex of the gonad is morphologically differentiated. It would therefore follow that early differentiation of the gonad depends primarily on genetic determiners of sex. The latter may, as Goldschmidt[4] has suggested, cause the formation of cortex and medulla by producing chemical substances with an enzyme-like action, which he terms "type I" substances. It seems likely, from the available evidence, that, as the cortex or medulla becomes more and more differentiated, its endocrine or inductive function becomes progressively better established, gradually replacing the direct products of the genes.

Mode of Action of Inductor Substances.—The available evidence does not unequivocally indicate whether inductor substances derived from one member of a parabiotic union modify sex differentiation in the heterosexual partner directly by stimulating the gonad primordium of the corresponding sex, or indirectly by suppressing the gonad primordium of the opposite sex. Observations in parabiotic and grafting experiments have been too variable to permit conclusions. In some, inhibition of the opposite sex primordium, in others stimulation of the corresponding one seems to constitute the initial effect. That the inductor substances act indirectly seems more likely, for it is more reasonable to suppose that the products of each inductor can suppress the opposite one, than that they can stimulate differentiation of tissue corresponding to that which produces them. Instances in which their first effect seemed to be stimulation of the corresponding gonad primordium do not conclusively prove that their action is direct. It is entirely possible that the primary alteration is suppression of the function of the opposite gonad primordium, but visible evidence of inhibition appears after the antagonistic inductor has begun to benefit visibly from the lowered level of its opponent's secretory products.

Relation of Inductor Substances to Hormonal Products of the Mature Gonad.—There is a difference of opinion as to whether the substances which control sex differentiation during embryonic life are identical with the hormones secreted by the mature gonad. Dantchakoff[12] maintains that substances identical with those elaborated by the mature gonad not only control differentiation of the sex characters but are also responsible for formation of the gonad primordia. An opposing hypothesis, to which Goldschmidt[4] and Witschi[8] subscribe, postulates the existence of three distinct types of substances, which act successively to carry sexual development to its normal climax. The first of these are the direct products of the genes and cause development of the medulla and cortex of the indifferent gonad. The second are produced by the medulla and cortex and control differentiation of the sex characters during embryonic life. Unlike the first type, they affect distant tissues, being carried by the blood or diffused through the tissues. The third group are the substances produced by the developed gonad. These are true hormones in the sense that they are borne by the blood stream. The last-mentioned substances exert what Halban[13] has termed a "protective" influence on the sex characters of the individual, bringing already differentiated tissues and organs to full maturity and function. In this respect they differ from the inductor substances, which exert a "formative" or morphogenetic effect on the sex characters.

In support of the view that the sex-differentiating substances and maturity sex hormones are distinct, it has been argued that the external sex characters of the free martin remain of the female type despite the masculinizing substances derived during embryonic life from the male co-twin, although the sex hormones of the mature male gonad are known to produce their most characteristic effect on these organs and tissues. Halban[13] has pointed out that if the sex-differentiating substances which produce such far reaching changes in the free martin were identical with the hormonal secretions of the mature male gonad, one might reasonably expect that in single males the embryonic testis would produce mature genitalia at birth. A further argument against their identity is provided by the observation that the sex characters of male human and horse embryos remain unmodified despite the considerable quantities of female sex hormones in the maternal circulation and placenta during gestation. Witschi[8] distinguishes between the embryonic and maturity hormones on the ground that the former behave, in certain species, more like inductors than like hormones, being spread by diffusion through the tissues rather than by way of the blood stream. Bridges[5] has questioned the validity of this argument on the ground that the inductor substances' tendency to be diffused through the tissues in some species may be due simply to their small quantity, which is not sufficient to insure their being taken up by the blood and carried to more distant tissues. As a further argument against the identity of the embryonic and maturity sex-controlling substances, Witschi[8] has stressed the fact that the antagonism, which exists between embryonic gonads in parabiotic partners of opposite sex, and is apparently dependent on the inductor substance produced by each, disappears after the partners reach maturity. Bridges'[5] answer to this is that the absence of antagonism between adult gonads may be due to a change in their reactivity to each other's secretions rather than to a change in the nature of those secretions.

Experimental Studies.—Since the embryonic sex-differentiating substances have not yet been isolated, their relation to the maturity hormones has been investigated by testing the latter's ability to duplicate the sex reversal effects observed in parabiotic animals and the cattle free martin. The results of such studies have thus far been inconclusive. Several investigators[12, 14–16] have found it possible to partially reverse the sex of *genetical male chicks* by introducing a relatively large quantity of ovarian sex hormone into the egg a few days after it is laid. With *estrogenic substances*, the histologic structure and form of the left testis of genetical males are markedly modified. It consists of a central core of medullary tissue on which a thick ovarian cortex is superimposed. The right testis remains testicular in structure but is often smaller than normal. With larger doses of estrogen, the left testis may show no trace of testicular tissue, the gonad being almost indistinguishable from a normal female ovary. Oviducts persist in such males, while the wolffian ducts remain unchanged. In *genetical females* injected with *androgenic substances*, the histologic structure of the right ovary is changed to that of a testis-like organ. The left ovary shows a thinning of the ovarian cortex, with hypertrophy of the ovarian medulla and its inversion to testis tissue. The oviducts show regressive changes while the wolffian ducts are greatly swollen. Though striking, these findings are not conclusive. The observation that nonspecific procedures, such as altered humidity, or grafting of nongonad tissues may modify the sex organs in chicks, indicates that sex differentiation in this species is readily disturbed. For this reason, we cannot be certain that the effects obtained with estrogenic and androgenic substances are specific, and not merely due to the fact that they constitute a disturbing influence.

Witschi[17] has attempted to solve this problem by comparing the changes noted in salamander larvae following parabiotic union with a heterosexual partner and those produced by administering crystalline estrogens or androgens. *Estrogens* produced sex reversal in genetical males, but *testosterone* propionate failed to have a corresponding effect on genetical females. As in adult animals, the secondary sex characters of the larvae responded to the sex hormones. The estrogens stimulated the larval müllerian ducts slightly, while testosterone caused an extensive and very precocious stimulation of the larval wolffian ducts and cloacal glands. In *parabiotic experiments*, the testes apparently released inductive substances which inhibited the development of the ovaries of female co-twins, and indirectly caused some genetical females to continue development in a male direction. There was no precocious stimulation of gonoducts or cloacal glands. These differences, Witschi believes, are proof that the sex hormones of the sterol class are not identical with the substances which normally act as inductors of sex differentiation. Like other environmental factors, they eventually produce sex transformation, not by replacing the products of the inductors, but by upsetting the cortico-medullary balance and thus influencing the direction of sex differentiation.

Studies in mammals, such as the rat,[18, 19, 20] mouse,[21] rabbit, guinea pig,[12] and opossum,[22] have failed to resolve this controversy. Attempts to influence sex differentiation by administering estrogenic or androgenic substances to the mothers before mating have yielded conflicting and unconvincing results.[23] A number of workers have investigated the effect of such substances when injected into the mother during gestation.[18-21] Under such conditions, the gonads of the offspring either remain unaltered or show evidence of repression. Various anomalies of the tubular tract have been induced, but these show no constant relationship to the type of sex hormone administered. In the opossum, for example, Moore[22] found that both sets of ducts in both sexes could be stimulated with either estrogens or androgens. In no case was he able to induce a free martin condition.

Control of Somatic Sex Differentiation by the Embryonic Gonad.— Observers have been puzzled by the fact that the external sex characters of the cattle free martin remain of the female type despite reversal of the gonad and internal genitalia in the male direction. Does this signify that the former differentiate independently of the embryonic gonad, or is some other expanation applicable? Danforth[3] has suggested that their resistance to masculinizing influences emanating from the male co-twin may be due to the stability of the genetically created bias, or to "fixation" of these sex characters during embryonic life and before the male inductors can act. Witschi[8] believes that the cortical and medullary inductors produce their stimulating and inhibiting effects through two distinct factors, and that only the inhibiting one is capable of passing over long distances. Consequently, in heterosexual cattle twins, there occurs only inhibition of the cortex with compensatory hypertrophy of the medulla, and suppression of the müllerian ducts with stimulation of the wolffian ducts. The action of the stimulating factors is not sufficiently strong to influence the external sex characters. According to Halban,[13] the external sex characters of the free martin remain of the female type because their differentiation is independent of the gonad. As proof of this independence, he offers the observation that in man external sex characters of one type may develop in the presence of gonads of the opposite sex or even in the complete absence of gonads (anorchism and aplasia of the ovaries). Reports of gonadless individuals are rare but well substantiated.[26, 27] Their occurrence suggests that the inductor substances emanating from the embryonic gonad are not indispensable for sex character differentiation, at least in the human being.

Summary.—Though many questions still remain unanswered, it seems likely, from the data at hand, that in man as in the lower forms, the sex of each cell in the entire body is primarily determined by its genic constitution, which is normally the same as that which characterizes the fertilized ovum. In the gonadless individual, who apparently lacks a special inductor organ capable of influencing sex differentiation, each cell differentiates according to its genetical constitution. In the normal individual, the inductor organ reflects the genic constitution of the fertilized ovum, producing inductive substances which reinforce the genetical bias of the individual cells. If, for some reason, as in the cattle free martin, inductor substances antagonistic to the genetical sex are introduced, the direction taken in differentiatoin will depend on the stability of the bias created within the individual cells, the stability of the balance between the cortex and medulla, and the strength of the opposing stimulus. Whether the con-

41

dition produced in nature in the cattle free martin is due to substances derived solely from the gonad or, as Moore[22] suggests, many or all the cells in the male co-twin contribute to this effect, is a question for the future.

BIBLIOGRAPHY

1. Lillie, F. R., in Sex and Internal Secretions, ed. by E. Allen. Baltimore, Williams & Wilkins Co., 1932, chap. 1, pp. 1–11.
2. Biedl, A.: Innere Sekretion, ed. 2. Berlin, Urban & Schwarzenberg, 1913, vol. 2, pp. 199–343.
3. Danforth, C. H., in Sex and Internal Secretions (*supra* 1), chap. 2, pp. 12–54.
4. Goldschmidt, R.: Arch. f. Entwicklngsmechan. d. Organ. *124*:618, 1931; Deutsche med. Wchnschr. *57*:1288, 1931; Quart. Rev. Biol. *12*:426, 1937.
5. Bridges, C. B.: Am. Naturalist *59*:127, 1925; Sex and Internal Secretions (*supra* 1), 1932, chap. 3, pp. 55–93.
6. Lebedeff, G. A.: Proc. Nat. Acad. Sci. *24*:165, 1938.
7. Riddle, O.: Sex and Internal Secretions (*supra* 1), chap. 6, pp. 246–280.
8. Witschi, E., in Sex and Internal Secretions, 2 ed. 1939, chap. 4, pp. 145–226.
9. Keller, K., and Tandler, J.: Wien. tierartzl. Monatschr. *3*:513, 1916.
10. Lillie, F. R.: Science, n.s. *43*:611, 1916; J. Exper. Zool. *23*:371, 1917; Biol. Bull. *44*:47, 1923.
11. Burns, R. K.: J. Exper. Zool. *42*:31, 1925; ibid. *55*:123, 1930; ibid. *60*:339, 1931; Anat. Rec. *63*:101, 1935.
12. Dantschakoff, V.: Bull. Biol. France et Belgique *71*:269, 1937; Compt. rend. Soc. de biol. *126*:177, 275, 851, 1937; ibid. *130*:1473, 1939.
13. Halban, J.: Arch. f. Gynäk. *70*:114, 1903; ibid. *130*:415, 1927; ibid. *163*:457, 1937.
14. Wolff, E., and Ginglinger, A.: Compt. rend. Soc. de biol. *120*:114, 901, 1312, 1314, 1935; ibid. *121*:1474, 1476, 1936; ibid. *126*:195, 275, 1937.
15. Willier, B. H., Gallagher, I. F., and Koch, F. C.: Physiol. Zool. *10*:101, 1938.
16. Greenwood, A., and Blyth, J. S.: Quart. J. Physiol. *28*:61, 1938.
17. Witschi, E.: Scientia *68*:146, 1940.
18. Hain, A. M.: Quart. J. Physiol. *25*:131, 1935: ibid. *26*:290, 1936.
19. Hamilton, J. B., and Wolfe, J. M.: Anat. Rec. *70* (Suppl.):433, 1938.
20. Greene, R. R., Burrill, M. M., and Ivy, A. C.: Science *87*:396, 1938; Physiol. Zool. *15*:1, 1942.
21. Raynaud, A.: C. R. Acad. Sci. *211*:572, 1940.
22. Moore, C. R.: J. Urol. *45*:869, 1941.
23. Fellner, O. O.: Med. Klin. *23*:1527, 1927.
24. Gostomirovic, D.: Biol. Zentralbl. *50*:599, 1930.
25. Koch, W.: Klin. Wchnschr. *13*:141, 1934.
26. Meyer, R.: Zentralbl. f. Gynäk. *45*:593, 1921.
27. Rössle, R., and Wallart, J.: Beitr. z. path. Anat. u. allg. Path. *84*:401, 1930.

CHAPTER XXXVIII

HERMAPHRODISM

Since ancient times, individuals with mixed sex characters have presented a fascinating medical, psychological and sociological problem. Not infrequently, these anomalous creatures seek the aid of the physician, requesting that he establish their "true" sex and remove or alter those characters which are inconsistent with the sex to which they are most closely akin psychologically. Often, the physician finds it difficult to decide whether the sex of the gonads or that of the external sex characters should be favored. Thanks to our ever increasing knowledge of the factors which control sex (see Chap. XXXVII), he is better qualified to classify and interpret these cases and recommend proper therapy.

Terminology.—Individuals with characters of both sexes have long been known as *hermaphrodites*. Two main forms are usually described: true and false. The true hermaphrodite is distinguished by the presence of gonadal tissue of both sexes, as for example, an ovary on one side and a testis on the other (lateral form), or an ovotestis on either (unilateral form) or both (bilateral form) sides. The *pseudohermaphrodite*, on the other hand, has unisexual glands, but some or all of the accessory genitalia and external sex characters are of the opposite sex. Such individuals are described as male or female according to the sex of the gonad.

Changing concepts regarding sex determination and differentiation of sex characters have led to the adoption of a new terminology. The older division into "true" and "false" hermaphrodites, based simply on the morphological findings, is giving way to a classification which emphasizes etiological differences. The terms *intersex* and *gynandromorph* have been evolved to distinguish individuals whose opposite sex characters have presumably developed at different times in the course of sex differentiation, from those whose opposite sex characters have developed simultaneously in different parts of the body. Recognition that both genetic and hormonal factors control sex character differentiation is the basis for a division into *zygotic or genetical intersexuality* and *hormonal intersexuality*. The full significance of these terms is best appreciated after considering the current theories as to the causes of hermaphrodism, and the interpretations which observers have placed on the various forms of abnormal sexuality.

CAUSES OF HERMAPHRODISM

It is now generally believed that sex in the lower mammals and man is controlled by genetical and hormonal factors. If this is true, it would follow that deviations from normal may be traced to some abnormality in either or both of these controlling mechanisms.

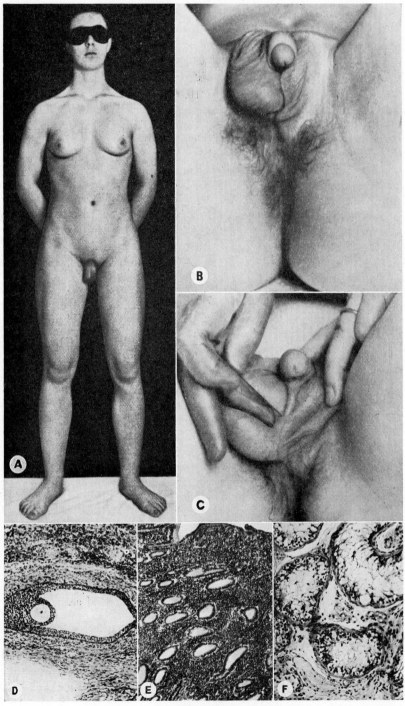

Fig. 162.

Genetical Causes.—According to Goldschmidt,[1-5] individuals with mixed sex characters fall into two groups: intersexes and gynandromorphs. He defines an *intersex* as an individual who, according to his genetic constitution, XX or XY (see Chap. XXXVII), is determined to be a male or a female. At the outset, sexual development proceeds in the direction of the genetical sex, but at a certain point in prenatal life, which varies in different intersexes, reversal occurs and development is completed according to the opposite sex. Since only those characters which have not yet differentiated are affected by the reversal, the final appearance of the intersex depends on when in the course of embryonic development the "turning point" falls. If the initial phase of sex differentiation was male, the individual is described as a *male intersex;* if the initial phase was female, as a *female intersex.* These so-called "intersexes in time" are to be distinguished from gynandromorphs, who have been described as "intersexes in space." *Gynandromorphs,* like intersexes, present a mosaic of parts of different sexes, but differ in two important respects. All the cells of the intersex are of the same genetical constitution, while in the gynandromorph, some parts are genetically determined to be male, others female. The intersex first passes through a purely male (or female) phase and then through a purely female (or male) phase, while in the gynandromorph one part is developing in the male direction at the same time that another is developing in the female direction.

Gynandromorphs.—As may be expected, these two forms are etiologically distinct. A gynandromorph may conceivably arise from any one of several causes. As Witschi[6] has suggested, there may be "(1) Double fertilization of binucleate eggs, resulting in XX and XY fusion-nuclei. (2) Loss of one X chromosome by some cell of an organism which had started development as an XX zygote. This may occur during the first cleavage division, resulting in half male embryos, or during the second division resulting in quarter male embryos, and so on. (3) Mutation, in one of the early embryonic cells, of a gene having influence on sex differentiation."

Gynandromorphs are rare; indeed, according to Goldschmidt,[3] a verified case in the human has not thus far been encountered. Lindvall and Wahlgren,[7] however, have recently reported a case which they interpret as an example of this type of hermaphrodism (see Fig. 162). Not only was there a female gonad on one side and a male gonad on the other, but on the female side only female internal genitalia were present and no derivatives of the wolffian ducts, while on the male side, male internal genitalia were found without any trace of müllerian derivatives. Externally, the sex characters on both the male and female side were of the female type. This they attribute to the fact that the female sex hormones exceeded the

---

Fig. 162.—True hermaphrodism (gynandromorphism). A, Note breast development, absence of body and facial hair. Blood noted in urine at monthly intervals since age of fifteen. B and C, External genitalia, showing insertion of sound into the urethral opening. Note penis and descent of one testicle. D, Section of ovary, found with uterus and tube on left side. Note follicle containing ovum. E, Section of uterus showing endometrium in the resting phase. F, Section of testicular tissue obtained by biopsy. Tissue atrophic with no evidence of spermatogenesis. (Lindvall, S., and Wahlgren, F.: Virchows Arch., Vol. 297.)

male sex hormones in the organism. They assume that when both hormones are present in equal quantities, cells determined to be XX react to the female hormone, while those determined to be XY respond to the male hormone. If one dominates, then both types of cells respond to the dominant hormone. To account for the paucity of human gynandromorphs, they suggest that this condition may be overlooked more readily in the human than in species, such as insects, whose sex is controlled by genic factors alone. To quote:

"In animals without endocrines influencing sex, each region shows its genotypical sex; but if hormones are present, whether each region will be so distinguishable depends on the degree to which male and female tissues in the particular species are specialized in their respective responses. In the complete absence of such specialization, it is unlikely that gynandromorphism would find a bilateral expression. Since most sex differences are differences of degree, it might be anticipated that in the amniotes, genetic gynandromorphism would be more or less completely masked, or represented by bilaterally occurring unusual combinations of normal units of organization with actual structural abnormalities limited chiefly to those parts, such as the reproductive organs, which cannot develop in two different ways."

Intersexes.—While there is general agreement as to the genesis of gynandromorphs, there is still some question as to how other forms of hermaphrodism arise. On the basis of his *observations in the gypsy moth, Lymantria dispar,* Goldschmidt[1, 3] proposed that intersexes come as a result of a too even balance of the male and female genes. Since the potency or "valency" of the dominant sex gene is only slightly greater than that of the opposite sex gene, development begins according to the genetic constitution, XX or XY as the case may be. Sooner or later, depending on how nearly equal is the potency of the two genes, the one which would normally be subordinated comes to the fore and gains control of differentiation. Goldschmidt speaks of *five grades of intersexuality:* beginning, weak, medium, strong, and complete sex reversal. The first three grades, in which the gonad is only partially transformed, include true hermaphrodites. This group, he believes, represents a lower grade of intersexuality than pseudohermaphrodites, whose gonads are unisexual because they have been completely transformed. The forms hitherto designated *pseudohermaphroditismus femininus, hermaphroditismus verus,* and *pseudohermaphroditismus masculinus,* and treated as distinct entities, are, according to Goldschmidt, three stages of the same process. He interprets the large majority of human intersexes as transformed genetical females and holds that there are no recognizable cases of male intersexuality in the human. This he attributes to the fact that the differentiated testis lacks a cortical rudiment and therefore cannot be transformed into an ovary unless the turning point occurs very early in embryonic life. Should such very early reversal occur, all the sex characters would be affected by it and its occurrence could then be ascertained only by reference to the chromosomal constitution of the cells. Moskowicz,[8] on the other hand, contends that the mammalian gonad is capable of reversal in either direction and that in man there are both male and female intersexes.

Some observers[9, 10] hold that a special gene, rather than abnormal valency of the male and female genes, is the cause of intersexuality. Lebedeff,[11] on the basis of *studies in Drosophila virilis,* concluded that the male and female factors are of equal potency, and that intersexuality is caused by a new mutant, a gene located in the third chromosome which he named "intersex (IX)." This gene has no effect on males but converts females into sterile males. In addition there are two modifying genes, A and B, which delay the transformation of these females into males, thereby producing hermaphrodites. He further found that the time law of intersexuality, which is applicable to Goldschmidt's Lymantria, applies also to Drosophila virilis. Individuals start to develop as females, then at the turning point, proceed in the male direction. The sexual organs whose imaginal discs are differentiated before the turning point is reached, develop into female organs, while the imaginal discs which appear after the turning point develop into male organs. The time of reversal determines the degree of intersexuality.

The question which chiefly concerns us here is whether the rules which Goldschmidt found applicable to the gypsy moth also apply to other species and especially man. A number of observers have expressed doubt as to whether rules may be laid down for the human on the basis of findings in insects, where sex differentiation is completely independent of the endocrines. Moskowicz holds that *hermaphrodism in man,* as in the lower animal, may be explained on the basis of reversal of sex occurring at some "turning point" during embryonic life. That Goldschmidt's rules are not universally applicable is indicated by the recent studies of Baltzer.[12] His findings in Bonellia led him to conclude that intersexuality in this species does not conform to a purely male development period followed by a purely female development period. Instead, the intersexual organs are so from the outset, male, female and intersexual organs being present at all stages of development. Baltzer's findings also failed to bear out Goldschmidt's rule that organs with early embryological development are least affected and those with late development most affected by sex reversal. In this connection, Bridges[13] has pointed out that Goldschmidt's concept of developmental sex transformation arises partly from a misconception of the genetic sex. Goldschmidt classifies an individual as a genetical male or female according to the genetical constitution XY and XX, regardless of whether or not the potency of the male and female factors is standard. Bridges believes this classification is justified only if the male and female factors are of standard potency. Should they deviate from standard values, either because of interracial breeding such as occurred in Lymantria in Goldschmidt's experiments, or for some other reason, they are more properly classed as genetical intersexes. On the whole, it is evident that caution must be exercised in establishing rules, applicable to man, by analogy from observations in any one or even in several species.

Hormonal Factors.—Intersexual conditions may arise not only if the balance of sex determiners is upset, but also if the action of normally balanced sex genes is interfered with or modified by conditions developing during the course of sex differentiation. In the lower mammals and man, these sex-modifying influences are hormonal in nature. The most obvious examples of hormonal intersexuality or hormonal sex reversal in the human are cases where heterosexual characters are associated with a hormone-producing tumor, and can be made to regress by removing the growth. Less obvious and indeed only recently proposed by Witschi[6] as possible examples of hormonal "ambisexuality" are cases of male pseudohermaphrodism. These he interprets as genetical males modified in the female direction by feminizing substances originating in the maternal organism during gestation.

Maternal Sex Hormones and Intersexuality.—Witschi's suggestion that the maternal sex hormones may be responsible for certain forms of intersexuality is interesting though not yet convincingly established. Unlike Goldschmidt, who interprets the majority of human intersexes as genetical females modified in the male direction, Witschi believes, with Bonnier[9] and Moebius,[10] that by far the most common hereditary type of human intersex is the genetical male who has been transformed in the female direction. In support of this view, he argues that if pseudohermaphrodites were branching off from the female sex, the most female-like types would be relatively frequent and the most male-like forms relatively rare. Actually, however, the reverse is true. As an additional argument, he points out that the relative proportion of males, females, and intersexes in families with hermaphroditic tendencies indicates that intersexes are developing at the expense of the males rather than of the females. Witschi also stresses the fact that in human intersexes, the morphological findings include fully or partially sterile testes and male gonoducts, a blind vagina, female type external genitalia, well-developed breasts, no beard and a high-pitched voice. These suggest that the first phase of sex differentiation was male but that this was followed by a period during which the last developed secondary sex characters differentiated in the female direction.

Witschi proposes that the cause of such feminization is partly genetical and partly hormonal. He postulates the existence in the maternal organism of a feminizing gene. This, he believes, is responsible for the production, during pregnancy, of female sex hormones which apparently differ either quantitatively or qualitatively from those present in the normal individual. The intersexuality is not due to the intersex's own genetical constitution but to that of the mother. To account for the fact that remasculinization occurs postnatally in some cases and not in others, he suggests that variations in the extent to which the gonad is affected by the feminizing influence may be explanatory. If the gonad is markedly affected, its endocrine function may be impaired to the extent that it produces female instead of male sex hormone, resulting in correspondingly female secondary sex characters. On the other hand, if it is only slightly modified, it may produce male sex hormones during postnatal life, thereby stimulating development of male sex characters. Thus, in accordance with Witschi's hypothesis, the many variants of male pseudohermaphrodism are determined by factors of time and intensity of maternal interference.

Comparative studies of the quality and quantity of the female sex hormones in pregnant females of families with hermaphroditic tendencies may eventually yield significant information. For the present Witschi's interpretation is largely theoretical. It is noteworthy that a possible influence of the maternal sex hormones on the male fetus was also earlier considered by Goldschmidt.[1, 3] More recently, Pich[14] has voiced the same thought, suggesting that the maternal sex hormones induce a reversal of sex only in male embryos in which the superior position of the male over the female factor is already somewhat insecure and therefore readily upset.

Hormone-Producing Tumors and Intersexuality.—Intersexuality may be traceable to hormone-producing tumors of the adrenal cortex or masculinizing tumors of the ovary, so-called arrhenoblastomata. The latter develop during postnatal life, usually after puberty. The masculinizing effects of adrenal tumors, on the other hand, usually become apparent at approximately the third month of fetal life, but at times may appear after birth or puberty.

According to Halban,[15] while the immediate cause of sex reversal is hormonal, the abnormality is, in the final analysis, as much genetically determined as that which develops during embryonic life without the intervention of hormonal agents. Individuals bearing sex-modifying tumors are *latent hermaphrodites*. In such individuals, the valency of the subordinate sex gene is above normal, but not sufficiently so to become manifest during embryonic life. It may express itself later if reinforced by an unusual hormonal stimulus emanating from an adrenal tumor or arrhenoblastoma. The tumor, according to Halban, is itself a manifestation of the abnormal balance of the sex genes. To account for the fact that arrhenoblastomata may occur with or without masculinization, and that adrenal tumors may cause either masculinization, feminization, or no change at all, this observer suggested that the response to the hormones produced by the tumor not only depends on the nature of the hormones, which in the case of the adrenals may perhaps be bisexual, but also on the genetical constitution of the receptor organs and tissues. If a latent hermaphrodism exists, heterosexual characters will develop in response to the tumor's influence. Thus, in accordance with Halban's reasoning, every person in whom contrasexual characters appear, no matter at what time of life, is a zygotic hermaphrodite. Because of marked differences in the valency of the contrasexual anlagen of zygotic hermaphrodites, not only is the turning point reached at different times, but, in some cases hormonal reinforcement is required before heterosexual characters can become phenotypically manifest.

CLINICAL MANAGEMENT OF INTERSEXUALITY

The diagnosis and treatment of sex reversal resulting from the postnatal activity of hormone-producing tumors is relatively simple. Once the presence of an adrenal tumor or an arrhenoblastoma has been established, its surgical removal is usually followed by regression of the heterosexual symptoms and a return to the individual's previous unisexual status. The task of the clinician is more difficult where the abnormality is congenital and unassociated with any tumor to which it may be ascribed, or, though associated with such neoplasm, has apparently arisen independently of it. According to Moskowicz,[16] the presence of a prostate is a valuable aid in distinguishing hermaphrodism arising independently of hormonal factors, from heterosexual characters due to adrenal cortical tumor. To distinguish between the male and female intersex, he is guided by the position of the prostate in relation to the portion of the urethra between the bladder and its junction with the vagina to form the urogenital sinus. It lies cranial to it in the male, and caudal to it in the female intersex.

The sex of the gonads in the pseudohermaphrodite cannot be determined from the external sex characters, nor even, as Witschi,[17] Kurzrok,[18] and others have shown, from the nature of the sex hormones present in the body fluids. Operation is often necessary to obtain this information, but even after this has been accomplished, the physician may find it advisable to be guided not so much by the sex of the gonad as by the attitude of the patient toward other individuals. Where the tendency is to seek intercourse with males, surgical means have been employed to elongate a blind vagina or remove a penis-like clitoris. Surgical methods, whose description is not within the province of the present writing, have been developed to correct hypospadias and thus enable handicapped individuals to take the male part in coitus. Obviously, where the gonads are sterile or important organs such as the uterus are absent, such individuals cannot be transformed into fertile males or females. The most that can be accomplished is an adjustment to permit the enjoyment of sexual relations with the sex to which they are most attracted, and freedom from the fear of appearing abnormal to those with whom they come in contact.

BIBLIOGRAPHY

1. Goldschmidt, R., The Mechanism and Physiology of Sex Determination, trans. by W. J. Dakin. London, Methuen & Co., 1923.
2. Goldschmidt, R.: Ztschr. f. indukt. Abstammungs- u. Verebungsl. *56:*275, 1930.
3. Goldschmidt, R.: Die Sexuellen Zwischenstufen. Berlin, J. Springer, 1931.
4. Goldschmidt, R.: Deutsche med. Wchnschr. *57:*1288, 1931.
5. Goldschmidt, R.: Bibliog. Genet. *11:*5, 1934.
6. Witschi, E., in Sex and Internal Secretions, ed. by E. Allen. Baltimore, Williams & Wilkins Co., 1939, chap. 4, pp. 145–226.
7. Lindvall, S., and Wahlgren, F.: Virchow's Arch. f. path. Anat. u. Physiol. *297:*1, 1936.
8. Moszkowicz, L.: Ergebn. d. allg. Path. *31:*236, 1936.
9. Pettersson, G., and Bonnier, G.: Hereditas *23:*49, 1937.
10. Moebius, H.: Ztsch. f. menschl. Vererb.- u. Konstitutionlehre *19:*456, 1935.
11. Lebedeff, G. A.: Proc. Nat. Acad. Sci. *24:*165, 1938.
12. Baltzer, F.: W. R. Arch. Ent. Org. *136:*1, 1937.
13. Bridges, C. B., in Sex and Internal Secretions, ed. by E. Allen. Baltimore, Williams & Wilkins Co., 1939, chap. 3, pp. 55–93.
14. Pich, G.: Beitr. z. path. Anat. u. z. allg. Path. *100:*460, 1938.
15. Halban, J.: Arch. f. Gynäk. *163:*457, 1937.
16. Moszkowicz, L.: Wien. klin. Wchnschr. *49:*545, 1936.
17. Mengert, W. F., and Witschi, E.: J. Clin. Endocrinol. *2:*279, 1942.
18. Kurzrok, R.: Endocrines in Obstetrics and Gynecology. Baltimore, Williams & Wilkins Co., 1937, chap. 26, pp. 405–420.

PART III

LABORATORY

CHAPTER XXXIX

DIAGNOSTIC AIDS

ENDOMETRIAL BIOPSY AND CURETTAGE

Histologic study of endometrial tissue is generally conceded to be the most simple, practical and accurate means of determining the functional status of the ovary.[62] Besides eliminating organic lesions of the uterus, it is of value in ascertaining whether an ovarian deficiency exists and whether the disturbance involves suppression of the follicular or luteal phase, or both.

Thorough *curettage* under anesthesia insures recovery of adequate tissue from all parts of the mucosa, and is preferable to the biopsy or suction method, particularly in cases of uterine bleeding and in women at the cancer age. The *biopsy* method on the other hand has several advantages. Since no anesthesia or dilatation is necessary, it may be carried out as an office procedure. Endometrial tissue may be obtained at frequent intervals throughout the cycle, thus enabling the investigator to follow successive events with a fair degree of precision. For this reason, endometrial biopsy may be used not only as a diagnostic aid, but also to ascertain the efficacy of therapy. Its disadvantage lies in the fact that it secures only minute fragments of tissue, so that malignancy, local areas of hyperplasia, or polyps may be missed.

Endometrial biopsy, as an office procedure, calls for an *instrument* which may be readily inserted into the uterine cavity without much dilatation and a minimum of discomfort. Some favor a small curette, with a thin, flexible shank, while others prefer a small caliber, long tube with an attached suction bulb or small punch curette.[1, 2, 3] Klinger and Burch[4] employ an instrument designed for both curettage and suction.

The *time of biopsy* should be chosen, where possible, in relation to the menstrual cycle. In women with approximately twenty-eight day cycles, the mucosal specimen should be obtained about the twenty-sixth day after the onset of the preceding flow, when the regenerative processes are normally complete. Some observers[5] advocate endometrial biopsy within two hours after the onset of menstruation to permit maximum endometrial modifications, and avoid possible disturbance of an existing early gestation. In cases of amenorrhea or prolonged uterine bleeding, where no menstrual rhythm exists, biopsy may be performed at any time and, where feasible, repeated at weekly intervals in order to establish or rule out the occurrence of cyclic endometrial changes.

Technique:

1. Place the patient in the lithotomy position.
2. Cleanse the vagina with soap and water or a mild antiseptic solution.
3. Expose the cervix by means of a bivalve speculum.
4. Paint the portio and vagina with 3 per cent tincture of iodine, tincture of merthiolate, or a solution of mercurochrome in acetone and alcohol.
5. Grasp the cervix gently with a tenaculum forceps and paint the cervical canal with tincture of iodine.
6. A uterine sound is gently passed into the uterine cavity.
7. When necessary, the cervical canal may be slightly dilated by means of Hegar dilators, numbers 1 to 3.
8. The curette, or instrument of choice, is introduced gently into the uterine cavity in the same manner as the sound.
9. Bits of endometrium are taken from the anterior, posterior, and lateral walls as well as the dome of the uterus.
10. Twenty-four hour paraffin sections are then made.

THE VAGINAL SMEAR

Stockard and Papanicolaou,[6] in 1917, called attention to the fact that the vaginal mucosa of the guinea pig undergoes cyclic alterations which may be correlated with events in the ovary. These observers introduced the vaginal smear as a means of following the vaginal changes and thus indirectly ascertaining the status of ovarian function. Allen[7] later described well defined cyclic changes in the vaginal mucosa of the mouse and, in collaboration with Doisy,[8] demonstrated the applicability of the vaginal smear in the rodent for the assay of estrogenic substances. Papanicolaou,[9] in 1933, on the basis of an extensive study, concluded that the human vaginal epithelium like that of the laboratory animal, undergoes cyclic changes which can be correlated with the ovarian and endometrial cycle (see Chap. I). Although a few observers have arrived at the same conclusion,[10, 11] others[12] maintain that the vaginal changes in the regularly menstruating woman are less striking than in the rodent and too inconstant to serve as a reliable index of the functional status of the ovary.

While the vaginal smear is inferior to endometrial biopsy or curettage as a means of following events in the ovary, it may nevertheless serve as a useful *adjunct in ascertaining the level of endogenous estrogen,* and gauging the efficacy of estrogen therapy. Studies of the vaginal mucosa before and after estrogen administration in children with gonorrheal vulvovaginitis, in hypomenorrheic and amenorrheic women, and those past the menopause, have shown that the human vagina responds with characteristic modifications. The difference between the estrogenic and the nonestrogenic or atrophic type of smear (see Fig. 163) is sufficiently marked for purposes of differentiation. The reliability of the smear as an index of the *level of progestin* in the body is not established. The effect of progestin is to inhibit the response to estrogen. Consequently, the typical premenstrual vaginal smear is much like that seen where no progestin is present and the estrogen level is dropping. According to Rubenstein,[10] luteal activity may be evaluated by the degree of desquamation, as evidenced by the folding and aggregation of the epithelial cells, and the degree of inhibition of cornification induced by estrogen. *Ovulation* is indicated by a sharp increase in the desquamation index with a simultaneous decrease from high levels of the cornification index. Krohn and his associates[11] found evidence of desquamation at all stages of the cycle, bordering at levels indistinguishable from progesterone effects. They conclude that this modification alone is not reliable evidence of ovulation, but believe that if inhibition of cornification is considered simultaneously, it is possible to distinguish between a true and false progesterone response. To avoid this source of error, they emphasize the importance of analyzing smears throughout the cycle.

Techniques.—*Vaginal smear Technique of Papanicolaou and Shorr.*[13]

1. Samples of vaginal fluid are obtained with a glen pipette, 8 inches long and ⅜ inch in diameter, to which is attached a strong rubber suction bulb.
2. Samples are obtained from a region 5 to 6 cm. within the vagina and are spread on a cover slide as a heavy film.
3. Soon after, and before the smear is dried, the slide is placed in a jar containing equal parts of 95 per cent alcohol and ether for quick fixation.
4. After fixing, the slide is carried through 80, 70, and 50 per cent alcohol into distilled water as a preliminary to staining.
5. The slide is stained with Ehrlich's hemotoxylin for about five minutes, and then washed in running water for at least a quarter of an hour.
6. Stain with 0.5 per cent eosin for about three to four minutes, and then rinse in water.
7. Pass the slide through 50, 70, 80 and 95 per cent alcohol and then through absolute alcohol. Pass into xylol and mount in Canada balsam.

Shorr[14] has devised a technic for staining smears, which he claims provides a sharp differentiation between cornified and non-cornified elements: the former stain a brilliant orange red, while the latter take a green stain which is deeper in the younger cells. The first three steps are essentially as in the technique of Papanicolaou and Shorr above. After fixing, the procedure is as follows:

1. Stain for approximately one minute in Solution S 3, made up as follows and used only after all ingredients are completely dissolved:

Ethyl alcohol (50%)	100 cc.
Biebrich Scarlet (water solution)	0.5 gm.
Orange G	0.25 gm.
Fast Green FCF	0.075 gm.
Phosphotungstic acid c.p.	0.5 gm.
Phosphomolybdic acid c.p.	0.5 gm.
Glacial acetic acid	1.0 cc.

2. Carry through 70 per cent, 95 per cent and absolute alcohol, dipping 10 times in each solution.
3. Clear in xylol and mount in damar.

Cytologic Classification.—The vaginal smear cytology, according to Geist and Salmon,[15] may be classified as follows (Fig. 163):

Reaction I.—Advanced estrogen deficiency (Fig. 163, A). This type of smear is characterized by (1) complete absence of squamous epithelial cells, (2) the presence of small, round or oval epithelial cells with rather large, darkly staining nuclei, known as "atrophy" or "deep" cells, and (3) varying numbers of leukocytes and erythrocytes.

Reaction II.—Moderate degree of estrogen deficiency (Fig. 163, B). The smear shows a variable number of rather irregularly shaped, large epithelial cells with relatively large nuclei.

"Atrophy" cells and leukocytes are interspersed among these cells. The relative proportion of the large epithelial cells to the "atrophy" cells is variable. The distinguishing feature of Reaction I and II is the association of the "atrophy" cells with the large epithelial cells.

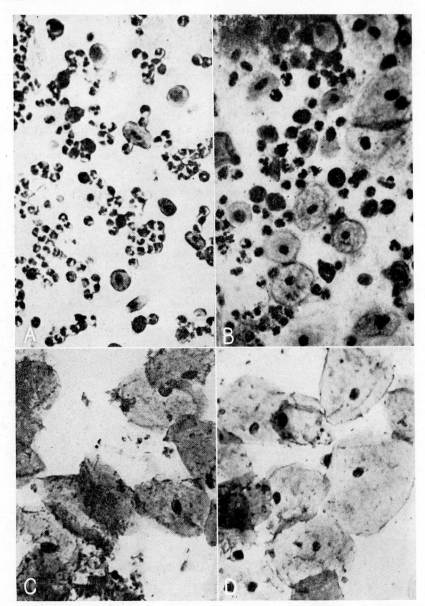

Fig. 163.—Human vaginal smear classification. A, Reaction I; B, Reaction II; C, Reaction III; D, Reaction IV. (S. H. Geist et al., in Am. J. Obst. & Gynec., Vol. 38.)

Reaction III.—Slight degree of estrogen deficiency (Fig. 163, C). A predominance of rather large, irregularly shaped epithelial cells is the characteristic feature. The cells vary in size and shape; their edges are somewhat irregular and their outline often indistinct, and they frequently appear in clumps. A few "atrophy" cells may be present.

Reaction IV.—Normal (Fig. 163, D). This smear is characterized by large, flat, clearly defined squamous epithelial cells which contain small deeply staining nuclei. They are larger, more clear cut and have relatively smaller nuclei than those in smear III. No "atrophy" cells and usually no leukocytes are present.

Iodine Vapor Method.—In 1942, Mack[58] introduced a method for the appraisal of estrogenic activity by the vaginal glycogen index. This is based on evidence that the glycogen content of the vaginal epithelium increases under the influence of estrogen and is deficient in the absence of this hormone. Their iodine vapor technique is as follows:

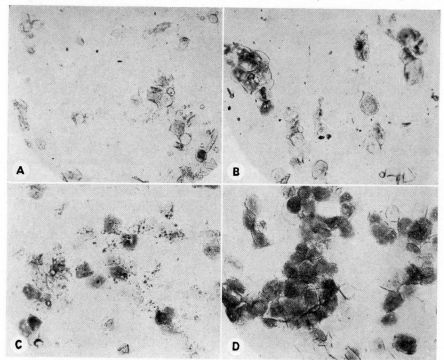

Fig. 164.—Vaginal smears stained for glycogen. A, Grade I; B, Grade II; C, Grade III; D, Grade IV. (Mack, H. C., and Ale, T.: J. Clin. Endocrinol. *2*:361, 1942.)

1. Insert a moistened cotton applicator into the vagina and twirl lightly (one complete rotation) against the vaginal wall.
2. Roll the cotton end of the applicator lengthwise over the surface of a clean glass slide. The film dries almost immediately and may be stained at once.
3. Staining is accomplished by laying the slide, face down, over a shallow dish containing a small amount of Lugol's solution. Iodine vapors stain the glycogen-containing cells in two or three minutes. Microscopic examination may be carried out immediately. The stain may fade in twenty-four to forty-eight hours, but it may be restained as desired.

Preparations for determining the glycogen index are graded as follows[59] (Fig. 164):

Grade I (Fig. 164, A).—This represents advanced vaginal atrophy characterized by complete glycopenia. The smear shows small yellow cells and amorphous debris. In extreme degrees, this grade is also distinguished by marked cytopenia.

Grade II (Fig. 164, B).—Smears of this grade show a greater abundance of cells than those of Grade I. Iodine vapor staining reveals glycogen in irregular brown deposits at the cell margins or scattered irregularly throughout the cytoplasm. Diffusely stained brown cells may also be present. Glycopenic yellow cells are also present in large numbers.

Grade III (Fig. 164, C).—A further increase in cell numbers is noted in this grade. The cells are larger and more regular in outline, and the majority are stained diffusely throughout the cytoplasm. They have a light brown color. Non-iodophilic yellow cells are also present in abundance.

Grade IV (Fig. 164, D).—This grade is distinguished by the presence, almost exclusively, of large, flat, deeply stained, brown, iodophilic cells present singly or in clumps. This grade represents maximal estrogenic effect, corresponding to the proliferative phase.

Pregnancy Changes.—It has been suggested that the vaginal smear may be of value in the diagnosis of pregnancy and allied conditions. Papanicolaou,[16] in 1925, observed that the vaginal smear changed markedly following conception and, as gestation advanced, there appeared highly differentiated cells which he named "pregnancy cells." In 1934, Smith and Brunner[17] reported that, though the pregnancy smear is distinguishable from that of the nonpregnant woman by the formation of *intracellular vacuoles,* the modifications are not sufficiently characteristic for the diagnosis of pregnancy. According to these observers, formation of intracellular vacuoles is *inhibited in the presence of marked pathologic modifications of the vaginal mucosa,* such as chronic vaginitis. In pathologic amenorrhea, on the other hand, the degree of vacuolation is greater than during the menstrual cycle and, though less marked than in pregnancy, occasionally is exaggerated to the point where it may be confused with the pregnancy smear. Confusion may also arise during and after the menopause, when the distal portion of the basal zone is rather highly vacuolated, although the cytological appearance of the intracellular spaces is not quite the same as during the child-bearing period.

On the whole, the value of the vaginal mucosa as a mirror of gonadal and reproductive function would seem to be limited. As recently emphasized by Mack,[60] the vaginal smear, as a method of diagnosis of ovarian dysfunction or failure, has very limited usefulness in clinical practice because of "(a) difficulties of interpreting the bizarre and highly variable histologic smear patterns, and (b) the frequency of normal smears in the presence of signs and symptoms of ovarian failure. . . . As a clinical method of determining the effectiveness of estrogen therapy, the vaginal smear technic may provide objective evidence of therapeutic results in limited instances in which vaginal atrophy accompanies other signs or symptoms of ovarian failure. . . . Until the technic of preparation and the criteria of interpretation of vaginal smears are simplified, use of the procedure will be restricted to research studies."

SEX HORMONE TESTS

Procedures designed for the quantitative study of the sex hormones in the blood and urine have been extensively employed as adjuncts in the diagnosis of gonadal and reproductive disorders. Failure to adopt a standard technique for each of the known sex hormones has made for widely divergent results and general disagreement as to the normal levels of excretion and the limits of normal variability. Because of this, and our incomplete knowledge of the factors which control the sex hormone concentration in the body fluids, it is difficult to interpret the results of the sex hormone tests in a given case. The practical application of these tests is consequently limited, and the information thus obtained is of value only when viewed in the light of the history, physical and pelvic findings, endometrial biopsy, and routine laboratory studies.

QUANTITATION OF ESTROGENS IN THE BLOOD AND URINE

The estrogen content of the blood and urine under normal and abnormal conditions has been intensively studied, by both biologic and chemical methods. Most of the biologic tests utilize the assay method of Allen and Doisy,[8] based on the ability of the injected material to induce the typical changes of estrus in the vagina of the castrate rat or mouse. Another assay method[18] utilizes the weight increase of the uterus in the immature rat, a reaction which reaches its height within six hours after injection. Space permits a description of only the more widely used procedures for the detection and measurement of estrogen in the blood and urine. These include tests designed for use where only small amounts of hormone are likely to be found, and those applicable in pregnancy and other conditions, where the estrogen concentration may be expected to be high.

Blood Estrogen Test of Frank and Goldberger (1935).[19]—This test is based on the observation that, in the regularly menstruating woman, the estrogen content of the circulating blood is materially increased a few days before the onset of the flow. The blood is obtained shortly before the expected flow in the regularly menstruating woman. Where the flow cannot be forecast, as in irregular bleeding or amenorrhea, the test is performed at weekly intervals for five weeks in order to detect a possible blood estrogen cycle. The procedure is as follows:

1. Draw 50 cc. of vein blood into a 50 cc. glass syringe.
2. Pour it at once into a petri dish, the bottom of which has just been covered evenly with 30 gm. of finely powdered anhydrous sodium sulphate.
3. Stir the blood and powder with a spatula until thoroughly dry, and the small lumps that form are then triturated in a mortar.
4. Extract the resulting powder twice with 200 cc. of 95 per cent alcohol; combine the alcohol fractions, evaporate to dryness on a water bath and take up the residuum in 5.0 cc. of oil.
5. The bio-assay is performed according to the Allen-Doisy method. The oil solution containing the hormone is administered in three equal doses at three to four hour intervals to an adult female white mouse, spayed two weeks before. A vaginal smear is taken twenty-four hours after the last injection and three more made at twelve hour intervals, with a final one on the third morning after the last injection. A positive estrogenic smear indicates that the blood contains at least 25 mouse units per liter.

Fluhmann's Mucification Test (1934).[20]—Fluhmann has proposed the following modification of the blood estrogen test which depends on the histologic demonstration of certain changes, particularly the formation of tall, columnar, mucus secreting cells, which precede cornification in the vaginal mucosa of recently spayed mice.

42

1. Take 25 to 40 cc. of blood by venipuncture and place immediately in a test tube for transmission to the laboratory. Secure the clear serum by centrifugalization and discard the cells.
2. Adult female mice, spayed six to seven days before the test is begun, are injected subcutaneously with 0.5 cc. of blood serum at 8 A. M., noon, and 5 P. M. on three consecutive days, each animal receiving a total of 4.5 cc. Kill the animals on the

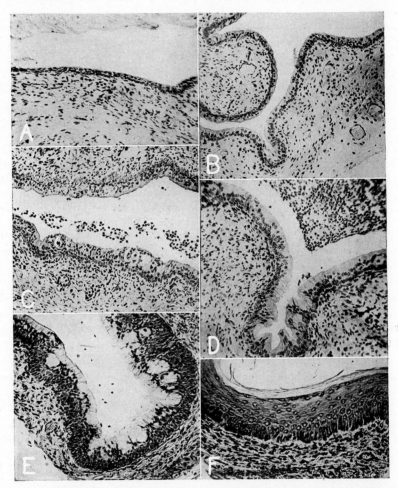

Fig. 165.—A, Atrophied vaginal mucosa of mouse spayed seven days previously. Negative reaction in Fluhmann mucification test for estrogen. B, Reaction I; C, Reaction II; D Reaction III; E, Reaction IV; F, Reaction V. (Fluhmann, C. F.: Endocrinol., Vol. 18.)

fourth day and carefully dissect the vagina free by making a long incision in the abdominal wall and separating the symphysis pubis. Fix the vagina in formalin mount it in paraffin, make transverse sections at different levels, and stain with hematoxylin-eosin.
3. According to Fluhmann, six reactions may be recognized (Fig. 165):
   0—Atrophy of vagina; the mucosa shows two layers of low cuboidal epithelium, and an occasional leucocyte.

I—Two layers are seen; a basal layer of low columnar cells; a few leukocytes appear.

II—The superficial cells are high, begin to show stratification and secrete mucus; there is a well marked increase in leucocytes which may also be found in the lumen of the vagina.

III—The epithelium is composed of several layers, the cells at the surface being of the mucified variety; folding in of the mucosa is a characteristic feature. The mucosa is invaded by numerous leucocytes, which are also present in the lumen along with epithelial debris.

IV—The mucosa is made up of six to ten or twelve rows of cells, the lower ones resembling the basal cells of squamous epithelium, while those at the surface are still of the tall mucified variety. In marked cases, early cornification may be observed between the stratified epithelium and the mucified cells. Leucocytes are greatly diminished or absent.

V—The vagina is now lined by fully developed squamous epithelium with cornified cells at the surface and no leucocytes.

4. No less than two or three mice should be used. After estimating the reaction of each animal the numbers are added and then divided by the number of animals used. An average reaction of 1 or less is negative; 1.1 to 1.5 is 1 plus, indicating only traces of estrogen; 1.6 to 2.5 is 2 plus and equivalent to plus or minus 3 mouse units of estrogen per 100 cc. of blood; 2.6 to 3.5 is 3 plus and equal to plus or minus 6 mouse units per 100 cc., while 3.6 to 4.5 is 4 plus and corresponds to plus or minus 12 mouse units per 100 cc. of blood.

Urine Estrogen Test of Kurzrok and Ratner (1932).[21]—This test is designed to detect small quantities of estrogen in the urine in conditions outside of pregnancy, and is designed for use in the diagnosis of menstrual disorders. The procedure is as follows:

1. Measure twenty-four hour urine specimen, place 900 cc. in a one liter Erlenmeyer flask, and acidify slightly with dilute acetic acid.

2. Saturate the urine with sodium chloride (approximately 50 grams) and then cover the treated urine with ethyl acetate to the top of the flask. Connect as in Fig. 166, A.

3. A second flask (B) of 300 cc. capacity is filled with 200 cc. ethyl acetate. Turn the hot plate to medium heat and the ethyl acetate distills over through the upper side arm, is condensed and drops to the bottom of flask (A), from which it returns through the lower side arm to flask (B). The drops of ethyl acetate extract the hormone as they pass upward through the urine. This provides continuous extraction for forty-eight hours.

4. Discard the extracted urine and concentrate the ethyl acetate which contains the hormone by vacuum distillation (see Fig. 166, B). Fill distilling flask (A) one-third full with ethyl acetate extract and connect it with condenser (B), a receiving flask (C), a second receiving flask (D), a trap (E) provided with a stopcock, and finally onto an aspirator type of suction pump.

5. After heating distilling flask in a steam bath, the suction is turned on. Allow remaining extract to drop into flask (A) through a thistle tube provided with a stopcock.

6. After adding all the ethyl acetate, concentrate it to as small a volume as possible and add 6 cc. of propylene glycol through the thistle tube. Continue the distillation until all the ethyl acetate has been removed. The oil now contains the hormone originally present in the 900 cc. of urine.

7. Use 6 cc. of oil containing hormone for biologic assay. Three ovariectomized rats are injected subcutaneously at 9 A. M. and 5 P. M. of the first day and 9 A. M. of the second day. One animal is given 0.5 cc. at each injection and the other two each receive 0.25 cc. at each injection. Take vaginal smears twenty-four and thirty-two hours after the last injection. The result is positive if cornified cells, characteristic of estrus, are present.

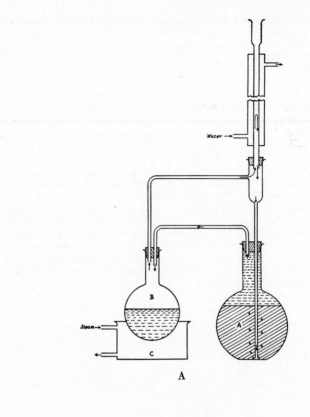

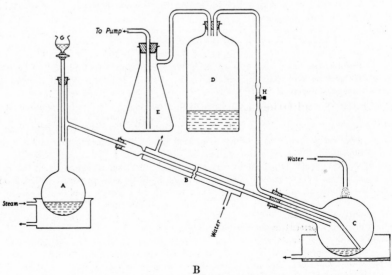

Fig. 166.—Apparatus employed in urine estrogen test of Kurzrok and Ratner. (Kurzrok, R.: Endocrines in Obstetrics and Gynecology, Williams and Wilkins Co.)

8. Calculate the hormone content of a liter of urine, in terms of rat units from the following formula:

$$\frac{6}{y} \times \frac{1000}{900} \text{ equals rat units per liter of urine}$$

when 6 equals the total amount of oil containing hormone injected into a single rat giving a positive result.

Urine Estrogen Test of Smith and Smith (1935).[22]—This procedure is designed to determine the "total" estrogen content of the urine by converting the inactive conjugated form of the hormone to the "free" or active form through acid hydrolysis:

1. Collect a twenty-four hour specimen of urine and measure. For each liter, measure 200 to 800 cc., depending on the amount of estrogen probably present, into an Erlenmeyer flask.
2. Add 15 volumes per cent of concentrated HCl; heat the mixture to boiling and boil vigorously for 10 minutes.
3. Transfer the material to a large extraction flask. This flask and the smaller one are both filled to the neck with benzene. Then extract for 24 hours.
4. Disconnect the large flask containing the urine and benzene, empty it, and put it back in place. Most of the benzene in the smaller flask may then be distilled over into it. The distilled benzene may be used repeatedly.
5. In the case of large specimens containing small amounts of estrogen, two runs must be made since the capacity of the apparatus is 1000 cc. In this case combine the benzene extracts and transfer to a smaller beaker, washing with benzene. Test 0.75 cc. of the olive oil extract on each of 2 castrated adult female rats. A positive estrogenic smear indicates 10 to 40 rat units of total estrin per 24 hours, depending on the amount of urine (200 to 800 cc.) extracted. If 200 to 800 cc. give a negative reaction, use progressively larger amounts.
6. *Calculation:* (24° volume ÷ cc. extracted) × 6 = rat units of estrogen in 24 hour volume of urine.

Smith and Smith studied the relative amount of "free" and "total" estrogen, but could demonstrate no constant ratio between the two. They therefore concluded that their method is superior to those carried out on untreated urines, which yield only part of the active principle and may give completely misleading values bearing no relation to the amount of estrogenic substance actually present.

Smith and Smith Method for Extraction and Separation of Estrone, Estriol, and Other Estrogens in the Urine (1939).[23]—Smith and associates have evolved a method for the hydrolysis, separation and extraction of estrogens from the urine of women. Their object is to obtain all the estrogen present and then separate and measure the estrone and estriol present. They argue that since, as shown by Pincus and Zahl,[24] progestin not only causes increased excretion of estrogen but also augments the conversion of estrone to estriol, it may be possible to obtain a quantitative index of progestin by measuring the total estrogen as well as the amount of estrone and estriol excreted. For this purpose, they employ the following procedure:

1. Use no preservative but keep urine in refrigerator during period of collection. When testing urine of nonpregnant women a twenty-four or forty-eight hour specimen is required, but when pregnancy urine is extracted, one-half to one-tenth of a twenty-four hour specimen is usually sufficient, depending on the stage of gestation.

2. When collection is complete, the urine is hydrolyzed and rendered approximately 1.5 N by adding 15 per cent concentrated hydrochloric acid. It is then placed under a reflux condenser, boiled vigorously for ten minutes, and cooled immediately under running tap water.

3. Extraction and separation of the estrogens is then carried out. After cooling, extract the urine four times with ether, using an amount equal to about one-fifth of the total volume of the material.

4. Wash the ether extract once with 20 to 30 cc. of 20 per cent sodium carbonate and discard washing.

5. Remove the strong phenolic fraction containing estriol from the ether by extracting four times with one-tenth normal sodium hydroxide (25 to 30 cc. per extraction).

6. Wash sodium hydroxide once with 30 cc. of ether to remove any estrone that may have been extracted, and add washing to ether.

7. Wash ethereal fraction 3 times with 10 to 15 cc. of water and evaporate to dryness.

8. Transfer residue to a separatory funnel with 100 cc. of toluene. Remove weak phenolic fraction containing estrone from toluene by extracting four times with 25 to 30 cc. of normal sodium hydroxide.

9. The one-tenth normal sodium hydroxide and normal sodium hydroxide fractions are then each made acid to congo red with hydrochloric acid and extracted for twenty-four hours in the Smith and Smith benzene extractor.

10. If pregnancy urine is being tested, the two fractions are then evaporated to dryness and the residues quantitatively transferred with small quantities of 95 per cent ethyl alcohol (and benzene if all the residue is not soluble in alcohol) to a test tube graduated at 20 cc.

11. The extract is then made up to volume with alcohol, tightly stoppered with rubber, and kept in a refrigerator to avoid evaporation.

12. Aliquot portions, removed for bio-assay, are added to a measured amount of olive oil and put on a steam bath to remove solvent. Use wide mouthed bottle large enough to permit frequent rotating during the evaporation, so no hormone will remain on the sides of the bottle.

13. If the urine of a nonpregnant woman is being tested, then, after evaporating to dryness, the estrone fraction is quantitatively transferred to a test tube graduated at 20 cc. with small amounts of 95 per cent ethyl alcohol and made up to volume with alcohol.

14. Exactly 10 cc. of this is measured into a 125 cc. Erlenmeyer flask for semicarbazide treatment to determine X estrogen (an as yet unidentified non-ketonic estrogen, probably estradiol).

15. The remaining 10 cc. is poured into a wide mouthed bottle containing olive oil, and the test tube rinsed out with alcohol which is then poured into the same bottle.

16. After the estriol fraction is evaporated to dryness, all of it is quantitatively transferred with small amounts of 95 per cent ethyl alcohol to another wide mouthed bottle containing olive oil.

17. The two bottles are then placed on a steam bath to evaporate off the alcohol.

18. Semicarbazide treatment of the estrone fraction for determining X estrogen.

19. An aliquot portion of the estrone fraction in 95 per cent ethyl alcohol (containing no more estrogenic potency than would be equivalent to 200 gamma of estrone) is measured into a 125 cc. Erlenmeyer flask and diluted to 10 cc. with alcohol.

20. 60 mgm. of semicarbazide hydrochloric acid and an equal amount of crystalline sodium acetate are weighed into a small test tube, dissolved in 1 cc. of water and added to the alcohol.

21. Refluxing is carried out for five hours. The extract is evaporated to dryness, the residue taken up in 3 to 5 cc. of alcohol, and the alcohol decanted from the precipitate into a wide mouthed bottle containing olive oil.

22. The precipitate is broken up with a stirring rod and washed several times with small amounts of alcohol which are decanted into the bottle. The alcohol is then evaporated off on the steam bath.

23. The extracts are assayed in mature spayed female rats. Each is injected in three divided doses at four-hour intervals and a vaginal smear taken forty-eight hours after the

first injection. A pre-estrous, full estrous or post-estrous smear is considered a positive reaction. One rat unit is the smallest amount which gives a positive smear in at least four out of six animals. By this method 1 microgram of estrone is equivalent to 2.0 R. U., 1 microgram of estriol to 2.5 R. U. and 1 microgram of estradiol to 20 R. U. Values are expressed in terms of rat units per twenty-four hour volume of urine.

Urine Estrogen Test for Pregnancy: Method of Mazer and Hoffman (1929).[25]

—This test is designed for the diagnosis of early pregnancy and allied conditions. It is based on the observation that estrogen excretion increases within a short time after conception. The technique is as follows:

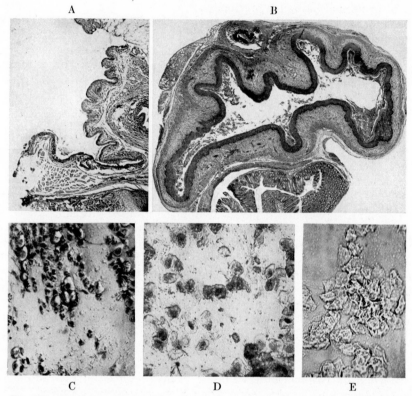

Fig. 167.—Vaginal reaction to human pregnancy urine in the castrate mature mouse. A, Vaginal mucosa of untreated castrate. B, Vaginal mucosa after injection of human pregnancy urine. C, D and E, Vaginal smears of the mouse. C, Anestrous smear: note leucocytes, mucus and an occasional epithelial cell. D, Proestrous smear: nucleated epithelial cells predominate. E, Estrous smear: note large cornified, non-nucleated epithelial cells.

1. Select four mature castrated female mice each weighing 20 to 25 grams.
2. Inject each subcutaneously with 12 cc. of slightly acidified filtered morning urine, in six divided doses over a period of two days.
3. Take a vaginal smear three times daily on the third and fourth days in order to detect the occurrence of estrus.
4. The test is positive if, on the fourth day after the first injection, the vaginal smear shows a preponderance of non-nucleated epithelial cells and the absence of leucocytes and mucus (see Fig. 167).

Sources of Error: This and other biologic tests for early pregnancy, based on the estrogen content of the body fluids, are not as reliable as the gonadotropic hormone tests, because the post-conceptional rise in estrogen excretion occurs later and is less marked than that of gonadotropin. This probably accounts for the fact that false negative estrogen tests for pregnancy are relatively common. A false positive estrogen test for pregnancy may sometimes be obtained in women with follicular cysts or a granulosa cell tumor, and occasionally also in patients in the polyfolliculin phase of the menopause. Such cases fortunately do not constitute a serious source of error, for the estrogen concentration in these conditions is usually below the lower normal limits for pregnancy.

Urine Estrogen Test for Adrenal Cortical Carcinoma: Method of Frank (1937).[26]—This test is designed for the diagnosis of adrenal cortical carcinoma and is based on Frank's observation that patients with malignancy of the adrenal cortex excrete large quantities of estrogenic substance. The procedure is as follows:

1. Obtain a fresh specimen of urine and inject a total of 1 and 2 cc. subcutaneously in 5 divided doses spread over forty-eight hours into adult castrated female mice (0.2 cc. $\times$ 5 and 0.4 cc. $\times$ 5).
2. After completion of injections, vaginal spreads are taken three times daily on three successive days in order to ascertain the occurrence of estrus. No significance may be attached to a positive reaction unless an Aschheim-Zondek or Friedman test for pregnancy (see below) has been performed and proves negative.

QUANTITATION OF PREGNANEDIOL IN THE URINE

Pregnanediol was first demonstrated in the urine of pregnant women by Marrian,[27] in 1929. This finding aroused no particular interest until 1934, when Butenandt and Schmidt[28] called attention to the fact that pregnanediol can be converted into progesterone. This, coupled with Browne and Venning's[29] observation that it appears in the urine of the nonpregnant woman coincident with the formation of the corpus luteum and after progesterone treatment, led the latter observers to believe it is an excretion product of progesterone. They suggested that conversion of progesterone into this biologically inactive compound probably accounts for the failure to detect appreciable amounts of the luteal hormone in the body fluids and tissues.

Method of Browne and Venning (1937).—In 1936, these observers isolated from human pregnancy urine a water soluble complex, sodium pregnanediol glucuronidate.[30] In the following year, they described a gravimetric method for measuring this excretion product, which is as follows: [31, 32]

1. Collect and measure a twenty-four hour specimen of urine and take an aliquot amount which may be expected to contain 20 to 40 mg. of the combined pregnanediol.
2. Extract urine four times with a total of about one-third of its volume of normal butyl alcohol in a separatory funnel. (If a liter of urine is taken, the volumes of butyl alcohol are 200, 85, 50 and 50 cc.)
3. Centrifuge the combined butyl alcohol extracts, or allow them to stand until clear.
4. Pour off the supernatant butyl alcohol into a distilling flask, wash the precipitate once with butyl alcohol, and add washings to flask.
5. Evaporate the butyl alcohol to dryness under reduced pressure and take up residue in 60 cc. of one-tenth normal sodium hydroxide. Extract this mixture four times with

butyl alcohol (20, 20, 10 and 10 cc.). Wash the butyl alcohol extract twice with 5 cc. of water and then centrifuge it and evaporate the clear butyl alcohol to dryness in a one liter distilling flask under reduced pressure.

6. Add exactly 5 cc. of water to flask with 10 cc. of acetone, warm it on a water bath about 50° C.

7. Dissolve the residue completely and transfer the contents to a 125 cc. Erlenmeyer flask. Wash out original flask several times with acetone and make up the final volume of the mixture to 100 cc. with acetone.

8. Allow to stand overnight in a refrigerator at 5 to 10° C. A white precipitate settles out and most of the supernatant fluid can then be drawn off by suction. Transfer the remainder to a 50 cc. centrifuge tube and after centrifuging, pour off acetone without disturbing precipitate.

9. Add a few drops of water to centrifuge tube and warm it on a water bath. Wash out original Erlenmeyer flask with hot 95 per cent ethyl alcohol and add it to the centrifuge tube to dissolve the contents. Filter the hot alcohol solution with suction into a weighed beaker, evaporate it to dryness on a water bath, and weigh the contents.

10. The first precipitate always contains from 10 to 30 per cent of impurities, depending on the volume of urine and the amount of combined pregnanediol extracted. If the urine contains blood, it is almost impossible to obtain a pure precipitate, but otherwise truly quantitative values can be obtained by making a second precipitation with acetone and water. In this event, the first residue obtained on addition of acetone is simply redissolved in water and acetone is added. The amount of water used depends upon the amount of compound present, 3 cc. being used for amounts between 5 and 10 mg., 5 cc. for amounts over 10 mg., and 2 cc. for less than 5 mg. An equal amount of acetone is added.

11. The calculated amount of sodium pregnanediol glucuronidate is converted into terms of pregnanediol excreted per twenty-four hours as follows:

Example: 800 cc. of a twenty-four hour specimen of urine of 1500 cc. volume are extracted. Two precipitations with water and acetone are carried out, 5 cc. of water being used in each case. The weight of the residue is 25 mg. which represents 85 per cent recovery, making the original amount 29.4 mg.

$$\text{Sodium pregnanediol glucuronidate excreted} = \frac{29.4 \times 1500}{800} \text{ mg. per 24 hours.}$$

$$\text{Pregnanediol excreted} = \frac{29.4 \times 1500 \times 0.597}{800} \text{ mg. per 24 hours.}$$

Studies since carried out have shown that pregnanediol is excreted in both free and combined form. In measuring the amount of combined pregnanediol excreted, error may arise from the fact that spontaneous hydrolysis of the combined pregnanediol into the free form may occur during collection of the urine. To insure maximum accuracy, Bucher and Geschichter[33] recommend that the total pregnanediol excretion be measured. For this purpose they employ a method by which it is possible to recover both the free and combined forms of pregnanediol from the same specimen of urine.

Method of Bucher and Geschichter (1940):

1. Determine the amount of sodium pregnanediol glucuronidate by the method of Venning (*supra*).

2. Free pregnanediol is also extracted quantitatively by this procedure and carried along with the conjugated form until the first acetone precipitation. At this stage, the conjugated form precipitates and is removed by centrifugation.

3. The acetone supernatant contains the free pregnanediol, which is removed by a modified form of Weil's method, as follows:

4. Decant the clear aqueous acetone from the centrifuge cup into a 125 cc. Erlenmeyer flask and allow to stand on a steam bath until it has evaporated to dryness.

5. Add 10 cc. of acetone and a few drops of 0.1 N sodium hydroxide and warm flask gently to dissolve residue. Introduce more sodium hydroxide, a few drops at a time while the mixture is kept warm, until a total of 40 cc. is added.

6. Allow to cool slowly and stand in ice-box overnight. The free pregnanediol precipitates and is filtered out by suction. The precipitate is washed with about 5 cc. of water and a small quantity of hexane and transferred back to the Erlenmeyer flask with hot acetone which is allowed to evaporate off on a steam bath.

7. Purify further by dissolving in 5 or 10 cc. of hot acetone and reprecipitating with three volumes of sodium hydroxide. Stand again in ice-box overnight and filter off.

8. Wash with water and transfer to 50 cc. Erlenmeyer flask. A third precipitation from 2, 3 or 5 cc. of ethyl alcohol by the addition of 2 volumes of water should complete purification. Repeat where desired.

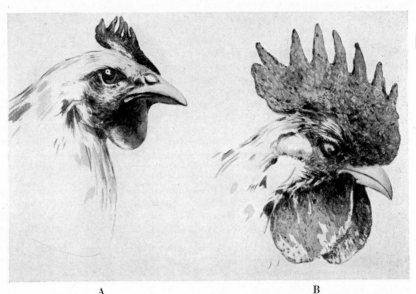

A
B

Fig. 168.—Capon before (A) and after (B) daily topical application of testosterone propionate for two weeks. Note marked growth of comb and wattles.

9. When carrying out above precipitations be careful to add water or sodium hydroxide very gradually while mixture is warmed gently on steam bath.

10. Filter off final precipitate, transfer with ethyl alcohol to a small flask and weigh after the alcohol has been evaporated off in a drying oven.

QUANTITATION OF ANDROGENS IN THE URINE

Both biologic and chemical methods have been devised for the measurement of androgens in the urine. The most widely used biologic assay method depends on the ability of androgenic material to induce comb growth in the caponized leghorn. Less extensively employed are the assay methods based on the ability of the androgens to induce comb growth in the baby chick, or alter the weight and histologic appearance of the prostate and seminal vesicles in the castrate male rat or mouse.

Method of Callow—Capon Comb Test (1936).—A test evolved by Callow,[34] which utilizes the capon, is as follows:

1. Take a 3 liter sample of urine and keep fresh by storing at 0° C. without preservative. Bring the urine to pH 1 with concentrated hydrochloric acid (about 20 ml. per liter when urine is fresh). After bringing it to pH 1, add an additional 20 ml. of hydrochloric acid per liter to render it strongly acid.
2. Place mixture in a flask fitted with a reflux condenser leading to an arrangement for absorbing fumes in alkali, bring it to a boil within one-half to one hour and boil for one hour.
3. Transfer urine to a continuous extraction apparatus and extract with benzene for twenty to twenty-four hours. Free the benzene solution from acid by extracting twice with 50 ml. portions of saturated sodium bicarbonate solution. Free it from phenols by extracting twice with 50 ml. portions of double normal sodium hydroxide, and then washing with water.
4. Evaporate the benzene solution to dryness and extract the residue 4 to 5 times with 10 ml. portions of redistilled ether.

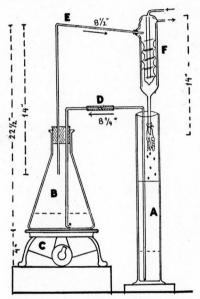

Fig. 169.—Apparatus for chloroform extraction of male and female sex hormones from urine.
(Frank, R. T., et al.: Endocrinol., Vol. 31.)

5. Filter the ethereal extracts through a coarse sintered-glass filter and evaporate the filtrate bit by bit in a small, weighed, flat-bottomed tube.
6. Add sufficient arachis oil from a syringe to the residue (100 to 300 mgm.) to make the volume up to 3 ml. Heat the mixture and stir until all the oil-soluble material has dissolved.
7. Inject 0.1 ml. daily for five days into each of five caponized leghorns. The reaction is positive if there is an average of 5 mm. increase in the length and height of the comb at the end of twenty-four hours after the last injection.

Chick Comb Assay Method of Frank and Associates (1942):[35]

1. Collect urine specimens over a twenty-four, forty-eight, or seventy-two hour period, depending on the purpose of the assay. Refrigeration is not necessary unless gonadotropic assays are also to be performed.
2. Acidify 1000 cc. of the urine with 100 cc. of 37 per cent hydrochloric acid and reflux at once for fifteen minutes. Place the flask containing the mixture in a container of cracked ice to stop further hydrolysis.

3. The hydrolyzed specimen is next extracted with chloroform in a continuous extractor (see Fig. 169). Place one-half of the urine-acid mixture (550 cc.) and 200 cc. of chloroform in a one-liter cylinder (A), and 500 cc. of chloroform in the two liter Erlenmeyer flask (B) which is provided with a two-holed stopper and rests on a hot plate (C). The flask and cylinder are supported as indicated in Fig. 169. A glass siphon tube, with a connecting portion of rubber tubing (D), passes from the bottom of the cylinder to the bottom of the flask; the end within the Erlenmeyer flask is provided with a "J"-shaped outlet as shown. A Hoffman clamp on the rubber portion (D) is left open throughout the process; it is closed only after the extraction is completed and during recovery of the chloroform from the sterol residue as described below. The glass tube (E), which transports the vapor from the flask to the condenser (F), has an inner diameter of 5–6 mm. and is covered with asbestos or cotton for thermal insulation. For finer dispersion of the drops of

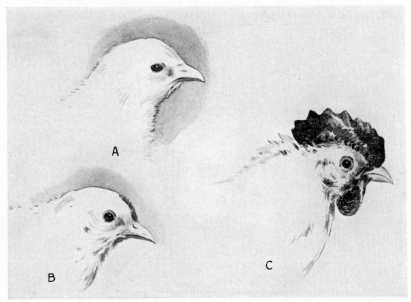

Fig. 170.—Effect of parenterally administered androgenic substance in white Leghorn chick. A, Untreated two and one-half week old chick. B, Untreated five and one-half week old chick. C, Five and one-half week old chick given total of 5 mg. testosterone propionate. Note complete development of comb and wattles.

chloroform which pass through the urine, a streamer of glass wool or gauze is attached to the condenser outlet. With this apparatus, the condensed vapor is allowed to drip through the urine at the rate of about 35 cc. per minute and is automatically siphoned back to the flask for repeated vaporization. The extraction is continued for four hours, two such assemblies being used for each one-liter specimen. After completion of the extraction, the tube (E) is disconnected from the condenser (F), suction is applied to the free end of the tube in order to transfer the chloroform layer from the cylinder to the flask, the screw clamp is closed and the tube (E) re-attached to the condenser. The cylinder containing the urine is then replaced by a receiving flask or bottle and all but about 50 cc. of the chloroform is distilled over. In this way, about 90 per cent of the extracting agent is recovered and can be used repeatedly.

4. The chloroform residues in the two flasks are transferred quantitatively to a single evaporating dish and the remaining chloroform driven off under a fan.

5. The residue is taken up in a total of 100 cc. of ether. If estrogen as well as androgen

assays are to be made on this material, the two are separated with sodium hydroxide at this stage. Otherwise, this separation is not necessary.

6. An aliquot part of this ether solution is transferred to a small Erlenmeyer flask and evaporated at once in an evaporating dish; the residue is preserved for future contingencies.

7. The residue from the aliquot part is taken up in 10 cc. of sesame oil and this solution is employed in the assay.

8. Use single-comb white leghorn chicks, two to three days old. Inject the material daily over a seven day period and kill the chicks with chloroform when nine to ten days old. Injections are made with an ordinary 1 cc. tuberculin syringe with hypodermic needle. Move needle lightly over the entire surface of the comb, applying slowly to minimize spreading to adjacent head feathers. Refrain from inunction to avoid possible mechanical stimulation of comb growth or loss of material. The portion of urine extract contained in the aliquot part of the ether solution is dissolved in 10 cc. of sesame oil. Of this, 0.05 cc. is used for each daily application to each chick; for sixteen chicks treated for seven days, the total volume required is 5.6 cc.

9. Comb size is determined by excision and weighing after the chicks have been killed and their body weights determined. Two parallel longitudinal incisions are made with a sharp scalpel, along the base of the comb at its juncture with the scalp. Remove the entire comb by undercutting directly on the skull. To avoid loss of tissue fluids by squeezing, comb is grasped only once with forceps during the entire procedure. Transfer it immediately to a suitable torsion balance and weigh to the nearest milligram. The initial body weight of each chick is measured to the nearest gram on the day of the first application of the extract. After excising the comb, determine the sex of each chick by laparotomy and inspection of the gonads.

10. Calculation of final result of assay involves use of work chart for which reader is referred to original article.[35]

Chemical Assay of Urinary Androgens and Related 17-ketosteroids.

—Colorimetric tests for the quantitative determination of urinary androgens and related non-phenolic 17-ketosteroids are now employed by several laboratories to replace or supplement the biologic assay methods. They are based on the fact that substances with an active methylene group, especially $CO-CH_2$, produce a red color in the presence of alkali and meta-dinitrobenzene. This reaction was applied to the sex steroids by Zimmermann,[36] in 1935. Observing that the intensity of the color was proportional to the amount of hormone present, this investigator proposed that the reaction be used for the quantitative assay of sex steroids, particularly the androgens. Zimmermann's color reaction has been developed for application to urinary extracts by Wu and Chou,[37] Oesting and Webster,[38] and Callow and associates.[39] The latter workers investigated the degree of specificity of the reaction to find whether it varied with the position of the keto-group in steroid compounds. Data obtained on various 3-, 6-, 17- and 20-ketones showed that, among the steroids, the production of an intense, broad absorption band with a maximum in the green, is characteristic of steroids with a ketone group on the seventeenth carbon atom. To this group of substances, Callow and his associates applied the now generally used term "17-ketosteroids." The 17-ketosteroids found in human urine are of two types, phenolic and non-phenolic. Those which are considered to be the degradation products of androgen metabolism are present in the non-phenolic or neutral fraction of urine extracts. It is therefore necessary, when preparing urine extracts for the assay of "androgens," to obtain the neutral fraction free from the phenolic and acidic fractions. The phenolic 17-ketosteroid, estrone, is removed by washing with alkali.

and is thus excluded from the chemical assay. The principal steroids in the androgen fraction of normal and most specimens of pathological human urines are the a-ketosteroids, androsterone and 3-a-hydroxy-etiocholanone-17, each of which comprises 40 to 45 per cent of the total, and the β-ketosteroids, dehydroisoandrosterone and isoandrosterone, which make up 2 to 15 per cent of the total.[40] Of these, all except 3-a-hydroxy-etiocholanone-17 possess varying degrees of androgenic activity.

The colorimetric tests of Oesting and Callow aroused wide interest and their publication was followed by the appearance of numerous modifications in the details of hydrolysis, extraction, purification, and production of color, aimed at eliminating interfering chromogens present in urine extracts and increasing the accuracy of chemical assay. A standard technique which satisfies all requirements has not yet been adopted. Limitations of space permit a description only of the procedure employed in the Endocrine Laboratory at the Jefferson Hospital. This is as follows:

Reagents:

1. Absolute alcohol.
2. Meta-dinitrobenzene, 2 per cent solution in absolute alcohol, to be kept in the dark.
3. Potassium hydroxide solution, aqueous, 5,000 Normal.
4. Standard androsterone solution in absolute alcohol.
5. Unknowns made to volume with absolute alcohol.

Reagents and solutions (2), (4) and (5) are made up in absolute alcohol at 25° C.

Procedure:

1. Measure out a desired volume of the unknown, but not more than 0.20 cc., placing it in a test tube (6-inch tubes).
2. Add enough absolute alcohol to make exactly 0.20 cc.
3. Add 0.20 cc. of reagent (2) at 25° C.
4. Add 0.20 cc. of reagent (3) and mix thoroughly.
5. Place in the water bath at 25° C. for sixty minutes (keep the water bath in the dark), and shake the tubes at ten-minute intervals.
6. To each tube add 10 cc. of freshly distilled 95 per cent ethyl alcohol, mix well and read at once in the Evelyn photoelectric colorimeter, using filter 540.
7. For the blank tube use 0.20 cc. of absolute alcohol, 0.20 cc. of reagent (2) and 0.20 cc. of reagent (3). Set at 100.
8. For the unknown run a color blank, which requires the following:
   (a) One tube exactly the same as the blank above.
   (b) A second tube with the same amount of the unknown as is used for the determination of the unknown, plus absolute alcohol to make exactly 0.20 cc., plus 0.20 cc. of absolute alcohol in place of the 0.20 cc. of reagent (2), plus 0.20 cc. of reagent (3). Place these tubes in the water bath along with the other tubes. Read tube (a) first by setting it at the point 100 in the Evelyn colorimeter; then mix content from tube (a) with the content of tube (b) and read again in the colorimeter. This is the reading for the color blank.

Determination of value for the constant K:

Blank micrograms of androsterone	Colorimeter (2-lg.G.) reading	Value for K	Average K
25			
" 50			
" 75			
" 100			

$$K—2—10 \text{ g } G \ / \text{ micrograms of androsterone.}$$

Calculation:

Record as follows:

Blank	Reading set at 100	2-log G.	$\dfrac{2\text{-}log.G - yA}{K}$	Net yA for unknown

Color blank
Unknown

Unknown

Unknown

The colorimetric tests for urinary androgens and related 17-ketosteroids are recommended for use as a diagnostic aid, particularly in disorders of gonadal and adrenal cortical function. Some observers also employ them as a means of checking the response to androgen and gonadotropin therapy. The reliability of these tests for diagnostic purposes is still uncertain. It must be emphasized that the Zimmermann color reaction is not specific for androgens as such. Since it is produced by biologically inactive as well as androgenic 17-ketosteroids present in the neutral fraction of urine extracts, the results of colorimetric assay methods tend to be appreciably higher than those obtained by bioassay. According to Callow and others, there exists a significant degree of correlation between the colorimetric assay, expressed in chromogenic equivalents of androsterone per liter of urine, and the biological assay expressed in international units of male hormone activity per liter. Consequently, though not an accurate measure, the colorimetric assay method may nevertheless serve as an index of the level of androgen production.

Application of the colorimetric assay of nonketonic 17-ketosteroids to *gonadal and adrenal cortical disorders* is based on the assumption that these substances are of both gonadal and adrenal cortical origin. This assumption finds support in the observation that they diminish but do not entirely disappear if the function of either the gonads or adrenals is suppressed, as in eunuchism and Addison's disease. On the other hand, an appreciable increase in the level of these compounds is demonstrable in most cases of adrenal cortical hyperfunction due to tumor or hyperplasia. Though their origin in the gonads and adrenals is fairly certain, the value of quantitative determinations of these substances in the diagnosis of gonadal and adrenal cortical disorders is limited because of wide individual variations in their level in both normal and abnormal subjects. The possibility of using assays of urinary androgens as a laboratory aid to diagnosis has been investigated by Callow's group.[41, 42] Their results in a group of patients with gonadal or adrenal cortical hypofunction, taken in conjunction with their earlier studies demonstrating the wide range of variation in the excretion of 17-ketosteroids in patients free from adrenal or sexual disorders, led them to conclude "that the method has, as yet, no diagnostic value, except in certain special cases. . . The estimation of 17-ketosteroids can be carried out with fair accuracy, and can replace biological estimation of androgens, but clear diagnostic significance can only be given to the very high figures which occur in cases of adrenal cortical tumor. In combination with other determinations and with clinical evidence it seems possible that assays of 17-ketosteroids can give some assistance in the diagnosis of pituitary insufficiency and of Addison's disease, in which low values would be confirmatory of other evidence, whilst average or high values would, in the absence of other strong evidence, be inconsistent with those diagnoses."[42] The occurrence of wide individual variations has also been stressed by Hamblen and associates.[43] Their review of reported 17-ketosteroid findings in normal and abnormal conditions up to 1941 led them to conclude that "the only consistently and inordinately increased values for 17-ketosteroids and androgens have been found in adrenal cortical carcinomata." In their own study of cases with simple hirsutism and virilizing syndromes, moderately elevated titers of 17-ketosteroids could be demonstrated in many of the cases, but "striking and unexplainable exceptions" were also encountered.

In general, therefore, it would seem that the chemical assay of urinary androgens and related 17-ketosteroids, like other available methods for the quantitative estimation of sex steroids in the body fluids, has only a limited sphere of usefulness.[61] It gives results which are of little value when taken alone, but may prove useful when viewed in the light of other laboratory and clinical evidence.

QUANTITATION OF GONADOTROPIC HORMONES IN THE BLOOD AND URINE

Quantitative determinations of the gonadotropin content of the blood and urine are widely employed as aids in the diagnosis of functional menstrual disorders, pregnancy, and allied conditions. In pregnancy, where the concentration of these hormones is high, they can readily be detected in the whole blood or urine. In conditions outside of pregnancy, where only small amounts are present, they must be extracted and concentrated before they can be detected and measured by the available biologic tests.

Blood Gonadotropin Tests for Use in Nonpregnant States.—*Fluhmann's Modification of the Aschheim-Zondek Test (1929).*[44]—Fluhmann devised a modification of the Aschheim-Zondek gonadotropin test (see p. 675), which is designed to detect the follicle-stimulating principle in the blood of castrate and postmenopausal women and those with primary ovarian failure. The technique is as follows:

1. Take 15 to 20 cc. of blood, under sterile precautions, from the arm vein of the patient, and centrifugate it or allow it to settle to obtain a clear serum.
2. An immature white mouse, between seventeen and twenty-two days old and weighing 6 to 8 grams, is injected subcutaneously with 0.5 cc. of the clear serum twice daily for four days, making a total of 4 cc.
3. Watch the animal over a period of five days, following the first injection of serum, for the establishment of the vaginal introitus. When this has occurred, make vaginal smears and examine them for the presence of cornified cells alone or with nucleated epithelium and an absence of leucocytes, modifications indicative of estrus. The animal is then killed and the genitalia inspected. To corroborate the smear picture, sections of the vaginal wall and ovaries are prepared for microscopic examination. The finding of mature, unruptured follicles (APR I) indicates the presence of the follicle-stimulating factor; hemorrhagic follicles (APR II), or mature corpora lutea (APR III), alone or in combination, signify the presence of the luteinizing factor (see Figs. 171, 172). A positive reaction indicates that the blood contains at least 50 m.u. per liter.

Fluhmann's test is recommended for the diagnosis of disorders of ovarian function. A negative reaction, if associated with a positive estrogen test, is taken to indicate that the ovary is responsive to pituitary stimulation and capable of utilizing the available gonadotropic hormones. On the other hand, a negative reaction associated with a negative estrogen test suggests ovarian depression secondary to pituitary hypofunction. A positive reaction associated with negative estrogen findings may be interpreted as evidence that the pituitary is functioning normally but the ovary fails to respond because of some inherent defect.

Blood Gonadotropin Test of Frank and Salmon (1936).[45]—To detect the minute quantities of gonadotropin present in the blood of the normal mature male or female, Frank and associates recommend a procedure, by

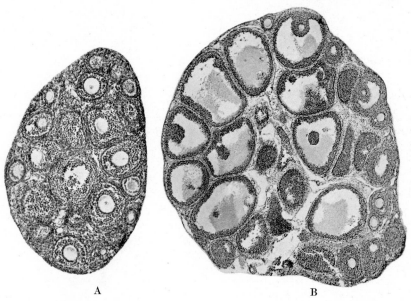

A   B

Fig. 171.—Anterior pituitary reaction I in immature mouse. A, Control ovary showing primordial follicles. B, Stimulated ovary containing numerous developing and mature follicles but no corpora lutea.

which it is possible to demonstrate both the follicle-stimulating and luteinizing principles:

1. Run 40 cc. of freshly drawn vein blood into 150 cc. of cold acetone. A fine precipitate forms, which settles to the bottom.
2. Shake the blood-acetone mixture in a mechanical shaker for twenty minutes, centrifuge it, and pour off the supernatant acetone.
3. Repeat this procedure twice more with 125 cc. of fresh cold acetone.
4. Dry the acetone precipitate under an electric fan, powder it and extract with 100 cc. of water, the mixture being acidified with dilute hydrochloric acid to pH 4.8 (brom-cresol-green).
5. Stir this mixture by hand for ten minutes, centrifuge it and decant the supernatant aqueous extract. Filter the aqueous extract through a single layer of gauze to remove suspended particles.

43

6. Add to the aqueous extract 400 cc. of cold acetone, a fine buff colored precipitate settling out. Allow the mixture to stand in the refrigerator overnight at 45 to 50° F.; centrifuge and discard the acetone.

7. Extract the precipitate with 5 cc. of water alkalinized with dilute sodium hydroxide to pH 8.5 (thymol-blue); centrifuge the mixture, decant the supernatant liquid and adjust to pH 7 with dilute hydrochloric acid (bromthymol blue).

8. Inject this extract in five divided doses over a period of sixty hours into an immature female rat weighing 24 to 26 grams. Sacrifice the animal at the end of ninety-six hours and study the ovaries in serial section. The finding of mature follicles signifies the presence of the follicle-stimulating factor; the finding of hemorrhagic follicles and mature corpora lutea, the presence of the luteinizing principle, their concentration being at least 25 rat units per liter of blood.

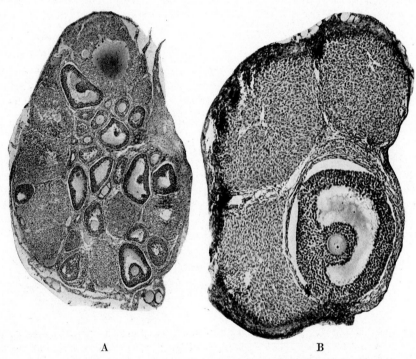

A   B

Fig. 172.—Anterior pituitary reactions II and III in immature mouse. A, Note hemorrhagic follicles ("blutpunkte") (APR II) and corpora lutea (APR III). B, Ovary contains three large corpora lutea (APR III).

Urine Gonadotropin Tests for Use in Nonpregnant States.—

Method of Zondek (1929).[46]—The aim of this test is to detect the small quantities of gonadotropic substance present in the urine outside of pregnancy. It may be of value in the diagnosis of primary ovarian failure.

1. Take 40 cc. of a first morning specimen of urine and, if alkaline, acidify with a few drops of acetic acid.

2. Add 200 cc. of 95 per cent alcohol, shake vigorously, and allow to stand overnight. A precipitate containing the hormone forms at the bottom.

3. Siphon off the supernatant fluid leaving a small amount, about 40 to 45 cc., with the precipitate.

4. Pour the precipitate into a centrifuge tube and centrifuge for about five minutes. Then pour off the alcohol.
5. Add about 30 cc. of ether to the precipitate and stir for about ten minutes, so as to remove estrogen and other impurities.
6. Centrifuge about five minutes and then pour off the ether. Repeat steps (5) and (6).
7. Spread the precipitate around the bottom of the tube with a glass rod and allow to dry, after which add 8 cc. of distilled water and allow to stand for several hours.
8. Centrifuge and discard the precipitate, then keep the clear fluid containing the hormone in a cold place.
9. Inject each of three mice five times within forty-eight hours with the dissolved extract, the first mouse getting 0.1 cc. at each injection, the second 0.2 cc., and the third 0.4 cc.
10. After 100 hours, sacrifice the mice and prepare sections of the ovaries for microscopic examination. Positive reactions with a total of 0.5 cc. of the extract indicate a concentration of 400 m.u. per liter; with a total of 1.0 cc., a concentration of 200 m.u. per liter, and with a total of 2.0 cc., 100 m.u. per liter.

This method achieves only a five-fold concentration of the urine and is therefore not adequate for the detection of the minute quantities of hormone present in normal men and women. For the study of such urines, various methods of concentration have been devised.

Urine Gonadotropin Test of Frank and Associates (1939).[47]—Frank has described a modification of Zondek's alcohol method, by which both the follicle-stimulating and luteinizing principles may be detected in the urine, in conditions outside of pregnancy. It is superior to Frank's earlier acetone extraction method because it requires smaller quantities of urine, thus lessening the toxicity of the extract. It is also an improvement over Zondek's original method, which detects only the follicle-stimulating principle. The procedure is as follows:

1. 400 cc. of fresh urine, or urine stored in the refrigerator at 4.5° C., is acidified with glacial acetic acid to pH 3.5 (bromcresol-green).
2. Four volumes (1600 cc.) of 95 per cent ethyl alcohol are added to the urine, and the preparation kept from six hours to overnight in a refrigerator at 4.5° C.
3. The clear supernatant liquid is poured off and the remainder centrifuged in a 250 cc. centrifuge tube.
4. Wash the precipitate three times with ether, using 75 cc. for each washing, to remove the estrogen.
5. Dry the precipitate under a fan or keep it in a refrigerator. Transfer the dry precipitate quantitatively to a 15 cc. centrifuge tube, using no more than 6 cc. of distilled water for the transfer.
6. Triturate the preparation thoroughly with a glass rod and then centrifuge for ten minutes. Pour the supernatant liquid into a graduated centrifuge tube and add distilled water to exactly the 6 cc. mark.
7. The solution is now ready for injection into immature female rats weighing 30 grams without further pH adjustment (average pH 6.7; widest variations found, 5.7 to 7.5). If the ovaries of the test animals contain mature follicles, hemorrhagic follicles and mature corpora lutea, it denotes the presence of the follicle-stimulating and luteinizing principles in the urine.

Urine Gonadotropin Test of Levin (1941).[48]—

1. Chloroform preserved urine is chilled (5° C.) and brought to pH 4.5 to 5.0 (methyl red or bromcresol green) by adding glacial acetic acid.

2. Add immediately a freshly prepared aqueous tannic acid solution, 50 cc. of 20 per cent solution usually being sufficient for a twenty-four-hour urine specimen. An immediate precipitate forms.

3. Stir mixture thoroughly and allow to stand in refrigerator for thirty to ninety minutes. Siphon off the supernatant solution, portions of it being used to quantitatively transfer the precipitate into 250 cc. centrifuge bottles. The supernatant solution is also used to facilitate collection of the precipitate into one centrifuge bottle after the centrifugation, which should be of only short duration.

4. After centrifuging the entire urine and collecting the precipitate in one bottle, suspend it immediately in 200 to 250 cc. of 95 per cent ethanol and completely break up all lumps.

5. Centrifuge the mixture and twice thoroughly extract the insoluble residue with 80 per cent ethanol, using 250 and 100 cc. volumes, respectively. Then wash with a small amount of acetone followed by washing with ether. It is finally freed of residual ether by reduced pressure. Bottle containing dry precipitate is stoppered and stored for assay.

6. To prepare dry powder for assay, extract with dilute alkali at pH 8.5 to 9.0 (phenolphthalein). The final volume of the extract is calculated (dependent on the volume of urine and concentration of gonadotropin expected) and slightly less than one-third of this volume of water is added to the pulverized precipitate.

7. Dilute alkali (0.5 to 1.0 NNaOH or NH_4OH) is added drop-wise until pH 8.5 to 9.0 is attained. Stir mixture thoroughly so all particles are completely broken up and remove residue by centrifugation. This residue is similarly re-extracted two more times, any material remaining insoluble after the third extraction being discarded.

8. Combine the three alkaline extracts and adjust to pH 7.5 (phenol red) by drop-wise addition of dilute acetic acid. Dilute the extract to the calculated volume and remove suspended material, if any, by centrifugation. This extract is to be used for injection and should be stored in a refrigerator at all times. No more than twenty-four hours should elapse between making the extract and injection.

9. *Assay method.*—Use five or more twenty-one- to twenty-three-day-old female mice, weighing 7 to 10 gm. The material is injected in three equal portions at twenty-four-hour intervals. The animals are killed seventy-two hours after the first injection. The reaction is positive if the uterus shows a weight increase of 100 to 150 per cent above that of the controls.

Levin maintains that the tannic acid precipitation method is more satisfactory than any other thus far proposed for the quantitative determination of urinary gonadotropin in normal men and women. He lists among its advantages that it is quantitative, yields extracts sufficiently nontoxic to permit large quantities of urine to be injected into the assay animal, and is sufficiently simple and rapid to make possible the handling of large numbers of urine samples.

Urine Gonadotropin Test of Varney and Koch (1942).[49]—

1. Chill urine and adjust to pH 4.8 to 5.2 with acetic acid. Then add four volumes of ethanol.

2. Collect the crude alcohol precipitate thus formed by settling and centrifugation in the freezing room. Where urine of castrate or postmenopausal women is being assayed, this crude precipitate can be injected without further treatment, but with less active urines it is necessary to remove the toxic substances.

3. Extract the crude alcohol precipitate with 50 per cent ethanol and reprecipitate the activity from the solution by adding four volumes of alcohol.

4. *Assay method.*—Use immature female white mice, weighing 6 to 8 gm., four or more animals being used at each dosage level. Levels injected are calculated so that a positive response in each successive dosage group of animals corresponds

to 10, 20 and 30 units per twenty-four-hour sample of urine from normal males and females. The material to be assayed is dissolved or suspended in 3 cc. of saline and 0.5 cc. is injected subcutaneously twice daily for three days. Kill the animals on the morning of the fifth day. The uteri are removed, freed of connective tissue and contained fluid, and weighed on a torsion balance. A mouse uterine unit is defined as the amount of activity necessary to cause a 100 per cent increase in uterine weight above that of the controls.

Varney and Koch claim that this method assures a higher yield of gonadotropin and less toxicity than the benzoic acid, tannic acid, or other procedures used by other investigators.

Gonadotropic Hormone Tests for Pregnancy and Allied Conditions.

—Most widely used for the diagnosis of early pregnancy and related conditions are the Aschheim-Zondek and Friedman tests, based on the presence of large amounts of luteinizing hormone in the urine.

Urine Gonadotropin Test of Zondek and Aschheim (1929).[50]—

1. Take a morning sample of urine and add one drop of tricresol per 25 to 30 cc. of urine. Acidify slightly with a few drops of 10 per cent dilute acetic acid.
2. Use five immature female white mice, each weighing 6 to 8 grams and three to four weeks old.
3. Inject the urine subcutaneously twice daily for three consecutive days as follows: in animal I, 6 × 0.2 cc.; in animal II, 6 × 0.25 cc.; in animal III, 6 × 0.3 cc.; in animal IV, 6 × 0.35 cc.; and in animal V, 6 × 0.4 cc.
4. Perform autopsy ninety-six hours after the first injection; examine the ovaries macroscopically and, where the reaction is doubtful, microscopically.
5. The test is positive if a single hemorrhagic follicle (APR II) or corpus luteum (APR III) is present in the ovary of any of the test animals.

To shorten the time required for a reaction, Zondek proposed the following modification:

1. Slightly acidify 66 cc. of morning urine with a few drops of 10 per cent acetic acid and then filter.
2. Add 240 cc. of 96 per cent ethyl alcohol and shake for five minutes, when a yellow white precipitate forms.
3. Allow to stand for thirty minutes and then centrifuge; take up the sludge, throw it down to 30 to 50 cc. of ether, and shake for three minutes.
4. Remove the ether and take up the residue in 11 cc. of distilled water; shake for five minutes and centrifuge. Preserve the supernatant fluid for injections. This contains the active principle and represents a six-fold concentration of the urine. Inject 0.4 cc. of this substance into each of four immature female mice, four times on the first day and twice on the second day.
5. Perform autopsy fifty-one to fifty-seven hours after the first injection. Since the corpora lutea do not form so early in this species, the presence of hemorrhagic follicles (APR II) constitutes a positive reaction.

Friedman Rabbit Test (1931).[51]—This is at once the most rapid and reliable modification of the Aschheim-Zondek pregnancy test thus far evolved. It is based on the observation that the mature female rabbit, unlike most other mammals, does not ovulate spontaneously but can be made to do so by the injection of an adequate amount of human pregnancy urine. Friedman observed that the intravenous injection of such urine in the mature unmated rabbit is followed within twenty-four to forty-eight hours by follicular rupture and corpus luteum formation. The procedure is as follows:

1. Take a first morning specimen of urine.
2. Select an adult female rabbit weighing no less than 4 pounds, which has been isolated for a period of three weeks before being used, to exclude the possibility of post-coital ovulation. The animal must be in estrus at the time of injection. Since the external criteria of estrus, namely reddening of the vulva and accessibility to the male, are not entirely reliable, Friedman prefers to use the postpartum animal to insure the existence of estrus.
3. Place the animal in a box with an opening on the side large enough to admit its ear or its entire head. Rub the ear with alcohol or xylol and then immediately inject the urine slowly into the marginal vein. Friedman's original method called for the injection of 4 cc. of urine three times on each of two successive days. The author prefers to inject 10 cc., followed twelve hours later by a second injection of 5 cc.
4. At the end of forty-eight hours after the first injection, kill the animal and remove the ovaries for examination. The test is positive if fresh corpora lutea or large corpora hemorrhagica are present.

When employing this test, skill in reading the reaction is most essential. In the words of Wilson and Corner,[52] "A positive test is determined by the presence in the ovaries of recently ruptured graafian follicles indicated by bright red elevations of conical form, a millimeter or two in diameter, having usually a small depression in the center. Inexperienced observers may possibly find it difficult to distinguish these ruptured follicles from large unruptured follicles which are somewhat engorged. The unruptured follicles are rounded rather than conical or mammillary in form, show no central stigma or depression, and are much paler and clearer. A hand lens may aid in the discrimination. Still more confusing are the rather frequently present hemorrhagic unruptured follicles, more or less peculiar to the rabbit. These are usually of dull red color approaching black, are generally smaller and less prominent than the ruptured follicles." They point out further that if there appear very large clear follicles verging on rupture, the result remains doubtful and a second test becomes advisable. Significance should not be attached to small black areas representing old corpora lutea, or to mere congestion of the uterus and ovaries. If macroscopic inspection leaves the technician in doubt, the ovaries should be microscopically examined.

Space does not permit a description of the numerous modifications of the Friedman test. Some prefer the immature to the mature rabbit, some favor single rather than multiple injections and some, laparotomy rather than autopsy; but aside from such minor alterations, the essentials of the test remain the same.

Frog (Xenopus laevis) Test for Pregnancy.—This test utilizes the South African clawed frog (*Xenopus laevis*) as a test animal. It is based on the observation that the mature female xenopus extrudes eggs after the injection of human chorionic gonadotropin. Though it has enjoyed some popularity abroad, it has only recently been introduced in this coun-

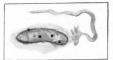
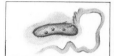
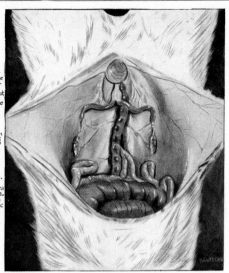

FRIEDMAN RABBIT TEST

Basis:- Marked increase in gonadotropic hormone content of the
urine following conception.
Test Animal:- Sexually mature
unmated female rabbits not
less than 4 months old and
isolated for one month before
test is performed.
Biologic Criteria:-
Ovulation and formation of
corpora lutea in ovary.
Procedure:-
(1) Inject into the marginal vein
of the ear 10 C.C. of morning
urine.
(2) Give second injection of
10 C.C. ten to fifteen hours
later.
(3) Autopsy at end of 48 hours
after first injection and
remove ovaries for inspection.
Reaction:- Positive when sub-serous
hemorrhagic areas or corpora
lutea are present in ovaries.
Negative if clear retention
follicles without hemorrhagic
areas are seen.

POSITIVE

NEGATIVE

ASCHHEIM-ZONDEK TEST

Basis:- Marked increase in gonadotropic hormone content of the
urine following conception.
Test Animal:- Infantile white mouse
weighing 6-8 lbs. or 3 to 4 weeks
old.
Biologic Criteria:- Production of hemorrhagic follicles or corpora lutea in
ovary.
Procedure:-
(1) Inject each of 5 animals subcutaneously with 2.4 C.C. morning urine in 9 divided doses in
the course of 3 days.
(2) Autopsy on fifth day after
the first injection and examine ovaries macroscopically
with a hand lens or if in
doubt microscopically.
Reaction:- Positive when the ovaries
show hemorrhagic follicles or
corpora lutea.

POSITIVE

NEGATIVE

ESTRIN TEST (MAZER-HOFFMAN)

Basis:- Marked increase in estrin content of urine following conception
Test Animal:- Sexually mature
castrated white mouse
Biologic Criteria:- Estrual changes in
the vaginal epithelium
Procedure:-
(1) Inject each of 3 animals subcutaneously with 12 C.C. morning
urine in 6 divided doses in the
course of 2 days.
(2) Take vaginal smears 3 times
daily on the third and fourth
day.
Reaction:- Positive when vaginal smear taken
66 hours after the first injection
shows estrual changes.

DI ESTRUM   PRO ESTRUM   ESTRUS

POSITIVE

NEGATIVE

Evaluation

	Total No. of Cases	Correct Results	Incorrect Results				Percent of error
			False Positives	Percent	False Negatives	Percent	
FRIEDMAN TEST	870	853	13	1.5	8	0.9	2.4
ASCHHEIM-ZONDEK TEST	511	487	8	1.6	15	2.9	4.5
MAZER-HOFFMAN TEST	526	429	5	0.9	92	17.4	18.3

Fig. 173.—Biologic tests for pregnancy.

try by Weisman and his associates,[53] who claim a high degree of accuracy (98 to 100 per cent) for it. Their procedure is as follows:

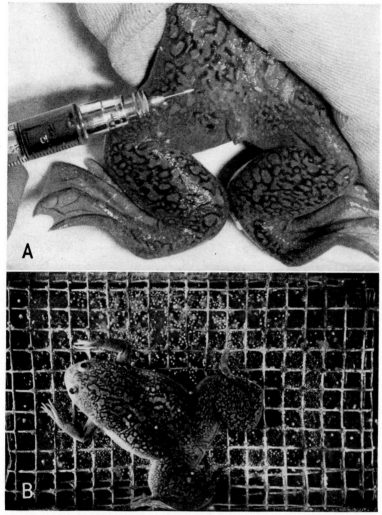

Fig. 174.—Frog (*Xenopus laevis*) test for early pregnancy. A, Position of needle during injection of 1 cc. of urine concentrate equivalent to 40 cc. of whole urine. B, Positive reaction. Note numerous extruded eggs. This may occur from four to eighteen hours after injection. (Courtesy of Dr. A. I. Weisman.)

1. Use three 12-gallon aquaria for each group of eight frogs. Tank A is used as "rest" tank, where animals recuperate for four weeks after having extruded eggs in a positive reaction. Tank B is the "negative reaction" tank in which frogs not reacting to urine rest for one week. Tank C is the "active" tank containing animals ready for use.

2. Water in tanks is kept at ordinary room temperature (70° F.) and maintained at level of 3 inches from bottom. Frogs are fed small strips of beef heart, calves liver and garden worms (if available) twice each week. Replace tank water with

fresh water of same temperature prior to each feeding and twenty-four hours after each feeding. Animals should not be fed for at least twenty-four hours before injection to avoid regurgitation which would interfere with reading the reaction.

3. For actual test, standard 2-gallon fish tanks are used. Half-inch wire mesh is bent to form a platform about 1 inch from bottom to prevent frog from devouring extruded eggs. Have 3 inches of water in tank and cover tank with glass plate kept firm by taping and weights to prevent exit of frog. Leave small space between glass plate and frame of tank to permit passage of air. The room should be of even temperature, bright and airy.

4. *Concentration of Urine.*—From 4-ounce specimen of morning urine take 80 cc. and add to it twice the volume of acetone. Stir mixture thoroughly and allow to stand for about fifteen minutes to allow hormones and proteins to precipitate and settle to bottom. Decant supernatant fluid and save for redistillation. Allow precipitate to dry, speeding drying with electric fan. Add 2 cc. of distilled water to dry precipitate and stir thoroughly. Pour mixture into small centrifuge tube, centrifuging to bring down insoluble proteins and other material, leaving gonadotropin in solution.

5. Immediately prior to injection, decant supernatant fluid and adjust with 10 per cent sulphosalicylic acid to pH 5.5 (nitrazine paper, Squibb). Use 1 cc. of concentrate for each injection. The remaining 1 cc. may be reserved for a later recheck or used simultaneously in a second animal. Each cubic centimeter of the final concentrate is equivalent to 40 cc. of whole urine.

6. Inject frog subcutaneously by means of a short insulin-type needle. To reach lymph space, thrust needle superficially into the left thigh muscle, directing point medially to the midline of the dorsum, $\frac{1}{2}$ inch above the upper cloacal fold. Throughout its course the needle should be seen clearly just beneath the skin. A firm gentle thrust carries through the connective tissue into the lymph space. Care must be taken to avoid puncturing lung.

7. After injection, place animal in separate waiting "test tank" and observe at intervals after the first four hours. Eggs may be extruded as early as four hours but usually appear in six to twelve hours.

Weisman and his associates claim 99.6 per cent accuracy in a series of 267 cases. Though the accuracy of this method is well established, its general adoption in this country has thus far been hampered by the difficulty of obtaining the test animals.

Two methods which utilize the immature white rat have recently been devised by Frank and Berman[63] and by Salmon and his associates.[64] Both claim the advantages of economy and speed, as compared with the Aschheim-Zondek and Friedman tests. In Frank's test, a positive reaction can be obtained within twenty-four hours; in that of Salmon's group, marked hyperemia of the ovaries, which is stated to be specific for human chorionic gonadotropin, is demonstrable as early as six hours after injection of the urine. The reliability of these methods awaits confirmation by other laboratories.

Blood Gonadotropin Test for Fetal Death: *Method of Rakoff (1940).*[53]—Rakoff recommends the following test for the diagnosis of fetal death:

1. Collect 25 cc. of blood and allow it to clot.
2. Separate the serum in the usual fashion.
3. Employ six infantile mice about seventeen days old, and weighing 8 to 10 grams.
4. Inject each of three mice with a total of 2 cc. of serum (0.66 cc. daily for three days);

inject each of the three remaining mice with a total of 1 cc. of serum (0.33 cc. daily for three days). Kill the animals on the fifth day.

5. The test is positive if at least one corpus hemorrhagicum or corpus luteum can be found in one ovary. If this appears in one or more of the animals receiving a total of 1 cc. of serum (100 m.u. per 100 cc.) it indicates the fetus is about to die. If a positive reaction is obtained only in one of the animals receiving a total of 2 cc. of serum (50 m.u. per 100 cc.), death of the fetus has already occurred.

Miscellaneous Tests for Pregnancy.—In the search for a simple, quick and inexpensive method, many tests besides those already described have been proposed for the diagnosis of early pregnancy. These include the *bitterling test*, which has been generally disappointing, and numerous skin tests and chemical or chemicohormonic reactions which have aroused particular interest because of their speed and the simplicity of their execution. Unfortunately, none of them has a degree of accuracy even approaching that of the gonadotropic hormone tests. A *skin test* recently evolved by Falls and associates[55] calls for the intradermal injection of a colostrum solution. Falls claims 96 per cent of the nonpregnant women tested reacted with a characteristic wheal and areola, while 98 per cent of his pregnant subjects showed no such reaction. In the hands of several competent observers,[56, 57] this test has thus far proved unreliable.

BIBLIOGRAPHY

1. Novak, E.: J.A.M.A. *104*:1497, 1935.
2. Sharman, A., and Sheehan, H. L.: Brit. Med. J. *1*:965, 1937.
3. Tamis, A. B.: Am. J. Obst. & Gynec. *32*:505, 1936.
4. Klinger, H. H., and Burch, J. C.: J.A.M.A. *99*:559, 1932.
5. Mason, L. W., and Black, W. C.: Am. J. Obst. & Gynec. *39*:1022, 1940.
6. Stockard, C. N., and Papanicolaou, G. N.: Am. J. Anat. *22*:225, 1917.
7. Allen, E.: Am. J. Anat. *30*:297, 1922.
8. Allen, E., and Doisy, E. A.: J.A.M.A. *81*:819, 1923.
9. Papanicolaou, G. N.: Am. J. Anat. *52*:519, 1933.
10. Rubenstein, B. B.: Endocrinol. *27*:843, 1940.
11. Krohn, L., Harris, J., and Hechter, O.: Am. J. Obst. & Gynec. *44*:213, 1942.
12. Hamblen, E. C., Cuyler, W. K., and Baptist, M.: Am. J. Obst. & Gynec. *44*:442, 1942.
13. Papanicolaou, G. N., and Shorr, E.: Am. J. Obst. & Gynec. *38*:392, 1939.
14. Shorr, E.: Science *94*:545, 1941.
15. Geist, S. H., and Salmon, U. J.: Am. J. Obst. & Gynec. *31*:806, 1936.
16. Papanicolaou, G. N.: Proc. Soc. Exper. Biol. & Med. *22*:436, 1925.
17. Smith, B. G., and Brunner, E. K.: Am. J. Anat. *54*:27, 1934.
18. Astwood, E. B.: Endocrinol. *23*:25, 1938.
19. Frank, R. T., and Goldberger, M. A.: Proc. Soc. Exper. Biol. & Med. *32*:1663, 1935.
20. Fluhmann, C. F.: Endocrinol. *18*:705, 1934.
21. Kurzrok, R., and Ratner, S.: Am. J. Obst. & Gynec. *28*:689, 1932.
22. Smith, G. V., and Smith, O. W.: Am. J. Physiol. *112*:340, 1935.
23. Smith, O. W., Smith, G. V., and Schiller, S.: Endocrinol. *25*:509, 1939.
24. Pincus, G., and Zahl, P. A.: J. Gen. Physiol. *20*:879, 1937.
25. Mazer, C., and Hoffman, J.: Am. J. Obst. & Gynec. *17*:186, 1929.
26. Frank, R. T.: J.A.M.A. *109*:1121, 1937; J. Mt. Sinai Hosp. *8*:514, 1942.
27. Marrian, G. F.: Biochem. J. *23*:1090, 1929.
28. Butenandt, A., and Schmidt, J.: Ber. d. deutsch. chem. Gesellsch. *67*:1901, 1934.
29. Venning, E. H., Henry, J. S., and Browne, J. S. L.: Canad. M. A. J. *36*:83, 1937.
30. Browne, J. S. L., and Venning, E. H.: Proc. Soc. Exper. Biol. & Med. *34*:792, 1936.
31. Venning, E. H.: J. Biol. Chem. *119*:473, 1937.

32. Venning, E. H.: J. Biol. Chem. *126*:595, 1938.
33. Bucher, N. L. R., and Geschickter, C. F.: Endocrinol. *27*:727, 1940.
34. Callow, R. K.: Lancet *2*:565, 1936.
35. Frank, R. T., Klempner, E., Hollander, F., and Kriss, B.: Endocrinol. *31*:63, 1942.
36. Zimmermann, W.: Ztschr. f. physiol. Chem. *233*:257, 1935.
37. Chou, C. Y., and Wu, H.: Chinese J. Physiol. *11*:413, 1937.
38. Oesting, R. B., and Webster, B.: Endocrinol. *22*:307, 1938.
39. Callow, N. H., Callow, R. K., and Emmens, C. W.: Biochem. J. *32*:1312, 1938.
40. Baumann, E. J., Metzger, N., and Sprinson, D. B.: Endocrinol. *30*:518, 1942.
41. Callow, N. H., Callow, R. K., Emmens, C. W., and Stroud, S. M.: J. Endocrinol. *1*:76, 1939.
42. Callow, N. H., Callow, R. K., and Emmens, C. W.: J. Endocrinol. *2*:88, 1940.
43. Hamblen, E. C., Cuyler, W. K., and Baptist, M.: J. Clin. Endocrinol. *1*:763, 1941.
44. Fluhmann, C. F.: J.A.M.A. *92*:1744, 1929; Am. J. Obst. & Gynec. *20*:1, 1930.
45. Frank, R. T., and Salmon, U. J.: Proc. Soc. Exper. Biol. & Med. *34*:363, 1936.
46. Zondek, B.: Endokrinol. *5*:425, 1929.
47. Frank, R. T., and Berman, R. L.: Endocrinol. *25*:996, 1939.
48. Levin, L.: Endocrinol. *28*:378, 1941.
49. Varney, R. F., and Koch, F. C.: Endocrinol. *30*:399, 1942.
50. Aschheim, S., and Zondek, B.: Klin. Wchnschr. *7*:1401, 1928.
51. Friedman, M. H., and Lapham, M. E.: Am. J. Obst. & Gynec. *21*:405, 1931.
52. Wilson, K. M., and Corner, G. W.: Am. J. Obst. & Gynec. *22*:513, 1931.
53. Rakoff, A. E.: Pennsylvania M. J. *43*:669, 1940.
54. Weisman, A. I., Snyder, A. F., and Coates, C. W.: Am. J. Obst. & Gynec. *43*:135, 1942; West. J. Surg. *50*:557, 1942.
55. Falls, F. H., Freda, V. C., and Cohen, H. H.: Canad. M. A. J. *41*:431, 1941.
56. Pulver, M., and Posner, L. B.: Am. J. Obst. & Gynec. *44*:690, 1942.
57. Goldman, L. M., Kessler, H. B., and Wilder, M. E.: J.A.M.A. *119*:130, 1942.
58. Mack, H. C.: Harper Hosp. Bull. *1*:54, 1942.
59. Mack, H. C., and Ale, T.: J. Clin. Endocrinol. *2*:361, 1942.
60. Mack, H. C.: J. Clin. Endocrinol. *3*:169, 1943.
61. Pincus, G.: J. Clin. Endocrinol. *3*:301, 1943.
62. Burch, J. C., and Phelps, D.: J. Clin. Endocrinol. *3*:475, 1943.
63. Frank, R. T., and Berman, R. L.: Am. J. Obst. & Gynec. *42*:492, 1941.
64. Salmon, U. J., Geist, S. H., Salmon, A. A., and Frank, I. L.: J. Clin. Endocrinol. *2*:166, 1942.

CHAPTER XL

SEX HORMONE FINDINGS IN THE BLOOD AND URINE

ESTROGEN FINDINGS IN NORMAL AND ABNORMAL CONDITIONS

Normal Children.—The newborn of both sexes excrete appreciable amounts of estrogen, which is probably derived from the maternal circulation since it disappears by the third or fourth day after birth. During childhood, minute quantities again appear in the urine. Zondek and Euler[1] demonstrated from 5 to 20 mouse units per liter in girls between six and eleven years of age. According to Dorfman and coworkers,[2] girls between eleven and thirteen excrete from 10 to 20 I.U. daily, and those between fifteen and sixteen, as much as 95 I.U.

Normally Menstruating Women.—*Blood Estrogen.*—Loewe, in 1925,[3] first demonstrated estrogen in the blood of normal mature women, and described cyclic variations in the level of this hormone in the course of the menstrual cycle. In the following year, Frank and Goldberger[4] noted that estrogen becomes demonstrable in 40 cc. of blood on the twenty-first day, rises to a peak one to two days before the onset of the flow, and then drops rapidly. Later, with a more sensitive test (see p. 655), they obtained a positive reaction with 40 cc. of blood (25 m.u. per liter) between the twenty-first and fourteenth day, and with 10 to 20 cc. (50 to 100 m.u. per liter) between the seventh day and the appearance of the flow.

Fluhmann,[5] by means of his mucification test (see page 655), demonstrated a peak of estrogen in the blood on the fourteenth or fifteenth day of the cycle, and a second one shortly before the flow. He believes the first to be related to ovulation, but attributes the second peak to release into the circulation of estrogen stored in the uterine mucosa.

Frank and Goldberger[6] believe that, in the mature woman who bleeds cyclically at monthly intervals, the presence of at least one mouse unit of estrogen in 40 cc. of vein blood obtained during the week preceding the flow, is a reliable index of normal ovarian function. According to the author's experience as well as that of Janney,[7] and Ford and Mueller,[8] this assumption does not seem altogether justified. Ford and Mueller found that 40 cc. of blood obtained premenstrually did not invariably give a positive Allen-Doisy reaction, while an equal amount of blood obtained during the early part of the cycle, when the estrogen concentration is presumably low, was not invariably negative. The author has simultaneously studied the estrogen content of the blood and the histologic appearance of endometrial tissue taken premenstrually. Pregravid secretory modifications, indicating functioning luteal tissue, were not always associated with a positive blood estrogen reaction. On the other hand, the estrogen test was not infrequently positive in women whose endometria showed varying degrees of proliferative activity but no luteal effect. Thus, while a positive estrogen reaction is fairly reliable evidence of follicular activity, it is not a dependable index of full ovaran function including ovulation and corpus luteum formation.

Urine Estrogen.—Studies of the estrogen content of the urine in the course of the menstrual cycle have yielded varied results. Cyclic increases in the concentration of the hormone have been noted by some observers only at the midperiod, while others have reported a second elevation shortly before the flow. According to Kurzrok and Ratner,[9] the normally menstruating woman excretes from 10 to 20 and sometimes as much as 30 rat units per liter (for technique see p. 657). Werner[10] has more recently reported values ranging from 5 to 50 rat units per twenty-four hour specimen. Zondek and Euler[1] found 50 mouse units per liter during the postmenstrum, and 300 units at the supposed time of ovulation. The lowest values have been obtained during the flow. Estimates of the total estrogen output during the entire menstrual cycle vary from less than 1,000 to over 2,000 m.u. At the peak of excretion, from 200 to 500 m.u. per twenty-four hour specimen have been reported. In a recent study, D'Amour[128] found the maximum peak of estrogen excretion to be 1000 I.U. in twenty-four hours. The total output in an entire cycle ranged from 5000 to 10,000 I.U.

The precise *relationship between the estrone and estriol* content of the urine in the normal mature woman is not established. Dingemanse and coworkers[11] found the proportion to be 1:1. Smith and his associates,[12] on the other hand, found that more estrone than estriol is excreted throughout the cycle, and that the absolute amount of estriol is greater during the luteal phase than during the follicular phase or menstruation. The estrone level rises with the onset of the flow, so that the estrone-estriol ratio on the first two days of menstruation is twice as high as at any other time of the cycle. According to Palmer,[13] estrogen is excreted in "free" form at the midperiod; a rise in "free" estrogen occurs before the onset of the flow, but none is demonstrable during menstruation.

Menstrual Disorders.—*Amenorrhea.*—On the basis of their estrogen findings in the blood and urine, Frank and his coworkers[14] divide cases of amenorrhea into four groups. *Group I* includes women with a subthreshold estrogen cycle. The estrogen level in the blood and urine here is below normal but shows the usual cyclic variations seen in the normally menstruating woman. In *group II* belong women who have a distinct blood estrogen cycle but whose urine contains less than 10 m.u. per liter. Women in *group III* show no estrogen cycle in the blood and less than 10 m.u. per liter in the urine. *Group IV* includes women with no estrogen in either the blood or urine. Zondek[15] has called attention to so-called *"polyfolliculin" amenorrhea*, in which the estrogen content of both the blood and urine is appreciably higher than in the normal nonpregnant woman. Frank's and Zondek's findings have been confirmed by the author and others.

Functional Uterine Bleeding.—In functional uterine bleeding, the estrogen content of the blood and urine may be normal or low,[16, 17] but is more often high. Seguy[18] found an excess of estrogen in the blood of cases of puberty and maturity bleeding associated with polycystic ovaries and endometrial hyperplasia. In uterine bleeding alternating with amenorrhea, Zondek[19] demonstrated above normal amounts of estrogen in the urine. Frank[20] found that some of his cases of excessive uterine bleeding excreted a total of 4,000 to 10,000 m.u. in the course of thirty days, though their blood estrogen values were subnormal. In five cases of abnormal uterine bleeding associated with endometrial hyperplasia, Seegar[21] found the urine estrogen within normal limits in three and excessive in two. The values varied widely between one individual and another and at different times in the same individual, ranging from less than 10 to 116 rat units in twenty-four hours. Smith and Smith[22] obtained high urine estrogen values in ten cases of abnormal uterine bleeding. All the hormone was excreted in the form of "X" estrogen, which they believe is probably estradiol. They interpret this as evidence of increased elaboration and destruction of estrogen, which is produced so rapidly that it spills over into the urine before it can be converted into estrone. The absence of estriol they attribute to a deficiency of progesterone.

Normal Pregnancy.—*Blood Estrogen.*—The blood estrogen gradually increases following conception. During the first eight weeks the hormone level is relatively low, but after this point it rises steadily to a peak just before term. Frank and Goldberger[6] could elicit a positive Allen-Doisy reaction with 10 to 15 cc. of blood (66 to 100 mouse units per liter) as early as the third week of gestation. More recently, these observers[23] found that the blood estrogen level remains approximately at the highest nonpregnant level (25 to 35 mouse units per liter) until the seventeenth week. After this point, there is a steady upward trend to a maximum of from 600 to 1300 mouse units per liter at term. Zondek[24] obtained values up to 300 m.u. per liter of blood during the fourth month, and from 800 to 1,000 m.u. at term, while Rakoff[25] found less than 1 m.u. in 4 cc. of blood serum before the eighth week and an average of 24 m.u. per 100 cc. from the eighth to the tenth week of gestation. A sudden rise occurred between the fourteenth and twentieth week and a second rise between the thirty-second and thirty-sixth week. At term, he obtained values of 500 m.u. or more per 100 cc. of blood.

Urine Estrogen.—The estrogen level of the urine rises steadily after conception, reaches its highest point at term, and rapidly disappears after delivery. Mazer and Hoffman[26] were the first to utilize the postconceptional rise in urinary estrogen as the basis for a test for early pregnancy (see p. 661). Zondek[27] found from 300 to 600 m.u. per liter of urine during the first eight weeks of gestation. After this the estrogen level rose until term, when the yield was as much as 20,000 m.u. per liter. In a more recent study, Browne and Venning[28] found the daily excretion of estrogen varied from 200 to 1,000 I.U. before the eighth week, and from 15,000 to 40,000 I.U. at term.

Human pregnancy urine contains estrogen, estriol, and probably also estradiol. The first two compounds are excreted in both "free" or active and "conjugated" or inactive form. Cohen and coworkers[29] found that only a very small proportion is excreted in the "free" form during the first eight months. A few weeks before the onset of labor the "free" estrogen rises appreciably, while the "combined" form diminishes, though it continues to make up the major part of the total urinary estrogen. Smith and Smith,[22] observed that, from the time of the second missed period, the excretion of estriol dropped off markedly. This coincided with an increase in the potency of the estrone fraction, due, they believe, to the presence of estradiol. Whether the pre-labor rise in "free" estrogen and change in the estrone-estriol ratio contribute to the initiation of labor is not established. Bachman,[30] who employed a colorimetric method in six normal pregnant women, found that apart from a gradual rise in estriol and estrone output with the approach of term, there were no constant patterns of hormonal excretion. The increases in estrogen excretion were too gradual and the individual variations in the peak levels too marked to make possible any forecast of the date on which labor would begin. Nor could he correlate the variations in the individual daily excretion with the length of the labors. He concluded that the rate at which estrogen or its end-products are excreted before parturition gives no clue to the role of the hormones in the processes of parturition.

Fetal Death.—Frank[31] was the first to point out that the level of urinary estrogen falls within twenty-four hours after fetal death. Evidence that death of the fetus is more rapidly reflected in the estrogen than in the gonadotropin content of the body fluids was provided by Bland and his associates,[32] who found the Mazer-Hoffman urine estrogen test (see p. 661) negative in eight cases of fetal death, at a time when the Aschheim-Zondek urine gonadotropin test (see p. 675) was still positive in four. This was subsequently confirmed by Spielman and his coworkers,[34] whose blood estrogen test for pregnancy was negative in all of their thirty-three cases of suspected abortion, whereas a urine gonadotropin pregnancy test performed simultaneously was positive in 50 per cent of the series. They concluded that tests based on the estrogen content of the body fluids are more reliable for the diagnosis of fetal death than the gonadotropin tests. The author's experience fully substantiates this conclusion.

Threatened and Habitual Abortion.—Estrogen findings in threatened and habitual abortion have been too varied to be of diagnostic or prognostic value. Smith and Smith[34] could demonstrate no significant deviation from normal. Browne and associates,[35] on the other hand, obtained low values in women who subsequently aborted. Where abortion threatened but did not occur, the estrogen level remained normal throughout, or fell to a low level at first and then rose again to normal values. In a third group with a history of habitual abortion, whose pregnancy was clinically normal, the estrogen values remained normal throughout. Palmer[36] has described a case aborting at the fourteenth week, in which the estrogen concentration rose steadily until the twelfth week. One week before abortion the total urinary estrogen dropped, but the proportion of the "free" form increased. Just before the abortion, the total estrogen, made up mainly of the "free" form, rose higher than at any previous time, but an abrupt drop soon followed.

Late Toxemias of Pregnancy, Hydatid Mole and Chorionepithelioma.—The blood estrogen tests are of little prognostic value in the late toxemias of pregnancy, for high, low and normal levels have been encountered (see Chap. XXXI). Studies of the estrogen level in mole and chorionepithelioma are limited. Jeffcoate[37] demonstrated large amounts of "free" estrogen in the blood in three cases of hydatid mole. While some workers[38] report low urine estrogen values in chorionepithelioma, Smith and Werthessen[39] found values up to 1,000 gamma of estrone and 100 gamma of estriol per twenty-four hours as compared with 100 gamma of estrone and 500 gamma of estriol in normal pregnancy. In one case observed by the author, the urine estrogen values were also appreciably elevated.

Castrate and Menopausal Women.—At the menopause, the estrogen content of the blood and urine shows marked individual variations which apparently depend on the degree of follicular activity present. Zondek[40] divides the menopause into a polyfolliculin and oligofolliculin phase, the former characterized by an excess, the latter by a deficiency of estrogen in the body fluids. During *the polyfolliculin phase*, he obtained values ranging from 200 to 500 m.u. daily. Recent studies indicate that though the cessation of menstrual function is usually followed within a short time by a marked drop in the estrogen content of the blood and urine, small amounts continue to appear in the body fluids many years after the menopause. This is also true of the surgical and x-ray castrate. Laroche and associates[41] found over 20 r.u. per liter of urine in bilaterally oophorectomized women, while Eng[42] obtained values ranging from 2 to 15 m.u. per liter. In two surgical castrates, Frank and his coworkers[14] found from 15 to 200 m.u. per liter. Over a period of one month they excreted a total of 255 and 720 m.u. respectively, as compared with 1500 in the normal cycle. No estrogen was demonstrable in the blood. It has been suggested that the estrogens found in the body fluids of castrate and postmenopausal women are derived from some extra-ovarian source, probably the adrenal cortex.

Granulosa Cell Tumors of the Ovary.—It is generally agreed that granulosa cell tumors are often associated with large quantities of estrogen in the blood and urine, and that their removal is soon followed by a return to normal values. For example, in a three year old girl studied by Glass and McKennon,[43] the urine yielded 400 m.u. per liter before operation and from 0 to 20 m.u. after removal of the tumor. Neumann[44] demonstrated 326 m.u. in a five day urine specimen from a patient who developed a granulosa cell tumor nine years after the menopause. In a forty-two year old woman observed by Stohr,[45] assays of the urine on the day immediately following removal of a granulosa cell tumor revealed an estrogen concentration of 172 mouse units per liter.

Normal Adult Males.—The presence of estrogen in male urine was first demonstrated by Laqueur,[46] in 1927. The estrogen level in the normal adult male approaches that in the normal nonpregnant woman, but cyclic variations are not demonstrable. Koch[47] obtained values ranging from 90 to 120 I.U. daily. The source of these estrogens is not clear. Eng's[42] observation that male castrates excrete only from 2 to 17 mouse units per liter, suggests that the major part of the hormone in the normal male is of testicular origin, the remainder being derived from some extra-gonadal source, probably the adrenal cortex.

Testicular Tumors.—There is some evidence indicating that estrogen excretion may be increased in males with testicular tumors containing chorionepithelial tissue. In two patients observed by Smith and Smith,[38] the amount of urinary estrogen exceeded that found in the normal male but was less than that excreted by the pregnant woman. Frank[20] obtained values ranging from 25 to 250 mouse units per liter of urine in five men with chorionepithelioma testis.

Adrenal Cortical Carcinoma.—Malignant adrenal cortical neoplasms, according to Frank,[48] are usually associated with high estrogen levels in the urine, the values exceeding 500 I.U. per liter. In the presence of benign tumors or hyperplasia of this gland, the values are below this level.

PREGNANEDIOL FINDINGS IN NORMAL AND ABNORMAL CONDITIONS

The pregnanediol content of the urine has been investigated in the normal nonpregnant woman, as well as in menstrual and reproductive disorders. The available data, though sufficiently consistent to constitute a satisfactory basis for further study, is still too limited to be of much practical value.

Normally Menstruating Women.—In a study of regularly menstruating women, Browne and Venning[49] could demonstrate pregnanediol only during that phase of the menstrual cycle when a functioning corpus luteum is presumably present in the ovary. In their series of cases, this substance was continuously excreted over a period of three to twelve days. The values at first were low, only 1 mg. being excreted in twenty-four hours. The peak was reached within a few days, when as much as 5 mg. could be extracted from a twenty-four hour specimen. The compound disappeared rather abruptly from one to three days before the flow. The total excretion in any one cycle varied from 30 to 54.6 mg. In a more recent study, D'Amour[128] obtained values ranging from 5 to 8 mgm. and occasionally as much as 11 mgm. daily. The total output in an entire cycle averaged 50 mgm., though values up to 86 mgm. were obtained.

Similar studies carried out by other investigators have shown that pregnanediol excretion is not always continuous, though it is never absent for more than one day during the period of excretion. In some cases it is present up to the onset of the flow or even beyond. Wilson and his co-workers,[50] who correlated the endometrial picture with the pregnanediol content of the urine, found that significant amounts first become demonstrable during the late proliferative phase of the cycle, that is, just before the appearance of secretory modifications of the mucosa.

Browne and Venning[49] believe that low pregnanediol values are a reliable index of deficient luteal activity. This they base on their observation that subnormal amounts of this compound were excreted by several regularly menstruating but sterile women. An association between low pregnanediol titers and subnormal luteal function has also been suggested by Wilson and his associates,[50] who obtained low values in fifteen of sixteen women whose endometria showed a mixture of hyperplastic and secretory changes. On the other hand, several investigators[51-54] have questioned the reliability of the pregnanediol level as an index of the amount of progesterone produced. They point out that low or negative values may be obtained where the endometrial picture indicates progestin is present, while, conversely, positive findings may be encountered where the endometrium[51, 54] and vaginal smears[133] show no evidence of luteal effect. Low or negative values despite the presence of progestin are readily explained. As Buxton[53] has pointed out, there are many variables concerned in the process of progesterone metabolism and pregnanediol excretion. Since the liver, kidney, and possibly other factors play a part in this transformation and excretion, a disturbance in any of these may lower pregnanediol excretion without necessarily affecting the secretion and utilization of progesterone. It is likely that such factors as the collection of the urine, its preservation, and technique of extraction, are partly responsible for the variable results obtained with the quantitative tests. Positive pregnanediol findings despite absence of luteal effect in the uterine and vaginal mucosa are less easily accounted for. It has been suggested that progestin is present in such cases but evokes no response in the endometrium or vaginal mucosa because of some inherent condition which makes them refractory. Of interest is Hechter's[134] suggestion that the material obtained in such cases is not sodium pregnanediol glucuronidate but another substance of similar solubility properties and macroscopically indistinguishable from small amounts of pure amorphous sodium pregnanediol glucuronidate. To distinguish between these two substances, this observer has devised a chemical method wherein sodium glucuronidate is determined by the estimation of copper reducing activity obtained after acid hydrolysis. It is to be hoped that improvements in technique and recognition of the presence of impurities will eventually minimize the sources of error inherent in pregnanediol determinations and increase their value as an aid in the diagnosis of luteal function. For the present, it would appear that the cyclic appearance of normal amounts of pregnanediol is strong presumptive evidence of ovulation and corpus luteum formation. Low values or complete absence of this substance, on the other hand, are suggestive, particularly if they recur on repeated tests,[54] but cannot be considered conclusive.

Menstrual Disorders.—Both low[54] and negative[52] values have been reported in women with anovulatory cycles. In primary and secondary amenorrhea, the findings have been negative in the vast majority of the cases.[51, 54] In one case observed by Hamblen,[51] however, amenorrhea of six years' duration was associated with a persistent estrogenic endometrium and the cyclic excretion of pregnanediol in amounts totaling from 13 to 24 mg. Excessive or irregular bleeding from an estrogenic endometrium has been found associated with high, low or negative findings.[21, 54, 135] It would thus appear, as Hamblen[51] has emphasized, that the excretion of pregnanediol cannot be regarded as proof that the endometrium is undergoing progestational modifications, while absence of secretory changes does not

44

necessarily exclude the occurrence of ovulation and corpus luteum formation.

Normal Pregnancy.—Browne and his associates,[35] in a study of nine normal pregnant women, found that the level of pregnanediol during the first sixty-nine days of gestation did not appreciably exceed that of the luteal phase of the infertile cycle, the daily excretion ranging from 4 to 10 mg. A rise occurred between the eightieth and one hundredth day and continued steadily to a maximum of 105 mg. per twenty-four hours by the eighth month. Variations in the rate of excretion were noted, but they could not determine whether these were of a cyclic nature. Other investigators have obtained up to 25 mg. daily during the early weeks of gestation, and as much as 155 mg. daily during its terminal phase. During the last weeks of gestation, Bachman[30] could demonstrate no marked or sudden changes in the pattern of pregnanediol excretion from which the date or character of the oncoming labor might be forecast.

It has been suggested that the pregnanediol excreted during the first three months of gestation is derived chiefly from the corpus luteum of pregnancy. After this point, the placenta is believed to be its main source. This assumption finds support in the observation that the compound disappears rapidly from the urine following delivery.

Abortion and Fetal Death.—The hope that studies of pregnanediol excretion may be an aid in the diagnosis and prognosis, and serve as a guide in the treatment of habitual or threatened abortion, is not borne out by the available data. Though several investigators have demonstrated subnormal values preceding abortion, cases have been encountered in which interruption of pregnancy occurred in the presence of normal pregnanediol values, or failed to occur despite subnormal values. According to Stover and Pratt,[55] negative or low values, even when associated with symptoms, do not necessarily signify that abortion is inevitable. The value of such studies as a diagnostic aid and therapeutic guide in habitual and threatened abortion has also been questioned by Hamblen.[56] Cope[57] believes that complete absence of pregnanediol is nearly always evidence of serious abnormality, suggesting in early pregnancy the imminence of abortion, and in late pregnancy, death of the fetus. Normal values, he maintains, do not definitely exclude the possibility of impending abortion or fetal death, while the significance of low values must remain uncertain for the present.

Toxemias of Pregnancy.—Subnormal values in the late toxemias of pregnancy have been reported by several investigators.[58, 59] Cope,[60] on the other hand, obtained values within normal limits in ten cases of toxemia uncomplicated by nephritis. Noting an absence of pregnanediol during the last week of gestation in one case of chronic nephritis, he concluded that deviations from normal pregnanediol titers are probably due to interference with its excretion and are not related to the toxemia.

Adrenogenitalism.—Venning and her associates[61] demonstrated pregnanediol in two cases of adrenogenitalism, while Finkler[62] found a persistently high concentration of this substance in one instance. In the latter case, 25.5 mg. was the average amount excreted daily. Finkler interprets this as evidence of excessive androgenic activity of the adrenal cortex, and suggests that high pregnanediol titers associated with amenorrhea in the nonpregnant woman point to a masculinizing ovarian neoplasm, or to hyperplasia or tumor of the adrenal cortex. According to Talbot and his associates,[129] the pregnanediol values are not consistently elevated in patients with adrenal cortical hyperplasia. Though above normal in some cases, they are within the limits of normal in others. These findings are particularly significant because they demonstrate that excretion of this compound is not associated exclusively with luteal or placental activity.

ANDROGEN FINDINGS IN NORMAL AND ABNORMAL CONDITIONS

Androgenic activity has been demonstrated in the urine of both sexes, and is at least partly attributable to the presence of androsterone and dehydroandrosterone. The reported values differ widely, due probably to variations in the techniques employed.

Normal Children.—The urine of children of both sexes contains small amounts of androgenic substance. Daily fluctuations occur but no cycle of excretion is demonstrable. The values in girls are somewhat lower than in boys. In both sexes, the androgen level tends to rise with the approach of puberty. The reported values range from less than 1 I.U. in young children to 20 I.U. at puberty.[2, 63, 64]

Normal Adult Males.—According to Gallagher's group,[65] the normal adult male excretes the equivalent of about 7 mg. (70 I.U.) of androsterone daily. Dingemanse and his associates[66] found from 15 to 170 units per liter, while Fraser and his coworkers,[67] who employed a colorimetric assay method, obtained values ranging from 8.1 to 22.6 mg., the average being 13.8 mg. daily. All observers agree there is no cyclic curve of excretion comparable to that of estrogen in the adult female. The androgen level is of no value as an index of spermatogenic function, but it may provide a clue to the incretory status of the testis and help in the differential diagnosis between psychic impotence and that due to a deficiency of the testicular hormone. The importance of interpreting androgen values in the light of other clinical evidence has been emphasized by D'Amour and Gustavson.[68] To quote: "In the early work on the testicular hormone, it was assumed that the androgenic material which could be extracted from normal urine was the 'male sex hormone' and that the biologic assay of urinary extracts would give an index to the level of testicular secretion. However, androgenic activity is not specific to one substance, and at least two related compounds with androgenic activity, androsterone and dehydroandrosterone, are present in the mixture of neutral compounds which can be prepared from urine. Further, these two compounds occur in the urine of both sexes. This distinction between hormones and excretory transformation products is confirmed by the discovery that testosterine is degraded in the human body to give androsterone and the sterioisomeric, inactive compound aetiocholan–3 (a)– ol–17–one. Androgenic substances in the urine may be derived from the adrenal cortex, since quantities of androgens and related steroids have been isolated from the urine in adrenal cortical disease. For these reasons, the comb-growth promoting activity of urinary extracts, which consists of a complex mixture of degradation products, may not be an index of the production of androgen."

Eunuchoid, Castrate and Senile Males.—Eunuchoid males excrete appreciably less androgen than normal men. In seven such individuals, Kenyon and his associates[69] obtained values which were one-third of those obtained in normal males, though in some cases the androgen level reached the lower limits of normal. In male castrates, Fraser's group[67] found an average of 7 mg. daily, as compared with 13.8 mg. in the normal male. Callow and Callow[70] found that the urine of a eunuch contained the same compounds, namely androsterone, transdehydroandrosterone, and etiocholan–3 (a)– ol–17–one, which are present in the urine of normal males, but the relative proportion of transdehydroandrosterone was greater. They suggest a possible adrenal cortical origin.

Kochakian[71] noted a gradual drop in androgen excretion after the forty-fifth year. Most workers agree that though the androgen level falls with advancing age, small amounts continue to be demonstrable in the senile individual.

Normal Mature Women.—The normal mature woman regularly excretes androgenic substances. Some investigators believe that such urine contains only epipregnanolon, a substance related to androsterone, but others[70, 72] maintain that the androgens in female urine are quantitatively and essentially similar to those in the male. In general, the values in the female approach those in normal men. Talbot and his associates[64] report values ranging from 1.4 to 47.3 mg. by colorimetric assay, and from 5 to 100 I.U., by the capon test. Werner's[10] values ranged from 5.4 to 19.6 mg. per twenty-four hour specimen. While it is generally agreed that marked daily fluctuations occur, it is not clear whether there is a monthly cycle of excretion. While several investigators report failure to demonstrate such a cycle,[10, 64, 65] others report a rise at the beginning of the cycle,[70] a drop during menstruation,[73] or a rise at this time.[74]

Normal Pregnant Women.—Studies of androgen excretion during gestation are limited. Dingemanse and his associates[11] demonstrated from 8 to 30 units per liter between the sixth and eighth month. According to Hain,[75] the amount tends to increase toward the end of pregnancy, but is at all times below the level for the nonpregnant woman.

Menstrual Disorders.—*Functional Uterine Bleeding.*—In irregular or excessive uterine bleeding, Drips and Osterberg[76] found the androgen values low or normal, except where the condition was associated with hirsutism. In the latter type of case, high values were obtained. Hamblen and his associates[73, 77] observed no significant deviation from normal values in irregular bleeding from an estrogenic endometrium. They noted a tendency to drop during the bleeding phase, when an average of 50 I.U. was excreted in contrast to 72 I.U. during the nonbleeding phase.

Amenorrhea.—In amenorrhea, Drips and Osterberg[76] found the values normal. Where there was an associated hirsutism, normal or high levels prevailed. Hamblen's group[78] report normal or slightly subnormal levels in primary amenorrhea with delayed or incomplete sexual maturation.

In secondary amenorrhea of six months or more, the values showed an elevation roughly proportional to the duration of the amenorrhea, the average range being from 21 to 101 I.U. per twenty-four hour specimen. Frasier's group[67] report subnormal levels in primary amenorrhea.

Castrate and Menopausal Women.—Androgen excretion tends to increase during the menopause and following x-ray or surgical castration. Hamblen and his coworkers,[78] and Ross[79] report increases of 50 to 100 per cent. This heightened excretion may persist for many years, but the level eventually returns to normal. Callow,[80] on the other hand, observed a drop in the androgen level following castration, though in some cases the values were within normal limits. Frasier's group[67] found the values essentially normal in the surgical and natural menopause. Hirschmann[81] has isolated dehydroisoandrosterone, androsterone, and etiocholan–3(a) – ol–17–one from the urine of ovariectomized women, and suggests a probable adrenal cortical origin.

Adrenal Cortical Disease and Masculinizing Ovarian Tumors.— *Adrenal cortical insufficiency,* according to Callow,[80] is associated with low androgen values. On the other hand, *adrenal cortical hyperfunction* due to hyperplasia or tumor, is usually accompanied by a marked increase in androgen excretion. Transdehydroandrosterone and etiocholan–3(a)– ol– 17–one have been isolated from the urine of such patients. Simpson[82] found that women with adrenal cortical hyperfunction excrete up to 200 and, in extreme cases, 500 capon units daily, as compared with 50 units, the upper limit of normal in the mature nonpregnant woman. In one case of adrenal cortical carcinoma, Kenyon and his associates[69] obtained values up to 480 I.U. daily. The rise in androgen excretion has been proposed as an aid in the differential diagnosis between Cushing's disease due to adrenal cortical tumor and that of pituitary origin, where the level is apparently within normal limits.[64, 83] According to Talbot and his associates,[129] the total 17–ketosteroid excretion is abnormally increased in patients with adrenal cortical hyperplasia or adrenal cortical carcinoma. Though the values in the latter condition tend to be higher, the highest values in adrenal cortical hyperplasia overlap the lowest values in carcinoma. These observers found, however, that the beta-alcoholic and nonalcoholic 17– ketosteroids are markedly increased in carcinoma and either normal or only slightly increased in hyperplasia. They therefore propose that the quantitative determination of those two fractions, rather than the total 17–ketosteroids is a reliable aid in the differential diagnosis.

In *virilism,* without gross pathologic changes in the adrenals, Kenyon[69] and Simpson[82] found normal or high levels. Talbot's group[64] could demonstrate no appreciable increase, and even where this occurred, the values were considerably less than in patients with adrenal cortical lesions. Ross and his associates[84] report above normal levels in thirty out of thirty-four cases of virilism. The average values ranged from 34 to 228 I.U. daily and tended to parallel the degree of virilization. As a rule, the highest levels were encountered in patients with verified adrenal cortical hyperplasia. In pseudohermaphroditism, normal or somewhat elevated levels have been found.

In *arrhenoblastoma,* it would appear from the limited evidence at hand, that androgen excretion is increased but less markedly than in adreno-genitalism.[85–87]

GONADOTROPIC HORMONE FINDINGS IN NORMAL AND ABNORMAL CONDITIONS

Since the gonadotropins of the adenohypophysis control sex function, their concentration in the blood and urine might be expected to serve as a reliable index of pituitary gonadotropic activity and thus aid in the diagnosis and prognosis of menstrual and reproductive disorders. The data obtained through quantitative studies of the gonadotropins in the body fluids have thus far only partially justified this expectation.

Normal Children.—The body fluids of the newborn contain appreciable amounts of predominantly luteinizing substances. These are apparently derived from the maternal circulation, since they disappear a few days after birth. Small amounts of predominantly follicle-stimulating hormone are demonstrable in the urine of both sexes during childhood. According to some workers, the hormone concentration is related to the developmental status rather than the choriological age of the individual. Frank[20] obtained 2 m.u. per liter of urine in a four-year-old girl and 4 m.u. per liter in another, aged nine. In children approaching the menarche he found about one-half the amount normally excreted by the adult. Freed[88] could detect little or no gonadotropin in children under five years of age, but after this it appeared in increasing amounts and by the tenth year he obtained values equivalent to those in the adult. Katzman and Doisy,[89] and McCullagh and Cuyler[90] also found the concentration of the hormone higher at puberty than during childhood.

Normal Mature Women.—Frank and Salmon[91] demonstrated a rise in the blood gonadotropin level between the ninth and twelfth day of the cycle, when 40 cc. of blood gave a positive reaction in the mouse (for technique see p. 671). On the ninth day, only the follicle-stimulating fraction was demonstrable, but by the twelfth day, a luteinizing reaction could also be obtained.

The available data indicate that small amounts of gonadotropin are continuously excreted by the normally menstruating woman. Some investigators have noted a peak of excretion only at the midperiod, while others observed a second one just before or during the menstrual flow. Zondek[92] could detect only the follicle-stimulating fraction in such urine. He obtained values up to 8 rat units in the postmenstruum, 25 units in the intermenstruum, 29 units in the premenstruum, and 25 rat units during the flow. Frank[93] found as much as 500 cc. of urine negative at all times of the cycle except the tenth to the fourteenth day, when a positive follicle-stimulating and luteinizing reaction could be obtained with amounts ranging from 40 to 500 cc. (2 to 25 rat units per liter) (for technique see p. 673). One of his patients excreted a total of 80 and 54 rat units in two successive cycles. Drips[94] observed that gonadotropic hormone was not always demonstrable and, when present, varied in amount from 5 to 15 rat units per liter. The time of its appearance showed wide individual variations. The hormone was usually demonstrable on the thirteenth day of the cycle, but at times could only be detected shortly before or during the flow. D'Amour and his coworkers[95] performed daily tests on five women in the course of 29 cycles. In four cycles no peak was demonstrable and they therefore suggested that these were probably of the anovulatory type. In the remaining twenty-five cycles, the peak occurred from twenty-one to sixteen days before the flow, regardless of variations in the length of the cycles. It is of interest that no case showed more than one peak, whereas in an earlier study, with a less sensitive test requiring the use of larger quantities of urine, they noted two peaks in many of the cases. In a more recent study, D'Amour[128] found that the total output varied greatly from cycle to cycle, values ranging from 4 to 150 I.U. being recorded. At the midcycle peak, most cases excreted 16 I.U. in twenty-four hours. According to Varney and his associates,[130] the normally menstruating woman excretes from less than 10 up to 50 m.u. daily (for technique see p. 674).

Disorders of Menstrual and Reproductive Function.—The gonadotropin content of the blood and urine increases appreciably in primary ovarian failure. Fluhmann,[96] the author[97] and others have found that the Fluhmann test (see p. 671), which depends on the presence of at least 50 mouse units of the follicle-stimulating hormone per liter of blood, is usually positive in such cases, though regularly negative in the normal mature woman. In a group of women with menstrual disorders accompanied by vasomotor symptoms and other manifestations of primary ovarian failure, Drips and associates[94] found from 20 to 66 rat units per liter of urine as compared with a maximum of 15 rat units in the normally menstruating woman. On the basis of these and other similar reports, it is now generally believed that a rise in the follicle-stimulating hormone content of the body fluids, particularly if associated with negative estrogen findings, is reliable evidence of primary ovarian failure. The Fluhmann test is therefore helpful in distinguishing between amenorrhea due to primary ovarian damage, and that traceable to pituitary deficiency, where little or no gonadotropin is demonstrable in the body fluids.

Normal Pregnancy.—In normal pregnancy, the body fluids contain large quantities of a predominantly luteinizing substance, the blood values roughly paralleling those in the urine. The hormone appears in ever increasing amounts within a few days after the first missed period. The peak of excretion is reached during the first third of gestation, after which the level gradually drops. Zondek[98] found an average of 10,000 mouse units per liter of blood during early pregnancy. Evans and associates[99] noted a sharp rise in the blood between the thirtieth and forty-sixth day of gestation. In one case, they found 100,000 rat units per liter on the thirty-seventh day and 500,000 rat units on the fortieth day. Rakoff[100] found an average of about 1600 mouse units per 100 cc. of blood between the fifth and sixth week. From the eighth to the tenth week the level rose to over 3,000 mouse units per 100 cc. By the twentieth to the twenty-fourth week it dropped to about 300 units, after which there was little change for the rest of gestation.

In the urine as in the blood, the concentration of gonadotropin rises rapidly following fertilization. According to Evans and associates,[99] the peak is reached at some time between the twentieth and the fiftieth, but most often on the thirtieth day after the first missed period. Their cases fell into two groups; those whose maximum daily output ranged from 75,000 to 150,000 rat units, and those in whom it varied from 750,000 to over 1,000,000 rat units. After the peak, the hormonal concentration decreased rapidly to 10,000 rat units by the sixty-fifth day, and this level was maintained for the rest of pregnancy. Browne and Venning[101] demonstrated a peak between the fifty-second and sixty-fourth day, when the urine contained from 133,000 to 400,000 rat units per liter. At the sixty-seventh day, the hormone level fell sharply to 40,000 rat units per liter, while after the one-hundred and twentieth day the values ranged from 1,500 to 5,000 rat units per liter.

The concentration of the gonadotropic hormones tends to be appreciably higher in multiple pregnancy. For example, Schoeneck[102] demonstrated 80,000 rabbit units per liter in a case of twin pregnancy, as compared with 20,000 rabbit units per liter in single pregnancy.

Ectopic Pregnancy.—Available data relating to the gonadotropin content of the blood and urine in ectopic pregnancy consists mainly of the results of pregnancy tests performed after the appearance of symptoms. This probably accounts for the large percentage of false negative tests. Aschheim and Zondek[103] obtained a negative reaction in four out of fourteen cases, and Goldberger and coworkers[104] in 32 per cent of forty-four cases. A negative pregnancy test is generally taken to signify that the chorion has ceased to discharge gonadotropin into the maternal circulation, either because it has degenerated and lost its secretory function or, though still secreting, is no longer in contact with the maternal circulation. It therefore follows that a negative pregnancy test does not necessarily exclude ectopic pregnancy. A positive test is of little assistance in distinguishing between intra- and extra-uterine pregnancy, but it is of distinct value in differentiating ectopic pregnancy from adnexal disease which may clinically simulate it.

Fetal Death.—The luteinizing hormone in the blood and urine during pregnancy is generally believed to be secreted by the viable chorionic elements. Death of the fetus does not necessarily immediately break the connection between the chorion and the maternal circulation; nor does placental degeneration cause an abrupt cessation of chorionic hormone secretion. For this reason, a positive gonadotropin pregnancy test is not per se reliable evidence that the fetus is still alive. On the other hand, a steady decline in the concentration of the chorionic gonadotropins, as ascertained by repeated quantitative determinations, may be of distinct diagnostic and prognostic value. According to Brindeau and his associates,[105] the presence of 1,000 to 4,500 rabbit units per liter of blood indicates normal pregnancy, while values under 500 rabbit units signify interrupted pregnancy. In a recent study, Rakoff[100] observed that after fetal death, the chorionic hormone content of the blood progressively dropped to subnormal values. He believes a drop below 100 m.u. per 100 cc. of blood indicates that the fetus is dead or about to die, while values below 50 m.u. per 100 cc. indicate that death has already occurred. Observing that the drop to values under 100 m.u. per 100 cc. of blood preceded a negative Friedman test of the urine by one week or more, Rakoff concluded that fetal death is more rapidly reflected in the serum gonadotropin. For this reason, he prefers the blood to the urine gonado-tropin tests (see p. 678) for the diagnosis of fetal death.

According to Chosson and Donnet,[106] from 1,000 to 4,500 rabbit units per liter of urine indicate normal pregnancy; 800 to 1,000 units raise a doubt as to whether pregnancy is normal or has been interrupted; while under 800 units indicate that gestation has been interrupted.

Toxemias of Pregnancy.—The blood of patients with hyperemesis gravidarum, according to Anselmino and Hoffmann,[127] and Rakoff[100] con-tains excessive amounts of gonadotropin. Brindeau and his coworkers,[105] Schoeneck,[102] and Ehrhardt[107] found that the urine contains twice the amount present in normal pregnancy. Evans' group,[99] on the other hand, observed that none of the minor disturbances common in early pregnancy occurred in cases where the early peak of gonadotropin excretion was be-tween 750,000 and 1,000,000 rat units daily, while women found to be excreting from 75,000 to 150,000 units experienced varying degrees of nausea and discomfort.

In preeclampsia and eclampsia, most observers report an abnormally high level of gonadotropin in the blood. Brindeau and his coworkers[105] found from 25,000 to 50,000 rabbit units per liter of blood, as compared with 10,000 to 12,000 units in normal pregnancy. Anker and Laland[108] demonstrated from 250,000 to 333,000 rat units per liter of blood. Studies of the urine in the late pregnancy toxemias have yielded high, normal or low values.[59]

Hydatid Mole and Chorionepithelioma.—Fels[109] and Rössler[110] were the first to point out that the body fluids of patients with hydatid mole and chorionepithelioma contain chorionic gonadotropin in amounts far exceeding those of normal pregnancy. Zondek,[98] on the basis of his earlier quantitative studies, concluded that 5,000 to 30,000 m.u. per liter of urine are the limits for normal pregnancy, over 50,000 m.u. suggest pathologic change, and values approaching 200,000 m.u. per liter make the diagnosis of mole or chorionepithelioma likely. In a more recent communication,[131] this observer stated that the presence of increased amounts of the follicle-stimulating factor is important in the diagnosis. Values up to 200,000 m.u. of this factor per liter of urine point to hydatid mole but malignant de-generation is unlikely. When the values rise to 500,000 m.u. per liter, chorionepithelioma may be suspected, while values in the millions make the diagnosis of malignant degeneration certain. The presence of 400 m.u. of the luteinizing factor per liter of spinal fluid is also significant. Because of the importance in the diagnosis of increased follicle-stimulating hormone in the body fluids, he recommends the use of the Aschheim-Zondek mouse test in preference to the Friedman rabbit test, which detects only the luteinizing factor. The values for mole and chorionepithelioma, reported by other investigators, range up to 800,000 mouse units per liter.[111] In studies employing the rabbit as the test animal, from 20,000 to 400,000 rabbit units per liter of urine have been found. The values in the blood in these conditions range from 2,000 to 333,000 units per liter.[111] In one case of chorionepithelioma observed by Zondek,[131] the blood contained 3,000,000 m.u. of the follicle-stimulating factor (APR I) per liter.

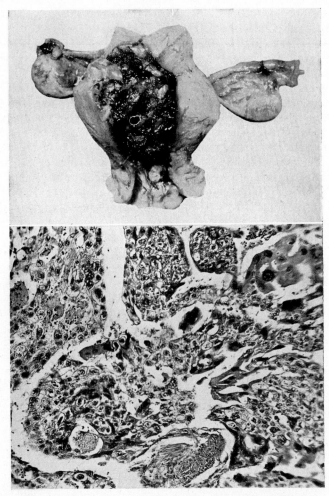

Fig. 175.—Chorionepithelioma of the uterus. Upper, Gross. Lower, Histologic appearance. Uterus and adnexa removed from a thirty-five year old female, four months after expulsion of a hydatid mole. Gonadotropin tests of both blood and urine, performed at short intervals following delivery of mole, gave abnormally high values. Estrogen values were within normal limits. Following operation, repeated gonadotropin tests negative.

The excretion of chorionic gonadotropin may persist for several weeks after mole delivery. If, after this time, the hormone continues to be demonstrable or its concentration increases, chorionepithelioma may be suspected, provided that a new gestation has been ruled out. The gonadotropic hormone tests may also aid in the prognosis, particularly where the diagnosis of chorionepithelioma has been established and the growth removed. If repeated quantitative estimations reveal no chorionic gonadotropin, it may be assumed that the growth has been completely eradicated. On the other hand, persistently high or rising excretion values point to recurrence and metastases.

Sources of Error.—The biologic tests for the diagnosis of hydatid mole and chorionepithelioma are not infallible. Values comparable to those encountered in mole and chorionepithelioma have been reported in normal pregnancy. Conversely, chorionic pathology may sometimes be associated with values equal to or below those of normal pregnancy.[112, 113, 132] A few observers have reported negative Friedman tests shortly before death in cases of chorionepithelioma with metastases.[114] A low gonadotropin level in the presence of mole may be due to degeneration of the growth or loss of contact with the maternal circulation. Low values in cases of malignant chorionepithelioma with metastases are difficult to explain. Fatal delay in removing the malignant growth, or unjustified abdominal section in cases of normal pregnancy, has been the experience of some observers who relied solely on the hormone findings. Such errors emphasize the importance of interpreting the results of the biologic tests in the light of the history, physical findings, and evidence yielded by endometrial curettage.

Castrate and Menopausal Women.—Menopausal women, and x-ray and surgical castrates excrete increased quantities of gonadotropin. The hormone concentration shows marked daily fluctuations but no cycle of excretion is demonstrable. Most workers report that the follicle-stimulating hormone content of the body fluids is increased, but Frank[115] maintains that a rise in luteinizing hormone is likewise demonstrable, provided that appropriate extraction methods are used (see p. 673). The rise is usually apparent within a short time after the extinction of ovarian function and may persist for many months or years. According to Fluhmann,[96] the blood contains at least 50 m.u. per liter. The values in the urine, as reported by Zondek[116] and others, exceed 110 m.u. and may sometimes reach 400 m.u. per liter. Drips and associates[94] demonstrated from 25 to 66 rat units per liter, and Katzman and Doisy[89] as much as 75 rat units per twenty-four-hour urine specimen. In a more recent study, Varney and his associates[130] found from 100 to 550 m.u. per twenty-four-hour specimen (for technique, see p. 674).

Tumors of the Female Genitalia.—Zondek[117] first pointed out that a large percentage of women with genital carcinoma excrete more than normal quantities of follicle-stimulating hormone. He suggested that this rise is related to the growth and may therefore serve as a diagnostic aid. In the light of recent findings, however, it seems likely that the increased excretion is not due to the tumor per se, but to the fact that many of the patients are at the menopausal age, or have suffered ovarian damage from x-rays directed to the pelvic region to control the growth.[118, 119]

A false positive gonadotropin pregnancy reaction (APR II and III) has been obtained in some women with genital tumors, and also occasionally in patients with retention, dermoid, or corpus luteum cysts of the ovary, hypernephroma of the ovary, granulosa cell tumor, and uterine or

TABLE 11

Sex Hormone Titers in the Blood and Urine*

	Gonadotropes		Estrogens		Pregnanediol	Androgens
	Blood	Urine	Blood	Urine	Urine	Urine
Childhood	Newborn—first 4–5 days—predominantly luteinizing hormone derived from maternal circulation.	Up to 10th year—2 to 4 m.u. of predominantly follicle stimulating hormone. From 10th to 15th year—gradual rise to adult values.		Before 10th year—5 to 15 m.u. per liter—no cyclic variations. From 10th to 15th year—gradual rise to adult values.		Before 13th year—1 to 3 I.U. daily. Between 13th and 15th year —5 to 20 I.U. daily.
Maturity	Cyclic variations—peak at mid-cycle—25 r.u. or more per liter of predominantly follicle stimulating hormone.	Cyclic variations—peak at mid-cycle—25 r.u. or more per liter of predominantly follicle stimulating hormone. Total output in cycle 50 to 80 r.u. (Frank)	21st day before flow—25 m.u. per liter. Between 21st and 14th day before flow—33.3 m.u. per liter. Between 7th day before flow and onset of flow—50 to 100 m.u. per liter. (Frank)	10 to 30 r.u. per liter. (Kurzrok) Total output during cycle—1000 to 2000 m.u. Peak at mid-cycle—200 to 500 m.u. per 24 hour specimen. Occasional second peak shortly before flow.	Appears only during luteal phase. Daily values from 1 to 5 mg. Disappears abruptly 1 to 3 days before onset of flow. Total output per cycle—30 to 54 mg. (Venning & Browne)	20 to 60 I.U. daily.
Normal Pregnancy	Predominantly luteinizing hormone present. Rapid rise begins soon after conception. Peak reached between 30th and 50th day—values up to 500,000 r.u. per liter—followed by gradual drop to term. (Evans) Between 5th and 6th week—average of 1600 m.u. per 100 cc. From 8th to 10th week—rise to over 3000 m.u. per 100 cc. Between 20th and 24th week—drop to 300 m.u. per 100 cc. Little change thereafter to term. (Rakoff)	Predominantly luteinizing hormone present. Rapid rise begins soon after conception. Peak reached between 20th and 50th day after missed period. Values at peak from 75,000 to 1,000,000 r.u. daily. Rapid drop to 10,000 r.u. daily by 65th day. Little change thereafter. (Evans)	Up to 17th week—25 to 35 m.u. per liter. Steady rise thereafter to peak at term—values from 600 to 1300 m.u. per liter. (Frank) At 4th month—up to 300 m.u. per liter. At term—800 to 1000 m.u. per liter. (Zondek) Up to 8th week—under 1 m.u. in 4 cc. Between 8th and 10th week—average of 24 m.u. per 100 cc. Sudden rise between 14th and 20th week, and again between 32nd and 36th week. At term—500 m.u. or more per 100 cc. (Rakoff)	Steady rise to peak at term. Up to 8th week—300 to 600 m.u. per liter. At term—up to 20,000 m.u. per liter. (Zondek) Before 8th week—200 to 1000 gamma daily. At term—15,000 to 40,000 gamma daily. (Venning & Browne)	First 2 months—4 to 25 mg. daily. Steady rise thereafter—values up to 155 mg. daily during last 2 months.	6th to 8th month—8 to 30 I.U. per liter.
Uterine Bleeding	Values usually within normal limits. Fluctuations but no cyclic variations.	Values usually within normal limits. Fluctuations but no cyclic variations.	Values vary widely from below to above normal. Fluctuations but no cyclic variations.	Values vary widely from below to above normal. Fluctuations but no cyclic variations.	Usually absent, but occasionally appears sporadically or at cyclic intervals.	Normal values as a rule.

Amenorrhea	Primary ovarian amenorrhea—above normal values—50 m.u. or more per liter of predominantly follicle stimulating hormone. (Fluhmann) Hypopituitary amenorrhea—below normal values. Polyfolliculin amenorrhea—within normal limits—no cyclic variations.	Primary ovarian amenorrhea—above normal values—up to 66 r.u. per liter of predominantly follicle stimulating hormone. (Drips) Hypopituitary amenorrhea—below normal values. Polyfolliculin amenorrhea—within normal limits—no cyclic variations.	Type 1—Subthreshold cycle—level below normal but usual cyclic variations. Type 2—Like type 1. Type 3—No estrogen cycle. Type 4—No estrogen cycle (Frank) Polyfolliculin amenorrhea—normal or above normal values—no cyclic variations.	Type 1—Subthreshold cycle—level below normal but usual cyclic variations. Type 2—Below normal (under 10 m.u. per liter)—no cyclic variations. Type 3—Like type 2. Type 4—No estrogen cycle (Frank) Polyfolliculin amenorrhea—normal or above normal values—no cyclic variations.	Absent as a rule.	Normal or above normal. Excess roughly proportional to duration of amenorrhea.
Natural and Artificial Menopause	Same as in primary ovarian amenorrhea—above normal values—50 m.u. or more per liter of predominantly follicle stimulating hormone. (Fluhmann)	Same as in primary ovarian amenorrhea—above normal values—up to 66 r.u. per liter of predominantly follicle stimulating hormone. (Drips)	Small quantities (adrenal cortical origin?)	Small quantities (adrenal cortical origin?)	Absent.	Low and high values.
Fetal Death	Steady drop to 100 m.u. or less per 100 cc. (Rakoff) Less rapid than drop in estrogen level.	Steady drop to less than 1000 m.u. or 200 rb.u. per 24 hour specimen. Less rapid than drop in estrogen level.	Rapid drop begins within 24 hours after fetal death.	Rapid drop begins within 24 hours after fetal death.	Usually diminished or absent but occasionally within normal limits.	
Toxemias of Pregnancy	Early toxemias—normal or high values. Late toxemias—normal or high values.	Early toxemias—normal or high values. Late toexnias—low, normal or high values.	Low, normal, and high values.	Low, normal, and high values.	Late toxemias—normal or low.	
Hydatid Mole and Chorionepithelioma	Far above normal as a rule but not invariably.	Far above normal as a rule but not invariably. Values up to 500,000 m.u. per liter.	Usually above normal values.	Usually above normal values.	Below normal values.	
Granulosa Cell Tumor	Values within normal limits. Usually no cyclic variations.	Values within normal limits. Usually no cyclic variations.	Tendency to above normal values. No cyclic variations, as a rule.	Tendency to above normal values. No cyclic variations, as a rule.		
Arrhenoblastoma	Normal or high	Normal or high	Below normal values.	Below normal values.	Variable amounts; acyclic.	Above normal values.
Adrenogenitalism	Normal or high	Normal or high	Below normal except in adrenal cortical carcinoma.	Below normal except in carcinoma (over 500 m.u./l.).	Variable amounts; acyclic.	Above normal—values up to 500 I.U. daily.
Virilism	Within normal limits	Within normal limits	Below normal values	Below normal values.		Normal or above—excess proportional to degree of virilism.

* Specific figures are omitted in most cases because of wide variations in the values obtained by different laboratories. Where given, they are based on the experience of the author and other investigators in large series of cases.

cervical carcinoma. Such cases are of interest because they constitute a potential source of error when employing the pregnancy tests based on the gonadotropic hormone content of the blood and urine.

Endocrine Disease.—False positive pregnancy tests have been reported in some cases with pituitary tumor, intracranial pressure, organic disease of the hypothalamus, hyperthyroidism, and hyperplasia or tumor of the adrenal cortex. While such cases are uncommon, their existence should be borne in mind when employing the gonadotropic hormone pregnancy tests.

Normal Adult Males.—The normal adult male excretes small amounts of gonadotropin, but there is no cyclic excretion of the hormone comparable to that in the normal adult female. Katzman and Doisy[89] demonstrated 4 to 19 mouse units daily in most of their cases, while up to 50 m.u. per liter of urine was found in normal males studied by Cutler and Owen.[120] Glass and McKennon[43] could demonstrate at least 25 m.u. per liter of the follicle-stimulating hormone in all their cases, but only a few excreted a comparable amount of the luteinizing fraction. Friedman and Weinstein[121] obtained values ranging from 6 to 36 rabbit units.

Castrate and Senile Males.—Increased excretion of the follicle stimulating hormone has been demonstrated in male castrates. A rise also occurs in old men, though less often than in menopausal women. According to Heller,[122] advancing age in the male is not associated with a rise in the gonadotropin level comparable to that observed in menopausal women. After surgical or x-ray castration, however, an appreciable increase is demonstrable.

Testicular Tumors.—Increased excretion of gonadotropic substances in teratoma testis was first noted by Zondek[117] in 1929. Ferguson,[123] in 1933, on the basis of a study of one hundred and seventeen cases of testicular tumor, concluded that the gonadotropic hormone concentration of the urine is related to the histologic character of the tumor. In choriocarcinoma he obtained 40,000 m.u. of the follicle-stimulating hormone per liter, and in embryonal carcinoma 10,000 to 40,000 units. In embryonal carcinoma with lymphoid stroma, the values ranged from 2,000 to 10,000 units, while in seminoma the urine contained from 400 to 2,000 units per liter. The lowest values, 50 to 500 units, were obtained in adult teratoma. Cutler and Owen[120] reported values of 50 mouse units per liter in patients with benign testicular neoplasms, and from 100 to 2,000 units in teratoma testis. According to Ehrhardt and Breitenbach,[124] a repeated positive follicle-stimulating reaction is presumptive evidence, while a positive luteinizing reaction (APR II and III) definitely points to testicular malignancy. Among 135 cases of testicular tumor collected from the literature by Gilbert,[125] chorionepitheliomatous elements were present in 103, and all showed high gonadotropin liters.

Ferguson's assumption that the gonadotropic hormone concentration is related to the histologic character of the tumor has recently been questioned by Twombly and associates.[126] In a study of 203 cases, they could demonstrate no close correlation between the rate of hormone excretion and the histologic character or clinical course of the neoplasm. In general, values under 1,000 m.u. were associated with relatively benign tumors and 10,000 m.u. or more with choriocarcinoma. They concluded that the quantitative Aschheim-Zondek test is of no value in disclosing the nature of the tumor or its clinical course. A negative test they believe is of little clinical significance, but the presence of chorionic gonadotropin (reaction APR II and III) is a bad prognostic sign and not infrequently constitutes the only evidence of the disease.

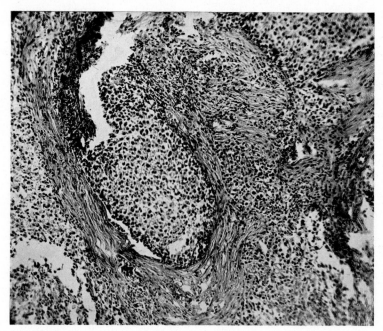

Fig. 176.—Malignant teratoma of the testis. Microphotograph of tissue obtained from a thirty-five year old male with high gonadotropin titers in the urine.

Furuhjelm[74] believes the prognosis is most favorable in cases excreting less than 165 m.u. of the follicle stimulating hormone, and considers it especially unfavorable if both the follicle-stimulating and luteinizing hormones are present.

BIBLIOGRAPHY

1. Zondek, B., and Euler, H.: Skandinav. Arch. f. Physiol. 67:259, 1934.
2. Dorfman, R. I., Greulich, W. W., and Solomon, C. I.: Endocrinol. 21:741, 1937.
3. Loewe, S.: Klin. Wchnschr. 4:1407, 1925.
4. Frank, R. T., and Goldberger, M. A.: J.A.M.A. 86:1686, 1926.
5. Fluhmann, C. F.: Endocrinol. 18:705, 1934.
6. Frank, R. T., and Goldberger, M. A.: Proc. Soc. Exper. Biol. & Med. 32:1663, 1935.
7. Janney, J. C.: Am. J. Obst. & Gynec. 18:807, 1929.
8. Ford, F. A., and Mueller, S. C.: Am. J. Obst. & Gynec. 24:329, 1932.
9. Kurzrok, R., and Ratner, S.: Am. J. Obst. & Gynec. 23:689, 1932.
10. Werner, S. C.: J. Clin. Investig. 20:21, 1941.
11. Dingemanse, E., Laqueur, E., and Mühlbock, O.: Monatschr. f. Geburtsh. & Gynäk. 109:37, 1939.
12. Smith, G. V., Smith, O. W., and Pincus, G.: Am. J. Physiol. 121:98, 1938.

13. Palmer, A.: Proc. Soc. Exper. Biol. & Med. *37*:273, 1937.
14. Frank, R. T., Goldberger, M. A., and Spielman, F.: J.A.M.A. *103*:393, 1934.
15. Zondek, B.: Acta obst. & gynec. Scandinav. *13*:309, 1934.
16. Hamblen, E. C.: J. Clin. Endocrinol. *1*:180, 1941.
17. Kurzrok, R.: J. Clin. Endocrinol. *1*:199, 1941.
18. Seguy, J.: Médicine *13*:277, 1932.
19. Zondek, B.: Clinical and Experimental Investigations on the Genital Functions and their Hormonal Regulators, Baltimore, Williams & Wilkins Co., 1941, p. 215.
20. Frank, R. T.: J.A.M.A. *104*:1991, 1935.
21. Seegar, G. E.: Am. J. Obst. & Gynec. *39*:469, 1940.
22. Smith, G. V., and Smith, O. W.: Am. J. Obst. & Gynec. *36*:769, 1938.
23. Frank, R. T., and Goldberger, M. A.: Am. J. Obst. & Gynec. *43*:865, 1942.
24. Zondek, B.: Hormone des Ovariums und Hypophysenvorderlappens, Berlin, J. Springer, 1935.
25. Rakoff, A. E.: Am. J. Obst. & Gynec. *38*:371, 1939.
26. Mazer, C., and Hoffman, J.: J.A.M.A. *96*:19, 1931.
27. Zondek, B., and Aschheim, S.: Klin. Wchnschr. *7*:485, 1928.
28. Browne, J. S. L., and Venning, E. H.: Am. J. Physiol. *116*:18, 1936.
29. Cohen, S. L., Marrian, G. F., and Watson, M.: Lancet *1*:674, 1935.
30. Bachman, C.: Am. J. Obst. & Gynec. *42*:599, 1941.
31. Frank, R. T., The Female Sex Hormone, Springfield, Ill., Charles C. Thomas, 1928.
32. Bland, P. B., First, A., and Roeder, P.: Am. J. Obst. & Gynec. *23*:83, 1932.
33. Spielman, F., Goldberger, M. A., and Frank, R. T.: J.A.M.A. *101*:266, 1933.
34. Smith, G. V., and Smith, O. W.: Surg., Gynec. & Obst. *61*:27, 1935.
35. Browne, J. S. L., Henry, J. S., and Venning, E. H.: Am. J. Obst. & Gynec. *38*:927, 1939.
36. Palmer, A.: Am. J. Obst. & Gynec. *36*:1005, 1938.
37. Jeffcoate, T. N. A.: Lancet *1*:1045, 1940.
38. Smith, G. V., and Smith, O. W.: Proc. Soc. Exper. Biol. & Med. *32*:847, 1935.
39. Smith, J. T., and Werthessen, N. T.: Am. J. Obst. & Gynec. *41*:153, 1941.
40. Zondek, B.: Klin. Wchnschr. *10*:2121, 1931.
41. Laroche, G., Simonnet, H., and Huet, J. A.: Compt. rend. Soc. de biol. *113*:286, 1933.
42. Eng, H.: Klin. Wchnschr. *15*:349, 1936.
43. Glass, S. J., and McKennon, B. J.: West. J. Surg. *45*:467, 1937.
44. Neumann, H. O.: Endokrinol. *12*:166, 1933.
45. Stohr, G.: Am. J. Obst. & Gynec. *43*:586, 1942.
46. Laqueur, E., Dingemanse, E., Hart, P. C., and de Jongh, S. E.: Klin. Wchnschr. *6*:1859, 1927.
47. Koch, F. C.: Ann. Int. Med. *11*:297, 1937.
48. Frank, R. T.: J. Mt. Sinai Hosp. *8*:514, 1942.
49. Browne, J. S. L., and Venning, E. H.: Endocrinol. *21*:711, 1937; J. Clin. Investig. *16*: 678, 1937.
50. Wilson, R. B., Randall, L. M., and Osterberg, A. E.: Am. J. Obst. & Gynec. *37*:59, 1939.
51. Hamblen, E. C.: Endocrine Gynecology, Springfield, Ill., Charles C. Thomas, 1939.
52. Cope, C. L.: Clin. Sc. *4*:217, 1940.
53. Buxton, C. L.: Am. J. Obst. & Gynec. *40*:202, 1940.
54. Siegler, S. L., and Bauer, D.: Am. J. Obst. & Gynec. *45*:277, 1943.
55. Stover, R. F., and Pratt, J. P.: Endocrinol. *24*:29, 1939.
56. Hamblen, E. C.: Am. J. Obst. & Gynec. *41*:664, 1941.
57. Cope, C. L.: Brit. Med. J. *2*:545, 1940.
58. Smith, G. V., and Smith, O. W.: Am. J. Obst. & Gynec. *39*:405, 1940.
59. Taylor, H. C., Jr., and Scadron, E. N.: Am. J. Obst. & Gynec. *37*:963, 1939.
60. Cope, C. L.: Lancet *2*:158, 1940.
61. Venning, E. H., Weil, P. G., and Browne, J. S. L.: J. Biol. Chem. *128*:cvii, 1939.
62. Finkler, R. S.: J. Clin. Endocrinol. *1*:151, 1941.
63. Oesting, R. B., and Webster, B.: Endocrinol. *22*:307, 1938.
64. Talbot, N. B., Butler, A. M., and MacLachlan, E. A.: New England J. Med. *223*:369, 1940.
65. Gallagher, T. F., Peterson, D. H., Dorfman, R. I., Kenyon, A. T., and Koch, F. C.: J. Clin. Investig. *16*:695, 1937.

66. Dingemanse, E., Borchardt, H., and Laqueur, E.: Biochem. J. *31*:500, 1937.
67. Fraser, R. W., Forbes, A. P., Albright, F., Sulkowitch, H., and Reifenstein, E. C.: J. Clin. Endocrinol. *1*:234, 1941.
68. D'Amour, F. E., and Gustavson, R. G.: J.A.M.A. *117*:188, 1941.
69. Kenyon, A. T., Gallagher, T. F., Peterson, D. H., Dorfman, R. I., and Koch, F. C.: J. Clin. Investig. *16*:705, 1937.
70. Callow, N. H., and Callow, R. K.: Biochem. J. *34*:276, 1940.
71. Kochakian, C. D.: Endocrinol. *21*:60, 1937.
72. Hamblen, E. C., Ross, R. A., Cuyler, W. K., Baptist, M., and Ashley, C.: Endocrinol. *25*:491, 1939.
73. Hamblen, E. C., Cuyler, W. K., and Baptist, M.: Endocrinol. *27*:16, 1940.
74. Furuhjelm, M.: Acta obst. & gynec. Scandinav. *20*:1, 1940.
75. Hain, A. M.: Edinburgh M. J. *45*:678, 1938.
76. Drips, D. G., and Osterberg, A. E.: Endocrinol. *27*:345, 1940.
77. Hamblen, E. C., Cuyler, W. K., and Baptist, M.: J. Clin. Endocrinol. *1*:772, 1941.
78. Hamblen, E. C., Cuyler, W. K., and Baptist, M.: J. Clin. Endocrinol. *1*:777, 1941.
79. Ross, R. A.: Am. J. Obst. & Gynec. *45*:497, 1943.
80. Callow, R. K.: Proc. Roy. Soc. Med. *31*:841, 1938.
81. Hirschmann, H.: J. Biol. Chem. *136*:483, 1940.
82. Simpson, S. L., de Fremery, P., and MacBeth, A.: Endocrinol. *20*:363, 1936.
83. Crooke, A. C., and Callow, R. K.: Quart. J. Med. *8*:233, 1939.
84. Ross, R. A., Hamblen, E. C., Cuyler, W. K., and Baptist, M.: Am. J. Obst. & Gynec. *42*:607, 1941.
85. Talbot, N. B., and Butler, A. M.: J. Clin. Endocrinol. *2*:724, 1942.
86. Kanter, A. E., and Klawans, A. H.: Am. J. Cancer *40*:474, 1940.
87. Szathmary, Z.: Arch. f. Gynäk. *164*:478, 1937.
88. Freed, S. C.: Proc. Soc. Exper. Biol. & Med. *33*:35, 1935.
89. Katzman, P. A., and Doisy, E. A.: J. Biol. Chem. *106*:125, 1934.
90. McCullagh, E. P., and Cuyler, W. K.: Am. J. Clin. Path. *10*:593, 1940.
91. Frank, R. T., and Salmon, U. J.: Proc. Soc. Exper. Biol. & Med. *32*:1237, 1935.
92. Zondek, B.: Klin. Wchnschr. *10*:2121, 1931.
93. Frank, R. T., in, Glandular Physiology and Therapy, Chicago, A.M.A., 1935, chap. 16, p. 219.
94. Drips, D. G., and Osterberg, A. E.: Endocrinol. *23*:703, 1938.
95. D'Amour, F. E., Funk, D., and Liverman, H.: Am. J. Obst. & Gynec. *37*:940, 1939.
96. Fluhmann, C. F.: Am. J. Obst. & Gynec. *20*:1, 1930.
97. Anspach, B. M., and Hoffman, J.: Am. J. Obst. & Gynec. *26*:147, 1933.
98. Zondek, B.: J.A.M.A. *108*:607, 1937.
99. Evans, H. M., Kohls, C. L., and Wonder, D. H.: J.A.M.A. *108*:287, 1937.
100. Rakoff, A. E.: Pennsylvania M. J. *43*:669, 1940.
101. Browne, J. S. L., and Venning, E. H.: Lancet *2*:1507, 1936.
102. Schoeneck, F. J.: Am. J. Obst. & Gynec. *39*:485, 1940.
103. Aschheim, S., and Zondek, B.: Klin. Wchnschr. *7*:1453, 1928.
104. Goldberger, M. A., Salmon, U. J., and Frank, R. T.: J.A.M.A. *103*:1210, 1934.
105. Brindeau, A., Hinglais, H., and Hinglais, M.: Presse Méd. *47*:281, 1939.
106. Chosson, J., and Donnet, V.: Presse Méd. *42*:892, 1934.
107. Ehrhardt, C.: Klin. Wchnschr. *15*:514, 1936.
108. Anker, H., and Laland, P.: Norsk. mag. f. laegevidinsk. *95*:1217, 1324, 1934.
109. Fels, E.: Zentralbl. f. Gynäk. *52*:466, 1929.
110. Rössler, H.: Ztschr. f. Geburtsh. u. Gynäk. *96*:516, 1929.
111. Payne, F. L.: Surg., Gynec. & Obst. *73*:86, 1941.
112. Fluhmann, C. F.: Am. J. Obst. & Gynec. *28*:668, 1934.
113. Schumann, E. A., and Voegelin, A. W.: Am. J. Obst. & Gynec. *33*:473, 1937.
114. Wilson, K. M., and Corner, G. W.: New York State J. Med. *33*:629, 1933.
115. Frank, R. T., Salmon, U. J., and Friedman, R.: Proc. Soc. Exper. Biol. & Med. *32*:1666, 1935.
116. Zondek, B.: Klin. Wchnschr. *9*:393, 1930.
117. Zondek, B.: Klin. Wchnschr. *9*:679, 1930.

45

118. Gostomirovic, D.: München. med. Wchnschr. *78*:1350, 1931.
119. Frank, R. T.: Am. J. Obst. & Gynec. *24*:932, 1932.
120. Cutler, M., and Owen, S. E.: Am. J. Cancer *24*:318, 1935.
121. Friedman, M. H., and Weinstein, G. L.: Endocrinol. *21*:489, 1937.
122. Heller, E. J., Heller, C. G., and Sevringhaus, E. L.: Endocrinol. *29*:1, 1941.
123. Ferguson, R. S.: Am. J. Cancer. *28*:269, 1933; J.A.M.A. *101*:1933, 1933.
124. Ehrhardt, K., and Breitenbach, H.: Deutsche. ztschr. f. Chir. *252*:549, 1939.
125. Gilbert, J. B.: J. Urol. *43*:722, 1940; ibid. *44*:345, 1940.
126. Twombly, G. H., Temple, H. M., and Dean, A. L.: J.A.M.A. *118*:106, 1942.
127. Anselmino, K. J., and Hoffmann, F.: Ztschr. f. Geburtsh. u. Gynäk. *114*:52, 1936.
128. D'Amour, F. E.: J. Clin. Endocrinol. *3*:41, 1943.
129. Talbot, N. B., Butler, A. M., and Berman, R. A.: J. Clin. Investig. *21*:559, 1942.
130. Varney, R. F., Kenyon, A. T., and Koch, F. C.: J. Clin. Endocrinol. *2*:137, 1942.
131. Zondek, B.: J. Obst. & Gynaec. Brit. Emp. *49*:397, 1942.
132. Benzadon, J., and Picena, J. P.: Bol. Soc. de obst. y ginec. de Buenos Aires *21*:583, 1942.
133. Krohn, L., Harris, J., and Hechter, O.: Am. J. Obst. & Gynec. *44*:213, 1942.
134. Hechter, O.: Proc. Soc. Exper. Biol. & Med. *49*:299, 1942.
135. Hamblen, E. C., Cuyler, W. K., and Baptist, M.: Am. J. Obst. & Gynec. *44*:442, 1942.

CHAPTER XLI

HORMONAL PREPARATIONS

Considerable progress has been made in the isolation and purification of hormonal substances adapted for the treatment of gonadal and reproductive disorders. There are now available estrogenic, progestational, androgenic, gonadotropic, lactogenic, and other hormonal preparations which are physiologically active in the lower mammal, subhuman primate, and to a limited extent in man.

ESTROGENIC SUBSTANCES

The term *estrogen* has been adopted to describe all substances, regardless of source or chemical composition, which can induce the typical modifications of estrus in the genitalia of the immature or spayed adult female rodent, and are in other respects (Chap. II) capable of simulating the action of the ovary during the follicular phase of the cycle. The estrogenic substances now available include naturally occurring hormones present in the animal body and certain plants, and synthetic estrogens prepared from ordinary laboratory reagents.

Naturally Occurring Estrogens.—The most important naturally occurring estrogens are estrone, estriol, and estradiol. Less potent and therefore less valuable as therapeutic agents are equilin, hippulin, equilenin, and dihydroequilenin, so named because of their equine origin.

Estrone.—Estrone (theelin, ketohydroxyestrin, 3–hydroxy 17–keto 1, 3,5–estratriene), the first natural estrogen isolated in crystalline form, is represented by the formula $C_{18}H_{22}O_2$. First obtained from human pregnancy urine, it has since also been found in the urine of pregnant mares, stallions and men, in human placenta, the adrenal cortex, horse testes, and sow's ovaries. A conjugated form, estrone sulfate, has been isolated from mare's urine.

Estriol.—Estriol (theelol, trihydroxyestrin, 3,16,17–trihydroxy, 1,3,5–estratriene), represented by the formula $C_{18}H_{24}O_3$, is physiologically less active than estrone and differs from it in that it possesses three hydroxyl groups instead of a ketone group. It can be converted into estrone by dehydration with potassium bisulfate. A physiologically inert, conjugated form, estriol glycuronide, has been obtained from the placenta and urine of pregnant women. Boiling human pregnancy urine with acid converts this combined form into free, physiologically active estriol.

Estradiol.—Estradiol (dihydrotheelin, dihydroxyestrin, 2,17–dihydroxy, 1,3,5–estratriene), represented by the formula $C_{18}H_{24}O_2$, is the most potent of the naturally occurring estrogens. It was first prepared in two isomeric forms by reducing the ketonic group of estrone to a secondary alcohol. The alpha form has been isolated from sow's ovaries, human placenta, horse testes, and the urine of pregnant women and mares. The beta form has been obtained from the urine of pregnant mares.

Equilin, Hippulin, and Dihydroequilenin.—These estrogens are found in the urine of pregnant mares. Conversion of equilenin into estrone has been achieved by Marker.[1] Its synthesis by Bachmann,[2] in 1939, marks the first total synthesis of a sex hormone.

Chemistry of the Natural Estrogens.—The naturally occurring estrogens are steroid compounds chemically related to such sterols as cholesterol, the bile acids, ergosterol, calciferol, and the androgens. They are essentially lipoid soluble, their solubility in water being comparatively

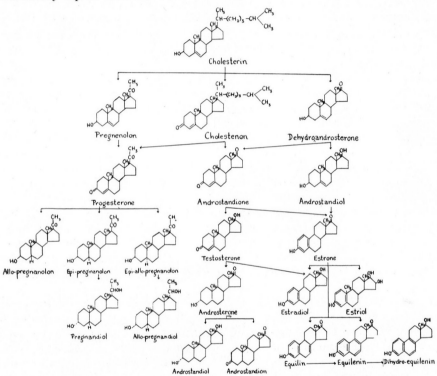

Fig. 177.—Relation of the sex hormones to cholesterin. (After Butenandt.)

low. Their separation from other lipoids is possible because of their relative insolubility in purified petroleum benzene. All the naturally occurring estrogens are phenolic. The phenolic hydroxyl group reacts with a variety of compounds to form esters. The estrogen esters, when administered subcutaneously or intramuscularly, exert a more prolonged effect than the free hormone, probably because of delayed absorption of the active principle. The observation that the naturally occurring estrogens give color reactions when combined with certain chemical compounds, forms the basis for various colorimetric methods of assay. Since these are cheaper, simpler and much less time consuming, they are employed by some laboratories to replace or supplement the biologic assay methods.

Metabolism of the Natural Estrogens.—The fate of endogenously and exogenously supplied estrogens in the organism is not yet fully established. It has been suggested that estradiol, most potent of the naturally occurring estrogens, is the true follicular hormone. This is thought to be converted to estrone, which in turn is transformed to estriol, least potent of the three estrogenic compounds. Estriol is then inactivated by conversion into estriol glycuronide, in which form it is excreted.

Studies of the hormonal content of the tissues and excreta of laboratory animals receiving estrogenic hormone have thrown some light on the complex mechanism which controls estrogen metabolism. There is evidence that 20 per cent or less of exogenously supplied estrogen is excreted in the urine and feces, partly in a physiologically inert and conjugated form.[3] The major part is recoverable during the first twenty-four hours after injection, practically none being demonstrable after forty-eight to ninety-six hours. Recent studies indicate that the unrecovered 80 or more per cent is not stored in the body but destroyed or inactivated, probably by the liver.[4, 5, 66] Dingemanse[6] found that in dogs the quantity of estrogen present in the organs after daily administration of estrone or estradiol benzoate was as a rule small compared with the quantity administered, the concentration being highest in the liver. A considerable amount was present in the combined form, while part of the estrogens were encountered either as keto-compounds or as nonketonic substances. Heller,[7] on the basis of in vitro studies, has suggested that liver tissue contains an estrone reducing enzyme system which converts estrone to estradiol, and an estradiol destroying system which inactivates the estradiol so formed. This, he believes, is accomplished through enzymatic destruction of an oxidative nature rather than through conjugation or conversion of estradiol to a less active form. He found that estriol is only mildly affected by the liver, and offers this as a possible explanation of why this compound is more efficacious orally than estrone or estradiol.

Role of the Ovary and Uterus.—The ovary and uterus, according to some workers, are concerned in estrogen metabolism. Pincus[8] believes functioning ovaries are essential for the conversion of estradiol to estrone, while the transformation of estrone to estriol requires the presence of a functioning uterus and is facilitated by progesterone or an active secretion of the corpus luteum. Heller[7] found the potency of estrone increased twenty-fold when incubated with minced uterine tissue. Incubation with spleen, lung, heart and kidney tissue was likewise effective in converting it to a more active form, which he believes is probably estradiol. On the other hand, removal of the ovary or uterus in the monkey does not affect the quantity of administered estrogen recoverable from the urine. In the bitch, according to Dingemanse and Tyslowitz,[9] hysterectomy does not appreciably alter the quantities and proportions of estrogenic activity present in the organs following daily injections of estradiol benzoate.

Synthetic Estrogens.—Dodds and associates,[10] in 1933, demonstrated varying degrees of estrogenic activity in certain phenanthrene and dibenzanthracene derivatives, chemically related to the naturally occurring estrogens. They later found that the phenanthrene ring system present in the natural sex hormones is not essential for estrogenic activity. In 1938, they described the synthesis of dihydroxydiethyl stilbene, a chemical compound possessing marked estrogenic activity, with the formula $C_{18}H_{22}O_2$ which resembles that of estrone.[11] The Council on Pharmacy and Chemistry[12] has adopted the name *stilbestrol* for the mother substance 4,4′–dihydroxystilbene, reserving the designation *diethylstilbestrol* for its more potent derivative 4,4′–dihydroxy–$a:\beta$–diethylstilbene. This substance is now included among New and Nonofficial remedies and has been judged by the Council to be a reliable therapeutic agent for those conditions recognized by it as suitable for estrogen therapy.[13] Formed from chemical compounds totally foreign to the body, these substances are not steroids, but, like the naturally occurring estrogens, have phenolic properties. Other less well-known synthetic estrogens are hexestrol (dihydrostilbestrol) and such compounds as triphenylethylene, triphenylchlorethylene and octofollin, which are not related to the natural estrogens or to the stilbenes.

Therapeutic Value: Potency and Toxicity.—The therapeutic value of the synthetic estrogens is now being investigated. Chief advantages are

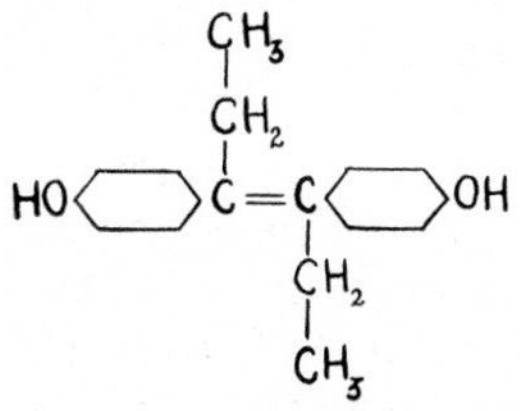

Diethylstilbestrol
(Alpha, alpha′-diethyl-4,4′-stilbenediol)

Fig. 178.

their relative cheapness and potency by the oral route. Though capable of simulating the action of the naturally occurring estrogens, they often produce unpleasant side effects, particularly nausea, vomiting and headache. The incidence and severity of toxic symptoms may be reduced to some extent by coating the pills, limiting the daily dose to 1 mgm. or less, and interrupting treatment with periods of rest. MacBryde and associates[67] recently reported that nausea was the only objectionable symptom and occurred in only 8.6 per cent of a group of 150 cases receiving 1 mg. of diethylstilbestrol daily for two to three weeks followed by a rest period of one to two weeks. Blood, urine and liver function studies revealed no evidence of toxic effect.

Diethylstilbestrol is estimated to be from one-half to one-sixth as effective by mouth as by injection in the human. Estimates of the comparative potency of the naturally occurring and synthetic estrogens vary considerably. According to Dodds and associates,[11] diethylstilbestrol is at least five times as potent as estrone by the oral route. Comparative studies of the potency of diethylstilbestrol by mouth and of estrone by injection have yielded values ranging from 1:5 to 2:1.

Triphenylethylene, triphenylchlorethylene, hexestrol, and *octofollin* have received comparatively scant attention. Some observers report that hexestrol is as potent but less toxic than diethylstilbestrol, while others find it not only less toxic but also less potent.[14, 15] Several investigators have found octofollin an effective estrogen and nontoxic in therapeutic doses, whether given by mouth or parenterally.[68, 69, 70] Its potency by the oral route, as judged by objective criteria, is one-fifth to one-tenth that of diethylstilbestrol.[70] Triphenylethylene and triphenylchlorethylene, according to Robson,[16] are active by both the oral and parenteral route. By mouth, the duration of their action, weight for weight, is approximately the same as that of estradiol benzoate and only slightly less than that of stilbestrol. When administered subcutaneously, the duration of their action, weight for weight, is about three times that of estradiol benzoate and five times that of stilbestrol. Robson found the toxicity of these compounds in animals extremely low.

Ethinyl estradiol, a derivative of estradiol, has been reported to be highly effective by the oral route, as compared with both natural and synthetic estrogens.[71, 72] As judged by subjective criteria, it is about ten times as effective as alpha-estradiol and from five to twenty times as potent as diethylstilbestrol by mouth.[72]

Standardization.—The estrogens were first standardized in terms of *rat and mouse units.* These were defined as the least amount of substance which, when given in three doses at four hour intervals to a spayed adult female rat or mouse, will produce a full change from the negative to the estrus vaginal smear in forty-eight to fifty-six hours after the first injection.[17] It soon became apparent that many factors influence the minimal effective dose, so that even minor differences in technique may make for wide discrepancies. To insure uniformity, an *international unit* was established in 1932 and defined as the specific estrus-producing activity contained in 0.1 gamma ($\frac{1}{10,000}$ mg.) of the international standard ketohydroxyestratriene (estrone), preserved at the National Institute for Medical Research in London. Standardization of a preparation entails a comparison between it and the international standard to determine the equivalent amounts which will induce vaginal cornification in adult castrate rats. The potency, in terms of international units, is ascertained by calculating from the physiologically determined relationship between standard and sample. It has been estimated that 1 international unit is equivalent to from one-third to one-tenth of a rat unit, depending on the method of bioassay used.

Following the introduction of esters of estrone and estradiol for clinical use, it became apparent that differences in rate of absorption make it impracticable to assay an ester in terms of the free hormone. For this reason an international unit for estradiol benzoate, the so-called *international benzoate unit (I.B.U.),* was established by the second Conference for the Standardization of Sex Hormones in 1935.[18] This is defined as the specific estrus-producing activity contained in 0.1 gamma ($\frac{1}{10,000}$ mg.) of the international standard dihydroxyestratriene (estradiol benzoate).

There is a growing conviction that the international estrone standard can be used only as a basis for comparison in the assay of estrone preparations, the international estradiol monobenzoate standard as a criterion only in the assay of estradiol monobenzoate preparations. With this in mind, several workers have stressed the desirability of limiting the production of estrogens "to pure preparations of the different forms of the hormone and its chemically defined derivatives or of mixtures thereof, so that the activity may be indicated in exact weights and indications in biological units may be abandoned."[19]

Efficacy of the Estrogens.—Accurate data relating to the efficacy of the estrogens in the human is not available at the present time. Estimates as to their relative potency in the laboratory animal vary widely, but even were the findings more uniform, there is nothing to warrant the assumption that the same holds for man. Comparative studies in man are still very limited. According to Werner,[20] estrone is more potent than estradiol benzoate in its effect on the human uterus. As proof he offers his observation that 84,000 I.U. of estrone was sufficient to prime the endometrium to respond to progesterone with pregravid modifications, whereas Elden[21] could not obtain this effect with 250,000 I.U. of estradiol benzoate and Kaufmann[22] found a total of 1,000,000 I.U. of the latter substance necessary for this purpose. In two castrate women with atrophic endometria, Herrnberger[73] found a total of 10 mgm. of diethylstilbestrol sufficient to produce changes equivalent to those normally found at the height of the proliferative phase of the menstrual cycle. Until additional evidence is forthcoming, the physician must rely on his own clinical experience in deciding the relative effectiveness of the various estrogens at his disposal.

Mode of Administration.—The naturally occurring and synthetic estrogens may be administered by the oral, parenteral, percutaneous, intravaginal, sublingual, or intranasal route, or may be implanted subcutaneously in pellet form. Some observers[23] consider the injection of estrone crystals suspended in water equivalent to pellet implantation. Before instituting estrogen therapy, the physician should first decide what he is trying to accomplish, what preparation is best adapted for his purpose, and by what route it should be administered to insure maximum efficiency.

Where a *local effect* is desired, as for example to develop the hypoplastic breast, topical application of the hormone in the form of an ointment is preferable to the oral or parenteral route. For the relief of senile vaginitis or gonorrheal vaginitis in children, vaginal suppositories of the hormone are the method of choice. Where a *systemic effect* is desired or the tissue to be affected is not directly accessible to the hormone, the oral, sublingual or parenteral route is indicated.

The naturally occurring estrogens, with the exception of estriol glycuronide, are many times more effective by injection than by the oral route. To obtain a *rapid, intense effect*, estrone or estradiol may be administered subcutaneously or intramuscularly. Ethinyl estradiol, diethylstilbestrol, diethylstilbestrol dipropionate, octofollin or hexestrol, if well tolerated, may likewise be employed for this purpose.

Where a *prolonged effect* is desired, the estrogen esters may be administered parenterally.[24] The estradiol esters such as the benzoate, propionate and dipropionate have a more intense and prolonged effect than the estrone esters, of which only the benzoate is now available for clinical use. For a *long continued, steady effect*, some observers recommend the subcutaneous implantation of pellets of pure crystalline estrogen.[25, 26] In the experience of some workers,[27] a single implantation may insure an estrogenic effect over a period of several weeks. This method is still in its experimental stage. Whether it will prove sufficiently practicable to warrant its general adoption remains to be seen.

In the *symptomatic menopause* or other conditions that require relatively small doses of the hormone over a protracted period of time, the oral route is desirable. For this purpose, estriol, estriol glycuronide, ethinyl estradiol, diethylstilbestrol, octofollin or hexestrol may be employed.

PROGESTATIONAL SUBSTANCES

The term *progestin* is applied to crude extracts of corpus luteum tissue which possess progestational activity. The name *progesterone* describes the crystalline form of the luteal hormone.[28] The active principle of the corpus luteum was prepared in crystalline form from sow corpora lutea in 1934. It has since been obtained from corpora lutea of other species, and also from ox adrenals.

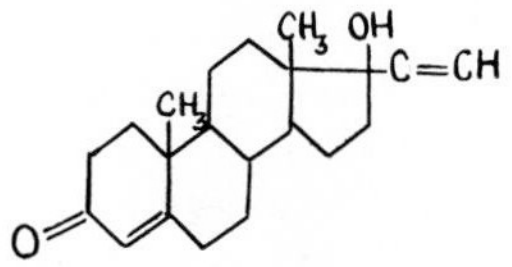

Pregneninolone
(Anhydro-hydroxy-progesterone)

Fig. 179.

Chemistry.—Progesterone has a phenanthrene nucleus and is chemically closely related to the estrogens, androgens and adrenal cortical hormones. It is an unsaturated diketone with the structural formula $C_{21}H_{30}O_2$, and exists in two forms: alpha-progesterone with a melting point of 128°C. (uncorr.), and beta-progesterone with a melting point of 121°C. (uncorr.). Progesterone has been synthesized from stigmasterol and pregnanediol, and also through oxidation of cholesterol.

Pregneninolone.—In addition to pregnanediol, human pregnancy urine yields allo-pregnanediol, epi-allopregnanediol, pregnanedione, and allopregnanolone,[29] all chemically closely related to progesterone, but with no progestational activity. Recent studies[74] indicate that many more compounds possess progestational activity than has hitherto been suspected, though their activity, as compared with progesterone, is relatively low. Of the various steroids shown to have luteoid activity only ethinyl testosterone has thus far been considered sufficiently active to merit production on a large scale for clinical use. This substance, which is also known as pregnenin–on–3–ol–17, anhydro-hydroxy-progesterone, and pregneninolone, has aroused particular interest because it is active by the oral route. Imhoffen and Hohlweg,[30] who first demonstrated its progestational activity, found that 4 mg. by mouth is as effective in eliciting progestational modifications of the uterine mucosa of the rabbit as 0.6 mg. of progesterone by injection. Courrier and Jost[31] found that when given parenterally or by mouth, pregneninolone maintained gestation in the ovariectomized rabbit. The importance of this compound can readily be appreciated when it is recalled that progesterone is orally inactive even in one hundred times the dose effective by injection. Where the parenteral route may conveniently be used, progesterone is preferable to pregneninolone, since the latter is only one-third as effective as progesterone by this route. The clinical efficacy of pregneninolone by the oral route is now being studied.[75, 76, 77] Investigations thus far carried[32] out indicate that, in terms of weight, six to seven times as much pregneninolone must be given by mouth to equal the effect of progesterone by injection. In the opinion of the Council on Pharmacy and Chemistry of the American Medical Association,[78] clinical studies have not yet convincingly proved that oral use of pregneninolone will accomplish all the effects obtainable with progesterone.

Standardization.—The progestational hormone was first standardized on the basis of its ability to induce progestational modifications in the estrogen primed endometrium of the rabbit. A *unit, as defined by Corner and Allen,*[33] is the minimum dose which, given in five equal doses on five successive days to adult female rabbits castrated when in heat, will produce by the sixth day progestational modifications of the uterine mucosa equivalent to those seen on the eighth day of gestation. A *Clauberg*[34] *unit,* estimated to equal from one-half to one-fifth of a Corner-Allen unit, is the amount of active substance required to induce progestational mucosal changes in the immature intact rabbit, weighing 600 grams and previously primed with estrogen. A *Clinical unit,* used abroad, is equal to one-third of a Clauberg unit. In 1935, the Standardization Committee of the League of Nations adopted an *international unit,* which is defined as the progestational activity present in 1 mg. of beta-progesterone. This equals approximately 1 Corner-Allen unit.[18]

Metabolism of Progesterone.—The discovery of pregnanediol and its identification as an excretion product of progesterone (see Chap. III) was the starting point for the investigation of the factors controlling progestin metabolism. It is not yet known by what complex process the diketone, progesterone, is reduced to the dihydroxy compound, pregnanediol, which is found conjugated with glucuronic acid in the urine of normal and pregnant women. Some believe the glucuronic complex is conjugated in the liver and excreted by the kidney. It has also been suggested that progesterone is partly excreted as physiologically inactive compounds, such as allopregnanediol and pregnanolone. The amount of sodium pregnanediol glucuronidate recoverable from the urine following progesterone administration is variable, and usually relatively small compared with the quantity of hormone injected. It was believed at first that a functioning uterine mucosa is essential for the conversion of progesterone to pregnanediol,[35] but recent studies indicate that the uterus favors but is not indispensable for such conversion.[36, 79] There is evidence that the recovery of pregnanediol following the injection of progesterone is facilitated by the presence of a functioning corpus luteum and a pregravid mucosa, as occurs in normal pregnancy or during the luteal phase of the menstrual cycle. It may also be increased by first building up the endometrium with estrogen, or by simultaneously administering this hormone.[35, 80]

ANDROGENIC SUBSTANCES

The term *androgen* describes substances possessing masculinizing activity. The naturally occurring androgens include androsterone and dehydroandrosterone, which have been isolated from the urine of men, normal, castrate and pregnant women, steers, bulls and pregnant cows. In addition, there are testosterone from bulls' testes, adrenosterone from adrenal cortical extract, and certain pregnane derivatives from the urine of patients with adrenal cortical tumors.

Chemistry of the Androgens.—The androgens are derivatives of androstane. Like the ovarian sex hormones, they contain the phenanthrene

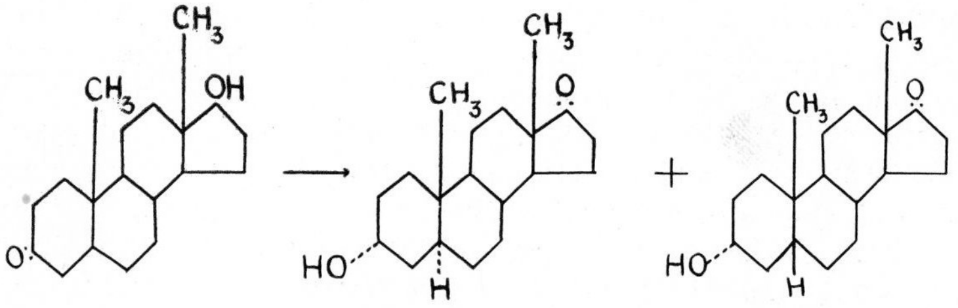

Testosterone   Androsterone   Etiocholan
$-3(\alpha)-$ ol-17–one

Fig. 180.—Scheme representing one course of the degradation of testosterone in the human organism. (After Callow and associates: J. Endocrinol., Vol. 1.)

nucleus. *Androsterone*, represented by the formula $C_{19}H_{30}O_2$, was the first androgen isolated in crystalline form by Butenandt and Tscherning[37] in 1931. It is a saturated compound, containing a secondary alcohol and a ketone group, and is chemically very stable. Ruzicka and coworkers[38] showed that oxidation of epicholesterol gives androsterone, thus establishing the relationship between the sex hormones and cholesterol.

Dehydroandrosterone is one-third as active as androsterone in promoting comb growth. It was synthesized from cholesterol in 1935 by Ruzicka and Wettstein,[39] who have also shown that it can be converted into $\triangle$ 4:5–androstene 17–ol–3–one, a compound shown to be identical with naturally occurring *testosterone*. The latter is about ten times as active as androsterone and has the formula $C_{19}H_{28}O_2$. It was isolated in crystalline form from bull's testes by David and coworkers.[40] Its synthesis was first accomplished by Butenandt[41] in 1935.

Standardization.—The *international unit,* established in 1935, is defined as the equivalent of 100 gamma (.0001 gram) of crystalline androsterone.

Metabolism of the Androgens.—Information relating to the metabolism of the androgens is still limited. It has been suggested that testosterone is the true testicular hormone, which is degraded in the organism to form androsterone and the inactive stereoisomeric compound etiocholan–3 (alpha) ol–17–one. In this connection Callow and coworkers[42] observed that the urine of patients injected with testosterone contained an increased amount of androsterone and etiocholan–3 (alpha) ol–17–one. Paschkis and his associates[81] observed estrogen excretion following the administration of androsterone and testosterone in the dog. This conversion of androgen into estrogen is independent of the adrenals and gonads for it occurs in their absence.

Method of Administration.—The clinical effectiveness of the androgens can be materially increased by delaying absorption of the active principle. This can be accomplished by injecting the hormone in an oily solution or by esterification. Miescher and coworkers[43] found the propionate to be one of the most potent of the various esters of *testosterone*. The high potency of testosterone and the fact that it can be commercially prepared from cholesterol is responsible for the general adoption of this compound and its propionate ester for clinical use.

Testosterone and testosterone propionate are commercially available in oily solution for subcutaneous or intramuscular use, and also in an ointment base for percutaneous administration. Salmon and his associates[44] recommend sublingual administration of testosterone in propylene glycol solution. Subcutaneous implants of the hormone in pellet form have been advocated by some workers where a continuous effect over a period of weeks or months is desired.[45] *Methyl testosterone* has recently been made available for oral use. This compound, represented by the formula $C_{20}H_{30}O_2$, is estimated to be from $\frac{1}{4}$ to $\frac{2}{5}$ as active by mouth as by injection. According to Vest and Barelare,[46] the optimal maintenance dose of methyl testosterone by mouth is from three to four times that of testosterone propionate by injection. These observers believe the ease of administering the methyl compound more than compensates for the large quantity of hormone required. To account for the fact that it is fairly active by mouth, Miescher and his associates[43] suggest that the methyl group in the 17 position protects the hydroxyl group from hydrolysis by intestinal ferments, so that the molecule is absorbed unchanged.

GONADOTROPIC SUBSTANCES

The terms *gonadotropic* and *gonad-stimulating* describe hormones capable of directly stimulating gonadal function. Such substances have been obtained from anterior lobe tissue, the body fluids and placenta of pregnant women (*chorionic gonadotropin*), and the serum of pregnant mares (*equine gonadotropin*).

Anterior Pituitary Gonadotropins.—There is evidence suggesting that the anterior pituitary gland elaborates at least two gonadotropic principles, one with follicle stimulating and a second with luteinizing properties (see Chap. XII). Their isolation in pure form has been attended by much difficulty, though considerable progress has been made in this direction.

Greep and associates[47] and Evans' group[48] have reported the preparation of the luteinizing hormone ("metakentrin") in relatively pure form. Mc-Shan[49] claims to have freed the follicle-stimulating factor from its luteinizing contaminant by tryptic digestion. Preparation of a fairly pure potent form of the follicle-stimulating factor from sheep pituitary has also been reported by Ceithaml and Koch.[82]

Chemistry.—Very little is known of the chemistry of the anterior pituitary gonadotropins or their fate in the organism. They are of a protein nature and belong to the group of glycoproteins. They are insoluble in alcohol, acetone and chloroform, and are readily destroyed by heating above 50° C., by dilute inorganic acids and bases, and by trypsin.

Standardization.—An international standard for the anterior pituitary gonadotropins has not yet been established. They are still assayed on the basis of the ovarian and uterine response in the immature rat. The degree of response is taken as the unit, which varies with each manufacturer. The follicle-stimulating hormone may be assayed on the basis of its ability to increase ovarian or uterine weight, stimulate the growth of follicles, or cause vaginal cornification. Levin and Tyndale[50] maintain that since the increase in uterine weight is the result of a functional response of the ovary, that is, increased estrogen secretion, it is of greater physiological significance than the increase in ovarian weight and would therefore appear a more logical test of the potency of predominantly follicle-stimulating extracts. The luteinizing hormone may be assayed on the basis of its ability to augment the effect of the follicle-stimulating hormone in the female, or to increase the weight of the seminal vesicles in the immature male rat. Frank and Berman,[51] who compared the four methods used for the assay of the gonadotropes, concluded that vaginal cornification is unreliable for bio-assay and that the ovarian and uterine weight increase indicates the amount of follicle-stimulating but not of luteinizing hormone present. In their opinion the most reliable assay method is that based upon the morphologic changes in the ovary. They define a unit of follicle-stimulating hormone as the amount of substance required to produce a full growth of 6 follicles in the immature rat, and a unit of luteinizing *hormone* as the amount required to produce contiguous corpora lutea.

Clinical Efficacy.—Most of the available commercial preparations of anterior lobe gonadotropin are derived from the glands of cattle and sheep. Their low unitage, and tendency to deteriorate rapidly on standing are probably at least partly responsible for their clinical ineffectiveness. There is as yet no clinical condition in which their usefulness has been adequately demonstrated. In a recent study, Parkes[83] observed that sheep pituitary gonadotropic extract could be rendered as much as twenty times more efficient in the rat by administering it over five days with excipient by the implantation route instead of by injection. Whether a similar result might be achieved in man remains to be seen.

Chorionic Gonadotropin.—The term "chorionic gonadotropin" designates gonadotropic substances, with predominantly luteinizing properties, present in the placenta and urine of pregnant women.

Standardization.—The active principle has recently been prepared in almost pure form, and an *international unit* established by the Third International Conference on the Standardization of Hormones.[52] This is defined as equivalent to the gonadotropic activity 0.1 mg. (100 gamma) of a standard dry powder prepared by members of the conference. It is approximately equal to the amount of hormone required to induce vaginal cornification in the immature rat. A method recently devised by Katzman and his associates,[84] for the extraction and purification of pregnancy urine gonadotropin, yields a preparation possessing a potency of 8500 I.U. per mg.

Clinical Efficacy.—Chorionic gonadotropin is effective only when administered parenterally. Observations in the laboratory animal indicate that its effectiveness may be increased by delaying absorption of the active principle through the use of multiple injections or the addition of a preciptant such as zinc sulphate. Though it is apparently capable of stimulating the function of the interstitial cells of the testis in man, it is otherwise of doubtful clinical value when used alone (see Chap. XII). A preparation which combines the anterior pituitary "synergist" (see Chap. XII) and chorionic gonadotropin has recently been made available for clinical use (see Synapoidin in Table 18). Marked stimulation of the human ovary has been described following its administration, but the reports thus far are still too limited for a fair judgment of its value.

Equine Gonadotropin.—The gonad-stimulating substances found in the serum of pregnant mares exert both a follicle-stimulating and luteinizing effect in the laboratory animal (see Chap. XII). In the monkey and man, their effect is primarily follicle stimulating.

Extraction and Purification.—Evans and associates,[53] in 1936, succeeded in obtaining a purified form of the hormone from acetone-dried protein material of blood serum. Gustus and associates[54] later extracted the active principle directly from the citrated plasma of the mare. Cartland and Nelson[55] prepared a highly purified extract of pregnant mare plasma, the hormone fractions being obtained as a dry, white, water-soluble, and remarkably stable powder. Rinderknecht and his associates[56] have described a method by which they extracted from pregnant mare's serum a white powder which is readily soluble in water and represents approximately a 1000-fold purification of the hormone in terms of solid content of the original serum. Goss and Cole[57] extracted serum of nonpregnant mares and purified it to the point where 1 mg. contained from 4000 to 7000 rat units.

The active principle is said to be of a polypeptid nature. It is active by the subcutaneous, intramuscular and intravenous route. Where intravenous injection is contemplated, sensitivity tests should be performed to avoid untoward effects. Failure to take this precaution may have serious consequences. On the whole, it is best to avoid the intravenous route.

Standardization.—The equine hormone was standardized at first by assay in the immature female rat, by the methods of Cartland and Nelson,[58] and of Cole and Saunders.[59] The *rat unit*, as defined by Cole and Saunders, is the amount of hormone which, when injected subcutaneously in a single dose into five immature female rats, twenty-one to twenty-three days old, will produce an average of three to ten large follicles or corpora lutea at the end of ninety-six hours; and which, if halved, will not produce this average in five rats similarly treated. Cartland and Nelson define a rat unit as the total dose of hormone which, when given subcutaneously in divided daily doses to twenty-one to twenty-three day old female rats weighing 30 to 40 grams, will produce in five days a pair of ovaries weighing 65 mg., which is five times the weight of the ovaries in the uninjected controls. One Cartland-Nelson unit equals approximately 10 Cole-Saunders units. The *international unit* is defined as the specific gonadotropic activity of 0.25 mg. (250 gammas) of a standard preparation held by the Health Organization of the League of Nations. It has been estimated to be equivalent to approximately one-half of a Cole-Saunders unit or about one-twentieth of a Cartland-Nelson unit. Cole and Erway[60] claim, however, that one Cole-Saunders rat unit is equivalent to one international unit.

LACTOGENIC SUBSTANCES

The terms *lactogen* and *lactogenic principle* are applied to substances of anterior pituitary origin which induce milk secretion in properly prepared breasts (see Chap. X).

Sources.—These substances are obtained mainly from the anterior pituitary glands of cattle and sheep. Substances possessing lactogenic properties have also been found in the urine of pregnant and postpartum women, and pregnant and lactating mares, in the young human placenta, the breast and milk of postpartum cows, and the livers of fishes and pigeons. None of these sources has yielded sufficient amounts for commercial purposes.

Physical Properties.—The lactogenic principle is protein in nature. It resists destruction by boiling for one hour at pH 7.5 to 8.5, but is readily inactivated at higher or lower pH, or in the presence of salts. It is stable when dry and may remain active in solution for some time if kept at low temperatures. Preparation from anterior lobe tissue of a homogeneous crystalline protein with high lactogenic potency has been reported by White and coworkers.[61] Li and his associates[85] have isolated from sheep and ox glands a chemically pure lactogenic preparation possessing a potency of 25 to 30 I.U. per mgm.

Standardization.—The lactogenic hormone may be assayed on the basis of its ability to induce milk secretion in the pseudopregnant rabbit or ovariectomized guinea pig,[62] or to increase the weight of the crop gland in the pigeon or dove. A *rabbit unit,* as defined by Gardner and Turner,[63] is the minimum amount of active substance which, when injected at daily intervals for seven days in rabbits previously pseudopregnant for twelve to sixteen days, will induce a plus 3 or 4 reaction, as determined by examination of the dissected glands. A *pigeon or dove unit,* as defined by Riddle and Bates,[64] is the minimum amount of substance which, when injected intramuscularly once daily for four days into birds two to three months old, will at the end of ninety-six hours after the first injection, cause a certain increase in the weight of the crop gland of the majority of a group of birds. The recently established *international unit* is defined as the lactogenic activity of 0.1 mg. (100 gamma) of Riddle's standard prolactin powder.

Clinical Efficacy.—The clinical effectiveness of the lactogenic hormone has not yet been convincingly demonstrated (see Chap. XXXII). Though a few favorable reports have appeared, critical observers[65] have been unable to stimulate milk secretion in hypogalactia with doses as high as 1000 pigeon units daily from the sixth to the ninth postpartum day.

ADRENAL CORTICAL SUBSTANCES

Of the many crystalline derivatives isolated from adrenal concentrates, seven are capable of replacing the functions of the adrenal cortex (see Fig. 48). The most active crystalline derivative thus far isolated from adrenal cortical tissue is a steroid compound with the formula $C_{19-21}H_{28-30}O_5$. From the commercial standpoint, the most important crystalline derivative is *desoxycorticosterone*, which can be synthesized from stigmasterol and is consequently available commercially in ample amounts. *Desoxycorticosterone acetate,* which is effective by the parenteral route, is now available for clinical use. Implantation of the hormone in pellet form has been tried by some observers but has proved less satisfactory than the injection method because of variation in the amount of material liberated. There is evidence that it is also effective by the sublingual route. Its clinical usefulness in conditions traceable to adrenal insufficiency is fairly well established (see Chap. XXXV).

TABLE 12

Source	a. Naturally occurring estrogens extracted from urine and placenta of pregnant women, and urine of pregnant mares.
	b. Synthetic estrogens derived from
	  1. Sterols
	  2. Common laboratory reagents (e.g. diethylstilbestrol)

Biologic Effects	In the female castrate animal: a. Directly stimulates growth of accessory genitalia and secondary sex characters. b. Develops uterine mucosa to proliferative phase; withdrawal followed by bleeding in monkey. c. Induces cornification of vaginal mucosa in rodent. d. Stimulates uterine and tubal motility. e. Stimulates growth of mammary duct system; in large doses inhibits milk secretion. f. Stimulates or inhibits anterior pituitary function, depending on intensity and duration of treatment. In the human female, effects essentially same as in lower mammal.
Standardization	Standardized in terms of: a. International unit, defined as estrogenic activity of 0.001 mgm. of ketohydroxyestrin (estrone). b. International benzoate unit, defined as estrogenic activity of 0.001 mgm. of benzoic acid ester of alpha-estradiol. c. Rat unit (1 R.U. is equivalent to 5–10 I.U., depending on assay method used). d. Weight, in milligrams, of active substance.
Route of Administration	Available for administration by: a. Subcutaneous or intramuscular injection (estrone, estradiol, and their esters; diethylstilbestrol). Diethylstilbestrol by injection in the rat is 1–3 times as active as equal quantity of estrone. b. Mouth (estriol, sodium estrone sulphate, ethinyl estradiol, diethylstilbestrol, hexestrol, octofollin). Diethylstilbestrol per os is $\frac{1}{2}$ to $\frac{1}{3}$ as active as equal quantity of estrone in oil by injection. Sodium estrone sulphate by mouth 3 times as active as equal quantity of estrone by mouth. c. Local application—percutaneous, intravaginal, intranasal (estrone, estradiol and their esters; diethylstilbestrol). d. Subcutaneous implantation (estrone, estradiol and their esters; diethylstilbestrol).
Commercial Preparations	Amniotin (Squibb), extract of pregnant mare's urine; contains estrone and small amounts of equilin, hippulin, and equilenin; in oil for intramuscular injection; ampuls contain 2000, 5000, 10,000, and 20,000 I.U. per cc. For administration per vaginam, pessaries containing 1000 and 2000 I.U. For oral use, capsules containing 1000, 2000, 4000, and 10,000 I.U. For intranasal application, oily solutions containing 10,000 I.U. per cc., and 20,000 I.U. in 30 cc.
	Ben-Ovocylin (Ciba), extract of human pregnancy urine; contains benzoic acid ester of alpha-estradiol; in oil for intramuscular injection; 1 cc. ampuls contain 0.083 mgm. (500 R.U.), 0.1 mgm. (600 R.U.), 0.166 mgm. (1000 R.U.), 0.2 mgm. (1200 R.U.), 0.333 mgm. (2000 R.U.), 1.0 mgm. (6000 R.U.), and 1.66 mgm. (10,000 R.U.).
	Dimenformon (Roche-Organon), extract of human pregnancy urine; contains crystalline alpha-estradiol; in solution containing 0.3 mgm. per cc.; in tablets containing 0.1 mgm. (1200 R.U.) and 0.2 mgm. (2400 R.U.); for use by mouth.

TABLE 12—*Continued*

ESTROGENIC SUBSTANCES

Commercial Preparations (*continued*)	Dimenformon Benzoate (Roche-Organon), extract of human pregnancy urine; contains benzoic acid ester of alpha-estradiol; in oil for intramuscular injection; ampuls contain 0.1 mgm. (600 R.U.), 0.166 mgm. (1000 R.U.), 0.333 mgm. (2000 R.U.), 1 mgm. (6000 R.U.), and 1.66 mgm. (10,000 R.U.).
	Dimenformon Dipropionate (Roche-Organon), extract of human pregnancy urine; contains propionic acid ester of alpha-estradiol; in oil for intramuscular injection; ampuls contain 0.1, 0.2, 1.0, 2.5, and 5.0 mgm. per cc.
	Di-Ovocylin (Ciba), extract of human pregnancy urine; contains propionic acid ester of alpha-estradiol; in oil for intramuscular injection; 1 cc. ampuls contain 0.1, 0.2, 1.0, 2.5, and 5 mgm.
	Emmenin (Ayerst), extract of human placenta; contains estriol glucuronide. In liquid form for oral use; 30 day-oral units per cc. (1 day-oral unit is amount given orally which will induce estrus in immature rat). Also in tablet form for oral use; 1 tablet = 1 teaspoonful of liquid = 120 day-oral units.
	Estinyl (Schering), synthetic ethinyl estradiol. (Not yet available commercially.)
	Estriol (Abbott), crystalline estriol from urine of pregnant women; in capsule form for oral use; capsules contain 0.06, 0.12, and 0.24 mgm.
	Estriol (Lilly), crystalline estriol from urine of pregnant women; in pulvules for oral use; pulvules contain 0.06, 0.12, and 0.24 mgm.
	Estrogenic Hormones (Upjohn), extract of pregnant mare's urine; in oil for intramuscular injection; ampuls contain 2000 and 10,000 I.U. per cc.
	Estrone (Abbott), crystalline estrone from urine of pregnant women; in oil for intramuscular injection; ampuls contain 1000, 2000, 5000, and 10,000 I.U. per cc. For administration per vaginam, suppositories containing 0.02 mgm. (200 I.U.), and 0.2 mgm. (2000 I.U.).
	Estrone (Lilly), crystalline estrone from urine of pregnant women, in oil for intramuscular injection; ampuls contain 1000, 2000, 5000, and 10,000 I.U. per cc. For administration per vaginam, suppositories containing 2000 I.U.
	Folestrin (Armour), extract of pregnant mare's urine; in oil for intramuscular injection; ampuls contain 2000, 5000, 10,000, and 20,000 I.U. per cc. For oral use, sealed gelatin capsules containing 1000, 2000, and 4000 I.U. per glanule. For administration per vaginam, suppositories containing 1000 and 2000 I.U.
	Menformon (Roche-Organon), extract of human pregnancy urine; contains estrone. In oil for intramuscular injection; ampuls contain 1000, 2000, 5000, and 10,000 I.U. per cc. In tablets containing 1000 I.U. for oral use. In ointment base for local application; dosules contain 2000 and 5000 I.U. For administration per vaginam, vaginal inserts containing 500 and 1000 I.U.
	Ovocylin (Ciba), extract of human pregnancy urine; contains alpha-estradiol. In tablet form for oral use; tablets contain 0.1, 0.2, and 0.5 mgm. For administration per vaginam, suppositories containing 0.04 and 0.4 mgm. For topical application, in ointment base containing 0.03 and 0.15 mgm. of estradiol per gram.
	Premarin (Ayerst), sodium estrone sulphate, conjugated estrogen; extracted from pregnant mare's urine; in tablet form for oral use; 1.25 mgm. tablets.
	Progynon (Schering), crude estrogen, in aqueous solution for intramuscular injection; 1 cc. ampuls contain 125 I.U. (25 R.U.), 225 I.U. (45 R.U.), 1000 I.U. (200 R.U.), and 3000 I.U. (600 R.U.).

TABLE 12—*Continued*

ESTROGENIC SUBSTANCES

Commercial Preparations (*continued*)	Progynon-B (Schering), contains benzoic acid ester of alpha-estradiol; in oil for intramuscular injection; ampuls contain 500, 1000, 2000, 6000 and 10,000 R.U. per cc.
	Progynon-DH (Schering), contains free alpha-estradiol for oral and topical use; tablets for oral use contain 0.1, 0.2, and 0.5 mgm. (1 mgm. more active than equal weight of estriol by mouth; is equivalent to 1200 I.U. estrone by injection). For administration per vaginam, suppositories containing 480 and 4800 R.U. For topical application, in ointment base, containing 360 and 1800 R.U. per gram. For oral use, also available in alcohol solution containing 3600 R.U. per cc. or 60 R.U. per drop. For intranasal administration, in solution containing 160 R.U. per cc.
	Progynon-DP (Schering), contains propionic acid ester of alpha-estradiol; in oil for intramuscular injection; 1 cc. ampuls contain 0.1, 0.2, 1.0, 2.5, and 5 mgm. (1 mgm. = 2000 R.U. or 30,000 I.U.).
	Theelin (Parke, Davis & Co.), extract of human pregnancy urine; contains crystalline estrone in oil for intramuscular injection; ampuls contain 1000, 2000, 5000, and 10,000 I.U. Also in aqueous suspension for intramuscular injection; 2 mgm. in 1 cc. of physiologic saline solution. For administration per vaginam, suppositories containing 2000 I.U.
	Theelol (Parke, Davis & Co.), crystalline estriol; in capsule form for oral use (1 I.U. by mouth equivalent to 5 I.U. of Theelin by injection); capsules contain 0.06, 0.12, and 0.24 mgm.
	Urestrin (Upjohn), extract of pregnant mare's urine; in capsule form for oral use; capsules contain 1000 and 2000 I.U.
(Diethylstilbestrol Preparations)	Diethylstilbestrol (Abbott), diethylstilbestrol in tablet form for oral use; tablets contain 0.1, 0.25, 0.5, 1.0 and 5.0 mgm. In oily solution for intramuscular injection; ampuls contain 0.5 and 1.0 mgm. per cc. In suppositories, for intravaginal administration, each containing 0.5 mgm.
	Diethylstilbestrol (Lakeside), diethylstilbestrol in tablet form, for oral use; tablets contain 0.25, 0.5, 1.0, 2.0 and 5.0 mgm. In oily solution for intramuscular injection; 1 cc. ampuls contain 0.1, 0.5, 0.25, 1.0, 2.0 and 5.0 mgm.
	Diethylstilbestrol (Lilly), diethylstilbestrol in tablet form for oral use; tablets contain 0.1, 0.25, 0.5, and 1.0 mgm.; also enteric-coated tablets containing 0.1, 0.25, 0.5, and 1.0 mgm. For administration per vaginam, suppositories containing 0.1 and 0.5 mgm. In oil for intramuscular injection; ampuls contain 0.5 and 1 0 mgm. per cc.
	Estrobene (Ayerst), diethylstilbestrol in oily solution contained in capsules for oral use; capsules contain 0.25, 0.5, 1 and 5 mgm.
	Estrobene-DP (Ayerst), propionic acid ester of diethylstilbestrol; in oil for intramuscular injection; ampuls contain 1 and 5 mgm. per cc.
	Stilbestrol (Armour) diethylstilbestrol in tablet form for oral use; tablets contain 1.0, 0.5, 0.25, and 0.1 mgm. In oil for intramuscular injection; 1 cc. ampuls contain 0.5 and 1.0 mgm.
	Stilbestrol (Breon), diethylstilbestrol in tablet form for oral use; tablets contain 0.2, 0.5 and 1.0 mgm. In oily solution for intramuscular injection, 1 cc. ampuls of 1.0 mgm.
	Stilbestrol (Merrell), diethylstilbestrol in tablet form for oral use; tablets contain 0.2 and 1.0 mgm.
	Stilbestrol (Sharp & Dohme), diethylstilbestrol in tablet form for oral use; tablets contain 0.1, 0.5 and 1.0 mgm. In oily solution for intramuscular injection; ampuls contain 0.5 and 1.0 mgm.

TABLE 12—*Continued*

Estrogenic Substances

	Stilbestrol (Squibb), diethylstilbestrol in form of tablets, uncoated and enteric-coated, for oral use; tablets contain 0.5, 1.0, and 5.0 mgm. In oil for intramuscular injection; 1 cc. ampuls contain 0.2, 0.5, 1.0, and 5 mgm. For administration per vaginam, pessaries containing 0.1 and 0.5 mgm.
	Stilbestrol (Upjohn), diethylstilbestrol, in form of perles for oral use; perles contain 0.1, 0.5, and 1.0 mgm. In sterile solution for intramuscular injection; 1 cc. ampuls contain 0.5 and 1.0 mgm.
	Stilbestrol (Winthrop), diethylstilbestrol in tablet form for oral use; tablets contain 0.1, 0.5, and 1.0 mgm. In oil for intramuscular injection; ampuls contain 0.5 and 1 mgm. per cc. For administration per vaginam, suppositories containing 0.1 and 0.5 mgm.
(Hexestrol Preparations)	Hexestrol (Merrell), hexestrol in tablet form for oral use; tablets contain 0.2, 1.0 and 3.0 mgm. In oily solution for intramuscular injection; ampuls contain 1.0 mgm. per cc.
(Octofollin Preparations)	Octofollin (Schieffelin), 2,4-di(p-hydroxyphenyl)-3-ethyl hexane in form of tablets, for oral use; tablets contain 0.5 mgm., 1.0 mgm., 2.0 mgm. and 5.0 mgm. In oily solution for intramuscular injection; ampuls contain 5 mgm. per cc. (1 mgm. by injection equals about 25,000 I.U. estrone by injection).

Indications and Dosage*	**Prepuberal Period:**
	  a. Vulvo-vaginitis of gonorrheal origin—local application of vaginal suppositories containing 500 I.U. nightly, until desired effect is achieved. In severe cases, some recommend combined local and parenteral therapy (1000–2000 I.U. intramuscularly every other day). Dose increased or decreased depending on response.
	Reproductive Period:
	  a. Uterine hypoplasia—5000 to 10,000 I.U. 2 to 3 times weekly until adequate growth is induced. In marked hypoplasia, higher doses and prolonged treatment may be required.
	  b. Amenorrhea (primary and secondary)—10,000 to 50,000 I.U. 2 to 3 times weekly for 2 weeks, followed by course of progesterone injections. Repeat as often as required.
	  c. Tubal hypoplasia—5000–10,000 I.U. 2 to 3 times a week during first half of cycle.
	  d. Dysmenorrhea due to uterine hypoplasia—1000–2000 I.U. 2 to 3 times a week during first half of cycle.
	  e. Mammary hypoplasia—topical application of estrogenic ointment daily; may supplement with 2000 to 10,000 I.U. intramuscularly 2 to 3 times a week.
	  f. Suppression of lactation—10,000 to 50,000 I.U. intramuscularly daily during first few days postpartum (or 5–10 mgm. diethylstilbestrol).
	  g. Uterine inertia associated with low estrogen levels—125,000 I.U. intramuscularly in five to ten injections over period of 12 hours.
	Climacteric:
	  a. Menopausal vasomotor symptoms—doses vary widely. Initial dose of 1000 I.U. intramuscularly daily; increase or decrease depending on response. After symptoms subside, maintain with 1 mgm. or less of stilbestrol by mouth; or other orally active estrogens.
	  b. Senile vaginitis and kraurosis vulvae—1000 to 2000 I.U. intramuscularly 2 to 3 times a week, or 1000 to 2000 I.U. per vaginam. In severe cases, the two forms may be combined.
	Miscellaneous Uses:
	  a. Atrophic rhinitis—after irrigating nose with alkaline wash and removing crusts, spray with estrogen in oil containing 10,000 I.U. per cc. then daily with oily solution containing 20,000 I.U. in 30 cc.

* Doses are based on those recommended in the literature. For evaluation, see text.

TABLE 13

PROGESTATIONAL SUBSTANCES

Source	Pure crystalline progesterone obtained
	  a. By extraction from corpora lutea of swine.
	  b. By synthesis from pregnanediol extracted rom human pregnancy urine.
	  c. By synthesis from stigmasterol obtained from the soy bean.
	Pregneninolone (anhydrohydroxy-progesterone), orally active compound obtained
	  a. By synthesis from progesterone.
	  b. By synthesis from testosterone.

Biologic Effects	In the lower mammal:
	  a. Induces pregravid modifications in estrogen-primed endometrium.
	  b. Inhibits uterine and tubal motility.
	  c. Induces mucification in estrogen-primed vaginal epithelium.
	  d. Stimulates development of mammary lobule-alveolar system.
	  e. Maintains pregnancy following ovariectomy.
	In the primate:
	  a. Induces pregravid modifications in estrogen-primed endometrium; withdrawal followed by bleeding.
	  b. Inhibits uterine (?) and tubal motility.
	  c. Antagonizes effect of estrogen on vaginal epithelium.
	  d. Stimulates development of mammary lobule-alveolar system.

Standardization	Standardized in terms of:
	  a. Corner-Allen rabbit unit (adult rabbit).
	  b. Clauberg rabbit unit (immature rabbit).
	  c. International unit (I.U), defined as progestational activity of 1 mgm. of pure crystalline progesterone.
	  d. By weight in milligrams (employed for both progesterone and pregneninolone).
	1 mgm. progesterone = 1 I.U. = 1 Corner-Allen unit = 2 Clauberg units.
	1 mgm. pregneninolone by mouth = $\frac{1}{5}$ mgm. progesterone by injection.

Route of Administration	Progesterone for intramuscular injection. Pregneninolone for oral use.
Commercial Preparations	Lipo-lutin (Parke, Davis & Co.), protein-free extract of fresh corpora lutea; in oil for intramuscular injection; 1 cc. ampuls contain 1 and 2 I.U. Lutocylin (Ciba), pure crystalline progesterone synthesized from stigmasterol; in oil for intramuscular injection; 1 cc. ampuls contain 1, 5, and 10 mgm. Nalutron (Winthrop), synthetic progesterone in oil for intramuscular injection; ampuls contain 1, 2 and 5 mgm. per cc. Progesterol (Smith) synthetic progesterone in oil for intramuscular injection; ampuls contain 1 I.U. per cc. Progesterone (Armour), synthetic crystalline progesterone; in oil for intramuscular injection; 1 cc. ampuls contain $\frac{1}{2}$, 1, 2, and 5 I.U. Progesterone (Upjohn), synthetic crystalline progesterone; in oil for intramuscular injection; 1 cc. ampuls contain 1 I.U. Progestin (Abbott), partially purified progesterone derived from oxidation of cholesterol; in oil for intramuscular injection; 1 cc. ampuls contain 1, 2, and 5 I.U. Progestin (Lilly), protein-free extract of fresh corpora lutea; in oil for intramuscular injection; 1 cc. ampuls contain 1, 5, and 10 mgm. Progestin (Roche-Organon), synthetic crystalline progesterone; in oil for intramuscular injection; 1 cc. ampuls contain 1 I.U. Progestin (Upjohn), protein-free extract of fresh corpora lutea; in oil for intramuscular injection; 1 cc. ampuls contain $\frac{1}{2}$ and 1 Corner-Allen unit.

TABLE 13—*Continued*

PROGESTATIONAL SUBSTANCES

(Pregneninolone Preparations)	Proluton (Schering), synthetic crystalline progesterone; in oil for intramuscular injection; 1 cc. ampuls contain $\frac{1}{5}$, 1, 2, 5, and 10 mgm. Lutocylin Linguets (Ciba), pregneninolone in tablet form for sublingual administration; tablets contain 5 mgm. Lutocylol (Ciba), pregneninolone, in tablet form for oral use; 5 and 10 mgm. tablets. Pranone (Schering), pregneninolone; in tablet form for oral use; 5 and 10 mgm. tablets. Progestoral (Roche-Organon), pregneninolone; in tablet form for oral use; 10 mgm. tablets.
Indications and Dosage*	Disorders of Menstruation: 　a. Amenorrhea—after course of estrogen for 2 weeks (total of 1,000,000 I.U. in primary amenorrhea, of 150,000 to 350,000 I.U. in secondary amenorrhea), give 35 to 50 I.U. progesterone over period of 7 days. 　b. Uterine Bleeding due to progesterone deficiency—in metrorrhagia, 1–5 I.U. daily until bleeding stops; in menorrhagia. 1–5 I.U. daily beginning 3 to 6 days before expected flow (in severe cases, 5–20 I.U. daily). 　c. Dysmenorrhea due to progesterone deficiency—1–5 I.U. or more daily beginning 3 to 6 days before expected flow. Disorders of Reproduction: 　a. Sterility due to inadequate preparation of nidatory bed—1–5 I.U. or more daily, beginning after ovulation (12th to 15th day of cycle) and continued until onset of flow or, if conception occurs, for several weeks after first miss. 　b. Habitual or threatened abortion—in habitual abortion, 5 I.U. 2 to 3 times a week, beginning after first miss or not later than 1 month before abortion tends to occur. After danger period is passed, continue with smaller doses for several months but not beyond the eighth month. May increase dose during missed periods. In threatened abortion, 10 or more I.U. daily until symptoms subside; then continue with 5 I.U. 2 to 3 times a week for several months, but not beyond eighth month. Miscellaneous Uses: 　a. After-pains—single injection of 1 or 2 I.U.; repeated if necessary. 　b. Hyperemesis gravidarum—1–5 I.U. daily for 3 to 4 days; then at longer intervals depending on response. 　c. Premenstrual tension—1–5 I.U. daily beginning about 1 week before expected flow.

* Doses are based on those recommended in the literature. For evaluation, see text. Figures given are for progesterone. Where pregneninolone is used by oral route, the dose is five times as much as that stated for progesterone.

TABLE 14

ANDROGENIC SUBSTANCES

Source	Pure crystalline testosterone obtained: a. By extraction from bull testes. b. By synthesis from the steroids. Methyl testosterone, orally active compound derived from testosterone.
Biologic Effects	In the male: a. Stimulates development of accessory genitalia and secondary sex characters. b. Inhibits anterior pituitary function when given in adequate doses. In the female: a. Antagonizes effects of estrogen. b. Stimulates masculine rudiments (in human, causes enlargement of clitoris, growth of facial and body hair, deepening of the voice). c. In primate, inhibits menstruation and lactation. d. Inhibits anterior pituitary function when given in adequate doses.
Standardization	Potency expressed in terms of weight (milligrams). An international unit is defined as the androgenic activity of 0.1 mgm. of crystalline androsterone. 1 mgm. of testosterone is 6 or more times as active as 1 mgm. of androsterone. 1 mgm. of methyl testosterone by mouth = $\frac{1}{3}$ to $\frac{1}{5}$ mgm. of testosterone by intramuscular injection.
Route of Administration	Testosterone (and its esters) for intramuscular injection. Methyl testosterone for oral use.
Commercial Preparations	Neo-Hombreol (Roche-Organon), propionic acid ester of testosterone; in oil for intramuscular injection; 1 cc. ampuls contain 5, 10, and 25 mgm. Oreton (Schering), propionic acid ester of testosterone; in oil for intramuscular injection; 1 cc. ampuls contain 5, 10, and 25 mgm. Perandren (Ciba), propionic acid ester of testosterone; in oil for intramuscular injection; 1 cc. ampuls contain 5, 10, and 25 mgm. Perandren Ointlets (Ciba), propionic acid ester of testosterone; in bland unguent base for topical application; each tube contains 4 mgm. of testosterone propionate. Metandren (Ciba), methyl testosterone; in tablet form for oral use; 10 mgm. tablets. Neo-Hombreol (M) Tablets (Roche-Organon), methyl testosterone; in tablet form for oral use; 10 mgm. tablets. Neo-Hombreol (M) Dosules (Roche-Organon), methyl testosterone, in ointment base for topical application; each dosule contains 4 mgm. of methyl testosterone. Oreton-M (Schering), methyl testosterone; in tablet form for oral use; 10 mgm. tablets. Oreton-M Toplicators (Schering), methyl testosterone; in ointment base for topical application; contains 2 mgm. of methyl testosterone per gram of ointment. Perandren Linquets (Ciba), methyl testosterone; in tablet form for sublingual administration.
Indications and Dosage*	In the male: a. Eunuchism and eunuchoidism—initial dose of 25 mgm. three times a week; gradually increase or decrease depending on response. b. Impotence—5 to 25 mgm. three times a week, depending on response. c. Male climacteric—begin with 10 mgm. three times a week and increase as required; for maintenance purposes, 5–10 mgm. methyl testosterone daily. d. Benign prostatic hypertrophy—5 to 25 mgm. three times a week depending on response.

TABLE 14—*Continued*

Androgenic Substances

In the female:
  a. Functional uterine bleeding—up to 25 mgm. every other day until bleeding is controlled.
  b. Functional dysmenorrhea—10 to 25 mgm. every other day beginning 3 to 6 days before the expected flow.
  c. After-pains—single injection of 10 or 20 mgm.; repeated if desired, after several hours.
  d. Breast engorgement—5–10 mgm. daily for 2 to 3 days.
  e. Premenstrual mammary pain—10 to 25 mgm. every other day until pain is relieved.
  f. Suppression of lactation—25 to 50 mgm. daily for two to three days.
  g. Female climacteric—initial dose of 10 mgm. twice weekly, increasing or decreasing depending on response.

* Doses are based on those recommended in the literature. For evaluation, see text.

TABLE 15

GONADOTROPIC SUBSTANCES (CHORIONIC GONADOTROFIN)

Source	By extraction from the urine and placenta of pregnant women.

Biologic Effects	In intact animal:
	  a. Female—induces ovulation and corpus luteum formation; effect predominantly luteinizing.
	  b. Male—stimulates interstitial cells with androgen production.
	In the human subject:
	  a. Female—no proof it stimulates hypofunctioning ovary; may augment existing luteal function; tends to promote follicular atresia.
	  b. Male—apparently promotes testicular descent and stimulates interstitial cells, thus indirectly causing growth of accessory genitalia.

Standardization	Standardized in international units, defined as the specific gonadotropic activity of 0.1 mgm. of the standard powder. 1 I.U. equals slightly less than 1 rat unit.
Route of Administration	For administration preferably by intramuscular injection, after dissolving dry powder in aqueous solution.
Commercial Preparations	Anterior Pituitary-Like Gonadotropic Hormone (Lakeside), extract of human pregnancy urine; in aqueous solution for intramuscular injection; ampuls contain 100 rat units per cc. Antuitrin-S (Apoidin) (Parke, Davis & Co.), extract of human pregnancy urine; in aqueous solution for intramuscular injection; vials contain 100 and 500 rat units per cc. "A.P.L." (Ayerst), extract of human placenta; in aqueous solution for intramuscular injection; vials contain 100, 500, 750, and 1000 I.U. per cc. Follutein (Squibb), extract of human pregnancy urine; ampuls contain 1000, 5000 and 10,000 I.U. in glycerin solution, to be diluted with distilled water, final mixture containing 100 I.U. per cc. Korotrin (Winthrop), extract of human pregnancy urine; in form of stable powder to be dissolved in distilled water for intramuscular injection; vials contain 100, 500, 1000, and 5000 I.U. Pregnyl (Roche-Organon), extract of human pregnancy urine; in powder form to be dissolved in distilled water for intramuscular injection; ampuls contain 100 and 500 rat units. Pranturon (Schering), extract of human pregnancy urine; in powder form to be dissolved in distilled water for intramuscular injection; ampuls contain 150 and 750 I.U.

Indications and Dosage*	In the female:
	  a. Amenorrhea (Primary and Secondary)—2 to 3 cc. of hypophyseal gonadotropin daily for 2 weeks to induce maturation of follicles; then follow with 200 or more I.U. of chorionic gonadotropin daily for 1 to 2 weeks. Repeat one or more times depending on response. If none, stop treatment to avoid antihormone formation. (Equine may replace hypophyseal hormone.)
	  b. Uterine bleeding due to progesterone deficiency—in metrorrhagia, 200 to 500 I.U. daily until bleeding is controlled; in menorrhagia, 200 units daily beginning several days before expected flow and continuing until bleeding is controlled.
	  c. Dysmenorrhea due to progesterone deficiency—500 I.U. for 2–4 days beginning at mid-point of cycle; or 200–300 units daily for several days preceding the flow.
	  d. Sterility due to inadequate preparation of the nidatory bed—100–500 I.U. three times a week during last two weeks of cycle.
	  e. Abortion due to progesterone deficiency—in habitual abortion, 100–500 U.I. three times a week during first half of gestation; or 100 units three times a week beginning 1 month before usual time of abortion and continuing for several months but

TABLE 15—*Continued*

GONADOTROPIC SUBSTANCES (CHORIONIC GONADOTROPIN)

	not beyond eighth month. In threatened abortion, 200–500 I.U. daily until danger passes; then continue with smaller doses for several months, but not beyond eighth month.
	In the male:
	  a. Cryptorchidism—100–500 I.U. three times a week until desired result is obtained.
	  b. Hypogonadism—100–200 I.U. 2–3 times weekly, increasing later, depending on response.

* Doses given are based on those recommended in the literature. For evaluation, see text.

TABLE 16

GONADOTROPIC SUBSTANCES (EQUINE GONADOTROPIN)

Source	By extraction from serum of pregnant mares.
Biologic Effects	In the lower mammal: a. Female—stimulates follicular maturation, ovulation, and corpus luteum formation in intact and hypophysectomized rodent. b. Male—stimulates interstitial cells of testis in intact immature and hypophysectomized animal. In the human subject: a. Female—some evidence that it stimulates follicular maturation and possibly also ovulation, but not conclusively established. b. Male—ability to stimulate hypofunctioning testis not established.
Standardization	Standardized in terms of: a. Cole-Saunders rat unit. b. Cartland-Nelson rat unit. c. International unit, defined as specific gonadotropic activity of 0.25 mgm. of the standard powder. 1 I.U. = $\frac{1}{2}$ Cole-Saunders unit = $\frac{1}{20}$ Cartland-Nelson unit.
Route of Administration	For administration by subcutaneous or intramuscular injection. Some recommend intravenous route.
Commercial Preparations	Anteron (Schering), in aqueous solution for subcutaneous or intramuscular injection; ampuls contain 400 and 2000 I.U. Also available in tablet form, to be dissolved in saline solution; tablets contain 400 and 2000 I.U. Gestyl (Organon), relatively protein-free extract of pregnant mare's serum; in tablet form to be dissolved in saline solution for intramuscular injection; ampuls of 200 and 400 I.U., with accompanying ampuls of solvent. Gonadin (Cutter), relatively protein-free extract of pregnant mare's serum; in saline solution for intramuscular injection; 1 cc. ampuls contain 500 I.U. Gonadogen (Upjohn), relatively protein-free extract of pregnant mare's serum; in tablet form to be dissolved in saline solution for intramuscular injection; tablets contain 10 and 20 Cartland-Nelson units.
Indications and Dosage*	In the female: a. Amenorrhea (Primary and Secondary)—if associated with genital hypoplasia, 200 I.U. daily until desired effect is achieved. If associated with some degree of genital development, 400 I.U. every other day for 6 injections followed by 2 weeks rest period or course of chorionic gonadotropin (see Table 15). b. Uterine bleeding due to deficient luteinizing impulse—single injection of 600 to 1200 I.U. at weekly intervals; or 200 to 400 I.U. three times a week for 1 to 2 weeks followed by 2 weeks rest period or by course of chorionic gonadotropin (see Table 15). c. Sterility—If due to suppression of both follicular and luteal function, 200–400 I.U. every other day for 2 weeks, followed by 2 week rest period. If due to failure of ovulation and corpus luteum formation, 200 to 400 I.U. on 7th, 8th, and 9th day of cycle, followed by single injection of 600 I.U. on 12th day. In the male: a. Cryptorchidism—200 I.U. 2 to 3 times a week until desired effect is achieved. b. Sterility due to hypogonadism secondary to pituitary deficiency —200–400 I.U. twice weekly.

* Doses given are based on those recommended in the literature. For evaluation, see text.

TABLE 17

Gonadotropic Substances (Hypophyseal Gonadotropin)

Source	By extraction from fresh anterior pituitary glands of cattle and sheep.

Biologic Effects	In the lower mammal:
	   a. Female—stimulates follicular maturation, ovulation, and corpus luteum formation in both intact and hypophysectomized animal.
	   b. Male—stimulates interstitial cells and the tubules, in both intact and hypophysectomized animal.
	In the human subject:
	   a. Female—ability to stimulate hypofunctioning ovary questionable.
	   b. Male—ability to stimulate hypofunctioning testis not established.

Standardization	Standardized in rat units, on basis of its ability to increase ovarian weight, induce morphologic alterations in ovary, increase uterine weight, or induce vaginal canalization. International unit not yet adopted.
Route of Administration	For administration preferably by intramuscular injection, after dissolving dry powder in sterile solution.
Commercial Preparations	Ambinon (Roche-Organon), contains follicle-stimulating, luteinizing and thyrotropic factors; in sterile solution for intramuscular injection; 1 cc. ampuls contain 50 rat units of gonadotropic hormone and 200 guinea pig units of thyrotropic hormone. Anterior Pituitary Extract (Squibb), alkaline aqueous extract from glands of cattle; contains growth, thyrotropic, and "sex complementary factor" (synergist); for intramuscular injection; vials contain 100 growth units per cc.; gonadotropic potency per cc. undetermined. Gonadophysin (Searle), extract of sheep anterior pituitary gland; in small doses predominantly follicle-stimulating, in large doses, has luteinizing effect; in powder form; vials contain 500 R.U. to be dissolved in 5 cc. of sterile solution. Gonadotropic Factor (Armour), extract from beef anterior pituitary gland; ampuls contain 300 rat units per cc. Gonadotropic Factor (Ayerst), extract from anterior pituitary gland of sheep; contains gonadotropic factors plus small amounts of other factors; predominantly follicle-stimulating; in sterile solution for intramuscular injection; vials contain 300 Collip rat units per cc. Prephysin (Chappel), contains follicle-stimulating factor plus small amount of luteinizing factor; in sterile solution for intramuscular injection; vials contain 25 R.U. per cc. Prephysin Special Potency—vials contain 100 R.U. per cc.

Indications and Dosage*	Hypogonadal conditions traceable to anterior pituitary deficiency.
	  a. Female—
	     1. Retarded sexual development.
	     2. Primary and secondary amenorrhea.
	     3. Sterility.
	     4. Habitual or threatened abortion due to deficient luteinization.
	     5. Functional uterine bleeding due to deficient luteinization.
	  b. Male—
	     1. Retarded sexual development.
	     2. Cryptorchidism.
	     3. Impotence.
	     4. Sterility.

* Doses recommended in the literature vary widely. Generally, 100 R.U. or more are used daily or every other day, depending on the individual case. Minimal effective dose in a given case uncertain because of questionable effect of hypophyseal gonadotropin on human gonad.

TABLE 18

COMBINED HYPOPHYSEAL AND CHORIONIC GONADOTROPIN

Commercial Preparations	Synapoidin (Parke, Davis & Co.), contains anterior pituitary follicle-stimulating factor ("synergist") and extract of human pregnancy urine; in sterile solution for intramuscular injection; vials contain 15 synergy rat units per cc. (1 synergy rat unit is the minimum total quantity, per rat, which, when injected subcutaneously in equally divided doses, twice daily for 3 days into normal immature rats, will produce in that time, an average ovarian weight five times that of untreated controls).
Indications and Dosage*	In the female: a. Amenorrhea (Primary and Secondary)—0.5 to 1.0 cc. three times a week for 3 weeks followed by one week rest period. Repeat as often as desired. b. Functional Uterine Bleeding—0.5 to 1.0 cc. daily or every other day until bleeding is controlled. c. Sterility due to failure of ovulation—0.5 to 1.0 cc. daily for one week preceding expected time of ovulation.

* Dosage recommended by manufacturer with warning against overdosage and recommendation of small initial dose because of difficulty of predicting response in specific case. Overdosage may result in formation of multiple hemorrhagic follicles sometimes associated with lower abdominal tenderness and pain, nausea, vomiting, chills and even fever. For evaluation, see text.

TABLE 19

LACTOGENIC SUBSTANCES

Source	A stable, dry, water-soluble powder extracted from bovine anterior pituitary gland tissue.
Biologic Effects	In the lower mammal, induces milk secretion in breast previously stimulated by estrogen and progestin. In the human subject, ability to stimulate milk secretion in the properly prepared breast not definitely established.
Standardization	Standardized in terms of: a. Bird unit (Riddle-Bates unit), defined as the smallest amount of substance which injected intramuscularly once daily for 4 days into pigeons 2 to 3 months old will cause an increase in the weight of the crop-glands at the end of 96 hours after the first injection. b. International unit, defined as the activity of 0.1 mgm. of the standard powder, assayed by the pigeon crop-gland response.
Commercial Preparations	Prolactin (Armour), in ampuls containing 100 Riddle units per cc., for intramuscular injection. Prolactin (Ayerst), in ampuls containing 100 Riddle units per cc., for intramuscular injection. Prolactin (Lilly), in ampuls containing 200 Bird units per cc., for intramuscular injection. Prolactin (Schering), in ampuls containing 100 I.U. per cc., for intramuscular injection.
Indications and Dosage*	Hypogalactia (primary and secondary), occurring in the presence of an adequately developed mammary tree; initial dose of 300 units twice during first 24 hours postpartum, followed by 200 units twice during the next 24 hours, making a total of 1000 units.

* For evaluation, see text.

BIBLIOGRAPHY

1. Marker, R. E.: J. Am. Chem. Soc. *60*:1897, 1938.
2. Bachmann, W. E., Cole, W., and Wilds, A. L.: J. Am. Chem. Soc. *61*:974, 1939; ibid. *62*:824, 1940.
3. Heard, R. D. H., and Hoffman, M. M.: J. Biol. Chem. *141*:329, 1941.
4. Pincus, G., and Martin, D. W.: Endocrinol. *27*:838, 1940.
5. Biskind, G. R., and Mark, J.: Bull. Johns Hopkins Hosp. *65*:212, 1939.
6. Dingemanse, E., and Laqueur, E.: Am. J. Obst. & Gynec. *33*:1000, 1937.
7. Heller, C. G.: Endocrinol. *26*:619, 1940.
8. Pincus, G., and Zahl, P. A.: J. Gen. Physiol. *20*:879, 1937.
9. Dingemanse, E., and Tyslowitz, R.: Endocrinol. *28*:450, 1941.
10. Dodds, E. C., Cook, J. W., Hewett, C. L., and Lawson, W.: Proc. Roy. Soc., London, s.B. *114*:272, 1934.
11. Dodds, E. C., Goldberg, L. Lawson, W., and Robinson, R.: Nature, London *141*:247, 1938.
12. Council on Pharmacy and Chemistry, A.M.A.: J.A.M.A. *117*:1625, 1941.
13. Council on Pharmacy and Chemistry, A.M.A.: J.A.M.A. *119*:632, 635, 1942.
14. Greenhill, J. P.: Am. J. Obst. & Gynec. *44*:475, 1942.
15. Bieren, R. E., and Compton, B. C.: Am. J. Obst. & Gynec. *44*:287, 1942.
16. Robson, J. M., and Schönberg, A.: Nature, London *150*:22, 1942.
17. Allen, E., and Doisy, E. A.: J.A.M.A. *81*:819, 1923.
18. Second Conference on Standardization of Sex Hormones, London, Jy., 1933, in Quart. Bull. Health Organiz., League of Nations, 1935, vol. 4, p. 618.
19. Doisy, E. A.: J.A.M.A. *116*:501, 1941.
20. Werner, A. A., and Collier, W. D.: J.A.M.A. *100*:633, 1933.
21. Elden, C. A.: Endocrinol. *20*:47, 1936.
22. Kaufmann, C.: Zentralbl. f. Gynäk. *56*:2058, 1932.
23. Freed, S. C., and Greenhill, J. P.: J. Clin. Endocrinol. *1*:983, 1941.
24. Emmens, C. W.: J. Endocrinol. *1*:142, 1939.
25. Deanesly, R., and Parkes, A. S.: Lancet *2*:606, 1938.
26. Bennett, H. G., Jr., Biskind, G. R., and Mark, J.: Am. J. Obst. & Gynec. *39*:504, 1940.
27. Salmon, U. J., Geist, S. H., and Walter, R. I.: Proc. Soc. Exper. Biol. & Med. *43*:424, 1940.
28. Reports of the Council on Pharmacy and Chemistry, A.M.A.: J.A.M.A. *106*:1808, 1936.
29. Pearlman, W. H., Pincus, G., and Werthessen, N. T.: J. Biol. Chem. *142*:649, 1942.
30. Imhoffen, H. H., and Hohlweg, W.: Naturwiss. *26*:96, 1938.
31. Courrier, R., and Jost, A.: Compt. rend Soc. de biol. *130*:1162, 1939.
32. Wiesbader, H.: Am. J. Obst. & Gynec. *42*:1013, 1941.
33. Corner, G. W., and Allen, W. M.: Am. J. Physiol. *88*:326, 1929.
34. Clauberg, C.: Zentralbl. f. Gynäk. *57*:1461, 1933.
35. Hamblen, E. C., Ashley, C., and Baptist, M.: Endocrinol. *24*:1, 1939.
36. Buxton, C. L., and Westphal, U.: Proc. Soc. Exper. Biol. & Med. *41*:284, 1939.
37. Butenandt, A., and Tscherning, K.: Ztschr. f. allg. Chem. *44*:905, 1931.
38. Ruzicka, L. M., Goldberg, M. W., Meyer, J., Brüngger, H., and Eichenberger, E.: Helvet. chim. Acta *17*:1395, 1934.
39. Ruzicka, L. M., and Wettstein, A.: Helvet. chim. Acta *18*:986, 1935.
40. David, K., Dingemanse, E., Freud, J., and Laqueur, E.: Ztschr. f. physiol. Chem. *233*:281, 1935.
41. Butenandt, A.: Deutsche. med. Wchnschr. *61*:781, 823, 1935.
42. Callow, N. H., Callow, R. K., and Emmens, C. W.: J. Endocrinol. *1*:99, 1939.
43. Miescher, K., Wettstein, A., and Tschopp, E.: Schweiz. med. Wchnschr. *66*:310, 1936; ibid. *68*:1258, 1938.
44. Salmon, U. J., Geist, S. H., Gaines, J. A., and Walter, R. I.: Am. J. Obst. & Gynec. *41*:991, 1941.
45. Abarbanel, A. R.: Endocrinol. *26*:765, 1940.
46. Vest, S. A., and Barelare, B., Jr.: J.A.M.A. *117*:1421, 1941.
47. Greep, R. O., Van Dyke, H. B., and Chow, B. F.: J. Biol. Chem. *133*:289, 1940.
48. Li, C. H., Simpson, M. E., and Evans, H. M.: Endocrinol. *27*:803, 1940.
49. McShan, W. H., and Meyer, R. K.: J. Biol. Chem. *135*:473, 1940.

50. Levin, L., and Tyndale, H. H.: Endocrinol. *21*:619, 1937.
51. Frank, R. T., and Berman, R. L.: Endocrinol. *25*:683, 1939.
52. Bull. Health Organiz., League of Nations, 1939, vol. 8, p. 862.
53. Evans, H. M., Korpi, K., Simpson, M. E., and Pencharz, R. I.: Univ. Calfornia Pub. in Anat. *1*:275, 1936.
54. Gustus, E. L., Meyer, R. K., and Woods, O. R.: Proc. Soc. Exper. Biol. & Med. *34*:54, 1936.
55. Cartland, G. F., and Nelson, J. W.: J. Biol. Chem. *119*:59, 1937.
56. Rinderknecht, H., Noble, R. L., and Williams, P. C.: Biochem. J. *33*:381, 1939.
57. Goss, H., and Cole, H. H.: Endocrinol. *26*:244, 1940.
58. Cartland, G. F., and Nelson, J. W.: Am. J. Physiol. *122*:201, 1938.
59. Cole, H. H., and Saunders, F. J.: Endocrinol. *19*:199, 1935.
60. Cole, H. H., and Erway, J.: Endocrinol. *29*:514, 1941.
61. White, A., Bonsnes, R. W., and Long, C. N. H.: J. Biol. Chem. *143*:447, 1942.
62. Lyons, W. R.: Endocrinol. *28*:161, 1941.
63. Gardner, W. U., and Turner, C. W.: Missouri Agr. Exp. Sta. Res. Bull. No. 196, 1933.
64. Riddle, O., Bates, R. W., and Dykshorn, S. W.: Am. J. Physiol. *105*:191, 1933.
65. Stewart, H. L., Jr., and Pratt, J. P.: Endocrinol. *25*:347, 1939.
66. Biskind, G. R., and Meyer, M. A.: Proc. Soc. Exper. Biol. & Med. *53*:91, 1943.
67. MacBryde, C. M., Castrodale, D., Helwig, E. B., and Bierbaum, O.: J.A.M.A. *118*:1278, 1942.
68. Freed, S. C., Eisin, W. M., and Greenhill, J. P.: J. Clin. Endocrinol. *2*:213, 1942.
69. Hufford, A. R.: J.A.M.A. *123*:259, 1943.
70. Roberts, H. K., Loeffel, E., and MacBryde, C. M.: J.A.M.A. *123*:261, 1943.
71. Salmon, U. J., Geist, S. H., Walter, R. I., and Mintz, N.: J. Clin. Endocrinol. *1*:556, 1941.
72. Soule, S. D.: Am. J. Obst. & Gynec. *44*:684, 1942; ibid. *45*:315, 1943.
73. Herrnberger, K.: Klin. Wchnschr. *20*:547, 1941.
74. Selye, H., and Masson, G.: Science *96*:358, 1942.
75. Joël, C. A.: J. Clin. Endocrinol. *2*:639, 1942.
76. Weber, H. W., Kurzrok, L., and Birnberg, C. H.: J. Clin. Endocrinol. *2*:392, 1942.
77. Allen, W. M., and Heckel, G. P.: Am. J. Obst. & Gynec. *44*:984, 1942.
78. Council on Pharmacy and Chemistry A. M. A.: J.A.M.A. *116*:1054, 1941.
79. Heard, R. D. H., Bauld, W. S., and Hoffman, M. M.: J. Biol. Chem. *141*:709, 1941.
80. Siegler, S. L., and Bauer, D.: Am. J. Obst. & Gynec. *45*:277, 1943.
81. Paschkis, K. E., Cantarow, A., Rakoff, A. E., Hansen, L. P., and Walkling, A. A.: Proc. Soc. Exper. Biol. & Med. *53*:213, 1943.
82. Ceithaml, J. J., and Koch, F. C.: Endocrinol. *31*:249, 1942.
83. Parkes, A. S.: J. Endocrinol. *3*:220, 1942.
84. Katzman, P. A., Godfrid, M., Cain, C. K., and Doisy, E. A.: J. Biol. Chem. *148*:501, 1943.
85. Li, C. H., Simpson, M. E., and Evans, H. M.: J. Biol. Chem., *146*:627, 1942.

BIBLIOGRAPHICAL INDEX

Note: Where two or more authors have made joint contributions to the literature, the complete entry is made only under the name of the first author in the group, and a cross-reference is attached to each of the others. *Italic* page numbers show where the full citations appear in the text.

Abarbanel, A. R., 142, *153*, 351, *361*, 383, *386*, 465, *474*, 493, *495*, 714, *732*
 and Goodfriend, M. J., 493, *495*
 and Klein, M. D., 493, *495*
Abelin, I., and Kursteiner, P., 237, *243*
Abrams, S. B. See *Adler, E. H.*
Abramson, D., and Hurwitt, E., Lesnick, G., 60, *63*, 462, *473*
 and Roberts, S. M., Wilson, P. D., 60, *63*, 462, *473*
Adair, F. A., 477, 487, *494*
Adair, J., and Chidester, F. E., 283, *284*
Adams, E., 104, *113*
Adams, M. See *Wilder, R. M.*
Addison, W. H. F., 196, *202*
Adler, E. H., and Abrams, S. B., 306, *324*
Adler, L. See *Hitschmann, F.*
Adler, M., 466, *474*
Adrian, J., 493, *495*
Aich, J., 309, *324*
Aird, R. B., *216*
Albright, F., 263, *267*, 431, *441*. See also *Fraser, R. W.,* and *Sturgis, S. H.*
 and Aub, J. C., Bauer, W., 266, *267*
 and Bloomberg, E., Drake, T., Sulkowitsch, H., 471, *474*
 and Butler, A. M., Hampton, A. O., Smith, P., 609, *619*
 and Ellsworth, R., 263, *267*
 and Parson, W., Bloomberg, E., 581, *617*
 and Smith, P. H., Fraser, R., 541, *614*
Alden, R. H., 58, *62*
Aldrich, T. B., 244, *259*. See also *Kamm, O.*
Ale, T. See *Mack, H. C.*
Allaben, G. R., and Owens, E., 39, *48*
Allan, H., and Wiles, P., 220, 221, *224*
Allen, E., 2, *30*, 33, 41, 46, *47*, *48*, *49*, 65, *74*, 76, 78, *98*, 433, *441*, 478, *494*, 518, *527*, 650, *679*. See also *Burr, H. S.,* *Chamberlin, T. L.,* *Duncan, P. A.,* *Gardner, W. U.,* *Hill, R. T.,* *Overholser, M. D.,* and *Pratt, J. P.*
 and Creadick, R. N., 2, *30*
 and Doisy, E. A., 650, 655, *679*, 709, *732*
 and Doisy, E. A., Francis, B. F., Gibson, H. V., Robertson, L. L., Colgate, C. E., Kountz, W. B., Johnston, C. G., 44, *49*
 and Gardner, W. U., Diddle, A. W., 150, *154*
 and Hisaw, F. L., Gardner, W. U., 80, *98*
 and Smith, G. M., Gardner, W. U., 35, *47*
Allen, E. B., and Henry, G. W., 309, *324*
Allen, E. V. See *Crisler, G. R.*

Allen, M. See *McCord, C. P.*
Allen, R., and Bourne, G., 256, *260*
Allen, W. M., 53, *62*. See also *Corner, G. W.,* *Heckel, G. P.,* *Lyon, R. A.,* and *Meyer, R. K.*
 and Corner, G. W., 56, *62*, 111, *114*
 and Heckel, G. P., 56, 57, *62*, 350, *361*, 712, *733*
 and Meyer, R. K., 59, *63*
Alperstein, B. B. See *Goldzieher, M. A.*
Althausen, T. L., and Stockholm, M., 236, *243*
Altman, F., 276, *280*
Altschule, M. P., and Iglauer, A., 525, *527*
Alvarez, W. C., 451, *455*
Ancel, P. See also *Bouin, P.*
 and Bouin, P., 104, *113*, 134, *151*
Andersen, D. H., 241, *243*, 275, *280*
 and Wolf, A., 608, *619*
Anderes, E., 58, *62*
Anderson, E. See also *Haymaker, W.*
 and Haymaker, W., 253, *260*
Anderson, E. M. See *Collip, J. B.*
Anderson, J. A., and Murlin, W. R., 221, *225*
Anderson, W. C. See *Loeb, L.*
Anker, H., and Laland, P., 457, *472*, 695, *703*
Anselmino, K. J., 456, *472*
 and Herold, L., Hoffmann, F., 142, *152*, 208, 209, *217*
 and Hoffmann, F., 210, 214, 215, 217, *218*, *219*, 241, *243*, 253, *260*, 457, 460, *472*, *473*, 509, 526, 695, *704*
 and Hoffmann, F., Herold, L., 467, *474*
 and Hoffmann, F., Kennedy, W. P., 224, *225*, 458, *472*
 and Hoffmann, F., Pencharz, R. I., 142, *152*
Anson, B. J. See *Kabat, H.*
Anspach, B. M., and Hoffman, J., 302, 315, 316, *324*, *325*, 345, 354, *360*, *361*, 398, 407, *410*, *411*, 429, 431, *441*, 693, *703*
Antopol, W. See *Finkler, R. S.*
Appel, M. See *Eisenstaedt, J. S.*
Arey, L. B., 129, *151*
Arnold, L. E., 461, *473*
Aron, M., 192, *202*, 239, *243*
 and Benoit, J., 241, *243*
 and Klein, M., 207, *217*
Artundo, A. See *Houssay, B. A.*
Ascheim, S. See also *Zondek, B.*
 and Zondek, B., 179, 180, *201*, 675, *680*, 694, *703*

Aschner, B., 45, *49*, 204, 211, *216, 218*, 229, *232*, 348, *360*
Asdell, S. A., 56, *62*. See also *Drummond-Robinson, G., Hammond, J.*
and Hammond, J., 115, *118*
and Seidenstein, H. R., 137, *152*
Asher, L., 274, 275, *280*
Ashley, C. See *Hamblen, E. C.*
Ashley-Montagu, M. F., 293, *296*
Askanazy, M., 608, *619*
Astwood, E. B., 60, *63, 655, 679*. See also *Jones, G. E. S.*
and Fevold, H. L., 178, 179, *200*
and Geschickter, C. F., 484, *494*
and Geschickter, C. F., Rausch, E. O., 137, *152*
Atchley, D. W. See *Ferrebee, J. W.,* and *Loeb, R. F.*
Atkins, H. J. B., 485, 487, *494*
Atkinson, A. J., and Ivy, A. C., 510, *526*
Atkinson, F. R. B., 549, 552, *615*
Atwell, W. J., 256, *260*. See also *Emery, F. E.*
Aub, J. C. See also *Albright, F.*
and Bauer, W., Heath, C., Ropes, M., *237, 243, 266, 267*
and Karnofsky, D., 324, *325*, 556, 564, *616*
Auchincloss, H., and Haagenson, C. D., 39, *48*
Auld, A. G., 278, *280*
Ault, C. C., and Hoctor, E. F., Werner, A. A., 439, *442*
Austin, P. R. See *Evans, H. M.*
Axelson, G. J. See *Hamblen, E. C.*

Babes, A. A., 338, *360*
Babinski, J., 556, *615*
Bach, E., 265, *267*
Bachman, C., 192, *202*, 684, 688, *702*. See also *Mortimer, H.*
and Collip, J. B., Selye, H., 36, *48*, 288, *290*
and Toby, G., 212, *218*
Bachmann, W. E., and Cole, W., Wilds, A. L., 706, *732*
Bailey, K. V., 318, *325*
Bailey, P. See also *Fulton, J. F.*
and Cushing, H., 552, *615*
Baker, B. L., 210, *217*
and Johnson, G. E., 162, *166*
Ball, H. A. See also *Samuels, L. T.*
and Samuels, L. T., Schott, H. F., 212, *218*
Baltzer, F., 645, *648*
Bamman, F. See *Jensen, H.*
Baptist, M. See *Davis, C. D., Hamblen, E. C.,* and *Ross, R. A.*
Bard, P., *233*
Barelare, B., Jr. See *Vest, S. A.*
Barger, G. See *Harrington, C. R.*
Barker, P. S. See *Freyberg, R. H.*
Barker, R. G. See also *Stone, C. P.*
and Stone, C. P., 295, *296*

Barnes, B. O., and Regan, J. F., 212, *218*
and Regan, J. F., Nelson, W. O., 270, *271, 509, 526*
Barnes, J., 493, *495*
Barnes, R. H. See also *MacKay, E. M.*
and Wick, A. N., Miller, E. S., McKay, E. M., 251, *260*
Barr, D. P. See *Bulger, J. A.*
Barraquer-Ferré, L., 611, *619*
Barris, R. W. See also *Ingram, W. R.*
and Ingram, W. R., 230, *232*
Bartel, M., 556, *615*
Bartelmez, G. W., 22, 25, *30*, 77, 90, 92, 93, 94, 96, *98*, 300, *324*
Bartholomew, R. A. See *Colvin, E. D.*
Bartlett, M. K. See *Rock, J.*
Barton, D. S. See *Burr, H. S.*
Basch, K., 272, *279*
Baskin, M. J., 394, *410*
Bassett, R. B. See *Loeb, L.*
Bates, R. W. See also *Riddle, O.,* and *Schooley, J. P.*
and Laanes, T., Riddle, O., 205, *216*
and Lahr, E. L., Riddle, O., 150, *154*
Bauer, D. See *Siegler, S. L.*
Bauer, J., 348, *360*, 498, 504, 505, *526*, 534, *536*, 562, 577, 579, *616*
Bauer, W. See *Albright, F.,* and *Aub, J. C.*
Bauld, W. S. See *Heard, R. D. H.*
Baumann, E. J. See also *Marine, D.*
and Hunt, L., 236, *243*
and Metzger, N., Sprinson, D. B., 668, *680*
Baumann, E., 235, *242*
Bayer, L. M., 528, *536*
Bayer, R., 413, *423*
Beall, D., 256, *261*
and Reichstein, T., 256, *261*
Beard, J., 50, *61*
Beckman, M., 338, *360*
Becks, H., and Roy, R. D., Simpson, M. E., Evans, H. M., 239, *243*
Beck, N. See *Newton, W. H.*
Beclere, 444, *455*
Behnke, A. R. See also *Welham, W. C.*
and Feen, B. G., Welham, W. C., 519, *527*
Belding, D. L., 394, *410*
Bell, A. C. See *Bourne, A. W.*
Bell, G. H., 104, *113*
and Robson, J. M., 104, *113*, 127, *128*
Bellerby, C. W. See *Parkes, A. S.*
Benda, C., 552, *615*
Benedict, E. B. See *Putnam, T. J.*
Benensohn, S. J. See *Falls, F. H.*
Bennett, H. G., Jr., and Biskind, G., Mark, J., 439, 440, *442*, 711, *732*
and TeLinde, R. W., 439, *442*
Bennett, L. L., 250, *260*. See also *Russell, J. A.*
Bennett, M. J., and Russell, P. B., Jr., 352, *361*
Bennhold, H., 581, *617*
Benoit, J. See *Aron, M.*
Bentivoglio, G. C., and Fumi, C., 273, 279, *279*
Benzadōn, J., and Piceña, J. P., 697, *704*

Berard, 17. See *Cotte, G.*
Berblinger, W., 491, *495*
Berg, M., 223, *225*
Bergman, A. J., and Turner, C. W., 140, *152*
Bergstrand, H., 579, 597, *617, 618*
Bergwall, A., and Kuschinsky, G., 434, *441*
Berkeley, W. N. See *Dana, C. L.*
Berlinger, V. See *McKenzie, F. F.*
Berman, L., 263, *267*
Berman, R. A. See *Talbot, N. B.*
Berman, R. L. See *Frank, R. T.*
Berman, S. See *Greenberg, B. E.*
Bernstein, P., and Feresten, M., 36, *48*
Berthold, A. A., 155, *164*
Best, C. H. See *Haist, R. E.*
Biassoti, A., 206, *217.* See also *Houssay, B. A.*
    and Houssay, B. A., 211, *218*
Bickenbach, W., and Fromme, H., 460, *473*
Bickers, W., 106, *114*, 370, *385*
    and Main, R. J., 103, 106, *113*
Biddulph, C., and Meyer, R. K., Gumbreck,
    L. G., 197, *202*
Biedl, A., 230, *232*, 561, *615*, 631, *640*
Bierbaum, O. See *MacBryde, C. M.*
Bieren, R. E., and Compton, B. C., 709, *732*
Bierring, K., 210, *217*
Bilderback, J. B. See *Rush, H. P.*
Biller, S. B. See *Spark, C.*
Billings, E. G., 37, *48*
Billingsley, L. W., 206, *217*
Binder, A., 58, *62*
Bing, J., and Globus, J., Simon, H., 605,
    607, 608, *618*
Bingel, A., 605, *618*
Birnberg, C. H., 73, *75.* See also *Kurzrok,*
    L., Livingston, S. H., and *Weber, H. W.*
    and Kurzrok, L., Klos, S. J., 493, *495*
    and Kurzrok, L., Weber, H., 59, *63*
Bishop, K. S. See *Evans, H. M.*
Bishop, P. M. F. See also *Brown, W. L.*
    and Boycott, M., Zuckerman, S., 476, *493*
Biskind, G. R. See also *Bennett, H. G., Jr,*
    and *Lisco, H.*
    and Escamilla, R. F., Lisser, H., 626, *630*
    and Mark, J., 707, *732, 733*
Bittenger, I. See *Moore, R. A.*
Black, J., and Heynes, O. H., Gillman, J.,
    53, *62*
Black, P. T., 287, *290*
    and Collip, J. B., Thomson, D. L., 241,
    219, 286, 289
Black, W. C. See *Mason, L. W.*
Blair-Bell, W., 119, *122,* 367, *385*
    and Datnow, M. M., Jeffcoate, T. N. A.,
    365, *385*
Bland, L. J. See *Pratt, J. P.*
Bland, P. B., and First, A., Roeder, P., 684,
    702
    and Goldstein, L., 605, *618*
Blandau, R. J. See *Boling, J. L.*
Blau, N. F., and McNamara, H., 434, *441*
Block, M., 503, *526*
Block, P. W. See *Traut, H. F.*
Bloom, M. A., and McLean, F. C., Bloom,
    W., 265, *267*

Bloom, W. See *Bloom, M. A.*
Bloomberg, E. See *Albright, F.*
Bloss, J. R., 420, *423*, 459, *473*
Blotevogel, W., and Poll, H., 323, *385*
Blotner, H., 214, *218*
Blumenfeld, C. W., 259, *261*
Blyth, J. S. See *Greenwood, A.*
Boas, C. van E., 69, *74*
Boas, F., 294, *296*
Boas, L. C. See *Collens, W. S.*
Bodansky, A., 236, *243*
Bogan, I. K. See *Wagner, R.*
Bohstedt, G. See *Kozelka, F. L.*
Boling, J. L. See also *Collins, V. J.*
    and Blandau, R. J., 60, *63*
Bolk, L., 292, *296*
Boll, R. G. See *Rowntree, L. G.*
Bollack, J. See *Roussy, G.*
Boller, R., 613, 614, *619*
Bomskov, C., and Holscher, B., 276, *280*
    and Lipps, H. G., 277, *280*
    and Schneider, E., 512, *527*
    and Sladovic, L., 276, 278, 279, *280*
    and Spiegel, R., 277, 279, *280*
Bonime, R. G., 321, *325*
Bonnier, G. See *Pettersson, G.*
Bonsnes, R. W. See *White, A.*
Boom, H., 289, *290*
Boothby, W. M. See *Deuel, H. J., Jr.*
Borchardt, H. See *Dingemanse, E.*
Borchardt, L., 223, *225*
Borduas, A. See *Selye, H.*
Born, G., 50, 56, *61*
Bottomley, A. C. See *Folley, S. J.*
Bouin, P. See also *Ancel, P.*
    and Ancel, P., 44, *49,* 50, *61*, 156, *165*
Bourg, R., and Legrand, G., 457, *472*
Bourgarel, R. See *Laffont, A.*
Bourne, A., and Burn, J. H., 247, *259*
Bourne, A. W., and Bell, A. C., 108, *114*,
    125, *128*
Bourne, G. See *Allen, R.,* and *Zuckerman,*
    S.
Bowers, L. M. See *Sherwood, T. C.*
Boycott, M. See *Bishop, P. M. F.*
Boynton, M. W. See *Davis, M. E.*
Boynton, R. E., and Winther, N., 375, 383,
    386
Bradbury, J. T., 180, *201.* See also *Browne,*
    W. E.
Brain, W. R., and Straus, E. B., 227, *232*
Brambell, F. W. R., and Parkes, A. S., 45,
    49
Brandstrup, E., 461, *473*
    and Okkels, H., 269, *271*
Brault, P., 70, *74*
Braun, C. See *Chiari, J.*
Brawner, J. N. See *Novak, E.*
Breipohl, W., 292, *296.* See also *Clauberg, C.*
Breitenbach, H. See *Ehrhardt, K.*
Brewer, J. I., *31,* 91, *99,* 318, *325,* 368, 373,
    385, 447, 453, *455*
    and Jones, H. O., Skiles, J. H., Jr., 176,
    200, 407, *411*
Brickner, R. M. See *Riley, H. A.*

Bridges, C. B., 634, 637, *640*, 645, *648*
Brindeau, A., and Hinglais, H., Hinglais, M.,
    119, *122*, 694, 695, *703*
Brissaud, E., and Meige, H., 546, *615*
Britton, S. W. See also *Corey, E. L.*
    and Silvette, H., 250, *259*
Brockway, G. See *Jaffe, I.*
Bronstein, I. P., *619*
    and Halpern, L. J., Brown, A. W., 562,
    616
Brookhart, J. M., and Dey, F. L., Ranson,
    S. W., 231, 232, *233*
Brooks, C. M., *233*
Brooksby, J. B., 197, *202*
Broster, L. R., 580, 585, *617*
    and Vines, H. W. C., 258, *261*, 585, *617*
Brougher, J. C., 266, *267*, 461, *473*
Brouha, L., 60, *63*
    and Desclin, L., 59, 60, *63*
Browman, L. G., 160, 161, *165*
Brown, A. See *Summerfeldt, P.*
Brown, A. D. See *Wolfe, J. M.*
Brown, A. W. See *Bronstein, I. P.*
Brown, W. E., and Bradbury, J. T., Metz-
    ger, I., 188, *201*
Brown, W. L., and Thompson, A. P., Bishop,
    P. M. F., 436, *441*
Brown-Séquard, C. E., 155, *164*
Browne, D., 622, *629*
Browne, J. S. L. See also *Henry, J. S.,
    Schacher, J., Selye, H.,* and *Venning,
    E. H.*
    and Henry, J. S., Venning, E. H., 416,
    418, 421, 422, *423*, 457, 460, *472, 473*
    and Venning, E. H., 41, *48*, 662, *679*, 683,
    686, 694, *702, 703*
Browne, O., and Torrens, D. S., 375, *386*
Brownell, K. A. See also *Hartman, F. A.,
    Pucher, G. W.,* and *Spoor, H.*
    and Lockwood, J. E., Hartman, F. A.,
    147, *153*
Bruch, H., 291, *296*, 562, *616*
    and Waters, I., 525, 526, *527*
Bruhl, R., 142, *153*
Brundage, J. T. See *Cantarow, A.*
Brungger, H. See *Ruzicka, L.*
Brunner, E. K., 416, *423*. See also *Hotch-
    kiss, R. S.,* and *Smith, B. G.*
Brunsting, L. A. See *Rowntree, L. G.*
Bryant, A. R., 238, 239, *243*
Bryce, T. H., and Teacher, J. H., 70, *74*
Bucher, N. L. R., and Geschickter, C. F.,
    484, 487, *494*, 663, *680*
Bucura, C. J., 92, *99*
Bucy, P. C., 228, *232*
Bugbee, E. P. See *Kamm, O.*
Bühler, F., 275, *280*, 450, *455*
Bulger, J. A., and Barr, D. P., 207, *217*
Bump, G. See *Clark, L. B.*
Bunde, C. A., and Greep, R. O., 178, *200*
Burch, J. C. See also *Klinger, H. H.,* and
    Phelps, D.
    and Phelps, D., 649, *680*
    and Wolfe, J. M., Cunningham, R. S.,
    336, *360*

Burch, L. E., 347, *360*
Burdick, H. O. See also *Whitney, R.*
    and Whitney, R., 36, *48*
    and Whitney, R., Emerson, B., 58, *62*
Burford, T., and Diddle, A. W., 116, 117,
    118
Burn, J. H. See *Bourne, A.*
Burns, E. L. See *Loeb, L.*
Burns, R. K., 635, *640*
Burnstein, C. L., 223, *225*
Burr, H. S. See also *Langman, L.*
    and Hill, R. T., Allen, E., 67, *74*
    and Musselman, L. K., 67, 68, *74*
    and Musselman, L. K., Barton, D. S.,
    Kelly, N. B., 67, *74*
Burrill, M. W. See also *Greene, R. R.*
    and Ivy, A. C., 274, *280*
Burrows, H., 484, *494*
Busso, R. R. See *Houssay, B. A.*
Butcher, E. O., and Persike, E. C., 276, *280*
Butenandt, A., 34, *47*, 156, *165*, *713*, *732*
    and Danenbaum, H., 156, *165*
    and Hanisch, G., 156, *165*
    and Kindzus, H., 161, *165*
    and Schmidt, J., 662, *679*
    and Tscherning, K., 156, *165*, *713*, *732*
Butler, A. M. See *Albright, F.,* and *Talbot,
    N. B.*
Butler, G. C. See also *Marrian, G. F.*
    and Marrian, G. F., 257, *261*
Butterworth, J. S. See *Furth, J.,* and *Traut,
    H. F.*
Büttner, W., 189, *201*
Buxton, C. L., 321, 322, *325*, 348, *360*, 687,
    702
    and Westphal, U., *713*, *732*
Byron, F. B., and Wilson, C., 458, *472*

Caffier, P., 58, *62*
Cahill, G. F., 585, 586, 610, *617, 619*
Cain, C. K. See *Katzman, P. A.*
Caire, A. See *Mendel, E. B.*
Calatroni, C. See *DeCastillo, E. R.*
Callow, N. H., and Callow, R. K., 690, *703*
    and Callow, R. K., Emmens, C. W., 258,
    261, 570, *616*, 667, 669, 670, *680*, 714,
    732
    and Callow, R. K., Emmens, C. W.,
    Stroud, S. M., 669, *680*
Callow, R. K., 258, *261*, 664, *680*, 691, *703*.
    See also *Callow, N. H.,* and *Crooke,
    A. C.*
    and Parkes, A. S., 256, 257, *261*
Calvet, J., 282, *284*
Cameron, A. T., and Carmichael, J., 236,
    243
Campbell, A. D., 365, 367, 375, 376, *385*,
    488, *494*
Campbell, D. See *Geiling, E. M. K.*
Campbell, R. E., and Hisaw, F. L., 382, *386*
    and Sevringhaus, E. L., 111, *114*, 420, *423*
Camus, L., and Roussy, G., 561, *615*
Cannon, D. J., 367, 384, *385, 386*
Cannon, W. B., 244, *259*

Cantarow, A., 266, 267. See also Gordon, B., Paschkis, K. E., and Rakoff, A. E. and Brundage, J. T., Housel, E. L., 264, 267

Cantilo, E., 435, 439, 441

Capitain. See Desmarest.

Carey, J. B. See Litzenberg, J. C.

Carlson, A. J. See Kunde, M. M.

Carmer, M. E. See Pucher, G. W.

Carmichael, J. See Cameron, A. T.

Carne, H. O. See MacKay, E. M.

Carnes, W. H., and Osebold, J., Stoerk, H. C., 210, 219

Carr, H. L., and Connor, L. C., 253, 260

Carter, H. D. See Pryor, H. B.

Cartland, G. F., and Nelson, J. W., 185, 201, 716, 733

Cary, W. H., 70, 71, 74

Casida, L. E., 174, 175, 200
and Hellbaum, A., 256, 260

Castallo, M. A., 321, 325

Castrodale, D. See MacBryde, C. M.

Catchpole, H. R. See also Marx, R., and Van Wagenen, A.
and Lyons, W. R., 183, 201

Ceithaml, J. J., and Koch, F. C., 715, 733

Cesa, I., 58, 63

Chadwick, M., 309, 324

Chaikoff, I. L., and Holtom, G. F., Reichert, F. L., 211, 218
and Lyons, W. R., 149, 153
and Reichert, F. L., Read, L. S., Mathes, M. E., 212, 218

Challans, J. S. See Johnson, G. E.

Chamberlin, P. E. See Hall, V. E.

Chamberlin, T. L., and Gardner, W. U., Allen, E., 137, 152

Chambers, W. H., and Sweet, J. E., Chandler, J. P., 250, 260

Chamorra, A. See Hohlweg, W.

Champy, C., and Keller, T., 57, 62

Chandler, J. P. See Chambers, W. H.

Chandler, S. B., 264, 267

Charipper, H. A., 195, 202. See Gordon, A. S.
and Haterius, H. O., 195, 202

Charny, C. W., and Meranze, D. R., 395, 410

Chaschinsky, P. C., and Jerschow, S. I., 609, 619

Cheatle, G. L., and Cutler, M., 129, 151, 481, 483, 494

Chen, G., and Geiling, E. M. K., 215, 219

Cheval, M., 117, 118

Chiari, J., and Braun, C., Spaeth, J., 491, 495

Chidester, F. E. See also Adair, J.
and Eaton, A. G., Thompson, E. P., 255, 260

Chiodi, H., 273, 275, 280

Chodkowska, S. See Tislowitz, R.

Chosson, J., and Donnet, V., 695, 703

Chou, C. Y., and Wu, H., 667, 680

Chow, B. F. See Greep, R. O., Shedlovsky, T., and Van Dyke H. B.

Chrisman, R. B., Jr., 525, 527

Church, C. F. See Henle, G.

Chvostek, F., 468, 474

Cinberg, B. L., 383, 386

Clark, A. R. See Gegerson, H. B.

Clark, G., and Magoun, H. W., Ranson, S. W., 231, 233

Clark, G. A., 223, 225

Clark, J. H. See also Rowntree, L. G.
and Steinberg, A., Rowntree, L. G., 276, 279, 280, 281

Clark, L. B., and Leonard, S. L., Bump, G., 162, 166

Clauberg, C., 35, 47, 53, 62, 348, 349, 360, 361, 420, 423, 712, 732
and Breipohl, W., 197, 198, 202

Clausen, H. J., 254, 260

Cleveland, D. See Davis, L.

Closs, W., and Loeb, L., McKay, E. M., 206, 217

Coates, C. W. See Weisman, A. I.

Cockrill, J. R. See Miller, E. G., Jr.

Coggeshall, C., and Root, H. F., 552, 554, 615

Cohen, H. H. See Falls, F. H.

Cohen, M. R. See also Stein, I. F.
and Stein, I. F., 422, 424

Cohen, S. L., and Marrian, G. F., Watson, M. C., 125, 128, 683, 702

Cohen-Solal, G. See Courrier, R.

Cohn, E. J. See Fevold, H. L.

Colcock, B. P., 384, 386

Cole, H. H. See also Goss, H., Hart, G. H., Saunders, F. J., and Van Wagenen, G.
and Erway, J., 717, 733
and Hart, G. H., 182, 201
and Saunders, F. J., 716, 733

Cole, V. V. See Enright, L.

Cole, W. See Bachmann, W. E.

Colgate, C. E. See Allen, E.

Collens, W. S., and Slo-Bodkin, S. G., Rosenbliett, S., Boas, L. C., 270, 271

Coller, F. A. See Freyberg, R. H.

Collett, M. E., and Smith, J. T., Wertenberger, G. E., 438, 442

Collier, W. D. See Werner, A. A.

Collin, R., 226, 228, 232

Collins, C. G., and Menville, L. J., Thomas, E. P., 440, 442

Collins, D. A., and Wood, E. H., 249, 259

Collins, R. M., 322, 325

Collins, V. J., and Boling, J. L., Young, W. C., 60, 63

Collip, J. B., 141, 152, 192, 202, 204, 209, 216, 217, 263, 267, 286, 287, 289. See also Bachman, C., Black, P. T., McEuen, C. S., Mortimer, H., Neufeld, A. H., O'Donovan, D. K., Selye, H., and Thomson, D. L.
and Anderson, E. M., 286, 287, 288, 289, 290
and Anderson, E. M., Thomson, D. L., 253, 260
and Selye, H., Thomson, D. L., 145, 153, 180, 181, 201

Colmer, M. J. See *Huberman, J.*

Columbo, E. O. See *Ramos, A. P.*

Colvin, E. D., and Bartholomew, R. A., 459, *473*
and Bartholomew, R. A., Grimes, W. H., 461, *473*

Compton, B. C. See *Bieren, R. E.*

Comte, L., 194, *202*

Conference (second) on Standardization of Sex Hormones, 709, 712, *732*

Conn, J. W. See *Newburgh, L. H.*

Connally, H. F., and Dann, D. I., Reese, J. M., Douglass, L. H., 493, *495*

Connor, L. C. See *Carr, H. L.*

Cook, J. W. See *Dodds, E. C.*

Cooper, W. D. See *Turner, C. W.*

Cope, C. L., 460, *473*, 687, 688, *702*

Copelman, L. See *Crainicianu, A.*

Corey, E. L., 254, *260*
and Britton, S. W., 221, *225*, 250, 251, *259*

Cori, C. F. See *Fisher, R. E.*

Corner, G. W., 57, *62*, 76, 78, 79, 82, 83, 84, *98*, *99*, 136, 138, *151*, 338, 360. See also *Allen, W. M.*, and *Wilson, K. M.*
and Allen, W. M., 34, *47*, 52, 60, *61*, *63*, 416, *423*, 712, *732*
and Bartelmez, G. W., Hartman, C. G., 338, *360*

Cornish, R. E. See *Reichert, F. L.*

Corsaro, J. See *Duffy, P. V.*

Cotte, G., 304, 316, 317, *325*, 384, *386*, 444, *454*
and Martin, J. F., Mankiewicz, E., 160, *165*
and Pallot, G., 483, 484, 487, *494*
and Pallot, G., Berard, M., 484, *494*

Cotte, G. J., and Martin, F., Mileff, 162, *166*

Council of Medical Women's Federation in England, 425, *441*

Council on Pharmacy and Chemistry A. M. A., 321, *325*, 407, *411*, 421, *423*, 708, 711, 712, *732*, *733*

Courrier, R., 55, *62*
and Cohen-Solal, G., 59, *63*
and Gros, G., 53, *62*, 161, *166*, 120, *122*
and Jost, A., 712, *723*
and Kehl, R., 55, *62*

Courville, C. B. See also *Gunther, L.*
and Mason, V. R., 551, *615*

Cowdry, E. V., 282, *284*

Cowsert, W. C. See *Ralston, N. P.*

Crafts, R. C. See *Engle, E. T.*

Crainicianu, A., and Copelman, L., 269, *271*

Cramer, H. J., 509, *526*

Cramer, W., and Horning, E. S., *202*, 488, *494*

Creadick, R. N. See *Allen, E.*

Crew, F. A., and Wiesner, B. P., 206, *217*

Cricklow, R. S., 450, *455*

Crisler, G. R., and Allen, E. V., 436, *441*

Crooke, A. C., 577, *616*
and Callow, R. K., 580, *617*, 691, *703*
and Russell, D. S., *260*

Crossen, H. S., and Crossen, R. G., 384, *386*

Crossen, R. G. See *Crossen, H. S.*

Crotti, A., 277, *280*

Crouch, R., and Elliott, W. H., Jr., *233*

Cunningham, B., and Kuhn, H. H., 121, *122*

Cunningham, R. S. See *Burch, J. C.*

Currier, F. P., and Frantz, C. H., Van der Meer, R., 548, *615*

Curschmann, H., 429, *441*
and Kramer, F., 612, *619*

Cushing, H., 226, *232*, 458, *472*, 573, 576, 579, 607, *616*, *618*. See also *Bailey, P., Teel, H. M., Thompson, K. W.*, and *Weed, H.*
and Davidoff, L. M., 553, *615*

Cuthbertson, W. F. J., and Drummond, J. C., 415, *423*

Cutler, H. H., and Power, M. H., Wilder, R. M., 590, *617*

Cutler, M., 484, *494*. See also *Cheatle, G. L.,*
and Owen, S. E., 700, *704*

Cuttle, T. D. See *Regester, R. P.*

Cutuly, E., and Cutuly, E. C., 157, *165*

Cutuly, E. C. See *Cutuly, E.*

Cuyler, W. K. See *Davis, C. D., Hamblen, E. C., McCullagh, E. P.*, and *Ross, R. A.*

DAELS, J., 107, *114*

Dale, H. H., 376, *386*

Daly, C. See *Dill, D. B.*

Dambrosi, R. G., 212, *218*

Damm, P., 432, *441*

Damm, P. N., 336, *360*

D'Amour, F. E., 67, *74*, 682, 686, 693, *704*. See also *D'Amour, M. C., Gustavson, R. G., Halpern, S.*, and *Kunde, M. M.*
and Dumont, C., Gustavson, R. G., 287, *290*
and Funk, D., Liverman, H., 693, *703*
and Gustavson, R. G., 110, *114*, 689, *703*
and Woods, L., 67, *74*

D'Amour, M. C., and D'Amour, F. E., 282, *284*

Dana, C. L., and Berkeley, W. N., 283, *284*

Dandy, W. E., 282, *284*, 285

Danenbaum, H. See *Butenandt, A.*

Danforth, C. H., 505, *526*, 633, 635, 639, *640*

Danforth, D. N., and Ivy, A. C., 125, *128*

Danforth, W. C., 465, *474*, 600, *618*

Dann, D. I. See *Connally, H. F.*

Dantschakoff, V., 636, 638, *640*

Darley, W. See *Draper, W. B.*

Daron, G. H., 58, *62*, 90, 91, 92, 93, 94, 96, *99*, 300, *324*

Das, K., 292, *296*

Datnow, M. M. See *Blair-Bell, W.*

David, K., and Dingemanse, E., Freud, J., Laqueur, E., 156, *165*, 713, *732*
and Freud, J., De Jongh, S. E., 43, *49*

David, K. J. See *Uyldert, I. E.*

Davidoff, L. M., 555, 581, *615*, *617*. See also *Cushing, H.*

Davidson, L. W. See *Zeckwer, I. T.*

Davies, W. L., and Moncrieff, A., 475, *493*

Davis, A. A., 374, 375, 384, *385, 386*
Davis, A. C., 552, 555, *615*
Davis, C. D., and Hamblen, E. C., Cuyler, W. K., Baptist, M., 420, *423*
  and Madden, J. H. M., Hamblen, E. C., 191, *203*
Davis, H. See *Reboul, J.*
Davis, H. P. See *Reece, R. P.*
Davis, K. B., 37, *48*
Davis, L., and Cleveland, D., Ingram, W. R., 230, *232*
Davis, M. E., 438, *442.* See also *Huber, C. P.*
  and Boynton, M. W., 493, *495*
  and Koff, A. K., 176, 188, 189, *200,* 321, *325*
Davison, C., and Selby, N. E., 231, *233*
Dawson, E. K., 130, *151*
Dean, A. L. See *Twombly, G. H.*
Dean, E. M. See *Russell, P. M. G.*
Deanesly, R., and Newton, W. H., 121, *122*
  and Parkes, A. S., 161, *165,* 711, *732*
Deaver, J., 129, *151*
de Fremery, P. See *Simpson, S. L.*
De Jongh, S. E. See also *David, K., Freud, J., Gaarenstroom, J. H.,* and *Laqueur, E.*
  and Laqueur, E., 144, *153*
Del Castillo, E. B. See also *Di Paolo, G.*
  and Calatroni, C., 270, *271*
De Lee, J. B., 462, *473*
Delfs, E. See *Lamar, J. K.*
Dempsey, E. W., 51, *61.* See also *Young, W. C.*
  and Hertz, R., Young, W. C., 60, *63*
  and Rioch, D. M., 231, *232*
Dennison, M. See *Korenchevsky, V.*
Denniston, R. H., II, 353, *361*
der Brucke, M. G. See *Matthews, H. B.*
Dercum, F. X., 612, 613, *619*
Desclin, L., 115, *118,* 137, *152.* See also *Brouha, L.*
  and Gregoire, C., 150, *154,* 199, *203*
Desmarest and Capitain, 487, *494*
de Snoo, K., 120, *122*
Deuel, H. J., Jr. See *Gulick, M.*
  and Sandiford, I., Sandiford, K., Boothby, W. M., 236, *243*
Dexter, L., and Weiss, S., 458, *473*
Dey, F. L., 231, *233.* See also *Brookhart, J. M.*
  and Fisher, C., Ranson, S. W., 127, *128,* 221, *225,* 233
  and Leininger, C. R., Ranson, S. W., *233*
Dickinson, R. L., 37, *48,* 66, *74,* 103, *113,* 444, *455*
Diddle, A. W. See *Allen, E. Burford, T.,* and *Gardner, W. U.*
Dieckmann, H., 130, *151*
Dierks, K., 27, *30*
Dietel, F. G., 241, *243*
Dietz, R., 348, *360*
Dill, D. B., and Johnson, R. E., Daly, C., 525, *527*
Dingemanse, E. See also *David, K.,* and *Laqueur, E.*

Dingemanse, E., and Borchardt, H., Laqueur, E., 689, *703*
  and Laqueur, E., 707, *732*
  and Laqueur, E., Mühlbock, O., 682, 690, *701*
  and Tyslowitz, R., 707, *732*
di Palma, J. R. See *Reynolds, S. R. M.*
Di Paola, G., and del Castillo, E. B., 79, *98*
Dippel, A. L., 117, *118*
Dockerty, M. B., 39, *48,* 599, *618*
  and MacCarty, W. C., 595, 598, *618*
Dodds, E. C., 35, *47*
  and Cook, J. W., Hewett, C. L., Lawson, W., 707, *732*
  and Goldberg, L., Lawson, W., Robinson, R., 708, *732*
  and Robertson, J. D., 306, 322, *324*
Dohan, F. C. See also *Lukens, F. D. W.*
  and Lukens, F. D. W., 213, *218,* 286, *289*
Dohrn, M. See *Hohlweg, W.,* and *Schoeller, W.*
Doisy, E. A., 710, *732.* See also *Allen, E.,* and *Katzman, P. A.*
  and Veler, E. D., Thayer, S., 34, *47*
Donnet, V. See *Chosson, J.*
Dorff, G. B., 543, *614*
Dorfman, R. I. See also *Gallagher, T. F.,* and *Kenyon, A. T.*
  and Greulich, W. W., Solomon, C. I., 681, 689, *701*
  and Wilson, H. M., Peters, J. P., 587, *617*
Dott, N. M., 221, *225*
Dotti, L. B. See *Riddle, O.*
Douglass, L. H. See *Connally, H. F.,* and *Savage, J. E.*
Drake, C. B., 620, 622, *629*
Drake, T. See *Albright, F.*
Draper, W. B., and Darley, W., Harvey, J. L., 224, *225*
Drips, D. G., and Osterberg, A. E., 690, 692, 693, 697, *703*
Drummond, J. C. See *Cuthbertson, W. F. J.*
Drummond-Robinson, G., and Asdell, S. A., 50, *61,* 142, *152*
Duckman, C., and Turino, T. R., 493, *495*
Duff, G. L. See *MacCallum, W. G.*
Duffy, P. V., and Corsaro, J., 493, *495*
Dumont, C. See *D'Amour, F. E.*
Duncan, D. R. L. See *Rubenstein, B. B.*
Duncan, G. G., and Fetter, F., 269, *271*
Duncan, P. A., and Allen, E., Hamilton, J. B., 81, *99,* 161, *165*
DuShane, G. P., and Levine, W. T., Pfeiffer, C. A., Witschi, E., 288, *290*
Duyvene de Wit, J. J., and Oppers, V. M., 56, *62,* 111, *114*
Dykshorn, S. W. See *Riddle, O.*

Eaton, A. G. See *Chidester, F. E.*
Ebbs, J. H., 489, *495*
Eckel, J. L. See *Winkelman, N. W.*
Ecker, A. D., 577, *616*
Eckhardt, C., 146, *153*

Edeiken, L., 353, *361*
Edmonds, E. W. See *Hertig, A. T.*
Effkemann, G. See also *Herold, L.*
and Müller-Jager, F., 567, *616*
Ehrhardt, C., 141, *152*, 695, *703*
and Breitenbach, H., 700, *704*
and Fischer-Wasels, H., 120, *122*
Ehrlich, H. E., 342, 343, *360*
Eichenberger, E. See *Ruzicka, L.*
Eidelsberg, J., and Ornstein, E. A., 626, *630*
Einhorn, N. H. See also *Rowntree, L. G.*
and Rowntree, L. G., 273, 274, *279, 280,* 622, *629*
Eisenberg, H. See *Thorn, G. W.*
Eisenhardt, L., and Thompson, K. W., 286, *289,* 573, 576, *616*
Eisenstaedt, J. S., and Appel, M., Fraenkel, M., 191, *202,* 622, 623, *629*
Eisin, W. M. See *Freed, S. C.*
Eisler, B. See *Schittenhelm, A.*
Eitel, H., and Krebs, H. A., Loeser, A., 206, *217*
and Loeser, A., 206, *217*
and Lohr, G., Loeser, A., 206, *217*
Elden, C. A., 710, *732*
and Wilson, K. M., 382, *386*
Elek, L., 509, *526*
Elekes, N. See *Urechia, C. I.*
Elliott, W. H., Jr. See *Crouch, R.*
Ellison, E. T. See also *Phelps, D.*
and Wolfe, J. M., 196, *202*
Ellsworth, H. C. See *Holman, D. V.*
Ellsworth, R. See *Albright, F.,* and *Mac-Callum, W. G.*
Ely, F., and Petersen, W. E., 490, *494*
Embleton, D., 502, *526*
Emerson, B. See *Burdick, H. O.*
Emerson, K., Jr. See *Thorn, G. W.*
Emery, F. E., and Atwell, W. J., 208, *217*
Emmens, C. W., 710, *732.* See also *Callow, N. H.*
Eng, H., 256, *260,* 685, *702*
Engel, L. L. See *Thorn, G. W.*
Engel, P., 283, *285,* 286, 288, *289, 290,* 608, *619.* See also *Silberstein, F.*
Engelhardt, H. T. See *Sodeman, W. A.*
Engelhart, E., 256, *261*
and Petzal, E., 348, *360*
and Tscherne, E., 431, *441*
Engelmann, G. J., 293, *296*
Engle, E. T., 78, 85, *98,* 99, 162, *166,* 172, 176, 180, 181, 182, 196, 199, *200, 201, 202, 203,* 292, *296.* See also *Smith, P. E.,* and *Wiesbader, H.*
and Crafts, R. C., 80, *99*
and Hamburger, C., 185, 189, *201*
and Shelesnyak, M. C., 292, 293, *296*
and Smith, P. E., 39, *48,* 53, 60, 62, 63, 79, 81, *98, 99*
and Smith, P. E., Shelesnyak, M. C., 85, *99*
Enneper, F., 414, *423*
Enright, L., and Cole, V. V., Hitchcock, F. A., 241, *243*

Epstein, A. A., 500, *526*
Erb, W., 468, *474*
Erdheim, J., 561, *615*
and Stumme, E., 194, *202*
Ersner, J. S., 525, *527*
Erving, H. W., and Sears, C., Rock, J., 189, *201,* 407, *411*
Erway, J. See *Cole, H. H.*
Escamilla, R. F. See also *Biskind, G. R.*
and Lisser, H., 565, 568, 569, 572, *616*
Escher, G. C. See *Geist, S. H.*
Estes, W. L., Jr., and Heitmeyer, P. L., 410, *411*
Euler, H. See *Zondek, B.*
Evans, F. A. See *Strang, J. M.*
Evans, H. M., 205, *216,* 277, 280, 543, *614.* See also *Becks, H., Fraenkel-Conrat, H. L., Li, C. H., Long, J. A., Lyons, W. R., Marx, W., Reichert, F. L., Reinhardt, W. O.,* and *Simpson, M. E.*
and Bishop, K. S., 406, *411,* 414, *423*
and Kohls, C. L., Wonder, D. H., 693, 694, 695, *703*
and Korpi, K., Pencharz, R. I., Simpson, M. E., 177, 186, *200, 201,* 716, *733*
and Korpi, K., Simpson, M. E., Pencharz, R. I., Wonder, D. H., 163, *166,* 173, *200*
and Long, J. A., 204, *216,* 546, 552, *615*
and Meyer, K., Simpson, M. E., 174, 176, 189, *200*
and Meyer, K., Simpson, M. E., Reichert, F. L., 515, *527*
and Moon, H., Simpson, M. E., Lyons, W. R., 276, 277, 279, *280*
and Pencharz, R. I., Simpson, M. E., 163, *166*
and Simpson, M. E., 136, *151,* 177, *200, 201,* 239, *243,* 276, 277, *280*
and Simpson, M. E., Austin, P. R., 183, *201*
and Simpson, M. E., Tolksdorf, S., Jensen, H., 173, 174, 177, *200*
and Swezy, O., 2, *30,* 192, *202*
Evans, L. T., 162, *166*
Everett, H. S. See *Novak, E.*
Eversole, W. J. See *Gaunt, R.*
Ewald, J. R. See *Goltz, F.*
Ewing, J., 456, *472*

Fabyan, M. See *MacCallum, W. G.*
Fagin, J., and Reynolds, S. R. M., 93, *99*
Falk, E. A., and Papanicolaou, G. N., 180, *201*
Falk, H. C., and Nahon, R., 101, *113*
Falls, F. H., and Freda, V. C., Cohen, H. H., 679, *680*
and Lackner, J. E., Krohn, L., 107, *114,* *424*
and Rezek, G. H., Benensohn, S. J., 420, *423*
Falta, W., 236, *243,* 513, *527,* 568, 569. *616*
Farber, J. E., and Gustina, F. J., Postoloff A. V., 607, *619*

Farquharson, R. F., and Hyland, H. H., 310, 325

Fawcet, E., 458, 459, 472, 473

Fazekas, J. F. See Himwich, H. E., Martin, S. J., and Nelson, W. O.

Fee, A. R., and Parkes, A. S., 231, 233

Feen, B. G. See Behnke, A. R.

Fein, M. J. See Siegler, S. L.

Feinstein, R. N., and Gordon, E. S., 216, 219

Fekete, E. See Woolley, G.

Fellner, O. O., 50, 61, 116, 118, 119, 122, 639, 640

Fellows, M. D., 287, 289

Fels, E., 51, 61, 197, 202, 695, 703
and Slotta, K. H., Ruschig, H., 57, 62

Fels, S. S. See Shay, H.

Felshin, G. See Frank, R. T.

Fenning, C., 109, 114

Feresten, M. See Bernstein, P., and Wimpfheimer, S.

Ferguson, R. S., 700, 704. See also Twombly, G. H.

Ferrebee, J. W., and Ragan, C., Atchley, D. W., Loeb, R. F., 593, 618

Fetter, F. See Duncan, G. G.

Fevold, H. L., 173, 174, 200. See also Astwood, E. G., Foster, M. A., Greep, R. O., Hisaw, F. L., and Nathanson, I. T.
and Hisaw, F. L., 176, 200
and Hisaw, F. L., Hellbaum, A., Hertz, R., 173, 176, 200
and Lee, M., Hisaw, F. L., Cohn, E. J., 173, 174, 179, 200

Fichera, G., 210, 217

Fielding, U. J. See Popa, G. L.

Fields, E. M. See Gordon, M. B.

Fieser, L. F. See Wolfe, J. K.

Finch, J. W., 456, 472

Finkler, R. S., 688, 702. See also Friedman, M.
and Antopol, W., 438, 442

Firor, W. M., 221, 225. See also Hartman, C. G., and Thorn, G. W.
and Grollman, A., 254, 260

First, A. See Bland, P. B.

Fischer, B. See Schultze, F.

Fischer, W. H. See Miescher, K.

Fischer-Wasels, H. See Ehrhardt, C.

Fishberg, A. M. See Vorzimer, J. J.

Fisher, C., 215, 219. See also Dey, F. L., Ingram, W. R., and Ranson, S. W.
and Ingram, W. R., 228, 232
and Ingram, W. R., Hare, W. K., Ranson, S. W., 229, 232
and Ingram, W. R., Ranson, S. W., 215, 219, 220, 225
and Magoun, H. W., Ranson, S. W., 127, 128, 221, 225

Fisher, R. E., and Russell, J. A., Cori, C. F., 211, 218

Fitzwilliams, D. C. L., 129, 151

Fleischmann, W. See also Wilkins, L.
and Goldhammer, H., 283, 285

Fliess, W., 376, 386

Florentin, P. See Watrin, J.

Fluhmann, C. F., 80, 99, 160, 165, 181, 201, 287, 288, 289, 316, 325, 341, 360, 367, 373, 383, 385, 429, 431, 441, 655, 671, 679, 680, 681, 683, 693, 697, 701, 703
See also Murphy, K. M.
and Morse, D. L., 327, 360
and Murphy, K. M., 309, 316, 319, 322, 325

Foo, C., 608, 619

Folley, S. J., 142, 154, 265, 267
and Kon, S. K., 142, 152
and Watson, H. M. S., Bottomley, A. C., 144, 153
and Young, F. G., 140, 152

Fomina, P. I., 128, 128

Fontes, J. M., 128, 128

Forbes, A. P. See Fraser, R. W.

Ford, F. A., and Mueller, S. C., 681, 701

Foster, C. See Henle, G.

Foster, F. I. See Reynolds, S. R. M.

Foster, M. A., 178, 200
and Fevold, H. L., 174, 175, 185, 200
and Foster, R. C., Fevold, H. L., 200
and Hisaw, F. L., 174, 180, 200

Foster, R. C. See Foster, M. A.

Fowler, W. M. See Gibson, R. B.

Fraenkel, L., 50, 56, 61, 307, 324

Fraenkel, M. See Eisenstaedt, J. S.

Frankel-Conrat, H. L. See also Simpson, M. E.
and Herring, V. V., Simpson, M. E., Evans, H. M., 210, 211, 218

Francis, B. F. See Allen, E.

Frank, I. L. See also Salmon, U. J.
and Geist, S. H., 38, 48

Frank, R. T., 66, 74, 82, 99, 257, 261, 348, 360, 404, 411, 438, 439, 442, 446, 448, 455, 587, 617, 662, 679, 683, 684, 686, 692, 697, 702, 703, 704. See also Goldberger, M. A., Salmon, U. J., and Spielman, F.
and Berman, R. L., 673, 677, 680, 715, 733
and Goldberger, M. A., 181, 201, 655, 679, 681, 683, 701, 702
and Goldberger, M. A., Salmon, U. J., 427, 434, 441
and Goldberger, M. A., Salmon, U. J., Felshin, G., 315, 325, 430, 441
and Goldberger, M. A., Spielman, F., 116, 118, 682, 685, 702
and Klempner, E., Hollander, F., Kriss, B., 665, 680
and Salmon, U. J., 431, 441, 692, 703, 671, 680
and Salmon, U. J., Friedman, R., 697, 703

Frankl, O., 80, 94, 99, 141, 143, 152, 304, 324, 339, 343, 360

Frankl-Hochwart, L., 466, 474

Franseen, C. C. See Nathanson, I. T.

Frantz, C. H. See Currier, F. P.

Fraser, R. W. See also Albright, F.
and Smith, P. H., 47, 49, 590, 616
and Forbes, A. P., Albright, F., Sulkowitch, H., Reifenstein, E. C., 689, 690, 691, 703

Frazier, W. R., 422, *424*
Freda, V. C. See *Falls, F. H.*
Fredet, P., 117, *118*
Freed, S. C., 692, *703.* See also *Greenhill, J. P.*
and Eisin, W. M., Greenhill, J. P., 709, *733*
and Greenhill, J. P., 710, *732*
Freedman, H. See *MacBryde, C. M.*
Freimann, S. C., 45, *49*
Fremery, P. de, and Luchs, A., Tausk, M., 55, *62*
and Scheygrond, B., 288, *290*
Freud, J., 178, *200.* See also *David, K.,* and *Uyldert, I. E.*
and De Jongh, S. E., Laqueur, E., 42, 43, *49*
and Levie, L. H., Kroon, D. B. L., 204, *216*
Freudenberger, C. B. See *Hashimoto, E. I.*
Freyberg, R. H., and Barker, P. S., Newburgh, L. H., Coller, F. A., 577, 581, *616*
Friedgood, H. B., 206, *216, 217,* 253, *260.* See also *Reboul, J.,* and *Wolfe, J. K.*
Friedman, A. B., and Seligman, B., 322, 323, *325*
Friedman, H. See *Loeb, L.*
Friedmann, M. See also *Zondek, B.*
and Finkler, R. S., 407, *411*
Friedman, M. H., 180, 182, *201.* See also *Makepeace, G. L., Reynolds, S. R. M.,* and *Weinstein, G. L.*
and Lapham, M. E., 675, *680*
and Weinstein, G. L., 700, *704*
Friedman, R. See *Frank, R. T.*
Friedman, S. M. See *Selye, H.*
Friedrich, H., 125, *128,* 463, *473*
Fröhlich, A., 556, *615*
Fromme, H. See *Bickenbach, W.*
Frommel, R., 491, *495*
Fry, E. G. See also *Long, C. N. H.*
and Long, C. N. H., Ritter, H. B., 250, *259*
Fuchs, H., 117, *118*
Fugo, N. F. See *Gross, E. G.*
Fujiwara, T. F., 585, *617*
Fulton, J. F., and Bailey, P., 561, *615*
Fulton, L. See *Palmer. A.*
Fumi, C. See *Bentivoglio, G. C.*
Funk, C., and Harrow, B., 156, *165*
Funk, D. See *D'Amour. F. E.*
Furth, J., and Butterworth, J. S., 596, *618*
Furuhjelm, M., 690, 701, *703*
Futcher, T. B. See *MacCallum, W. G.*

GAARENSTROOM, J. H., and De Jongh, S. E., 180, *201*
and Levie, L. H., 543, *614*
Gabriel, J. E. See *Hartman, F. A.*
Gaebler, O. H., 216, *219*
and Galbraith, H. W., 216, *219*
Gagel, O., 231, *233*
Gaines, J. A., 480, *494.* See also *Geist, S. H.,* and *Salmon, U. J.*

Gaines, J. A., and Geist, S. H., Salmon, U. J., 350, *361*
and Salmon, U. J., Geist, S. H., 160, 161, *165*
Galbraith, H. W. See *Gaebler, O. H.*
Gallagher, I. F. See *Willier, B. H.*
Gallagher, T. F. See also *Kenyon, A. T.,* and *Nelson, W. O.*
and Koch, F. C., 156, *164*
and Peterson, D. H., Dorfman, R. I., Kenyon, A. T., Koch, F. C., 689, 690, *702*
Gamarra, N., and Schouten, G. B., 394, *410*
Garbutt, H. R. See *Thorn, G. W.*
Gardiner-Hill, H., 268, *271*
and Smith, J. F., 306, *324*
Gardner, W. U., 137, *152.* See also *Allen, E., Chamberlin, T. L., Landauer, W., Pfeiffer, C. A.,* and *Turner, C. W.*
and Allen, E., Smith, G. M., Strong, L. C., 39, *48*
and Allen, E., Strong, L. C., 37, *48*
and Diddle, A. W., Allen, E., Strong, L. C., 136, *151*
and Gomez, E. T., Turner, C. W., 138, *152*
and Turner, C. W., 717, *733*
Gargill, S. L. See *Greenberg, B. E.*
Garvin, C. F., and Reichle, H. S., 590, *617*
Gauld, A. G. See *Rock, J.*
Gaunt, R. See also *Nelson, W. O.*
and Eversole, W. J., Kendall, E. C., 148, 153
and Tobin, C. E., 147, *153,* 259, *261*
Geber, H., 376, *386*
Gebert, W., 452, *455*
Geesink, A., and Koster, S., 209, *217*
Gegerson, H. B., and Clark, A. R., Kurzrok, R., 286, 287, *289*
Geiling, E. M. K. See also *Chen, G., Grollman, A.,* and *Hartman, C. G.*
and Campbell, D., Ishikawa, Y., 222, *225*
and Robbins, L. L., 220, *224*
Geist, S. H., 29, *31,* 160, 161, 164, *165,* 188, 201, 383, *386,* 448, *455,* 487, *494,* 599, 603, *618.* See also *Frank, I. L., Gaines, J. A., Mintz, M., Salmon, U. J.,* and *Walter, R. I.*
and Gaines, J. A., 580, *617*
and Gaines, J. A., Escher, G. C., *49,* 596, *618*
and Gaines, J. A., Pollock, A. D., 45, *49*
and Gaines, J. A., Salmon, U. J., 42, *48,* 161, *165,* 190, *202,* 322, *325,* 351, *361,* 427, 434, 439, *441, 442,* 651, *679*
and Mintz, M., 440, *442*
and Salmon, U. J., Mintz, M., 36, *48,* 58, *62,* 161, *166*
and Spielman, F., 602, *618*
and Walter, R. I., Salmon, U. J., 440, *442*
Geller, F. C., 43, *49*
Gellhorn, G., 528, *536*
Gemmell, H. A., and Jeffcoate, T. N. A., 39, *48*
Genther, I., 45, 47, *49*
Gerard-Lefebre, M., 579, *617*
Gerschman, R., 209, *217*

Gersh, I., and Grollman, A., 257, *261*
    and Tarr, A., 220, *224*
Gershon-Cohen, J. See *Shay, H.*
Geschickter, C. F., 482, 487, 484, *944*. See
    also *Astwood, E. B., Bucher, N. L. R.,*
    and *Lewis, D.*
Gessler, C. J., and Halsted, J. A., Stetson,
    R. P., 435, 439, *441*
Geuer, C., 241, *243*
Gey, G. O. See also *Seegar, G. E.*
    and Seegar, G. E., Hellman, L. M., 121,
    122
Gey, M. K. See *Seegar, G. E.*
Gibson, H. V. See *Allen, E.*
Gibson, R. B., and Fowler, W. M., 268, *217*
Gierhake, E. See *Wehefritz, E.*
Gilbert, C., 53, *62*
Gilbert, J. B., 700, *704*
Gill, A. M., 581, *617*
Gillman, J., 82, 83, 99, 370, 385, 421, *424,*
    446, 448, *455*. See also *Black, J.*
    and Stein, H. B., 53, *62*
Ginglinger, A. See *Wolff, E.*
Giusti, L. See *Houssay, B. A.*
Glanzmann, E., 274, *280*
Glass, S. J. See *Marx, R.*
    and McKennon, B. J., 685, 700, *702*
Gley, E., 234, *242*, 262, *266*
Gley, P., 51, *61*
Globus, J. See *Bing, J.*
Goddard, H. H., 283, *284*
Godfrid, M. See *Katzman, P. A.*
Goecke, H., 579, 580, *617*
Goldberg, L. See *Dodds, E. C.*
Goldberg, M. B., and Lisser, H., 555, *615*
Goldberg, M. W. See *Ruzicka, L.*
Goldberger, M. A. See also *Frank, R. T.,*
    and *Spielman, F.*
    and Frank, R. T., 125, *128*, 463, *473*
    and Peck, S. M., 348, *360*
    and Salmon, U. J., Frank, R. T., 694, *703*
Goldblatt, H., 249, *259*
Golden, J. B. See *Lauson, H. D.*
Goldhammer, H. See *Fleischmann, W.*
Golding, G. T., and Ramirez, F. T., 42, *48*
Goldman, A. M. See *Mendel, E. B.*
Goldman, L. M., and Kessler, H. B., Wilder,
    M. E., 679, *680*
Goldner, M. See *von Bergmann, G.*
Goldschmidt, R., 633, 636, 637, *640*, 643,
    644, 647, *648*
Goldstein, L. See *Bland, P. B.*
Goldwasser, M., 377, *386*
Goldzieher, M. A., 251, *260*. 266, *267*, 322,
    325, 449, *455*, 543, *614*, *615*. See also
    Gusman, H.
    and Sherman, I., Alperstein, B. B., 214,
    218
Goltz, F., and Ewald, J. R., 146, *153*
Gomez, E. T., 149, *153*. See also *Gardner,*
    W. U., Lewis, A. A., and *Turner, C. W.*
    and Turner, C. W., 137, 140, *152*
    and Turner, C. W., Reece, R. P., 137, *151*
Goodall, J. R., and Power, R. M. H., 376,
    386

Goodfriend, M. J. See *Abarbanel, A. R.*
Goodman, B. A., 479, 488, *494*
Gordon, A. S., and Kleinberg, W., Char-
    ipper, H. A., 288, *290*
    and Levenstein, I., Charipper, H. A., 288,
    290
Gordon, B., and Cantarow, A., 264, *267*
Gordon, E. S. See also *Feinstein, R. N.*
    and Sevringhaus, E. L., Stark, M. E.,
    591, *617*
Gordon, F. F., 292, *296*
Gordon, M. B. See also *Handelsmann, M. B.*
    and Fields, E. M., 623, *630*
Goss, H., and Cole, H. H., 716, *733*
Gossip, W. H., 451, *455*
Gostomirovic, D., 640. 697, *704*
Gradinescu, A., 255, *260*
Grafenberg, E., 393, *410*
Graham, W. R., Jr., 148, *153*. See also *Her-*
    man, A.
Grant, G. A., 147, *153*
Gray, H. I., 30, 382, *386*
Gray, L. A., 189, *201*, 321, *325*, 349, *361*,
    383, *386*, 448, *455*
    and Manly, W. F., 383, *386*
Greenberg, B. E., and Berman, S., Gargill,
    S. L., Griffin, R. C., 396, *411*
Greenblatt, R. B., 446, 448, *455*. See also
    Greenhill, J. P.
    and McCall, E., Torpin, R., 370, 382, *385*
    and Pund, E. R., 322, *325*
Greene, J. A., and Johnson, J. A., 543, *614*
Greene, R. See *Hart, F. D.*
Greene, R. R., and Burrill, M. W., Ivy, A.
    C., 605, *618*, 638, 639, *640*
Greenhill, J. P., 409, *411*, 465, *474*, 709,
    732. See also *Freed, S. C.*
    and Freed, S. C., 161, *165*, 446, 447, 448,
    455
    and Greenblatt, R. B., 599, *618*
Greenwald, I., 263, *266*
Greenwood, A., and Blyth, J. S., 638, *640*
Greep, R. O., 41, *48*, 156, *165*, 178, 180, *200*,
    201. See also *Bunde, C. A., Hisaw, F.*
    L., Shedlovsky, T., and *Van Dyke,*
    H. B.
    and Fevold, H. L., 162, *166*
    and Fevold, H. L., Hisaw, F. L., 163, *166*
    and Stavely, H. E., 138, *152*
    and Van Dyke, H. B., Chow, B. F., 46,
    49, *200*, 715, *732*
Gregoire, C. See *Desclin, L.*
Grenley, P. See *Hotchkiss, R. S.*
Greulich, W. W. See *Dorfman, R. I.*
Griffin, R. C. See *Greenberg, B. E.*
Griffith, L. S., and McBride, W. P. L., 398,
    406, *410*
Griffith, F. R., Jr. See *Pucher, G. W.*
Griffiths, M., 223, *225*
    and Marks, H. P., Young, F. C., 270, *271*
Grimes, W. H. See *Colvin, E. D.*
Groebbels, F., 275, *280*
Grollman, A., 248, 254, 256, 257, 259, *260*,
    585, *617*. See also *Firor, W. M.,* and
    Gersh, I.

Grollman, A., and Geiling, E. M. K., 222, 225

Gros, G. See *Courrier, R.*

Gross, E. G., and Ingram, W. R., Fugo, N. F., 223, 225

Grosser, O., 71, *75*

Grote, I. W. See *Kamm, O.*

Grueter, F., 148, *153*. See also *Stricker, P.*

Grumbrecht, P., 434, *441*

Grundlach, R. See *Hess, W. R.*

Grynfeltt, E., 475, *493*

Gudernatsch, J. F., 236, *242*, 274, *280*. See also *Hoffman, O.*

Gueissaz, M. E., 444, *455*

Guggisberg, H., 509, 525, *526*

Guldberg, E., 134, *151*

Gulick, M., and Samuels, L. T., Deuel, H. J., Jr., 270, *271*, 509, *526*

Gull, W., 234, *242*

Gumbreck, L. G. See *Biddulph, C.*

Gunther, L., and Courville, C. B., 568, *616*

Gurney, R., 505, 511, *526*

Gusman, H., and Goldzieher, M. A., 407, *411*

Gustavson, R. G. See also *D'Amour, F. E.,* and *Kunde, M. M.*
  and Mason, L. W., Hays, E. E., Wood, T. R., D'Amour, F. E., 67, *74*
  and Van Dyke, H. B., 111, *114*

Gustina, F. J. See *Farber, J. E.*

Gustus, E. L. See also *Meyer, R. K.*
  and Meyer, R. K., Woods, O. R., 716, *733*

Guthert, H., 210, *217*

Guthmann, H., and Voelcker, L., 258, *261*

Guttmacher, A. F. See also *Wang, G. H.*
  and Shettles, L. B., 59, *63*, 409, *411*

Guttman, P. H., 589, *617*

HAAGENSON, C. D. See *Auchincloss, H.*

Haden, R. L., and Singleton, J. M. S., 307, *324*

Haffner, J., 120, *122*

Hagen, W., 452, *455*

Hageman, P. O., and McCordick, H. A., 206, *216*

Hagquist, C. W. See *Young, W. C.*

Hain, A. M., 460, 464, *473*, 638, 639, *640*, 690, *703*

Haines, S. F. See also *Mussey, R. D.*
  and Mussey, R. D., 322, *325*

Haist, R. E., and Best, C. H., 210, *217*

Halban, J., 119, *122*, 133, 141, *151*, 152, 637, 639, *640*, 647, *648*
  and Koehler, R., 65, *73*

Hall, J. F. See *Sherwood, T. C.*

Hall, K. See *Korenchevsky, V.*

Hall, V. E., and Chamberlin, P. E., Muller, O. H., 256, *260*

Halpern, L. J. See *Bronstein, I. P.*

Halpern, S., and D'Amour, F. E., 198, *202*

Halsted, J. A. See *Gessler, C. J.*

Ham, G. C., and Landis, E. M., 459, *473*

Hamblen, E. C., 41, *48*, 188, 189, *201, 202,* 319, 321, *325,* 327, 337, 340, 349, 357, *360, 361,* 407, *411,* 421, 422, *423,* 446, *455,* 682, 687, 688, *702.* See also *Davis, C. D., Pullen, R. L.,* and *Ross, R. A.*
  and Ashley, C., Baptist, M., 712, 713, *732*
  and Cuyler, W. K., Baptist, M., 259, *261,* 434, *441,* 585, *617,* 650, 670, *679, 680,* 687, 690, 691, *703, 704*
  and Cuyler, W. K., Pattee, C. J., Axelson, G. J., 421, *424*
  and Cuyler, W. K., Wilson, J. A., Pullen, R. L., 47, *49*
  and Hirst, D. V., Cuyler, W. K., 350, *361*
  and Ross, R. A., Cuyler, W. K., Baptist, M., Ashley, C., 690, *703*
  and Sprunt, D. H., 353, 354, *361*

Hamilton, J. B., 157, 165. See also *Duncan, P. A.,* and *Wolfe, J. M.*
  and Hubert, G., 620, 622, *629*
  and Wolfe, J. M., 638, 639, *640*

Hamburger, C., 163, *166.* See also *Engle, E. T.*

Hammar, J. A., 276, *280*

Hammett, F. S., 264, *267*

Hammond, J., 50, *61,* 70, *74,* 111, *114,* 142, *152.* See also *Asdell, S. A.,* and *Walton, A.*
  and Asdell, S. A., 70, 74, 135, *151*
  and Marshall, F. H. A., 146, *153*
  and Walton, A., 70, *74*

Hampton, A. O. See *Albright, F.*

Handelsmann, M. B., and Gordon, M. B., 525, *527*

Hanisch, G. See *Butenandt, A.*

Hannan, J. H., 434, *441*

Hansen, L. P. See *McCahey, J. F.,* and *Paschkis, K. E.*

Hansmann, F. S., 277, *280*

Hanson, A. M., 263, *267.* See also *Rowntree, L. G.*

Hare, W. K. See *Fisher, C.*

Harington, C. R., 235, *242*
  and Barger, G., 235, *242*
  and Rowlands, I. W., 286, *289*

Harlow, C. See *Selye, H.*

Harne, O. G., and Painter, E. E., 102, 103, *113*

Harnik, M. See *Novak, J.*

Harrington, M. M., 498, *526*

Harris, J. M. See *Hechter, O.,* and *Krohn, L.*

Harris, R. G., and Pfiffner, J. J., 56, *62*

Harrison, K. S., 207, *217*

Harrop, G. A. See also *Thorn, G. W.*
  and Pfiffner, J. J., Weinstein, A., Swingle, W. W., 252, *260*
  and Soffer, L. J., Nicholson, W. M., Strauss, M., 248, *259*
  and Weinstein, A., Soffer, L. J., Threscher, J. H., 248, *259,* 590, *617*

Harrow, B. See *Funk, C.*

Hart, E. B. See *Kozelka, F. L.*

Hart, F. D., and Greene, R., 554, *615*

Hart, G. H. See also *Cole, H. H.*
  and Cole, H. H., 119, *122*

Hart, P. C. See *Laqueur, E.*
Hartley, E. C., 264, *267*
Hartman, C. G., 66, 69, 70, 71, *74, 75,* 77, 84, 85, 95, *98, 99, 100,* 161, *165,* 185, *201,* 294, *296,* 305, *324,* 359, *361,* 407, *411.* See also *Ivy, A. C.*
and Firor, W. M., 85, 91, *99*
and Firor, W. M., Geiling, E. M. K., 84, *99*
and Geiling, E. M. K., 85, 91, *99*
and Speert, H., 53, 59, *62, 63,* 134, *151.*
Hartman, F. A., 251, 252, *260.* See also *Thorn, G. W., Brownell, K. A.,* and *Spoor, H.*
and Lewis, L. A., Gabriel, J. E., 288, *290*
and Lockwood, J. E., Brownell, K. A., 259, *261*
Hartmann, H., and Störring, F., 103, *113*
Harvey, J. L. See *Draper, W. B.*
Hashimoto, E. I., and Freudenberger, C. B., 273, 275, *280*
Haslhofer, L. See *Tapfer, S.*
Haterius, H. O., 120, *122,* 144, *153.* See also *Charipper, H. A.*
Hathaway, I. R. See *Reece, R. P.*
Haussmann, D., 71, *75*
Haymaker, E., and Anderson, W., 578, 579, *616*
Haymaker, W. See *Anderson, E.*
Hays, E. E. See *Gustavson, R. G.*
Hays, H. W. See *Swingle, W. W.*
Hayward, S. J. See *Loeb, L.*
Heard, R. D. H., and Bauld, W. S., Hoffman, M. M., 713, *733*
and Hoffman, M. M., 707, *732*
Heath, C. See *Aub, J. C.*
Hechler, R. See *Lucke, H.*
Hechter, O., 687, 704. See also *Krohn, L.*
and Krohn, L., Harris, J. M., 58, *62*
Heckel, G. P., 115, *118.* See also *Allen, W. M.*
and Allen, W. M., 41, *48,* 110, *114,* 121, *122*
Heckel, N. J., 42, *48,* 159, 164, *165, 166.* See also *Thompson, W. O.*
Heffernan, R. J. See *Sullivan, C. L.*
Heiberg, B., and Heiberg, P., 39, *48*
Heiberg, P. See *Heiberg, B.*
Heim, K., 460, *473*
Heimann, J., and Krehbiel, O. F., 484, *494*
Heinbecker, P., and White, H. L., 215, *219,* 221, *225,* 230, *232,* 517, *527,* 561, *615*
and White, H. L., Rolf, D., 222, *225*
Heinberg, C. J., 452, *455*
Heitmeyer, P. L. See *Estes, W. L., Jr.*
Hellbaum, A. See *Casida, L. E.,* and *Fevold, H. L.*
Heller, C. G., 707, *732.* See also *Heller, E. J.,* and *Lauson, H. D.*
and Heller, E. J., 432, *441*
and Heller, E. J., Sevringhaus, E. L., 432, 439, *441*
Heller, E. J. See *Heller, C. G.*
and Heller, C. G., Sevringhaus, E. L., 700, *704*

Heller, H., 222, 223, *225*
Hellman, L. M. See *Gey, G. O.,* and *Moore, R. A.*
Helwig, E. B. See *MacBryde, C. M.*
Hemmingsen, A. M., 36, *48*
Hemphill, R. E., and Reiss, M., 572, *616*
Henderson, W. R., and Rowlands, I. W., 193, *202,* 429, 431, *441*
Henkel, M., 413, *423*
Henle, G. See also *Henle, W.*
and Church, C. F., Foster, C., 394, *410*
Henle, W., and Henle, G., 394, *410*
Henley, W., 270, *271*
Henriksen, E., 384, *386,* 444, 455, 605, *618.* See also *Wharton, L. R.*
Henry, G. W. See *Allen, E. B.*
Henry, J. S. See also *Browne, J. S. L.,* and *Venning, E. H.*
and Browne, J. S. L., 96, *100,* 106, *114*
Herlant, M., 116, *118*
Herman, H. A. See *Ralston, N. P.*
and Graham, W. R., Jr., Turner, C. W., 148, *153*
Hermann, W. See *Neumann, R.*
Herold, L. See also *Anselmino, K. J.*
and Effkemann, G., 484, *494*
Herrell, W. E., 39, *48*
Herring, J. S. See *King, E. L.*
Herring, P. T., 220, *222, 224, 225*
Herring, V. V. See *Fraenkel-Conrat, H. L.*
Herrmann, E., 50, *61*
Herrnberger, K., 710, *733*
Hertig, A. T., and Edmonds, E. W., 413, *423*
Hertz, R. See also *Dempsey, E. W.,* and *Fevold, H. L.*
and Hisaw, F. L., 174, 192, *200, 202*
and Meyer, R. K., Spielman, M., 60, *63*
Hertz, S. See also *Means, J. H.*
and Kranes, A., 209, *217*
and Roberts, A., *216*
Hertzler, A. E., 374, *385*
Hertzman, J. See *Lurie, L. A.*
Hess, W. R., and Grundlach, R., 223, *225*
Hesseltine, H. C., and Spear, W. M., 307, *324*
Hetenyi, G., 503, *526*
Hetherington, A. W., 517, *527*
and Ranson, S. W., 230, *232,* 517, *527,* 561, *615*
Hewett, C. L. See *Dodds, E. C.*
Heydemann, E. R. See *Lucke, H.*
Heynemann, T., 347, *360*
Heynes, O. H. See *Black, J.*
Hicks, G. S., and Matters, R. F., 256, *260*
Hildebrand, A. G. See *Rynearson, E. H.*
Hill, M., and Parkes, A. S., 180, *201*
Hill, R. T., 47, *49.* See also *Burr, H. S.,* and *Reece, R. P.*
and Allen, E., Kramer, T. C., 67, *74*
Himsworth, H. P., and Scott, D. B. M., 250, *260*
and Scott, D. D. M., 213, *218*
Himwich, H. E., 212, *218.* See also *Nelson, W. O.*

Himwich, H. E., and Fazekas, J. M., Martin, S. J., 250, 251, *259*
and Keller, A. D., 230, *232*
Hinglais, H. See *Brindeau, A.*
Hinglais, M. See *Brindeau, A.*
Hinsey, J. C. See *Markee, J. E.*
Hirschmann, H., 691, *703*
Hirst, D. V. See *Hamblen, E. C.*
Hirst, J. C., 456, *472*
Hirtz, G., 116, *118*
Hisaw, F. L., 52, 53, 60, *61, 63,* 78, 79, 80, 81, 82, *98, 99,* 161, *166,* 344, *360.* See also *Allen, E., Campbell, R. E., Fevold, H. L., Foster, M. A., Hertz, R.,* and *Greep, R. O.*
and Greep, R. O., 82, 83, *99*
and Greep, R. O., Fevold, H. L., 53, 59, 60, *62, 63,* 159, *165,* 176, *200*
and Lendrum, F. C., 59, *63*
and Leonard, S. L., 55, *62*
Hitchcock, F. A. See *Enright, L.,* and *Thorn, G. W.*
Hitschmann, F., and Adler, L., 16, *30, 34, 47, 64, 73,* 76, *85, 98*
Hoctor, E. F. See *Ault, C. C.*
Hoet, M., 207, *217*
Hofbauer, J., 458, 459, 461, *473*
Hoffman, F. G. See *Schmidt, I. G.*
Hoffman, J., 172, 193, *200.* See also *Anspach, B. M.,* and *Mazer, C.*
Hoffman, M. M. See *Heard, R. D. H.*
Hoffman, O., and Gudernatsch, J. F., 274, *280*
Hoffmann, F., 466, *474,* 489, 490, 493, *494, 495.* See also *Anselmino, K. J.*
Hohlweg, W., 198, *202.* See also *Imhoffen, H. H.,* and *Schoeller, W.*
and Chamorro, A., 198, *202*
and Dohrn, M., 197, *202*
and Junkmann, K., 199, *203,* 238, 239, *243*
Holden, F. C., and Sovak, F. W., 410, *411*
Hollander, E., 612, *619*
Hollander, F. See *Frank, R. T.*
Holman, D. V., and Ellsworth, H. C., 223, *225*
Holscher, B. See *Bomskov, C.*
Holst, S., and Turner, C. W., 141, *152*
Honda, K., 288, *290*
Horie, K. See *Mujuda, T.*
Horney, K., 375, *386*
Horning, E. S. See *Cramer, W.*
Horrax, G., 282, *284,* 608, *619*
Hosemann, H., 415, *423*
Hoskins, R. G., 224, *225,* 283, *284*
and McClure, C. W., 245, *259*
Hoskins, W. H. See *Webster, B.*
Hotchkiss, R. S., 395, *410*
and Brunner, E. K., Grenley, P., 395, *410*
Housel, E. L. See *Cantarow, A.*
Houssay, B. A., 148, *153,* 212, 213, *217, 218,* 250, *260.* See also *Biasotti, A.*
and Artundo, A., 215, *219*
and Biassotti, A., 212, *218*
and Biasotti, A., Mazzocco, P., 208, *217*

Houssay, B. A., and Biasotti, A., Mazzocco, P., Sammartino, R., 207, *217*
and Busso, R. R., 211, *218*
and Giusti, L., 231, *233*
and Hug, E., 220, *224*
and Lascano-Gonzalez, J. M., 211, *218,* 276, *280*
and Mazzocco, P., 208, *217*
and Potick, D., 212, *218*
and Sammartino, R., 209, *217,* 467, *474*
Howard, J. E., 543, *614*
and Whitehill, M. R., 585, *617*
Howard, N. J., 488, *494*
Howard, R. P. See *Thorn, G. W.*
Howitz, F., 234, *242*
Huber, C. P., and Davis, M. E., 189, *201*
Huberman, J. and Colmer, M. J., 431, *441*
Hubert, G. See *Hamilton, J. B.*
Huet, J. A. See *Laroche, G.*
Hufford, A. R., 709, *733*
Hug, E. See *Houssay, B. A.*
Hughes, E. C., 456, 459, *472, 473*
Hühner, M., 398, *410*
Hunt and associates, 418, *423*
Hunt, H. See *White, P.*
Hunt, H. F. See *Patterson, W. B.*
Hunt, L. See *Baumann, E. J.*
Hunter, D., 496, *526*
Hunter, J. L. See *Singleton, J. M.*
Hurd, G. B. See *Novak, E.*
Hurwitt, E. See *Abramson, D.*
Hurxthal, L. M., 548, *615*
Hyland, H. H. See *Farquharson, R. F*

Iglauer, A. See *Altschule, M. P.*
Imhoffen, H. H., and Hohlweg, W., 712, *732*
Ingelbrecht, P., 146, *153*
Ingle, D. J., 248, *261,* 270, *271, 279, 281*
Ingram, W. R. See also *Barris, R. W., Davis, L., Fisher, C., Gross, E. G.,* and *Ranson, S. W.*
and Barris, R. W., 230, *232*
and Fisher, C., 206, *233*
Isenschmid, R., 231, *233*
Ishikawa, Y. See *Geiling, E. M. K.*
Israel, S. L., 446, 448, *455.* See also *Mazer, C.,* and *Scarf, M.*
and Meranze, D. R., 415, *423*
Ito, P. K., 292, *296*
Ivy, A. C. See also *Atkinson, A. J., Burrill, M. W., Danforth, D. N.,* and *Greene, R. R.*
and Hartman, C. G., Koff, A., 108, *114*

Jaboulay, M., 384, *386*
Jacobi, J., and Tigges, F., 577, 580, *616*
Jacobsohn, D. See *Westman, A.*
Jacobson, A. W., and Kramer, A. J., 479, *494*
Jacobson, C. See *Weed, H.*
Jacobson, E., and Lackner, J. E., Sinykin, M. B., 101, *113*
Jaffe, I., and Brockway, G., 623, *630*

Jailer, W., and Leathem, J. H., 289, *290*
Jamenson, E. M., 307, *324*
Janeway, M. M., 448, *455*
Janney, J. C., 681, *701*
Jares, J. J., 136, *151*
Jaschke, R. T., 490, *494*
Jeffcoate, T. N. A., 125, *128*, 349, *361*, 398, 406, *410*, 417, *423*, 463, 465, *473*, *474*, 685, *702*. See also *Blair-Bell, W.*, and *Gemmell, A. A.*
   and Potter, A. L., 38, *48*
Jensen, H. See also *Evans, H. M.*, and *Tolksdorf, S.*
   and Tolksdorf, S., 206, *217*
   and Tolksdorf, S., Bamman, F., 173, *200*
Jerschow, S. I. See *Chaschinsky, P. C.*
Joachimowits, R., 92, *99*
Joël, C. A., 25, *30*, 58, *62*, 712, *733*
Johnson, G. E. See also *Baker, B. L.*
   and Challans, J. S., 56, *62*
Johnson, J. A. See *Greene, J. A.*
Johnson, P. E. See *Swann, H. G.*
Johnson, R. E. See *Dill, D. B.*
Johnson, W. W., 620, 622, *629*
Johnston, C. G. See *Allen, E.*
Johnstone, R. W., and Wiesner, B. P., Marshall, P. G., 422, *424*
Joll, C. A. See *Levy-Simpson, S.*
Jonáš, V., 206, *217*, 575, 576, *616*
Jones, E. I., 224, *225*
Jones, G. E. S., and Astwood, E. B., 59, *63*
   and Te Linde, R. W., 347, 350, *361*
Jones, H. O. See *Brewer, J. I.*
Jones, H. W., 354, *361*
   and Weil, P. G., 120, *122*
Jores, A., 577, 580, *616*
Jorpes, E. See *Westman, A.*
Joslin, E. P. See also *White, P.*
   and Root, H. F., White, P., Marble, A., 268, *271*
Jost, A. See *Courrier, R.*
Junghans, E., 344, *360*
Junkmann, K. See *Hohlweg, W.*

Kabat, H., *233*. See also *Ranson, S. W.*
   and Anson, B. J., Magoun, H. W., Ranson, S. W., 232, *233*
Kaiser, W. See *Stähler, F.*
Kalb, S. W., 235, *243*
Kaminester, S. See *Reynolds, S. R. M.*
Kamm, O., and Aldrich, T. B., Grote, I. W., Rowe, L. W., Bugbee, E. P., 222, *225*
Kane, H. F., 421, *423*
Kanter, A. E., and Klawans, A. H., 587, *617*, *703*
Kaplan, I. I., 322, *325*, 352, 353, *361*, 407, *411*
Karnofsky, D. See *Aub, J. C.*
Karplus, I. P., and Peczenik, O., 230, *232*
Katzin, B., and Long, C. N. H., 250, *259*
Katzman, P. A., and Doisy, E. A., 109, *114*, 692, 697, 700, *703*
   and Godfrid, M., Cain, C. K., Doisy, E. A., 716, *733*

Kaufmann, C., 52, *61*, 81, *99*, 319, 320, *325*, 336, *360*, 710, *732*
Kausch, E. See *Mikulicz-Radecki, F. von.*
Kearns, W. M., 164, *166*, 626, *630*
Keck, W. N. See *Witschi, E.*
Kehl, R., 109, *114*. See also *Courrier, R.*
Kehrer, E., 101, *113*, 266, *267*
Keiffer, H., 91, 92, *99*, 117, *118*, 369, *385*
Keller, A. D. See *Himwich, H. E.*
Keller, K., and Tandler, J., 635, *640*
Keller, R. See *Schickele, G.*
Keller, T. See *Champy, C.*
Keller, T. B. See *Zeckwer, I. T.*
Kelly, G. L., 109, *114*
Kelly, N. B. See *Burr, H. S.*
Kemp, T., 211, *218*, 276, *280*
Kemp, W. N., 279, *281*, 456, *472*
Kendall, E. C., 235, *242*, 250, 251, *259*, *260*. See also *Gaunt, R.*, and *Wilder, R. M.*
Kennard, J. H., 112, *114*. See also *Smith, G. Van S.*
Kennedy, R. B., and Shelton, C. F., 349, *361*
Kennedy, W. P., 373, *385*. See also *Anselmino, K. J.*
Kenny, M., and King, E., 490, *495*
Kenyon, A. T. See also *Gallagher, T. F.*, and *Varney, R. F.*
   and Gallagher, T. F., Peterson, D. H., Dorfman, R. I., Koch, F. C., 690, 691, *703*
Kepler, E. J. See *Robinson, F. J.*, and *Wilder, R. M.*
Kepp, R. K., 465, *474*
Kern, R. See *Kunde, M. M.*
Kessler, H. B. See *Goldman, L. M.*
Kessler, R. See *Schröder, R.*
Kido, I., 121, *122*
Kindzus, H. See *Butenandt, A.*
King, E. See *Kenny, M.*
King, E. L., and Herring, J. S., 418, *423*
King, J. C., 353, *361*
King, J. E., 351, *361*
King, J. T. See *Myers, W. K.*
King, L. S. See *Wislocki, G. B.*
Kippen, A. A. See *Loeb, L.*
Kirklin, B. R., and Seedorf, E. E., 224, *225*
Kirsch, R., 123, *128*
Kirschbaum, A. See *Pfeiffer, C. A.*
Klaften, E., 198, *202*, 269, *271*, 466, *474*
Klawans, A. H. See *Kanter, A. E.*
Kleefisch, J. See *Koloth, J.*
Kleegman, J. S., 319, *325*
Klein, F., 276, *280*
Klein, H., 612, *619*
Klein, J. D. See *Pucher, G. W.*
Klein, M., 55, 56, *62*, 115, *118*. See also *Aron, M.*
Klein, M. D. See *Abarbanel, A. R.*
Klein, W. See *Lapin, J. H.*
Kleinberg, W. See *Gordon, A. S.*
Klempner, E. See *Frank, R. T.*
Klingelhofer, W., 346, *360*
Klinger, H. H., and Burch, J. C., 649, *679*
Klinkenberg, H., 344, *360*
Kloppner, K., 307, *324*, 426, *441*, 551, *615*

Klor, S. J. See *Birnberg, C. H.*
Klose, H., and Vogt, H., 272, 273, *279*
Knauer, E., 133, *151*
Knaus, H., 66, 68, 69, 71, *74*, 101, 103, 104, 108, *113*, *114*
Kneer, M., 106, *114*, 126, 128, 344, *360*
Koch, F. C., 685, *702*. See also *Ceithaml, J. J., Gallagher, T. F., Kenyon, A. T., Varney, R. F.,* and *Willier, B. H.*
Koch, W., *640*
Kochakian, C. D., 690, *703*
Kocher, T., 234, *242*
Koehler, R. See *Halban, J.*
Koff, A. See *Ivy, A. C.*
Koff, A. K., 1, 3, *30*. See also *Davis, M. E.*
Kohn, A., 262, *266*
Koller, T., and Zoller, C. M., 519, *527*
Koloth, J., and Kleefisch, J., 397, *410*
Kon, S. K. See *Folley, S. J.*
Koneff, A. A. See *Wainmain, P.*
König, F., 483, *494*
Korenchevsky, V., and Dennison, M., 42, *49*
and Dennison, M., Hall, K., 162, *166*
and Dennison, M., Simpson, S. L., 161, *165*
and Hall, K., 161, *166*
Korpi, K. See *Evans, H. M.*
Koster, S., 211, *218*. See also *Geesink, A.*
Kountz, W. B. See *Allen, E.*
Kozelka, A. W., 283, *284*
Kozelka, F. L., and Bart, E. B., Bohstedt, G., 466, *474*
and Hart, E. B., Bohstedt, G., 264, *267*
Kraatz, C. P., and Nice, L. B., 286, 287, *289*
Krabbe, K. H., 257, *261*, 284, *285*, 585, *617*
Kramer, A. J. See *Jacobson, A. W.*
Kramer, F. See *Curschmann, H.*
Kramer, T. C. See *Hill, R. T.*
Krane, W., 116, *118*
Kranes, A. See *Hertz, S.*
Kraul, L., 493, *495*
and Simon, S., 103, 107, *113*
Kraus, E. J., 144, *153*, 253, *260*, 552, *615*
Krebs, H. A. See *Eitel, H.*
Krehbiel, O. F. See *Heimann, J.*
Kreis, J., 108, *114*
Krigbaum, R. E., 399, *410*
Kriss, B. S. See *Frank, R. T.*
Krock, F. See also *Taylor, J. M.*
and Wolfermann, S. J., 600, *618*
Krohn, L. See also *Falls, F. H., Hechter, O.,* and *Lackner, J. E.*
and Harris, J. M., 422, *424*
and Harris, J., Hechter, O., 30, *31*, 403, *411*, 650, 651, *679*, *704*
and Lackner, J. E., Soskin, S., 103, 107, *113*, *114*
Krohn, P. L., and Zuckerman, S., 510, *526*
Kroon, D. B. L. See *Freud, J.*
Kross, I., 117, *118*
Kross, P. L., 124, *128*
Kuder, A. See *Traut, H. F.*
Kueter, K. See *Richards, R. K.*
Kuhn, H. H. See *Cunningham, B.*
Kun, H., 43, *49*

Kunde, M. M., and D'Amour, F. E., Carlson, A. J., Gustavson, R. G., 241, *243*
and Oslund, R., Kern, R., 266, *267*
Kupperman, H. S., and Mellish, C. H., McShan, W. H., 287, *290*
Kuramitsu, C., and Loeb, L., 146, 151, *153, 154*
Kurdinowski, E. M., 125, *128*
Kurland, A. A. See *Rubinstein, H. S.*
Kursteiner, P. See *Abelin, I.*
Kurzrok, L. See also *Birnberg, C. H.,* and *Weber, H. W.*
and Birnberg, C. H., Livingston, S., 382, 383, *386*, 440, *442*
Kurzrok, R., 66, *74*, 188, *201*, 270, *271*, 337, *360*, 399, *411*, 431, *441*, 648, *648*, 682, *702*. See also *Gegerson, H. B., Lass, P. M., Miller, E. G., Jr., Riley, H. A., Watson, B. P.,* and *Wilson, L.*
and Bates, R. W., Riddle, O., Miller, E. G., 490, *494*
and Lass, P. M., Smelser, J., 149, *153*, 298, *324*
and O'Connell, C. P., 161, *165*, 493, *495*
and Ratner, S., 657, *679*, 682, *701*
and Rothbart, H., 440, *442*
and Wiesbader, H., Mulinos, M. G., Watson, B. P., 106, *114*, 370, *385*, 421, *424*
and Wilson, L., 354, *361*
Kuschinsky, G. See *Bergwall, A.*
Küstner, H., 491, *495*
Kylin, E., 571, 579, *616, 617*
Kyriakis, L., 298, *324*

Laanes, T. See *Bates, R. W.*
LaBarre, J. See *Zunz, E.*
Lacassagne, A., 37, *48*, 478, *494*
Lackner, J. E. See also *Falls, F. H., Jacobson, E.,* and *Krohn, L.*
and Krohn, L., Soskin, S., 369, 370, 371, 382, *385*
and Tulsky, A. S., 103, *113*
and Wachtel, H., Soskin, S., 107, *114*
Laferty, J. M., 124, *128*
Laffont, A., and Bourgarel, R., 393, *410*
Lahm, W., 92, *99*
Lahr, E. L. See *Bates, R. W.,* and *Riddle, O.*
and Riddle, O., 150, *154*
Laland, P. See *Anker, H.*
Lamar, J., and Shettles, L. B., Delfs, E., 59, 63, 401, *411*
Lammli, K. A., 553, *615*
Landauer, W., Pfeiffer, C. A., Gardner, W. U., Man, E. B., 265, *267*
and Pfeiffer, C. A., Gardner, W. U., Shaw, J. C., 265, *267*
Landis, E. M. See *Ham, G. C.*
Lane, C. E., 198, *202*
Lang, F. J., 568, *616*
Lange, F., 450, *455*
Langecker, H., and Schenk, F., 141, *152*
Langer, K., 546, *615*
Langman, L., and Burr, H. S., 68, *74*
Langrock, E. G. See *Vorzimer, J. J.*

Lanz, W., 509, *526*
Lapham, M. E. See *Friedman, M. H.*
Lapin, J. H., and Klein, W., 622, 623, *630*
Laprida, E., 241, *243*
Laqueur, E. See also *David, K., DeJongh,
    S. E., Dingemanse, E.,* and *Freud, J.*
    and Dingemanse, E., Hart, P. C., De Jongh,
        S. E., 605, *702*
Larkin, W. L., 369, *385*
Laroche, G., and Simmonet, H., 286, *289*
    and Simmonet, H., Huet, J. A., 685, *702*
Larson, P. S. See *Chaikoff, K. L.*
Lascano-Gonzalez, J. M. See *Houssay, B. A.*
Lass, P. M., 493, *495.* See also *Kurzrok, R.*
    and Smelser, J., Kurzrok, R., 298, *324*
Laszt, L. See *Verzar, F.*
Latz, L. J., and Reiner, E., 66, 69, *74*
Laughlin, K. A. See *Mengert, W. F.*
Lauson, H. D., and Golden, J. B., Sevring-
        haus, E. L., 196, *202*
    and Heller, C. G., Sevringhaus, E. L., 275,
        280
Lawrence, R. D., 586, *617*
    and Madders, K., 270, *271*, 435, 439, *441*
    and Oakley, W., 269, 270, *271*
Lawson, W. See *Dodds, E. C.*
League of Nations Bulletin Health Organiza-
        tion, 716, *733*
Leathem, J. H. See *Jailer, W.*
Lebedeff, G. A., 634, *640*, 645, *648*
Leblond, C. P., 141, 145, *152*
Lee, M. See *Fevold, H. L.*
Legrand, G., 456, *472.* See also *Bourg, R.*
Lehmann, P., 318, *325*
Lehmann, W. See *Soskin, S.*
Lein, A., 177, *200*
Leiner, G., 214, *218*
Leininger, C. R. See *Dey, F. L.*
Le Marquand, H. S., and Russell, D. S., 608,
        619
Lendrum, F. C. See *Hisaw, F. L.*
Lenhart, C. H. See *Marine, D.*
Leonard, O. L. See *Leonard, S. L.*
Leonard, S. L., 174, *200.* See also *Clark,
    L. B., Hisaw, F. L., Reece, R. P., Sager,
    V., Smith, P. E.,* and *White, W. E.*
    and Leonard, O. L., 185, *201*
    and Reece, R. P., 138, *152*
    and Smith, P. E., 180, *201*
Lepper, E. H., and Pratt, C. L. G., Pratt,
    F. B., Vaux, D. M., 484, *494*
Lerman, J. See *Means, J. H.*
    and Stebbins, H. D., *217*
Leschke, E., 295, *296*, 514, 527, 561, *615*
Lesnick, G. See *Abramson, D.*
Lessman, F., 141, *152*
Levenstein, I., 147, *153.* See also *Gordon,
    A. S.*
Leventhal, M., 303, *324.* See also *Stein, I. F.*
Levie, L. H. See *Freud, J.,* and *Gaaren-
    stroom, J. H.*
Levin, L., 673, *680*
    and Tyndale, H. H., 182, *201*, 715, *733*
Levine, R. See *Soskin, S.*
Levine, W. T. See *Du Shane, G. P.*

Levy-Simpson, S., and Joll, C. A., 257, *261*,
        583, *617*
Lewis, A. A., and Gomez, E. T., Turner,
        C. W., 138, *152*
    and Turner, C. W., 133, 137, 144, *151*,
        152, 153
Lewis, D., and Geschickter, C. F., 487, 488,
        494
Lewis, L. A. See *Hartman, F. A.,* and *Toby,
    C. G.*
Lewis, L. L., 70, *74*
Lewis, R. A. See *Thorn, G. W.*
Lewis, T., 368, *385*
Lewis, W. K., 65, *74*
Li, C. H. See *Simpson, M. E.*
    and Simpson, M. E., Evans, H. M., *200*,
        208, *219*, 715, 717, *732, 733*
Lichter, 376, *386*
Liegner, B., 269, *271*
Lilienfeld, A., 590, *617*
Lillie, F. R., 631, 635, *640*
Limon, 44, *49*
Lindner, E. See *Werner, S. C.*
Lindvall, S., and Wahlgren, F., 643, *648*
Lipps, H. G. See *Bomskov, C.*
Lipschutz, A., 38, 42, *48*
Lisco, H., and Biskind, G. R., 42, *49*
Lisser, H. See *Biskind, G. R., Escamilla,
    R. F.,* and *Goldberg, M. B.*
Little, C. C. See *Woolley, G.*
Litzenberg, J. C., 418, 420, *423*
    and Carey, J. B., 306, *324*, 407, *411*
Liverman, H. See *D'Amour, F. E.*
Livingood, C. S. See *Zeckwer, I. T.*
Livingston, S. See *Kurzrok, L.*
Livingston, S. H., and Birnberg, C. H., Kurz-
        rok, L., 319, *325*
Lockwood, J. E. See *Brownell, K. A.* and
    Hartman, F. A.
Loeb, L., 41, 48, 50, 53, 54, *61, 62*, 83, *99*,
        115, 116, *118*, 135, 143, *151, 153.* See
        also *Closs, W.,* and *Kuramitsu, C.*
    and Anderson, W. C., Saxton, J., Hayward,
        S. J., Kippen, A. A., 177, *200*
    and Bassett, R. B., 206, *216*
    and Burns, E. L., Suntseff, V., Moskop,
        M., 41, *48*
    and Friedman, H., 206, *216*, 286, *289*
Loeb, R. F., 248, 249, *259.* See also *Ferre-
    bee, J. W.*
    and Atchley, D. W., Parson, W., 251, *260*
    and Atchley, D. W., Stahl, J., 248, *259*,
        594, *618*
Loeffel, E. See *MacBryde, C. M.,* and
    Roberts, H. K.
Loeffler, E., and Priesel, A., 598, *618*
Loeser, Alfred, 53, 62, 320, *325*, 351, *361*
Loeser, Arnold, 206, *216*, 238, 243. See also
    Eitel, H.
Loewe, S., 681, *701*
    and Voss, H. E., 156, *165*
Loewy, A., and Richter, P. F., 509, *526*
Lohr, G. See *Eitel, W.*
Lollinger, R., and Vaughan, W. W., 440,
        442

Long, C. N. H., 216, *219*, 250, *259.* See also *Fry, E. G., Katzin, B., Shipley, R. A.,* and *White, A.*
and Fry, E. G., Thompson, K. W., 250, *259*
and Lukens, F. D. W., 211, 213, *218,* 250, *259*
and Zuckerman, S., 79, *98*
Long, J. A. See *Evans, H. M.*
and Evans, H. M., 33, *47*
Long, J. H. See *Novak, E.*
Lopez, F. S., 253, *260*
Lopez, R. E., 460, *473*
Lorand, S., 101, *113*
Lubin, S., and Waltman, R., 420, *423,* 465, *474*
Luchetti, S. E. See *Waldorp, C. P.*
Luchs, A. See *Fremery, P. de*
Lucke, H., and Heydemann, E. R., Hechler, R., 212, *218*
Lukens, F. D. W. See *Dohan, F. C.* and *Long, C. N. H.*
and Dohan, F. C., 250, *259*
Lurie, L. A., and Hertzman, J., 543, *614*
Lyon, R. A., and Allen, W. M., 55, *62*
Lyons, W. R., 179, *201,* 717, *733.* See also *Catchpole, H. R., Chaikoff, I. L., Evans, H. M.* and *Pencharz, R. I.*
and Pencharz, R. I., 137, *152*
and Sako, Y., 137, *152*
and Simpson, M. E., Evans, H. M., 150, *154,* 179, *203,* 298, *325*

MacBeth, A. See *Simpson, S. L.*
MacBryde, C. M., 471, *474,* 476, 477, *493.* See also *Roberts, H. K.*
and Castrodale, D., Helwig, E. B., Bierbaum, O., *733*
and Freedman, H., Loeffel, E., Castrodale, D., 476, *494*
MacCallum, W. G., and Fabyan, M., 238, *243*
and Futcher, T. B., Duff, G. L., Ellsworth, R., 579, *617*
and Voegtlin, C., 262, *266,* 467, *474*
MacCarty, W. C. See *Dockerty, M. B.*
MacDonald, A. D. See *Sharpey-Schafer, E.*
MacDonald, I. G., 484, *494*
MacGregor, T. N., 350, *361*
Mack, H. C., 653, 654, *680*
and Ale, T., 653, *680*
MacKay, E., 513, *527*
and Barnes, R. H., 251, *260*
and Carne, H. O., 251, *260*
MacKay, E. M. See also *Barnes, R. H.,* and *Closs, W.*
and Sherrill, J. W., 503, *526*
MacKenzie, 620, *629*
Mackintosh, J., 364, *385*
MacLachlan, E. A. See *Talbot, N. B.*
Madden, J. H. M. See *Davis, C. D.*
Madders, K. See *Lawrence, R. D.*
Maddox, K., 613, *619*
Magnus, R., 101, *113*

Magnus-Levy, A., 235, 237, *242, 243*
Magoun, H. W. See also *Clark, G., Fisher, C., Kabat, H.,* and *Ranson, S. W.*
Mahnert, A., 51, *61*
Mahoney, W., and Sheehan, D., 237, *243*
Main, R. J. See *Bickers, W.*
Makepeace, A. W., and Weinstein, G. L., Friedman, M. H., 51, *61,* 178, *200*
Man, E. B. See *Landauer, W.*
Mankiewicz, E. See *Cotte, G.*
Manley, O. T. See *Marine, D.*
Manly, W. F. See *Gray, L. A.*
Manning, G. R. See *Reuben, M. S.*
Manzi, L., 36, *47*
Marangoni, P., 274, *280*
Marañón, G., 425, *441,* 610, 613, *619*
Marble, A. See *Joslin, E. P.*
Marburg, O., 561, 608, 612, *615, 619*
Marchetti, A. A. See *Traut, H. F.*
Marcus, E. See *Rogoff, J. M.*
Marie, P., 548, 552, *615*
Marine, D., 238, 242, *243.* See also *Shapiro, S.*
and Baumann, E. J., 252, 254, *260,* 278, *280*
and Lenhart, C. H., 235, *242*
and Rosen, S. H., 206, *217*
Mark, J. See *Bennett, H. G., Jr.*
Markee, J. E., 79, 85, 90, 91, 93, 94, 96, 97, 99, *100,* 300, *324,* 351, *361,* 372, *385,* 453, *455*
and Hinsey, J. C., 124, *128*
Marker, R. E., 706, *732*
Marks, H. P. See *Griffiths, M.*
and Young, F. G., 210, 211, *217, 218*
Marlow, A. See *Weinstein, A.*
Marlow, F. W., 92, *99*
Marrian, G. F., 662, *679.* See also *Butler, G. C.* and *Cohen, S. L.*
and Butler, G. C., 585, *617*
and Newton, W. H., 103, *113*
Marshall, F. H. A. See *Hammond, J.*
Marshall, P. G. See *Johnstone, R. W.*
Martin, D. W. See *Pincus, G.*
Martin, J. F. See *Cotte, G.*
Martin, S. J. See *Himwich, H. E.*
and Fazekas, J. F., 253, *260*
Martins, T., and Rocha, A., 163, *166,* 197, *202*
Martzloff, K. H. See *Novak, E.*
Marvin, H. N. See *Wells, B. B.*
Marx, R., and Catchpole, H. R., McKennon, B. S., 117, *118*
and Glass, S. J., Shulman, A., 38, *48*
Marx, W. See *Reinhardt, W. O.*
and Simpson, M. E., Evans, H. M., 205, 207, *217, 219*
and Simpson, M. E., Reinhardt, W. O., Evans, H. M., 498, *526*
Mason, L. W., 420, *423.* See also *Gustavson, R. G.*
and Black, W. C., 649, *679*
Mason, V. R. See *Courville, C.*
Masson, G. See *Selye, H.*
Mathes, M. E. See *Chaikoff, K. L.*

Mathieu, F., 265, 267
Matson, D. See Rock, J.
Matters, R. F. See Hicks, C. S.
Matthews, H. B., and der Brucke, M. G., 519, 527
May, E., and Robert, P., 567, 571, 616
Mayer, A., 534, 536
Mayer, L., 117, 118
Mazer, C., 484, 494
  and Hoffman, J., 409, 411, 661, 679, 683, 702
  and Israel, S. L., 189, 202, 319, 325
  and Ravetz, E., 321, 325, 349, 361, 407, 411
  and Spitz, L., Jr., 322, 325
Mazzocco, P. See Houssay, B. A.
McBride, W. P. L. See Griffith, L. S.
McCahey, J. F., and Soloway, D., Hansen, L. P., 288, 290
McCall, E. See Greenblatt, R. B.
McClellan, R. H., 396, 410
McClugage, H. B. See Strang, J. M.
McClure, C. W. See Hoskins, R. G.
McClure, R. D. See Park, E. A.
McCord, C. P., and Allen, M., 283, 284
McCordick, H. A. See Hageman, P. O.
McCullagh, D. R., 159, 164, 165, 166
McCullagh, E. P., and Cuyler, W. K., 692, 703
  and McGurl, F. J., 543, 614
  and Rossmiller, H. R., 164, 166, 543, 614, 626, 629, 630
  and Ryan, E. J., 191, 202
McCullough, N. B. See McGinty, D. A.
McEuen, C. S. See Selye, H.
  and Selye, H., Collip, J. B., 39, 48
McGavack, T. H., 587, 594, 617, 618
McGee, L. C., 156, 164
McGinty, D. A., and McCullough, N. B., Wolter, J. G., 120, 122
McGregor, T. N., and Stewart, C. P., 111, 114
McGurl, F. J. See McCullagh, E. P.
McHenry, E. W. See Watson, M. C.
McIsaac, P., 466, 474
McKennon, B. J. See Glass, S. J., and Marx, R.
McKenzie, F. F., and Berlinger, V., 9, 30
  and Terrill, C. E., 71, 75
McKeown, T. See Selye, H.
  and Zuckerman, S., 150, 154
McLean, F. C. See Bloom, M. A.
McLellan, A., 106, 114
McNamara, H. See Blau, N. F.
McPhail, M. K., 55, 62, 208, 217, 417, 423
McQueen-Williams, M. See Reese, J. D.
McShan, W. H. See Kupperman, H. S.
  and Meyer, R. K., 715, 732
McSweeney, D. J., and Wood, F. O., 443, 454
Meaker, S. R., 389, 393, 409, 410
  and Vose, S. N., 387, 389, 410
Means, J. H., and Hertz, S., Lerman, J., 207, 217, 570, 616
Meige, H. See Brissaud, E.

Meigs, J. V., 384, 386. See also Nathanson I. T. and Sturgis, S. H.
Meites, J. See Turner, C. W.
  and Turner, C. W., 140, 141, 144, 145, 152, 153, 489, 494
Mellish, C. H. See Kupperman, H. S.
Mendel, E. B., and Goldman, A. M., Caire, A., 493, 495
Mengert, W. F., and Laughlin, K. A., 269, 271
  and Witschi, E., 648, 648
Menninger-Lerchenthal, E., 161, 165
Menville, L. J. See Collins, C. G.
Meranze, D. R. See Charny, C. W., Israel, S. L. and Shay, H.
Meranze, T. See Shay, H.
Metzger, I. See Brown, W. E.
Metzger, N. See Baumann, E. J.
Meyer, H. See von Arvay, A.
Meyer, H. H., 231, 233
Meyer, J. See Ruzicka, L.
Meyer, K. See Evans, H. M.
Meyer, M. A. See Biskind, G. R.
Meyer, R., 3, 12, 16, 22, 30, 34, 45, 47, 49, 52, 61, 64, 70, 73, 74, 76, 94, 98, 99, 335, 360, 595, 596, 600, 601, 618, 639, 640
Meyer, R. K. See Allen, W. M., Biddulph, C., Gustus, E. L., Hertz, R., McShan, W. H., Rothschild, I., and Wolfe, H. R.
  and Allen, W. M., 120, 122
  and Gustus, E. L., 286, 289
  and Sevringhaus, E. L., 289, 290
Meyer, W., 252, 260
Miescher, K., and Fischer, W. H., Tschopp, E., 257, 261
  and Wettstein, A., Tschopp, E., 714, 732
Migliavacca, A., 197, 202, 256, 260, 270, 271
Mikulicz-Radecki, F. von, and Kausch, E., 294, 296
Mileff. See Cotte, G.
Millen, R. S. See Twombly, G. H.
Miller, A. G., 66, 74
Miller, E. G. See Kurzrok, R.
  and Cockrill, J. R., Kurzrok, R., 103, 113
Miller, E. S. See Barnes, R. H.
Miller, H. R., 231, 233
Miller, M. L. See Moore, R. A.
Miller, N. F., and Willson, J. R., 318, 325
Mills, C. A., 292, 295, 296
  and Ogle, C., 293, 296
Minkowski, O., 552, 615
Mintz, M. See Geist, S. H., and Salmon, U. J.
  and Geist, S. H., 585, 617
Mintz, M. E., 409, 411
Mirsky, I. A., 211, 216, 218
Mishell, D. R., 439, 442
  and Motyloff, L., 116, 118
Mittelmann, B., 562, 615
Moebius, H., 644, 646, 648
Moench, G. L., 70, 71, 74, 393, 396, 410
Moffat, W. M., 222, 225
Moir, C., 93, 99, 101, 103, 104, 108, 113, 114, 151, 154, 367, 373, 385

Møller-Christensen, E., and Pedersen-Bjergaard, K., 463, *473*
Moncrieff, A. See *Davies, W. L.*
Moon, H. See *Evans, H. M.*
Moore, C. R., 156, 164, *165, 166*, 183, *203*, 275, *280*, 622, *629*, 638, 640, *640.* See also *Wells, L. J.*
Price, D., 42, *48*, 157, *165*
and Quick, W. J., 620, *629*
and Samuels, L. T., 162, *166*
Moore, R. A., and Bittenger, I., Miller, M. L., Hellman, L. M., 415, *423*
Moran, C. S. See *Riddle, O.*
Morgan, T. N., 102, 103, 111, *113, 114*, 374, *385*
Moricard, R., 46, *49*, 172, *203*
Morrell, J. A. See *Swingle, W. W.*
Morse, A. H. See *Zuckerman, S.*
Morse, D. L. See *Fluhmann, C. F.*
Mortimer, H., and Wright, R. P., Bachman, C., Collip, J. B., 452, *455*
Mosinger, M. See *Roussy, G.*
Moskop, M. See *Loeb, L.*
Mossman, H. W., 44, *49*
Moszkowicz, L., 644, 647, *648*
Motyloff, L. See *Mishell, D. R.*
Mueller, R. S. See *Potter, P. C.*
Mueller, S. C. See *Ford, F. A.*
Mühlbock, O. See *Dingemanse, E.*
Mujuda, T., and Horie, K., 406, *411*
Mulinos, M. G. See *Kurzrok, R.*
Müller, H., 112, *114*
Müller-Jager, F. See *Effkemann, G.*
Muller, O. H. See *Hall, V. E.*
Murlin, W. R. See *Anderson, J. A.*
Murphy, D. L., 101, 109, *113*
Murphy, K. M. See *Fluhmann, C. F.*
and Fluhmann, C. F., 431, *441*
Murray, G. R., 234, *242*
Musselman, L. K. See *Burr, H. S.*
Mussey, R. D., 242, *243.* See also *Haines, S. F.*
and Haines, S. F., 351, *361*
Myers, H. I. See *Young, W. C.*
Myers, W. K., and King, J. T., 434, *441*

Nahon, R. See *Falk, H. C.*
Nakamura, U., 241, *243*
Nathanson, I. T., and Fevold, H. L., 150, *154*
and Franseen, C. C., Sweeney, A. R., 160, 161, *165*
and Meigs, J. V., Parsons, L., 487, *494*
Nelson, E. E., 113, *114.* See also *Paine, W. G.*
Nelson, J. W. See *Cartland, G. F.*
Nelson, K. R. See *Thorn, G. W.*
Nelson, W. O., 37, *48*, 130, 137, 142, 144, 148, *151, 152, 153*, 159, *165*, 196, *202*, 259, *261.* See also *Barnes, B. O.* and *Segaloff, A.*
and Gallagher, T. F., 197, *202*
and Gaunt, R., 140, 147, *152, 153*
and Himwich, H. E., Fazekas, J. F., 149, *153*
and Tobin, C. E., 148, *153*

Neufeld, A. H., and Collip, J. B., 215, *219*, 223, *223*, 263, *267*
Neugebauer, K., 117, *118*
Neulenberg, P., 245, *259*
Neumann, H. O., 256, *260*, 685, *702*
Neumann, R., and Hermann, W., 509, *526*
Neustaedter, T., 320, *325*
Neuweiler, W., 241, *243*, 265, 267
Newburgh, L. H., 496, 505, *526.* See also *Freyberg, R. H.*
and Conn, J. W., 502, *526*
Newell, Q. U. See *Pratt, J. P.*
Newton, W. H., 103, *113.* See also *Deanesly, R.,* and *Marrian, G. F.*
and Beck, N., 121, *122*
and Richardson, K. C., 121, *122*
Nice, L. B. See *Kraatz, C. P.*
and Schiffer, A. L., 255, *260*
Nicholson, W. M. See *Harrop, G. A.*
Nicodemus, R. E. See *Patterson, W. B.*
Nicolle, G., 568, *616*
Nitschke, A., 279, *281*
Nixon, N. K., 505, *526*
Noble, R. L. See *Rinderknecht, H.*
Nogayama, A., 121, *122*
Nordmann, O., 273, *279*
Nothmann, M., 269, *271*
Novak, E., 76, *98*, 341, *360*, 367, *385*, 398, *410*, 431, 436, 438, *441*, 597, 599, *618*, 649, 679
and Brawner, J. N., 598, 605, *618*
and Everett, H. S., 25, *30*
and Hurd, G. B., 349, *361*
and Long, J. H., 602, *618*
and Martzloff, K. H., 338, *360*
and Reynolds, S. R. M., 365, 370, 374, 383, *385*
and Richardson, E. H., Jr., 426, 427, 434, *441*
and TeLinde, R. W., 16, *30*, 65, *74*
Novak, J., and Harnik, M., 375, *386*

Oakley, W. See *Lawrence, R. D.*
Ochsner, E. H., 304, *324*
O'Connell, C. P. See *Kurzrok, R.*
O'Connor, F. E., and Taylor, J. S., 413, *423*
O'Donovan, D. K., and Collip, J. B., 215, *219*
Oehme, C., 254, *260*
Oesting, R. B., and Webster, B., 667, *680*, 689, *702*
Ogilvie, R. F., 502, 509, 513, *526*
Ogino, K., 65, 68, 69, *74*
Ogle, C. See *Mills, C. A.*
Ohlin, C. A., 71, *75*
Okkels, H., 289, *290.* See also *Brandstrup, E.*
Oliver, G., and Schäfer, E. A., 244, 245, *259*
Oppers, V. M. See *Duyvene de Wit, J. J.*
Orbin, F., and Watrin, J., 181, *201*
Ord, W. M., 234, *242*
Orias, O., 211, *218*
Ornstein, E. A. See *Eidelsberg, J.*
Osebold, J. See *Carnes, W. H.*
Oslund, R. See *Kunde, M. M.*

Osterberg, A. E. See *Drips, D. G.* and *Wilson, R. B.*
Osterreicher, W., 316, *325*
Oswald, A., 235, *242*
Ott, I., and Scott, J. C., 148, *153*
Oudet, P., 288, *290*
Overholser, M. D., 265, *267*
  and Allen, E., 39, *48*
Owen, S. E. See *Cutler, M.*
Owens, E. See *Allaben, G. R.*

Pace, N. M., 620, *629*
Page, E. W., 458, *472*
Pages, R. See *Roussy, G.*
Paine, W. G., and Nelson, E. E., 224, *225*
Painter, E. E. See *Harne, O. G.*
Pallos, K., and Treite, P., 345, 355, *360*
Pallot, G. See *Cotte, G.*
Palmer, A. 126, *128*, 682, 684, *702*
  and Fulton, L., 118, *118*
Papanicolaou, G. N., 29, *31*, 51, *61*, 314, *325*,
  650, 654, *679*. See also *Falls, E. A.,
  Shorr, E.,* and *Stockard, C. R.*
  and Ripley, H. S., Shorr, E., 161, *165*
  and Shorr, E., 29, *31*, 436, 439, *442*, 651,
  679
Park, E. A., and McClure, R. D., 273, 275,
  276, *279*
Parkes, A. S., 45, *49*, 109, *114*, 136, 146, 149,
  151, 153, 336, *360*, 715, 733. See also
  Callow, R. K., Deanesly, R., Fee, A. R.,
  and *Hill, M.*
  and Bellerby, C. W., 51, *61*, 109, *114*, 125,
  128
  and Rowlands, I. W., 287, *290*
Parkins, W. M. See *Swingle, W. W.*
Parson, W. See *Albright, F.* See also *Loeb,
  R. F.*
Parsons, L. See *Nathanson, I. T.*
Paschkis, K. E., 216, *219*. See also *Rakoff,
  A. E.* and *Shay, H.*
  and Cantarow, A., Rakoff, A. E., Hansen,
  L. P., Walkling, A. A., 714, *733*
  and Rakoff, A. E., Cantarow, A., 581, *617*
Patey, D. H., 486, *494*
Patterson, W. B., and Nicodemus, R. E.,
  Hunt, H. F., 459, *473*
Patton, H. See *Starr, P.*
Payne, F. L., 38, *48*, 695, 696, *703*
Pearl, R., 528, *536*
Pearlman, W. H., and Pincus, G., Werthessen, N. T., 711, *732*
Peck, S. M. See *Goldberger, M. A.*
Peczenik, O. See *Karplus, J. P.*
Pedersen-Bjergaard, K. See *Møller-Christensen, E.,* and *Rydberg, E.*
Pedrini, I., 307, *324*
Pehl, B. See *Stähler, F.*
Pencharz, R. I., 41, *48*. See also *Anselmino,
  K. J., Evans, H. M.,* and *Lyons, W. R.*
  and Lyons, W. R., 140, *152*, 417, *423*
Pende, N., 528, *536*
Peperkorn, R., 270, *271*
Persike, E. C. See *Butcher, E. O.*
Peters, J. P. See *Dorfman, R. I.*

Petersen, W. E. See *Ely, F.,* and *Samuels,
  L. T.*
Peterson, D. H. See *Gallagher, T. F.,* and
  Kenyon, A. T.
Pettersson, G., and Bonnier, G., 644, 646,
  648
Petzal, E. See *Engelhart, E.*
Pfeiffer, C. A., 47, *49*, 180, *201*. See also
  DuShane, G. P., and *Landauer, W.*
  and Gardner, W. U., 265, *267*
  and Kirschbaum, A., 157, *166*
Pfiffner, J. J. See *Harris, R. G., Harrop,
  G. A., Swingle, W. W.,* and *Webster, B.*
Phelps, D., 373, *385*. See also *Burch, J. C.*
  and Burch, J. C., Ellison, E. T., 161, *165*
  and Ellison, E. T., Burch, J. C., 199, *203*
Philipp, E., 195, *202*, 417, *423*
Phillips, R. A., and Robb, P., 212, *218*
Phillips, E. W., 350, *361*
Phillips, W. A., 51, *61*
Picena, J. P. See *Benzadón, J. P.*
Pich, G., 647, *648*
Pick, L., 596, 601, *618*
Pincus, G., 670, *680*. See also *Pearlman, W.
  H.,* and *Smith, G. V. S.*
  and Martin, D. W., 707, *732*
  and Werthessen, N. T., 57, *62*, 241, *243*
  and Zahl, P. A., 60, 61, *63*, 659, *679*, 707
  732
Plate, W. P., 596, 602, *618*
Poll, H. See *Blotevogel, W.*
Pollock, A. D. See *Geist, S. H.*
Pollock, F., 612, *619*
Pompen, A. W. M., 102, *113*
Popa, G. L., *232*
  and Fielding, U. J., 228, *232*
Posner, L. B. See *Pulver, M.*
Postoloff, A. V. See *Farber, J. E.*
Potick, D. See *Houssay, B. A.*
Pottenger, F. M., and Simonsen, D. G., 256,
  261
Potter, A. L. See *Jeffcoate, T. N. A.*
Potter, C. J. See *Hamblen, E. C.*
Potter, P. C., and Mueller, R. S., 223, *225*
Power, M. H. See *Cutler, H. H.,* and *Robinson, F. J.*
Power, R. M. H. See *Goodall, J. R.*
Pratt, C. L. G. See *Lepper, E. H.*
Pratt, J. P., 56, *62*, 75, 164, *166*, 188, *201*,
  438, *442*, 564, *616*, 629, *630*. See also
  Stewart, H. L., Jr., and *Stover, R. F.*
  and Allen, E., Newell, Q. U., Bland, L. J.,
  65, *74*
  and Thomas, W. L., 438, *442*
Pratt, P. C., 415, *423*
Preissecker, E., 484, 490, *494, 495*
Prenant, A., 50, *61*
Price, D. See *Moore, C. R.*
Priesel, A., 542, *614*. See also *Loeffler, E.*
Priestley, W. O., 443, *454*
Probstner, A., 119, *122*
Prout, T. P., and Thomson, C. S., 572, *616*
Pryor, H. B., 292, 294, *296*
  and Carter, H. D., 292, *296*, 478, 479, *494*
  and Smith, R. T., 292, *296*

Pucher, G. W., and Griffith, F. R., Jr., Brownell, K. A., Klein, J. D., Carmer, M. E., 447, *455*
Pullen, R. L. See *Hamblen, E. C.* and Hamblen, E. C., 362, *385*
Pulver, M., and Posner, L. B., 679, *680*
Pund, E. R. See *Greenblatt, R. B.*
Putnam, T. J., and Benedict, E B., Teel, H. M., 208, *217*, 552, 615
and Wilcox, H. B., 552, 615

QUICK, W. J. See *Moore, C. R.*

RAAB, W., 214, *218*, 223, 225, 230, *232*, 509, *524*, 576, *616*
Ragan, C. See *Ferrebee, J. W.*
Ragsdale, A. C. See *Ralston, N. P.*
Rakoff, A. E., 456, 457, 460, *472*, *473*, 677, 678, *680*, 683, 694, 695, *702*, 703. See also *Paschkis, K. E.*
and Cantarow, A., Paschkis, K. E., 581, *617*
Ralston, N. P., and Cowsert, W. C., Ragsdale, A. C., Herman, H. A., Turner, C. W., 148, *153*
Ramirez, F. T. See *Golding, G. T.*
Ramos, A. G. P. See *Schteingart, M.*
Ramos, A. P., and Columbo, E. O., 493, *495*
Randall, L. M. See *Wilson, R. B.*
Ranson, S. W. See *Brookhart, J. M.*, *Clark*, *G.*, *Dey, F. L.*, *Fisher, C.*, *Hetherington*, *A. W.*, and *Kabat, H.*
and Fisher, C., Ingram, W. R., 231, *233*
and Kabat, H., Magoun, H. W., 232, *233*
and Magoun, H. W., 227, *232*
Rappaport, E. M. See *Vorzimer, J. J.*
Rasmussen, A. T., 194, *202*, 227, 231, *232*, 433, *441*, 458, *472*, 577, *616*
Ratner, S. See *Kurzrok, R.*
Rausch, E. O. See *Astwood, E. B.*
Ravetz, E. See *Mazer, C.*
Raybaud, A., 556, *615*
Raynaud, A., 638, 639, *640*
Rea, C. E., 620, *629*
Read, L. S. See *Chaikoff, I. L.*
Reboul, J. See *Rock, J.*
and Davis, H., Friedgood, H. B., 67, *74*
Reclus, P., 483, *494*
Reeb, M., 491, *495*
Reece, R. P. See *Gomez, E. T.*, and *Leonard*, *S. L.*
and Hathaway, I. R., Davis, H. P., 141. *152*
and Leonard, S. L., 137, *152*
and Turner, C. W., 141, 144, 146, *152*, *153*
and Turner, C. W., Hill, R. T., 137, *152*
Reese, J. D. See *Wainman, P.*
and McQueen-Williams, M., 163, *166*
Reese, J. M. See *Connally, H. F.*
Reforzo-Membrives, J., 206, *219*. See also *Waldorp, C. P.*
Regan, J. F. See *Barnes, B. O.*
Regester, R. P., and Cuttle, T. D., 571, *616*

Reiche, F., 571, *616*
Reichert, F. L. See *Chaikoff, I. L.*, and *Evans, H. M.*
and Simpson, M. E., Cornish, R. E., Evans, H. M., *216*, 615
Reichle, H. S. See *Garvin, C. F.*
Reichstein, T., 258, *261*, 586, *617*. See also Beall, D.
Reid, D. E. See *Teel, H. M.*
Reifenstein, E. C. See *Fraser, R. W.*
Reinecke, R. M. See *Samuels, L. T.*
Reineke, E. P. See *Turner, C. W.*
Reiner, E. See *Latz, L. J.*
Reinhardt, W. O. See *Marx, W.*
and Marx, W., Evans, H. M., 277, *280*
Reiss, M. See *Hemphill, R. E.*
Reuben, M. S., and Manning, G. R., 605, 607, *618*
Reycraft, J. L., 318, *325*
Reynolds, S. R. M., 102, 103, 104, 108, 112, *113*, *114*, 124, 125, *128*, 336, *360*, 444, *455*. See also *Fagin, J.*, *Novak, E.*, and *Weinstein, G. L.*
and di Palma, J. R., 447, 453, *455*
and Foster, F. I., 452, *455*
and Friedman, M. H., 101, 111, *113*
and Kaminester, S., 125, *128*
and Kaminester, S., Foster, F. I., Schloss, S., 435, 441, 448, 452, 454, *455*
and Kaminester, S., Schloss, S., 79, *98*
Rezek, G. H. See *Falls, F. H.*
Richards, R. K., and Kueter, K., 543, *614*
Richardson, E. H., Jr. See *Novak, E.*
Richardson, J. S., 254, *260*
Richardson, K. C. See *Newton, W. H.*
and Young, F. G., 210, *217*
Richter, P. F. See *Loewy, A.*
and Wislocki, G. B., 211, *218*
Richter, P. E. See *Loewy, A.*
Riddle, O., 205, 213, *216*, *218*, 270, 271, 634, *640*. See also *Bates, R. W.*, *Kurzrok*, *R.*, *Lahr, E. L.*, *Schooley, J. P.*, and *Wells, B. B.*
and Bates, R. W., 150, *154*
and Bates, R. W., Dykshorn, S. W., 140, *152*, 717, *733*
and Dotti, L. B., 209, *217*, 265, *267*
and Lahr, E. L., Bates, R. W., Moran, C. S., 150, *154*
and Smith, G. C., Bates, R. W., Moran, C. S., Lahr, E. L., 215, *219*
Rieser, C., 622, 623, *629*
Riley, G. M. See *Witschi, E.*
Riley, H. A., and Brickner, R. M., Kurzrok, R., 449, *455*
Rinderknecht, H., and Noble, R. L., Williams, P. C., 716, *733*
Rioch, D. M. See *Dempsey, E. W.*
Ripley, H. S. See *Papanicolaou, G. N.*
Ritter, H. B. See *Fry, E. G.*
Robb, P. See *Phillips, R. A.*
Robbins, L. L. See *Geiling, E. M. K.*
Roberg, O. T., Jr., 97, *100*, 117, *118*
Robert, P. See *May, E.*
Roberts, A. See *Hertz, S.*

Roberts, H. K., and Loeffel, E., MacBryde, C. M., 709, *733*
Roberts, S. M. See *Abramson, D.*
Robertson, J. D. See *Dodds, E. C.*
Robertson, L. L. See *Allen, E.*
Robinson, F. J., and Power, M. H., Kepler, E. J., 590, *617*
Robinson, M. R., 318, *325, 352, 361*
Robinson, R. See *Dodds, E. C.*
Robson, J. M., 41, *48, 53, 56, 62,* 103, 108, 111, *113, 114,* 126, *128,* 160, 161, *165, 166.* See also *Bell, G. H.*
and Schönberg, A., 709, *732*
Robson, K., and Todd, J. W., 609, *619*
Rocha, A. See *Martins, T.*
Rochat, R. L., 310, *325,* 571, *616*
Rock, J. See *Erving, H. W.*
and Bartlett, M. K., 65, 69, *74,* 305, *324*
and Bartlett, M. K., Gauld, A. G., Rutherford, R. N., 407, *411*
and Bartlett, M. K., Matson, D., 398, *410*
and Reboul, J., Wiggers, H. C., 67, *74*
Rockstroh, H., 355, 358, *361*
Rodecurt, M., 415, *423*
Roeder, P. See *Bland, P. B.*
Rogers, A. See *Rash, H. P.*
Rogoff, J. M. See *Stewart, G. N.*
and Marcus, E., *259*
and Stewart, G. N., 254, 255, *260*
Rogowitsch, N., 238, *243*
Rohmer, P., and Woringer, P., 263, *267*
Rokitansky, C., 595, *618*
Rolf, D. See *Heinbecker, P.*
Rolly, 509, *526*
Romeis, B., 274, *280*
Rony, H. R., 496, 498, 500, *526*
Root, H. F. See *Coggeshall, C.,* and *Joslin, E. P.*
Ropes, M. See *Aub, J. C.*
Rosen, S. H. See *Marine, D.*
Rosenbliett, S. See *Collens, W. S.*
Rosenburg, A., 130, *151,* 483, *494*
Rosenkranz, K. D., 127, *128,* 464, *473*
Ross, J. R., 490, *495*
Ross, R. A., 691, *703.* See also *Hamblen, E. C.*
and Hamblen, E. C., Cuyler, W. K., Baptist, M., 691, *703*
Rössle, R., and Wallart, J., 639, *640*
Rössler, H., 695, *703*
Rossman, I., 54, *62*
Rossmiller, H. R. See *McCullagh, E. P.*
Rothbart, H. See *Kurzrok, R.*
Rothen, A. See *Shedlovsky, T.,* and *Van Dyke, H. B.*
Rothermich, N. O., 161, *165*
Rothschild, I., and Meyer, R. K., 54, 55, *62*
Roussy, G. See *Camus, L.*
and Bollack, J., Pages, R., *616*
and Mosinger, M., 228, *232,* 568, 608, *616, 619*
Rowe, L. W. See *Kamm, O.*
Rowlands, I. W., 287, *289.* See also *Harington, C. R., Henderson, W. R.,* and *Parkes, A. S.*

Rowlands, I. W., and Singer, E., 414, *423*
and Spence A. W., 289, *290*
and Young, F. G., 288, *290*
Rowntree, L. G. See *Clark, J. H., Einhorn, N. H., Schaffer, N. K.* and *Steinberg, A.*
and Boll, R. G., 591, *618*
and Brunsting, L. A., 505, *526*
and Clark, J. H., Hanson, A. M., Steinberg, A., 274, 275, *280,* 283, *284,* 608, *619*
and Clark, J. H., Steinberg, A., Einhorn, N. H., 274, *280*
and Clark, J. H., Steinberg, A., Hanson, A. M., Einhorn, N. J., Shannon, W. A., 284, *285*
and Steinberg, A., Einhorn, N. H., Schaffer, N. K., 274, *280*
Roy, R. D. See *Becks, H.*
Rozin, S. See *Zondek, B.*
Rubenstein, B. B., 29, *31,* 650, *679*
and Duncan, D. R. L., 29, *31*
Rubin, I. C., 401, 409, *411*
Rubinstein, H. S., and Kurland, A. A., 159, *165*
and Solomon, M. L., 543, *614*
Runge, E., 71, *74*
Rupp, H., 452, *455*
Ruschig, H. See *Fels, E.*
Rush, H. P., and Bilderback, J. B., Slocum, D., Rogers, A., 609, *619*
Russell, D. S. See *Crooke, A. C.* and *Le Marquand, H. C.*
Russell, J. A., 213, *218.* See also *Fisher, R. E.*
and Bennett, L. L., 212, 213, *218*
Russell, P. B., Jr. See *Bennett, M. J.*
Russell, P. M. G., and Dean, E. M., 374, *386*
Rutherford, R. N., 493, *495.* See also *Rock, J.*
Rutishener, E., 47, *49*
Ruzicka, L., and Goldberg, M. W., Meyer, J., Brungger, H., Eichenberger, E., 156, *165,* 713, *732*
and Wettstein, A., 156, *165,* 713, *732*
Ryan, E. J. See *McCullagh, E. P.*
Rydberg, E., and Pedersen-Bjergaard, K., 321, *325*
Rynearson, E. H. See *Wilder, R. M.*
and Hildebrand, A. G., 268, 269, *271*

Sackett, N. B., 462, *473*
Sagar, V., and Leonard, S. L., 111, *114*
Saiki, S., 85, *99*
Saito, O., 22, *30*
Sako, Y. See *Lyons, W. R.*
Salen, E. B., 376, *386*
Salmon, A. A. See *Salmon, U. J.*
Salmon, U. J., 160, 164, *165,* 257, *261,* 440, *442.* See also *Frank, R. T., Gaines, J. A., Geist, S. H., Goldberger, M. A.,* and *Walter, R. I.*
and Frank, R. T., 426, 427, 434, *441*
and Geist, S. H., Gaines, J. A., Walter, R. I., 714, *732*
and Geist, S. H., Salmon, A. A., 257, *261,* 587, *617*

Salmon, U. J., and Geist, S. H., Salmon,
  A. A., Frank, I. L., 677, *680*
  and Geist, S. H., Walter, R. I., 320, 321,
  325, 439, *442*, 711, *732*
  and Geist, S. H., Walter, R. I., Mintz, N.,
  709, *733*
Salter, W. T., and Bassett, M. A., Sapping-
  ton, T. S., *203*
Saltykow, S., 536, *536*
Salus, F., 491, *495*
Sammartino, R. See *Houssay, B. A.*
Samuels, L. T., 356, 357, *361*. See also
  Ball, H. A., Gulick, M, and *Moore,
  C. R.*
  and Ball, H. A., 212, *218*
  and Reinecke, R. M., Petersen, W. E., 137,
  152
Sandiford, I. See *Deuel, H. J., Jr.*
  and Wheeler, T., 241, *243*
Sandiford, K. See *Deuel, H. J., Jr.*
Sandstrom, I. V., 262, *266*
Santo, E., *217*
Saphir, O., 603, *618*
Saphir, W., 284, *285*
Saunders, F. J. See *Cole, H. H.*
  and Cole, H. H., 176, 186, *200, 201*
Savage, J. E., and Wylie, H. B., Douglass,
  L. H., 460, *473*
Savage, M. See *Sherwood, T. C.*
Sawizki, W., 493, *495*
Saxton, J. See *Loeb, L.*
Scadron, E. N. See *Taylor, H. C., Jr.*
Scaglione, S., 25, *30*
Scarf, M., and Israel, S. L., 579, *617*
Scarff, R. W., and Smith, C. P., 484, *494*
Schacher, J., and Browne, J. S. L., Selye, H.,
  276, *280*
Schachter, M., 295, *296*
Schaefer, R. L., 438, *442*
Schaeffer, R., 292, *296*
Schäfer, E. A. See *Oliver, G.*
Schaffer, N. K. See *Rowntree, L. G.*
  and Ziegler, W. M., Rowntree, L. G., 274,
  280
Schenk, F., 196, *202*. See also *Langecker, H.*
Scheps, M., 458, *472*
Scherf, D., 439, *442*
Scheyer, H. E., 292, *296*
Scheygrond, B. See *Fremery, P. de*
Schickele, G., 65, *73*
  and Keller, R., 365, *385*
Schiffer, A. L. See *Nice, L. B.*
Schiller, S. See *Smith, O. W.*
Schiller, W., 605, *618*
Schimmelbusch, C., 483, *494*
Schittenhelm, A., and Eisler, B., 206, *216*
Schloss, S. See *Reynolds, S. R. M.*
Schmidt, I. G., and Hoffman, F. G., 2, *30*
Schmidt, J. See *Butenandt, A.*
Schneider, E. See *Bomskov, C.*
Schneider, P. F., 431, *441*
Schockaert, J. A., 162, *166, 201*
Schoeller, W., and Dohrn, M., Hohlweg, W.,
  163, *166*
Schoeneck, F. J., 457, *472*, 694, 695, 697, *703*

Schönberg, A. See *Robson, J. M.*
Schonemann, A., 238, *243*
Schonfeld, W. A., 622, *629*
Schooley, J. P., and Riddle, O., Bates, R. W.,
  216
Schott, H. F. See *Ball, H. A.*
Schouten, G. B. See *Gamarra, N.*
Schrire, I., and Sharpey-Schafer, E., 555,
  615
Schröder, R., 16, 17, 22, *30*, 34, *47*, 64, 65,
  73, 74, 76, 85, *98*, 300, *324*, 335, 341,
  343, *360*, 365, 385
  and Kessler, R., Tietze, K., 304, *324*, 356,
  361, 557
Schteingart, M., and Ramos, A. G. P., 394,
  410
Schultz, V., 365, *385*
Schultze, F., and Fischer, B., 553, *615*
Schultze, G. K. F., 104, *113*
Schultze, K. W., 413, *423*, 511, *527*
Schumacher, P. H., 69, *74*
Schumann, E. A., 461, *473*
  and Voegelin, A. W., 697, *703*
Schurger, S., 465, *474*
Scipiades, E., 161, *166*
Scott, D. B. M. See *Himsworth H. P.*
Scott, J. C. See *Ott, I.*
Scowen, E. F., 159, *165*, 207, *217*
  and Spence, A. W., 286, 288, *289*
Sears, C. See *Erving, H. W.*
Seckinger, D. L., and Snyder, F. F., 36, *47*
Seedorf, E. E. See *Kirklin, B. R.*
Seegar, G. E., 340, 350, *360, 361*, 683, 687,
  702. See also *Gey, G. O.*
  and Gey, G. O., Gey, M. K., 120, 121,
  122
Segaloff, A., and Nelson, W. O., 273, 274,
  279, *280, 281*
Seguy, J., 444, 455, 683, *702*
  and Simmonet, H., 59, *63*
  and Vimeux, J., 59, *63*
Seidenstein, H. R. See *Asdell, S. A.*
Seiferle, E., 45, *49*
Seitz, L., 45, *49*
  and Wintz, H., 51, *61*
Selby, N. E. See *Davison, C.*
Seligman, B. See *Friedman, A. B.*
Selye, H., 51, 53, *61, 62*, 134, 142, 146, *151,
  153*, 160, *166, 278*, 279, *280*, 287, *290*.
  See also *Bachman, C., Collip, J. B.,
  McEuen, C. S.*, and *Schacher, J.*
  and Borduas, A., Masson, G., 55, *62*
  and Browne, J. S. L., Collip, J. B., 51, *61*
  and Collip, J. B., 47, *49*
  and Collip, J. B., Thomson, D. L., 46, *49*,
  56, *62*, 120, *122*, 123, 124, *128*, 141, 142,
  143, 145, 146, *152, 153*, 181, 192, *201*
  and Friedman, S. M., 159, 160, *165*
  and Harlow, C. M., Collip, J. B., 275, *280*
  and Harlow, C., McKeown, T., 149, *153*
  and Masson, G., 711, *733*
  and McEuen, C. S., Collip, J. B., 162, *166*
  and McKeown, T., 146, 149, 150, *153, 154*
Severinghaus, A. E., 169, 194, 195, 196, 200,
  202

Severinghaus, A. E., and Thompson, K. W., 287, *290*, 577, 579, *616*
Sevringhaus, E. L., 431, *441*. See also *Campbell, R. E., Gordon, E. S., Heller, C. G., Heller, E. J., Lauson, H. D.,* and *Meyer, R. K.*
Sexton, D. L. See *Vogt, W. H.*
Seymour, F. I., 70, *74*, 395, *410*
Shaefer, R. L., and Strickroot, F. L., 543, *614*
Shannon, W. A. See *Rowntree, L. G.*
Shapiro, H. A., and Zwarenstein, H., 265, *267*
Shapiro, S., and Marine, D., 254, *260*
Sharman, A., and Sheehan, H. L., 649, *679*
Sharpey-Schafer, E. See *Schrire, I.*
   and MacDonald, A. D., 222, *225*
Shaw, H. N., 117, *118*
Shaw, J. C. See *Landauer, W.*
Shaw, W., 16, *30*, 76, *98*, 384, *386*
Shay, H., and Gershon-Cohen, J., Fels, S. S., Meranze, D. R., Meranze, T., 273, 275, *279*
   and Gershon-Cohen, J., Paschkis, K. E., Fels, S. S., 158, *165*
Shedlovsky, T., and Rothen, A., Greep, R. O., VanDyke, H. B., Chow, B. F., *200*
Sheehan, D. See *Mahoney, W.*
Sheehan, H. L., 567, *616*. See also *Sharman, A.*
Sheldon, J. H., 310, *325*, 564, *616*
Sheldon, W. H., and Stevens, S. S., Tucker, W. B., 528, *536*
Shelesnyak, M. C. See *Engle, E. T.*
Shelling, D. H., 263, *267*
Shelton, C. F. See *Kennedy, R. B.*
Shelton, E. K., 543, *614*. See also *Tager, B. N.*
Sherman, I. See *Goldzieher, M. A.*
Sherrill, J. W. See *MacKay, E. M.*
Sherwood, T. C., 241, *243*
   and Bowers, L. M., 241, *243*
   and Savage, M., Hall, J. F., 241, *243*
Sherrod, T. R., and Struck, H. C., 274, *281*
Shettles, L. B. See *Guttmacher, A. F.* and *Lamar, J. K.*
Shipley, R. A., and Long, C. N. H., 214, 215, *219*
Shorr, E., 29, *31*, 348, *360*, 435, 439, *441*, 651, *679*. See also *Papanicolaou, G. N.*
   and Papanicolaou, G. N., 29, *31*
   and Papincolaou, G. N., Stimmel, B. F., 440, *442*
   and Stimmel, B. F., Papanicolaou, G. N., 432, *441*
Shulman, A. See *Marx, R.*
Shute, E. V., 383, *386*, 406, *411*, 414, 417, *423*
Siebert, W. J., and Smith, R. S., 206, *216*
Siebke, H., 79, *98*
Siegel, P. W., 65, *74*
Siegert, F., 148, *153*
Siegler, S. L., 398, *410*
   and Bauer, D., 687, *702*, 713, *733*
   and Fein, M. J., *200* 321, *325*, 406, *411*
   and Silverstein, L. M., 493, *495*

Siegmund, H., 117, *118*, 120, *122*, 188, 192, 196, *201, 202*
Silberberg, M., and Silberberg, R., 204, **216**
Silberberg, R. See *Silberberg, M.*
Silberstein, F., and Engel, P., 284, *285*
Silver, S., 567, 577, 587, *616, 617*
Silverstein, L. M. See *Siegler, S. L.*
Silvette, H., 223, *225*. See also *Britton, S. W.*
Simkins, C. S., 4, *30*
Simmonds, M., 564, *616*
Simmonet, H. See *Laroche, G.*
Simmons, F. A. See *Williams, W. W.*
Simon, H. See *Bing, J.*
Simon, S. See *Kraul, L.*
Simonnet, H. See *Seguy, J.*
Simonsen, D. G. See *Pottenger, F. M.*
Simpson, M. E. See *Becks, H., Evans, H. M., Fraenkel-Conrat. H. L., Li, C. H., Lyons, W. R., Marx, W.,* and *Reichert, F. L.*
   and Evans, H. M., Fraenkel-Conrat, H. L., Li, C. H., 42, *48*
Simpson, S. L. See *Korenchevsky, V.*
   and de Fremery, P., MacBeth, A., 691, *703*
Singer, E. See *Rowlands, I. W.*
Singleton, J. M., 420, *423*. See also *Haden, R. L.*
   and Hunter, J. L., 409, *411*
Sinykin, M. B. See *Jacobson, E.*
Sjövall, A., 27, *30*, 58, *63*
Skiles, J. H., Jr. See *Brewer, J. I.*
Sladovic, L. See *Bomskov, C.*
Slo-Bodkin, S. G. See *Collens, W. S.*
Slocum, D. See *Rush, H. P.*
Slotta, K. H. See *Fels, E.*
Smelser, C. L., 238, *243*
Smelser, J. See *Kurzrok, R.,* and *Lass, P. M.*
Smith, B. G., Brunner, E. K., 29, *31*, 654, *679*
Smith, C. P. See *Scarff, R. W.*
Smith, G. C. See *Riddle, O.*
Smith, G. M. See *Allen, E.* and *Gardner, W. U.*
Smith, G. V. S. See *Smith, O. W.*
   and Kennard, J. H., 120, *122*
   and Smith, O. W., 61, *63*, 66, *74*, 120, *122*, 126, *128*, 142, 143, 144, *152*, 269, *271*, 372, *385*, 457, 460, 461, *472, 473*, 659, *679*, 683, 684, 685, 686, *702*
   and Smith, O. W., Pincus, G., 61, *63*, 682, *701*
   and Smith, O. W., Schiller, S., 460, *473*
Smith, J. F. See *Gardiner-Hill, H.*
Smith, J. T., 9, *30*. See also *Collett, M. E.* and Werthessen, N. T., 685, *702*
Smith, O. W. See also *Smith, G. V. S.*
   and Smith, G. V. S., Schiller, S., 127, *128, 352, 385*, 659, *679*
Smith, P. E., 149, *153*, 162, *166*, 183, *203*, 208, 209, 211, *216*, 217, *218*, 221, *225*, 231, *233*, 514, *527*, 571, *616*. See also *Engle, E. T., Leonard, S. L., Watson, B. P.,* and *Wiesbader, H.*
   and Engle, E. T., 95, *99*, 172, 181, 192. *200, 201, 202*

Smith, P. E., and Leonard, S. L., 181, *201*
and Tyndale, H. H., Engle, E. T., 85, *99,*
156, 165
Smith, P. H. See *Albright, F.* and *Fraser, R.*
W.
Smith, R. E., 620, 622, *629*
Smith, R. S. See *Siebert, W. J.*
Smith, R. T. See *Pryor, H. B.*
Snell, A. M. See *Wilder, R. M.*
Snyder, A. F. See *Weisman, A. I.*
Snyder, F. F., 25, *30.* See also *Seckinger,*
D. L.
Sodeman, W. A., and Engelhardt, H. T., 224,
225
Soffer, L. J. See *Harrop, G. A.*
Sokoloff, A., 103, *113*
Solomon, C. I. See *Dorfman, R. I.*
Solomon, M. L. See *Rubinstein, H. S.*
Soloway, D. See *McCahey, J. F.*
Soskin, S. See *Krohn, L., Lackner, J. E.* and
Taubenhaus, M.
and Levine, R., Lehmann, W., 214, *218*
Sotiriadu, E., 183, *203*
Soule, S. D., 382, *386,* 422, *424,* 709, *733*
Sovak, F. W. See *Holden, F. C.*
Spaeth, J. See *Chiari, J.*
Spark, C., 458, *472*
and Biller, S. B., 554, *615*
Spear, W. M. See *Hesseltine, H. C.*
Speert, H., 131, *154,* 257, *261.* See also *Hart-*
man, C. G.
Spence, A. W. See *Rowlands, I. W.* and
Scowen, E. F.
Spiegel, R. See *Bomskov, C.*
Spiegelman, A. R., 270, 271, *271*
Spielman, F. See *Frank, R. T.* and *Geist,*
S. H.
and Goldberger, M. A., Frank, R. T., 684,
702
Spielman, M. See *Hertz, R.*
Spitz, L., Jr. See *Mazer, C.*
Spoor, H., and Hartman, F. A., Brownell,
K. A., 147, *153, 261*
Sprinson, D. B. See *Baumann, E. J.*
Sprunt, D. H. See *Hamblen, E. C.*
Stahl, J. See *Loeb, R. F.*
Stähler, F., and Kaiser, W., 414, *423*
and Pehl, B., 414, *423*
Stander, H. J., 412, *423*
Stanley, A. J. See *Walker, S. M.*
Stapfer, 66, *74*
Stark, M. E. See *Gordon, E. S.*
Starr, P., and Patton, H., 241, *243*
Stavely, H. E. See *Greep, R. O.*
Stebbins, H. D. See *Lerman, J.*
Stehle, R. L., 222, *225*
Stein, H. B. See *Gillman, J.*
Stein, I. F. See *Cohen, M. R.*
and Cohen, M. R., 303, 318, *324,* 390, *410*
and Leventhal, M., 303, *324*
Steinberg, A. See *Clark, J. H.* and *Rowntree,*
L. G.
Stella, G., 246, *259*
Stephens, D. J., *217,* 492, *495*
Sternberg, M., 546, *615*
48

Stetson, R. P. See *Gessler, C. J.*
Stevens, S. S. See *Sheldon, W. H.*
Stewart, C. P. See *McGregor, T. N.*
Stewart, G. N. See *Rogoff, J. M.*
and Rogoff, J. M., 245, 246, *259*
Stewart, H. L., Jr., and Pratt, J. P., 491,
495, 718, *733*
Stieve, H., 29, *30,* 58, *63*
Stimmel, B. F. See *Shorr, E.*
Stockard, C. R., and Papanicolaou, G. N.,
27, *30,* 33, *47,* 650, *679*
Stockholm, M. See *Althausen, T. L.*
Stoerk, H. C. See *Carnes, W. H.*
Stohr, G., 685, *702*
Stokes, E. H., 509, *526*
Stokes, W. R., 70, *74*
Stolkind, E., 438, *442.* See also *Brown, W. L.*
Stolz, F., 244, *259*
Stone, C. P. See *Barker, R. G.*
and Barker, R. G., 294, *296*
Störring, F. See *Hartmann, H.*
Stover, R. F., and Pratt, J. P., 688, *702*
Strang, J. M., and Evans, F. A., 500, *526*
and McClugage, H. B., 500, *526*
Strassmann, E. O., 9, *30*
Stratz, C. H., 294, *296*
Straus, E. B. See *Brain, W. R.*
Strauss, M. See *Harrop, G. A.*
Stricker, P., and Grueter, F., 136, 138, 139,
151
Strickroot, F. L. See *Shaefer, R. L.*
Strong, L. C. See *Gardner, W. U.*
Stroud, S. M. See *Callow, N. H.*
Strouse, S. See *Wang, C. C.*
Struck, H. C. See *Sherrod, T. R.*
Stumme, E. See *Erdheim, J.*
Sturgis, S. H., 56, *62*
and Albright, F., 370, *385*
and Meigs, J. V., 22, *30,* 382, *386*
Suden, C. T. See *Wyman, L. C.*
Sulkowitsch, H. See *Albright, F.* and *Fraser,*
R. W.
Sullivan, C. L., and Heffernan, R. J., 458,
472
Sulman, F. See *Zondek, B.*
Summerfeldt, P., and Brown, A., 609, *619*
Suntseff, V. See *Loeb, L.*
Sussman, W., 457, *472*
Swann, H. G., and Johnson, P. E., 237, *243*
Sweeney, A. R., Jr. See *Nathanson, I. T.*
Sweeney, J. S. See *Thomas, W. A.*
Sweet, J. E. See *Chambers, W. H.*
Swezy, O. See *Evans, H. M.*
Swingle, J. J. See *Webster, B.*
Swingle, W. W. See *Harrop, G. A.*
and Parkins, W. M., Taylor, A. R., Hays,
H. W., Morrell, J. A., 258, *261*
and Pfiffner, J. J., 249, 252, *259, 260*
Szathmary, Z., *703*

TACHEZY, R., 104, *114*
Tager, B. N., and Shelton, E. K., 164, *166,*
626, *630*
Takahashi, K., 287, *289*
Takakusu, S., 116, *118*

Takamine, J., 244, *259*

Talbot, N. B., and Butler, A. M., Berman, R. A., 689, 691, *704*
  and Butler, A. M., MacLachlan, E. A., 689, 690, 691, 692, *702, 703*

Tamis, A. B., 322, *325*, 431, *441*, 649, *679*

Tandler, J., 50, 61, 528, 536. See also *Keller, K.*

Tapfer, S., and Haslhofer, L., 60, *63*

Tarkham, A. A., 284, *285*

Tarr, A. See *Gersh, I.*

Taubenhaus, M., and Soskin, S., 231, *233*

Tausk, M. See *Fremery, P. de*

Taussig, E. J., 412, *423*

Taylor, A. R. See *Swingle, W. W.*

Taylor, H. C., Jr., 130, *151*, 461, *473*, 482, 483, 484, 485, 488, *494*
  and Scadron, E. N., 460, *473*, 688, 695, *702*
  and Waltman, C. A., 484, *494*

Taylor, H. M., 376, *386*

Taylor, J. M., and Wolfermann, S. J., Krock, F., 602, *618*

Taylor, J. S. See *O'Connor, F. E.*

Taylor, Z. E., 381, *386*

Teacher, J. H. See *Bryce, T. H.*

Teel, H. M. See also *Putnam, T. J.*
  and Cushing, H., 215, *219*
  and Reid, D. E., 458, *473*

Te Linde, R. W. See *Bennett, H. G., Novak, E., and Jones, G. E. S.*

Temesvary, N., 112, *114*

Temple, H. M. See *Twombly, G. H.*

Terrill, C. E. See *McKenzie, F. F.*

Thaddea, S., 254, 258, *260, 261*

Thayer, S. See *Doisy, E. A.*

Theobald, G. W., 370, *385*

Thiessen, N. W., and Walters, W., 620, 622, *629*

Thomas, E. P. See *Collins, C. G.*

Thomas, W. A., and Sweeney, J. S., 510, *526*

Thomas, W. L. See *Pratt, J. P.*

Thompson, E. P. See *Chidester, F. E.*

Thompson, K. W., 287, *290*. See also *Eisenhardt, L., Long, C. N. H.*, and *Severinghaus, A. E.*
  and Cushing, H., 287, *289, 290*, 515, 516, *527, 617*

Thompson, W. O., and Heckel, N. J., 622, *629*

Thomson, A. P. See *Brown, W. L.*

Thomson, C. S. See *Prout, T. P.*

Thomson, D. L. See *Black, P. T., Collip, J. B.* and *Selye, H.*
  and Collip, J. B., 466, *474*

Thorn, D. W. See *Thorn, G. W.*

Thorn, G. W., 484, *494, 618*
  and Engel, L. L., Eisenberg, H., 593, *618*
  and Engel, L. L., Lewis, R. A., 251, *260*, 593, *618*
  and Garbutt, H. R., Hitchcock, F. A., Hartman, F. A., 591, *617*
  and Harrop, G. A., 510, *526*
  and Howard, R. P., Emerson, K., Jr., Firor, W. M., *618*

Thorn, G. W., and Nelson, K. R., Thorn, D. W., 254, *260*, 447, 450, *455*, 510, *526*

Threscher, J. H. See *Harrop, G. A.*

Tietze K., 84, *99*, 310, *324*, 336, *360*. See also *Schröder, R.*
  and Wegener, R., 51, *61*

Tigges, F. See *Jacobi, J.*

Tilney, F., and Warren, L. F., 282, *284*

Timme, W., 449, *455*

Tinklepaugh, O. L., 37, *48*

Tislowitz, R., and Chodkowska, S., 279, *281*

Titus, P., 410, *411*

Titus, R. S. See *White, P.*

Tobin, C. E., 147, 150, *153, 154*, 255, *260*. See also *Gaunt, R.* and *Nelson, W. O.*

Tobler, M., 365, *385*

Toby, C. G., and Lewis, L. A., 286, *289*

Toby, G. See *Bachman, C.*

Todd, J. W. See *Robson, K.*

Tolksdorf, S. See *Evans, H. M.*, and *Jensen, H.*
  and Jensen, H., *200*

Tonkes, E., 117, *118*

Topkins, P., 298, *325*

Torpin, R. See *Greenblatt, R. B.*

Torrens, D. S. See *Browne, O.*

Traut, H., and Marchetti, A. A., 46, *49*, 600, *618*

Traut, H. F., 408, *411*
  and Block, P. W., Kuder, A., 29, *31*
  and Butterworth, J. S., 597, 603, *618*
  and Kuder, A., 354, *361*

Treite, P. See *Pallos, K.*

Trentin, J. J., and Turner, C. W., 137, *152*

Triepel, H., 70, *74*

Trizzino, E., 613, *619*

Trousseau, A., 468, *474*

Tschaikowsky, W. K., 109, *114*

Tscherne, E. See *Engelhart, E.*

Tscherning, K. See *Butenandt, A.*

Tschopp, E. See *Miescher, K.*

Tsunoda, T., 211, *218*

Tsutsulopulos, G., 104, *113*, 463, *473*

Tucker, W. B. See *Sheldon, W. H.*

Tuft, L., 376, *386*

Tulsky, A. S. See *Lackner, J. E.*

Turino, T. R. See *Duckman, S.*

Turner, C. W., 132, 136, *151*. See also *Bergman, A. J., Gardner, W. U., Gomez, E. T., Herman, A., Holst, S., Lewis, A. A., Meites, J., Ralston, N. P., Reece, R. P., Trentin, J. J.*
  and Cooper, W. D., 149, *153*, 490, *494*
  and Gardner, W. U., 136, *151*
  and Gomez, E. T., 141, 145, *152*, 488, 492, *494*
  and Meites, J., 141, 145, *152*
  and Reineke. E. P., 146, *153*

Twombly, G. H., 288, *290*
  and Ferguson, R. S., 286, *289*
  and Millen, R. S., 439, *442*
  and Temple, H. M., Dean, A. L., 700, *704*

Tyndale, H. H. See *Levin, L.* and *Smith, P. E.*

Tyslowitz, R. See *Dingemanse, E.*

UHLENHUTH, E., 279, *281*
Ulrich, H., 554, 577, *615, 616*
Uotila, U. U., 199, *203*
Urbach, E., 376, *386*
Urechia, C. I., and Elekes, N., 568, *616*
Urner, J. A., 414, *423*
Uyldert, I. E., and David, K. J., Freud, J., 137, *152*
  and Freud, J., 276, *280*

VAN BOGAERT, A., 230, *232*
van der Hoeven, H., 352, *361*
Van der Meer, R. See *Currier, F. P.*
Van Dyke, H. B. See also *Greep, R. O., Gustavson, R. G.,* and *Shedlovsky, T.*
  and Chow, B. F., Greep, R. O., Rothen, A., 222, *225*
Van Horn, W. M., 239, *243,* 352, *361,* 418, *423*
van Leeuwen, H. C., 611, *619*
Van Wagenen, G., 96, *100*
  and Catchpole, H. R., 116, *118*
  and Cole, H. H., 287, *290*
  and Zuckerman, S., 96, *100*
Varney, R. F., and Kenyon, A. T., Koch, F. C., 693, 697, *704*
  and Koch, F. C., 674, *680*
Vassale, G., and Generali, F., 262, *266*
Vaughan, W. W., 555, *615.* See also *Lollinger, R.*
Vaux, D. M. See *Lepper, E. H.*
Veler, E. D. See *Doisy, E. A.*
Venning, E. H., 662, *679, 680.* See also *Browne, J. S. L.*
  and Browne, J. S. L., 67, *74,* 315, *325,* 404, *411*
  and Henry, J. S., Browne, J. S. L., 662, *679*
  and Weil, P. G., Browne, J. S. L., 688, *702*
Verzar, F., 251, *260*
  and Laszt, L., 251, *260*
Vest, S. A., and Barelare, B., Jr., 714, *732*
Vilas, E., 3, *30*
Vimeux, J. See *Seguy, J.*
Vinals, E., 284, *285*
Vines, H. W. C. See *Broster, L. R.*
Voegelin, A. W. See *Schumann, E. A.*
Voegtlin, C. See *MacCallum, W. G.*
Voelcker. L. See *Guthmann, H.*
Voelker, H., 467, *474*
Vogt, E., 270, *271,* 394, *410*
Vogt, H. See *Klose, H.*
Vogt, W. H., and Sexton, D. L., 321, *325*
Vollmann, R., 70, *74,* 305, *324*
von Arvay, A., and Meyer, H., 241, *243*
Von Bergmann, G., 564, 571, *616*
  and Goldner, M., 503, *526*
Von Drigalski, W., 548, *615*
von Economo, E., 231, *233*
von Farkas, G., 438, *442*
von Grafe, E., 501, 504, *526*
von Hann, F., 215, *219*
von Jaschke, R. T., 132, *151*
Von Kahlden, C., 595, *618*

von Noorden, C., 504, 513, *526, 527*
von Probstner, A., 304, *324*
von Storch, T. J. C., 450, *455*
Von Werdt, F., 595, *618*
Vorzimer, J. J., and Fishberg, A. M., Langrock, E. G., Rappaport, E. M., 459, 462, *473*
Vose, S. N. See *Meaker, S. R.*
Voss, H. E. See *Loewe, S.*
Votquenne, M., 149, *154*

WACHSTEIN, M., *217*
Wachtel, H. See *Lachner, J. E.*
Watchel, M., 493, *495*
Wade, N. J., 283, 284, *285*
Wagner, G. A., 318, *325*
Wagner, R., and White, P., Bogan, I. K., 268, *271*
Wahlgren, F. See *Lindvall, S.*
Wainman, P., and Reese, J. D., Koneff, A. A., 159, *166*
Wainwright, J. M., 486, *494*
Wakeham, G., 509, *526*
Waldorp, C. P., 613, *619*
  and Reforzo-Membrives, J., Luchetti, S. E., 543, *614*
Waldstein, E., 119, *122*
Walker, S. M., and Stanley, A. J., 144, *153*
Walkling, A. A. See *Paschkis, K. E.*
Wallart, J., 45, *49.* See also *Rössle, R.*
Wallen-Lawrence, Z., 173, *200*
Walter, R. I. See also *Geist, S. H.,* and *Salmon, U. J.*
  and Geist, S. H., Salmon, U. J., 300, *324,* 429, 431, *441*
Walters, W. See *Thiessen, N. W.*
Waltman, C. A. See *Taylor, H. C., Jr.*
Waltman, R. See *Lubin, S.*
Walton, A. See *Hammond, J.*
  Hammond, J., 9, *30*
Wang, C. C., and Strouse, S., 500, *526*
Wang, G. H., and Guttmacher, A. F., 117, *118*
Wangensteen, O. H., 623, *629*
Wanke, R., 487, *494*
Warren, J. C., 483, *494*
Warren, L. F. See *Tilney, F.*
Warren, S., 361, 486, *494*
Waterman, 43, *49*
Waters, I. See *Bruch, H.*
Watkins, C. H., 348, *360*
Watrin, J. See *Orbin, F.*
  and Florentin, P., 211, *218,* 276, 277, *280*
Watson, B. P. See *Kurzrok, R.*
  and Smith, P. E., Kurzrok, R., 193, *202,* 429, *441*
Watson, C., 59, *63.* See also *Cohen, S. L.*
  and McHenry, E. W., 84, 94, *99,* 344, *360*
Watson, H. M. S. See *Folley, S. J.*
Weber, F. P., 611, *619*
Weber, H., 488, *494.* See also *Birnberg, C. H.*
  and Kurzrok, L., Birnberg, C. H., 320, *325,* 712, *733*
Webster, B. See *Oesting, R. B.*

Webster, B., and Hoskins, W. H., 543, *614*
  and Pfiffner, W. W., Swingle, J. J., 252, *260*
Weed, H., and Cushing, H., Jacobson, C., 230, *232*
Wegener, R. See *Tietze, K.*
Wehefritz, E., and Gierhake, E., 307, *324*
Weichert, C. K., 54, *62*, 150, *154*, 298, *324*, 416, *423*
Weil, A., 270, *271*
Weil, P. G. See *Jones, H. W.* and *Venning, E. H.*
Weinstein, A., 555, *615*. See also *Harrop, G. A.*
  and Marlow, A., 254, *260*
Weinstein, G. L. See also *Friedman, M. H.,* and *Makepeace, A. W.*
  and Reynolds, S. R. M., Friedman, M. H., 376, *386*
Weinstock, F., 66, *74*
Weir, W. H., 384, *386*
Weisman, A. I., 464, *473*, 620, *629*
  and Snyder, A. F., Coates, C. W., *680*
Weiss, S. See *Dexter, L.*
Welham, W. C. See *Behnke, A. R.*
  and Behnke, A. R., 519, *527*
Wells, B. B., and Riddle, O., Marvin, H. N., 277, 279, *280*
Wells, L. J., and Moore, C. R., 159, *165*
Wendell, A., 374, *385*
Wenner, R., 350, *361*, 420, *423*
Werner, A. A., 134, *151*, 164, *166*, 476, 477, *493*. See also *Ault, C. C.*
  and Collier, W. D., 710, *732*
Werner, S. C., 191, *202*, 288, 290, 564, *616*, 682, 690, *701*
  and Lindner, E., 452, *455*
Wertenberger, G. E. See *Collett, M. E.*
Werthessen, N. T. See *Pearlman, W. H., Pincus, G.,* and *Smith, J. T.*
Westman, A., 41, 43, *48*, 58, *63*, 93, *99*, 187, 188, *201, 233*, 444, *455*
  and Jacobsohn, D., 41, *48*, 231, *233*
  and Jorpes, E., Widstrom, G., 58, *62*
Westphal, U. See *Buxton, C. L.*
Wettstein, A. See *Miescher K.,* and *Ruzicka, L.*
Weysser, C., 420, *423*, 462, *473*
Wharton, L. R., and Henriksen, E., 444, *454*
Wheeler, T. See *Sandiford, I.*
White, A., and Bonsnes, R. W., Long, C. N. H., 717, *733*
White, H. L. See *Heinbecker, P.*
White, P. See also *Joslin, E. P.,* and *Wagner, R.*
  and Hunt, H., 269, *271*, 460, 461, *473*
  and Titus, R. S., Joslin, E. P., 269, *271*
White, W. E., and Leonard, S. L., 180, *201*
Whitehill, M. R. See *Howard, J. E.*
Whitehouse, B., 365, 366, 367, 375, *385*, 430, *441*, 483, 484, 487, *494*
Whitney, R. See *Burdick, H. O.*
  and Burdick, H. O., 36, *47*
Whittenberger, J. L. See *Williams, R. H.*
Wick, A. N. See *Barnes, R. H.*

Widstrom, G. See *Westman, A.*
Wiesbader, H., 350, *361*, 712, 732. See also *Kurzrok, R.*
  and Engle, E. T., Smith, P. E., 82, *99*
Wiesner, B. P. See *Crew, F. A.* and *Johnstone, R. W.*
Wiggers, H. C. See *Rock, J.*
Wilbur, D. L. See *Wilder, R. M.*
Wilcox, H. B. See *Putnam, T. J.*
Wilder, M. E. See *Goldman, L. M.*
Wilder, R. M. See *Cutler, H. H.*
  and Kendall, E. C., Snell, A. M., Kepler, E. J., Rynearson, E. H., Adams, M., 590, *617*
  and Wilbur, D. L., 503, *526*
Wilds, A. L. See *Bachmann, W. E.*
Wiles, P. See *Allan, H.*
Wilkins, L., and Fleischmann, W., 206, 207, *217*
Williams, P. C., 41, *48*. See also *Rinderknecht, H.*
Williams, R. H., and Whittenberger, J. L., 572, *616*
Williams, W. W., 396, *410*
  and Simmons, F. A., 399, *411*
Willier, B. H., and Gallagher, I. F., Koch, F. C., 638, *640*
Willson, J. R. See *Miller, N. F.*
Wilson, H. M. See *Dorfman, R. I.*
Wilson, J. A. See *Hamblen, E. C.*
Wilson, J. G., and Young, W. C., 430, *441*
Wilson, K. M. See *Elden, C. A.*
  and Corner, G. W., 676, *680*, 697, *703*
Wilson, L., 109, *114*. See also *Kurzrok, R.*
  and Kurzrok, H., 96, *100*, 103, 106, *113*, *114*, 342, *360*, 369, 370, 373, 375, *385*, *386*
Wilson, P. D. See *Abramson, D.*
Wilson, R. B., and Randall, L. M., Osterberg, A. E., 686, 687, *702*
Wimpfheimer, S., and Feresten, M., 36, *47*
Winchester, C. F., 240, *243*
Winge, M., and Winkel Smith, C. C., 25, *30*
Winkel Smith, C. C. See *Winge, M.*
Winkelman, N. W., and Eckel, J. L., 613, *619*
Winkelstein, L. B., 407, *411*
Winters, E. W., 116, *118*, 256, *260*, 432, 441, 492, *495*
Winther, N. See *Boynton, R. E.*
Wintz, H. See *Seitz, L.*
Wirth, W., 284, *285*
Wislocki, G. B. See *Richter, G. P.*
  and King, L. S., 228, *232*
Witherius, E. P., 269, *271*
Witherspoon, J. T., 38, *48*
Witschi, E., 634, 635, 637, 638, 639, *640*, 643, 646, *648*. See also *Du Shane, G. P.* and *Mengert, W. F.*
  and Keck, W. N., 162, *166*
  and Riley, G. M., 429, 431, *441*
Wittenbeck, F., 103, *113*
Wohl, M., 505, *526*
Wolf, A. See *Andersen, D. H.*
Wolfe, H. R., and Meyer, R. K., 288, *290*

Wolfe, J. K., and Fieser, L. F., Friedgood, H. B., 585, *617*
Wolfe, J. M., 193, 195, 196, *202, 203*. See also *Burch, J. C.*, and *Ellison, E. T.*
and Brown, A. D., 199, *203*
and Hamilton, J. B., 197, *202*
Wolfermann, S. J. See *Krock, F.*, and *Taylor, J. M.*
Wolff, E., and Ginglinger, A., 161, *165*, 638, *640*
Wollner, A., 25, 27, *30*, 37, *48*, 58, 59, *62, 63*
Wolter, J. G. See *McGinty, D. A.*
Wonder, D. H. See *Evans, H. M.*
Wood, E. H. See *Collins, D. A.*
Wood, F. O. See *McSweeney, D. J.*
Wood, T. R. See *Gustavson, R. G.*
Woods, L. See *D'Amour, F. E.*
Woods, O. R. See *Gustus, E. L.*
Woolley, G., and Fekete, E., Little, C. C., 258, *261*
Woringer, P. See *Rohmer, P.*
Wright, R. P. See *Mortimer, H.*
Wu, H. See *Chou, C. Y.*
Wyatt, H. G., 266, *267*
Wylie, H. B. See *Savage, J. E.*
Wyman, L. C., and Suden, C. T., 220, *224*

Yerby, L. D., 82, *99*
Young, F. G., 210, 212, 213, *217, 218*, 286, *289*, 513, *527*, 553, *615*. See also *Folley, S. J., Griffiths, M., Marks, H. P., Richardson, K. C.*, and *Rowlands, I. W.*
Young, J., 422, *424*, 460, *473*
Young, R. H., 428, *441*
Young, W. C., 70, *74*. See also *Collins, V. J., Dempsey, E. W.*, and *Wilson, J. G.*
and Dempsey, E. W., Myers, H. I., 71, *75*

Young, W. C., and Dempsey, E. W., Myers, H. I., Hagquist, C. W., 37, *48*

Zacherl, 196, *202*
Zahl, P. A. See *Pincus, G.*
Zalesky, M., 242, *243*
Zangemeister, W., 65, *74*
Zeckwer, I. T., and Davidson, L. W., Keller, T. B., Livingood, C. S., 239, *243*
Zeller, W., 291, *296*
Ziegler, W. M. See *Schaffer, N. K.*
Zimmerman, H. M., 231, *233*
Zimmermann, W., 667, *680*
Ziskin, D. E., 452, *455*
Zoller, C. M. See *Koller, T.*
Zondek, B., 37, 39, 45, 48, *49*, 181, 182, 192, 195, 198, 199, *202*, 265, *267*, 302, 313, 318, 320, *324, 325*, 336, 352, *360, 361*, 430, *441*, 543, *614*, 672, *680*, 682, 683, 685, 692, 693, 695, 696, 697, *702, 703, 704*. See also *Aschheim, S.*
and Aschheim, S., 44, *49*, 172, 174, *200*, 683, *702*
and Euler, H., 681, 682, *701*
and Friedmann, M., 28, *30*
and Rozin, S., 82, *99*
and Sulman, F., 287, 288, *289, 290*
Zondek, H., 504, *526*
Zuckerman, S., 37, 38, 39, *48*, 59, *63*, 79, 81, 83, 84, *98*, 99 160, *165*, 257, 261. See also *Bishop, P. M. F., Krohn, P. L., Long, C. N. H., McKeown, T.*, and *Van Wagenen, G.*
and Bourne, G., 80, *98*
and Morse, A. H., 336, *360*
Zuelzer, G., 246, *259*
Zunz, E., and La Barre, J., 270, *271*
Zwarenstein, H. See *Shapiro, H. A.*

SUBJECT INDEX

ABDOMINAL distention, postoperative, pitressin treatment of, 223
Abortion, debilitating condition and, 414
etiology of, 412
  anterior hypophysis in, 417
  debilitating conditions in, 414
  endocrine factors in, 416
  estrogen in, 416
  fetal faults in, 412
  germ cells in, 413
  maternal faults in, 413
  nutritional causes in, 414
  progestin in, 416
  psychic factors in, 415
  thyroid gland in, 418
  trauma in, 414
  uterine abnormalities in, 413
from corpus luteum ablation, 56
from progestin deficiency, 56
habitual, definition of, 412
idiopathic, definition of, 412
impending, treatment of, 422
incidence of, 412
organotherapy in, preconceptional, 419
  postconceptional, 420
pregnanediol level in, 688
prevention of, 111
spontaneous and habitual, 412
  definition of, 412
threatened and habitual, estrogen levels in, 684
treatment of, 419
  chorionic gonadotropin, 727
  postconceptional, 420
  preconceptional, 419
  progesterone, 724
trophoblastic activity in, 413
Accessory genitalia, effects of androgens on, in female, 160
  in male, 157
  in climacteric, 426
Acromegaly, 548
basal metabolic changes in, etiology of, 553
course and prognosis of, 555
definition of, 556
diabetes mellitus in, etiology of, 553
diagnosis of, 554
differentiation from giantism, 555
  from Paget's disease, 554
  from pulmonary osteo-arthropathy, 555
endocrine alterations in, 552
etiology and pathology, 552
hyperpituitarism in, experimental evidence, 552
incidence of, 549
manifestations, formative phase, 551
  terminal phase, 551

Acromegaly, metabolic disturbances in, 550
pathology of, 552
precipitating causes, 554
prognosis of, 555
sexual manifestations in, 551
  etiology of, 553
skeletal alterations in, 549
soft parts in, 550
symptomatology of, 549
thymus gland in, 276
treatment of, 555
voice in, 550
Addison's disease, 588
adenohyphophysis in, 253
amenorrhea in, 254
asthenia in, 588
blood pressure in, 588
clinical characteristics, 588
course and prognosis, 591
definition of, 588
diagnosis of, 590
  through therapy, 591
etiology and pathology of, 589
gastro-intestinal symptoms in, 588
gonadal function in, 255
Harrop's salt-deprivation test in, 590
manifestations of, 253
  nervous and psychic, 589
organotherapy of, 592
ovarian atrophy in, 254
pathology of, 589
prognosis, 591
reproductive function in, 254
sexual function in, 589
skin changes in, 588
surgical risk in, 592
treatment of, 592
  diet in, 592
  general care of patient, 592
  hormonal, 592
  sodium chloride, 594
  underlying cause, 594
Adenohypophysis. See also *Anterior hypophysis* and *Hypophysis*.
effects of adrenal cortical disease on, 253
in myometrial activity, 111
in pregnancy, 121
role of, in effects of androgen in female, 160, 161
  in mammary activity in late pregnancy, 135
  in menstruation, 84
synergism with progesterone, 112
Adenoma tubulare testiculare, 601. See also *Arrhenoblastoma*.
Adiposis dolorosa. See *Dercum's disease*.
Adiposity, Fröhlich's type, 621

Adiposity, in adiposogenital dystrophy, 556
Adiposogenital dystrophy, 556
  adiposity in, 556
  clinical characteristics of, 556
  course and prognosis, 563
  definition of, 556
  diagnosis of, 562
  etiology of, 560
  genitalia in, 557
  metabolic disturbances in, 559
  nervous and psychic manifestations, 559
  Neurath-Cushing type, 556
  pathology of, 560
  prognosis, 563
  sexual development in, 557
  skeletal findings in, etiology of, 561
  somatic alterations in, 558
  treatment of, 563
  with skeletal overgrowth, 566
Adolescence, 291
  definition of, 291
  sexual alterations in, 291
  somatic alterations in, 294
  troublesome manifestations in, 295
Adolescent sterility, 293
Adrenal-anterior hypophyseal relationship, 208, 252
  role of, in gonadal function, 253
Adrenal cortex, androgenic activity of, 257
  antidotal properties of, 252
  carcinomatous lesions of, 255
  effects of, detoxicating, 252
    gonads on, 258
    on estrogen stimulation, 79
    on gonadal function, 256
    thyroid hormone administration on, 254
  -gonadal relationship, 254
  histologic appearance of, 254
  -hypophyseal relationship, 250
  in pituitary disease, 253
  influence of, on basal metabolic rate, 252
    on sex characters, 254
  -pancreas relation, 250
  physiology of, 248
  relation of, to sexual sphere, 254
  role of, in arterial tension, 249
    in blood volume, 249
    in capillary tone, 249
    in carbohydrate metabolism, 249
    in electrolyte balance, 248
    in fat metabolism, 251
    in gonad stimulation, 253
    in gonadal function, 258
    in lactation, 147, 259
    in oxygen consumption, 252
    in renal function, 251
    in reproductive function, 258
    in vascular circulation, 249
    in wound healing, 252
  vitamin C content of, 254
  cortical ablation, effects of, on fat metabolism, 251
    carcinoma, urine estrogen in, 686
      test for, 662

Adrenal cortical compounds, 248
  effect of, on carbohydrate metabolism, 251
  disease, androgen and related 17-ketosteroid tests in, 669
  androgen levels in, 691
  effects of, on adenohypophysis, 253
  sex alterations in, 254
    experimental evidence, 255
  extracts, effects of, 255
    on gonadal function, 256
    on metabolism, 254
    on ovaries after hypophysectomy, 256
    on status thymicolymphaticus, 279
    estrogenic activity of, 256
    progestational activity of, 256
  function, effects of castration on, 258
  hormone, relationship of progesterone to, 255
  hyperfunction, androgen levels in, 691
    sex characters in, 255
  hyperplasia after thyroid feeding, 254
    masculinization from, 257
  implants, effects of, 255
  insufficiency. See also *Addison's disease.*
    androgen levels in, 691
    sex characters in, 254
  neoplasms, urine in, 257
  substances, 718
  glands, allopregnanolone isolation from, 256
  effects of hypophysectomy on, 253
  estrone isolation from, 256
  in acromegaly, 552
  progesterone isolation from, 256
  role of, in climacteric, 434
    in obesity, 511
  injury, role of thyroid gland in basal metabolic rise after, 252
  effects of, on thyroid gland, 254
  insufficiency, effects of, thyroid extract in, 254
Adrenal medulla, function of, theories regarding, 244
  physiology of, 244
  role of, in carbohydrate metabolism, 246, 247
  -thymus relationship, 278
  -thyroid relationship, 253
  virilism, 257
Adrenalectomy, carbohydrate metabolism after, 251
  during pregnancy, 254
  effects of, 251, 252
    on blood sugar, 250, 251
    on hypophysis, 253
    on metabolism, 254
    on ovaries, 255
    on thymus gland, 278
    thyroidectomy after, 254
  experiments, 255
  in hypertension, 249
Adrenalin, administration in insulin poisoning, 247
  effects of, on basal metabolic rate, 247

Adrenalin, effects of, on bronchial musculature, 246
   on cardiovascular system, 246
   on metabolism, 247
   on mucous membranes, 247
   on myometrial activity, 112
   on myometrium, 246
   on skin, 247
   on smooth muscle, 246
   on striated muscle, 247
   toxic, 247
 first production of, 244
 insulin antagonism, 247
 synergistic action of thyroid hormone with,
   236
 therapeutic application of, 248
Adrenin. See *Adrenalin* and *Epinephrine.*
Adrenocorticotropic factor of anterior hypophysis, 208
Adrenogenital syndrome, 581
   adult form, 583
   androgen levels in, 691
   climacteric form, 584
   clinical characteristics, 582
   congenital form, 582
   definition of, 581
   diagnosis of, 586
   differentiation from arrhenoblastoma, 587
     from macrogenitosomia praecox, 586
     from ovarian tumor, 587
     from pituitary basophilism, 580
     from pseudohermaphrodism, 586
   etiology of, 584
     adrenal cortical factors, 584
     androgenic factors, 585
   juvenile form, 582
   pathology of, 584
   pregnanediol levels in, 688
   prognosis of, 587
   treatment of, 587
Adrenoluterin, induction of luteinization by, 256
   isolation of, 256
Adrenomedullotropic principle of anterior
   hypophysis, 208
After-pains, treatment of, androgen, 726
   progesterone, 724
Agonadism. See *Eunuchism.*
Alimentary castration, 308
Allergy, role of, in migraine, 449
Allopregnanolone isolation from adrenal
   glands, 256
Amenorrhea and lactation, 149
   androgen levels in, 316, 690
   blood estrogen in, 315, 682
   blood gonadotropin in, 316
   classification of, 313, 314
     according to estrogen findings, 682
   definition of, 297
   diagnosis of, 310
     differential, 316
   during lactation, 298
   during pregnancy, 297
   endometrium in, 314
   estrogen excretion in, 315
   functional, 300

Amenorrhea, history in, 311
   hyperhormonal, 302
   hypohormonal, 301
   in Addison's disease, 254
   in tuberculosis, 307
   infectious diseases and, 307
   laboratory studies in, 313
   nonendocrine causes of, 306
   obesity and, 309
   oligomenorrhea and hypomenorrhea. 297
   organotherapy in, 318
     contraindications, 319
   pathologic, etiology of, 298
     ovarian causes of, 300
     uterine causes of, 299
   pelvic examination in, 312
   physical examination in, 313
   physiologic, 297
   polyfolliculin, 302
     estrogen levels in, 682
   polylutein, 304
   postpartum, 298
   pregnanediol excretion in, 315, 687
   primary, definition of, 297
     ovarian, 300
   prognosis, 317
   radiation of anterior hypophysis in, 323
     of ovaries in, 323
   role of adenohypophysis in, 305
     of adrenal glands in, 306
     of malnutrition in, 307
     of thyroid gland in, 306
   secondary, definition of, 297
     ovarian, 301
   sex hormone findings in, 315
   symptomatology of, 310
   treatment of, 317
     estrogen and progesterone, 319
     estrogenic substances, 319
       contraindications, 319
     gonadotropic hormones, 320
     gonadotropin, chorionic, 727
       equine, 729
       hypophyseal and chorionic, 321, 731
     gynecologic, 318
     medical, 318
     thyroid substance, 322
     x-ray, 322
     Zondek's simplified, 320
   urine estrogen in, 682
   vaginal smear in, 314, 650, 654
   x-ray studies in, 313
     treatment, 322
   Zondek classification of, 313
Androgen administration, method of, 714
   route of, 725
   biologic effects of, 725
   chemistry of, 713
   clinical application of, 164
   commercial preparations, 725
   description of, 713
   effects of, in experimental animals, 157
     in female, 160
     in male, 157
     on anterior hypophysis in animals, 159

Androgen, effects of, on endometrium, 161
    on female accessory genitalia, 160
    on female secondary sex characters, 160
    on mammary gland, 161
    on menstruation, 161
    on ovary, 160
    on spermatogenesis in animals, 158
    on testis, 157
  estrogen-like effects of, in female, 161
  excretion during pregnancy, 690
    in amenorrhea, 316
    in arrhenoblastoma, 692
    in castrate males, 690
    in castrate women, 691
    in children, 689
    in differential diagnosis of Cushing's disease, 691
    in eunuchoid males, 690
    in menopause, 691
    in normal mature woman, 690
    in senile males, 690
  factors influencing effects of, 159
  findings in normal and abnormal conditions, 689
    in sterility, 404
  in male hypogonadism, 160
  in placenta, 121
  in urine, quantitation of, 664. See also *Urine androgen tests.*
  in urine of normal women, source of, 258
  indications and dosage, 725
  level as spermatogenic function index, value of, 689
    in adrenal cortical disturbances, 691
    in amenorrhea, 690
    in differential diagnosis of impotence, 689
    in masculinizing ovarian tumors, 691
    in menstrual disorders, 690
    in virilism, 691
  masculinizing effects of, in female, 161
  mechanism of effects of, 159
  metabolism, 714
  progesterone-like effects of, in female, 161
  secretion of, by ovary, 47
  source of, 725
  standardization of, 713, 725
Androgenic activity of adrenal cortex, 257
  substances, 713, 725
Androsterone, chemistry of, 713
  excretion in adult male, 689
  isolation of, from human, 156
  level in male urine, 689
  potency of, 156
Anestrus, lactation, 149
Antagonistic factor of anterior hypophyseal hormone, action of, 177
Anterior hypophyseal extract and chorionic gonadotropin, combined therapy, 189
Anterior hypophyseal extract, effects of, on blood sugar level, 212
    on insulin sensitivity in hypophysectomized animal, 212
    on liver glycogen in hypophysectomized animal, 212

Anterior hypophyseal extract, effects of thyroidectomy on, 238
    in treatment of hypophyseal infantilism, 542
    of obesity, 525
Anterior hypophysis. See also *Adenohypophysis* and *Hypophysis.*
  antagonistic factor, action of, 177
  -adrenal relationship, 208, 252
    role in gonadal function, 253
  adrenocorticotropic factor of, 208
  adrenomedullotropic principle of, 208
  and testis, 162
  carbohydrate metabolism and, relationship, 211
  cytology of, 167
    during pregnancy, 194
  diabetogenic extracts of, 210, 212
    factor of, theories on nature and identity of, 213
  effects of adrenalectomy on, 253
    of androgen on, in animals, 159
    of estrogen on function of, 197
    of gonads on, 194
    of hypothalamus on, 230
    of testes on, 163
    of thyroid feeding on, 239
    on thyroid function, 239
    of thyroidectomy on, 238
  fat metabolism and, 214
  function of cells of, 169
  glycostatic principle of, 213
  glycotropic factor of, 213
  gonadotropes from, 187, 714, 715
  gonadotropic hormone of, after thyroidectomy, 238
  growth promoting activity of, role of thyroid in, 239
  hormonal content of, during pregnancy, 195
  hypothalamic effects on, 230
  in climacteric, 431
  in growth and metabolism, 204
  ketogenic factor of, 214
  lactogenic principle of, 211
  luteotrophic factor, 172
  mammogenic principle of, 211
  metabolic principle, specific, 215
  -ovarian relationship, disturbance of, 449
  ovulation-inducing factors of, 174
  -pancreas relationship, 210
  pancreatic principle of, 210
  parathyroid relationship, 209, 266
  parathyrotropic principle of, 209
  percentage of acidophils in, 168
    of basophils in, 168
  physiology of, 167
  pineal gland relationship, 211
  proportion of cell types of, 168
  protein metabolism and, 216
  relationship of ketogenic and diabetic factors of, 215
  role of hypothalamus in gonadotropic function of, 230, 231

Anterior hypophysis, role of, in amenorrhea, 305
 in body growth, 204
 in carbohydrate metabolism, 211
 in fat metabolism, 214
 in gonad stimulation, 253
 in gonadal function, 169
 in incretory function of testis, 162
 in production of diabetes insipidus, 215, 221
 in protein metabolism, 216
 in spermatogenesis, 162
 in sterility, 390
 in water metabolism, 215
 sex hormones of, 172
 synergic factor, action of, 177
 -thymic relationship, 276
 -thyroid relationship, 205, 238
 thyrotropic principle of, 205, 239
 water metabolism and, 215
Antidiuretic principle of posterior hypophysis, 220
 role of, in diabetes insipidus, 224
Antidotal properties of adrenal cortex, 252
Anti-hormones, 286
 clinical significance of, 289
 mode of action of, 289
 nature of, 286
 source of, 288
Anti-luteogenic principle of anterior hypophysis, 178
Appetite, excessive, causes of, 498
 factors controlling, 498
Arrhenoblastoma, 600
 androgen excretion in, 692
 atypical, 601
 clinical characteristics, 602
 diagnosis of, 602
 histogenesis of, 601
 histology of, 601
 masculinization from, 47
 prognosis, 602
 treatment of, 602
Arterial tension, role of adrenal cortex in, 249
Aschheim-Zondek test for pregnancy, 675
 Fluhmann's modification of, 671
Asthenic types, treatment of, 536
Ateliosis. See *Hypophyseal infantilism.*
Atresia, follicular, 15
 cystic form, 15
 in pregnancy, 16
 obliterative form, 15
Atresin. See *Antagonistic Factor.*
Autosomes, role of, in sex determination, 632

Basal metabolic rate, effects of adrenal injury on, 252
 of adrenalin on, 247
 of thyrotropic extracts on, 206
 in hyperthyroidism, 235
 in obesity, 499
 in pregnancy, 241
 influence of adrenal cortical extract on, 252

Biopsy, endometrial, advantages of, over curettage, 649
 technique of, 650
 time of, 649
Blood calcium after hypophysectomy, 209
 effects of parathyroid extracts on, 263
 in eclampsia, 266
 in parathyroid deficiency, 262
 dyscrasias, menstrual function in, 307
 effects of thyrotropic extracts on iodine in, 206
 estrogen and gonadotropin content, 66
 estrogen during menstruation, 681
  during pregnancy, 683
  in amenorrhea, 315
  in castrate women, 685
  in functional uterine bleeding, 682
  in granulosa cell tumors, 685
  in menopause, 685
  in menstrual disorders, 682
  in normally menstruating women, 681
  in premenstrual tension, 446
  role in uterine bleeding, 80
Blood estrogen tests, 655
  Fluhmann's mucification, 655
  in chorionepithelioma, value of, 685
  in hydatid mole, value of, 684
  in late pregnancy toxemias, value of, 685
  of follicular activity, value of, 684
  of Frank and Goldberger, 655
  of ovarian function, value of, 682
Blood gonadotropin in eclampsia, 695
 in normal mature woman, 692
 in pregnancy toxemias, 695
 tests for nonpregnant states, 671
Blood phosphorus in parathyroid deficiency, 262
 pressure in Addison's disease, 588
  role of adrenal medulla in, 245
 sex hormone findings in, 681
 sugar after adrenalectomy, 251
  after adrenalin administration, 247
  effect of adrenalectomy on, 250, 251
  of anterior hypophyseal extracts on, 212
  of posterior hypophyseal extract on, 223
 thyrotropic substances in, 206, 207
 volume, role of adrenal cortex in, 249
Body weight, effects of thyrotropic extracts on, 206
Breast. See also *Mammary.*
 abnormalities of, 475
 engorgement, treatment of, androgen, 493, 726
  estrogen, 493
  postpartum, 492
 physiology of, 129
Bronchial musculature, effects of adrenalin on, 246

Cachexia strumipriva, etiology of, 234
 treatment of, with thyroid extract, 234
 thyropriva, pituitary hypertrophy in, 238

Calcium metabolism, effects of thymectomy on, 279
  in dysmenorrhea, 264
  role of parathyroids in, 263
  role of thyroid gland in, 237
Callow capon comb test, 664
Cancer, estrogen and, 38
Capillary tone, role of adrenal cortex in, 249
Carbohydrate metabolism. See *Metabolism, carbohydrate.*
Cardiac. See *Heart.*
Cardiovascular system, effects of adrenalin on, 246
  of thyroid gland on, 238
Castrate and menopausal urine gonadotropes, 181
  male, androgen excretion in, 690
    gonadotropin excretion in, 700
  women, androgen excretion in, 691
    effect of estrogen on myometrium of, 103
    estrogen levels in, 685
    gonadotropin excretion in, 697
Castration, effects of, on adrenal cortical function, 258
  on parathyroid glands, 265
  hypophyseal modifications following, 196
Cervical mucosa, cyclic changes in, 25
Cervix, cyclic changes in, 58
  effects of ovarian sex hormones on, 58
  of progestin on, 58
  hyperplasia of, 37
Chorionepithelioma, biologic test for, 675
  sources of error, 697
  blood estrogen tests in, value of, 685
  gonadotropic levels in, 695
Chorionic and hypophyseal gonadotropes, comparison of, 181
  gonadotropin, 715, 727
    action of, 180
    anterior hypophyseal extract and, combined therapy, 189
    biologic effects of, 727
    clinical efficacy of, 716
    commercial preparations, 727
    effects of, 187
    indications and dosage, 127
    route of administration of, 727
    source of, 727
    standardization of, 727
Chromosomes, role of, in sex determination, 632
Chronic adrenal insufficiency, 588. See also *Addison's disease.*
Climacteric, 425
  anterior hypophysis in, 431
  blood pressure in, 427
  cardiac symptoms in, 427
  circulatory symptoms in, 427
  definition of, 425
  diagnosis of, 436
  digestive disturbances in, 429
  etiology of, 429
    adrenal gland in, 434
    estrogen-deprivation theory, 431
    hyperestrogen theory, 430

Climacteric, etiology of, nervous and psychic factors, 435
    pancreas in, 434
    thyroid gland, 433
  female, treatment of, androgen, 726
  genital changes in, 426
  hot flush in, 427
  incidence of symptomatology, 425
  male, treatment of, androgen, 725
  menstrual function in, 425
  metabolic disturbances in, 429
  nervous and psychic manifestations in, 428
  organotherapy in, 436
  ovary in, 430
  ovulation in, 425
  prophylaxis in, 436
  secondary sex characters in, 427
  senile vaginitis and kraurosis vulvae, estrogen treatment of, 722
  skin changes in, 429
  symptomatology, 425
  treatment of, 126, 436, 726
    hormonal, 436
    medical 436
    with androgens, 440, 725, 726
    with estrogens, 438
    with x-ray, 440
  vasomotor symptoms in, treatment of, estrogen, 722
Climax praecox, 297
Coitus, effect of, on ovulation, 71
Conception, control of, 68
  following single coitus, analysis of cases, 65
  prerequisites for, 387
  vaginal smear after, 654
Constitution, definition of, 528
  gynecologic significance of, 534
Constitutional inferiority, organotherapy in, 536
  treatment of, 535
  types, 528
    hypertonic, 532
    hypotonic, 529
    normal, 528
Contraception, 68. See also *Conception.*
Corpus luteum ablation during pregnancy, 110
  effects of estrogen on, 41
  endocrine role of, 50
  extract, 34, 57
  formation, correlation with endometrial changes, 52
  histologic appearance of, 254
  of animals after uterine implants, 116
  of menstruation, 14
  of pregnancy, 15, 32
  role of, in mammary gland in late pregnancy, 135
  vitamin C content of, 254
Creatine excretion, effects of thyrotropic extract administration on, 206
Cretinism, etiology of, 234
  pituitary hypertrophy in, 238
  treatment of, with thyroid extract, 234

Cryptomenorrhea, 312
Cryptorchidism, 620
　accessory genitalia in, 156, 620
　definition of, 620
　diagnosis of, 622
　efficacy of gonadotropes in, 190
　etiology of, 620
　incidence of, 620
　male hypogonadism and, 630
　organotherapy in, 622
　secondary sex characters in, 156
　sexual development in, 620
　spermatogenesis in, 156
　treatment of, 620
　　chorionic gonadotropin, 727
　　equine gonadotropin, 729
　　hormonal, 622
　　medical, 623
Curettage, endometrial, 649
　advantages of, over biopsy, 649
　effect on sterility, 72
　technique of, 650
Cushing's syndrome, 573–581
　adiposity in, cause of, 579
　blood in, 253
　bone changes in, 575
　cardiac symptoms, 576
　course and prognosis of, 581
　cranial symptoms, 575
　definition of, 573
　diagnosis of, 580
　differential diagnosis of, androgen ex-
　　cretion in, 691
　etiology of, 576
　　adrenal cortex in, 576
　　hypophysis in, 576
　gonadal depression in, 579
　hypertension in, 575
　　cause of, 579
　incidence of, 573
　metabolic disturbances in, 575
　obesity of, 574
　pathology of, 576
　prognosis of, 581
　sexual disturbances in, 575
　skeletal changes in, cause of, 579
　skin and hair changes in, 574
　symptomatology of, 574
　　causes of, 579
　treatment of, 581

DECIDUA, dependency of, on corpus luteum,
　54
Deciduoma in experimental animals, 54
Dehydroandrosterone, chemistry of, 713
　isolation of, from human, 156
Dercum's disease, 612
　course and prognosis, 614
　diagnosis, 614
　etiology, 613
　symptomatology, 612
　treatment, 614
Desoxycorticosterone, effects of, on genitalia,
　257
　on urinary sodium, 221

Diabetes, experimental pancreatic, effect of
　hypophysectomy on, 212
　insipidus after hypophyseal injury, effects
　　of thyroid ablation on, 237
　etiology of, 224
　　role of anterior hypophysis in, 215, 221
　　of hypothalamus in, 229
　　of posterior hypophysis in, 215, 220,
　　　224, 229
　treatment of, with pitressin, 224
　mellitus, adrenal medulla in, 246
　age incidence of, 270
　effect of thyroid treatment on, 236
　　of thyroidectomy on, 236
　fetal mortality in, 269
　genital retardation in, 268
　growth in, 268
　in acromegaly, etiology, 553
　maternal mortality in, 269
　obesity in, 513
　pregnancy in, 269
　reproductive function in, 268
　sexual development in, 268
　disturbances in, 269
　function in, 268
Diabetogenic extracts of anterior hypophysis,
　210, 212
　factor of anterior hypophysis, nature and
　　identity of, 213
　relation of ketogenic factor to, 215
Diagnostic aids, 649
Diethylstilbestrol. See also Estrogens, syn-
　thetic.
　commercial preparations, 721
　therapeutic value of, 708
Dilatation and curettage, effect on sterility,
　72
　in amenorrhea, 313, 314
　in dysmenorrhea, 383
　in uterine bleeding, 345, 347, 357, 359
Dinitrophenol therapy, contraindications, 525
Diuresis from thyrotropic extract administra-
　tion, 206
Dysmenorrhea, functional, 362
　definition of, 362
　diagnosis of, 378
　due to hypoplasia, treatment of, 722
　etiology of, 101, 264, 362, 364, 378
　　allergy in, 376
　　anterior hypophysis in, 374
　　cervical factors, 369
　　constitutional factors in, 377
　　extra-uterine causes of, 370
　　hormonal, 370
　　mucosal factors, 365
　　myometrial factors, 365
　　nasal mucosa in, 376
　　"obstructive theory," 364
　　ovary in, 370
　　psychic and nervous factors, 374
　　thyroid gland in, 374
　　uterine, 364
　　vascular, 367
　incidence of, 362
　organotherapy of, 382

Dysmenorrhea, functional, progesterone in, 107
   role of calcium metabolism in, 264
   symptomatology of, 362
   treatment of, 380
     calcium gluconate, 264
     chorionic gonadotropin, 727
     drugs, 381
     gynecologic, 383
     hormonal, 382, 722, 726
     medical measures, 381
     progesterone, 724
     with androgenic substances, 383
Dysmenorrhea, organic, definition of, 362
   etiology of, 364
   incidence of, 362
Dystocia, definition of, 461
   diagnosis of, 464
   endocrine aspects of, 461
   etiology of, 461
     endocrine disturbances in, 461
     fetal and maternal, 461
   organotherapy of, 465
   treatment of, 464
Dystrophia adiposogenitalis, 556. See also
   Adiposogenital dystrophy.

Eclampsia and hyperemesis gravidarum,
   etiology of, 456
   and parathyroid glands, 266
   blood calcium in, 266
     gonadotropin in, 695
   etiology of, 266
   treatment of, 266
Effusion seminis, 408
Electrical potential, changes related to follicular rupture, 67
Electrolytic balance, effect of parathyroidectomy on, 262
   role of adrenal cortex in, 248
Embryo, development of, 1
   sex primordia in, 634
Emotional expression, role of hypothalamus
   in, 232
Endocrine system, relationship of, to vegetative nervous system, 226
Endocrinopathies, 537
Endometrial biopsy, 649
   curettage, 649
   cycle, blood vessel changes in, 22
     early proliferative phase, 16
     early secretory phase, 18
     glandular changes in, 20
     interval phase, 17
     late proliferative phase, 17
     late secretory phase, 19
     menstrual phase, 22
     phases of, 16
     postmenstrual phase, 16
     pregravid phase, 19
     premenstrual phase, 19
     stromal changes in, 22
   findings in sterility, 403, 404
Endometrioma from estrogenic stimulation,
   38

Endometrium, arteries of, in ovulatory cycle,
   90
   atrophic, abnormal bleeding from, 353–354
   blood vessels of, role in menstrual bleed-
     ing, 92
   changes in, correlation with formation of
     corpus luteum, 52
   cyclic changes in, 16
   effects of androgen on, 161
     of progestin on, 55
   examination of, 65
   glandular changes in, in anovulatory
     uterine bleeding, 332
   hyperplasia of, 37
   in amenorrhea, 314
   in anovulatory uterine bleeding, 332, 333,
     338
   progestational modifications of, 52, 53
   response of, to progesterone, 53
     to testosterone, 81
   stimulation of, by estrogen, 53
   stromal changes in, in anovulatory uterine
     bleeding, 332
   vascular changes in, in anovulatory uterine
     bleeding, 333
Energy expenditure, control of, 499
   intake, control of, 498
Epinephrine. See also *Adrenalin.*
   effects of, on sympathetic nervous system,
     246
   isolation of, 244
   pharmacology of, 246
Epiphyses, effect of, hypophyseal ablation
   on, 204
Equilin, description of, 706
Equine gonadotropin, 716, 729. See also
   Pregnant mare's serum.
   biologic effects, 729
   commercial preparations, 729
   extraction and purification of, 716
   indications and dosage, 729
   route of administration, 729
   source, 729
   standardization of, 716, 729
Estradiol, description of, 705
   excretion during pregnancy, 683
Estrin-deprivation theory of menstruation,
   78
Estrinpriva hypothesis in anovulatory uterine
   bleeding, 342
Estriol, conversion from estrone, 61
   description of, 705
   excretion during pregnancy, 683
Estrogen, action of, on lactogenic hormone,
   144
   administration in menopause, 711
   and cancer, 38
   and gonadotropes, 41
   and gonadotropin content of blood, 66
   and male sex hormone, 43
   and progestin, experiments on menstrual
     rhythm, 81, 82, 83
   biology of, 34, 719
   carcinogenic action of, in animals, 38
     in humans, 39

Estrogen, commercial preparations of, 719
  content of blood, Frank and Goldberger
    tests, of, 655
  definition of, 705
  diethylstilbestrol preparations, 721
  effects of, after ovariectomy, 275
    in the male, 42
    on anterior hypophyseal function, 197
    on blood calcium, 265
    on corpus luteum, 41
    on fallopian tubes of animals, 35
    on fallopian tubes of women, 36
    on gonadal function, 41
    on male accessory genitalia, 42
    on mating instinct, 36, 60
    on myometrial activity, 102, 125
    on ovary, 41 r
    on pancreas, 270
    on parathyroid function, 265
    on pituitary gland, 41
    on secondary sex characteristics, 36
    on testis, 42
    on thyroid function, 241
    on uterine cervix, 58
    on uterus of human castrate, 35
      of animals, 34
    on vagina, 37
      of animals, 35
  efficacy of, 710
  excretion after hysterectomy, 116
    in amenorrhea, 315, 682
    in childhood, 681
    in functional uterine bleeding, 682
    in menstrual disorders, 682
    in newborn, 681
    in normal menstrual cycle, 315
    in pregnancy, 683
    tests, 655, 657
  findings in normal and abnormal condi-
    tions, 681
    in sterility, 404
  hexestrol preparations, 722
  hyperglycemic effect of, 271
  in blood and urine, quantitation of, 655.
    See also Blood estrogen tests, Urine
    estrogen tests.
  in placenta, 119
  indications and dosage, 722
  interference of, in effects of progesterone,
    53
  levels in abortion, 684
    in adrenal cortical carcinoma, 686
    in castrate women, 685
    in fetal death, 684
    in granulosa cell tumors, 685
    in male urine, 685
      in testicular tumors, 685
    in menopause, 685
    in menstrual disorders, 682
    in normal children, 681
    in normally menstruating women, 681
    in pregnancy, 683
    vaginal smear as index of, 650, 653
  metabolism, 707
    effects of progestin on, 61

Estrogen, metabolism, role of ovary in, 707
    of uterus in, 707
  mode of administration, 710
  natural, 705
    chemistry of, 706
    metabolism of, 707
  octofollin preparations, 722
  relationship to carcinogenic carbons, 40
  role of, in mammary gland, 133
    in lactation inhibition, 142
    in myometrial activity in pregnancy,
      109
    in parturition, 125
  route of administration of, 719
  secretion, 43
    during menstrual cycle, 682
    function of adenohypophyseal hormones
      in, 173
  site of production, 43
  skeletal effects of, 265
  source of, 719
  standardization of, 709
  stimulation, chronic, cause of bleeding in,
      80
      effects of, 37
  stimulation of hypophyseal function by,
      198
  synthetic, 707
    potency and toxicity of, 708
    therapeutic value of, 708
  treatment, chronic, effects of, on pituitary
    gland, 198
Estrogenic activity of adrenal cortical ex-
    tracts, 256
  substances, 705, 719
Estrone, conversion, 61
  description of, 705
  isolation from adrenal glands, 256
  -estriol ratio in urine of normal mature
    woman, 682
Estrual cycle after parturition, 149
Ethinyl estradiol, therapeutic value of,
    709
Eunuchism, 623
  clinical manifestations of, 623
  definition of, 623
  treatment of, androgen, 725
    before puberty, 625
    dosage, 626
    in adult, 626
Eunuchoid female, 33
  male, androgen excretion in, 690
Eunuchoidism, 624
  clinical manifestations of, 624
  definition of, 623
  etiology of, 624
  sexual development in, 625
  somatic manifestations of, 625
  treatment of, androgen, 725
    before puberty, 627
    in adults, 629
Exophthalmos from thyrotropic extract ad-
    ministration, 206
Extragenital hemorrhage, periodic, 451. See
    also "Vicarious menstruation."

FALLOPIAN TUBES. See also *Tubal, Uterine tubes.*
cyclic variations in, 58
effects of estrogen on, 35, 36
Fat metabolism, anterior hypophysis and, 214
effects of adrenal cortical ablation on, 251
hormone. See *Ketogenic factor.*
role of adrenal cortex in, 251
of hypothalamico-hypophyseal system in, 230
of lipoitrin in, 223
of posterior hypophysis in, 223
of thyroid gland in, 236
Fertile days of menstrual cycle, 66, 68
Fetal death, diagnosis of, 678
blood gonadotropin test, 678
estrogen test in, 684
gonadotropin after, 684
gonadotropin level in, 694
pregnanediol level in, 688
urine estrogen after, 684
mortality in diabetes mellitus, 269
Fetus, role of, in abortion, 413
in maintaining labor, 123
Fibromyoma from estrogen stimulation, 38
Fluhmann's mucification test, 655
modification of Aschheim-Zondek test, 671
Follicle, graafian. See also *Graafian.*
stimulating and luteinizing hormones, action of, 173, 174
excretion of, 692
role in ovulation, 176
tests for, 670
Follicular activity, blood estrogen test of, value of, 684
atresia, 15
in pregnancy, 16
cysts with uterine hypoplasia, 303
rupture with intraperitoneal hemorrhage. See *Intermenstrual pain.*
Frank and Goldberger blood estrogen test, 655
chick comb assay method, 665
Free martin, 635
Friedman rabbit test, 675
Fröhlich's syndrome, 556. See also *Adiposogenital dystrophy.*
Functional uterine bleeding, 326

GALACTORRHEA, 491
definition of, 491
etiology of, 491
treatment of, 492
Genes, sex-determining, 633
Genital development, role of parathyroid glands in, 264
function, role of parathyroid glands in, 264
hypoplasia in adiposogenital dystrophy, 556
tumors, female, gonadotropin excretion in, 697
Genitalia, accessory, effects of estrogen on, in the male, 42

Genitalia, accessory, in cryptorchidism, 156
external, during puberty, 6
in embryo, 4
internal, during puberty, 6
hyperplasia of, 37
Genetical sex, 633
Gestation, abnormal manifestations during, 456
gonadotropes' function in, 418
vaginal smear during, 654
Giantism. See *Hypophyseal giantism.*
Glutathione, 274
Glycostatic principle of anterior hypophysis, 213
Glycotropic factor of anterior hypophysis, 213
Gonad (s) and osteomalacia, 265
effects of estrogen on, 41
of hyperparathyroidism on, 264
on adrenal cortex, 258
on anterior hypophysis, 194
on metabolism, 509
on pancreas, 270
on parathyroid glands, 265
on thymus gland, 275
on thyroid function, 240
embryonic, 633
sex differentiation, somatic, control of, 639
male. See *Testis.*
role of, in obesity, 509
stimulation, role of adrenal cortex in, 253
of anterior hypophysis in, 253
Gonadal-adrenal cortical relationship, 254
Gonadal disorders, diagnosis of, tests in, 654
urine androgen and related 17-ketosteroid tests in, 669
function, adrenal-anterior hypophyseal role in, 253
and lactation, 149
effects of adrenal cortex on, 256
of hypophysectomy on, 169
of hypothalamic lesions on, 230
of insulin on, 269
of pancreas on, 268
of pineal extracts on, 283
of thyroid ablation on, 239
of thyroid feeding on, 240
in Addison's disease, 255
mechanism of thyroid influence on, 240
role of adrenal cortex in, 258
of hypothalamus in, 230
of thymus gland in, 274
tests of, 654
vaginal smear as index of, 654
hormones, relationship of, to parathyroid function, 264
-pancreatic relationship, 268
-parathyroid relationship, 264
-thymus relationship, 274
-thyroid relationship, 239
Gonadectomy, effects of, in male animals, 155
in the male, effects of, on hypophysis, 163
prolan A in urine after, 163
Gonadotropes, age factor in response to, 191

Gonadotropes and estrogen, 41
  during gestation, function of, 418
  effects of, on testes, 182
  from anterior hypophyseal tissue, 187
  of extrahypophyseal origin, 179
  ovarian effects of, 181
  response of human ovary to, 187
    of immature mammals to, 192
    of juvenile animals to, 193
    of postmature and senile animals to, 193
    of women of various ages to, 194
Gonadotropic function of anterior hypophysis,
  role of hypothalamus in, 230, 231
  hormones, description of, 714
    findings in normal and abnormal condi-
      tions, 692
    in blood and urine, quantitation of, 670.
      See also *Blood gonadotropin tests* and
      Urine gonadotropin tests.
    of anterior hypophysis after thyroidec-
      tomy, 238
    tests for pregnancy and allied conditions,
      675
  substances, 714, 727
Gonadotropin. See also *Gonadotrope, Anterior hypophyseal gonadotropins, Chorionic gonadotropin, Equine gonadotropin,
  Hypophyseal gonadotropin.*
  and estrogen content of blood, 66
    of urine, 66
  body fluids containing, 179
  chorionic, action of, 180
    and stilbestrol, 42
    combined hypophyseal and chorionic, 731
  excretion, after cervical dilatation, 73
    in castrate male, 700
    in castrate women, 697
    in genital tumors in women, 697
    in male urine, 700
    in menopause, 697
    in menstrual cycle, 692
    in normal adult male, 700
    in senile male, 700
    in testicular tumors, 700
  level during pregnancy, 693
    in amenorrhea, 316
    in children, 692
    in diagnosis of fetal death, 694
    in eclampsia, 695
    in ectopic pregnancy, 694
    in endocrine disease, 700
    in hydatid mole, 695
    in menstrual disorders, 693
    in newborn, 692
    in reproductive disorders, 693
    in sterility, 404
Gonadotropin, pregnant mare's serum, 182
  effects of, 183, 188
    on ovarian function, 188
    follicular response to, 186, 188
    induction of ovulation from, 188
    luteinizing extract from, 186
    source of, 183
  therapy, combined equine and human
    chorionic, 189

Gonorrheal vulvovaginitis, vaginal smear in,
  650
Graafian follicle. See also *Follicular.*
  adenoma, 595. See also *Granulosa cell
    tumor.*
  endocrine role of, 32, 34
  generative phase of development, 51
  hormone production by, 34
  vegetative phase of development, 51
Granulosa cell carcinoma, 595
  destruction by x-ray, in rodents, 45
  role of, in estrogen production, 43
  tumor, 595
    blood estrogen in, 685
    classification and histology, 595
    clinical characteristics, 597
    course and prognosis, 597
    cylindroid, 596
    diagnosis of, 598
    diffuse, 596
    folliculoid, 596
    formation after x-ray, 596
    histogenesis, 596
    histology of, 595
    prognosis of, 597
    sarcomatoid, 596
    treatment of, 598
    urine estrogen in, 685
    virilism in, 597
Granulosa lutein cell, 12
Graves' disease, adrenal cortical hormone
  therapy in, 254
  etiology of, 254
  osteoporosis in, 237
  sugar tolerance in, 236
  treatment of, with adrenal cortical ex-
    tract, 254
Growth and thymus gland, 272
  effects of pineal extracts on, 283
    of thymocrescin on, 274
  role of anterior hypophysis in, 204
    of thyroid gland in, 235, 239
Gynandroblastoma, 602
Gynandromorph, definition of, 641, 643
Gynandromorphism, causes of, 643

Harrop's salt-deprivation test in Addison's
  disease, 590
Headache in climacteric, 428
Heart in climacteric, 427
  in puberty, 295
  rate, effects of thyrotropic extracts on, 206
Height, relationship of, to sexual development, 295
Hemorrhage, postpartum, treatment of, with
  pitocin, 224
Hermaphrodism, 641. See also *Intersexuality
  and Pseudohermaphrodism.*
  causes of, 641
    hormonal factors, 645
    genetical, 643
  terminology of, 641
Hermaphroditismus verus, 644
Heterosexual type, 533
  treatment of, 536

Hexestrol, therapeutic value of, 709
Hormonal preparations, 705
Hormone, sex, tests, 654
Hot flush, 427
Huhner test, 398
Human chorionic gonadotropin. See *Chorionic gonadotropin.*
Hydatid mole, biologic tests for, 675, 695
   sources of error, 697
  blood estrogen tests in, value of, 684
  gonadotropin levels in, 695
Hydrophilia, 504
Hymen, development of, in embryo, 3
Hyperemesis gravidarum, 456
  and eclampsia, etiology of, 456
  blood gonadotropin in, 695
  definition of, 456
  etiology of, hormones in, 456
  treatment of, 457, 724
Hyperesthesias in climacteric, 428
Hyperinsulinism, experiments in effects on reproductive system, 269
  obesity from, 513
Hyperirritability from thyrotropic extract administration, 206
Hyperparathyroidism, effects of, on gonads, 264
  thyroid feeding in, 266
  libido in, 265
  menstruation in, 265
Hyperpituitarism, menstrual function in, 305
Hyperplastic bleeding. See *Uterine bleeding.*
Hypertension, effects of adrenal cortical ablation on, 249
Hyperthyroidism, basal metabolic rate in, 235
  effects of, on calcium excretion, 237
  on cardiovascular system, 238
  on phosphorus excretion, 237
  nervous irritability in, 238
  thyrotropic content of blood in, 207
  of urine in, 207
Hypogalactia, definition of, 489
  diagnosis of, 490
  etiology of, 489
  treatment of, 490, 731
Hypogenitalism, efficacy of gonadotropes in, 190
Hypogonadism, male, 623. See also *Eunuchism* and *Eunuchoidism.*
  and cryptorchidism, 620
  androgens in, 160
  treatment of, chorionic gonadotropin, 729
Hypo-insulinism, experiments in effects on reproductive system, 269
Hypomenorrhea, definition of, 297
  etiology of, 300
  pregnanediol excretion in, 315
  vaginal smear in, 650
Hypophyseal activity, theories regarding, 163
  and chorionic gonadotropin, combined, 731
    commercial preparations, 731
    comparison of, 181
  cachexia. See also *Simmonds' disease.*
    blood in, 206

Hypophyseal function, estrogenic stimulation of, 198
  role of thymus gland in, 276
giantism, definition of, 544
  diagnosis of, 547
  differentiation from eunuchoid tallness, 547
    from macrogenitosomia praecox, 547
    from physiological giantism, 547
  etiology of, 546
  pathology of, 546
  prognosis in, 548
  sexual development in, 545, 546
  symptomatology of, 545
  treatment of, 548
gonadotropin, 730
  biologic effects of, 730
  commercial preparations, 730
  indications and dosage, 730
  route of administration of, 730
  source of, 730
  standardization of, 730
hormone, effect of, on myometrial activity, 102
-hypothalamic system, 277. See also *Hypothalamico-hypophyseal system.*
infantilism, 537
  body proportions in, 538
  clinical characteristics of, 538
  course and prognosis of, 542
  definition of, 537
  diagnosis of, 540
  differentiation from achondroplasia, 541
    from Albright's syndrome, 542
    from Fröhlich's syndrome, 541
    from infantile hypothyroidism, 541
  etiology of, 540
  genital retardation with, treatment of, 543
  incidence of, 537
  sex characters in, 539
  skeletal characteristics in, 539
  treatment of, 542
    hormonal, 543
Hypophysectomy, effects of, on adrenal glands, 253
  on blood calcium level, 209
  on cytology of parathyroid glands, 210
  on experimental pancreatic diabetes, 212
  on gonads, 169
  pituitary extracts after, 172
  implants after, 172
Hypophysis-adrenal cortex relation, 250
  after castration, 196
  cytology of, effects of thyroidectomy on, 239
  description of, 167
  effects of male gonadectomy on, 163
  modifications of, during pregnancy, 194
  relationship of, to hypothalamus, 226
  role of, in effects of androgen on ovary, 160
  in fat metabolism, 230
  in hypothalamic function, 229
  in menstruation, 85

49

Hypophysis, role of, in myometrial activity during pregnancy, 111
  in obesity, 514
  in ovarian effects of androgen, 160
Hypopituitarism, menstrual function in, 305
Hypothalamico-hypophyseal system, 227
  anatomy of, 227
  role of, in carbohydrate metabolism, 230
    in fat metabolism, 230
    in water metabolism, 229
  tract, anatomy of, 227
Hypothalamus and hypophysis, vascular connections between, 228
  effects of, on anterior hypophysis, 230
  functions of, 229
  role of hypophysis in, 229
  relationship of, to hypophysis, 226
  role of, in carbohydrate metabolism, 229
    in diabetes insipidus, 229
    in emotional expression, 232
    in gonadal function, 230
    in obesity, 516
    in sleep, 231
    in temperature regulation, 231
    in wakefulness, 232
    in water metabolism, 229
Hypothyroidism, effects of, on cardiovascular system, 238
  primary, definition of, 206
    importance of distinguishing from secondary, 207
  secondary, definition of, 206
    importance of distinguishing from primary, 207
Hysterectomy, estrogen excretion after, 116
  experiments, 115
  ovarian function after, 116
  sequelae, 117
  with ovarian tissue implant, 117
  with retention of ovaries, 117
  with uterine implants and extracts, in animals, 116
    in humans, 117

Ileus, paralytic, pitressin treatment of, 223
Immunologic theory, 287
Impotence, androgen level in differential diagnosis of, 689
  treatment of, androgen, 725
Inanition, effects of, on spermatogenesis, 162
Infantile type, 530
  treatment of, 536
Infantilism, pituitary. See *Hypophyseal infantilism.*
Infectious diseases, amenorrhea in, 307
Infertile period, 64
Inhibin, 164
Insomnia in climacteric, 428
Insulin-adrenalin antagonism, 247
  effect of, on gonadal function, 269
    on reproductive function, 269
  poisoning, treatment of, with adrenalin, 247

Insulin-adrenalin, sensitivity after hypophysectomy, 212
  role of hypophysis in, 222
Intermenstrual pain, 443
  definition of, 443
  diagnosis of, 444
  differentiation from appendicitis, 444
    from ruptured tubal pregnancy, 445
  etiology of, 443
  ovulation and, 443
  symptomatology of, 443
  treatment of, 445
Intersex, 644
  definition of, 641, 643
Intersexuality, causes of, 644
  clinical management of, 647
  genetical, 641
  grades of, 644
  hormonal, 641
  hormone-producing tumors and, 647
  maternal causes of, 646
  zygotic, 641
Interstitial cell stimulating hormone, 173
Intoxications, menstrual function in, 307
Iodothyrin, isolation of, 235
Iodothyroglobulin, isolation of, 235
Itching in climacteric, 428

Joint pains in climacteric, 428

Ketogenic factor of anterior hypophysis, 214
  relation of diabetogenic factor to, 215
Knaus-Ogino theory, 68
  summary of, 73
Knaus' test, 66, 69
Kurzrok and Ratner urine estrogen test, 657

Labor. See also *Parturition.*
  factors initiating and maintaining, 123
  mechanism of, 101
Lactation. See also *Suckling.*
  amenorrhea during, 149, 298
  amount of secretion in, factors controlling, 146
  anestrus, 149
  duration of, factors controlling, 146
  effect of, on reproductive organs, 149
  gonadal function, 149
  hormonal prerequisites for, 138
  inhibition, factors responsible for, 141
    role of estrogen in, 142
      of placenta in, 141
      of progesterone in, 142
  lactogenic hormone in, 140
  maintenance of, factors controlling, 145
  mammary gland after, 132
  role of adrenal cortex in, 147, 259
    of pancreas in, 149
    of parathyroid glands in, 149
    of pituitary gland in, 148
    of thyroid gland in, 148
  suppression of, androgen in, 726
    estrogen in, 722
  undesired, 492
  uterine involution, 151

Lactogenic extracts, effects of, in **animals**, 150
  hormone, 136
    action of estrogen on, 144
    in absence of hypophysis, 140
      of ovary, 139
    in hypogalactia, 490, 731
    in initiation of lactation, 140
  substances, 717, 731
    biologic effects of, 730
    clinical efficacy of, 718
    commercial preparations, 731
    indications and dosage, 731
    physical properties of, 717
    sources of, 717, 731
    standardization of, 717, 731
Lateral hypotonic type, 529
  sthenic type, 533
Laurence-Moon-Biedl syndrome, 520
Libido. See also *Mating Instinct*.
Linear asthenic type, 529
  sthenic type, 532
Lipodystrophia progressiva, 610
  diagnosis, 612
  etiology of, 611
  symptomatology, 610
  treatment, 612
Lipoitrin, role of, in fat metabolism, 223, 230
Luteal cell tumor, 603. See also *Luteoma*.
Luteinizing and follicle stimulating hormones, action of, 173, 174
  extract from pregnant mare's serum gonadotropin, 186
  hormone, effects of suckling on, 150
Luteoma, clinical characteristics of, 605
  histogenesis of, 603
  prognosis of, 605
Luteosterone C, 57
  D, 58
Luteotrophin, action of, 179

MACROGENITOSOMIA praecox, 284, 605. See also *Precocious puberty*.
Male sex hormone. See also *Androgen, Testicular Extract, Testosterone*.
  source of, 156
Mammary function, abnormalities in, 489
  gland, abnormalities in growth of, 475
    after lactation, 132
    after parturition, 132
    anatomy of, 129
    at maturity, 130
    at menopause, 132
    cyclic changes in, 130
    development of, endocrine control of, 132
    during lactation, 132
    during pregnancy, 131
    effects of androgen on, 161
    from birth to puberty, 130
    function of, endocrine control of, 132
    growth of, endocrine control of, 132
    in adolescence, 292
    in early pregnancy, 134
      endocrine control of, 134

Mammary gland, in late pregnancy, role of corpus luteum in, 135
    in prenatal life, 129
    role of anterior hypophysis in growth and function of, 211
      of estrogen in, 133
      of progesterone in, 133
    senile involution of, 132
  growth, age variations in, 478
  hyperplasia, 480
    adult, 482
    and cancer, 485
    clinical characteristics of, 482
    cystic, 481
    diagnosis of, 486
    differentiation from cancer, 486
    etiology of, 483
      hormonal factors in, 483
      nervous factors in, 485
      vascular factors in, 484
    treatment of, hormonal, 487
      x-ray, 488
    types of, 481
  hypertrophy, 479
  hypoplasia, 476, 480
    treatment of, 476
      estrogen, 722
  pain, premenstrual, hormonal treatment of, 726
  pseudohypertrophy, 479
Mammogen I and II, 136
Masculinization, androgen levels in, 691
  from adrenal cortical hyperplasia, 257
  from androgen administration, 161
  from arrhenoblastoma, 47, 601
  from granulosa cell tumors, 47
  from theca cell tumors, 47, 597
Mastitis adolescentium, 482
  adult, 482
  chronic. See *Mammary hyperplasia*.
  neonatorum, 474
Maternal mortality in diabetes mellitus, 269
  sex hormones and intersexuality, 646
  tetany, acute or manifest, 467
    chronic, 468
      diagnosis of, 469
    clinical manifestations of, 467
    course and prognosis of, 470
    definition of, 466
    diagnosis of, 468
    differential diagnosis of, 469
    etiology of, 466, 472
    latent, 468
    manifest, 468
    treatment of, 470
Mating instinct, cyclic variation, 36
  difficulties of investigation in human, 36
  effects of estrogen on, 36, 60
    of progestin on, 60
Mazer and Hoffman urine estrogen pregnancy test, 661
Melancholia in climacteric, 428
Membranous dysmenorrhea, 366
Menarche, 292

Menopausal and castrate urine gonadotropes, 181
Menopause, androgen excretion in, 691
  blood estrogen in, 685
  definition of, 425
  estrogen administration in, 711
    levels in, 685
  gonadotropin excretion in, 697
  mammary gland at, 132
  treatment of, androgen, 726
  urine estrogen in, 685
  uterine bleeding in, treatment of, 346
  vaginal smear in, 654
Menorrhagia, definition of, 327
  etiology of, 354
  treatment of, hormonal, 358, 724
Menstrual cycle, blood estrogen during, 681
  fertile period of, 68
  gonadotropin excretion in, 692
  myometrial activity at follicular phase of, 103
  postovulatory phase of, 69
  pregnanediol excretion during, 686
  progestin and estrogen in, 81
  reestablishment after parturition, 149
  thyroid activity and, 241
  troublesome manifestations, 443
  urine estrogen during, 682
  variability in length of, 71, 72
  disorders, androgen levels in, 690
    blood estrogen in, 682
    gonadotropin levels in, 693
    pregnanediol excretion in, 687
    treatment of, progesterone, 724
    urine estrogen in, 682
  flow, amount and duration of, 92
    at adolescence, 294
    uterine factors in, 92
  function, effect of nervous and psychic influences on, 309
    effects of uterine injuries on, 300
    in climacteric, 425
    in hypopituitarism, 305
    in obesity, 309
  rhythm, changes in after marriage, 72
Menstruation and pseudomenstruation, comparison of, 94
  as a negative phenomenon, 78
  as positive phenomenon, 84
  bleeding of. See *Menstrual flow.*
  blood estrogen during, 681
    vessel destruction in, 94
  causation of, 77
  central nervous system and, 96
  cessation of bleeding, 91
  corpus luteum of, 14
  definitions of, 76
  effects of androgen on, 161
    of progestin and estrogen on, 81, 82, 83
    on pancreatic function, 270
  endocrine factors in, 76
    summary of, 97
  endometrium in, 91, 107
  estrin-deprivation theory, 78
  factors precipitating, 91

Menstruation, hormonal factors in, 78
  in hyperparathyroidism, 265
  interrelation of vascular and myometrial activity in, 93
  myometrial activity in, 96
  nasal mucosa in, 376
  progestin-deprivation theory of, 81
  regression of corpus luteum in, 78
  role of adenohypophysis in, 84
    parathyroid glands in, 264
    posterior hypophysis in, 85
  significance of, 76
  source of bleeding in, 91
  tissue loss in, 94
  uterine changes preceding, 90
    events before and after, 85
  uterus during bleeding of, 90
  vascular changes during, 107
  vicarious, 451. See also *Vicarious menstruation.*
Menstruation-like bleeding. See *Pseudomenstruation.*
Metabolism, androgen, 714
  calcium, effects of thymectomy on, 279
    role of estrogen in, 265
      in dysmenorrhea, 264
      parathyroid glands in, 263
      thyroid gland in, 237
  carbohydrate, effects of adrenal cortical compounds on, 251
    of adrenalectomy on, 251
    role of adrenal cortex in, 249
      adrenal medulla in, 246, 247
      anterior hypophysis in, 211
      hypothalamico-hypophyseal system in, 230
      hypothalamus in, 229
      thyroid gland in, 236
  effects of adrenal cortical extract on, 254
    of adrenalectomy on, 254
    of adrenalin on, 247
    of posterior hypophyseal extract on, 223
    of thyroxin on, 254
  estrogen, role of uterus in, 707
  fat, effects of adrenal cortical ablation on, 251
    role of adrenal cortex in, 251
      anterior hypophysis in, 214
      hypothalamico-hypophyseal system in, 230
      lipoitrin in, 223, 230
      thyroid gland in, 236
  influence of gonads on, 509
  phosphorus, role of parathyroid glands in, 263
  progesterone, 712
  progestin, 712
  protein, role of anterior hypophysis in, 216
    thyroid gland in, 237
  role of anterior hypophysis in, 204, 211
    in sex differentiation, 634
    posterior hypophysis in, 222
    thyroid gland in, 235
  water, role of anterior hypophysis in, 215

Metabolism, water, role of hypothalamico-hypophyseal system in, 229
  of hypothalamus in, 229
  of posterior hypophysis in, 229
  of thyroid gland in, 237
Metakentrin, 715
Methyl testosterone, commercial preparations, 725
  method of administration, 714
Metropathia haemorrhagica. See *Uterine bleeding, anovulatory.*
Metrorrhagia, definition of, 327
Migraine, 449
  definition of, 449
  diagnosis of, 450
  etiology of, 449
  hormonal causes of, 449
  treatment of, 450
Milk secretion, deficient, 489. See also *Hypogalactia.*
Miller-Kurzrok test, 399
  modification of, 401
Mittelschmerz, 443. See also *Intermenstrual pain.*
Mucification test, Fluhmann's, 655
Mucous membranes, effects of adrenalin on, 247
Müllerian ducts, embryonic, 2, 633
Muscle, smooth, 246
  striated, 247
Myometrial activity after menopause, 103
  after ovarian ablation, 103
  during follicular phase of menstrual cycle, 103
  during menstruation, 104
  effects of adrenalin on, 112, 246
    of pituitrin on, 104, 107, 112
      during menstrual cycle, 106
    of progestin on, 104
    of thymus extract on, 112
  endocrine control of, 101
  in anovulatory uterine bleeding, observations on, 344
  in pregnancy, 108
    effect of oxytocin on, 108
      of pituitrin on, 108, 109, 112
      of vasopressin on, 109
    role of adenohypophysis in, 111
      estrogen in, 109, 125
      posterior hypophysis in, 112
      progesterone in, 110
  methods of study of, 101
  role of hormones in, 102
Myometrium, activity of. See *Myometrial activity.*
  at parturition, 124
  hyperplasia of, 37
  response to estrogen and progestin, 94
  role in menstrual bleeding, 92
Myxedema, etiology of, 234
  first reports of, 234
  nervous irritability in, 238
  pituitary hypertrophy in, 238
  sugar tolerance in, 236
  treatment of, with thyroid extract, 234

Nanosomia pituitaria. See *Hypophyseal infantilism.*
Neoplasms from estrogen stimulation, 38
Nervous fatigue in climacteric, 428
  system, effect of thyroid gland on, 238
  role of, in amenorrhea, 309
    in obesity, 517
Neurath-Cushing type of adiposogenital dystrophy, 566
Newborn, estrogen excretion in, 681
  gonadotropin in, 692
  witches' milk, 475

Obesity, 496. See also *Adiposity.*
  and amenorrhea, 309
  and diabetes mellitus, 513
    pituitary hyperfunction in, 513
  basal metabolic rate in, 499
  complications and sequels, 518
  definition and classification of, 496
  diagnosis of, 519
  dietotherapy in, 522
  endocrine glands in, 506
  endogenous *vs.* exogenous, 496
  energy intake in, 498
  etiology of, 496
    appetite in, 498
    energy expenditure in, 499
    energy intake in, 498
    luxury consumption theory, 501
    muscular and nervous activity in, 502
    specific dynamic action of foodstuffs, 500
    sugar and fat metabolism in, 502
    water metabolism in, 504
  Fröhlich's type, 521
  heredity and constitution in, 505
  history in, 519
  hypogonadal, diagnosis of, 520
  in Cushing's syndrome, 574
  neural factors in, 516
  neurogenic, diagnosis of, 521
  organotherapy in, 523
  physical examination in, 519
  pituitary hyperfunction in, 513
  prognosis of, 519
  prophylaxis in, 520
  role of adrenal glands in, 511
    of gonads in, 509
    of hypophysis in, 514
    of hypothalamico-hypophyseal system in, 230
    of hypothalamus in, 516
    of pancreas in, 513
    of pineal gland in, 514
    of thymus gland in, 514
    of thyroid gland in, 506
  thyrogenic, diagnosis of, 520
  treatment of, 520
    anterior hypophyseal extracts, 525
    benzedrine sulfate, 525
    diet, 522
    dinitrophenol, 525
    diuretics in, 523
    fluid intake, 522
    hormonal, 523

Obesity, treatment of, ovarian extracts, 525
  thyroid substance, 523
  water-salt, 504
Octofollin, therapeutic value of, 709
Oligomenorrhea, 304
  definition of, 297
  pregnanediol excretion in, 315
Orophysin. See *Ketogenic factor*.
Osteomalacia, etiology of, 265
  gonads and, 265
  parathyroid hyperplasia in, 265
  treatment of, by ovariectomy, 265
Ova, recovery of, from fallopian tubes, 65
Ovarian atrophy in Addison's disease, 254
  cycle, 7
    corpus luteum phase, 12
    follicular phase of, 7
    maturity of corpus luteum in, 13
    phases of, 7
    proliferation of corpus luteum in, 12
    retrogression of corpus luteum in, 14
    vascularization of corpus luteum in, 13
  extracts, 33
    in treatment of obesity, 525
  follicle, endocrine role of, 34
  function, blood estrogen test, as index of,
      682
    blood gonadotropin tests of, 671
    vaginal smear as index of, 314
  neoplasms, 595
  transplants, 33
  tumors, masculinizing, androgen levels in,
      691
Ovariectomy, effects of, 33
  on parathyroid glands, 265
  on skeleton, 265
  on urine androgen, 258
  in treatment of osteomalacia, 265
  thymus gland after, 275
Ovary after conception, 32
  after hypophysectomy, effects of adrenal
      cortical extracts on, 256
  after infertile ovulation, 32
  bimanual palpation of, 66
  cells secreting estrogen, 43
  cyclic modifications, at maturity, 7
  development of, from birth to puberty, 4
    in embryo, 1
  effects of adrenalectomy on, 255
    of androgens on, 160
    of estrogen on, 41
    of gonadotropes on, 181, 187
    of mare's serum gonadotropin on, 188
  endocrine role of, 32
  examination of, 64, 66
  excretory function of, 32
  hormone production, 33
  hormone-secreting tumors of, 595
  in animals, effects of x-ray on, 45, 46
  incretory function of, 132
  role of, in estrogen metabolism, 707
  secretion of androgen by, 47
  transplantation of, 33
Ovulation, 9
  coitus-induced, 71

Ovulation, diagnosis of, by pregnanediol
    test, 404
  by vaginal smear, 651
  effects of thyroid feeding on, 240
  in climacteric, 425
  in ovarian cycle, 7, 9
  inducing factors of anterior hypophysis,
      175
  induction of, from mare's serum gonado-
      tropin, 188
  inhibition of, 50
  observation of, in animals, 9
  optimal conditions for, 176
  role of follicle stimulating and luteinizing
      hormones in, 176
  time, 64
    calculation of, 64, 69
Ovum, fertilized, potential bisexuality of,
    633
  unfertilized, life span of, 70
Oxygen consumption, effects of thyrotropic
    extracts on, 206
  role of adrenal cortex in, 252
Oxytocic factor of posterior hypophysis, 221
  role of, in parturition, 221
Oxytocin, effect of, on myometrial activity,
    106
  in pregnancy, 108
  gastrointestinal effects of, 223
  role of, in parturition, 127

PANCREAS-adrenal cortex relation, 250
  antagonism between thyroid gland and, 236
  effects of estrogen on, 270
    of gonads on, 270
    on gonadal function, 268
      experiments in, 269
    on reproductive function, 268
      experiments in, 269
  -gonadal relationship, 268
  -hypophyseal relationship, 210
  in acromegaly, 552
  role of, in climacteric, 434
    in lactation, 149
    in obesity, 513
  -thymus relationship, 279
Pancreatic function, effects of menstruation
    on, 270
  of pregnancy on, 270
Pancreatropic principle of anterior hypophy-
    sis, 210
Panhypopituitarism, 541. See also *Hypo-
    physeal infantilism.*
Parabiotic experiments, 288
Parathormone, pharmacology of, 263
Parathyroid-anterior hypophyseal relation-
    ship, 209, 266
  deficiency, blood calcium in, 262
    blood phosphorus in, 262
  extracts, effects of, 263
    blood calcium, 263
  function, experimental studies of, 262
    relationship of, to gonadal hormones,
        264
  glands and eclampsia, 266

Parathyroid glands, effects of castration on, 265
  of gonads on, 265
  of hypophysectomy on cytology of, 210
  of thyroidectomy on, 266
  in acromegaly, 552
  physiology of, 262
  role of, in calcium metabolism, 263
    in genital development, 264
    in genital function, 264
    in lactation, 149
    in menstruation, 264
    in phosphorus metabolism, 263
    in tetany, 262
    in thyroid function, 266
  -gonadal relationship, 264
  hormone, effects of, on bone, 263
    on renal threshold, 263
  hyperplasia in osteomalacia, 265
  -thyroid interrelationship, 266
  -thymus relationship, 279
Parathyroidectomy, dietary influence on effects of, 262
  effect of, 262, 264
    on electrolytic balance, 262
    on thyroid gland, 266
Parathyrotropic principle of anterior hypophysis, 209
Parenchymatous goiter, pituitary hypertrophy in, 238
Paresthesias in climacteric, 428
Parturition, 123
  estrual cycle after, 149
  mammary gland after, 132
  menstrual cycle after, 149
  myometrium in, 124
  nervous factors in, 124
  role of estrogen in, 125
    of oxytocic factor of posterior hypophysis in, 127, 221
    of placenta in, 124, 128
    of progesterone in, 127
    of uterus in, 124
Pelvic ligaments, effects of corpus luteum on, 59
  of relaxin on, 59
Peristalsis, effect of pitressin on, 223
Phosphorus metabolism, role of parathyroid glands in, 263
Pick's testicular adenoma, 601. See also *Arrhenoblastoma.*
Pineal body, physiology of, 282
  extracts, effects of, on gonadal function, 283
    on growth, 283
  feeding, effects of, 283
  function, experimental studies of, 282
  gland, role of, in development, 284
    in obesity, 514
    in sexual development, 284
  -hypophyseal relationship, 211
  implants, effects of, 283
Pinealectomy, effects of, 282
Pitocin, clinical uses of, 223, 224
  pharmocologic effects of, 222

Pitressin administration in diabetes insipidus, 224
  in pyelitis, 224
  in shock, 224
  cardiovascular effects of, 222
  clinical uses of, 223
  contraindications for use of, 223
  gastrointestinal effects of, 223
  in renal function tests, 224
  pharmacologic effects of, 222
Pituitary basophilism. See also *Cushing's syndrome.*
  resemblance of, to adrenogenitalism, 253
  disease, adrenal cortex in, 253
  dwarfism, 537. See also *Hypophyseal infantilism.*
  extracts, effects of, after hypophysectomy, 172
  giantism, 544. See also *Hypophyseal giantism.*
  gland. See also *Hypophysis, Anterior Hypophysis, Hypophyseal, Posterior Hypophysis.*
    and myometrial activity, 112
    effects of estrogen on, 41
    role of, in lactation, 148, 150
      in menstruation, 78
    size of, after thyroidectomy, 238
  hypertrophy in cachexia thyropriva, 238
    in cretinism, 238
    in myxedema, 238
    in parenchymatous goiter, 238
  implants, effects of, after hypophysectomy, 172
Pituitrin, effect of, on myometrial activity, 104, 107
    in pregnancy, 108, 109
  uterine reactivity to, 66. See also *Knaus test.*
Placenta, androgen in, 121
  endocrine role of, 119
  estrogen in, 119
  gonadotropic hormones in, 121
  pregnancy gonadotropes in, 121
  progesterone in, 120
  role of, in lactation inhibition, 141
    in parturition, 124, 128
Polydipsia, pitressin treatment of, 224
Polymenorrhea, definition of, 327
  diagnosis of, 357
  etiology of, 356
Polyuria, treatment of, with pitressin, 224
Postencephalitis lethargica, obesity in, 520
Posterior hypophyseal extract, effect of, metabolic, 223
    on blood sugar, 223
    on insulin sensitivity in hypophysectomized animal, 222
    on lactation, 148
    on urinary sodium, 221
    pharmacologic, 222
    renal, 222
Posterior hypophysis, antidiuretic factor of, 220
    diseases of, clinical aspects, 224

Posterior hypophysis, hyperfunction of, 224
  incretory function of, 220
  oxytocic factor of, 221
  physiology of, 220
  properties of extracts from, 220
  role of, in diabetes insipidus production, 229
    in fat metabolism, 223
    in metabolism, 222
    in production of diabetes insipidus, 215, 220, 224
    in water metabolism, 229
  syndrome due to hyperfunction of, 224
Precocious puberty, 605
  cerebral causes of, 608
  constitutional, 609
  definition of, 605
  diagnosis of, 609
  etiology of, 605
    adrenal cortical, 606
    cerebral, 608
    gonads in, 605, 607
    hypophysis in, 607
    pineal gland in, 607
  hypothalamus in, 608
  prognosis, 610
  treatment, 610
Pregnancy, adenohypophysis in, 121
  adrenalectomy during, 254
    effects of, 255
  amenorrhea during, 297
  androgen excretion during, 690
  basal metabolic rate in, 241
  blood estrogen during, 683
  corpus luteum of, 32
  early, mammary gland development in, 134
  ectopic, gonadotropin level in, 694
  effects of, on pancreatic function, 270
  estrogen excretion during, 683
  gonadotropin level during, 693
  hypophyseal modifications during, 194
  in diabetes mellitus, 269
  late toxemias of, 457. See also Preeclampsia, Eclampsia.
    etiology, 457
      adrenal cortex in, 459
      parathyroid glands in, 459
      placenta in, 461
      posterior hypophysis in, 458
      thyroid gland in, 459
    treatment of, 461
  mammary gland during, 131, 134
  myometrial activity in, 108
  pregnanediol excretion during, 688
  relation of body weight and oxygen consumption in, 241
  response to corpus luteum ablation during, 110, 120
  role of corpus luteum in maintenance of, 56
  test for, bitterling, 679
    estrogen, Mazer-Hoffman, 661
    false, 697, 700
    Friedman rabbit, 675

Pregnancy, test for, frog, 676
    gonadotropic, 675
    skin, 679
    Zondek-Aschheim, 675
  thymus gland during, 276
  thyroid gland in, 241
    hypertrophy, mechanism of, 242
  toxemias, blood gonadotropin in, 695
    estrogen tests in, value of, 685
    pregnanediol excretion in, 688
  urine estrogen in, 683
    test for, 661
      sources of error in, 662
  gonadotropin level as index of state of, 695
    test for, Zondek and Aschheim, 675
  vaginal smear in, 654
Pregnanediol excretion during menstrual cycle, 686
  during pregnancy, 688
  in abortion, 688
  in amenorrhea, 315, 687
  in fetal death, 688
  in hypomenorrhea, 315
  in menstrual disorders, 687
  in normally menstruating woman, 686
  in oligomenorrhea, 315
  in pregnancy toxemias, 688
  in urine, quantitation tests of, 662. See also Urine pregnanediol tests.
  excretion studies, 67, 120, 127
  findings in sterility, 404
  level as index of progesterone production, value of, 687
  in adrenogenitalism, 688
  sodium glucuronidate, determination of, 687
Pregnant mare's serum gonadotropin, 182. See also Equine gonadotropin.
    effects of, 183, 188
    follicular response to, 186
    induction of ovulation from, 188
    source of, 183
Pregneninolone, 59
  chemistry of, 711
  preparations, 724
Premenstrual distress, 446
  tension, 446
    blood estrogen in, 446
    definition of, 446
    diagnosis of, 448
    edema in, 447
    etiology, 446
      nervous system in, 448
      ovarian sex hormones in, 446
      progestin deficiency in, 446
    symptomatology, 446
    treatment of, 448
      progesterone, 724
    weight in, 447
Progestational activity of adrenal cortical extracts, 256
  hormone, standardization of, 712
  substances, 711, 723
    pregneninolone preparations, 724

Progesterone. See also *Progestin*.
and adenohypophysis, role of, in myometrial activity, 112
biology of, 50, 723
chemistry of, 711
commercial preparations of, 723
description of, 711
effect of, on vagina, 59
in placenta, 120
indications and dosage, 724
isolation of, 50
from adrenal glands, 256
metabolism, 712
production, pregnanediol level as index of,
687
relationship of, to adrenal cortical hormone, 255
role of, in mammary gland, 133
in lactation inhibition, 142
in myometrial activity of pregnancy,
110
in parturition, 127
route of administration, 723
source of, 723
standardization of, 712, 723
Progestin. See also *Progesterone*.
action of, on follicular growth, 51
on hypophysis, 51
and estrogen, experiments on menstrual
rhythm, 81, 82, 83.
deficiency as cause of abortion, 416
in premenstrual tension, 446
-deprivation theory of menstruation, 81
description of, 711
effects of, in monkeys, 60
on mating instinct, 60
on myometrial activity, 104
on uterine blood vessels, 56
on uterine cervix, 58
on uterine musculature, 57
on uterine tubes, 58
in placenta, 120
in prevention of abortion, 111
isolation of, 50
level, index of, vaginal smear as, 650
limitations of endometrial response to, 55
metabolism, 712
Prolan A. See also *Follicle stimulating hormone*.
in male urine after gonadectomy, 163
Prostatic hypertrophy, benign, treatment of,
androgen, 725
Protein metabolism, anterior hypophysis and,
216
role of thyroid gland in, 237
Pseudocyesis, 310
Pseudohermaphrodite, 641
Pseudohermaphroditismus femininus, 644
masculinus, 644
Pseudomenstruation after estrogen deprivation, 78, 82
and menstruation, comparison of, 94
blood vessel destruction in, 94
definition of, 76
myometrial activity in, 96

Pseudomenstruation, tissue loss in, 94
Pseudoparturition, 124
Pseudopregnancy, suckling, 150
Puberal manifestations, etiology of, 296
treatment of, 296
troublesome, 295
Pubertas praecox. See *Precocious puberty*.
tarda, 297
Puberty, 292. See also *Adolescence*.
anovulatory bleeding in, treatment of, 347
heart in, 295
ovary during, 5
physical manifestations of, 295
psychic manifestations of, 295
Pyelitis, treatment of, with pitressin, 224
Pyknic type. See *Lateral hypotonic type*.

RAKOFF blood gonadotropin test for fetal
death, 678
Rathke's pouch, 167
Relaxin, 59, 123
Renal function, role of adrenal cortex in, 251
tests, pitressin in, 224
threshold, effects of parathyroid hormone
administration on, 263
Reproductive disorders, diagnostic tests, 654
gonadotropin level in, 693
treatment of, progesterone, 724
function, vaginal smear as index of, 654
effect of insulin on, 269
of pancreas on, 268
of thyroid feeding on, 240
in Addison's disease, 254
role of adrenal cortex in, 258
tests, 654
Rhinitis, atrophic, estrogen treatment of, 722
Rhythm method, 64
Rubin test, 401

"SAFE period," 64
"Schwergiebigkeit," 489
Secondary sex characters, 291
in climacteric, 427
in cryptorchidism, 156
in female, effects of androgen on, 160
Sella turcica, x-ray of, in amenorrhea, 314
Semen, collection of, 394
ejaculate, volume, 395
spermatozoa count in, 395
temperature for keeping, 395
Senile male, androgen excretion in, 690
gonadotropin excretion in, 700
Serum cholesterol, effects of thyrotropic extract administration on, 206
Sex characters, classification of, 631
differentiation, 631
in adrenal cortical hyperfunction, 255
in adrenal cortical insufficiency, 254
influence of adrenal cortex on, 254
secondary, effects of estrogen on, 36
control of, theories on, 632
determination, 631
chromosomal theory, 632
and differentiation of sex characters
631

Sex determination, definition of, 631
    genetical, 632
    differentiation, definition of, 631
        experimental studies in, 637
        hormonal factors in, 634
            unsettled questions regarding, 635
        inductor substances, mode of action of,
            636
            relation of, to gonadal hormones,
                636
        metabolic factors in, 634
        role of inductor system in, 634, 636
        somatic, control of, by embryonic gonad,
            639
        substances, embryonic, site of origin,
            635
    genetical, determining factors, 632
    hormone findings in blood and urine, 681
        maternal, and intersexuality, 646
        of anterior hypophysis, 172
        relation of, to sex differentiation induc-
            tor substances, 636
        tests, 654
        titers in blood and urine, table of, 698
    organs, primary, definition of, 631
        secondary, definition of, 631
Sexual alterations in adolescence, 291
    in adrenal cortical disease, experimen-
        tal evidence of, 255
    characteristics, secondary, definition of, 631
    development and cryptorchidism, 620
        relationship of, to height, 295
    role of pineal gland in, 284
    precocity. See *Precocious puberty.*
Shock, treatment of, with pitressin, 224
Simmonds' disease, 564. See also *Hypo-
    physeal cachexia.*
    clinical characteristics, 565
    course and prognosis of, 571
    definition of, 564
    diagnosis of, 568
    differentiation from Addison's disease,
        569
        from anorexia nervosa, 568
        from glandular sclerosis, 568
        from primary hypothyroidism, 570
    etiology and pathology, 567
        anterior hypophysis in, 567
        hypothalamus in, 568
    incidence of, 564
    manifestations of, 253
    metabolic disturbances in, 566
    pathology of, 567
    prognosis of, 571
    somatic alterations in, 565
    subjective symptoms of, 567
    thymus gland in, 276
    treatment of, 571
Skeletal effects of estrogen, 265
    of ovariectomy, 265
    of parathyroid hormone administration,
        263
Skin, capillaries of, premenstrually, 91
    changes in climacteric, 429
    effects of adrenalin on, 247

Skin in Addison's disease, 588
Sleep, role of hypothalamus in, 231
Smith   and   Smith,   estrogen   separation
        method, 659
    urine estrogen test, 659
Smooth muscle, effects of adrenalin on, 246
Sodium   pregnanediol   glucuronidate,   deter-
    mination of, 687
Spermatogenesis, 155
    deficiency, gonadotropes in, 191
    effects of androgens on, in animals, 158
        of gonadotropes on, 182, 183
    in cryptorchidism, 156
    nonendocrine factors influencing, 162
    role of anterior hypophysis in, 162, 171,
        181
Spermatozoa, life span of, 70
    morphology of, 396
    motility of, 395
    survival of, in female genitalia, 70
Status thymicolymphaticus, 275
    effects   of   adrenal   cortical   extract   on,
        279
Sterility, 387
    adolescent, 293
    androgen findings in, 404
    causes of genital nonunion in, 392
    definition of, 387
    diagnosis of, 394
        semen collection in, 394
    effect of dilatation and curettage on, 72
    endometrial biopsy in, 403
        curettage in, 403
        findings in, 403, 404
    etiology of, barriers to cervical insemina-
        tion, 393
        dyspareunia in, 392
        frigidity in, 392
        germ cell incompatibility in, 393
        hymenal atresias in, 392
        immunity to spermatozoa in, 394
        vagina in, 392
        vulval, 392
        uterine faults in, 393
    female role in, 389
    gonadotropin findings in, 404
    history of female partner in, 397
    Huhner test in, 398
    impotence in, 389
    in Addison's disease, 254
    incidence of, 387
    investigation of female partner in, 397
        male partner in, 394
    male role in, 389
        treatment of, gonadotropin in, 729, 730
    menstrual history in, 397
    Miller-Kurzrok test in, 399
        modified, 401
    organotherapy in, 406
    pelvic examination in, 398
    physical examination of female in, 398
    physiologic, definition of, 387
    pregnanediol findings in, 404
    primary, definition of, 387
    radiotherapy of, 407

Sterility, Rubin test, 401
  secondary or acquired, definition of, 387
  sex hormone studies in examination of female, 403
  spermatogenic faults in, 389
  spermatozoal motility in, 395
    morphology in, 396
  treatment of, 405
    chorionic gonadotropin, 727
    gonadotropin, 731
    gynecologic, 406
    hormonal, 406
    progesterone, 724
    sex hygiene instruction, 408
    surgical, 408
    tubal insufflation, 409
    x-ray, 407
  tubal insufflation test, 401
  uterine causes of, 393
  vaginal smear in, 403
Stilbestrol. See also *Diethylstilbestrol* and *Estrogens, synthetic.*
  and chorionic gonadotropin, 42
Striated muscle, effects of adrenalin on, 247
Stroma-lutein cells. See *Theca cells.*
Suckling and maintenance of lactation, 145
  effects of, on luteinizing hormone, 150
Sugar excretion after adrenalin administration, 247
Suprarenal glands, physiology of, 244
Suprarenalin. See *Adrenalin.*
Sympathetic nervous system, effects of epinephrine on, 246
Sympathomimetic substance, 246. See *Adrenalin* and *Epinephrine.*

TEMPERATURE regulation, role of hypothalamus in, 231
Testicular extract experiments, 155
  hormone production, time of onset of, 157
  tumors, gonadotropin excretion in, 700
    urine estrogen in, 685
Testis, active principle of. See *Testosterone.*
  and anterior hypophysis, 162
  effects of androgens on, 157
    of estrogen on, 42
    of gonadotropes on, 182
    on anterior hypophysis, 163
  endocrine function of, 155
  incretory function of, role of anterior hypophysis in, 162
  physiology of, 155
  response of, to gonadotropes, 190
Testosterone, commercial preparations of, 725
  isolation of, from bull's testes, 156
  method of administration, 714
  potency of, 156
  propionate, 156
  response of endometrium to, 81
  route of administration of, 725
Tetany, maternal. See *Maternal tetany.*
  treatment of, with parathyroid extracts, 263

Theca cell tumor, 598. See also *Thecoma.*
Theca cells, role of, in estrogen production, 43
Theca-lutein cells. See *Theca cells.*
Thecoma, 598
  clinical characteristics of, 599
  diagnosis of, 600
  histogenesis of, 599
  histology of, 599
  prognosis of, 600
Thymectomy, effects of, 272
  gonadal, 274
  on calcium metabolism, 279
Thymophysin. See *Thymus extract.*
Thymocrescin, 274
Thymus-adrenal relationship, 278
  -anterior hypophyseal relationship, 211, 276
  gland after adrenalectomy, 278
    and growth, 273
    effects of gonads on, 275
    extracts, effects of, 273
      gonadal, 275
      on myometrial activity, 112
    functions of, 272
    in acromegaly, 276, 552
    in pregnancy, 276
    in Simmonds' disease, 276
    isolation of hormone of, 276
    physiology of, 272
    relationship to other glands, 276
    role of, in gonadal function, 274
      in hypophyseal function, 276
      in obesity, 514
  -gonadal relation, 274
  implants, effects of, 273
  -pancreas relationship, 279
  -parathyroid relationship, 279
  -thyroid relationship, 277
Thyroid ablation, effects of, after posterior hypophyseal injury, 237
  on anterior hypophysis, 238
  on diabetes insipidus, 237
  on gonads, 239
  experiments, 234
  -adrenal relationship, 253
  -anterior hypophyseal relationship, 205, 238
  extract, effects of, in adrenal insufficiency, 254
  feeding, adrenal cortical hyperplasia after, 254
    effects of, in hyperparathyroidism, 266
    on anterior hypophysis, 238
    on gonadal function, 240
    on reproductive function, 240
    on ovulation, 240
  function, biochemical investigations of, 235
    effects of anterior hypophysis on, 239
    of estrogen on, 241
    of gonads on, 240
    experimental studies of, 234
    present concept of, 235
    role of parathyroid glands in, 266
  gland and menstrual cycle, 241

Thyroid gland, antagonism between pancreas and, 236
   effects of adrenal injury on, 254
      of parathyroidectomy on, 266
      of thyrotropic extracts on, 206
      on cardiovascular system, 238
      on nervous system, 238
   extracts for clinical use, 235
      in acromegaly, 552
      in climacteric, 433
      in pregnancy, 241
   physiology of, 234
   role of, in basal metabolic rise after adrenal injury, 252
      in calcium metabolism, 237
      in carbohydrate metabolism, 236
      in fat metabolism, 236
      in growth-promoting activity of anterior hypophysis, 239
      in lactation, 148
      in metabolism, 235
      in obesity, 506
      in protein metabolism, 237
      in skeletal growth, 239
      in somatic growth, 235
      in specific dynamic action of foodstuffs, 236
      in water metabolism, 237
   globulin, comparison of, with other thyroid extracts, 235
   -gonadal relationship, 239
   hormone administration, effects of, on adrenal cortex, 254
      synergistic action of adrenalin with, 236
   hypertrophy in pregnancy, mechanism of, 242
   -parathyroid interrelationship, 266
   -parathyroidectomy, effects of, 264
   -posterior hypophyseal antagonism, 237
   replacement experiments, 234
   -thymus relationship, 277
   treatment of obesity, 524
Thyroidectomy. See also *Thyroid ablation.*
   bones after, 237
   "cells" in adenohypophysis, 238
   effects of, 234
      after adrenalectomy, 254
      on anterior hypophysis, 238
      on diabetes mellitus, 236
      on gonadotropic hormone of anterior hypophysis, 238
      on hypophyseal cytology, 239
      on parathyroid glands, 266
   size of pituitary gland after, 238
Thyrotropic extracts, effects of, 206
   factor of anterior hypophysis, 205
   hormone, 205, 276
      therapeutic considerations of, 207
   substances in blood and urine, 206
Thyroxin, effects of, on metabolism, 254
   isolation of, 234
   properties of, 235
Thyroxine, production of, 235
Toxemia of pregnancy. See also *Eclampsia* and *Hyperemesis gravidarum.*

Toxemia of pregnancy, role of vasopressin in, 224
Triphenylchlorethylene, 709
Triphenylethylene, therapeutic value of, 709
Tubal hypoplasia, treatment of, estrogen, 722
   insufflation, 401
   motility, effect of castration on, 36
      of estrogen on, 35
      of progestin on, 58
   mucosa, cyclic changes in, 25
      effect of estrogen on, 35
      of progestin on, 58
Tuberculosis, amenorrhea in, 307
Tubular tract, uterine, fetal development of, 3

Urine androgens and related 17-ketosteroids, chemical assay of, 667
      colorimetric tests for, 668
      diagnostic uses of, 669
   in children, 689
   tests, 664
      capon comb method of Callow, 664
      chick comb method of Frank and associates, 665
   androsterone in male, 689
   effects of posterior hypophyseal extract on, 221
   estrogen after fetal death, 684
      and gonadotropin content, 66
      before abortion, 684
      extraction and separation method, 659
      in adrenal cortical carcinoma, 686
      in castrate women, 685
      in childhood, 681
      in functional uterine bleeding, 682
      in granulosa cell tumors, 685
      in menopause, 685
      in menstrual disorders, 682
      in newborn, 681
      in pregnancy, 683
      male, 685
      tests, 655, 657
         for adrenal cortical carcinoma, 662
         for pregnancy, Mazer and Hoffman method, 661
            Kurzrok and Ratner, 657
            Smith and Smith, 659
   gonadotropin in, 179, 181
      after fetal death, 684
      as index of state of pregnancy, 695
      male, 700
      tests for nonpregnant states, 672
         of Frank and associates, 673
         of Levin, 673
         of Varney and Koch, 674
         of Zondek, 672
         of Zondek and Aschheim, 675
   of castrates, gonadotropins in, 181
   of menopause, gonadotropins in, 181
   of pregnancy, gonadotropins in, 179
   pregnanediol in normally menstruating women, 686
      tests, 662
         method of Browne and Venning, 662

Urine, pregnanediol tests, method of Bucher and Geschichter, 663
  sex hormone findings in, 681
  thyrotropin content of, 207
  substances in, 206
Uterine bleeding, functional, age distribution of, compared with organic, 326
  anovulatory, 328
    age incidence of, 334
    anatomical and histological characteristics, 328
    blood estrogen in, 682
    clinical characteristics of, 334
    clinical course of, 346
    cyclic and acyclic, 335
    desquamation in, 343
    diagnosis of, 345
    differential diagnosis of, 345
    endometrial changes in, 332
    endometrium in, 331
    estrinpriva hypothesis in, 342
    etiology of, 335
      adrenal glands in, 340
      anterior hypophysis in, 340
      corpus luteum in, 338
      endometrial resistance to progesterone in, 338
      estrogen stimulation in, 335
      follicular activity in, 335
      nonendocrine factors in, 340
      ovary in, 335
      pancreas in, 340
      parathyroid glands in, 340
      thyroid glands in, 340
      uterus in, 341
    in maturity, treatment of, 347
    in menopause, treatment of, 346
    in puberty, treatment of, 347
    myometrial activity in, 344
    organotherapy in, 348
    ovarian changes in, 328
    prognosis, 346
    radiotherapy in, 352
    treatment of, 346
      medical, 348
      surgical, 352
      with androgens, 351, 726
      with estrogen and progesterone, 350
      with gonadotropes, 349, 727, 729, 731
      with progesterone, 350, 724
      with thyroid substance, 351
      with x-ray, 352
    uterine changes in, 331
    vascular changes in, 342
  atrophic endometrium in, 353
  definition and nomenclature, 327
  endometrial findings in, 327
  hyperplastic, definition of, 327
  incidence of, 326
  intermenstrual, 358
  ovulatory, 354
  treatment of, 346, 354, 357, 359, 724, 727, 729, 731

Uterine bleeding, organic, age distribution of, compared with functional, 326
Uterine extracts and implants in animals, 116
  hormone, 117
  hypoplasia, follicular cysts with, 303
    treatment of, estrogen, 722
  implants and extracts in animals, 116
  inertia, 463
    treatment of, estrogen, 722
  injuries, effects of, on menstrual function, 300
  involution and lactation, 151
  mucosa, cyclic changes in, 16
  tubes, cyclic changes in, 25
  effect of sex hormones on, 35, 36, 58
Uterus. See also *Uterine.*
  before and after menstruation, 85
  bimanual palpation of, 66
  bleeding from. See *Uterine bleeding.*
  cyclic modifications at maturity, 7
  during puberty, 6
  effects of estrogen on, 34
  endocrine role of, 115
  examination for size and consistency of, 66
  in climacteric, 426
  involution of, and lactation, 151
  motility of. See *Myometrial activity.*
  mucosa of. See *Endometrium.*
  reactivity of, to pituitrin, 66. See also *Knaus test.*
  response of, to oxytocin, 106
    to vasopressin, 106
  role in controlling menstrual flow, 92
    in estrogen metabolism, 707
    in parturition, 124
  veins of, role in menstrual bleeding, 92

Vagina, effects of estrogen on, 35, 59
  of progesterone on, 59
Vaginal epithelium, cyclic changes in, 650
  glycogen index, 653
  mucosa, cyclic changes in, 27
    interpretation of, 30
  smear, cytologic classification of, 651
    interpretation of, 651
    iodine vapor method, 653
    pregnancy changes in, 654
    premenstrual, 650
    techniques of, 651
    uses of, 650
Vaginitis, chronic, vaginal smear in, 654
  senile, treatment of, estrogen, 722
Vasalgia, 428
Vascular circulation, role of adrenal cortex in, 249
Vasoconstriction before menstrual bleeding, 85, 91
Vasomotor instability in migraine, 449
Vasopressin, 222. See also *P'tressin.*
  effects of, on myometrial activity in pregnancy, 109
    respiratory, 222
  response of uterus to, 106

Vasopressin, role of, in pregnancy toxemias, 224
Vegetative nervous system, relationship of, to endocrine system, 226
Vertigo in climacteric, 428
"Vicarious menstruation," 451
　　clinical characteristics of, 451
　　definition of, 451
　　diagnosis of, 454
　　etiology of, 451
　　　estrogen in, 451
　　　progesterone in, 452
　　　psychogenic factors in, 453
　　skin capillaries in, 452
　　treatment of, 454
Virilism. See *Adrenogenital syndrome* and *Masculinization.*
Vitamin C content of adrenal cortex, 254
　　of corpus luteum, 254

Vitamin deficiency, effects of, on spermatogenesis, 162
　in abortion, 414
Voice in adolescence, 292
Vulvovaginitis, gonorrheal, estrogen treatment of, 722

WAKEFULNESS, role of hypothalamus in, 232
Water metabolism. See *Metabolism, water.*
Water-salt obesity, 504
Wolffian ducts, embryonic, 633
Wound healing, role of adrenal cortex in, 252

YELLOW body. See *Corpus luteum.*

ZONDEK urine gonadotropin test, 672
Zygote, sex determiners in, 633